CURRENT
Diagnosis & Treatment
Neurology

SECOND EDITION

Edited by

John C.M. Brust, MD
Professor of Clinical Neurology
Columbia University College of Physicians & Surgeons
New York, New York

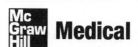

New York   Chicago   San Francisco   Lisbon   London   Madrid   Mexico City
Milan   New Delhi   San Juan   Seoul   Singapore   Sydney   Toronto

The McGraw·Hill Companies

Current Diagnosis & Treatment: Neurology, Second Edition

Copyright © 2012 by The McGraw-Hill Companies, Inc. All rights reserved. Printed in the United States of America. Except as permitted under the United States Copyright Act of 1976, no part of this publication my be reproduced or distributed in any form or by any means, or stored in a data base or retrieval system, without prior written permission of the publisher.

1 2 3 4 5 6 7 8 9 0   DOC/DOC   15 14 13 12 11

ISBN 978-0-07-170118-1
MHID 0-07-170118-4
ISSN 1932-1074

This book was set by Cenveo Publisher Services.
The editors were Anne M. Sydor and Harriet Lebowitz.
The production supervisor was Catherine Saggese.
Cover photos: (clockwise from top left) CT scans of intracranial aneurysm on computer screen, credit: Centre Hospitalier Universitaire de Poitiers/Photo Researchers, Inc; reflex testing, credit: Will and Deni McIntyre/Photo Researchers, Inc; computer art based on a sagittal MRI brain scan, credit: Photo Researchers, Inc
RR Donnelley was printer and binder.

This book is printed on acid-free paper.

Cataloging-in-Publication data for this title is on file with the Library of Congress.

McGraw-Hill books are available at special quantity discounts to use as premiums and sales promotions, or for use in corporate training programs. To contact a representative please e-mail us at bulksales@mcgraw-hill.com.

Contents

9. Dementia & Memory Loss   78

Karen Marder, MD, MPH (editor), Karen Bell, MD, Jennifer L. Williamson, MS, Sarah C. Janicki, MD, MPH, Lawrence S. Honig, MD, PhD, Nikolaos Scarmeas, MD, MS, James M. Noble MD, & Clinton B. Wright, MD

10. Cerebrovascular Disease: Ischemic Stroke   102

Brian-Fred M. Fitzsimmons, MD, & Marc Lazzaro, MD

11. Cerebrovascular Disease: Hemorrhagic Stroke   128

Richard A. Bernstein, MD, PhD

12. Central Nervous System Neoplasms   149

Christopher E. Mandigo, MD, & Jeffrey N. Bruce, MD

13. Paraneoplastic Neurologic Syndromes   165

Lakshmi Nayak, MD, Alfredo D. Voloschin, MD, & Andrew B. Lassman, MD

14. Trauma   177

Katja E.Wartenberg, MD, PhD, & Stephan A. Mayer, MD

15. Movement Disorders   201

Amanda Deligtisch, MD, Blair Ford, MD, Howard Geyer, MD, & Susan B. Bressman, MD

Color insert appears between pages 18 and 19.

Authors

Karen Bell, MD
Clinical Professor of Neurology, Taub Institute, Columbia University Medical Center, New York, New York
Dementia & Memory Loss

Richard A. Bernstein, MD, PhD
Associate Professor of Neurology, Feinberg School of Medicine of Northwestern University, Chicago, Illinois
Cerebrovascular Disease: Hemorrhagic Stroke

Susan B. Bressman, MD
Professor, Department of Neurology, Albert Einstein College of Medicine; Alan and John Mirken Chair, Department of Neurology, Beth Israel Medical Center, New York, New York
Movement Disorders

Jeffrey N. Bruce, MD
Edgar M. Housepian Professor of Neurological Surgery, Columbia University College of Physicians & Surgeons, New York, New York
Central Nervous System Neoplasms

John C.M. Brust, MD
Professor of Clinical Neurology, Columbia University College of Physicians & Surgeons, New York, New York
Coma; Aphasia, Apraxia, & Agnosia; Disorders of Cerebrospinal Fluid Dynamics; Alcoholism; Drug Dependence

Claudia A. Chiriboga, MD, MPH
Associate Professor of Clinical Neurology and Clinical Pediatrics, Division of Pediatric Neurology, Department of Neurology, Columbia University College of Physicians & Surgeons, New York, New York
Neurologic Disorders of Childhood & Adolescence

Bruce A.C. Cree, MD, PhD, MCR
Assistant Professor of Neurology, University of California, San Francisco, San Francisco, California
Multiple Sclerosis & Demyelinating Diseases

Amanda Deligtisch, MD
Assistant Professor, Department of Neurology, University of New Mexico, Albuquerque, New Mexico
Movement Disorders

Lydia B. Estanislao, MD
Instructor, Department of Neurology, Mt. Sinai School of Medicine, New York, New York
HIV Neurology

Tanya Fatimi, MD
Clinical Instructor in Neurology, Weill Cornell Medical College, Attending Neurologist, Department of Neurology, Lenox Hill Hospital, New York, New York
Peripheral Neuropathies

Brian-Fred M. Fitzsimmons, MD
Assistant Professor of Clinical Neurology, Medical College of Wisconsin, Milwaukee, Wisconisn
Cerebrovascular Disease: Ischemic Stroke

Blair Ford, MD
Professor, Department of Neurology, Columbia University College of Physicians & Surgeons, New York, New York
Movement Disorders

Jennifer A. Frontera, MD
Assistant Professor, Department of Neurology, Mount Sinai School of Medicine, New York, New York
Viral Infections of the Nervous System

Howard L. Geyer, MD, PhD
Assistant Professor, Department of Neurology, Albert Einstein College of Medicine, Bronx, New York
Movement Disorders

Soha N. Ghossaini, MD
Associate Professor, Department of Otolaryngology-Head and Neck Surgery, Pennsylvania State Hershey Medical Center, Hershey, Pennsylvania
Hearing Loss & Dizziness

Clifton L. Gooch, MD
Professor and Chair, Department of Neurology, University of South Florida, Tanpa, Florida
Peripheral Neuropathies

Mark W. Green, MD
Professor, Department of Neurology, Mount Sinai School of Medicine, New York, New York
Headache and Facial Pain

Todd Hayano, BS
Research Assistant, Department of Neurology, Metropolitan Hospital, New York, New York
Bacterial, Fungal, & Parasitic Infections of the Nervous System

Claire Henchcliffe, MD, DPhil
Associate Professor, Department of Neurology and Neuroscience, Weill Cornell Medical College, New York, New York
Ataxia & Cerebellar Disease

Michio Hirano, MD
Professor, Department of Neurology, Columbia University College of Physicians & Surgeons, New York, New York
Motor Neuron Diseases; Mitochondrial Diseases

Lawrence S. Honig, MD, PhD
Professor of Clinical Neurology, Department of Neurology/Taub Institute, Columbia University College of Physicians & Surgeons, New York, New York
Dementia & Memory Loss; Prion Diseases

Sarah C. Janicki, MD, MPH
Instructor, Department of Neurology, Columbia University Medical Center, New York, New York
Dementia & Memory Loss

Cheryl A. Jay, MD
Clinical Professor, Department of Neurology, University of California, San Francisco, San Francisco, California
Systemic & Metabolic Disorders

Petra Kaufmann, MD, MSc
Associate Professor of Neurology, Columbia University College of Physicians & Surgeons, New York, New York
Myasthenia Gravis & Other Disorders of the Neuromuscular Junction

Barbara S. Koppel, MD
Professor of Clinical Neurology, New York Medical College, New York, New York
Bacterial, Fungal, & Parasitic Infections of the Nervous System

Andrew B. Lassman, MD
Assistant Professor, Department of Neurology, Hospital for Special Surgery/Weill Cornell Medical College, New York, New York
Paraneoplastic Neurologic Syndromes

Marc Lazzaro, MD
Neurointerventional Fellow, Department of Neurology, Medical College of Wisconsin, Milwaukee, WI
Cerebrovascular Disease: Ischemic Stroke

Dora Leung, MD
Assistant Professor of Clinical Neurology, Hospital for Special Surgery/Weill Cornell Medical College, New York, New York
Electromyography, Nerve Conduction Studies, & Evoked Potentials

John P. Loh, MD
Assistant Professor, Department of Radiology, New York University School of Medicine, New York, New York
Neuroradiology

Christopher E. Mandigo, MD
Department of Neurological Surgery, Columbia University College of Physicians & Surgeons, New York, New York
Central Nervous System Neoplasms

Eric R. Marcus, MD
Professor of Clinical Psychiatry, Columbia University College of Physicians & Surgeons, New York, New York
Psychiatric Disorders

Karen Marder, MD, MPH
Professor of Neurology, Columbia University College of Physicians & Surgeons, New York, New York
Dementia & Memory Loss

Stephan A. Mayer, MD, FCCM
Associate Professor of Clinical Neurology, Columbia University College of Physicians & Surgeons, New York, New York
Trauma

Lakshmi Nayak, MD
Fellow, Department of Neurology, Memorial Sloan-Kettering Cancer Center, New York, New York
Paraneoplastic Neurologic Syndromes

James M. Noble, MD, MS
Assistant Professor of Clinical Neurology, Department of Neurology and the Taub Institute, Columbia University Medical Center, New York, New York
Dementia & Memory Loss; Viral Infections of the Nervous System

Santiago Ortega-Gutierrez, MD
Neurology ICU Clinical Fellow, Department of Neurology, Columbia University College of Physicians & Surgeons, New York, New York
Neurologic Intensive Care

Marc C. Patterson, MD, FRACP
Professor, Departments of Neurology, Pediatrics, and Medical Genetics, Mayo Clinic College of Medicine, Rochester, Minnesota
Neurologic Disorders of Childhood & Adolescence

Shanna Kathlyn Patterson, MD
Assistant Director of Electromyography, Department of Neurology, St. Luke's-Roosevelt Hospital Center, New York, New York
Myasthenia Gravis & Other Disorders of the Neuromuscular Junction

Anne Helena Remmes, MD
Assistant Professor (retired), Department of Neurology, Columbia University College of Physicians & Surgeons, New York, New York
Sleep Disorders

Jeffrey Rumbaugh, MD, PhD
Assistant Professor, Department of Neurology, Emory
University, Atlanta, Georgia
HIV Neurology

Ned Sacktor, MD
Professor, Department of Neurology, Johns Hopkins
University School of Medicine, Baltimore, Maryland
HIV Neurology

Nikolaos Scarmeas, MD, MSc
Associate Professor, Department of Neurology, Sergievsky
Center, Taub Institute, Columbia University College of
Physicians & Surgeons, New York, New York
Dementia & Memory Loss

Alan Z. Segal, MD
Associate Professor of Clinical Neurology, New York
Presbyterian-Weill Cornell Medical College, New York,
New York
Neurologic Intensive Care

Jeffrey J. Sevigny, MD
Assistant Professor of Neurology, Department of Neurology,
Beth Israel Medical Center, Albert Einstein College
of Medicine, New York, New York
Viral Infections of the Nervous System; HIV Neurology

Tina Shih, MD
Assistant Professor of Clinical Neurology, Department
of Neurology, University of California, San Francisco,
California
Electroencephalography; Epilepsy & Seizures

Marisa Schiller Sosinsky, MD
Attending Physician, Four Peaks Neurology, Scottsdale,
Arizona
*Myasthenia Gravis & Other Disorders of the Neuromuscular
Junction*

Michelle Stern, MD
Associate Professor, Department of Physical Medicine
and Rehabilitative Medicine, Albert Einstein College
of Medicine, New York, New York
Nontraumatic Disorders of the Spinal Cord

Alfredo D. Voloschin, MD
Assistant Professor, Department of Hematology and
Oncology, Emory University, Atlanta, Georgia
Paraneoplastic Syndromes

Katja Elfriede Wartenberg, MD, PhD
Co-Director, Neurocritical Care Unit, Department of
Neurology, Martin Luther University Halle Wittenberg,
Halle, Germany
Trauma

Jack J. Wazen, MD, FACS
Director of Research, Ear Research Foundation, Silverstein
Institute, Sarasota, Florida
Hearing Loss & Dizziness

Louis H. Weimer, MD
Associate Clinical Professor, Department of Neurology,
Columbia University College of Physicians & Surgeons,
New York, New York
Autonomic Disorders

Olajide Williams, MD, MSc
Associate Professor of Neurology, Columbia
University College of Physicians & Surgeons,
New York, New York
*Nontraumatic Disorders of the Spinal Cord; Diseases
of Muscle*

Jennifer Williamson, MPH, MS, CGC
Senior Staff Associate of Research, Sergievsky Center,
Columbia University College of Physicians & Surgeons,
New York, New York
Dementia & Memory Loss

Clinton B. Wright, MD
Associate Professor, Departments of Neurology,
Epidemiology, and Public Health, University of Miami,
Miami, Florida
Dementia & Memory Loss

Benjamin J. Wycherly, MD
Fellow, Ear Research Foundation, Silverstein Institute,
Sarasota, Florida
Hearing Loss & Dizziness

Preface

Five years after the first edition of this book, neurological conundrums and controversies continue to perplex. What is the difference between vegetative state and minimally conscious state? What is the most appropriate anticonvulsant drug for a patient with epilepsy? What is "tension-type headache"? How often does "mild cognitive impairment" in the elderly progress to Alzheimer dementia? How long after an ischemic stroke can tissue plasminogen activator therapy be given safely? Should a patient with carotid artery atherosclerosis receive endarterectomy or vascular stenting? Should a ruptured saccular aneurysm be clipped or coiled? Following severe head injury, how should increased intracranial pressure be managed? What is postconcussion syndrome"? Should patients with Parkinson disease receive levodopa or a dopamine agonist as initial therapy? When are natalizumab or mitoxantrone indicated in the treatment of multiple sclerosis? How effective are the many medications marketed for treatment of painful diabetic polyneuropathy? Is riluzole of any benefit in the treatment of amyotrophic lateral sclerosis? Which patients with myasthenia gravis should receive thymectomy? Does moderate alcohol consumption increase or decrease risk for stroke or cognitive impairment? What defines "autistic spectrum disorder"?

As with the first edition, the focus of this book is practical, and the principal intended audience is primary care physicians, including internists and family practitioners. Nurses and physicians' assistants are also invited, as are surgeons and specialists (including neurologists). With the exception of a few chapters addressing particular symptoms or diagnostic procedures, each chapter is disease specific and adheres to a standard format, beginning with Essentials of Diagnosis—wherein a puzzled clinician can get an up-front sense of being in the right ballpark—followed by sections on Symptoms and Signs, Diagnostic Studies, Differential Diagnosis, Treatment, and Prognosis. Relatively arcane material is relegated to tables. References have been updated with annotation and PMID numbers.

Clinicians in every branch of medicine regularly encounter patients with neurological symptoms. Too often, the response to such encounters ranges from unease to outright phobia. Steering a course between oversimplicification and mind-crushing detail, this book is designed to instill clinical confidence and improve patient care.

John C.M. Brust, MD

Electroencephalography

1

Tina Shih, MD

General Considerations

Although brain electrical activity is very low in voltage (on the order of microvolts) in comparison with ambient noise (on the order of volts), electroencephalography (EEG) uses the technique of differential amplification to cancel out noise and increase the amplitude of the waveforms of interest. EEG compares the voltages recorded in two different regions and plots this result over time. A standard array of metal electrodes is placed on the scalp of the patient, and over a 30-minute period, brain electrical activity sampled from different regions of the cortex is recorded simultaneously. EEG thus provides both spatial and temporal information.

In the past, EEG was recorded on paper, and the electrical activity was displayed in a static manner. Today, the activity is recorded digitally, allowing the data to be displayed in multiple ways after the recording has been completed. EEG recordings use standard montages, which compare the recordings from individual electrodes with either adjacent electrodes or distant electrodes (Figure 1–1). Montages provide a means of viewing the data in an organized fashion; some montages enhance localized findings, whereas others highlight global or diffuse findings.

For routine outpatient EEGs, an ideal recording environment is quiet, allowing the patient to achieve relaxed wakefulness and to fall asleep (Figure 1–2). During the EEG recording, hyperventilation (having the patient exhale repeatedly and deeply for 180 seconds) and photic stimulation (strobe light flashes for 10 seconds at a time, at different frequencies ranging from 1–25 Hz) are also performed, as both techniques can elicit abnormal EEG activity in certain patients.

When to Order

The EEG has multiple clinical applications. It can be used to confirm the diagnosis of seizures or epilepsy, either by demonstrating interictal (between seizures) epileptiform activity or, serendipitously, by directly recording a seizure. The EEG is important in the classification of seizures and epilepsy syndromes, and it can uncover a previously unknown structural, functional, or metabolic abnormality, even when imaging is normal. The EEG is also useful in diagnosing nonconvulsive status epilepticus (interminable seizure activity during which the patient appears comatose from an unknown cause), revealing intermittent seizure activity as a potential factor in unexplained coma, confirming electrocerebral inactivity (ie, so-called *brain death*, see Chapter 4 for discussion concerning more reliable tests to confirm electrocerebral inactivity), diagnosing certain neurologic syndromes (eg, Creutzfeldt-Jakob disease, subacute sclerosing panencephalitis), and monitoring cerebral perfusion during carotid endarterectomy.

Findings

The EEG report generally includes several observations:

1. Is the background activity normal or abnormal for age and state of the patient (wakefulness versus sleep)? Is the mixture of frequencies appropriate? Is there a normal organization of the waveforms?

2. Are there any focal features? Do the two hemispheres of the brain appear electrically symmetric?

3. Are there any epileptiform discharges (also known as *spikes* or *sharp waves*)?

4. Is the sleep architecture appropriate?

5. Does hyperventilation or photic stimulation bring out any abnormalities?

The EEG report ends with the interpreter's impression of whether the tracing is normal or abnormal and how these findings correspond to the patient's clinical picture.

It is important to realize that despite the application of EEG in certain clinical settings, findings are often nonspecific. The abnormality referred to as *diffuse background*

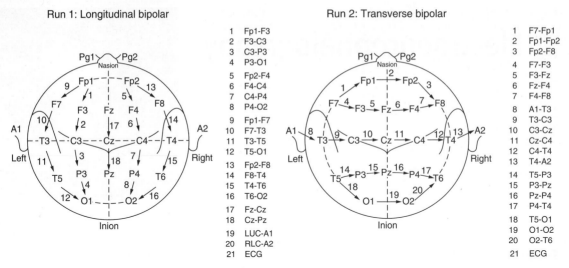

Run 1: Longitudinal bipolar

1	Fp1-F3
2	F3-C3
3	C3-P3
4	P3-O1
5	Fp2-F4
6	F4-C4
7	C4-P4
8	P4-O2
9	Fp1-F7
10	F7-T3
11	T3-T5
12	T5-O1
13	Fp2-F8
14	F8-T4
15	T4-T6
16	T6-O2
17	Fz-Cz
18	Cz-Pz
19	LUC-A1
20	RLC-A2
21	ECG

Run 2: Transverse bipolar

1	F7-Fp1
2	Fp1-Fp2
3	Fp2-F8
4	F7-F3
5	F3-Fz
6	Fz-F4
7	F4-F8
8	A1-T3
9	T3-C3
10	C3-Cz
11	Cz-C4
12	C4-T4
13	T4-A2
14	T5-P3
15	P3-Pz
16	Pz-P4
17	P4-T4
18	T5-O1
19	O1-O2
20	O2-T6
21	ECG

▲ **Figure 1–1.** Two commonly used EEG montages: longitudinal bipolar and transverse bipolar. (C = central; F = frontal; Fp = frontal polar; O = occipital; P = parietal; T = temporal. Odd numbers denote "left"-hemisphere electrodes and even numbers denote "right"-hemisphere electrodes.)

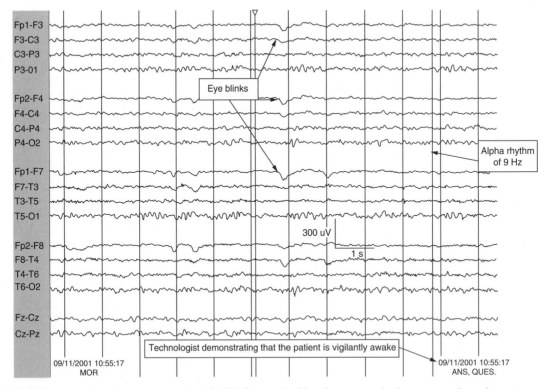

▲ **Figure 1–2.** Normal awake EEG of a 7-year-old child (longitudinal bipolar montage). This 11-second epoch is presented using the longitudinal bipolar montage with the first four channels representing the left parasagittal electrodes and the next four channels representing the right parasagittal electrodes. Channels 9 through 11 are left temporal electrodes; channels 13 through 16 are right temporal electrodes. Channels 17 and 18 are over the vertex of the head. Note the V-like deflections in the bifrontal channels, which are secondary to eye blinks and the 8–9 Hz "alpha" rhythm in the occipital channels.

slowing and disorganization can result from metabolic derangements, intoxication, or brain structural abnormalities involving both hemispheres (eg, head trauma, strokes, hydrocephalus, multiple sclerosis, or Alzheimer dementia). The EEG can also lack sensitivity, even in the face of glaring clinical abnormalities. Patients with clear memory impairment, language difficulties, and poor attention and concentration in mild-to-moderate Alzheimer dementia may have a normal EEG. Persistently normal tracings do not exclude the possibility of underlying epilepsy.

▶ Continuous EEG Monitoring

Because it is rare that a seizure will occur during a 30-minute recording, long-term EEG monitoring (with or without simultaneous video monitoring) has been developed to record and characterize seizures and other paroxysmal spells. In a specialized nursing unit in the hospital or as an ambulatory outpatient recording, long-term monitoring is becoming more widely available. Concurrent video and EEG monitoring is considered the gold standard for diagnosis of seizures, epilepsy, and psychogenic nonepileptic seizures and for distinguishing other paroxysmal spells from seizures (eg, syncope, hypoglycemia, or breath-holding spells). Another major indication is for epilepsy presurgical evaluation—to determine whether a patient is a candidate for focal brain resection.

Long-term monitoring is also increasingly used in the critical care arena, most commonly in cases of status epilepticus, but also in patients after craniotomy, stroke, or head trauma. Prolonged EEG recordings provide another means of monitoring the neurologic status of patients.

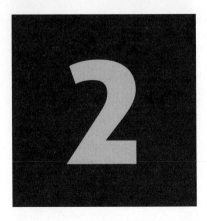

Electromyography, Nerve Conduction Studies, & Evoked Potentials

Dora Leung, MD

Nerve conduction studies and needle electromyography (EMG) provide objective physiologic assessment of peripheral nerves and muscles. These two parts of the examination are performed sequentially, and when a patient is referred to an EMG laboratory, the understanding is that electrodiagnostic evaluation will include both nerve conduction studies and EMG. Special studies are performed in selected patients when clinically indicated.

NERVE CONDUCTION STUDIES

1. Routine Studies

General Considerations

Studies are performed on motor and sensory nerves, but only large myelinated fibers can be evaluated in nerve conduction studies (Figure 2–1). Most studies use surface recording electrodes because of ease and convenience.

Technique

In motor conduction studies, an electrical stimulus is delivered to a skin location known to overlie a peripheral nerve, and motor responses are recorded from muscles supplied by that nerve (Table 2–1). For example, the median nerve can be stimulated at the wrist and then more proximally at the elbow, with the recording electrode placed over the abductor pollicis brevis muscle in the thenar eminence. The evoked response obtained from the electrical stimulation is called the *compound motor action potential* (CMAP) (Figures 2–2 and 2–3). By measuring the distance between the two stimulating sites and the difference between latency onset of the resultant CMAPs, the examiner can calculate the motor conduction velocity of the nerve.

Sensory nerve conduction studies directly assess sensory axons by recording a sensory nerve action potential (SNAP) proximal or distal to the site of stimulation (Figure 2–4; see also Table 2–1). If the stimulus site is distal and the recording electrode is proximal, the impulse is directed toward the spinal cord (orthodromic study). If the stimulation site is proximal and recording site is distal, the impulse is directed away from the spinal cord (antidromic study). SNAP responses usually have small amplitudes in the order of microvolts (as compared with millivolts in the motor responses), and multiple responses with averaging are required to separate background noise from the desired waveforms.

Electrodiagnostic Data

Components that are evaluated in nerve conduction studies include distal latency, conduction velocity, amplitude, and duration.

A. Distal Latency

Distal latency is measured in milliseconds and is the time between the onset of the stimulus to the onset of resulting action potential.

Distal latencies of motor nerves are compared with standardized values and can indicate distal nerve lesions if prolonged as a result of demyelination. However, because of the conduction time required for a nerve impulse to cross the neuromuscular junction and generate the CMAP response, distal latency alone cannot be used to calculate motor conduction velocity. Motor conduction velocity requires an additional stimulation at a more proximal segment of the nerve. The conduction velocity is calculated by the measured distance between the two stimuli divided by the difference in the distal latencies of the motor evoked potentials (see Figure 2–3).

In sensory nerves, because of the absence of neuromuscular junctions, velocity can be calculated directly from sensory latency; the measured distance between stimulation and recording sites is divided by the distal latency of the sensory potential (see Figure 2–4).

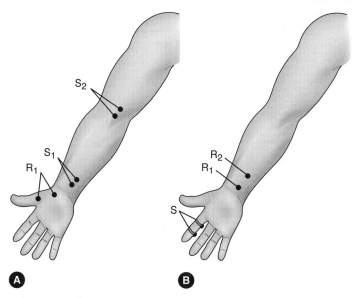

▲ **Figure 2–1.** Technique of nerve conduction studies. Electrode setup for **(A)** motor and **(B)** sensory conduction studies of the median nerve. (R_1 = recording electrode; R_2 = reference electrode; S = stimulation sites.)

Table 2–1. Nerves Commonly Tested in Nerve Conduction Studies

Location	Nerves
Commonly Studied	
Arms	Median (sensory and motor) Ulnar (sensory, and motor recording from abductor digiti minimi)
Legs	Tibial (motor) Peroneal (motor recording from extensor digiti brevis) Sural (sensory)
Less Commonly Studied	
Motor	Ulnar (recording from first dorsal interossei) Radial Musculocutaneous Axillary Peroneal (recording from tibialis anterior) Femoral
Sensory	Radial Dorsal ulnar cutaneous Lateral antebrachial cutaneous Superficial peroneal Deep peroneal Saphenous

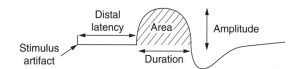

▲ **Figure 2–2.** Components of the motor action potential.

B. Conduction Velocity

Conduction velocity studies measure the speed of impulse conduction in the largest and fastest fibers in the nerve tested. They may therefore fail to detect abnormalities in small sensory fibers.

C. Amplitude

Amplitude is the height of the evoked responses, which is on the order of millivolts in motor responses and microvolts in sensory responses. In a CMAP, the amplitude reflects both the number of fibers generating the action potential and the efficiency of neuromuscular transmission. The CMAP amplitude often correlates clinically with patients' symptoms; weakness and sensory loss caused by large fiber peripheral neuropathy may have low CMAP and SNAP amplitudes. In advanced peripheral neuropathy, sensory or motor responses may be absent.

D. Duration

Duration refers to the total duration of an evoked response measured in milliseconds. It reflects the different conduction rates of axons traveling in the nerve and contributing to the

$$MCV = \text{Distance between } S_2 - S_1/DL_2 - DL_1 = m/s$$

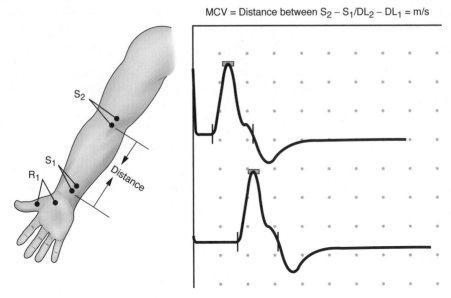

▲ **Figure 2–3.** Motor conduction study of the median nerve. (MCV = motor conduction velocity; R = recording site; S_1 = distal stimulation site; S_2 = proximal stimulation site.)

evoked response. Axons that contribute to the beginning of a motor response are the fastest. If the spread of velocities in the axons within a nerve increases, the duration of response will also increase, with a corresponding drop in amplitude because of dispersion and phase cancellation. However, the area of the response (CMAP or SNAP), which is a product of duration and amplitude measured in millivolt-millisecond (mV·ms) or microvolt-millisecond (μV·ms), reflects the number of activated axons and should be unchanged or only slightly decreased.

▶ **Advantages**

Sensory nerve conduction studies are especially useful because sensory nerves are affected earlier than motor nerves in most peripheral neuropathies. Sensory studies also help differentiate lesions proximal and distal to the dorsal root ganglion. Sensory responses are normal if a lesion is proximal to the dorsal root ganglion. Therefore, even when there is nerve root avulsion from trauma with corresponding

$$SCV = \text{Distance between } R - S/DL = m/s$$

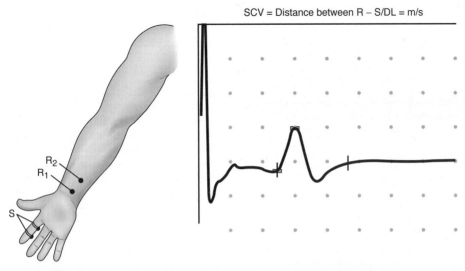

▲ **Figure 2–4.** Sensory conduction study of the median nerve. (DL = distal latency; R = recording site; S = stimulation site; SCV = sensory conduction study.)

anesthesia in that dermatome, sensory responses are normal as long as the dorsal root ganglion is intact.

► Disadvantages

The limitation of sensory conduction is that results are easily affected by other physiologic factors such as age, limb temperature, or limb edema (Table 2–2). In addition, the studies evaluate more proximal portions of the sensory nerve and not the most distal segments.

Often in patients with focal or unilateral lesions, the contralateral limb is used as an internal control. The amplitude of a CMAP or SNAP is considered abnormal if it is less than 50% of the value in the contralateral side. Therefore, studies are usually performed bilaterally.

► When to Order

Motor and sensory conduction studies can be used to identify focal lesions and to distinguish peripheral neuropathy from myopathy and motor neuron disease. They can also detect subclinical lesions (eg, Charcot-Marie-Tooth disease, carpal tunnel syndrome) and differentiate among inherited, acquired, and autoimmune demyelinating polyneuropathy.

► Findings

1. Axonal neuropathy—In axonal neuropathy, motor and sensory action potentials show low amplitudes, with conduction velocity either preserved or only mildly slowed. With nerve transection, distal motor and sensory responses are normal during the first 2 days, but as wallerian

Table 2–2. Sources That Can Affect Nerve Conduction Studies

Factor	Type of Change or Error
Limb temperature	Artificially slow nerve conduction velocity, caused by excessively cool limb temperature
Patient age	Mild decrease in nerve conduction amplitudes and velocities associated with aging
Nerve anomalies	Errors in interpretation due to anatomic variation
Technical problems	Lack of standardization Mistakes in electrode placement Variation in interelectrode distance
Stimulation problems	Submaximal stimulation Excessive stimulation Reversal of cathode/anode Movement artifact
Measurement errors	Errors in measuring distance due to change in limb position between time of stimulation and measurement, resulting in inaccurate calculation of conduction velocity

degeneration proceeds, the response amplitude diminishes and becomes absent 7–10 days after injury.

2. Demyelinating neuropathy—In demyelinating neuropathy, CMAP and SNAP amplitudes can be normal with distal stimulation. If there is focal demyelination, the CMAP amplitude can be markedly reduced on proximal stimulation due to conduction failure across the demyelinated segment. Demyelination can also cause slowing without complete conduction failure or block; the CMAP will then have lower amplitude with longer than normal duration as a result of excessive temporal dispersion within the nerve. However, the area under the negative peak is less affected than the amplitude, indicating that the amplitude decrease is a result of dispersion rather than axonal loss.

2. Late Responses

Routine nerve conduction studies can evaluate only distal segments of the nerve. In the leg, conduction studies evaluate the peroneal and tibial nerves up to the knee. Therefore, late responses such as F waves and H-reflex are used to evaluate the less-assessable proximal portions of the nerve.

A. F Waves

F waves are low-amplitude responses produced by antidromic stimulation of a small number of motor neurons during motor conduction studies. Because the nerve acts as an electric cable, stimulation not only results in CMAP response in the distal muscle, but the impulse is also transmitted proximally toward the spinal cord. A small population of motor neurons (about 2–3% of total at that level) may then become activated and transmit a motor impulse back along the nerve to the recording muscle. The resulting evoked response, which can be viewed as "backfiring," is much smaller in amplitude than the CMAP. Because each electrical stimulation activates a different subpopulation of motor neurons, consecutively recorded F waves will vary in latency, amplitude, and duration. The F-wave latency is the time between the stimulus and onset of an F wave, and the minimal F-wave latency is the most commonly recorded parameter. Prolonged or absent F-wave latency can reflect a proximal lesion when distal nerve conduction is normal. F-wave study is especially useful if there is suspicion of demyelinating neuropathy in proximal segments. In Guillain-Barré syndrome, abnormal or absent F waves may be the earliest finding on nerve conduction studies. If the motor nerve conduction study is slowed distally due to underlying peripheral or entrapment neuropathy, F-wave latency can also be prolonged.

B. H-Reflex

The H-reflex is the electrophysiologic equivalent of the Achilles tendon reflex. By early childhood it is present only in gastrocnemius-soleus and flexor carpi radialis muscles. It is a motor-evoked response that is elicited by stimulating sensory fibers in a peripheral nerve, usually the tibial nerve. A

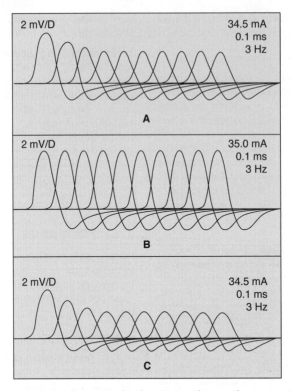

▲ Figure 2–5. Procedure for repetitive stimulation. Study of patient with myasthenia gravis is depicted here. **A: Baseline repetitive stimulation:** (1) Stabilize limb and obtain supramaximal response in distal nerve-muscle pain (eg, median-thenar or ulnar-hypothenar); (2) deliver 10 supramaximal stimuli at 3 Hz; (3) calculate % decrement between first and fourth potentials (shown here, 30% decrement). **B: Postexercise facilitation:** (1) Perform voluntary maximal contraction of muscle being tested for 15 seconds; (2) deliver 10 stimuli at 3 Hz immediately after exercise; (3) calculate % decrement (here 2%) and look for increment. **C: Postexercise exhaustion:** (1) Exercise using maximal force for 1 minute; (2) repeat train of stimulation at 3 Hz at 1, 2, 3, and 4 minutes after exercise; (3) calculate % decrement (here 45%) and, if no decrement, repeat study in the proximal system (accessory-trapezius or facial-nasalis).

high-duration (1 millisecond), low-voltage stimulus is used to activate large-diameter, fast-conducting sensory fibers at an intensity that is below the activation threshold of motor fibers. The action potential then propagates to the dorsal root ganglion and subsequently into the dorsal root, and through a monosynaptic pathway, anterior horn cells are activated, in turn activating the corresponding muscle (the soleus). Because the H-reflex is mediated primarily through the S1 root, asymmetry of latency between sides is often used to support a diagnosis of S1 radiculopathy or a proximal tibial nerve lesion. However, an H-reflex is not present in all normal people.

3. Repetitive Stimulation

Repetitive stimulation of motor nerves is indicated when there is suspicion of a neuromuscular junction disorder such as myasthenia gravis (Figure 2–5). In normal subjects, persistent stimulation at rates less than 5 Hz will cause progressive decline in release of acetylcholine vesicles into the synaptic cleft. Because there is a large excess of vesicles and

neurotransmitters compared with the number of receptors, the decline does not result in reduced numbers of activated muscle fibers. In myasthenia gravis, reduced number of functional acetylcholine receptors results in failure of neuromuscular transmission with repetitive stimulation. Fewer activated fibers result in progressively smaller CMAP amplitude, referred to as *decremental response to repetitive stimulation.*

In myasthenia gravis, the drop in amplitude is progressive from the first to the fourth response, and more than 10% decline in amplitude is considered abnormal. Subsequent responses may show a slight recovery in amplitude. Usually a stimulation rate of 2–3 Hz is adequate to produce maximal decrement. Sustained maximal activation of the muscle being tested is similar to repetitive stimulation at high frequency and can also result in a decremental response, usually maximal 3–4 minutes after the exercise (postexercise exhaustion). Repetitive stimulation immediately after brief (15-second) exercise at maximal effort will have the opposite effect and reverse the decrement that is seen at baseline before exercise (postexercise facilitation). In normal subjects, postexercise facilitation never causes increased response (increment) greater than 50% of baseline. However, in patients with Lambert-Eaton myasthenic syndrome, a presynaptic disorder, the increment increase from postexercise facilitation can be more than two- to threefold. This amplitude increase can also be seen with repetitive stimulation at a high rate (50 Hz).

NEEDLE ELECTROMYOGRAPHY

▶ General Considerations

The needle study is an extension of clinical muscle testing. Almost any muscle can be examined, although to do so is not always practical or useful.

▶ Electrodiagnostic Data

Needle EMG includes assessment of spontaneous activity; evaluation of motor unit amplitude, duration, and appearance; and recruitment pattern of the muscle.

A. Spontaneous Activity

At rest, a normal muscle is electrically silent except in the region of the neuromuscular junctions, where spontaneous endplate potentials result from spontaneous continuous release of vesicles containing acetylcholine. Abnormal spontaneous activity includes fibrillation potentials, positive sharp waves, and fasciculations (Figure 2–6).

Fibrillations and **positive sharp waves** are spontaneous discharges of individual muscle fibers and have characteristic configurations. They are present in both denervation and myopathic diseases, and they have similar pathologic significance. Fibrillations and positive sharp waves are seen about 2 weeks after nerve injury, indicating muscle denervation. In chronic neurogenic diseases such as peripheral neuropathy or motor neuron disease, these potentials can be persistent. Fibrillations and positive sharp waves are also present in myopathic conditions, especially inflammatory myopathies and muscular dystrophy, in which muscle necrosis can separate remaining muscle fibers from their nerve axons and effectively denervate them. Thus these abnormal spontaneous potentials by themselves cannot distinguish neuropathic

from myopathic processes, and information from nerve conduction studies as well as motor unit and recruitment analysis are crucial for diagnosis.

Fasciculations are abnormal, large, spontaneous discharges of single motor units. Their firing pattern is slow and irregular, and although their configuration may be identical to an activated motor unit, they are not under voluntary control. A fasciculation represents a motor unit (all the muscle fibers innervated by a motor neuron); its configuration is therefore larger in amplitude and more complex than a fibrillation or a positive sharp wave. Often visible on skin surface as small muscle movements that are insufficient to move the joint, fasciculations are characteristic of motor neuron diseases such as amyotrophic lateral sclerosis. They can also occur in chronic neurogenic conditions such as peripheral neuropathy or radiculopathy, and they can be a normal finding in small foot muscles and in patients with benign fasciculation syndrome.

In addition to documenting the presence of abnormal spontaneous activity, it is important to note the frequency and abundance of these activities. The abundance of fibrillations and positive sharp waves on EMG corresponds with the severity of denervation.

Other abnormal spontaneous activities occur in certain diseases. **Myotonic discharges** are high-frequency repetitive discharges that wax and wane in amplitude to produce a sound similar to revving up of a motorcycle engine. Myotonic discharges are seen in myotonic dystrophy, myotonia congenita, paramyotonia, familial periodic paralysis, and acid maltase deficiency. **Complex repetitive discharges** are high-frequency discharges that begin and end abruptly without the waxing and waning quality of myotonic discharges. They can be seen in both muscle and nerve diseases. **Myokymia** are grouped discharges occurring in a semirhythmic manner separated by periods of silence. Corresponding to continuous rippling or quivering in the muscle, they are often seen in facial muscles, especially in patients with multiple sclerosis, brainstem tumors, hypocalcemia, or polyradiculopathy. **Cramps** are painful involuntary muscle contractions that on EMG are seen as high-frequency motor unit action potential discharges. **Cramps** can be benign (eg, nocturnal or postexercise cramps), but they are also associated with neuropathic and metabolic abnormalities.

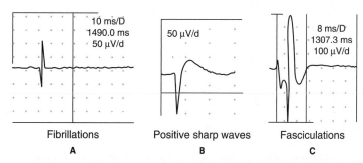

▲ **Figure 2–6.** Abnormal spontaneous potentials. **A:** Fibrillations. **B:** Positive sharp waves. **C:** Fasciculations.

B. Motor Unit Potentials

Following evaluation of insertional and spontaneous activity, motor unit potentials (MUPs) are assessed (Figure 2–7). The normal extracellularly recorded MUP is a triphasic waveform with a duration of 5–15 milliseconds. Its amplitude varies with the size of the motor unit and its proximity to the recording needle. The number of fibers in each motor unit varies, from very few in muscles requiring fine control (eg, eye muscles) to hundreds in large muscles. Each motor unit territory measures about 5–10 mm in diameter, with many units overlapping each other. When a nerve impulse travels down a motor axon, all the muscle fibers in that motor unit fire almost simultaneously, producing the characteristic triphasic waveform. In initial voluntary contraction at low effort, small motor units are activated first, with initial increase in power from higher firing frequency. However, as more force is required, this increased firing frequency is insufficient and larger motor units are recruited on stronger contraction.

To characterize whether a muscle is normal or whether it reflects a myopathic or a neurogenic disorder, quantitative EMG (QEMG) is needed. In QEMG, at least 20 MUPs are collected from one muscle and analyzed, and their values are compared with standardized MUPs. Shorter mean duration and lower amplitudes suggest loss of motor fibers in the motor unit, as seen in myopathies. In neurogenic diseases, amplitude and duration increase due to reinnervation and expansion of MUP territory. Polyphasic MUPs result from temporal dispersion of the individual muscle fibers in the motor unit and can be seen in both myopathic and neuropathic conditions.

C. Recruitment Pattern

The recruitment pattern is the electrical summation of activated MUPs during a submaximal or maximal contraction (Figure 2–8). On maximal effort, the needle recording from a muscle will show a dense band of motor units that completely obliterates the baseline (full recruitment pattern; see Figure 2–8A). The amplitude of the recruitment pattern (the so-called *envelope*) normally is in the range of 2–4 mV.

In myopathy, the number of motor units is unchanged, but the number of muscle fibers in each unit is decreased. Therefore, the density of the recruitment pattern is unchanged, but the amplitude of the envelope during maximal force is low. In addition, because motor units are small in myopathy, more units are recruited at low force, creating an early recruitment pattern.

In neurogenic disease, the number of muscle fibers in a motor unit can be either normal or increased, depending on whether sprouting and reinnervation have occurred. However, there are fewer motor units in the affected muscle,

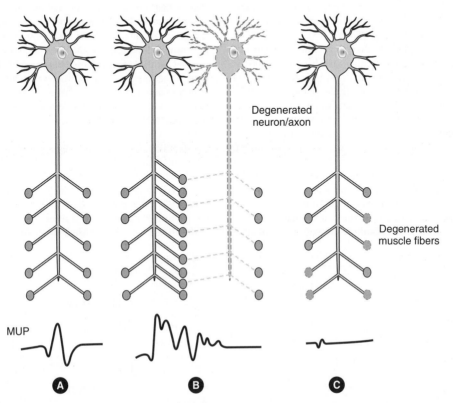

Degenerated neuron/axon

Degenerated muscle fibers

MUP

A   **B**   **C**

▲ **Figure 2–7.** Comparison of **(A)** normal muscle fiber and motor unit potential with changes seen in **(B)** neuropathic and **(C)** myopathic diseases.

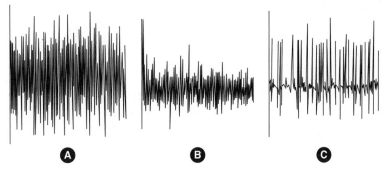

▲ **Figure 2–8.** Recruitment patterns. **A:** Full. **B:** Reduced. **C:** Discrete.

and fewer MUPs are recorded by EMG on maximal effort. The recruitment pattern in neurogenic disease is usually less dense, or "reduced" (see Figure 2–8B). In severe neurogenic disease, very few motor units may remain in the muscle, and increase in muscle power depends on increased firing frequency. In extreme cases, recruitment patterns may show only one or two motor units firing at high frequency (up to 40 Hz), resulting in a "discrete" pattern (see Figure 2–8C).

▶ **Findings**

1. Acute axonal loss—In acute axonal loss, wallerian degeneration occurs in the first week, with denervation of muscle fibers of the affected motor units and appearance of fibrillations and positive sharp waves (Table 2–3). Surviving axons then sprout collateral fibers to reinnervate the muscle fibers over the course of weeks or months. The resultant MUP reflects an increased number of fibers and shows an increase in amplitude, duration, and polyphasia; however, the recruitment pattern is reduced because of loss of motor units.

2. Demyelinating neuropathy—In demyelinating neuropathy, the underlying axons are intact; therefore, no denervation or reinnervation is seen on needle EMG study. Motor unit amplitude, duration, and configuration are normal, and unless conduction block occurs with failure of axonal transmission, the recruitment pattern should be full.

3. Acute myopathy—In acute myopathy, fibrillations and positive sharp waves may be present, with fewer muscle fibers remaining for each motor unit. MUPs show low amplitude and decreased duration. The recruitment pattern can show early recruitment to compensate for decreased motor fibers by activating more motor units for each level of force.

4. Chronic myopathy—In chronic myopathy, such as polymyositis and muscular dystrophies, reinnervation by other motor axons may occur as the muscle fibers regenerate, and MUPs may have larger than expected amplitude and duration as well as polyphasia. However, the recruitment pattern will still be full in a clinically weak muscle. In end-stage myopathy, with severe damage to all muscle fibers, there may be loss of entire motor units, with small, short-duration MUPs and decreased recruitment in clinically weak muscles.

▼ EVOKED POTENTIALS

Evoked potentials are electrical responses of the nervous system to motor or sensory stimuli. Classically, the evoked responses in clinical testing involve the sensory pathways of the visual, auditory, and somatosensory systems. The sensory stimuli that are used in the clinical laboratory include electrical stimulation of certain sensory nerves, flashing lights or checkered board patterns, and brief clicks. The recordings are from surface electrodes placed over the limbs, spinal cord, and scalp. The recorded potentials are of extremely low amplitudes when compared with ongoing spontaneous cortical electrical activity. Only through the time-locked summation of hundreds or thousands of stimulus-response trials can the cortical and subcortical responses be recorded. Changes in evoked potentials as a result of neurologic lesions reflect conduction delay along the corresponding pathways and thus in the latency of response. When the waveform component is attenuated or lost, it can indicate a conduction block in the pathway.

Evoked potentials are most sensitive in detecting lesions in the spinal cord and brain, including lesions that are not

Table 2–3. Electromyographic Criteria for Neuromuscular Disease

	Neurogenic Disease	Myopathic Disease
Spontaneous activity	+	+
Polyphasia	Increased	Increased
MUP amplitude	Increased	Decreased (nonpolyphasic units)
Mean MUP duration	>120% normal	<80% normal
Recruitment/maximal effort	Reduced/discrete	Early/full
Envelope amplitude (normal = 2–4 mV)	Normal or increased	Normal or decreased

MUP = motor unit potential; + = present.

clinically apparent. Their primary use in the past was in the detection of silent lesions in patients suspected of having multiple sclerosis. With the advent of magnetic resonance imaging, evoked potentials are now rarely required in the diagnosis of multiple sclerosis. Evoked potentials are currently used for intraoperative monitoring of the integrity of the nervous system during spinal cord and some brain surgeries. It has also been used to aid prognosis for comatose patients.

VISUAL EVOKED POTENTIALS

To test for visual evoked potentials (VEPs), a checkered board pattern is flashed in front of an individual with each eye tested separately. This rapid pattern reversal produces a positive signal recording at the occiput with a latency of about 100 milliseconds after stimulus onset, called the *P100*. A significant asymmetry of the P100 is strongly indicative of an abnormality of the optic nerve. A bilateral delayed response is less specific, and is seen in bilateral optic nerve disease, widespread brain disease, or abnormality of the chiasm.

VEPs are very sensitive in detecting demyelinating lesions of the optic nerve, but they can also be abnormal in patients with glaucoma, cataracts, retinopathy, refractive error, and compressive or ischemic lesions of the optic nerve.

BRAINSTEM AUDITORY EVOKED POTENTIALS

Brainstem auditory evoked potentials (BAEPs) are generated by the auditory nerve and the brainstem in response to a stimulus, usually a click. Three components of the BAEP are of clinical interest: wave I is from the peripheral auditory nerve, wave III is generated in the caudal pons, and wave V is generated in the region of the inferior colliculus (Figure 2–9).

Abnormal BAEPs are almost always associated with abnormalities in the brainstem generator sites. BAEPs are especially sensitive in detecting the presence of an acoustic neuroma or other cerebropontine angle tumors and for monitoring the integrity of the brainstem during tumor debulking surgery in this anatomic area. As with VEPs, abnormal BAEPs can detect clinically silent demyelinating lesions in the brainstem.

SOMATOSENSORY EVOKED POTENTIALS

Somatosensory evoked potentials (SSEPs) are obtained with electrical stimulation of nerves in arms and legs and reflect sequential activation of the posterior column sensory pathways. For SSEPs of the arm, the stimulation is delivered at the wrist, and the volleys are simultaneously recorded with electrodes at the clavicle (Erb point), neck, and parietal scalp, reflecting activity generated from the brachial plexus, upper cervical cord (N13), lower brainstem (P14), thalamus (N18), and primary sensory cortex (N20).

Because the somatosensory pathway is more physically widespread than that of other evoked potentials, SSEPs are sensitive to many different lesions. Similar to the other evoked potentials, SSEPs can detect subclinical lesions in patients with multiple sclerosis. Currently, SSEPs are used for

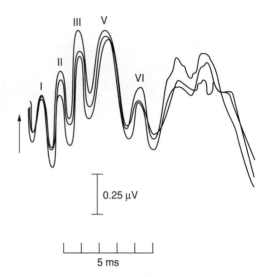

0.25 μV

5 ms

▲ **Figure 2–9.** Components of the brainstem auditory evoked potential (BAEPs). Waves I through VI indicate BAEPs generated by the peripheral auditory (eighth) nerve (I), cochlear nucleus (II), superior olivary complex (III), high pons, low midbrain (lateral lemniscus and inferior colliculus) (IV and V).

intraoperative monitoring of the spinal cord during neurosurgical and orthopedic surgeries. SSEPs can also be used to help guide prognosis in comatose patients due to anoxic injury. Studies have shown that postanoxic patients who have absent cortical SSEP (N20) response uniformly have poor neurologic outcome.

Bouwes A, et al. Somatosensory evoked potentials during mild hypothermia after cardiopulmonary resuscitation. *Neurology* 2009;73:1457–1461. [PMID: 19884573]

Fisher MA. H reflexes and F waves. Fundamentals, normal and abnormal patterns. *Neurol Clin North Am* 2002;20:339–360. [PMID: 12152439]

Katirji B. The clinical electromyography examination. An overview. *Neurol Clin North Am* 2002;20:291–303. [PMID: 12152437]

Kothbauer KF, Novak K. Intraoperative monitoring for tethered cord injury: An update. *Neurosurg Focus* 2004;16:E8. [PMID: 15209491]

Preston DC, Shapiro BE. Needle electromyography. Fundamentals, normal and abnormal patterns. *Neurol Clin North Am* 2002;20:361–396. [PMID: 12152440]

Wang JT, Young GB, Connolly JF. Prognostic value of evoked responses and event-related brain potentials in coma. *Can J Neurol Sci* 2004;31:438–450. [PMID: 15595246]

Wilbourn AJ. Nerve conduction studies. The components, abnormalities and value in localization. *Neurol Clin North Am* 2002;20:305–338. [PMID: 12152438]

Young GB, Wang JT, Connolly JF. Prognostic determination in anoxic ischemic and traumatic encephalopathies. *J Clin Neurophysiol* 2004;21:379–390. [PMID: 15592010]

Neuroradiology

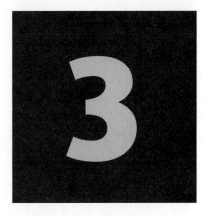

John P. Loh, MD

The basic modalities available for imaging the central nervous system are plain films, computed tomography (CT), magnetic resonance imaging (MRI), myelography and post-myelography CT, catheter angiography, ultrasonography, and nuclear medicine techniques. The strengths and weakness of each modality, and guidelines regarding the "right" test to order, are included in the following discussion.

PLAIN FILMS

▶ General Considerations

Although largely replaced by CT and MRI, plain films of the skull and spine are still used for screening purposes in various clinical situations (Figure 3–1). The term *plain films* is becoming increasingly anachronistic in the digital age. *Plain radiographs* is more accurate.

▶ Advantages

Plain films are inexpensive and easy to obtain. Portable x-ray machines can be moved to the patient's bedside and into operating rooms. The entire spine can be rapidly surveyed. Plain films provide good detail of bone in an easily understood format.

▶ Disadvantages

Overlapping structures obscure pathology and complicate film interpretation. As plain films are replaced by CT and MRI, expertise in their interpretation is disappearing. Plain films provide virtually no soft tissue information.

▶ When to Order

1. Foreign bodies—Plain films can identify and locate metallic foreign bodies in the skull or spine. They often are used to screen patients suspected of having metallic foreign bodies near vital structures before MRI examination.

2. Spinal alignment and stability—Plain films are used to evaluate spinal alignment in patients with spinal trauma, rheumatoid arthritis, and scoliosis. Comparison of films taken in flexion and extension is a good method of ascertaining spinal stability.

3. Spinal fractures, infections, and metastases—Plain films are sometimes used in the initial evaluation of patients with suspected fractures, infections, and metastases of the spine.

4. Spinal anomalies—Plain films are also used to identify congenital spinal anomalies, such as segmentation anomalies, hemivertebrae, and spina bifida.

5. Degenerative disk disease—Many physicians use plain films as an inexpensive survey of degenerative changes in patients with chronic back or neck pain.

6. Bone lesions—Plain films remain the mainstay in the diagnosis of focal primary bone lesions of the skull and spine.

7. Ventriculoperitoneal shunt—A shunt series, consisting of plain films of the skull and neck, chest, and abdomen, is often used in the initial evaluation of the integrity of a shunt.

COMPUTED TOMOGRAPHY

▶ General Considerations

The soft tissue contrast resolution of CT allows direct cross-sectional imaging of the brain and spine. An x-ray tube emitting a thin, collimated x-ray beam is rotated around the region of interest. X-ray detectors rotating in tandem at the opposite side of the patient measure how much the x-ray beam is attenuated at the various positions of the x-ray tube. A relative attenuation coefficient is calculated for every volume element, called a voxel, within the patient, directly correlating with the ability of the tissue to block x-rays, which, in turn, is directly related to the electron density of the tissue. This coefficient is assigned a shade on a gray scale, and an image of a slice of brain or spine is created.

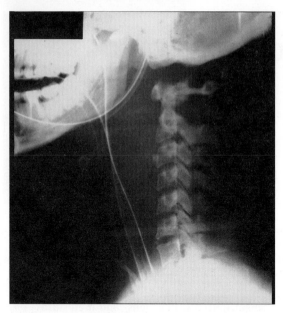

▲ **Figure 3–1.** Lateral plain film of the cervical spine reveals traumatic occipitovertebral dissociation manifested by separation of the occipital condyles from the atlas (C1) and marked prevertebral soft tissue swelling.

To decrease scan time, continuous scanning of the patient as he or she is moved through the x-ray beam (ie, helical scanning) is performed. Modern scanners have multiple rows of x-ray detectors. Depending on the scanner configuration, 64, 128, 256, or even 320 image slices can be created in one rotation of the x-ray tube. Slices as thin as 0.5 mm can be obtained. This large volume of high-quality data can be used to create sagittal, oblique, and coronal reformations and three-dimensional (3D) volume-rendered images. New dual-energy CT scanners with two x-ray tubes instead of one, each emitting different energies, can distinguish bone, blood, and contrast material, allowing for bone-subtracted CT angiograms as well as even shorter scan times.

▶ Use of Contrast Agents

Iodinated nonionic water-soluble materials, the principle contrast agents used for CT scans, are considered reasonably safe. Contrast material is administered intravenously. It rapidly circulates throughout the body and enters the interstitial space everywhere except within the central nervous system, where it is contained within the vascular system by the blood–brain barrier.

Many lesions enhance and become brighter and more conspicuous than surrounding tissue on CT scans after the intravenous administration of iodinated contrast material. This enhancement greatly increases the sensitivity of the examination.

There are two mechanisms by which contrast enhancement of lesions occurs. First, intravascular contrast enhances normal and abnormal blood vessels. This is the mechanism by which aneurysms, vascular malformations, and some hypervascular neoplasms enhance. Second, intravascular contrast material leaks into a lesion if the blood–brain barrier is disrupted, as it occurs in a wide variety of clinical conditions, including demyelinating disease, infarction, abscess, and neoplasm. The timing and pattern of enhancement can offer important clues to the diagnosis, increasing the specificity of the examination.

The fast scanning times of modern scanners allow imaging of a contrast bolus as it passes through the vascular system and the creation of 3D images of the vascular system (ie, CT angiography). The ability of modern scanners to perform rapid repeated imaging of the same location of the brain allows time-attenuation curves to be generated for each and every voxel, from which CT perfusion blood volume, blood flow, time-to-peak density, and mean transit time maps can be generated. The measurement of the upward slope of the curve as the contrast arrives at the voxel is an approximation of blood flow. The area under the curve is proportional to blood volume. The mean transit time is blood volume divided by blood flow. The time-to-peak is the time between the time of injection and the time of maximum or peak attenuation.

Adverse reactions to contrast agents do occur. The most common category of reaction is idiosyncratic, including flushing, nausea, and vomiting; skin rashes, including urticaria; and anaphylactoid reactions, including bronchospasm, hypotension, cardiac arrhythmia, syncope, and death. There is no reliable way of predicting whether any given patient will suffer an adverse idiosyncratic reaction. Contrast administration may be uneventful even in patients with a history of severe contrast reaction; conversely, severe contrast reactions may occur in patients who have never previously been exposed to contrast material or who have previously received contrast material uneventfully. It is a good rule of thumb to premedicate with corticosteroids any patient whose history suggests that a severe contrast reaction is possible; a history of severe allergies, bronchospasm, or laryngospasm warrants premedication. A widely used premedication regimen is prednisone 50 mg given by mouth at 13 hours, 7 hours, and 1 hour before the examination.

A second major category of adverse reaction is renal toxicity. Patients at risk include those with abnormal renal function, diabetes mellitus, congestive heart failure, dehydration, or multiple myeloma. Particular care should be taken that such patients are adequately hydrated and that the lowest possible amount of contrast is used. Renal failure, manifested by a rise in serum creatinine levels and oliguria, is usually transient. Metformin, an oral agent for the treatment of diabetes mellitus, should be stopped and not restarted until 48 hours after contrast administration because of the rare occurrence of acute lactic acidosis, which has a mortality rate approaching 50%.

Advantages

CT is inexpensive and widely available compared with MRI. A complete examination of the head or spine or both can be obtained in seconds. Because of the very short scan time, emergency patients can easily be "squeezed" into the schedule. Patients can be brought safely into the CT room with the full armamentarium of the intensive care unit or emergency department staff without the screening for metallic foreign bodies that is required for MRI. The studies are relatively easy to interpret.

Disadvantages

CT scanners use ionizing radiation. The radiation dose is relatively high, particularly in evaluating the lumbar spine. Variability in the thickness of the skull, particularly in the posterior fossa adjacent to the petrous pyramids, leads to unequal absorptions of the x-ray beam. This phenomenon, called *beam hardening*, causes streak artifacts that obscure detail. In the brain, certain white matter lesions are poorly seen, particularly demyelinating lesions. In the lower cervical and thoracic spine, very poor spatial and soft tissue resolution of the contents of the spinal canal is obtained.

When to Order

1. Head trauma—The utility of CT scans of the head in head trauma is well established. Epidural, subdural, subarachnoid, and parenchymal hematomas and contusions are readily identified (Figure 3–2).

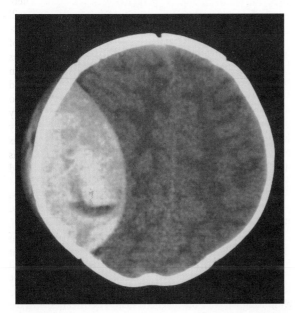

▲ **Figure 3–2.** Nonenhanced axial CT scan of the head shows a large, biconvex, high-density epidural hematoma compressing the adjacent cerebral hemisphere.

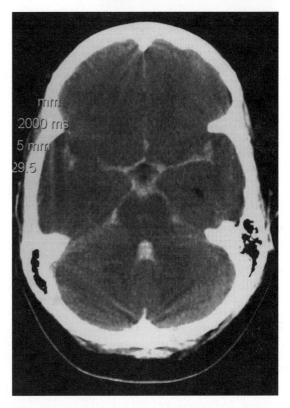

▲ **Figure 3–3.** Nonenhanced axial CT scan of the head shows high-density material in the suprasellar cistern consistent with subarachnoid hemorrhage. Subsequent cerebral angiography disclosed an aneurysm of the right posterior communicating artery.

2. Acute headache—CT is the test of choice to diagnose acute intracranial hemorrhage, particularly subarachnoid hemorrhage (Figure 3–3). Its sensitivity for subarachnoid hemorrhage is very high, exceeding 95% on the first day of hemorrhage but dropping off rapidly after that. Lumbar punctures are required in cases of suspected subarachnoid hemorrhage if the initial imaging study is negative.

3. Acute cerebral infarction—A stroke series or stroke protocol followed at many stroke centers consists of the following. A nonenhanced CT is obtained to rule out intracranial hemorrhage before the administration of tissue plasminogen-activating factor (Plate 1A). CT perfusion is performed to establish the presence and size of a penumbra of ischemic yet potentially salvageable tissue around a core of infracted tissue. Blood volume measurements are usually used to identify the infarction core (Plate 1B). Blood flow, mean transit time, and, to a lesser extent, time-to-peak measurements are used to identify the ischemic penumbra (Plate 1C,D). CT angiography is performed to detect the precise location of the occlusion in the brain (Figure 3–4) and to

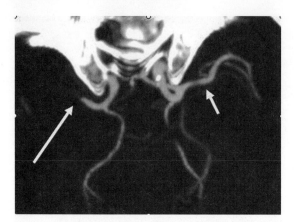

▲ **Figure 3–4.** Maximum-intensity projection (MIP) axial image of the circle of Willis shows occlusion of the proximal right middle cerebral artery (long arrow). The left middle cerebral artery is normal (short arrow).

evaluate the cervical arteries (Plate 2). CT perfusion and CT angiographic results may lead to aggressive neurointerventional procedures when a substantial ischemic penumbra and an accessible occlusion, such as in the proximal middle cerebral artery, exist.

4. Chronic headache, suspicion of raised intracranial pressure, and suspicion of intracranial mass—A CT scan is obtained before lumbar puncture in patients suspected of having meningitis or pseudotumor cerebri. In the emergency department, CT can be used to triage patients with suspected intracranial masses. Positive scans might mandate immediate admission and emergent MRI. Negative scans may allow outpatient follow-up and an elective MRI.

5. Intracranial calcifications—The detection of calcifications within a lesion often increases diagnostic accuracy. MRI is notorious for missing calcifications.

6. Bone lesions—The high spatial resolution of CT scans provides exquisite detail of osseous lesions, improving diagnostic accuracy in these lesions even when detected by other modalities such as plain film, MRI, or nuclear medicine scans.

7. Temporal bone lesions—CT can detect congenital anomalies, lytic or blastic changes, inflammatory disease such as otomastoiditis and cholesteatoma, fractures, and ossicular dislocations. MRI is preferred for sensorineural hearing loss to rule out acoustic schwannoma and other lesions of the internal auditory canal or cerebellopontine angle cistern.

8. Spinal trauma—In the initial evaluation of severe spinal trauma, CT can demonstrate fractures and alignment abnormalities. In many instances, CT can demonstrate hematomas and disk herniations within the spinal canal.

9. Postoperative spine—In postoperative patients, CT provides an accurate assessment of the alignment of the spine and the position of surgical hardware, such as pedicle screws, surgical cages, and bone grafts. The use of very thin slices sharply reduces the amount of streak artifacts arising from metallic devices.

10. Degenerative spinal disease—CT can identify disk bulges and herniations, particularly in the lumbar spine, and it can be more accurate than MRI in demonstrating ossific or calcific abnormalities such as osteophytes or ossification of the anterior or posterior longitudinal ligament.

11. MRI not obtainable—In patients in whom an MRI examination is contraindicated (eg, by the presence of a pacemaker or intracranial ferromagnetic aneurysm clip) or who cannot tolerate an MRI (eg, due to claustrophobia), or in circumstances in which an MRI is unavailable, a CT examination may be an adequate substitute.

12. CT angiography—Although catheter angiography remains the gold standard, modern scanners can generate very high-quality angiographic images. The safety and widespread availability of CT angiography compared with catheter angiography often makes it the initial diagnostic test in a variety of clinical circumstances, including subarachnoid hemorrhage and stroke (Plate 3). Image quality is often such that catheter angiography can be forgone. CT angiography does not suffer from the turbulence-related artifacts that affect magnetic resonance (MR) angiography.

MAGNETIC RESONANCE IMAGING

▶ General Considerations

MRI offers further improvements in soft tissue resolution. The patient is placed in a strong magnetic field. Hydrogen protons within the patient tend to align themselves with the magnetic field. A radiofrequency pulse stimulates these protons to emit a radio signal. This signal or echo differs in strength, frequency, and phase from point to point, depending on differences in the local molecular environment. Using radio receivers, the strength and location of these signals or echoes are mapped on a matrix of tissue volumes called *voxels*. The strength of the signal is displayed on a gray scale, and an image is generated. The entire combination of stimulating radiofrequency pulse, secondary radiofrequency pulses, and applied magnetic field gradients constitutes the pulse sequence.

The strength of the echo signal depends on many factors intrinsic to the tissues examined. These include proton density, brownian motion, flow, magnetic susceptibility, and time constants, called *T1* and *T2*. T1 correlates with the time it takes for the stimulated protons to return to their rest condition aligned with the magnetic field. T2 correlates with the time it takes for signal to be lost because of dephasing.

By manipulating the various components of the pulse sequence, the relative contribution to echo signal strength of

Table 3–1. Magnetic Resonance Pulse Sequences

Pulse Sequence	Tissue Contrast Based on Differences in	Comments
T1-weighted	Time constant T1	Good anatomic display Used for contrast-enhanced examinations Fat, methemoglobin, contrast material, and proteinaceous fluid are high signal on T1-weighted pulse sequences
T2-weighted	Time constant T2	Many CNS lesions are high signal on T2-weighted pulse sequences; these include vasogenic edema, cytotoxic edema (infarction), demyelinating plaques, cysts, necrosis, subacute hemorrhage, and encephalomalacia
Spin density-weighted	"Spin" or proton density	Balance between T1-weighted and T2-weighted pulse sequences
FLAIR	Time constant T2	T2-weighted pulse sequence with signal from CSF nullified High T2-signal lesions rendered more conspicuous than on regular T2-weighted pulse sequence
Magnetic susceptibility (gradient echo)	Susceptibility of tissue to becoming magnetized in magnetic field of scanner	Deoxyhemoglobin, methemoglobin, and hemosiderin (found in acute, subacute, and chronic hematomas, respectively) are particularly susceptible to magnetization; this distorts the local magnetic field, causing conspicuous loss of signal
Diffusion-weighted	Ability of water molecules to diffuse	Restricted diffusion in acute or subacute infarction causes very bright signal; this finding is confirmed by calculation of apparent diffusion coefficients (ADC), a quantitative measure of diffusivity, for every voxel, which are then displayed on an ADC map
Time-of-flight and phase contrast	Blood flow velocity	Used to create MR angiograms and venograms

CNS = central nervous system; CSF = cerebrospinal fluid; FLAIR = fluid-attenuated inversion recovery; MR = magnetic resonance.

these various factors can be enhanced or minimized (Table 3–1). These different pulse sequences, each achieving tissue contrast by different mechanisms, give rise to the complexity and power of MRI.

▶ Use of Contrast Agents

Chelated gadolinium, a paramagnetic material that shortens T1 and T2 values, is used as an intravenously administered contrast agent in MRI examinations. Lesions enhancing after gadolinium appear bright or hyperintense on T1-weighted pulse sequences (Figure 3–5). Chelated gadolinium is probably the safest contrast agent used in radiology. Reactions ranging from mild to severe occur, but they are much less common than with CT contrast material. Patients in renal failure, particularly those patients on hemodialysis, are at risk for a potentially severe, potentially fatal disorder called nephrogenic systemic sclerosis. Careful screening and use of new contrast agents at reduced dosages have dramatically diminished the incidence of this complication.

Chelated gadolinium is not administered to pregnant women because of its known accumulation in the amniotic fluid and the risk of teratogenic effects. Chelated gadolinium is considered safe to administer in lactating women because of the extremely low amounts transmitted to and subsequently absorbed by the breast-feeding infant.

As with CT, MR contrast agents enhance vascular structures, both normal and abnormal, but because the tumbling motion of the hydrogen protons in pulsatile flowing blood leads to unpredictable signal changes, this vascular enhancement is somewhat inconsistent and unpredictable. The most common mechanism of abnormal enhancement is disruption of the blood–brain barrier, allowing leakage of contrast into the interstitial space. As with CT, this mechanism is seen in a wide variety of conditions, with the pattern of enhancement aiding in the diagnosis of the lesion.

As with CT, MR perfusion values of relative blood flow, relative blood volume, mean transit time, and time-to-peak can be obtained by rapid repetitive scanning at the same location as the infused chelated gadolinium passes through the brain. Instead of generating a time-attenuation curve, a time-signal intensity curve is generated from which perfusion values are generated in a manner analogous to that of CT perfusion.

▶ Safety

The strong magnetic field required by MRI constitutes its main hazard. Floor buffers, crash carts, "sand bags" filled with BB pellets, and oxygen tanks have been pulled into the scanner, sometimes with fatal results. MRI-compatible stretchers, oxygen tanks, trays, foot-stools, intravenous poles, backboards, ventilators, monitoring devices, and fire extinguishers are commercially available. Scissors, clamps, and other surgical instruments held in the pockets of medical personnel must be removed or secured before entry into the vicinity of the MRI scanner.

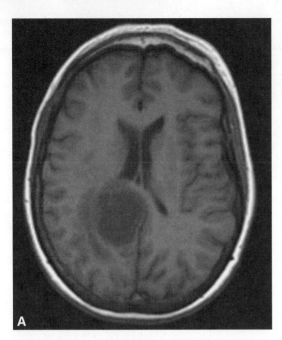 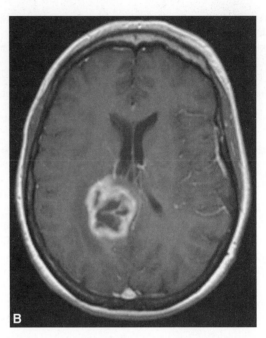

▲ **Figure 3–5.** **A:** Nonenhanced MRI of the brain shows a low T1-signal right deep parietal mass. **B:** Postcontrast MRI of the brain shows avid enhancement of the lesion with nonenhancing central components suggesting necrosis. The lesion is a surgically proven glioblastoma.

Patients must be screened for the presence of metallic foreign material before placement on the MRI table. Such material includes ferromagnetic aneurysm clips, cardiac pacemakers, implanted cardiac defibrillators, cochlear implants, and neurostimulation systems. Plain films or CT scans help identify and localize foreign bodies. Online reference services such as *www.MRIsafety.com* are helpful in determining the safety of foreign bodies or devices.

▶ Advantages

The large number of pulse sequences, each creating contrast by different mechanisms, greatly increases sensitivity and specificity.

Sagittal and coronal images are routinely obtained by manipulating the magnetic field gradients without changing the patient's position.

MRI scans do not involve ionizing radiation, which is of particular importance when imaging children and pregnant women.

Chelated gadolinium is a safer contrast agent than the agents used with CT examinations.

Excellent soft tissue resolution is obtained in evaluating the brain and spinal cord. Portions of the brain adjacent to the skull base, which are often obscured by streak artifacts on CT, are well seen on MRI scan. The central gray matter of the spinal cord can be identified and small spinal cord lesions seen. MRI is very sensitive for bone marrow abnormalities, including metastases and bone edema.

Certain pulse sequences exceed the sensitivity of CT for specific questions. For example, with fluid-attenuated inversion recovery (FLAIR), high T2-signal white matter lesions, including vasogenic edema, infiltrating tumors, and demyelinating plaques, are more conspicuous than with CT (Figure 3–6).

MRI often detects nonspecific white matter lesions not seen with CT. These hyperintense lesions, best seen using FLAIR and unassociated with mass effect or abnormal enhancement, are variously described as unidentified bright objects (UBOs), areas of leukoaraiosis, microvascular disease, or chronic ischemia. They are found most often in elderly, diabetic, and hypertensive patients.

Diffusion-weighted imaging (DWI) can detect cerebral infarctions within minutes of symptom onset.

MR angiograms (Plate 4) and venograms can be obtained without contrast material.

Magnetic susceptibility gradient echo pulse sequences are very sensitive in detecting acute, subacute, or chronic brain or spinal cord hemorrhages.

▶ Disadvantages

Because of the large number of pulse sequences now considered an essential part of every examination, MRI scan times are significantly longer as compared with CT.

Many patients experience claustrophobia in the closed environment of the MRI scanner. This problem can sometimes be overcome with sedation. So-called *open MRI*

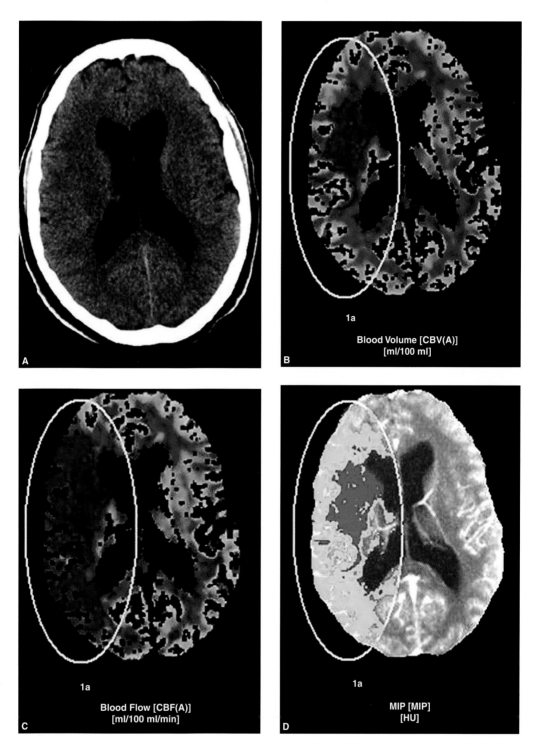

▲ **Plate 1. A:** Nonenhanced axial CT scan of the head shows no evidence of hemorrhage. **B:** Perfusion CT blood volume map shows a core of infracted tissue in the right basal ganglia. **C:** Perfusion CT blood flow map shows a much larger ischemic zone of reduced blood flow. **D:** The size of the mismatch is shown on this overlay map of blood volume and blood flow. (Used with permission from Dr. Ke Lin)

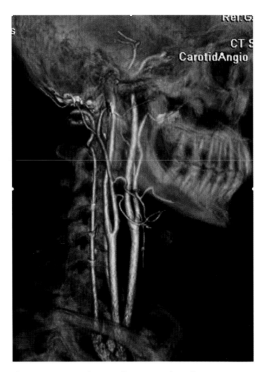

▲ **Plate 2.** Normal 3D-volume rendered CT angiogram of the neck. (Used with permission from Emilio Vega, RT)

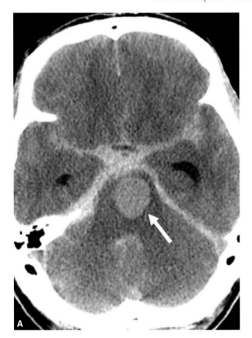

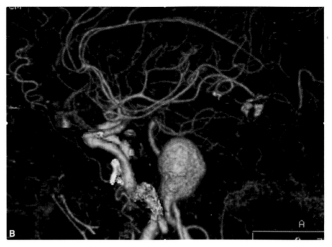

▲ **Plate 3. A:** Nonenhanced axial CT of the head shows subarachnoid hemorrhage and a high density in the pons, which might mistakenly be interpreted as a hematoma. **B:** 3D-volume rendered image of the CT angiogram of the brain viewed from the patient's left side shows a large proximal basilar aneurysm, which had invaginated into the pons from below.

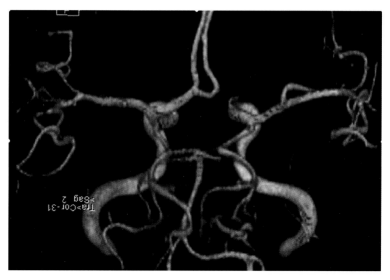

▲ **Plate 4.** Normal MIP 3D-volume rendered MR angiogram of the circle of Willis. The A1 segment of the right anterior cerebral artery is hypoplastic. (Used with permission from Kelly Anne Mcgorty, BS, RT [R] [M] [MR])

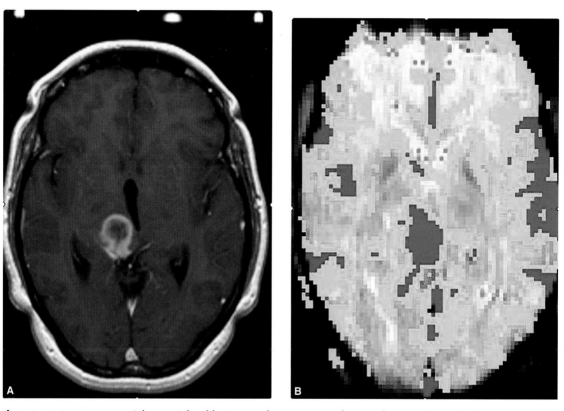

▲ **Plate 5. A:** Postcontrast axial T1-weighted brain MRI shows a ring-enhancing lesion in the right thalamus. **B:** MR relative blood volume perfusion map shows marked hyperfusion of this lesion. This is a surgically proven glioblastoma.

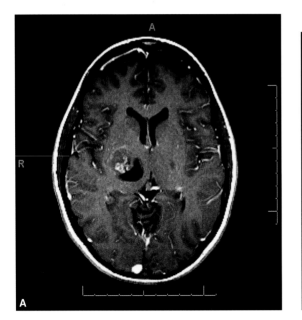
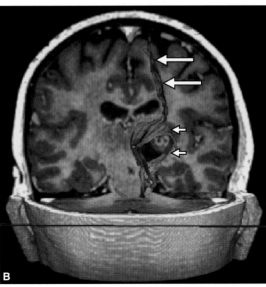

▲ **Plate 6.** **A:** Postcontrast T1-weight axial image shows a right thalamic pilocytic astrocytoma. **B:** MR tractography viewed from behind the patient shows the position of myelin tracts (long arrows) and their displacement by the mass (short arrows).

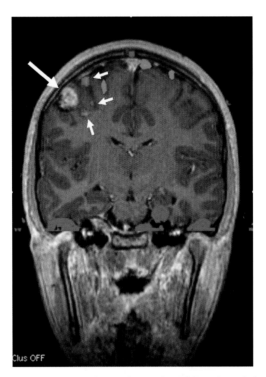

▲ **Plate 7.** Functional MRI shows the relationship of this patient's enhancing cavernoma (long arrow) to the motor cortex (short arrows) using a finger-tapping paradigm.

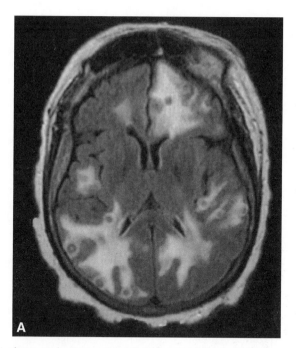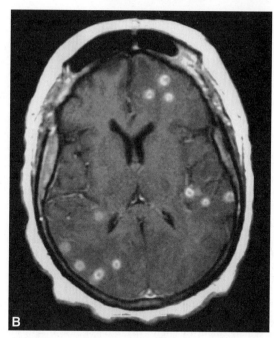

▲ **Figure 3–6. A:** Axial FLAIR MRI scan of the brain shows multiple areas of vasogenic edema. **B:** Contrast-enhanced axial T1-weighted image of the brain shows multiple small ring-enhancing lesions that were subsequently proven at surgery to be tuberculomas.

scanners are available, but these are generally less versatile than standard scanners.

The dangers of the magnetic field are a threat, especially to patients in whom an adequate history is unavailable. This threat also exists for health care personnel accompanying the patient.

The numerous types of the pulse sequences that give MRI its power at the same time add to the complexity of scan interpretation. Thus a description of a lesion on MRI may seem long-winded: "Isointense signal on T1-weighted pulse sequences, low signal on T2-weighted pulse sequences, hypointense on FLAIR, markedly hypointense on gradient echo. . . ." (The same patient's CT report reads: "There is a hyperdense mass consistent with an acute hematoma in. . . .")

Calcifications are notoriously difficult to appreciate on MRI. Bone detail is poor.

▶ **When to Order**

A. Brain

1. Stroke—DWI is a fast and accurate method of detecting acute infarction (Figure 3–7). Signal abnormalities on diffusion-weighted images appear within minutes of symptom onset and can persist for weeks. Magnetic susceptibility pulse and FLAIR sequences can detect hemorrhage and exclude other lesions mimicking strokes. Because of its speed, accessibility, and sensitivity in detecting hemorrhage,

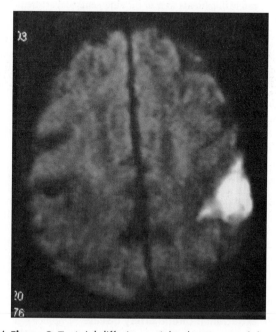

▲ **Figure 3–7.** Axial diffusion-weighted MRI scan of the brain shows a conspicuous, high-signal acute infarction in the distribution of the right middle cerebral artery. The nonenhanced CT scan of the brain obtained at the same time was normal.

a CT is the test of choice before the intravenous administration of tissue plasminogen activator. A CT is, however, less effective than MRI in confirming the diagnosis of acute ischemic infarction. In the first 3 hours, it may be normal or may exhibit only very subtle abnormalities. An MR angiogram can be obtained to determine the site of occlusion. MR perfusion is discussed later.

2. Chronic headache—Most patients with headaches do not require imaging. However, when imaging is required, MRI is the test of choice. In some circumstances, a CT scan can be used as an initial screening examination (eg, before lumbar puncture). If pseudotumor cerebri is a clinical suspicion, MR venography can exclude dural sinus thrombosis, stenosis, or occlusion.

3. Seizures—CT performed acutely can exclude hemorrhage and large mass lesions. MRI is more sensitive, particularly in patients with partial complex seizures.

4. Tumors—MRI is the test of choice for both primary and metastatic lesions. After tumor resection, MRI with and without contrast should be promptly obtained to detect any residual tumor. (If MRI is delayed, postoperative enhancement of gliotic tissue may cause diagnostic confusion.)

5. Infection—MRI is the test of choice; however, the speed and availability of CT often make it the first diagnostic test for acutely ill patients seen in the emergency department.

6. Trauma—CT is the first examination. MRI may be useful in patients in whom the severity of the neurologic deficit is not fully explained by the findings on CT. Diffuse axonal injury, in particular, is much better demonstrated on MRI than on CT scan.

7. Demyelinating disease—MRI is the test of choice. A sagittal FLAIR pulse sequence is usually added, to search for lesions of the corpus callosum, which, if found, are highly suggestive of multiple sclerosis.

8. Vascular malformations—These are best evaluated with MRI and sometimes MR angiography.

9. Aneurysms—Catheter angiography is the gold standard, although high-quality CT angiography is comparable. MR angiography sometimes can be of high quality, although less consistently so because of signal loss due to turbulence. MR angiography or CT angiography may be used as a screening procedure in patients at risk for aneurysm (eg, those with polycystic kidney disease) or in the evaluation of an equivocal finding on CT or MRI.

10. Extracranial carotid artery disease—Doppler sonography and MR angiography are both good screening methods, particularly when used as complementary procedures.

11. Vasculitis—MR angiography may, on rare occasions, detect lesions, but catheter angiography is more sensitive.

12. Temporal bone—MRI can detect lesions of the brainstem, cerebellopontine angle cisterns, and seventh or eighth cranial nerves. The vestibulocochlear apparatus is well seen. CT is recommended for evaluation of lesions of the temporal bone itself, such as congenital anomalies and inflammatory conditions, including otomastoiditis, osteomyelitis, and cholesteatoma.

13. Leptomeningeal lesions—MRI with gadolinium can reveal enhancement of the leptomeninges in patients with meningeal metastases, lymphoma, leukemia, tuberculosis and other leptomenigitides, and sarcoidosis.

14. Pituitary masses—MRI with gadolinium is the test of choice. Dynamic MRI scans, in which images at the same locations are obtained repeatedly over time after the injection of gadolinium, are often useful in detecting microadenomas. Initially, normal pituitary tissue will enhance and the microadenoma will not. Over time, the enhancement pattern reverses: contrast in the normal pituitary tissue "washes out" while contrast accumulates in the microadenoma.

15. Congenital malformations—MRI is the test of choice. Gadolinium is generally not required. Prenatal MRI examination can detect congenital malformations in utero (Figure 3–8).

16. Nonspecific neurologic complaints—MRI without gadolinium is a suitable screening procedure.

B. Spine

1. Lumbar degenerative spinal disease—If imaging is required, MRI without gadolinium is the test of choice. CT is an adequate substitute, unless symptoms suggest a conus medullaris lesion. In the postoperative spine, MRI with gadolinium can differentiate postoperative epidural fibrosis and residual or recurrent disk herniation, because fibrosis usually enhances and disk herniations do not.

2. Cervical degenerative spinal disease—MRI is the test of choice. CT can add precise information regarding osteophytic encroachment on the spinal canal and neuroforamina or ossification of the posterior longitudinal ligament and ligamentum flavum.

3. Infections—MRI with and without contrast is the test of choice in detecting disk space infections, osteomyelitis, and epidural abscess.

4. Congenital anomalies and scoliosis—MRI is probably the test of choice, although CT provides better resolution of any bony anomalies. Syrinx cavities, often associated with Chiari malformations, are best seen with MRI.

5. Tumors—MRI with and without gadolinium is the test of choice for the evaluation of brain tumors. It is particularly important to use gadolinium when searching for brain metastases. Small brain metastases are easily missed on a nonenhanced MRI scan.

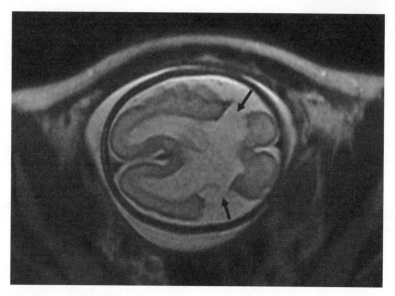

▲ **Figure 3–8.** Fetal MRI shows in utero bilateral schizencephalic clefts (arrows). (Used with permission from Dr. Sarah Milla.)

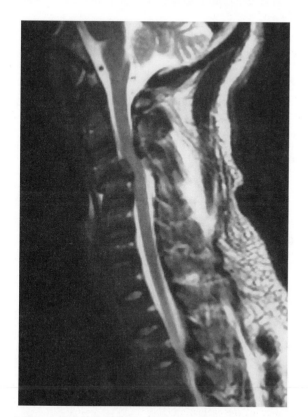

▲ **Figure 3–9.** Sagittal T2-weighted image of the cervical spine demonstrates an anterior subluxation of C3 on C4, a C3–C4 disk herniation, and spinal cord compression.

6. Trauma—Plain films and CT can be the initial studies for the evaluation of fractures and alignment. MRI can identify spinal cord compression and injury (Figure 3–9).

7. Demyelinating lesions—MRI is the test of choice. It is vastly superior to CT in the detection of lesions. A nonenhanced scan can be used to detect the lesions. A postcontrast scan aids in refining the diagnosis. Multiple white matter lesions, some of which enhance and others of which do not, are highly suggestive of multiple sclerosis.

ADVANCED MAGNETIC RESONANCE IMAGING TECHNIQUES

MR perfusion, MR spectroscopy, MR tractography, and functional magnetic resonance imaging (fMRI) can now be performed using commercially available scanners.

▶ Magnetic Resonance Perfusion

The rapid acquisition of images that new MR scanners can achieve allows for repeated imaging of a volume of brain over time as contrast material enters and leaves. In a manner analogous to CT perfusion techniques, dynamic MR perfusion study allows for calculation of relative blood flow, relative blood volume, mean transit time, and time-to-peak perfusion. MR perfusion can be used to identify areas of ischemia in the brain. In patients with stroke, a mismatch is said to exist if the size of the ischemic zone is larger than the size of the infarcted brain as determined by DWI. If such an ischemic penumbra exists, more aggressive therapeutic interventions can be implemented to salvage the ischemic but not infarcted tissue.

MR perfusion can also be used to characterize brain tumors. Enhancing primary brain tumors can be distinguished from enhancing metastatic deposits by differences in perfusion values in the area of the brain surrounding the lesion. T2/FLAIR-hyperintense vasogenic edema surrounding a metastatic deposit shows normal to decreased relative blood volume, whereas T2/FLAIR-hyperintense infiltrating nonenhancing tumor surrounding an enhancing primary neoplasm shows increased relative blood volume due to associated tumor angiogenesis. The tumor grade of primary brain tumors can be predicted by perfusion values. Increased relative blood volume indicates a high-grade lesion (Plate 5). Normal or near-normal relative blood volume indicates a low-grade lesion. MR perfusion can be used to distinguish tumor recurrence, which has high relative blood volume, from radiation necrosis, which has low relative blood volume.

Magnetic Resonance Spectroscopy

MR spectroscopy provides information on the biochemical nature of the tissues within a given volume of interest and is available on many commercially available scanners. The spectrum of normal brain tissue includes peaks for *N*-acetyl aspartate, considered to be a neuronal marker; creatine, associated with cellular energy metabolism; and choline, associated with cell membrane synthesis. Other identifiable biochemicals include lactate, myoinositol, lipids, and alanine. Different spectral patterns can suggest specific diagnoses (Figure 3–10).

Magnetic Resonance Tractography

Diffusion of water molecules in the brain occurs preferentially in a direction paralleling the direction of the axons in a myelin tract. By obtaining MR diffusion data in multiple directions, a tensor can be described that reflects the strength and net direction of diffusion within a voxel. By combining these data, one voxel to the next, a map of the myelin tract can be obtained. The disruption or displacement of the tracts by a mass may offer useful diagnostic or surgically relevant information (Plate 6).

Functional Magnetic Resonance Imaging

fMRI, in which focal areas of increased blood flow are associated with the performance of specific tasks, is an established research tool with as yet limited clinical utility. fMRI studies

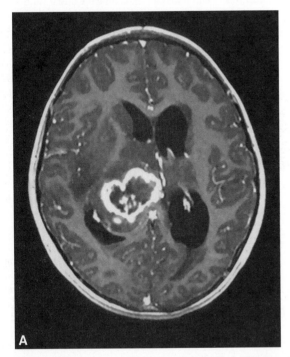
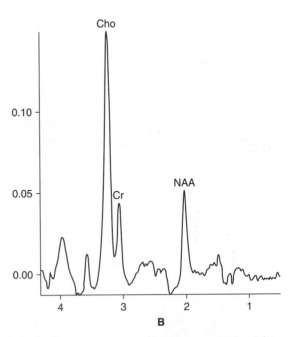

▲ **Figure 3–10. A:** Postcontrast axial T1-weighted image of the brain demonstrates an enhancing mass in the right thalamus. **B:** MR spectrum of a voxel of tissue adjacent to the mass is abnormal. *N*-acetyl aspartate (NAA) is decreased consistent with neuronal destruction. Choline (Cho) is markedly increased consistent with membrane turnover. (Cr = creatine; Cr2 = second creatine peak.) Final diagnosis: Grade III/IV astrocytoma. (Reproduced with permission from Law M, et al. Differentiating surgical from non-surgical lesions using perfusion MR imaging and proton spectroscopic imaging. *Technol Cancer Res Treat* 2004;3:557. Adenine Press, Inc. http://www.tcrt.org.)

can be used to identify the motor cortex and speech areas in patients being considered for surgical resection of mass lesions or epileptogenic foci in close proximity to these eloquent areas of the brain (Plate 7).

MYELOGRAPHY & POSTMYELOGRAPHY COMPUTED TOMOGRAPHY

▶ General Considerations

Myelography is a modified plain-film technique in which water-soluble contrast material is introduced into the subarachnoid space via a lumbar puncture. Multiple plain films in different projections are then obtained. The spinal cord and nerve roots in the subarachnoid space are seen as filling defects in the opacified cerebrospinal fluid. Deformities in the configuration of the subarachnoid space, spinal cord, and nerve roots can localize the lesion into one of three spaces: epidural, intramedullary (inside the spinal cord), and intradural-extramedullary (inside the dura but outside the spinal cord). Leakage of contrast material outside the dura can be used to identify the site of dural tears or to confirm the diagnosis of brachial plexus avulsion.

A CT myelogram, often called a *myelo-CT,* is a CT scan of the spine obtained soon after a myelogram while sufficient contrast material is still present to opacify the cerebrospinal fluid. Axial images can be reformatted into coronal and sagittal images (Figure 3–11). Nerve roots, spinal cord, blood vessels, and other normal structures are sharply outlined by the contrast material. In most institutions, postmyelography CT is obtained after every myelogram.

Adverse reactions to the spinal tap and to the irritating effects of the contrast medium can include headaches, nausea, and vomiting. Rare, severe reactions include mental status changes, seizures, and focal neurologic deficits.

Routine postmyelography orders include instructions to elevate the head (to minimize the rate at which contrast reaches the surface of the brain), drink fluids, and avoid phenothiazines and other medications that lower the seizure threshold (in particular prochlorperazine, which might be given when the patient complains of nausea).

▶ Advantages

Some surgeons are more comfortable with the more familiar anatomic display of myelography and the excellent spatial resolution of CT myelography compared with MRI.

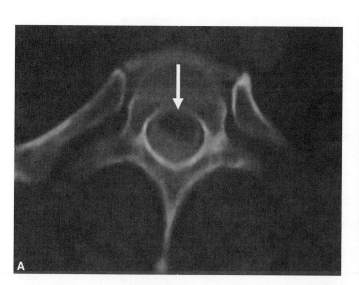

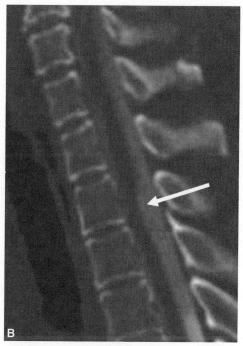

▲ **Figure 3–11. A:** One axial image of a cervical CT-myelogram shows the spinal cord displaced forward and rotated slightly to the left (arrow). The subarachnoid space is opacified by contrast material instilled via a lumbar puncture. **B:** A sagittal image of the CT-myelogram reformatted from the axial images shows a focal deformity of the spinal cord at C6 and C7 (arrow), originally thought to be due to herniation of the spinal cord through a defect in the dural sac, but proven at surgery to be due to a dorsal intradural arachnoid cyst.

Disadvantages

Myelography and CT myelography are invasive procedures. The contrast agent is relatively neurotoxic, and side effects are common, especially headache, nausea, and vomiting. The possibility of iatrogenic infection or hemorrhage related to the spinal tap also exists.

Compared with MRI, myelography and CT myelography are relatively insensitive for intramedullary lesions, which are difficult to characterize even when found because of the inherently poor resolution of structures within the spinal cord.

When to Order

1. Degenerative spinal disease—A myelogram or CT myelogram can be ordered in degenerative spinal disease if the initial CT or MRI scan is inconclusive.

2. MRI not obtainable—A myelogram or CT myelogram should be ordered in patients in whom spinal cord compression is suspected and an MRI scan cannot be obtained in a timely fashion or in patients in whom an MRI scan is refused by the patient or is contraindicated.

3. Interference from surgical artifacts—A myelogram should be considered in patients in whom artifacts from surgical hardware would render the CT or MRI scan uninterpretable.

4. CSF leak—The site of a suspected CSF leak can be identified on myelography or CT myelography by the extravasation of intrathecal contrast material through the defect in the thecal sac. The site and extent of brachial plexus avulsion injuries can be ascertained by the visualization of such leaks, occurring as they do at the site of avulsed nerve roots.

CATHETER ANGIOGRAPHY

General Considerations

Catheter angiography is an invasive, potentially high-risk procedure in which a small catheter is introduced into the arteries supplying the brain. The arterial system is usually accessed via a puncture in the femoral artery. Under fluoroscopic guidance, the catheter is passed up the aorta into the aortic arch and then into the specific arteries of interest. Contrast material is then injected, and multiple films in different projections are obtained.

Although this test has largely been supplanted by MR angiography and CT angiography, it remains the gold standard in the evaluation of intracranial, extracranial, and spinal vascular lesions (Figure 3–12).

It is performed routinely in patients with subarachnoid hemorrhage or unexplained intracranial hemorrhage. Occasionally it is performed to evaluate the intracranial blood vessels for vasculitis.

The blood supply to the spinal cord can be investigated using catheter spinal angiography. Vessels supplying the spinal cord are individually catheterized, usually to diagnose spinal vascular malformations.

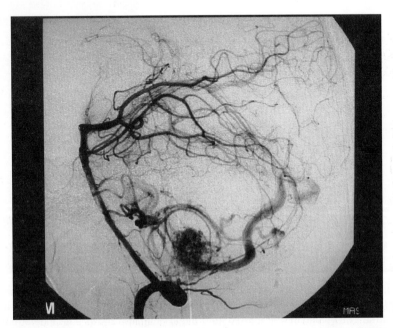

▲ **Figure 3–12.** Lateral image from a vertebral angiogram shows an arteriovenous malformation fed by branches of the basilar artery draining into the straight sinus.

Major complications involve blood vessel damage. Bleeding and thrombosis can occur at the puncture site, sometimes requiring surgical intervention. Vascular dissections can occur at any level. Small plaques dislodged by the catheter and small clots forming around the catheter tip may embolize, leading to cerebral or spinal cord infarction. The overall serious complication rate is about 1%.

Major risk factors for complications include age, hypertension, diabetes, peripheral vascular disease, and coronary artery heart disease.

▶ Advantages

Catheter angiography provides extremely high spatial resolution and remains the gold standard in the evaluation of the vascular system, whether in the head, neck, or spine.

▶ Disadvantages

There is a small but real risk of morbidity and mortality. The procedure is long and uncomfortable and often requires conscious sedation. The procedure and the postprocedure observation period may involve an overnight hospital stay.

▶ When to Order

1. Subarachnoid or parenchymal hemorrhage—Angiography should be considered in any patient with unexplained subarachnoid or parenchymal hemorrhage.

2. Vasculitis—Angiography should be considered in patients with symptoms of a vasculitis, although neither sensitivity nor specificity is high.

3. Spinal vascular malformation—Spinal angiography is the definitive test in patients suspected of harboring a spinal vascular malformation.

INTERVENTIONAL NEURORADIOLOGY

Superselective catheterization of individual blood vessels of the brain allows for several advanced therapeutic techniques. For strokes, intra-arterial thrombolytics can be administered directly into the occluded vessels, and clots can be mechanically disrupted or retrieved. For aneurysms, metallic coils can be used to fill the aneurysm, or stents can be used to divert blood flow from the aneurysm (Figure 3–13). Both procedures will lead to thrombosis of the aneurysm. For arteriovenous malformations, various agents can be used to partially obliterate the malformation—generally a preoperative procedure. For arteriovenous fistulas, various devices can be used to close the fistula. All these procedures are a technical tour de force requiring a high level of experience and expertise.

Vertebroplasty and kyphoplasty are procedures in which glues are instilled into collapsed vertebrae to stabilize the collapse and reduce the associated pain.

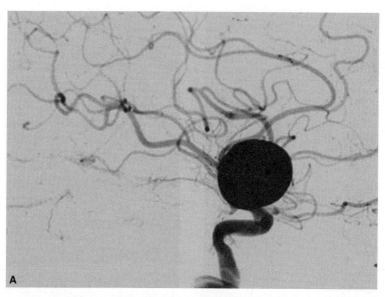

▲ Figure 3–13. A: Lateral image from an internal carotid catheter angiogram shows a large ophthalmic artery aneurysm. **B:** Lateral scout image of a catheter angiogram shows embolization coils in a large ophthalmic artery aneurysm and a stent in the adjacent internal carotid artery. **C:** Lateral image after the injection of contrast material into the internal carotid artery shows patency of the internal carotid artery and non-filling of the aneurysm.

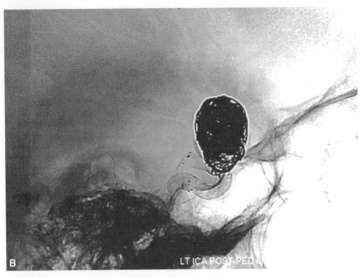

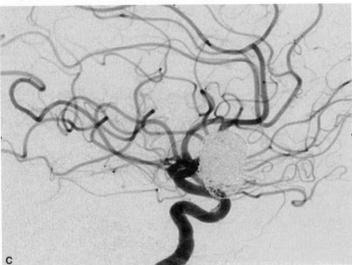

▲ **Figure 3–13.** (*Continued*)

ULTRASONOGRAPHY

▶ General Considerations

Ultrasonography is an imaging technique that uses reflected sound waves to create images of blood vessels, brain, and spine. Ultrasonography displays the strength and location of the echoes as a cross-sectional image.

The Doppler effect on sound waves reflected off moving blood cells can be used to calculate flow velocities, which in turn can be used to calculate the degree of vascular stenosis. A tight stenosis is associated with increased flow rate, much like the increased flow of water through the end of a garden hose when a finger is placed over it. The flow rate and direction can be displayed as a graph (ie, duplex Doppler) or as colors superimposed on the cross-sectional images (ie, color Doppler).

▶ Advantages

Equipment is inexpensive and readily available. Portable machines can be brought to the patient's bedside. Using only sound waves, the examination is safe. In utero evaluation of central nervous system structures can be performed. Intracranial and spinal anomalies can be detected. Perinatal intracranial hemorrhage can be seen.

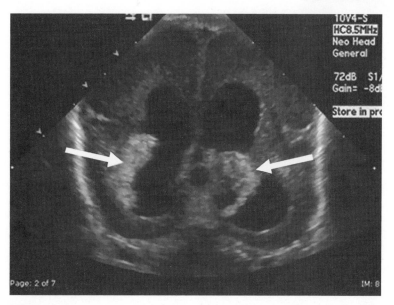

▲ **Figure 3–14.** Neonatal ultrasound shows hydrocephalus and hyperechoic intraventricular hemorrhage (arrows). (Used with permission from Dr. Sarah Milla.)

▶ Disadvantages

The technique is operator dependent. The skull and vertebrae block sound waves. In infants, this problem is overcome by scanning through open fontanelles.

▶ When to Order

1. Prenatal examination of the brain and spine—Ultrasound is routinely used for intrautero examination of the brain and spine. Subdural hematoma, hydrocephalus, and many anomalies of the brain and spine can be detected and, in some cases, treated before birth.

2. Postnatal examination of the brain and spine—Open fontanelles are an excellent window for ultrasonic evaluation of the brain. Subdural hematoma, germinal matrix hemorrhage, periventricular leukomalacia, and many brain anomalies can be identified (Figure 3–14). Often, ultrasound can obtain good information about the condition of the spinal cord in the neonate.

3. Intraoperative use—Ultrasound can be used to locate lesions detected by MRI that are deep within the brain or spinal cord and initially invisible to the surgeon. A properly draped ultrasound probe is used after the skull or vertebrae covering the lesion has been removed.

4. Bifurcation of the common carotid artery—Both the morphology of the common carotid bifurcation as well as the severity of stenoses can be determined by ultrasound.

5. Vasospasm and vascular stenosis—Transcranial Doppler ultrasonography can be performed in adults through the thin temporal squamosa to evaluate vasospasm in patients with subarachnoid hemorrhage and to detect intracranial vascular stenosis in patients with sickle cell anemia.

NUCLEAR MEDICINE

Various radioactive tracers may be instilled into the body and then detected and imaged with scintillation cameras.

Technetium pertechnetate is injected intravenously for confirmation of *brain death*; failure of the tracer to accumulate in the brain indicates absence of cerebral blood flow. Indium 111 DTPA can be injected into the subarachnoid space via a lumbar puncture to demonstrate cerebrospinal fluid leaks through basal skull defects and fractures. This procedure is also used to demonstrate communicating and normal pressure hydrocephalus, in which there is a lack of normal tracer accumulation over the cerebral convexities.

Positron emission tomography (PET) uses positron-emitting isotopes of chemical elements produced in a cyclotron. Fluorine 18–labeled deoxyglucose is used to determine glucose utilization. PET can distinguish metabolically active tumor from metabolically inactive radiation necrosis. It can also localize epileptic foci in the temporal lobe. Combined PET and CT scanners are now available; this combination helps to overcome the problems of low spatial resolution inherent in nuclear imaging.

Single-photon emission computed tomography (SPECT) uses iodinated radiotracers or technetium 99m agents as cerebral perfusion and extraction agents. It is used to study stroke, epilepsy, and dementia.

Coma

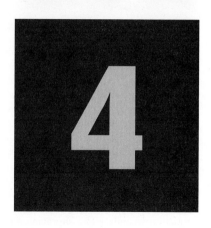

John C.M. Brust, MD

▶ General Considerations

Stupor and **coma** are reduced states of alertness that differ from syncope in being sustained and from sleep in being less easily reversed. They are clinically defined in terms of response to stimulation, and because terms such as lethargy, obtundation, stupor, and coma are not rigorously defined, an examiner should record both the minimal stimulus that produces a response (eg, voice, passive movement, pain) and the response itself (eg, groaning, purposeful movement, extensor posturing, no response).

Delirium refers to severe inattentiveness, altered mental content, and sometimes hyperactivity. Delirium can presage or alternate with stupor or coma.

▶ Pathogenesis

Consciousness requires both arousal and mental content. Coma can be caused by any lesion—structural or metabolic—that disrupts the brainstem reticular activating system, the cerebral hemispheres to which it projects, or both. The causes of coma are usefully divided into supra- and infratentorial structural lesions and diffuse or metabolic disorders. By concentrating the neurologic examination on motor responses to stimuli, respirations, pupils, and eye movements, the clinician can usually identify which type of lesion is present.

▶ Clinical Findings

A. Initial Examination and Immediate Interventions

The examination begins with the detection and treatment of any immediate life-threatening condition (eg, hemorrhage, airway obstruction, hypotension, or cardiac arrhythmia). Fifty percent dextrose is given intravenously without waiting for blood glucose level determination or relying on fingerstick estimation. Thiamine (and other multivitamins) is given with the glucose to prevent precipitation of Wernicke-Korsakoff syndrome. If opioid overdose is a possibility, naloxone is administered. If trauma is suspected, injury to internal organs or the neck must be considered.

B. General Examination

Examination includes skin, nails, and mucous membranes (cyanosis, pallor, cherry redness, jaundice, petechiae, decubiti, uremic frost, hypo- or hyperpigmentation, signs of trauma), breath (acetone, alcohol), and fundi (papilledema, hypertensive or diabetic retinopathy, Roth spots, subhyaloid hemorrhage). Fever might reflect infection or heat stroke. Hypothermia might indicate cold exposure, hypothyroidism, hypoglycemia, or sepsis. Urinary or fecal incontinence might signify an unwitnessed seizure. The scalp should be palpated for signs of trauma and the ears and nose examined for blood or cerebrospinal fluid. Resistance to passive neck flexion suggests meningitis or subarachnoid hemorrhage; resistance in all directions suggests bone or joint disease, including fracture.

C. Neurologic Examination

1. Motor responses—Inspection identifies limb position and spontaneous movements, either voluntary or involuntary (eg, seizure or myoclonus). Asymmetric movements or postures can signify either hemiparesis or focal seizures. Asymmetry of muscle tone suggests a structural lesion, but it may not be clear which side is abnormal.

Motor response to stimuli can be appropriate, inappropriate, or absent. Appropriate responses to painful stimuli (eg, sternal rubbing, nailbed pressure) include limb withdrawal, fending off, grimacing, or vocalization. Inappropriate responses include so called *decorticate posturing* (flexion of arms and extension of legs) and *decerebrate posturing* (extension of arms and legs). In both decorticate and decerebrate posturing, there is usually internal rotation of the upper arms, and the limbs are flaccid and not moving in the absence of external stimulation. Spontaneous posturing should suggest seizures or an unrecognized stimulus such as airway obstruction. Decorticate and decerebrate postures are generated by lower brainstem structures and most often indicate upper brainstem damage, especially during transtentorial herniation secondary to a supratentorial mass lesion. They can also occur, however, in patients with metabolic derangement, including hepatic coma and sedative overdose.

Lack of any motor response might simply reflect the depth of coma, but should also raise the possibility of paralysis caused by cervical trauma, Guillain-Barré polyneuropathy, or the locked-in state.

2. Respiratory pattern—Abnormal respiratory patterns include Cheyne-Stokes respiration (CSR), hyperventilation, and ataxic breathing. In CSR, hyperventilation and apnea alternate in a crescendo-decrescendo fashion. CSR occurs with bilateral cerebral disease, upper brainstem lesions, and metabolic encephalopathy. It usually signifies that the patient is not in imminent danger and does not, by itself, mandate artificial ventilation.

Sustained hyperventilation is usually due to metabolic acidosis, hypoxia, pulmonary congestion, hepatic encephalopathy, or stimulation by analgesic drugs. So-called *primary hyperventilation*, with respiratory alkalosis, can follow upper brainstem damage, which may occur during the course of transtentorial herniation.

Ataxic breathing refers to variably irregular rate and amplitude. A variant of this pattern, called *cluster breathing*, includes periods of apnea but without the crescendo-decrescendo cycling of CSR. Ataxic breathing signifies damage to the lower brainstem and mandates immediate ventilatory support.

3. Pupillary responses—Although many people have slight anisocoria, unequal pupils should be considered abnormal in a comatose patient. As with other neurologic asymmetries, anisocoria by itself does not indicate which side is abnormal. A larger pupil could indicate parasympathetic dysfunction involving the oculomotor nerve (including compression by the inferomedial temporal lobe during transtentorial herniation or by a posterior communicating/internal carotid artery aneurysm). A smaller pupil could indicate sympathetic dysfunction either intraparenchymally (eg, infarction of the lateral medulla) or extraparenchymally (eg, destruction of the superior cervical ganglion by lung cancer).

Oculomotor nerve damage becomes obvious when the pupil becomes fully dilated and unreactive to light or when extraocular muscles innervated by the oculomotor nerve are affected. Sympathetic damage is evident when miosis is accompanied by other features of a Horner syndrome. Bilateral pinpoint (but reactive) pupils occur with pontine lesions (eg, hemorrhage) that transect descending sympathetic pathways. Unilateral or bilateral midposition and unreactive pupils occur with midbrain lesions that destroy both parasympathetic and sympathetic projections.

Because the pupillary light reflex is consensual, retinal or optic nerve damage does not cause anisocoria. Rather, there is reduced response bilaterally when light is directed at the affected eye, but whether the light is directed at either the good or the bad eye, the pupils remain equal (the so-called *afferent pupillary defect*).

With few exceptions, metabolic disorders do not cause unequal or unreactive pupils. Fixed, dilated pupils after anoxic-ischemic injury carry a bad prognosis. Anticholinergic drugs, including amitriptyline, antiparkinsonian agents, and recreational use of *Datura stramonium*, can abolish pupillary reactivity. Hypothermia and severe sedative intoxication can cause not only unreactive pupils but a reversible state resembling brain death. Unreactive pupils can accompany or outlast a seizure. Opioid drugs do not abolish pupillary light reactivity, but miosis can be so severe that reactivity is difficult to discern. Some pupillary abnormalities are local in origin (eg, trauma or synechiae).

4. Eye movements—Abnormal eye movements can be conjugate or dysconjugate. Eyes conjugately deviated away from hemiparetic limbs indicate a destructive cerebral lesion on the side toward which the eyes are directed. Eyes turned toward paretic limbs favor a pontine lesion or an adversive seizure. Eyes dysconjugate at rest indicate paresis of individual muscles, internuclear ophthalmoplegia, or preexisting tropia or phoria.

Eyes roving from side to side with a slow smooth velocity indicate nonwakefulness and an intact brainstem. Jerky movements suggest saccades and relative wakefulness. If on inspection the eyes are seen to move conjugately and fully in both horizontal directions, further testing is usually unnecessary. If eye movements are unilaterally or bilaterally limited, then oculocephalic (so-called *doll's-eye*) or caloric testing is performed.

In a nonawake person with an intact reflex arc (vestibular-brainstem-eye muscles), passive head turning causes the eyes to deviate conjugately in the opposite direction. Similarly, irrigation of each ear with 30–100 mL of ice water when the head is elevated 30 degrees will produce conjugate deviation of the eyes toward the stimulus. Oculocephalic or caloric testing may reveal intact eye movements, gaze palsy, individual muscle paresis, internuclear ophthalmoplegia, or no response. Either extensive brainstem damage (including transtentorial herniation) or metabolic coma can cause complete ophthalmoplegia, but eye movements are usually intact in early metabolic encephalopathy. Dysconjugate eyes suggest a brainstem or cranial nerve lesion (including abducens palsy due to increased intracranial pressure).

Downward eye deviation suggests a lesion of the rostral midbrain or thalamus; it may be accompanied by loss of pupillary light reactivity (Parinaud syndrome). Vertical divergence of the eyes (so-called *skew deviation*) follows brainstem or cerebellar lesions.

Comatose patients rarely have rhythmic nystagmus, but a variety of abnormal spontaneous eye movements are encountered. So-called *ocular bobbing*—conjugate brisk downward movements several times per minute—usually reflect lesions of the pons. Periodic alternating or *ping-pong gaze*—rapid regular conjugate side-to-side horizontal movements—indicate extensive cerebral or cerebellar lesions with an intact brainstem.

5. Symptoms associated with specific lesions—Supratentorial, infratentorial, and metabolic or diffuse lesions produce characteristic symptoms that can aid in diagnosis.

A. SUPRATENTORIAL STRUCTURAL LESIONS—Unilateral supratentorial structural lesions can produce coma if they are acute (thereby functionally disrupting the contralateral cerebral hemisphere) or if they cause significant lateral brain displacement.

With transtentorial herniation, there is downward brain displacement and rostrocaudal brainstem dysfunction, including interruption of the reticular activating system. Respirations may progress from Cheyne-Stokes to hyperventilation to ataxic breathing to apnea.

Decorticate posturing may progress to decerebrate posturing and then to unresponsiveness. Unilateral oculomotor palsy may progress to complete ophthalmoplegia and pupillary unreactivity. Eventually there is circulatory collapse and death. Lesions causing transtentorial herniation include trauma (epidural, subdural, or intraparenchymal hemorrhage), stroke (ischemic or hemorrhagic), infection (including lesions associated with acquired immunodeficiency syndrome), and neoplasm (primary or metastatic).

B. INFRATENTORIAL STRUCTURAL LESIONS—Infratentorial structural lesions can cause downward herniation through the foramen magnum with compression of the medulla, apnea, and circulatory collapse. In coma, a primary infratentorial structural lesion is suggested by bilateral weakness or sensory loss, crossed cranial nerve and long-tract signs, miosis, dysconjugate gaze, ophthalmoplegia, or ataxic breathing.

C. METABOLIC OR DIFFUSE LESIONS—In metabolic, diffuse, or multifocal encephalopathy, mental and respiratory abnormalities tend to occur early. There may be tremor, asterixis, or multifocal myoclonus. Except in anticholinergic poisoning and diffuse anoxic-ischemic brain damage, the pupils remain reactive. Focal seizures and lateralizing neurologic signs, however, can be due to metabolic disease, especially hypo- and hyperglycemia.

D. Laboratory Findings and Imaging Studies

Computerized tomography (CT) or magnetic resonance imaging (MRI) is performed promptly in patients with unexplained coma. If meningitis is suspected and the patient is deteriorating, antimicrobial therapy is given without delay, and imaging should precede lumbar puncture. If imaging reveals frank transtentorial or foramen magnum herniation, the risk of performing a spinal tap must be weighed against the risk of treating for meningitis without cerebrospinal fluid (CSF) confirmation.

Additional emergency laboratory studies include blood levels of glucose, sodium, calcium, and urea nitrogen or creatinine; arterial pH, PO_2, and PCO_2; blood or urine toxicology testing including blood ethanol concentration; cultures of blood and CSF; and liver function tests. Arterial blood gases are of particular value in patients with metabolic coma. For example, metabolic acidosis in a comatose patient narrows diagnostic considerations to diabetic ketoacidosis, lactic acidosis, uremia, and exogenous toxins such as methanol, ethylene glycol, ethanol, or aspirin. Other metabolic tests are based on index of suspicion.

The electroencephalogram (EEG) can distinguish coma from psychic unresponsiveness or locked-in state, but its chief usefulness is to identify nonconvulsive seizures. Patients may have subtle focal jerking movements of fingers or face yet widespread epileptiform activity on EEG. On the other hand, focal seizures or postanoxic or postmyoclonus may be evident in patients whose EEGs show only diffuse slowing, or EEG epileptiform activity may be intermittent and detected only with continuous monitoring.

▶ Differential Diagnosis

A. Psychogenic Unresponsiveness

Psychogenic (conversion) unresponsiveness is rare. Typical features include eupnea or hyperpnea; closed eyelids that resist passive opening or, when released, close abruptly or jerkily; and eyes that do not slowly rove but move with saccadic jerks and respond to ice-water caloric testing with nystagmus rather than slow deviation.

B. Locked-in State

Infarction of the basis pontis can transect the descending corticospinal tracts while preserving tegmental sensory and respiratory pathways and the reticular activating system. The result is paralysis of lower cranial nerve and limb muscles with preserved alertness and respirations (*locked-in state*). Vertical eye movements, controlled by the oculomotor nerve, are normal, and sometimes there are horizontal eye movements and voluntary blinking.

Communication becomes possible through blinking or eye movements and yes-no questions.

C. Vegetative State

Comatose patients either die or improve, and their improvement may consist of sleep-wake cycles, intact cardiorespiratory function, and primitive response to stimuli (including reflexes mediated through the brainstem and behavioral fragments such as screaming or even single-word utterances) but no

Table 4–1. Determination of Brain Death

General Guidelines/Recommended Testing	Specific Findings
	Criteria
Prerequisites 1. Clinical or neuroimaging evidence of acute CNS catastrophe compatible with clinical diagnosis of brain death 2. Exclusion of complicating medical conditions that may confound clinical assessment (no severe electrolyte, acid-base, or endocrine disturbance) 3. No drug intoxication or poisoning 4. Core temperature of 32°C (90°F) **Cardinal findings** 1. Coma	
2. Absence of brainstem reflexes	No cerebral motor response to pain in all extremities (nailbed pressure and supraorbital pressure) **Pupils** • No response to bright light • Size—midposition (4 mm) to dilated (9 mm) **Ocular movement** • No oculocephalic reflex (testing only when no fracture or instability of the cervical spine is apparent) • No deviation of the eyes to irrigation in each ear with 50 mL of cold water (allow 1 min after injection and at least 5 min between testing on each side) **Facial sensation and facial motor response** • No corneal reflex to touch with a throat swab • No jaw reflex • No grimacing to deep pressure on nailbed, supraorbital ridge, or temporomandibular joint **Pharyngeal and tracheal reflexes** • No response after stimulation of the posterior pharynx with tongue blade • No cough response to bronchial suctioning
3. Apnea testing **Prerequisites** • Core temperature of 36.5°C or 97°F (can achieve with warm blanket) • Systolic blood pressure of 90 mm Hg • Euvolemia (option: positive fluid balance in the previous 6 h) • Normal arterial Po_2 (option: preoxygenation to obtain arterial Po_2 of 200 mm Hg) **Procedure** • Connect pulse oximeter and disconnect ventilator • Deliver 100% O_2 at rate of 6 L/min into trachea (option: Place a cannula at level of the carina) • Look closely for respiratory movements (abdominal or chest excursions that produce adequate tidal volumes) • Measure arterial Po_2, Pco_2, and pH after approximately 8 min and reconnect ventilator (CO_2 partial pressure increases at a rate of approximately 3 mm Hg/min)	• If respiratory movements are absent and arterial Pco_2 is 60 mm Hg (option: 20 mm Hg increase in Pco_2 over a baseline normal Pco_2), the result of apnea testing is positive (ie, it supports diagnosis of brain death) • If respiratory movements are observed, the result of apnea testing is negative. If deoxygenation or cardiac arrhythmia requires termination of apnea testing before $Paco_2$ of 60 mm Hg is reached, test is indeterminate and another confirmatory test should be considered
	Pitfalls
Several conditions may interfere with clinical diagnosis of brain death, so that diagnosis cannot be made with certainty on clinical grounds alone. Confirmatory tests are recommended.	• Severe facial trauma • Preexisting pupillary abnormalities • Toxic levels of any sedative drugs, aminoglycosides, tricyclic antidepressants, anticholinergics, antiepileptic drugs, chemotherapeutic agents, or neuromuscular blocking agents • Sleep apnea or severe pulmonary disease resulting in chronic retention of CO_2

(Continued)

Table 4–1. Determination of Brain Death (*Continued*)

Clinical observations compatible with brain death	
Certain observations compatible with diagnosis of brain death are occasionally noted and should not be misinterpreted as evidence of brainstem function	• Tendon reflexes, superficial abdominal reflexes, triple flexion response • Babinski reflex • Respiratory-like movements (shoulder elevation and adduction, back arching, expansion of intercostal muscles without significant tidal volumes) • Spontaneous movements of limbs other than pathologic flexion or extension; response including facial twitching, flexion at waist, slow turning of head, undulating movements of toes, and shoulder adduction with arm flexion. Such movements sometimes occur during apnea testing or following pronunciation of brain death and disconnection from ventilator (so-called *Lazarus sign*) • Sweating, blushing, tachycardia • Normal blood pressure without pharmacologic support or sudden increases in blood pressure • Absence of diabetes insipidus
Repeat examinations	
• Adults—perform repeat examination 6 h later except for subjects with anoxic-ischemic brain damage, who should be reexamined after 24 h • Children—for those younger than 2 months of age, perform repeat examination after 48 h; for those aged 2 mo to 1 y, after 24 h; and for those between 1 y and 18 y of age, after 12 h	
Confirmatory laboratory tests (optional)	

Children younger than 2 mo of age should have two confirmatory tests; those aged 2 mo to 1 y of age should have one confirmatory test. For children older than 1 y of age and adults, confirmatory tests are optional	• Conventional angiography—no intracerebral filling at level of carotid bifurcation or circle of Willis; external carotid circulation is patent, and filling of superior longitudinal sinus may be delayed
	• Electroencephalography—no electrical activity during at least 30 min of recording
	• Transcranial Doppler ultrasonography
	  — Ten percent of patients may not have temporal insonation windows; therefore, initial absence of Doppler signals cannot be interpreted as consistent with brain death
	  — Small systolic peaks in early systole without diastolic flow or reverberating flow, indicating very high vascular resistance associated with greatly increased intracranial pressure
	• **Technetium-99m hexamethylpropylene-amine-oxime brain scan**—no uptake of isotope in brain parenchyma (so-called *hollow skull phenomenon*)
	• **Somatosensory evoked potentials**—bilateral absence of N20–P22 response with median nerve stimulation

evidence of inner or outer awareness (so-called *vegetative state*). Some patients recover further; others do not. Persistent vegetative state (PVS) is defined as a vegetative state present for at least 1 month, and with a high degree of probability, PVS in adults and children can be considered permanent 12 months after traumatic injury and 3 months after nontraumatic injury (usually anoxic-ischemic brain damage).

Some patients evolve into a "minimally conscious state," and are able to follow commands yet unable to communicate interactively. Difficulty in distinguishing voluntary from reflexive behavior can blur the distinction between a vegetative and a minimally conscious state. In a small proportion of vegetative or minimally conscious patients, functional imaging has identified brain activation consistent with some degree of awareness and cognition. Magnetic resonance diffusion tensor imaging is more sensitive than conventional MRI in identifying brain abnormalities in vegetative and minimally conscious patients.

D. Brain Death

In brain death, unlike vegetative state, neither the cerebrum nor the brainstem is functioning. The only spontaneous activity is cardiovascular, apnea persists in the presence of hypercarbic respiratory drive, and the only reflexes are those mediated by the spinal cord (Table 4–1). In adults brain death rarely lasts more than a few days and is always followed by circulatory collapse. In the United States, brain death is equated with legal death, and artificial respiratory and blood pressure support are appropriately terminated whether or not organ donation is intended.

Coleman MR, et al. Towards the routine use of brain imaging to aid the clinical diagnosis of disorders of consciousness. *Brain* 2009;132:2541–2552. [PMID: 19710182] (Describes the prognostic usefulness of functional magnetic resonance imaging in certain patients diagnosed as vegetative.)

Monti MM, et al. Willful modulation of brain activity in disorders of consciousness. *N Engl J Med* 2010;362:579–589. [PMID: 20130250] (Provides evidence consistent with awareness in a small proportion of vegetative or minimally conscious patients.)

Newcombe VF, et al. Aetiological differences in neuroanatomy of the vegetative state: Insights from diffusion tensor imaging and functional implications. *J Neurol Neurosurg Psychiatr* 2010;81:552–561. [PMID: 20460593] (Demonstrates the sensitivity of diffusion tensor imaging in identifying the extent of pathology in vegetative patients, as well as differences between those with anoxic/ischemic injury and these with traumatic brain injury.)

Wijdicks EF. The case against confirmatory tests for determining brain death in adults. *Neurology* 2010;75:77–83. [PMID: 20603486] (A persuasive argument that confirmatory tests serve no useful purpose.)

Wijdicks EF, et al. Evidence-based guideline update: Determining brain death in adults. Reports of the Quality Standards Subcommittee of the American Academy of Neurology. *Neurology* 2010;74:1911–1918 [PMID: 20530327] (Provides a detailed brain death evaluation and discusses areas of uncertainty.)

Aphasia, Apraxia, & Agnosia

John C.M. Brust, MD

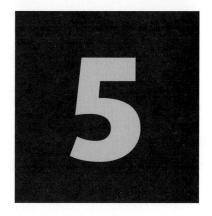

APHASIA

ESSENTIALS OF DIAGNOSIS

▶ Language disturbance unexplained by articulatory impairment or sensory loss

▶ Variable abnormalities of verbal expression, speech comprehension, naming, repetition, writing, and reading

▶ Cerebral damage present, either focal or widespread

▶ General Considerations

Approximately 90% of people are right-handed, and approximately 95% of them process language in the left cerebral hemisphere (ie, have left-cerebral dominance). Of the 10% of people who are left-handed, approximately 60% have left-cerebral dominance for language. Aphasia occurs with structural lesions of the language-dominant hemisphere that involve regions critical for language processing—especially the frontal, parietal, and temporal areas of the operculum (cerebral areas surrounding the sylvian fissure). Such lesions can be small but critically located (eg, cerebral contusion or infarction), or they can be part of more widespread damage (eg, Alzheimer disease).

Aphasia affects more than speech. A disturbance of language in its broadest sense, aphasia is not explained by articulatory impairment (dysarthria) or sensory loss.

▶ Clinical Features

A. Symptoms and Signs

Language assessment involves six components: verbal expression, speech comprehension, naming, repetition, writing, and reading.

1. Verbal expression—Verbal expression refers to the speech a patient generates spontaneously, for example, full sentence responses to questions. A variety of abnormalities might be detected in an aphasic's spontaneous speech (Table 5–1). There may be a reduction in **fluency**, the amount of speech produced over time. Word-finding difficulty can produce hesitations in otherwise fluent speech; by contrast, the speech of Broca aphasia (discussed later) is labored and hesitant throughout, independent of word-finding per se. Reduced **prosody** refers to impairment of the musical qualities of speech—rhythm, accent, and pitch. **Paraphasias** are word errors, either real but unintended words (semantic paraphasias, eg, "hotel" for "hospital") or substituted syllables within words (phonemic paraphasias, eg, "hosicle" for "hospital"). Paraphasias may be occasional contaminants of speech or they may nearly replace it, rendering it incomprehensible (jargon).

Even in the absence of paraphasias, the content of aphasic speech may be difficult to grasp, with fluent prosodic sentences and seemingly intact grammar (**paragrammatism**) but limited or empty content. By contrast, the nonfluent, nonprosodic speech of Broca aphasia may consist only of nouns and verbs, with loss of grammatical words (ie, telegraphic speech, **agrammatism**). Some aphasic patients tend to repeat a single phrase or word over and over (**recurrent utterance**).

2. Speech comprehension—Assessment of speech comprehension must take into account abnormalities of verbal expression or other cognitive disturbance.

For example, an incorrect answer to a question could be the result of a paraphasic error or memory impairment. Following a simple command (eg, "Show me two fingers") indicates that the command was understood, but failure to follow a command could have other explanations (eg, pain, depression, or apraxia). Alternative strategies for assessing speech comprehension include indicating objects ("Where is the ceiling?"), answering yes-no questions ("Am I wearing a hat?"), and for syntactical comprehension, object manipulation ("Put the keys on top of the book").

Table 5–1. Abnormalities Encountered in Aphasic Speech

Reduced fluency
Reduced prosody
Paraphasias
Paragrammatism
Agrammatism
Recurrent utterance

3. Naming—Naming can be tested by showing a patient various objects, body parts, or colors. Abnormal naming may consist of paraphasic substitutions, word-finding hesitations (often with the word correctly selected from a list—so-called *tip-of-the-tongue misnaming*), or descriptive misnaming (eg, "what you tell time with" rather than "wristwatch"). Some aphasics successfully name seen objects but have difficulty listing names within a category (eg, animals, items of clothing).

4. Repetition—Repetition is tested by having the patient repeat a sentence (eg, "The train came into the station an hour late"). Syntactically complex sentences can be especially difficult.

5. Writing—Assessment of writing can begin by having patients write their own names, but for many people a signature is an "overlearned" motor act no longer dependent on language processing. Writing to dictation (sentences, words, or letters) or generating a spontaneous written sentence

more sensitively detects language dysfunction. The great majority of aphasics of any type have impaired writing, and over time, aphasia can improve such that agraphia is the only residual abnormality.

6. Reading—Reading is tested both orally and for comprehension. The patient reads aloud sentences, words, or letters. Written comprehension is tested employing the same strategies used for speech comprehension. Striking dissociations in reading ability can occur, with impaired oral reading but normal reading comprehension and vice versa.

B. Classification

Aphasic syndromes have been classified in many different ways, with conflicting views regarding their anatomical specificity. Table 5–2 shows a classification that may be linguistically simplistic but is clinically useful. Most patients with nonfluent, nonprosodic Broca aphasia have moderate-to-severe hemiparesis, whereas most patients with fluent, prosodic aphasias do not. The term *global aphasia* refers to severely nonfluent, nonprosodic speech coupled with severely impaired speech comprehension. Such patients have extensive damage to the language-dominant cerebral hemisphere (eg, infarction in the entire territory of the middle cerebral artery), and they nearly always have additional cognitive impairment not explained by their aphasia.

▶ Treatment

It was long believed by many neurologists that speech therapy was of benefit in aphasia chiefly by teaching patients to make the best of their preserved language function; actual improvement was attributed to natural history. Functional

Table 5–2. Subtypes of Aphasia

Syndrome	Spontaneous Speech	Comprehension	Naming	Repetition	Writing	Reading	Hemiparesis	Lesion Localization
Broca	Nonfluent	Relatively preserved	Poor	Poor	Poor	Variable	Common	Includes frontal operculum
Wernicke	Fluent, paraphasic	Poor	Poor	Poor	Poor	Usually poor	Infrequent	Includes posterior superior temporal lobe
Conduction	Fluent, paraphasic	Relatively preserved	Variable	Poor	Poor	Variable	Infrequent	Includes angular and supramarginal gyri (inferior parietal lobule)
Anomic	Fluent	Preserved	Poor	Preserved	Poor	Variable	Infrequent	Includes angular and supramarginal gyri
Transcortical motor	Nonfluent	Relatively preserved	Poor	Preserved	Poor	Variable	Common	Frontal convexity
Transcortical sensory	Fluent	Poor	Poor	Preserved	Poor	Usually poor	Infrequent	Parietal convexity
Global	Nonfluent	Poor	Poor	Poor	Poor	Poor	Common	Frontal, parietal, and temporal operculum

imaging reveals considerably more plasticity in neuronal circuitry than hitherto recognized, and it is plausible that speech therapy assists in developing not only compensatory strategies, but also new connectivities and neurologic improvement. Patients rendered aphasic by acute, self-limited injuries (usually cerebral trauma or stroke) should be referred to a speech therapist as early as possible.

APRAXIA

ESSENTIALS OF DIAGNOSIS

▶ Impaired motor activity not explained by weakness, incoordination, abnormal tone, bradykinesia, movement disorder, dementia, aphasia, or poor cooperation

▶ Cerebral damage present, either focal or widespread

▶ General Considerations

The term *apraxia* has been used over the years to describe very different phenomena, and conventional definitions list motor abnormalities that are not apractic. Lesions potentially capable of causing apraxia often cause aphasia or dementia as well, and in such patients identifying apraxia can be difficult.

▶ Clinical Findings

A. Symptoms and Signs

Apraxia is impaired motor activity not explained by weakness, incoordination, abnormal tone, bradykinesia, movement disorder, dementia, aphasia, or poor cooperation. Failure to perform an act at all is not apractic; the act must be performed incorrectly. Parts of the act might be omitted or performed out of sequence or incorrectly oriented in space. Three types of testing are conventionally employed (Table 5–3); these might involve limb or buccofacial gestures (eg, hitchhiking, sticking out the tongue), object manipulation (eg, opening a door with a key, blowing out a match), or serial acts (eg, folding a letter, putting it in an envelope, sealing the envelope, and placing a stamp on it).

Table 5–3. Testing for Apraxia

Type of Test	Example
Pantomime	"Show me how you would …."
Imitation	"Watch how I …, then you do it"
Use of an actual object	"Here is a …. Show me how you would use it"

Table 5–4. Apraxia Subtypes

Subtype	Description
Ideomotor	Inability to perform, by pantomime or imitation, learned or complex motor acts (gesture or object use) even though the individual components of the act can be performed and the idea of the act is intact.
Conceptual	Loss of the idea of the act.
Ideational	Inability to sequence task elements correctly.
Limb-kinetic	Preservation of the idea of the act, but loss of ability to perform either the act or its individual components.

B. Classification

Apraxia is conventionally categorized into several subtypes (Table 5–4). In **ideomotor apraxia,** gestures or object use can be accurately described but cannot be pantomimed on verbal command; often the act can be performed correctly when a real object (eg, a key) is provided. Thus both the idea of the act and its individual motor components are intact. In **conceptual apraxia,** the idea of the act is lost; patients cannot describe what they are trying to do, and presentation of a real object produces no improvement. In **ideational apraxia,** there is failure to sequence task elements correctly. In **limb-kinetic apraxia,** the idea of the act is preserved, and the problem appears to involve the executive apparatus insufficiently to produce weakness or bradykinesia but sufficiently to impede performance of either the act or its individual components; hand and finger movements are principally affected.

Ideomotor apraxia most often follows lesions of the language-dominant parietal or temporal lobes (and thus is often confounded by aphasia), and the limbs are usually affected bilaterally. Damage to the anterior corpus callosum can result in left-limb ideomotor apraxia, presumably by disconnecting the right motor cortex from left-hemispheric language areas or, alternatively, areas storing motor representations (engrams).

AGNOSIA

ESSENTIALS OF DIAGNOSIS

▶ Failure of recognition not explained by impaired primary sensation or cognitive impairment

▶ Cerebral damage present, either focal or widespread

General Considerations

Agnosia has been described as "perception stripped of its meaning." Primary sensation (tactile, visual, auditory) is unaffected, but patients neither name nor recognize what they feel, see, or hear. Impaired cognition, if present, is insufficient to account for the agnosia.

Clinical Findings

Agnosia may involve individual sensory modalities such that nothing touched, seen, or heard is recognized; these are termed, respectively, **tactile agnosia** (astereognosis), **auditory agnosia,** and **visual agnosia**. Agnosia can also be more restrictive or complex; for example, **simultanagnosia** (inability to recognize the meaning of a whole scene or object even though its individual components are recognized), **prosopagnosia** (inability to recognize faces), **topographagnosia** (difficulty reading maps or finding one's way about), or **anosognosia** (inability to recognize a neurologic deficit, usually hemiplegia but sometimes memory loss, aphasia, or blindness). Patients with right-sided cerebral lesions (or, less often, left-sided) can demonstrate hemineglect; they may not only have anosognosia for hemiplegia, but they fail to recognize the contralateral limb as their own, and they ignore the contralateral half of their own bodies and of extracorporeal space. Hemineglect can be either mild or severe, and it can be detected by asking patients to bisect a line (left hemineglect will result in bisection to the right of midline) or copy simple pictures (parts on the left will be omitted).

Dobkin BH. Clinical practice: Rehabilitation after stroke. *N Engl J Med* 2005;352:1677–1684. [PMID: 15843670] (Persuasively argues that speech therapy makes a difference and should be started as soon as possible.)

Kelly H, Brady MC, Enderby P. Speech and language therapy for aphasia following stroke. *Cochrane Database Syst Rev* 2010;CD000425. [PMID: 20464716] (Summarizes 30 trials involving 1,840 participants. The reviewers conclude that evidence supports a benefit from speech and language therapy but is insufficient to recommend one form of therapy over another.)

Wheaton LA, Hallett M. Ideomotor apraxia: A review. *J Neurol Sci* 2007;260:1–10. [PMID: 17507030] (Describes ideomotor apraxia in relation to other apraxia subtypes and discusses a possible clinicopathologic correlation.)

Hearing Loss & Dizziness

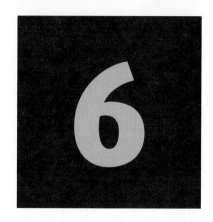

Jack J. Wazen, MD, FACS, Soha N. Ghossaini, MD, FACS, & Benjamin J. Wycherly, MD

HEARING LOSS

ESSENTIALS OF DIAGNOSIS

- ▶ Duration of symptoms
- ▶ Sudden onset of hearing loss
- ▶ Fluctuation of hearing
- ▶ Associated tinnitus or vertigo
- ▶ Previous ear surgeries
- ▶ Family history of hearing loss

▶ General Considerations

Approximately 28 million Americans experience some degree of hearing loss. Hearing loss is divided into two types: conductive and sensorineural. Conditions that include both types are classified as mixed hearing loss. Pathologies limited to the external auditory canal or the middle ear result in conductive hearing loss. Lesions involving the cochlea or the retrocochlear structures (cranial nerve [CN] VIII, or the central auditory pathways) produce sensorineural hearing loss.

▶ Clinical Findings

A. Symptoms and Signs

Hearing loss can be congenital or acquired. Patients with congenital hearing loss may have other associated congenital malformations. Family history of hearing loss may be present. Delay in speech acquisition is common in children with bilateral congenital hearing loss and is often the presenting complaint.

Acquired hearing loss may be sudden or insidious in onset. Ear pain in such patients usually reflects an acute infection involving the external or the middle ear. Otorrhea in the absence of ear pain is common in patients with chronic middle ear infections. Painless, progressive hearing loss, without a history of previous ear infection or surgery, may be secondary to otosclerosis or pathologies involving the inner ear. Associated aural fullness, tinnitus, or vertigo is common in patients with inner ear pathologies. Sudden onset hearing loss should be evaluated immediately to rule out the presence of sensorineural hearing loss.

Patients with hearing loss should undergo a complete examination of the head and neck. Impacted cerumen, if present, should be removed to allow for better visualization of the tympanic membrane. Erythema and edema of the external auditory canal are signs of acute otitis externa. The status of the tympanic membrane reflects the status of the middle ear. An erythematous, bulging tympanic membrane is indicative of an acute infection in the middle ear. Otorrhea in association with an abnormal appearance of the tympanic membrane suggests a possible perforation. Patients with dull tympanic membranes should be assessed for the presence of fluid in the middle ear. Retraction of the tympanic membrane with no signs of acute infection could be a sign of eustachian tube dysfunction. The ear examination is usually normal in patients with sensorineural hearing loss.

Tuning-fork testing, using a 256-Hz or 512-Hz tuning fork, can sometimes differentiate conductive from sensorineural hearing loss. Sound presented to the patient by air conduction is perceived as louder than bone conduction (positive Rinne test) in patients with normal hearing or sensorineural hearing loss. Patients with conductive hearing loss, on the other hand, perceive bone conduction as louder than air conduction (negative Rinne test). When the tuning fork is placed at the center of the forehead (Weber test), the sound lateralizes to the better hearing ear in patients with sensorineural hearing loss and to the affected ear in conductive hearing loss.

B. Diagnostic Studies

1. Audiometric examination—All patients with hearing loss, tinnitus, or vertigo require audiometric examination in a soundproof booth. Pure tones presented by air conduction and by bone conduction at various frequencies (250–8000 Hz) can identify the presence of conductive, sensorineural, or a mixed hearing loss. Word recognition scores (percentage of correctly repeated monosyllabic words presented at suprathreshold levels) are an important audiologic measure of the patient's ability to understand speech.

2. Auditory brainstem response audiometry (ABR or BSER)—A test for synchrony along the cochlear nerves. Abnormalities in the latencies of the measured waves or abnormal interaural differences suggest retrocochlear or brainstem pathologies, such as an acoustic neuroma, or multiple sclerosis.

3. Electrocochleography (Ecog)—measures the cochlear microphonics and cochlear N1 potentials. Abnormalities in the SP/AP ratio of the N1 potential have been linked to endolymphatic hydrops and Meniere disease.

4. Electronystagmography (ENG)—to assess the inner ear vestibular responses it is required in patients with associated vertigo, dizziness, or disequilibrium.

5. Imaging studies—Computed tomographic (CT) scans of the temporal bones are helpful in patients with middle ear pathology to rule out cholesteatoma and bony erosion. Magnetic resonance imaging (MRI) of the brain and the internal auditory canals with gadolinium can identify retrocochlear (CN VIII, or central nervous system) pathology such as an acoustic neuroma in a patient presenting with sudden or insidious asymmetric sensorineural hearing loss.

▶ Differential Diagnosis

A. Conductive Hearing Loss

Conductive hearing loss results from pathologies of the external or middle ear, which interfere with the conduction of sound to the inner ear. Most causes of conductive hearing loss are amenable to correction by medications or surgery or by the use of hearing aids.

1. External auditory canal pathology—Complete obstruction of the external auditory canal can result in conductive hearing loss. The most common cause is cerumen impaction. Other causes include foreign bodies, exostosis or osteomas, otitis externa, congenital aural atresia, and tumors.

2. Infections of the middle ear—Acute infections of the middle ear can cause transient hearing loss or can progress to more chronic forms of infection, with middle ear effusion, otorrhea, or tympanic membrane perforation. Eustachian tube dysfunction is believed to be a contributing factor in patients with recurrent ear infections. If not properly treated, chronic middle ear infections may result in the development of cholesteatoma with potential bony erosion and ossicular discontinuity, or in tympanosclerosis with stiffening of the ossicular chain. Surgery may be required for the control of refractory middle ear infection and for the removal of

cholesteatoma. Once the cholesteatoma is removed and the infection is controlled, ossicular reconstruction using autologous grafts or ossicular prostheses is performed to correct the hearing deficit.

3. Otosclerosis—Otosclerosis is a bony disorder of the otic capsule, which most commonly involves the oval window resulting in fixation of the footplate. It manifests clinically as conductive or mixed hearing loss. Surgical treatment, a stapedectomy, which involves replacement of the fixed stapes with a prosthesis, is highly successful in correcting the conductive component of the hearing loss. Hearing aids are also a useful alternative.

B. Sensorineural Hearing Loss

Sensorineural hearing loss may result from sensory or neural causes. Sensory hearing loss usually results from pathologies affecting the cochlea. These include injury to hair cells secondary to excessive exposure to noise, ototoxic medications, viral or bacterial infections, complications of meningitis, and age-related cochlear degeneration (presbycusis). Neural hearing loss results from retrocochlear pathology affecting the cochlear nerve, central nervous system pathways, or both. Cochlear nerve pathologies include compression by tumors such as vestibular schwannomas (acoustic neuromas) or neural forms of presbycusis. Lesions affecting the central nervous system, such as recurrent small strokes or multiple sclerosis, infrequently can produce sensorineural hearing loss if the auditory pathways are affected.

Further audiologic and radiologic testing is required to differentiate sensory and neural causes of hearing loss. Patients with sensory hearing loss are able to maintain better speech discrimination scores relative to their pure tone thresholds than patients with neural hearing loss and are therefore more likely to benefit from amplification.

Rehabilitation using hearing aids is the solution, and the benefits depend on the severity of hearing loss and the preservation of speech discrimination abilities. Surgical procedures for the treatment of sensorineural hearing loss include cochlear implantation in cases of severe bilateral loss or implantable hearing devices.

1. Presbycusis—Presbycusis (age-related hearing loss) is one of the most common causes of sensory hearing loss. Higher frequencies are usually most affected. Hearing loss is usually symmetric, progressive, and associated with difficulty understanding speech in noisy environments. In neural forms of presbycusis, the speech discrimination loss is greater than the pure tone loss, making amplification using hearing aids more challenging.

2. Sudden sensorineural hearing loss—Sudden sensorineural hearing loss is defined as a loss greater than 30 dB in three contiguous frequencies, occurring over a period of less than 3 days. The incidence appears to increase with age, and most patients are 40 years of age or older. The etiology of this disease is unknown. Viral and vascular etiologies have been suggested. Early initiation of treatment with prednisone, 1 mg/kg/day, is recommended. MRI of the internal auditory canals is obtained to rule out the presence of vestibular schwannoma.

3. Vestibular schwannoma (acoustic neuroma)—
Vestibular schwannomas are benign tumors arising from the Schwann cells sheath of the CN VIII. They are by far the most common tumor of the cerebellopontine angle (CPA). Patients usually present with unilateral, progressive sensorineural hearing loss and tinnitus. Early diagnosis, using MRI of the internal auditory canals with gadolinium, is crucial for early diagnosis and preservation of hearing and facial nerve function.

4. Other causes—
Other causes of sensorineural hearing loss include infection (measles, rubella, mumps, syphilis, and Lyme disease), metabolic disorders (diabetes, hyperlipoproteinemia, renal failure, and hypothyroidism), autoimmune disorders, vasculitis, multiple sclerosis, and radiotherapy.

▶ Treatment

Persistent hearing loss with its various etiologies results in a handicap proportionate to the severity of the loss. In children, there is an additional effect on speech acquisition. Early diagnosis using newborn hearing screening is therefore important. Early institution of hearing rehabilitation using hearing aids or cochlear implants is recommended in an attempt to alleviate the hearing disability and its effects. Early intervention yields better outcomes at any age.

Most conductive hearing losses are treatable by either surgical reconstruction or with the use of hearing aids. Most patients with sensorineural hearing loss can also be helped by amplification using hearing aids. Advances in hearing aid technology have resulted in smaller and more efficient devices. Digitally programmable hearing aids allow patients to choose between different programs to optimize their hearing in different environments. The latest development in this field has been the introduction of semi-implantable and totally implantable hearing aids.

Bone-anchored cochlear stimulators (eg, BAHA and Ponto Oticon systems) are available for patients with conductive hearing loss who are unable to use conventional hearing aids because of anatomic deformities of the ear canal or persistent ear drainage. They are also used in patients with unilateral sensorineural hearing loss, the severity of which can render conventional hearing aids ineffectual. In such patients, the cochlear stimulator (implanted on the deaf side) transmits sound transcranially to the normal contralateral cochlea.

Cochlear implants have revolutionized the care of patients with bilateral profound hearing loss who show no benefit from hearing aids. Cochlear implants stimulate the auditory nerve fibers directly via an electrode array that is inserted into the cochlea, bypassing the damaged hair cells. Children who use cochlear implants have been mainstreamed into regular schools, and adults have resumed gainful employment.

Basura GJ, Eapen R, Buchman CA. Bilateral cochlear implantation: Current concepts, indications, and results. *Laryngoscope* 2009; 119:2395–2401. [PMID: 19894280]

Kim JS, Lee H. Inner ear dysfunction due to vertebrobasilar ischemic stroke. *Semin Neurol* 2009;29:534–540. [PMID: 19834865]

Lee H, et al. Sudden deafness and anterior inferior cerebellar artery infarction. *Stroke* 2002;33:2807–2812. [PMID: 12468774]

Lee H, Yi HA, Baloh RW. Sudden bilateral simultaneous deafness with vertigo as a sole manifestation of vertebrobasilar insufficiency. *J Neurol Neurosurg Psychiatry* 2003;74:539–541. [PMID: 12640087]

Lee H, et al. Infarction in the territory of anterior inferior cerebellar artery: Spectrum of audiovestibular loss. *Stroke* 2009;40: 3745–3751. [PMID: 19797177]

Nelson HD, Bougatsos C, Nygren P. Universal newborn hearing screening: Systematic review to update the 2001 US Preventive Services Task Force Recommendation. *Pediatrics* 2008;122: e266–276. [PMID: 18595973]

Park P, et al. Unilateral sensorineural hearing loss after spine surgery: Case report and review of the literature. *Surg Neurol* 2006;66:415–418. [PMID: 17015127]

Wazen JJ, et al. Transcranial contralateral cochlear stimulation in unilateral deafness. *Otolaryngol Head Neck Surg* 2003;129: 248–254. [PMID: 12958575]

Wellman MB, Sommer DD, McKenna J. Sensorineural hearing loss in postmeningitic children. *Otol Neurotol* 2003;24:907–912. [PMID: 14600473]

TINNITUS

ESSENTIALS OF DIAGNOSIS

▶ Duration and precipitating factors
▶ Unilateral or bilateral
▶ Pulsatile or nonpulsatile
▶ Associated symptoms
▶ Effect on daily activities

▶ General Considerations

Tinnitus is the perception of sound in the ear or the head in the absence of an external signal source. For some patients tinnitus constitutes a mild annoyance, but it can be devastating to others, interfering with sleep, concentration, and daily activities.

▶ Clinical Findings

A. Signs and Symptoms

Tinnitus may be unilateral or bilateral, insidious or sudden in onset, and pulsatile or nonpulsatile in nature. Precipitating factors include loud noise, head trauma, and sudden sensorineural hearing loss. The presence of other otologic complaints, especially hearing loss and vertigo, should be assessed. Unilateral tinnitus may be an early symptom of a vestibular schwannoma. The ear should be examined to rule out cerumen impaction and middle ear pathology, such as acute or chronic otitis media, eustachian tube dysfunction, or previous ear surgery. Auscultation of the ear and adjacent head and neck areas should be performed in patients with pulsatile tinnitus. Pulsatile tinnitus associated with headaches or blurred vision may signify pseudotumor cerebri syndrome.

B. Diagnostic Studies

Complete audiologic examination is the next step in the evaluation of patients with tinnitus. MRI of the brain and internal auditory canals with gadolinium is recommended for patients with pulsatile tinnitus to rule out vascular abnormalities such as glomus (tympanicum or jugulare) tumors or arteriovenous malformations, or for patients with unilateral tinnitus to rule out a vestibular schwannoma. Magnetic resonance angiography or venography should be considered in patients with pulsatile tinnitus and normal MRI results.

▶ Differential Diagnosis

A. Tinnitus

Tinnitus can result from pathologic conditions at different levels along the auditory pathways. It is hypothesized that central auditory pathways are involved in the maintenance of chronic tinnitus. Most often the cause of tinnitus remains unknown; however, loud noise exposure, hearing loss secondary to degenerative changes, and Ménière disease are some of the more commonly identified causes.

B. Tinnitus Generated by Para-auditory Structures

This form of tinnitus usually results from sounds generated by the body and detected by the auditory system. Mechanisms include vascular turbulence; movements of the soft palate, temporomandibular joint, or eustachian tube; and increased blood flow. Examples include arteriovenous malformations of the head and neck, carotid stenosis, glomus jugulare tumors, aneurysms, high-riding jugular bulb, high blood pressure, and intracranial hypertension.

▶ Treatment

Management of patients with tinnitus depends on detection of the cause. In patients with chronic idiopathic tinnitus, therapy depends on the level of annoyance. Most patients are managed well with cognitive therapy, counseling, and reassurance. Masking of the tinnitus with music, hearing aids (in patients with hearing loss), or commercially available tinnitus maskers can provide relief. Biofeedback therapy and tinnitus retraining therapy have been successfully used in patients with severe tinnitus. The Neuromonics tinnitus treatment system, the latest in the tinnitus treatment protocols, shows good results in tinnitus control without resorting

to medications. Among the many medications that have been used, alprazolam (0.25–0.5 mg orally up to three times a day), amitriptyline (25 mg orally up to three times a day), and gabapentin (100–300 mg orally three times a day) appear to be effective in some patients.

Bartels H, Staal MJ, Albers FW. Tinnitus and neural plasticity of the brain. *Otol Neurotol* 2007;28:178–184. [PMID: 17255884]

Davis PB, Wilde RA, Lyndall GS, et al. Treatment of tinnitus with a customized acoustic neural stimulus: A controlled clinical study. *Ear Nose Throat J* 2008;87:330–339.

Gopinath B, et al. Incidence, persistence, and progression of tinnitus symptoms in older adults: The Blue Mountains Hearing Study. *Ear Hear* 2010;31:407–412. [PMID: 20124901]

Mattox DE, Hudgins P. Algorithm for evaluation of pulsatile tinnitus. *Acta Otolaryngol* 2008;128:427–431. [PMID: 18368578]

Michaelides EM, et al. Pulsatile tinnitus in patients with morbid obesity: The effectiveness of weight reduction surgery. *Am J Otol* 2000;21:682–685. [PMID: 10993458]

Moller AR. Pathophysiology of tinnitus. *Otolaryngol Clin North Am* 2003;36:249–266. [PMID: 12856295]

Møller AR. Tinnitus: Presence and future. *Prog Brain Res* 2007;166:3–16. [PMID: 17956767]

Rudnick E, Sismanis A. Pulsatile tinnitus and spontaneous cerebrospinal fluid rhinorrhea: Indicators of benign intracranial hypertension syndrome. *Otol Neurotol* 2005;26:166–168. [PMID: 15793399]

Seidman MD, Standring RT, Dornhoffer JL. Tinnitus: Current understanding and contemporary management. *Curr Opin Otolaryngol Head Neck Surg* 2010;18:363–368. [PMID: 20625292]

Sindhusake D, et al. Risk factors for tinnitus in a population of older adults: The Blue Mountains Hearing Study. *Ear Hear* 2003;24:501–507. [PMID: 14663349]

DIZZINESS

ESSENTIALS OF DIAGNOSIS

- ▶ Differentiate between vertigo, light-headedness, syncope, and imbalance
- ▶ Episodic or constant
- ▶ Precipitating factors
- ▶ Duration of the dizzy episode
- ▶ Associated nausea or vomiting
- ▶ Associated hearing loss, tinnitus, or aural fullness
- ▶ Neurologic symptoms

▶ General Considerations

The sense of balance is provided by the integration of inputs from the visual, proprioceptive, and vestibular systems into the brain. Pathologies along these pathways result in dizziness

Table 6–1. Subtypes of Dizziness and Their Characteristics

Type	Characteristics	Ask About[a]
Vertigo	Sensation of movement in the absence of stimuli: spinning, rocking, tilting	Episodic—duration of spell, change with head position, associated nausea and vomiting Constant—associated disequilibrium
Disequilibrium	Unsteadiness or imbalance, occurring mainly when standing up or walking and better when sitting or lying down	Associated neurologic symptoms, difficulty ambulating in the dark, other types of vestibular symptoms
Dizziness hypotension	Presyncope, light-headedness, foggy head, spatial disorientation	Associated heart diseases, postural (symptoms that occur upon standing), palpitation, medication use, anxiety, hyperventilation

[a]Asking about these symptoms and conditions at the time of history taking will help in the differential diagnosis of the dizzy patient.

with its various forms and severity. Dizziness is a vague symptom, which in the patient's dictionary may include vertigo, light-headedness, disequilibrium, fainting, or syncope. In patients whose dizziness is considered vertiginous, the evaluation should be directed toward differentiating between peripheral and central vestibular pathology.

► Clinical Findings

A. Symptoms and Signs

A thorough history is of prime importance in the evaluation of the dizzy patient. Often patients have difficulty describing their symptoms; hence questions should be directed at describing the quality of symptoms (vertigo, dizziness, or disequilibrium), duration of a typical episode, associated symptoms, precipitating factors, and current use of medications.

Dizziness, as a general term, can be subdivided broadly into vertigo, disequilibrium, and dizziness (Table 6–1). Vertigo is a true sensation of motion, classically spinning, which can be caused by lesions within the peripheral or the central vestibular system. Absence of vertigo, however, does not rule out the possibility of primary vestibular pathology. Dizziness, which also could be described as a vague sensation in the head, nonspecific light-headedness, disorientation, or wooziness, is usually secondary to vasovagal reaction, postural hypotension, or hypoperfusion of the central nervous system secondary to cardiovascular pathology. Other less common causes of light-headedness include central vestibular pathology, poorly compensated peripheral vestibular pathology, or general medical disorders. Imbalance or disequilibrium is observed in bilateral vestibular weakness, poorly compensated acute vestibular injury, or progressive vestibular pathology.

Inquiring about precipitating factors can help in the differential diagnosis of the dizzy patient (see Table 6–1). Examples include head movement and head position in benign paroxysmal positional vertigo, stress in Ménière disease, food intake in migraine, and trauma in perilymphatic fistula.

Recurrent acute episodes of vertigo associated with nausea and vomiting are characteristic of peripheral vestibular pathology; vertigo in central nervous system disease, although it can be acute in onset, is more likely to be prolonged and persistent. Falling, difficulty ambulating with eyes closed, or difficulty ambulating in the dark suggests decreased vestibular function. The presence of associated ear symptoms such as tinnitus or hearing loss usually suggests a pathologic process in the peripheral vestibular system. On the other hand, the presence of visual field defect, diplopia, limb ataxia, dysarthria, paresthesia, or other neurologic symptoms favors central vestibular abnormalities. In episodic vertigo, the duration of the attacks can assist in the differential diagnosis (Table 6–2).

In the absence of middle ear pathology, the basic head and neck examination is usually negative in the dizzy patient. Physical examination of the dizzy patient focuses on the cranial nerves, limb coordination, stance, and gait, including the ability to walk tandem and to stand with feet together and eyes closed (Romberg test). Nystagmus is a common finding and is usually horizontal and rotatory in peripheral vestibular disorders. Vertical nystagmus favors central pathology. Suppression of nystagmus with visual fixation is characteristic of peripheral lesions. The Fukuda stepping test, in which the patient marches in place with eyes closed, helps in detecting a subtle vestibular disturbance. Patients with vestibular pathology are often unable to maintain their position and turn toward the affected side.

Table 6–2. Differential Diagnosis of Vertigo Based on Duration of Attacks

Duration	Hearing Loss	
	Absent	**Present**
Seconds	Benign paroxysmal positional vertigo	Perilymphatic fistula
Minutes to hours	Migraine	Ménière disease
Days	Vestibular neuronitis	Labyrinthitis

B. Diagnostic Studies

1. Vestibular testing—In addition to a complete audiologic evaluation, patients with dizziness, disequilibrium, or vertigo should undergo vestibular testing. **Electronystagmography (ENG)** measures the vestibulo-ocular response to various stimuli, including gaze, positional, tracking, saccadic, optokinetic, and bithermal caloric testing. ENG helps in differentiation of central and peripheral pathology and in the detection of unilateral vestibular pathology.

Rotatory chair testing measures the vestibulo-ocular reflex in response to varying speeds of chair rotation. A limitation of the rotatory chair is that it cannot lateralize pathology.

The **static and dynamic posturography** test evaluates the interaction of the vestibular system with the visual and proprioceptive systems in maintaining balance. It measures postural sway and shift in the center of gravity on a moving computerized platform under various conditions in which visual and somatosensory input is altered. This allows for measurement of the contribution of each sense on balance control. It is frequently used to assess the rate of improvement with vestibular rehabilitation therapy.

2. Imaging studies—CT or MRI scan of the brain and internal auditory canals with and without contrast is necessary whenever hemorrhage, infarction, or tumor is suspected.

▶ Differential Diagnosis

Dizziness, in its various forms, can be caused by numerous disease processes (Table 6–3). The primary challenge in the management of the dizzy patient is to determine whether the complaint is vestibular or nonvestibular in origin. Patients usually have difficulty explaining their symptoms and differentiating among vertigo, light-headedness, imbalance, and other symptoms of dizziness. Traditionally, vertigo is thought to be caused mainly by vestibular pathology and nonvertiginous dizziness by nonvestibular diseases. In reality, vertigo can occur with nonvestibular pathology, and its absence does not rule out the possibility of primary vestibular pathology. Dizziness or light-headedness, in the context of vestibular problems, is the chief indicator of poor vestibular compensation. Therefore, the differentiation between vestibular and nonvestibular origin of various types of dizziness based solely on the nature of the complaint is an artificial one. Nevertheless, there are certain diseases that present more commonly with vertigo and others with disequilibrium or dizziness (see Table 6–3).

A. Benign Paroxysmal Positional Vertigo

Benign paroxysmal positional vertigo (BPPV) is characterized by recurrent episodes of vertigo lasting for seconds and precipitated by changes in head position, especially neck extension, bending down, lying supine with the affected ear down, rising from bed, and rolling over in bed to the affected side. A prior history of trauma or labyrinthitis is common. In most patients, spontaneous resolution of symptoms occurs within a few weeks to months, during which avoidance of the precipitating head position is helpful. However, recurrence of symptoms is common.

In patients with BPPV, otoliths (calcium carbonate crystals), normally found in the utricle and saccule, are thought to dislodge into one of the semicircular canals, making the canal sensitive to gravity. The result is hair cell stimulation and the perception of motion when the head is put in the dependent position with the affected ear down. The posterior semicircular canal is most commonly involved.

Symptoms can be reproduced by performing the Dix-Hallpike test. Rotatory nystagmus beating toward the floor is elicited after a latency of a few seconds in posterior semicircular canal BPPV. Symptoms of BPPV are fatigable and abolished with repeated testing.

Vertigo can be relieved by a variety of positioning maneuvers, including the Epley, Semont, and Brandt-Daroff maneuvers (Figure 6–1). Refractory symptoms can be abolished surgically by sectioning of the posterior ampullary nerve (singular neurectomy) or a transmastoid posterior semicircular canal occlusion.

B. Ménière Disease

Ménière disease, in its classic form, causes episodic attacks of vertigo, tinnitus, and low-frequency fluctuating hearing loss. Aural fullness or pressure is characteristic. Patients may initially present with vertigo and no hearing loss or with fluctuation in hearing in the absence of vertigo. The classic triad, however, follows as the condition progresses. Vertigo usually lasts several minutes to hours and is often associated with

Table 6–3. Common Causes of Dizziness

Type	Cause
Vertigo	Benign paroxysmal positional vertigo, Ménière disease, labyrinthitis, vestibular neuronitis, inner ear autoimmune disease, perilymphatic fistula, migraine,[a] labyrinthine concussion,[a] transverse temporal bone fracture, vertebrobasilar ischemia, lateral medullary infarct (Wallenberg syndrome), cervical injury
Disequilibrium	Peripheral neuropathy, acoustic neuroma,[a] ototoxic drugs, cerebellar atrophy, cerebellar infarction, tumors of the posterior fossa, aging, multiple sclerosis,[a] Wernicke encephalopathy
Dizziness, light-headedness	Cardiac arrhythmia, vasovagal reaction, postural hypotension, systemic viral or bacterial infection, hypoglycemia, hyperglycemia, electrolyte disturbances, thyrotoxicosis, anemia, psychophysiologic,[b] adverse drug reaction, ocular dizziness due to rapid vision change (after cataract surgery, a change in a corrective prescription)

[a]May also present with dizziness.
[b]May also present with vertigo.

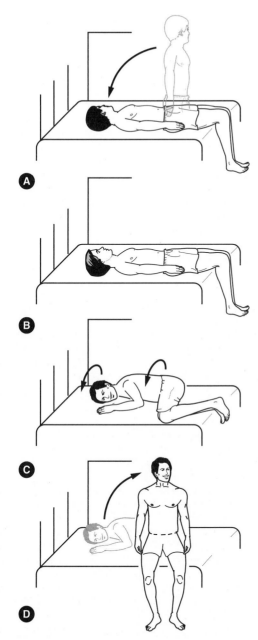

▲ **Figure 6–1.** The Epley maneuver starts with the patient in the seated position. **A:** The patient's head and body are moved into the Dix-Hallpike position with the affected ear downward. **B:** After resolution of the elicited nystagmus or the symptoms, the patient's head is turned to the neutral position. **C:** The head and body are then turned away from the affected ear. The patient should stay in each position for 60 seconds. **D:** To conclude the maneuver, the patient is raised to a sitting position with the head tilted 20 degrees forward.

nausea and vomiting. Cold sweating, pallor, and diarrhea may occur during severe spells. Movement exacerbates the symptoms. The pathophysiology of Ménière disease is an increase in the endolymphatic fluid pressure and volume. Causes are multiple and include trauma, infection, immune-mediated disorders, and genetic predisposition. The disease is unilateral in the majority of patients. Bilateral disease, however, occurs in 20–30% of patients, commonly in the immune-mediated category. Most patients respond to conservative medical management with dietary salt restriction and diuretics, antihistamines, corticosteroids, and labyrinthine suppressants such as meclizine. Limiting caffeine intake, reducing alcohol consumption, and stress management are advisable. Patients who fail to respond to the medical management are treated with intratympanic steroids or gentamycin perfusion, endolymphatic shunt surgery, labyrinthectomy, or vestibular neurectomy.

C. Vestibular Neuronitis

Vestibular neuronitis presents with sudden and severe vertigo associated with nausea and vomiting lasting a few days. Physical examination reveals nystagmus and inability to maintain balance. ENG reveals a unilateral reduced response to caloric stimulation. Audiologic evaluation is usually normal. A history of viral illness is common. Vestibular neuronitis is a self-limited disorder, and vestibular suppressants can be used for symptomatic treatment. Patients may complain of unsteadiness for a few weeks after the acute attack. Early ambulation should be encouraged to facilitate vestibular compensation for the unilateral sudden loss of vestibular function. Recurrent attacks occur in some patients.

D. Perilymphatic Fistula

Perilymphatic fistula is an abnormal communication between the perilymph-filled inner ear and the air-filled middle ear. It can be caused by various kinds of trauma (head injury, barotrauma) or can occur spontaneously secondary to increased intracranial pressure (coughing, sneezing, straining, or lifting). Perilymphatic fistula usually manifests with vertigo in association with a unilateral sensorineural hearing loss. Conservative management with bed rest should be initiated. Refractory patients require surgery to patch the fistula.

E. Labyrinthine Concussion

Labyrinthine concussion follows head trauma with or without temporal bone fracture; vertigo and imbalance appear immediately after injury. Audiometry is usually normal but sometimes reveals a high-frequency sensorineural hearing loss. Spontaneous resolution of symptoms usually occurs over 6 months to 1 year. Vestibular exercises can hasten recovery.

F. Whiplash Injury

Dizziness is reported to be one of the most frequent symptoms of a whiplash injury. Positional nystagmus can be observed on physical examination and recorded by ENG. Audiologic testing is usually normal. Spontaneous resolution usually occurs over weeks to months; diazepam with its dual effect as a vestibular suppressant and muscle relaxant can offer symptomatic relief. Cervical neck collar and vestibular rehabilitation can be helpful.

G. Migraine-Associated Vertigo

Migraine is a common cause of episodic vertigo. Vertiginous episodes may precede or occur simultaneously with the headache and may also occur during headache-free periods. Patients often have a positive family history of migraine. Treatment of migraine-associated vertigo is the same as for migraine.

H. Superior Semicircular Canal Dehiscence

Vertigo may be caused by dehiscence of bone over the superior semicircular canal. Patients usually complain of vertigo induced by loud noise or pressure in the external auditory canal. Other symptoms may include autophony (hearing one's own voice as loud in the affected ear) or conductive hearing loss with a normal middle ear system. CT scan of the temporal bone with oblique views of the superior semicircular canal usually shows the bony dehiscence. The treatment for severe symptoms is surgical plugging of the affected semicircular canal via a temporal craniotomy or transmastoid approach.

I. Tumors

Vertigo in association with cranial nerve palsy, seizures, ataxia, or signs of increased intracranial pressure warrant further investigation to rule out a space-occupying lesion. Vestibular schwannoma (acoustic neuroma) and other tumors of the cerebellopontine angle can present with vestibular symptoms in association with hearing loss and tinnitus. Imbalance is far more common than true vertigo in patients with vestibular schwannoma. Early diagnosis is crucial for preservation of postoperative hearing and facial nerve function.

J. Nonvestibular Causes of Dizziness

Evaluation of the dizzy patient is not complete without ruling out general medical disorders that most commonly present with nonvertiginous dizziness. These disorders include hypothyroidism, anemia, orthostatic hypotension, cardiac arrhythmias or failure, carotid sinus syncope, diabetes mellitus, hypoglycemia, psychophysiologic disorders, and medications side effects.

▶ Treatment

Although definitive treatment of the dizzy patient depends on etiology, symptomatic treatment with vestibular suppressants provides relief in acute attacks. Meclizine hydrochloride, 25 mg orally up to three times daily or during acute attacks; lorazepam, 0.5–1 mg; or diazepam, 5–10 mg orally can reduce the intensity of the vertigo. Antiemetics may be needed to control associated nausea and vomiting. In chronic

forms of vertigo, vestibular rehabilitation therapy is prescribed to enhance the ability of the central nervous system to compensate for the vestibular loss or weakness.

Intratympanic therapy has evolved as a potential alternative to surgical therapy in patients with intractable vertigo. Medication instilled into the middle ear is absorbed via the round window into the perilymph of the inner ear. The most commonly used medication is gentamycin because of its vestibulotoxic effect, creating a chemical labyrinthectomy. With judicious use, the drug has an 80–90% success rate in controlling the vertigo while preserving hearing.

Surgery is reserved for patients with refractory vertigo. Those with serviceable hearing can be treated surgically by vestibular neurectomy; endolymphatic sac decompression and shunt is an alternative for patients with Ménière disease. Labyrinthectomy (removal of the vestibular part of the inner ear) is the procedure of choice in patients with severe to profound sensorineural hearing loss.

Baloh RW. Vestibular neuritis. *N Engl J Med* 2003;348:1027–1032. [PMID: 12637613]

Bhattacharyya N, et al. Clinical practice guideline: benign paroxysmal positional vertigo. *Otolaryngol Head Neck Surg* 2008; 139(Suppl 4):S47–81. [PMID: 18973840]

Cesarani A, et al. The treatment of acute vertigo. *Neurol Sci* 2004; 25(Suppl 1)S26–30. [PMID: 15045617]

Chan Y. Differential diagnosis of dizziness. *Curr Opin Otolaryngol Head Neck Surg* 2009;17:200–203. [PMID: 19365263]

Chawla N, Olshaker JS. Diagnosis and management of dizziness and vertigo. *Med Clin North Am* 2006;90:291–304. [PMID: 16448876]

Fife TD. Benign paroxysmal positional vertigo. *Semin Neurol* 2009;29:500–508. [PMID: 19834861]

Korres S, et al. Occurrence of semicircular canal involvement in benign paroxysmal positional vertigo. *Otol Neurotol* 2002;23 926–932. [PMID: 12438857]

Lee H, et al: Nodulus infarction mimicking acute peripheral vestibulopathy. *Neurology* 2003;60:1700–1702. [PMID: 12771273]

Lempert T, Neuhauser H. Epidemiology of vertigo, migraine and vestibular migraine. *J Neurol* 2009;256:333–338. [PMID: 19225823]

Minor LB. Labyrinthine fistulae: pathobiology and management. *Curr Opin Otolaryngol Head Neck Surg* 2003;11(5):340–346. [PMID: 14502064]

Neuhauser HK. Epidemiology of vertigo. *Curr Opin Neurol* 2007;20:40–46. [PMID: 17215687]

Pappas DG Jr. Autonomic related vertigo. *Laryngoscope* 2003;113: 1658–1671. [PMID: 14520090]

Sloane PD, et al. Dizziness: State of the science. *Ann Intern Med* 2001;134(9 Pt 2):823–832. [PMID: 11346317]

Straube A. Pharmacology of vertigo/nystagmus/oscillopsia. *Curr Opin Neurol* 2005;18:11–14. [PMID: 15655396]

Strupp M, Arbusow V. Acute vestibulopathy. *Curr Opin Neurol* 2001;14:11–20. [PMID: 11176212]

Strupp M, Brandt T. Vestibular neuritis. *Semin Neurol* 2009;29: 509–519. [PMID: 19834862]

Epilepsy & Seizures

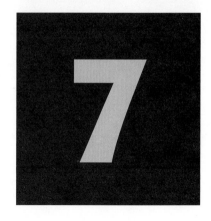

Tina Shih, MD

INCIDENCE & PATHOGENESIS

Seizures are episodes of temporary brain dysfunction secondary to abnormal electrical activity. They are common, affecting approximately 10% of individuals at some point in their lives. Approximately 25% of seizures have a clearly identifiable, temporally associated cause. These seizures, labeled *acute symptomatic seizures* or *provoked seizures*, do not have a tendency to recur, unless the underlying condition returns.

In contrast, **epilepsy** is defined as two or more *unprovoked* seizures (ie, having no identifiable acute, proximal cause). Individuals with epilepsy have a significantly increased risk of recurrent seizures. According to the World Health Organization, epilepsy is the most common primary disorder of the brain. More than 2.3 million people in the United States have epilepsy, and an estimated 181,000 Americans are diagnosed with the disorder each year.

In industrialized countries, epilepsy has an age-specific incidence, highest in the very young and the very old (Figure 7–1). This finding has important implications. As the US population ages, it is expected that the prevalence of epilepsy will also increase. This finding also mirrors what are well-established risk factors for epilepsy. Disorders manifesting in the very young (eg, cerebral palsy and mental retardation) and diseases of the elderly (eg, clinically detected stroke and Alzheimer dementia) increase an individual's risk of epilepsy by more than 10-fold (Figure 7–2).

Seizures are a common final pathway in a myriad of diseases of the central nervous system (CNS); however, not all individuals with clinically evident brain injury develop epilepsy. Further confounding the situation, many individuals without any clinical evidence of structural or functional brain abnormalities have epilepsy. *Epileptogenesis,* defined as the process by which a region of brain, over time, becomes hyperexcitable and develops the ability to spontaneously generate seizures, is not well understood. Clinicians still have no means by which they can prevent the development of epilepsy in high-risk individuals, and for almost two thirds of patients, no cause for their epilepsy can be identified.

Some regions of the brain, for example, the hippocampus, entorhinal cortex, and amygdala (which constitute the mesial or middle temporal lobe), appear to be more vulnerable to the epileptogenic process. Abnormalities in synaptic transmission and neuronal excitability have been implicated, but the pathophysiology of epilepsy is much more complex than any single pathway. Much current research has focused on the molecular level, with studies examining voltage-gated ion channels, neurotransmitters, neuronal proteins and trophic factors, and alterations in gene expression within neurons.

SEIZURE TYPES

Despite advances in the genetics and the molecular and cellular biology of epilepsy, seizure classification remains firmly rooted in the phenomenology of the seizure episode. Seizures can be subtle, involving merely behavioral arrest or rhythmic eye blinking, or they can be dramatic, with yelling and shaking of the limbs.

The International League Against Epilepsy (ILAE) first established a classification schema in 1960, based on the clinical manifestations and the ictal (during a seizure) and

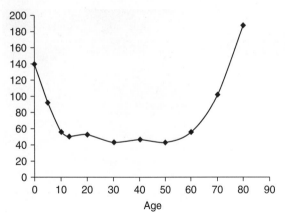

▲ **Figure 7–1.** Age-specific incidence of epilepsy in the United States. (y-axis incidence/100,000)

Table 7–1. International League Against Epilepsy (ILAE) Classification of Seizures (Simplified Version)

Focal seizures
Generalized Seizures
Absence
• Typical absence
• Atypical absence
Myoclonic
Clonic
Tonic
Tonic-clonic (in any combination)
Atonic or astatic ("drop")
May be focal, generalized, or unclear
Epileptic spasms

interictal (between seizures) electroencephalographic (EEG) pattern. They recently revised the terminology and organization (Table 7–1). Seizures are either **focal** (coming from one area of the brain, with or without spread to other areas; "partial" in the old classification schema) or **generalized** (involving both hemispheres of the brain simultaneously).

1. Focal Seizures

ESSENTIALS OF DIAGNOSIS

▶ Characteristics depend on the involved cortical region

▶ Varying manifestations, ranging from the patient reporting an altered subject experience to dramatic, bilateral limb shaking with falling

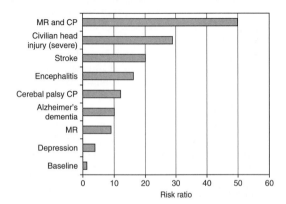

▲ **Figure 7–2.** Risk factors for epilepsy. A risk ratio of 1 (baseline) indicates that there is no increased risk. (CP = cerebral palsy; MR = mental retardation.)

These seizures may affect the temporal lobe, frontal lobe, occipital lobe, or parietal lobe.

▶ General Features

The behavioral manifestations or subjective experience of a focal seizure are largely determined by the area of cortex that is involved. For example, seizures involving the primary motor cortex cause rhythmic movements of the contralateral hand or foot, whereas seizures involving the visual cortex can cause patients to see complex figures or colors in a part of their visual field. In the past, focal seizures were divided into "simple partial," "complex partial," and "secondarily generalized" seizures, depending on whether the patient experienced an impairment of awareness and/or uncontrolled shaking and stiffness of the limbs. Reflecting the scientific imprecision and inconsistent application of this terminology, the new classification system no longer makes such a distinction; however, pragmatically speaking, these clinical manifestations have immediate safety and societal implications (eg, for driving competence). The current teaching is less of a reliance on classification and a return to better descriptions of the actual seizures.

Lay individuals still use the terminology *aura,* which is the patient's subjective experience at the onset of a seizure. An aura is a focal seizure, and depending on the area of brain involved, its description can vary widely from a burning odor (olfactory cortex) to a sense of fear (limbic cortex) or tingling in a limb (primary sensory cortex).

▶ Temporal Lobe Seizures

Data from video and EEG monitoring suggest that the majority of focal seizures arise from the temporal lobe. These seizures often begin with an aura, ranging from an epigastric rising sensation (involvement of the cortex with projections to the autonomic nervous system) to a stereotyped sense of fear (involvement of the amygdala). Such seizures are often clinically bland or quiet. Witnesses, when

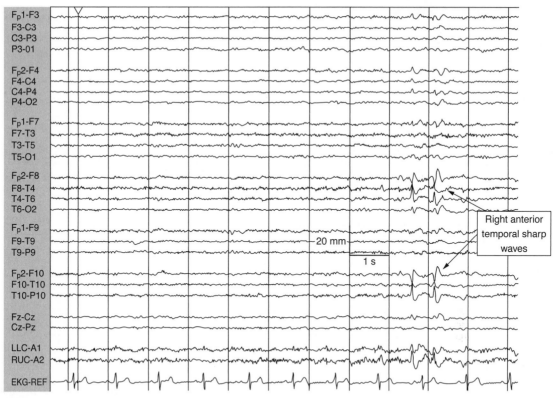

▲ **Figure 7–3.** Interictal (between-seizure) EEG in a patient with temporal lobe epilepsy. Note the sharp waves in channels 13–15 and 20–22 approximately 9 seconds into this epoch. These are typical anterior temporal epileptiform discharges and are highly suggestive of an epileptogenic lesion in the right mesial temporal lobe (amygdala and hippocampus).

prompted, may report oral automatisms (lip smacking or chewing), manual automatisms (eg, picking at clothes repeatedly, patting), or subtle dystonic posturing of a limb (sustained contortion of the hand or foot), but often the most consistent feature is the patient's unresponsiveness for a period of time. Afterward, the patient may describe fatigue, confusion, or difficulty speaking and comprehending, which can last for several minutes. The interictal EEG may be normal, or it may demonstrate focal slowing and epileptic-form discharges (Figure 7–3). The ictal EEG is often a rhythmic discharge best developed in the temporal channels (Figure 7–4).

▶ **Frontal Lobe Seizures**

The second most common focal seizures are frontal lobe seizures. These seizures, in contrast to temporal lobe seizures, are typically dramatic and have prominent motor manifestations. They are often nocturnal, arising from sleep, and are usually brief in duration (15–45 seconds). Witnesses may describe loud vocalizations, shaking of limbs, forced head turning to one side, or bicycling movements. *Jacksonian*

march seizures involve progression of the abnormal electrical activity along the primary motor cortex. Clinically, the patient may describe involuntary rhythmic jerking of the thumb, followed by spread to the hand and wrist, then to the arm and face, all on the same side of the body. If the seizure involves the supplementary motor cortex on the medial surface of the frontal lobe, the patient may assume an asymmetric dystonic posture (so-called *fencer position*), with the head turned to one side, one arm extended, and the other arm bent with the hips abducted and the legs flexed. With this type of seizure, the patient may have bilateral motor manifestations, yet retain awareness and consciousness throughout. The interictal EEG may be normal or it may show parasagittal focal slowing. Often, the ictal EEG is obscured by muscle artifact, but the postictal EEG may show focal attenuation of cerebral activity or diffuse background slowing or attenuation.

▶ **Occipital Lobe Seizures**

These seizures frequently begin with sudden visual changes. If the primary visual cortex is implicated, the patient sees poorly formed colors or lights. With seizures of the supplementary

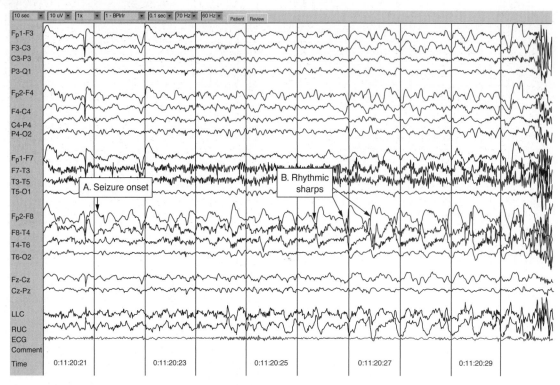

▲ **Figure 7–4.** Ictal (during a seizure) EEG demonstrating repetitive and rhythmic activity in channels 13–15, beginning 2 seconds (seizure onset) into this epoch, with evolution of the discharge in amplitude and rhythmicity. By the sixth second of this epoch, there are definite, rhythmic 2-Hz discharges arising from the right anterior temporal lobe.

visual cortex, patients may report seeing complex figures, detailed scenes, or other visual hallucinations, which are usually stereotyped. The electrical activity may then spread to the temporal lobe or frontal and parietal lobes; motor manifestations therefore can vary from subtle to dramatic.

▶ **Parietal Lobe Seizures**

These seizures are uncommon and are associated with subjective tingling or numbness of the contralateral limb or body or, rarely, with pain involving the contralateral limb or body.

2. Generalized Seizures

ESSENTIALS OF DIAGNOSIS

▶ Both hemispheres of the brain are involved simultaneously

▶ Variable subtypes, ranging from subtle staring spells (absence seizures) to brief lightning-like jerks (myoclonic seizures) to dramatic, bilateral limb shaking with falling (generalized tonic-clonic seizures)

This category includes generalized tonic-clonic seizures, absence seizures, myoclonic seizures, tonic seizures, and atonic or astatic seizures.

▶ **Generalized Tonic-Clonic Seizures**

For the general public, generalized tonic-clonic seizures are the seizures most commonly associated with epilepsy. They are dramatic in appearance and often associated with self-injury.

Generalized tonic-clonic seizures involving both hemispheres from the onset usually do not begin with any aura or warning, but some individuals describe a nonspecific, vague feeling that can occur minutes to hours before the event. There is a sudden loss of consciousness, a loud cry (as air is being forced out of the lungs through contracted vocal cords), *tonic* contraction of appendicular muscles, and loss of postural control, resulting in falling to the ground. Tonic contractions are then replaced by rhythmic *clonic* movements of the limbs, and loud inspiratory breath sounds are heard. The duration is variable, lasting between 30 seconds and 2–3 minutes, and there is often a protracted period of unconsciousness or decreased consciousness. During the seizure, fecal or urinary incontinence and tongue biting may occur. Patients are amnestic for the event. For patients who live alone, the only sign may be oral trauma, evidence of incontinence, or awakening with unexplained bruising, dislocated shoulder, or bony fracture. The interictal EEG may demonstrate generalized spike-and-wave discharges, and the ictal EEG at the onset will show generalized epileptiform discharges that are rapidly obscured by muscle artifact.

▶ Absence Seizures

These seizures begin with sudden behavioral arrest, staring, and unresponsiveness, lasting 10–20 seconds. There may be rhythmic eye blinking (eye flutter) or subtle head nodding. Sudden return to normal activity without postevent confusion is typical of absence seizures. Because of their subtle behavioral manifestations and lack of postevent confusion, these seizures are commonly missed for long periods of time, and the patients, who are most often young children, are accused of daydreaming or being inattentive. Typical absence seizures can be elicited in the clinic or at the bedside by having the patient hyperventilate for 2–3 minutes. On EEG,

typical absence seizures correlate with a regular, generalized 3-Hz (three cycles per second) spike-and-wave pattern (Figure 7–5). Atypical absence seizures, which are usually seen in children with static encephalopathy or developmental delay, are more likely to produce an irregular, generalized 2–3-Hz spike-and-wave pattern.

▶ Myoclonic Seizures

Myoclonic seizures are sudden, brief, and lightning-like in speed. They occur singly or repetitively and consist of jerky movements involving the entire body or one part of the body, usually without loss of consciousness. If the myoclonus involves the entire body, the patient may fall and sustain injury. Examples of physiologic myoclonus (not epileptic), which convey the speed and rhythm of the movement, include hiccups (myoclonus of the diaphragm) and hypnic jerks (sleep startles, which occur in early sleep). EEG may be necessary to differentiate myoclonic seizures from physiologic, segmental, or spinal myoclonus, which does not originate

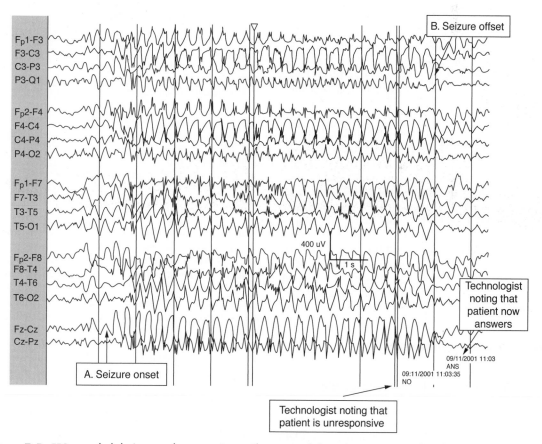

▲ **Figure 7–5.** EEG recorded during an absence seizure. The onset of the seizure occurs within the first 2 seconds of this epoch (**A**) Note the three-cycles-per-second spike-and-wave pattern over all the channels. Seizure offset (**B**) is noted by the crisp return to baseline.

from the cerebral cortex. Myoclonic seizures are associated with brief bursts of high-amplitude, generalized, irregular spike- or polyspike-and-wave activity on EEG.

▶ Tonic Seizures

In this seizure subtype, the patient manifests sudden loss of consciousness and rigid posture of the entire body, which lasts 10–20 seconds, with rapid return of consciousness or awareness. Sometimes, the head or eyes are deviated to one side. These seizures are uncommon, typically arise from sleep, and can occur repeatedly throughout the night. They are often seen in individuals with static encephalopathy or mental retardation and are commonly associated with other seizure types. The ictal EEG demonstrates a low-amplitude, generalized, fast (>15 Hz or >15 cycles per second) discharge during the clinical event.

▶ Atonic or Astatic Seizures

These seizures are also uncommon, typically occur in individuals with static encephalopathy or mental retardation, and are often accompanied by other seizure types. There is a sudden loss of consciousness and postural tone, resulting in dramatic falls and severe self-injury. A hard-shell helmet with face guard is often prescribed for these patients. The interictal EEG often shows generalized or multifocal spike- or polyspike-and-wave activity, whereas the ictal EEG may show a burst of spike-and-wave activity, followed by a brief, generalized attenuation of cortical activity (or "flattening" of the EEG).

EPILEPSY SYNDROMES

Once the patient's seizures have been characterized, the clinician attempts to classify the epilepsy syndrome, with therapeutic and prognostic implications. Many epilepsy syndromes are age-dependent and incorporate the patient's developmental and medical history, neurologic status, seizure subtypes, and ictal and interictal EEG.

The epilepsy classification schema has also been revised (Table 7–2) to reflect the changing understanding with advances in neuroimaging, genetics, molecular biology, and epidemiology. The following summary merely highlights the more common or better understood syndromes and should not be considered comprehensive.

1. Electroclinical Syndromes Arranged by Age at Onset

▶ Infancy: West Syndrome & Infantile Spasms

Infantile spasms typically occur in the first year of life (between the ages of 3 months and 1 year) and are characterized by stereotyped clusters of brief axial contractions (either flexion or extension, occurring symmetrically or asymmetrically). Oftentimes, these clusters occur when the infant

Table 7–2. International League Against Epilepsy (ILAE) Classification of Epilepsies (Simplified Version)

Electroclinical syndromes arranged by age at onset
Neonatal
• Benign familial neonatal seizures (BFNS)
• Early myoclonic encephalopathy (EME)
Infancy
• West syndrome
• Dravet syndrome
• Benign infantile seizures
• Myoclonic epilepsy in infancy (MEI)
Childhood
• Childhood absence epilepsy (CAE)
• Early-onset benign childhood occipital epilepsy (Panayiotopoulos type)
• Lennox-Gastaut syndrome
• Benign epilepsy with centrotemporal spikes (BECTS)
• Autosomal-dominant nocturnal frontal lobe epilepsy (ADNFLE)
• Epileptic encephalopathy with continuous spike-and-wave during sleep (CSWS)
• Lennox-Gastaut syndrome (LGS)
• Epilepsy with myoclonic-atonic seizures
• Epilepsy with myoclonic absences
Adolescence-Adult
• Juvenile absence epilepsy (JAE)
• Juvenile myoclonic epilepsy (JME)
• Progressive myoclonic epilepsies (PME)
• Epilepsy with generalized tonic-clonic seizures
• Autosomal dominant partial epilepsy with auditory features (ADPEAF)
Distinctive Constellations
• Mesial temporal lobe epilepsy with hippocampal sclerosis (MTLE with HS)
• Rasmussen syndrome
• Gelastic seizures with hypothalamic hamartoma

awakens and are followed by irritability or crying. Infantile spasms are most often associated with West syndrome, which consists of the triad of *infantile spasms, neurologic or psychomotor deterioration,* and an interictal EEG pattern known as *hypsarrhythmia* (chaotic, high-amplitude recording with multifocal spike-and-slow wave discharges). Infantile spasms are frequently difficult to diagnose and require confirmation by simultaneous video and EEG recording. Treatment regimens include adrenocorticotropic hormone, prednisone, vigabatrin (especially in West syndrome secondary to tuberous sclerosis, a neurocutaneous disorder), and topiramate. Prognosis depends on the underlying etiology.

▶ Childhood: Childhood Absence Epilepsy (CAE)

This epilepsy syndrome has an onset between 4 and 8 years of age, usually in children with a normal birth and developmental history. Up to 45% of patients have a family history of epilepsy. Typical absence seizures, with regular 3-Hz generalized spike-and-wave activity, are the predominant seizure type and are easily elicited with hyperventilation. Many patients also have a history of generalized tonic-clonic seizures. Medications to treat CAE include ethosuximide, valproic acid, and lamotrigine. A significant proportion of children with CAE will ultimately "outgrow" their epilepsy; a more favorable prognosis is associated with an earlier age of onset and an absence of generalized tonic-clonic seizures.

Childhood: Benign Epilepsy With Centrotemporal Spikes (BECTS)

In this epilepsy syndrome, onset is typically between 4 and 8 years of age, and patients have a normal birth and developmental history. There is a well-described familial tendency for seizures; up to 40% of cases have a positive family history of febrile seizures, epilepsy, or epileptiform EEG findings. Typical characteristics of the seizures include:

1. Unilateral paresthesias involving tongue, lip, gum, and cheek
2. Unilateral clonic activity involving face, lip, and larynx, resulting in speech impairment
3. Drooling
4. Intact consciousness initially, then secondary generalization
5. Occurrence shortly after the child has fallen asleep

The EEG is often pathognomonic, with highly stereotyped unilateral or bilateral spikes over the centrotemporal region during drowsiness and light sleep. MRI scan of the brain is invariably normal. Seizures and the interictal EEG findings usually remit by adolescence, whether or not medical treatment is initiated. If medical treatment is warranted, appropriate anticonvulsants include gabapentin, oxcarbazepine, or carbamazepine. Seizures generally are well-controlled with low-dose medication. The prognosis for patients with this syndrome is generally excellent.

Childhood: Lennox-Gastaut Syndrome (LGS)

The triad of mental retardation, slow-spike-and-wave activity on EEG, and multiple seizure types (must include either tonic or atonic seizures) are the cardinal features of LGS. Onset is usually before the age of 8 years, with the diagnosis generally made between ages 3 and 5 years. This seizure syndrome is associated with poor prognosis, and the typical history elicits frequent, medically refractory seizures and severe developmental delay. Almost 90% of patients have tonic seizures; atypical absence seizures, atonic seizures, and generalized tonic-clonic seizures can all be observed in patients with LGS. Medications include lamotrigine, valproic acid, topiramate, and felbamate.

Because medication treatment has been generally disappointing, nonpharmacologic treatments are frequently considered, including vagal nerve stimulation, ketogenic diet, and corpus callosotomy.

Adolescence: Juvenile Myoclonic Epilepsy (JME)

JME is a common epilepsy syndrome, comprising an estimated 5–10% of all the epilepsies. Onset is usually in adolescence, between 13 and 18 years of age, but onset as early as age 8 and as late as 26 years has been reported. About one third of patients diagnosed with JME have a family history of epilepsy. The cardinal seizure type is a myoclonic seizure, usually involving the arms and shoulders symmetrically and preferentially occurring in the morning. Often, the clinician elicits a history of morning "clumsiness" (eg, tremors with the morning coffee or frequently dropping soap in the shower). Generalized tonic-clonic seizures and absence seizures are also frequently seen in this syndrome. Between 15% and 42% of patients with JME are photosensitive, which can be confirmed by strobe-light testing during EEG recording. Valproic acid, lamotrigine, or topiramate are generally considered first-line medications, although there are reports that myoclonic seizures may not be completely controlled with lamotrigine. Zonisamide, levetiracetam, and felbamate are other possibilities. In contrast to CAE patients, those with JME generally do not have remission of their seizures and require anticonvulsant treatment throughout their lives.

2. Distinctive Constellations

Mesial Temporal Lobe Epilepsy With Hippocampal Sclerosis

Before high-resolution magnetic resonance imaging (MRI) of the brain was available, most cases of mesial temporal lobe seizures were categorized as "cryptogenic" because there was no obvious lesion on brain imaging. Once patients underwent surgery, however, it was discovered that they had *mesial temporal sclerosis,* a term that pathologically describes loss of hippocampal neurons and gliosis in the CA1 and hilar regions.

Currently, mesial temporal sclerosis can be accurately predicted with MRI; this syndrome consists of focal seizures, often beginning with an experiential warning and unresponsiveness and EEG recordings suggesting anterior temporal localization.

Although it is widely believed that febrile seizures are strongly associated with this syndrome, population-based studies have failed to confirm the correlation. For individuals who continue to have seizures despite therapeutic trials of two anticonvulsant medications, resective surgery is today considered standard-of-care, with a relatively low risk of subsequent morbidity. There are reports that 80–90% of patients can be rendered free of disabling seizures through removal of the abnormal hippocampus and most of the amygdala, sparing lateral neocortical structures. A recent randomized, controlled trial comparing mesial temporal resection with best medical therapy demonstrated that surgery resulted in a significantly greater chance for freedom from seizures.

3. Special Situations

Although febrile seizures and neonatal seizures are considered age-specific acute symptomatic seizures, they are included in this chapter because of their relevance in epilepsy prognosis and because of similarities in diagnostic evaluation.

▶ Febrile Seizures

Febrile seizures are an age-specific event, occurring in children between 3 months and 5 years of age, in the setting of high fever not due to a CNS infection (meningitis or encephalitis). Febrile seizures are generally divided into two categories: **simple febrile seizures,** which last less than 15 minutes and are characterized by generalized shaking, and **complex febrile seizures,** which are prolonged in duration, occur repetitively, or are focal in semiology (eg, forced head turning or eye deviation, unilateral shaking or stiffening, or weakness on one side of the body after the seizure). In evaluating the pediatric patient with febrile seizures, it is important to exclude the possibility of CNS infection or any other acute precipitant (trauma, toxic overdose). For a child with a normal developmental history and a simple febrile seizure, who recovers rapidly after the seizure, it is important to stress to the parents that brief febrile seizures do not cause permanent brain damage and are not predictors of future epilepsy; however, there is an increased risk of future febrile seizures, and parents or caretakers should be educated in the administration of seizure first aid. Treatment with an anticonvulsant is typically not recommended, although in cases of severe parental anxiety, intermittent oral diazepam can be administered at the start of a febrile illness and may be effective in preventing febrile seizures. Alternatively, rectal diazepam (Diastat) can be administered by parents during a prolonged febrile seizure lasting longer than 10 minutes.

▶ Neonatal Seizures

Defined as seizures occurring in the first month of life, neonatal seizures are common and are often the only sign of neurologic dysfunction in this age group. Clinical presentation of neonatal seizures is often subtle, making diagnosis difficult. Focal repetitive movements or stiffening of the limbs, face, or trunk; pedaling or bicycling movements; roving eye movements; and repetitive sucking or chewing movements are some of the various possible clinical manifestations. Continuous, simultaneous video and EEG recording may be critical to confirming a diagnosis of seizures in this age

Table 7–3. Causes of Neonatal Seizures (Abbreviated)

Hypoxic-ischemic encephalopathy
Trauma
Congenital abnormalities (malformations of cortical development)
• Ohtahara syndrome
Genetic syndromes
• Benign familial neonatal seizures (BFNS)
Metabolic (hypocalcemia, hypoglycemia, hyponatremia, hypernatremia)
Inborn errors of metabolism
• Early myoclonic encephalopathy (EME)
Infections
Drug withdrawal
Pyridoxine dependency
Toxins (bilirubin, maternal cocaine)

group. Possible etiologies of neonatal seizures include hypoxic-ischemic injury, CNS infection, intracranial hemorrhage, ischemic stroke, systemic metabolic abnormalities, congenital abnormalities of the brain, and familial or genetic syndromes (Table 7–3). Treatment is controversial, because there is little evidence in support of the common practice of using phenobarbital or phenytoin. Prognosis depends on the underlying etiology.

Berg AT, et al. Revised terminology and concepts for organization of seizures and epilepsies: Report of the ILAE Commission on Classification and Terminology, 2005-2009. *Epilepsia* 2010;51: 676–685. [PMID: 20196795] (Commission report detailing the new epilepsy classification schema.)

CLINICAL FINDINGS

For specific symptoms and signs of various seizure types and epilepsy syndromes, refer to the earlier section on classification. This segment focuses on components of the clinical evaluation and diagnostic studies that can be used to confirm the diagnosis, classify the type of seizure, and determine the cause.

▶ Initial Evaluation

Patients with an initial presentation of seizures often seek care in the emergency department. The evaluation and management of such individuals should proceed in tandem. Assurance that the seizure activity has been terminated and controlled must first be attained, and the search for an underlying serious CNS disorder as a cause of the seizure(s) must begin. A seizure is presumed to be of acute symptomatic origin until all provocative causes have been excluded.

The other common clinical scenario is one in which the patient is seen in a physician's office a few days after a seizure.

In this case, the evaluation proceeds differently, with the clinical history, physical examination, and clinical testing aiming to fulfill the following:

1. Confirm that the episode was a seizure
2. Classify the seizure(s)
3. Determine whether the case meets criteria for the diagnosis of epilepsy
4. Classify the epilepsy syndrome
5. Search for any underlying cause

▶ History

The clinical history is the crucial first step in the diagnostic evaluation. Family members and friends are often key witnesses to the seizure and can provide information such as a description of the seizure, any potential inciting or provocative causes, and any underlying medical or neurologic conditions.

1. Features to suggest a focal onset—Was there shaking on one side of the body? Was there forced gaze or head deviation to one side? Was there postseizure focal weakness or problems speaking (also known as a Todd paralysis)? Could the patient interact or speak during the seizure?

2. Search for an acute, proximate cause—Was there a history of recent fever, change in mental status, or headache? Has there been recent intoxication with alcohol, cocaine, methamphetamine, or other drugs? Did the seizure follow significant trauma? Does the patient have diabetes, HIV or AIDS, or renal failure?

▶ Physical & Neurologic Examinations

The physical and neurologic examination should focus on the following features: skull deformities or signs of external trauma (suggesting old or new trauma), abnormal head circumference (microcephaly or macrocephaly), dysmorphism (suggests chromosomal defect), birthmarks or dermatologic stigmata (sign of underlying neurocutaneous disorder or chronic alcoholism), and limb asymmetry in terms of size, strength, reflexes, or tone.

▶ Diagnostic Studies

Focal features on history or examination suggest structural abnormalities of the CNS and direct the clinician to seek early brain imaging with computerized tomography (CT) or MRI of the head and brain. Any history of fever, mental status change, or headache prompts an emergent lumbar puncture to look for underlying CNS infection. Blood tests examining serum sodium, glucose, blood urea nitrogen and creatinine, complete blood count, and blood alcohol level, as well as urine for toxicology screening, should be routinely obtained.

A. Electroencephalography

This study is an essential tool for the diagnosis and classification of seizures and epilepsy syndromes (see Chapter 1). Both interictal (between seizures) findings, such as focal slowing or epileptiform discharges, and ictal (during a seizure) findings are used in the classification of seizures and epilepsy. EEG is also a crucial diagnostic tool. If the diagnosis of seizures or epilepsy is being considered, epileptiform potentials on an EEG can help confirm the diagnosis. A normal EEG, however, does not exclude the possibility of epilepsy and seizures. If the diagnosis is in doubt, recording a seizure using EEG remains the gold standard for diagnosis. Occasionally, the EEG can be normal during a focal seizure because the orientation of the electrical activity and/or the volume of brain involved in the abnormal electrical activity are not well-reflected by scalp recordings.

B. Structural Imaging

MRI is currently the preferred means of structural imaging for patients with underlying epilepsy. It is highly sensitive at revealing brain tumors, vascular malformations, stroke, mesial temporal sclerosis, and developmental abnormalities, which are all common causes of seizures and epilepsy. However, specific sequences are better than others at demonstrating certain abnormalities; for example, mesial temporal sclerosis is best seen using coronal T2 and fluid-attenuated inversion recovery (FLAIR) sequences, whereas gradient echo (GRE) images are necessary to determine prior hemorrhage and the extent of hemosiderin deposition in cases of vascular malformation.

C. Functional Imaging

Interictal positron emission tomography (PET performed between seizures) uses radiolabeled glucose to study the metabolic function of different regions of the brain. In the field of epilepsy, focal areas of decreased metabolism may be important in elucidating the hemisphere and the lobe responsible for a patient's seizures, even if structural imaging is normal.

Ictal single-photon emission tomography (SPECT performed during a seizure) is an imaging process using a radioisotope that binds on first pass through the brain. Its role in epilepsy evaluations is based on the presumption that areas of increased blood flow during a seizure correspond to the region of the brain responsible for the patient's seizures. The ictal SPECT and interictal PET are primarily used in the evaluation of patients for resective surgery, especially if structural imaging is normal.

D. Other Tests

Depending on the clinical history, neurologic status, and physical examination of the patient, further testing may be warranted, including referral to a geneticist for chromosomal karyotyping (eg, fragile X, Down syndrome) or specific genetic testing (eg, certain progressive myoclonic epilepsies, neurofibromatosis). Metabolic serum, urine, or cerebrospinal fluid testing (eg, to uncover abnormalities in glucose transport or in amino acid or organic acid metabolism) may also be considered. A comprehensive survey is beyond the scope of this chapter.

DIFFERENTIAL DIAGNOSIS

Because seizures are paroxysmal, often lead to loss of consciousness or awareness on the part of the patient, and are rarely witnessed by the examining physician, the diagnosis relies on third-party observation and the ability to elicit a description of the events. As a result, other paroxysmal events and spells may be easily confused with or mistaken for epileptic seizures. Conversely, if a patient presents with an unexplained paroxysmal event, the diagnosis of seizure should be entertained. What distinguishes seizures, generally, from other events, is the strong similarity of the manifestations comparing one spell to the next.

▶ Syncope

The most common diagnostic error is mistaking syncope for seizures, the classic "fit" versus "faint" dilemma. Syncope is defined as a transient decrease in blood flow to the brain, resulting in a loss of consciousness. To distinguish seizures from syncope, the following questions should be asked:

1. *What brings on your spells?* Epileptic seizures usually occur without precipitant, although patients may report an increase in certain periods (nocturnal predilection, catamenial [menstrual cycle] association, and sometimes psychologic stress), whereas syncope tends to be associated with changes in position, exertion, and certain environmental or external factors (hot room, pain, or anticipation of pain).

2. *What do you feel like during your spell?* Patients with epileptic seizures may report an aura (again this should be stereotyped) or they may report complete amnesia for the event. Patients with vasovagal or orthostatic syncope often report feeling light-headed, with diaphoresis and palpitations, and they may describe hyperventilation.

3. *What does your spell look like?* With seizures, witnesses may describe shaking of the limbs, chewing or manual automatisms, or staring with unresponsiveness. With syncope, patients often appear pale and sweaty. Occasionally, some rapid generalized jerky movements or even generalized convulsive movements (so-called *convulsive syncope*) can occur. There should not be any focal features with a syncopal event.

4. *How long do the spells last?* Seizures generally last 30 seconds to 2 minutes, and then are often followed by a period of protracted confusion or sleepiness. Syncopal events tend to be briefer, lasting 10–30 seconds and are accompanied by a rapid return to normal mental status.

▶ Transient Ischemic Attack

Transient ischemic attacks (TIAs) are brief periods of decreased perfusion of a region of brain leading to focal, paroxysmal neurologic dysfunction. The predominant features distinguishing TIAs from seizures involve positive versus negative phenomena, confusion, and the number of events.

1. *Positive versus negative phenomena*—TIAs are associated with negative phenomena (numbness, weakness, loss of vision in part of the visual field), whereas seizures are associated with positive phenomena (tingling, shaking, lights or colors in a part of the visual field, hallucinations).

2. *Confusion*—With most TIAs, there should not be any loss of awareness or confusion.

3. *Number of events*—The underlying etiology of most TIAs is either focal stenosis of a blood vessel or emboli being released into distal blood vessels. It would be highly unusual for an individual to present with a protracted history of multiple, recurrent, stereotyped events and not have demonstrated some evidence of cerebral infarction on MRI scan of the brain.

▶ Migraine

The most reliable and distinctive feature separating migraine from seizure is the time course. Migraine auras tend to last minutes rather than seconds, and the experiential phenomena and neurologic dysfunction are slow in evolution.

▶ Psychogenic Nonepileptic Seizures

Psychogenic nonepileptic seizures are easily mistaken for epileptic seizures but are not associated with any change in brain electrical activity. These spells are notoriously difficult to distinguish from epileptic seizures. The gold standard in diagnosis remains simultaneous video and EEG monitoring. The etiology is unknown, but it is believed to be a conversion disorder, with a higher prevalence in women and in individuals with a history of physical or sexual abuse. Prognosis is variable, although a history of underlying psychiatric diagnosis is usually associated with a worse prognosis.

▶ Other Diagnoses

In children, a wide variety of spells are often mistaken for seizures. The most common include breath-holding spells (behavioral events in which a 2–4-year-old child cries secondary to some painful stimulus, and then holds his or her breath, leading to momentary loss of consciousness), gastroesophageal reflux (also known as Sandifer syndrome, in which a child has paroxysmal repetitive back arching due to the discomfort), tics, or other movement disorders. The parasomnias (eg, periodic limb movements, rapid eye movement sleep disorder) rarely are also considered in the differential diagnosis.

TREATMENT

▶ General Management

Most of the treatments available for seizures and epilepsy are symptomatic and aim to reduce the recurrence of seizures; none of the available treatments, except perhaps resective brain surgery, has been shown to change the natural course of the disease.

A. Acute Seizures

For acute symptomatic seizures from a toxic or metabolic cause, the treatment consists of avoiding the acute precipitant or normalizing the metabolic disturbance. For acute symptomatic seizures resulting from intracranial lesions, removal of the lesion may stop the seizures, but not always, even in lesions that are nonprogressive. Gliosis or changes in synaptic connections in the adjacent tissue may form new epileptogenic foci for continued seizure generation.

B. Unprovoked Seizures and Epilepsy

The fundamental treatment for unprovoked seizures and epilepsy remains pharmacologic. Between 1993 and 2009, twelve new anticonvulsant medications were introduced in the United States; despite the tremendous increase in choices, the proportion of patients who remain medically refractory has not definitively changed. There are few head-to-head comparisons between the newer and older anticonvulsants. The commonly used older medications include carbamazepine, ethosuximide, phenobarbital, phenytoin, and valproic acid. The newer medications are listed, here and in the accompanying tables, in the order of their introduction to the US market: felbamate, gabapentin, lamotrigine, topiramate, tiagabine, levetiracetam, oxcarbazepine, zonisamide, pregabalin, lacosamide, rufinamide, and vigabatrin. In general, the goal of therapy is to reduce frequency and severity of seizures with minimal adverse effects. The choice of a particular anticonvulsant continues to be based on the epilepsy syndrome (Tables 7–4 and 7–5). Currently, it is generally considered that the newer anticonvulsants are better tolerated and have fewer adverse side effects, but the cost differential is considerable. Despite advances in molecular biology, there still does not exist a rational, scientific basis for individual selection of treatment, and trial and error remains the modus operandi.

▶ Common Treatment Errors & Pitfalls

A. Drug–Drug Interactions

Many anticonvulsant medications are metabolized in the liver and affect cytochrome P-450 enzyme metabolism. Valproic acid inhibits cytochrome P-450 and can cause increases in lamotrigine, phenytoin, carbamazepine, zonisamide, and oxcarbazepine levels. Valproic acid can cause skyrocketing prothrombin times in individuals receiving warfarin, whereas carbamazepine and phenytoin cause decreased efficacy of warfarin. Erythromycin is notorious for causing toxic levels of carbamazepine.

B. Treating the Serum Level Rather Than the Patient

Although therapeutic drug levels have been identified for older medications (eg, valproic acid, carbamazepine, and phenytoin), there is a great degree of individual variability regarding tolerance, toxicity, and efficacy. Some individuals require valproic acid levels of 130 μg/mL to control their seizures; in others, toxicity may be seen at 90 μg/mL. Drug levels are only a guide and are most useful in monitoring compliance. For many of the newer anticonvulsants, no meaningful clinical relationships have yet been established between serum levels and efficacy or toxicity. Seizure control and dose-related neurotoxicity (ataxia, double vision, dizziness, lethargy) should be the primary end points of anticonvulsant titration. Generally, treatment with one drug at higher doses is preferable to treatment with two drugs at lower doses because of the reduced risk of adverse events with monotherapy.

C. Unbound Level of Highly Protein-Bound Medications

Phenytoin and valproic acid are highly protein-bound medications, and the active component of these medications is the unbound fraction. In cases of hypoalbuminemia and renal failure, the ratio of unbound to bound forms becomes less predictable, and toxicity may be seen with low total serum levels. Also, of importance, when individuals take both phenytoin and valproic acid, valproic acid displaces phenytoin protein binding, rendering a higher fraction of the drug in its active form.

D. Zero-Order Pharmacokinetics of Phenytoin

Phenytoin is unique in having a nonlinear pharmacokinetic profile (Figure 7–6). At higher oral doses, serum levels of the drug can sharply increase, leading to toxicity. Thus when increasing phenytoin doses in individuals who receive typical doses (~300 mg/day in most full-sized adults) or have serum levels in the therapeutic range (10–20 μg/mL), the clinician should do so in small increments (eg, 30 or 50 mg).

E. Patient Noncompliance or Compliance Variability

It is well-known that patient compliance with chronic medications decreases inversely to the number of daily dose requirements. Once-a-day medications or at most twice-a-day formulations allow for maximal compliance.

Table 7–4. Efficacy of Anticonvulsant Agents Based on Seizure Type

Drug	Tonic-Clonic	Partial	Absence	Myoclonic
Efficacy for				
Older Agents				
Carbamazepine[a]	Yes	Yes	May worsen	May worsen
Clonazepam	Yes	Yes	Yes	Yes
Ethosuximide[a]	No	No	Yes	Sometimes
Phenobarbital[a]	Yes	Sometimes	No	Sometimes
Phenytoin[a]	Yes	Yes	May worsen	May worsen
Primidone[a]	Yes	Yes	No	Sometimes
Valproic acid[a]	Yes	Yes	Yes	Yes
Newer Agents				
Felbamate[a]	Yes	Yes	Yes	Yes
Gabapentin	Probably no	Yes	May worsen	May worsen
Lamotrigine[b,c]	Yes	Yes	Yes	Sometimes
Topiramate[a,c]	Yes	Yes	Yes	Yes
Levetiracetam	Yes	Yes	Yes	Yes
Oxcarbazepine[a]	Yes	Yes	No	May worsen
Zonisamide	Yes	Yes	Yes	Yes
Pregabalin	Unclear	Yes	Unclear	Unclear
Rufinamide[c]	Yes	Unclear	Yes	Yes
Lacosamide	Unclear	Yes	Unclear	Unclear
Vigabatrin[d]	Yes	Yes	Unclear	Unclear

[a]Approved by the Food and Drug Administration (FDA) for monotherapy.
[b]FDA-approved for conversion to monotherapy from another agent.
[c]FDA-approved as adjuvant therapy for Lennox-Gastaut syndrome
[d]Only available through special restricted distribution program, FDA-approved as adjuvant therapy and for infantile spasms

▶ Treatment of Generalized Convulsive Status Epilepticus

Although traditionally, generalized convulsive status epilepticus (GCSE) is defined as 30 minutes of continuous seizure activity or two seizures in a 30-minute period without recovery of consciousness in between, the emerging consensus is that any convulsive seizure exceeding 5–10 minutes or any attack that persists at the time of evaluation should be considered status epilepticus.

GCSE requires immediate treatment and evaluation, occurring concurrently (Table 7–6). Considerable evidence suggests that the earlier treatment is begun, the more likely it will be effective. Intravenous lorazepam (4 mg or 0.1 mg/kg) is the first-line medication. Second-line treatment is generally considered to be intravenous fosphenytoin (20 mg/kg). If both of these medications fail to terminate the seizure, then the status epilepticus is considered refractory to medications. Continuous intravenous sedation is then required, and at this point, the patient must be intubated and mechanically ventilated.

Many physicians advocate the use of fosphenytoin even if the initial status epilepticus has terminated, because the duration of efficacy of lorazepam is only 4–24 hours, possibly leaving patients with an increased risk of seizure recurrence. For refractory status epilepticus that has not responded to first- or second-line therapy, most epileptologists now advocate aggressive treatment with continuous intravenous sedation rather than intravenous valproate or intravenous phenobarbital, and the use of continuous EEG monitoring to

Table 7–5. Characteristics of Anticonvulsant Agents

Drug	Typical No. of Daily Doses[a]	Protein Bound (%)	Side Effects Not Related to Dose	Other FDA-Approved Indications
Older Agents				
Carbamazepine	2–3	60	Rash, hyponatremia, bone marrow suppression, hepatotoxicity	Bipolar disorder, trigeminal neuralgia
Clonazepam	2	50	Lethargy, cognition	Anxiety
Ethosuximide	2	Small	Rash, gastrointestinal symptoms, bone marrow suppression	—
Phenobarbital	1	40–60	Lethargy, impaired cognition, fetal malformation	—
Phenytoin	1–2	90	Gum hyperplasia, coarse features, osteomalacia, rash, fetal malformation	—
Primidone	1–2	Small	Lethargy, impaired cognition	—
Valproic acid	1–3	80–90	Hepatotoxicity, weight gain, dyslipidemia, anovulation, hair loss, fetal malformation	Bipolar disorder, migraine
Newer Agents				
Felbamate	2	25	Aplastic anemia, hepatotoxicity, anorexia	—
Gabapentin	3–4	None	Weight gain	Postherpetic neuralgia
Lamotrigine	1–2	55	Rash, insomnia	Depression in bipolar type II
Topiramate	2	9–17	Impaired cognition, anorexia, kidney stones	Migraine
Levetiracetam	2	None	Irritability, insomnia	—
Oxcarbazepine	2	25	Hyponatremia	—
Zonisamide	1	40	Irritability, anorexia, kidney stones	—
Pregabalin	2	None	Weight gain	Anxiety, neuropathic pain, and diabetes
Rufinamide	2	35	Shortened QT interval on ECG	—
Lacosamide	2	<15	Asymptomatic first-degree AV block	—
Vigabatrin	2	None	Permanent visual field defect	

[a]Dosing regimens may be more frequent in children younger than 12 years of age.

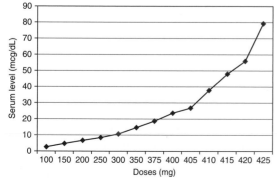

▲ **Figure 7–6.** Zero-order pharmacokinetics of phenytoin.

monitor for breakthrough seizures. If intravenous pentobarbital is required, continuous EEG monitoring to determine dose adequacy (titration of pentobarbital to burst-suppression on EEG) is required and may prompt transfer of the patient to a quaternary care center.

▶ Neurosurgical Treatment of Epilepsy

If a patient has received two or more conventional anticonvulsants pushed to toxic levels and continues to have frequent, disabling seizures, epilepsy surgery should be considered. For patients who show mesial temporal sclerosis in the nondominant (nonlanguage) hemisphere on MRI scan, concordant ictal and interictal EEG data, and evidence that the contralateral hemisphere can support memory, the

Table 7–6. Treatment Protocol for Generalized Convulsive Status Epilepticus (GCSE)

Time	Action
0–5 min	Diagnose; give O_2; maintain airway, breathing, and circulation with frequent vital sign monitoring; obtain IV access; begin ECG monitoring; draw blood for CBC, sodium, glucose, magnesium, calcium, phosphate, LFTs, antiepileptic drug levels, ABGs, and toxicology screen. Give thiamine, 100 mg IV, with 50 mL of 50% dextrose IV.
6–10 min	Give **lorazepam, 4 mg IV** over 2 min. If seizures persist, repeat in 5–10 min. If patient is not already intubated, consider rapid sequence induction with endotracheal intubation.
10–20 min	Give **fosphenytoin, 20 PE/kg IV** at 150 PE/min, with blood pressure and ECG monitoring.
20–60 min	If seizures persist, give one of the following (intubation is necessary with all medications except for valproate): • **Continuous IV (cIV) midazolam**—Load 0.2 mg/kg; repeat 0.2–0.4 mg/kg boluses every 5 min until seizures stop, up to a maximum total loading dose of 2 mg/kg. Initial cIV rate is 0.1 mg/kg/h; cIV dose range is 0.05–2 mg/kg/h. If seizures persist, proceed to pentobarbital. • **cIV propofol**—Load 1 mg/kg; repeat 1–2 mg/kg boluses every 3–5 min until seizures stop, up to a maximum total loading dose of 10 mg/kg. Initial cIV rate is 2 mg/kg/h; cIV dose range is 1–15 mg/kg/h. If seizures persist, proceed to pentobarbital. • **IV valproate**—40 mg/kg over approximately 10 min. If seizures persist, give 20 mg/kg over approximately 5 min. If seizures persist, proceed to cIV midazolam or propofol. • **IV phenobarbital**—20 mg/kg IV at 50–100 mg/min. If seizures persist, proceed to cIV midazolam, propofol, or pentobarbital.
>60 min	Give **cIV pentobarbital**—load 5–10 mg/kg up to 50 mg/min. Repeat 5 mg/kg boluses until seizures stop. Initial cIV rate is 1 mg/kg/h; cIV dose range is 0.5–10 mg/kg/h. Traditionally titrated to suppression-burst on EEG. Begin EEG monitoring as soon as possible if patient does not rapidly awaken or if any cIV treatment is used.

ABGs = arterial blood gases; CBC = complete blood count; ECG = electrocardiogram; EEG = electroencephalogram; IV = intravenous; LFTs = liver function tests.

chance for seizure freedom may be as high as 80–90% with resective surgery, with low risk of morbidity. Class I evidence now supports resective surgery (as opposed to best medical therapy) for many patients with medically refractory temporal lobe epilepsy. In general, favorable surgical candidates have a single epileptogenic focus, temporal lobe seizures, well-defined lesions on MRI scan, and concordant data.

▶ Vagal Nerve Stimulator

Developed in the late 1980s and available since 1997 as an add-on form of treatment for medically refractory epilepsy, the programmable stimulator requires surgical placement in the left chest region with wires wrapped around the left vagus nerve. It is believed that intermittent stimulation of the afferent fibers of the vagus nerve causes desynchronization of cortical electrical activity, thereby decreasing the frequency and severity of seizures. Although the vagal nerve stimulator has never rendered an individual seizure-free, it appears to be as effective as adding another anticonvulsant agent, with different and possibly fewer side effects (hoarseness, intermittent cough). The medically refractory candidates who should be considered for treatment with the vagal nerve stimulator include patients with

Lennox-Gastaut syndrome and those who have more than one seizure focus.

▶ Ketogenic Diet

Used for the treatment of epilepsy since the 1920s, the ketogenic diet was rediscovered in the mid-1990s after treatment attempts with the newer anticonvulsant medications proved disappointing. The diet in practice requires strict calculation of caloric requirements and ratios of fat, protein, and carbohydrate. It is generally recommended for children between the ages of 1 and 15 years who have multifocal or generalized epilepsy syndromes not responsive to anticonvulsant medications. A typical meal consists of 28-g ham, 23-g applesauce, 30-g heavy cream, and 30-g butter. The mechanism of action and the long-term effects are not known. About one-third of patients become seizure-free and another third demonstrate significant decrease in the frequency of their seizures.

▶ Special Situations

A. Perioperative Period (Supratentorial Craniotomy)

Approximately 5% of patients who undergo craniotomy have seizures in the immediate perioperative period (first 2 weeks).

The types of surgery associated with increased risk of seizures in this period include aneurysm (ruptured with subarachnoid hemorrhage or unruptured, but with significant cortical retraction during surgery), meningiomas, gliomas, arteriovenous malformations, intracerebral hemorrhage requiring evacuation, and infection (subdural empyema, intracerebral abscess).

Patients with the highest risk of perioperative seizures may be treated prophylactically with phenytoin or fosphenytoin for up to 2 weeks after surgery. A standard treatment regimen includes serum loading with fosphenytoin (15–20 phenytoin equivalents [PE] per kilogram) followed by oral daily dosing of 5 PE/kg/day to keep serum levels between 10 and 20 mcg/mL.

B. Head Trauma

Patients with severe head trauma (defined as intracranial hemorrhage, depressed skull fracture, penetrating head injury, and altered mental status or coma for 24 hours or more) are at increased risk for seizures in the period immediately after injury. It is generally recommended that these patients receive prophylactic anticonvulsants for the first 7 days after head trauma, following the regimen outlined for perioperative patients after supratentorial craniotomy (described in the preceding paragraph). Prolonged treatment with anticonvulsants is not recommended and may actually impede rehabilitation.

Seizures that occur at the time of impact or in the first week after mild-to-moderate head trauma are not predictive of future unprovoked seizures; however, severe head trauma is a risk factor for epilepsy, and patients with severe head trauma have a 15–30 times greater risk of developing epilepsy compared with the general population.

C. Seizures in the Elderly

Treatment of seizures in the elderly is fraught with potential complications. Little is known about the pharmacokinetics of anticonvulsants in individuals 55 years of age and older. Additionally, the elderly are more likely to have comorbid medical conditions, take multiple medications, have decreased hepatic and renal clearance of anticonvulsants, and be more sensitive to adverse effects. Data also suggest that serum levels of anticonvulsants may be more prone to fluctuations in this population.

D. Epilepsy in Women of Childbearing Age or During Pregnancy

There is evidence that some antiepileptic medications (especially oxcarbazepine, but also phenytoin, carbamazepine, primidone, phenobarbital, and topiramate) may lower the efficacy of oral contraceptives. It is recommended that women with epilepsy take a formulation containing at least 50 μg of ethinyl estradiol or mestranol.

Women with epilepsy are also at greater risk of bearing a child with major malformations. It is unclear whether this can be attributed to seizures, to medications, or to the underlying cause of the epilepsy syndrome. Current data published by multiple prospective observational studies suggest that valproic acid (alone or in combination with other medications) and phenobarbital are associated with higher rates of major birth defects. Data are not sufficient to recommend any one seizure medication. It is also recommended that folic acid supplementation (1–4 mg/day) be prescribed to all women with epilepsy throughout their reproductive years.

During pregnancy, compliance with anticonvulsant medication is paramount because generalized convulsions may result in temporary decreased placental blood flow and increased risk of miscarriage. Evidence exists that total and unbound anticonvulsant serum levels may decrease considerably during pregnancy and that close monitoring in the second and third trimester is necessary. Prenatal testing for α-fetoprotein at 14–16 weeks of gestation, structural ultrasounds at 16–24 weeks of gestation, and amniocentesis for α-fetoprotein and acetylcholinesterase levels may be necessary.

E. Renal Failure

On dialysis days, antiseizure medications should generally be administered after dialysis. The bound and unbound levels should be monitored if the individual is taking phenytoin, carbamazepine, or valproic acid. Dose adjustments may be necessary in individuals taking levetiracetam, gabapentin, zonisamide, topiramate, pregabalin, lacosamide, and vigabatrin.

F. HIV and AIDS

For individuals taking highly active antiretroviral therapy, maintaining adequate serum levels is important for long-term survival and the prevention of resistant viral strains. It is, therefore, preferable to avoid medications that induce the hepatic cytochrome P-450 enzymes.

Glauser TA, et al. Ethosuximide, valproic acid and lamotrigine in childhood absence epilepsy. *N Engl J Med* 2010;362:790–799. [PMID: 20200383] (Important randomized controlled trial demonstrating superiority of ethosuximide and valproic acid in treatment of absence seizures.)

Harden CL, et al. Practice parameter update: Management issues for women with epilepsy—focus on pregnancy (an evidence-based review): Teratogenesis and perinatal outcomes: Report of the Quality Standards Subcommittee and Therapeutics and Technology Assessment Subcommittee of the American Academy of Neurology and American Epilepsy Society. *Neurology* 2009; 73:133–141. [PMID: 19398681] (Practice parameter guiding treatment of pregnant patients with epilepsy.)

Ramsay RE, Rowan AJ, Pryor FM. Special considerations in treating the elderly patient with epilepsy. *Neurology* 2004;62:S24–S29. [PMID: 15007161] (A concise review on diagnostic and pharmacologic issues in the elderly; includes recent data from a Veterans Affair study comparing carbamazepine, lamotrigine, and gabapentin in elderly men.)

Wiebe S, et al. A randomized, controlled trial of surgery for temporal-lobe epilepsy. *N Engl J Med* 2001;345:311–318. [PMID: 11484687] (Landmark paper definitively demonstrating that surgical treatment is superior to best medical therapy in medically refractory temporal lobe epilepsy.)

PROGNOSIS

The risk of sudden death in individuals with medically refractory epilepsy is 24 times that of the general population. The cause of sudden unexplained death in epilepsy (SUDEP) is unclear. Hypotheses include arrhythmias, asphyxiation, and respiratory failure. It is estimated that between 2% and 17% of all deaths in individuals with epilepsy may be due to SUDEP. Risk factors for SUDEP include poorly controlled seizures, early onset of seizures, and a history of generalized tonic-clonic seizures.

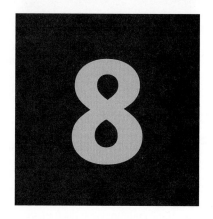

Headache & Facial Pain

Mark W. Green, MD

Headache is a common malady experienced by 90% of the US population. Half of the population has suffered from a severe headache, and 25% experience recurrent disabling attacks. Four percent endure chronic daily headaches.

Head pain can be elicited by inflammation or traction of pain-sensitive structures, vasodilation, and muscle contraction (Table 8–1). Nearly all pain-sensitive intracranial structures are innervated by trigeminovascular neurons, mainly of the ophthalmic division. For this reason, most forms of head pain are referred to the eye or temple. Trigeminovascular neurons are bipolar neurons whose cell bodies reside in the trigeminal ganglion. A peripheral branch innervates pain-producing dural blood vessels and the dura itself, and a branch projects centrally into the trigeminal nucleus caudalis. The trigeminal nucleus caudalis also receives afferents from upper cervical pain fibers. The superior salivatory nucleus, a parasympathetic nucleus, ultimately has synaptic connections with the trigeminal nucleus caudalis, probably accounting for the autonomic symptoms of nasal congestion and lacrimation that accompany many headache syndromes.

APPROACH TO THE PATIENT WITH HEADACHE

Clinical descriptions of headache and the neurologic examination usually suffice to diagnose headache types, and further testing is not useful in most cases of primary headache syndromes. Increasing frequency or severity of attacks, subjective dizziness or incoordination, pain increasing by Valsalva maneuver, awakenings with headaches from sleep, new attacks in the elderly, and new attacks in those with cancer or HIV infections increase the chance of detecting a structural abnormality. Magnetic resonance imaging (MRI) scanning is more sensitive than computed tomography (CT) in detecting abnormalities relevant to headache, with the exception of apoplectic headaches, whereas the presence of intracerebral hemorrhage is better detected by CT.

Electroencephalography is rarely useful in the evaluation of headache, except in rare patients in whom fleeting focal complaints could be secondary to a seizure disorder. Thermography does not provide additional useful information.

PRIMARY HEADACHE SYNDROMES

MIGRAINE

ESSENTIALS OF DIAGNOSIS

Migraine Without Aura (80% of patients)

► At least five attacks

► Headache attacks lasting 4-72 hours (unless successfully treated)

► At least two of the following pain characteristics:
  · Unilateral location
  · Pulsating quality
  · Moderate to severe intensity
  · Aggravated by or causes avoidance of routine physical activity

► During headache at least one of the following:
  · Nausea or vomiting
  · Photophobia and phonophobia

Migraine With Aura (15–20% of patients)

► Same features as migraine without aura

► Visual symptoms, including positive features (eg, flickering lights, spots, or lines) or negative features (eg, blind spots, loss of vision), or both

► Sensory symptoms, including negative features (eg, pins and needles) or negative features (eg, numbness), or both

► Dysphasic speech disturbance
► Symptoms of aura that develop over at least 5 minutes and last less than 1 hour; headache, if present, that follows within the hour

General Considerations

Migraine is the most important cause of disabling headaches, and most medical visits for headache are due to migraine. Although the cause of migraine is unknown, it is most commonly a familial and probably a polymorphic genetic condition. Eighteen percent of women and 6% of men experience migraines. Only 50% of these individuals receive the diagnosis of migraine, generally believing that they suffer from tension headaches or sinus headaches. More than 37% of women of reproductive age sitting in a physician's waiting room have migraine. The most sensitive criterion for migraine is headache worsening with activity.

Pathogenesis

The so-called *vascular theory of migraine,* which had widespread acceptance until the 1970s, held that migraine symptoms were a function of hyperemia and ischemia. This perspective led to the development of potent vasoconstrictors, which, in retrospect, were less safe and less effective than most of the current therapies.

Biologically, migraineurs have a hyperexcitable cerebral cortex, which probably underlies migraine auras and the frequent comorbid depression, mania, and anxiety. There is no evidence that auras are ischemic in nature. Pain appears to be related to sensitization of peripheral perivascular nerve terminals, possibly a consequence of distended meningeal blood vessels, leading to activation and sensitization of the central trigeminal system. Neuropeptide release results in neurogenic inflammation of meningeal vessels and to further activation of trigeminal sensory fibers. Neuropeptides, such as substance P and calcitonin gene–related peptide, initiate

Table 8-1. Pain Sensitivity of Structures of the Head

Pain-Sensitive Structures	Structures Largely Insensitive to Pain
Venous sinuses and their tributaries	Brain parenchyma
Dural and meningeal arteries, arteries at the base of the brain	Ventricular ependyma
Portions of the meninges	Most of the dura
Upper cervical nerve roots	Pia arachnoid
Scalp muscles and aponeurosis	

this inflammatory response, and medications targeted to these neuropeptides are being developed. A self-sustaining process of further pain, inflammation, and sensitization of central trigeminal neurons occurs, with sensitization of glial cells in the periaqueductal gray, for which there appears to be a central generator, located in the rostral brainstem. By the time these central structures become sensitized, they are activated independently of peripheral stimuli, explaining why triptans, which do not enter the central nervous system, are ineffective at this stage.

There appears to be an important genetic contribution to the development of migraine. Eight percent of migraineurs have first-degree relatives with migraine. Both identical twins are twice as likely to have migraine as fraternal twins. Only three migraines genes have been positively identified, all associated with forms of familial hemiplegic migraine, which are rare.

Prevention

Although the underlying state of migraine is likely to be genetically based, the frequency and severity of attacks can often be altered by patient behaviors. Sleep should be regular, even on weekends and vacations, because oversleeping or undersleeping can increase the likelihood of an attack. So-called *antimigraine diets* are occasionally useful, but a diet diary can be helpful even if strict adherence to the diet is not. Patients should be instructed to avoid missing meals and to minimize caffeine intake and keep amounts consistent throughout the week. Stress should be controlled, if possible. Psychiatric comorbidities such as depression, mania, social phobias, and anxiety should be evaluated and appropriately treated.

Clinical Findings

A. Symptoms and Signs

Attacks can be bilateral and nonpulsatile; the severity alone does not define a migraine. Neck pain, often unilateral, is common with migraine and often leads to an erroneous diagnosis of tension headache. Associated lacrimation and rhinorrhea, due to the activation of cranial parasympathetic nerves, often lead to the erroneous diagnosis of sinus headache.

Most migraineurs have migraine without aura (formerly known as *common migraine*). The attack frequency and degree of disability is higher in migraine without aura than in migraine with aura. In addition to migraine with aura and migraine without aura, several variant forms are encountered (Table 8–2).

Migraine with its variants accounts for 94% of primary care visits for the complaint of recurrent disabling headache. Tension-type headaches are the most common headache type, but these headaches are rarely disabling and therefore generally are self-treated. Patients in whom tension headache

Table 8–2. Subtypes of Migraine

Migraine Variant	Symptoms
Acephalic	Typical migraine auras without subsequent headache
Basilar	Auras with dysarthria, vertigo, diplopia, and decreased consciousness with bilateral numbness
Childhood periodic symptoms	Paroxysmal vertigo, periodic abdominal pains, and cyclic vomiting
Chronic	Migraines without aura for at least half of the days, present for at least 2 mo, in the absence of medication overuse
Hemiplegic	Familial and sporadic cases with reversible aura of hemiplegia
Status migrainosus	Debilitating migraine attacks lasting >72 h

appears to be disabling most often also have migraine; the "tension headaches" are best understood as part of the spectrum of an individual's migraine and treated as other forms of migraine.

B. Diagnostic Studies

Individuals with a normal neurologic examination and a stable pattern of periodic attacks that fulfill criteria for migraine rarely benefit from additional testing.

▶ Differential Diagnosis

"Migraine" is a biologic state, and individuals with migraine who develop additional medical problems (infections, neoplasms, etc.) often manifest them by a change in the character and frequency of their preexisting migraines. Therefore, if attacks do not fulfill the criteria for the diagnosis of migraine, if the neurologic examination is abnormal, or if the attack frequency and character of a preexisting headache syndrome are clearly worsening, further testing is appropriate.

▶ Complications

Some migraineurs experience a progressive frequency and severity of attacks. Many, but not all, cases of chronic migraine result from the overuse of concomitant medications. Whether aggressive symptomatic and prophylactic treatment of attacks in those with pervasive migraines will alter this natural history remains to be seen.

▶ Treatment

A. Acute Attacks

The goal of therapy for patients experiencing acute attacks is to fully terminate the head pain and its associated symptoms of light and sound sensitivity and nausea, without causing additional disability. It is preferable to avoid sedation, a common disabling side effect of some medications, allowing one to return to normal functioning. The fundamental principal of symptomatic therapy is early intervention. "False alarms" in patients with migraine are relatively uncommon. For this reason, migraineurs should be instructed to identify and aggressively treat their attacks at the earliest stages. Delayed treatment often leads to incomplete resolution of the attacks and repeated dosing because of headache recurrences.

1. Nonsteroidal anti-inflammatory drugs (NSAIDs)—If used early in an attack and at high doses, these agents are often effective. They are nonsedating and do not increase nausea, which, along with decreased gastric motility, can complicate migraine therapy. However, oral agents may not be well absorbed. Risks of gastrointestinal bleeding and hepatic disease, as well a risk of enhancing the development of cardiovascular disease, limit their frequent use. Frequent use has also been associated with an increased risk of cardiovascular and cerebrovascular disease.

2. Triptans—Most migraineurs presenting for management of their headaches are experiencing disabling attacks, for which triptans are the preferred therapy. Multiple products are available, which differ in their efficacy and delivery systems (Table 8–3). Nasal sprays (sumatriptan and zolmitriptan) or injections (sumatriptan) are preferred in attacks with a rapid onset of nausea and head pain where gastric stasis may delay the absorption of pills. Orally dissolving tablets are not sublingual and are no faster than their regular tablet counterparts, although they are convenient and therefore may encourage early intervention. Triptans with longer

Table 8–3. Commonly Prescribed Triptans

Drug	Half-Life	Metabolism	Available Formulations
Almotriptan	3 h	Hepatic CYP3A4, renal, MAO	Tab 6.25, 12.5 mg
Eletriptan	4 h	Hepatic CYP3A4	Tab 40 mg
Frovatriptan	26 h	Hepatic CYP1A2	Tab 2.5 mg
Naratriptan	6 h	Renal, hepatic P450	Tab 1, 2.5 mg
Rizatriptan	2 h	Renal, MAO, hepatic	Tab 5,10 mg; orally dissolving tab 5,10 mg
Sumatriptan	2 h	Hepatic, MAO, renal	Tab 25, 50, 100 mg; NS 20 mg; injection 4-6 mg
Zolmitriptan	3 h	Hepatic CYP-450, MAO	Tab 2.5, 5 mg; orally dissolving tab 2.5, 5 mg; NS 5 mg

half-lives (naratriptan and frovatriptan) appear to be somewhat less effective than the other products in terminating migraines. They are often used "off label" for short-term prophylaxis of predictable forms of migraine.

Recurrences refer to situations in which the headache is relieved but returns within 24 hours. Many triptan studies show high rates of headache recurrences. A longer half-life does not ensure a longer duration of action or a lower risk of headache recurrence. Early treatment with a high-dose triptan, and often the concomitant administration of an NSAID, reduces rates of recurrence in patients experiencing this treatment problem. As noted, if nausea occurs early in an attack, the absorption of oral medications may be impaired. If nausea occurs later in the attack, triptan tablets are usually satisfactory, because they relieve the nausea, vomiting, photophobia, and phonophobia in parallel with the headache.

All triptans are contraindicated in patients with coronary artery disease, although the chance of a triptan actually triggering a cardiac event is exceedingly rare. There is no evidence of a safety difference between these products. So-called *triptan sensations* (chest and neck tightness and pressure) are not due to cardiac ischemia; these effects are probably caused by esophageal constriction, pulmonary arterial constriction, or abnormalities in the energy metabolism of chest wall muscles. Triptans are also contraindicated in cerebrovascular disease. Because cerebral ischemic events are commonly associated with headache, cases of migraine with aura can be confused with stroke.

Injectable sumatriptan, when administered during an aura, does not prolong the aura but is less effective in treating the subsequent headache. This association has not been investigated with other forms of sumatriptan or other triptan products, but in patients with this response, treatment can be appropriately withheld until the pain actually begins. Moreover, migraine headaches do not invariably follow an aura. Therefore, although there is no safety concern of treating during an aura, it is recommended that treatment begin at the earliest stages of head pain. Caution is recommended when coprescribing triptans and selective serotonin reuptake inhibitors or selective norepinephrine reuptake inhibitors, as cases of a serotonin syndrome with hyperthermia, confusion, muscle stiffness, and sweating, has been reported. However, well-documented cases are very rare.

3. Ergots—Ergot medications are generally less effective than triptans in relieving all migraine symptoms. Ergotamine tartrate is a powerful arterial vasoconstrictor; dihydroergotamine (DHE), although a less powerful arterial vasoconstrictor, is a powerful venoconstrictor. These drugs have affinities for the same 5-HT$_1$ receptors as triptans, but also have affinities for additional receptors, most of which contribute to side effects rather than efficacy. Their high affinity for the 5-HT$_2$ receptor, the major serotonin receptor involved in coronary artery constriction, suggests that they are more likely than triptans to cause coronary ischemia. Ergotamine tartrate is now rarely used, but DHE remains a useful agent

Table 8–4. Intravenous Agents Used in the Treatment of Severe and Prolonged Migraine

Drug	Dose
Dexamethasone	10 mg, administered with an analgesic, prochlorperazine, valproic acid, dihydroergotamine, or subcutaneous sumatriptan to reduce risk of headache recurrence in status migrainosus
Dihydroergotamine (DHE)	1 mg in normal saline over 5 min, following an intravenous antiemetic
Ketorolac	30 mg
Prochlorperazine	10–30 mg in normal saline administered over 60 min
Valproic acid	1000 mg in 50-mL normal saline over 5 min

in migraine therapy, particularly in the treatment of status migrainosus and the inpatient management of patients with intractable and medication-induced headaches. DHE is available as a nasal spray but is most effective when administered intravenously in conjunction with an antiemetic (see Table 8–4).

Triptans and ergots cannot be used concomitantly or within 24 hours of each other.

4. Analgesics—Analgesics containing butalbital are often satisfactory for treatment when they are not overused. Despite a short duration of action, the half-life of butalbital is long, and even modest use can result in the accumulation of the barbiturate. Rebound or medication overuse headache is common with these agents. Depression can occur with prolonged use, and convulsions have been reported after abrupt continuation.

5. Opioid analgesics—These agents generally yield disappointing results. Head pain is mediated through trigeminovascular neurons, which possess a relative scarcity of opioid receptors. Moreover, migrainous pain is associated with neurogenic inflammation, and opioids are proinflammatory agents, as evidenced by the frequent complaint of itching after their use. The clearance of glutamate (an excitatory amino acid involved in the pathogenesis of migraine) from the cerebral cortex is blocked by opioids.

6. Corticosteroids—These agents shorten the duration of prolonged migraines and reduce rates of headache recurrence but do not work acutely and are inappropriate for frequent administration.

B. Prolonged Attacks

Prolonged migraine attacks (status migrainosus) are far more difficult to manage than the early stages of an attack. If unrelieved, neurogenic inflammation and sensitization of second- and third-order trigeminal neurons lead to the

Table 8–5. Drug Stabilization of Migraine

Drug	Tablet Size (mg)	Daily Dose Range (mg)	Most Common Side Effects
Propranolol	10, 20, 40, 60, 80, 90; sustained release: 60, 80, 120, 160	40–320	Fatigue, insomnia, light-headedness, impotence
Amitriptyline	10, 25, 50, 75, 100	10–175 blood levels required to determine maximum dose	Sedation, dry mouth, appetite stimulation
Verapamil	40, 80, 120; sustained release: 120, 180, 240	120–480	Constipation, nausea, fluid retention, lightheadedness, hypotension
Valproate	125, 250, 500	500–2000	Nausea, tremor, alopecia, appetite stimulation
Phenelzine	15	30–90	Sedation, orthostatic hypotension, constipation, urinary retention
Topiramate	25,100	75–200	

development of cutaneous allodynia, a marker of an advanced attack. Allodynic individuals report that brushing their hair is painful and that their glasses, clothes, and jewelry are uncomfortable. Medications used for acute attacks, when taken late, tend to relieve only the pulsatile pain in the trigeminal distribution, not the generalized head pain. Intravenous corticosteroids (eg, dexamethasone), valproic acid, ketorolac, dihydroergotamine, or neuroleptics (eg, prochlorperazine) appear to afford the best relief for patients experiencing prolonged attacks (Table 8–4).

C. Preventive Therapies

There is some evidence that migraine attacks can lead to structural changes in the brain, possibly related to the progressive nature of the disorder in some patients. For this reason, preventive therapy is appropriate when attacks are frequent, although the exact frequency of attacks prompting this therapy is controversial. If attack frequency exceeds two attacks or three times weekly, prophylactic medications are almost always used (Table 8–5). However, frequency of attacks is not the sole determinant of their use. Some migraineurs have few attacks, but these are refractory to symptomatic treatment. In this setting, prevention may not only reduce the attack frequency, but also render attacks more responsive to symptomatic therapies. Those appearing to overuse acute medications require preventive medications as well as education on their appropriate use. Preventive therapies are often only modestly effective; a 50% reduction in headache frequency occurs in roughly 50% of migraineurs.

1. Pharmacotherapy—The comorbidities of migraine often drive the choice of prophylactic medications. These include depression, bipolar disease, panic attacks, anxiety disorder, and epilepsy. Tricyclic antidepressants, notably amitriptyline, nortriptyline, and doxepin, can be useful but are rarely tolerated at doses that have antidepressant properties. Selective serotonin reuptake inhibitors, although occasionally useful in migraine, are as likely to trigger headache attacks as improve them, particularly when initiating therapy. It is important to assess the presence of mania or hypomania in those who appear to have comorbid migraine and depression. Bipolar disease is frequently seen in migraineurs, and the use of antidepressants in these individuals can trigger an acute manic episode.

Some β-blockers, notably propranolol, nadolol, metoprolol, atenolol, timolol, and nebivolol, can reduce migraine frequency, but they can trigger or worsen depression. Calcium channel blockers, in particular verapamil, are occasionally effective, but can trigger attacks.

Some antiepileptic agents are useful in migraine prevention. Valproate and topiramate are approved by the US Food and Drug Administration for migraine prophylaxis. Gabapentin, and zonisamide, and levetiracetam may also be of value for migraine prevention.

The chronic use of NSAIDs can be helpful but is often limited by adverse reactions. Onabotulinum toxin botulinum neurotoxin type A injections of the forehead and neck have been widely used to treat migraine, although studies suggest that the optimal doses, number, and locations of injection sites and frequency of readministration need to be clarified. Recent studies show efficacy only in chronic migraines (15 or more days of headache monthly). It has recently been approved by the US FDA for the treatment of chronic migraine, and is the only agent to receive that approval. Angiotensin-converting enzyme inhibitors and angiotensin receptor blockers may have efficacy in the prevention of migraine attacks, but the studies at this time are small.

2. Alternative and complementary therapies—"Natural" remedies that have received some scientific support include high-dose riboflavin, feverfew, coenzyme Q10, magnesium, and *Petasites hybridus*. Relaxation training, biofeedback, and cognitive-behavioral therapies can be useful in the management of migraine and may confer additional benefits over preventive medications alone. Improvement in migraine with cervical manipulation, hypnosis, occlusal adjustments, transcutaneous nerve stimulation, and acupuncture is less well-documented. Greater and lesser occipital nerve blocks or stimulation may be of value.

3. Supplementary estrogen—The drop in estrogen levels that occurs during the menstrual cycle can trigger migraine, and supplemental estradiol during the late luteal phase, with blunting of that decline, can prevent or delay the attack. These migraines are best understood as estrogen-withdrawal headaches. Because decreases in the levels of estrogen and progesterone during the late luteal phase are not identical, menstruation is not an accurate marker of estrogen withdrawal. This explains why supplemental estrogen treatment to prevent menstrual migraines often fails.

Migraine relief is common with the continuous elevations of estrogens seen in pregnancy, particularly in the second and third trimesters. This improvement is less likely to occur in women with a history of menstrually associated migraine. Breast-feeding decreases the recurrence of migraines in the postpartum period. Migrainous women who take estrogen-containing oral contraceptives often experience a significant migraine attack during the days that "blanks" are used. In those instances, replacing the blanks with active hormones for 2 of 3 months is advised.

Migraine often improves with menopause, but this relief may not occur if estrogen replacement therapy is used. Percutaneous estradiol produces sustained estrogen levels and is often the most satisfactory estrogen replacement for a migrainous woman.

▶ Prognosis

The peak prevalence of migraine occurs around the fourth decade in both men and women. Younger patients often experience a resolution of migraine attacks with advancing age. A subgroup of women begins to experience migraine only after menopause. Those who experience so-called *chronic migraine* may not experience remissions with age.

Ashina S, Jensen R, Bendtsen L. Pain sensitivity in pericranial and extracranial regions. *Cephalalgia* 2003;23:456–462. [PMID: 001280725]

Burstein R, Jakubowski M. Analgesic triptan action in an animal model of intracranial pain: A race against the development of central sensitization. *Ann Neurol* 2004;55:27–36. [PMID: 0014705109] (Reviews a current theory of why early treatment with migraine therapy is more likely to fully terminate an attack and explains the anatomic correlates of head pain as a migraine attack progresses.)

Gillman P. Triptans, serotonin agonists, and serotonin syndrome (serotonin toxicity): A review. *Headache* 2010;50:264–272. [PMID: 19925619]

Headache Classification Committee. The International Classification of Headache Disorders, 2nd edition. *Cephalalgia* 2004;24:1–160. [PMID: 0014979299] (The most recent classification of headache disorders.)

Kruit MC, van Buchem MA, Hofman PA. Migraine as a risk factor for subclinical lesions. *JAMA* 2004;291:427–434. [PMID: 0014747499]

Lipton RB, Pan J. Is migraine a progressive brain disease? *JAMA* 2004;291:493–494. [PMID: 0014747508]

Lipton RB, et al. Sumatriptan for the range of headaches in migraine sufferers: Results of the spectrum study. *Headache* 2000;40:783–791. [PMID: 0011135021] (Documents that the various types of head pain experienced by migraineurs are part of the spectrum of a single disorder, often with a single treatment.)

Mathew N. Antiepileptic drugs in migraine prevention. *Headache* 2001;41(Suppl 8):18–25. [PMID: 0011903536]

Silberstein SD. Migraine. *Lancet* 2004;363:381–391. [PMID: 15447713]

Tobin J, Flitzman S. Occipital nerve blocks: When and what to inject? *Headache* 2009;49:1521–1533. [PMID: 19674126]

TENSION-TYPE HEADACHE

 ESSENTIALS OF DIAGNOSIS

- ▶ At least 10 episodes occurring on less than 1 day per month, on average
- ▶ Headache lasting from 30 minutes to 7 days
- ▶ At least two of the following pain characteristics:
  - Bilateral location
  - Pressing or tightening (nonpulsating) quality
  - Mild to moderate intensity
  - Not aggravated by routine physical activity
- ▶ Absence of nausea of vomiting
- ▶ Photophobia or phonophobia, but not both

▶ General Considerations

Tension-type headaches are the most common form of headache, experienced by 35–78% of adults. They are rarely severe and are generally responsive to over-the-counter medications. For this reason, they do not commonly prompt a medical visit, accounting for fewer than 5% of patient visits for recurring headaches in primary care practice. There is little evidence to support the theory that contracted pericranial muscles cause these headaches, although pericranial tenderness is common. Nor is there any evidence to suggest that tension-type headaches are caused by physical or emotional stress. When tension-type headaches are disabling, they typically occur in conjunction with migraine, respond to migraine therapies, and are best understood as part of the so-called *spectrum of migraines*.

Clinical Findings

Tension-type headaches are generally described as "band-like" head pain without significant accompanying autonomic phenomenology. They may be short- or long-lasting. As in other forms of primary headaches, a chronic form can develop over time, often as a consequence of medication overuse.

Treatment

Chronic tension-type headache is difficult to manage and responds best to a combination of pharmacologic and non-pharmacologic therapies. In patients with chronic headaches, the possibility of underlying depression and sources of secondary headaches should be explored. Medications include tricyclic antidepressants. Some headaches may respond to centrally active muscle relaxants or selective serotonin reuptake inhibitors. Botulinum neurotoxin type A injections to the face and neck may be effective in the treatment of tension-type headache. Physiotherapy, biofeedback, and acupuncture appear to be useful in some chronic tension-type headache sufferers.

Ashina M. Neurobiology of chronic tension-type headache. *Cephalalgia* 2004;24:161–172. [PMID: 0015009009]

Bussone G. Chronic migraine and chronic tension-type headache: Different aspects of the chronic daily headache spectrum. Clinical and pathogenetic considerations. *Neurol Sci* 2002;24:S90–S93. [PMID: 0012811601]

Jensen R. Diagnosis, epidemiology, and impact of tension-type headache. *Curr Pain Headache Rep* 2003;7:455–459. [PMID: 0014604504]

Kaniecki R. Migraine and tension-type headache. An assessment of challenges in diagnosis. *Neurology* 2002;58(Suppl 6):S15–S20. [PMID: 0012011269]

Torelli P, Jensen R, Olesen J. Physiotherapy for tension-type headache: A controlled study. *Cephalalgia* 2004;24:29–36. [PMID: 0014687010]

TRIGEMINAL AUTONOMIC CEPHALGIAS

1. Cluster Headache

ESSENTIALS OF DIAGNOSIS

▶ Multiple attacks of severe unilateral orbital, supraorbital, or temporal pain lasting 15–180 minutes if untreated

▶ During headache at least one of the following:
- Unilateral conjunctival injection, lacrimation, or both
- Ipsilateral nasal congestion, rhinorrhea, or both
- Ipsilateral eyelid edema
- Ipsilateral forehead and facial sweating
- Ipsilateral miosis, ptosis, or both
- A sense of restlessness or agitation

▶ Attack frequency ranging from one every other day to eight per day

General Considerations

Cluster headache is the most painful cause of primary headaches. Its hallmark is its striking circadian periodicity. It occurs predominantly in men, with a 4:1 male-to-female ratio. The prevalence is approximately 15 cases per 100,000 people.

Pathogenesis

Activation of the posterior hypothalamus has been demonstrated on positron emission tomographic (PET) scans in spontaneous attacks. This is in contrast to the activation of mesencephalic structures in migraine and hemicrania continua. This finding is not surprising, considering the striking rhythmicity of cluster attacks and the role of the hypothalamus in mediating circadian rhythms.

Clinical Findings

Attacks tend to cluster over time, including daily headaches for weeks to months, followed by long periods of remission. During the active cluster period, sufferers tend to have one to four attacks daily, lasting 20 minutes to 3 hours. Onset of attacks is more rapid than with migraine, reaching full intensity over minutes, but not seconds. The pain is invariably unilateral and often affects the same side with recurrent attacks. Drinking alcohol during this period nearly always triggers an attack. Unlike migraineurs, who seek dark, quiet environments and prefer to keep still during attacks, patients who experience cluster headaches often pace relentlessly, seeking cold and other distractions. Attacks are commonly nocturnal, rendering sufferers sleep deprived. The quality of the pain is described as "boring" and "knifelike." Cluster attacks are associated with ipsilateral lacrimation and rhinorrhea. The rhinorrhea is clear and profuse, but not infected. Nausea and vomiting are uncommon. A partial Horner syndrome (without anhidrosis) is common and may persist after recurrent attacks.

▶ Treatment

Treatment involves both symptomatic and prophylactic medications. Nonmedicinal therapies are of no value in this condition.

Symptomatic management of acute attacks includes administration of inhaled oxygen (8–12 L/min until the attacks resolve). Injectable sumatriptan, 2–6 mg, is highly effective, but its use is limited to a maximum of 12 mg daily. Because these attacks are more rapid in onset but shorter in duration than migraines, no other form of sumatriptan or other triptan tends to be effective.

Preventive management generally involves polytherapy. Corticosteroids are effective in high doses and generally work rapidly but are inappropriate for long-term treatment in a cluster period. They are most appropriately used as a bridge therapy while the other preventive agents become effective. Verapamil is often effective, largely at high doses of 480–720 mg/day. Use of divalproex, lithium carbonate, or topiramate in conjunction with verapamil can provide additional benefit. β-Blockers are ineffective and may even be unsafe, as some cluster attacks are associated with significant bradycardia resulting from the dramatic parasympathetic involvement seen during an attack. Should the attacks respond to pharmacotherapy, preventive therapy should continue for the predicted period of a cluster and then be slowly withdrawn. During a cluster period, patients are aware of *forme frustes,* which are abortive forms of attacks. Although these symptoms remain, preventive drugs should be continued. In highly refractory cases of cluster, hypothalamic stimulation, occipital nerve stimulation, and sphenopalatine ganglion stimulation have had some success.

There is significant use of cigarettes and alcohol in the population affected by cluster headaches. Some cluster headache patients appear to improve after smoking cessation. Cigarette use increases the risk of cardiovascular disease, and care should be taken to exclude significant coronary artery disease in patients before administering sumatriptan or any medication that causes vasoconstriction. Because alcohol reliably triggers attacks during the cluster period, its use should be curtailed.

▶ Prognosis

Improvement with age is far less certain in patients with cluster headaches than in migraineurs. Some patients undergo complete remissions after suffering recurring attacks for years.

Bahra A, May A, Goadsby P. Cluster headache: A prospective clinical study with diagnostic implications. *Neurology* 2002;58: 354–361. [PMID: 0011839832]

May A, Leone M. Update on cluster headache. *Curr Opin Neurol* 2003;16:333–340. [PMID: 0012858070]

2. Chronic Paroxysmal Hemicrania

ESSENTIALS OF DIAGNOSIS

▶ At least 20 attacks

▶ Attacks of severe unilateral orbital, supraorbital, or temporal pain lasting 2–30 minutes

▶ During headache at least one of the following:
- Ipsilateral conjunctival injection, lacrimation, or both
- Ipsilateral nasal congestion, rhinorrhea, or both
- Ipsilateral eyelid edema
- Ipsilateral forehead and facial sweating
- Ipsilateral miosis, ptosis, or both

▶ Attack frequency of about five per day for more than half of the time, although periods with lower frequency can occur

▶ Prevented by therapeutic doses of indomethacin

Attacks of chronic paroxysmal hemicrania (CPH) are similar to and often confused with cluster headache attacks, but there are some significant differences. Most patients with CPH are female. Attacks are short-lived, but frequent, and respond dramatically to indomethacin, usually 75–150 mg daily, administered in divided doses. Patients may experience a first attack at any age. Positive family histories are not seen. Attacks may undergo spontaneous remission or may persist lifelong.

Trucco M, et al. Chronic paroxysmal hemicrania, hemicrania continua and SUNCT syndrome in association with other pathologies: A review. *Cephalalgia* 2004;24:173–184. [PMID: 0015009010] (A current review of the trigeminal autonomic cephalgias.)

3. Hemicrania Continua

ESSENTIALS OF DIAGNOSIS

▶ Headache lasting more than 3 months

▶ All of the following pain characteristics:
- Unilateral pain without side shift
- Daily and continuous headache, without pain-free periods
- Moderate intensity, but with exacerbations of severe pain

- ▶ At least one of the following autonomic features occurring during exacerbations and ipsilateral to the side of pain:
  - • Conjunctival injection, lacrimation, or both
  - • Nasal congestion, rhinorrhea, or both
  - • Ptosis, miosis, or both
- ▶ Prevented by therapeutic doses of indomethacin

Hemicrania continua is another indomethacin-responsive headache syndrome with a female preponderance. Patients describe a continuous head pain that fluctuates in intensity, with more severe paroxysms superimposed. Needle-like pains in the eye and temple are often present. PET scans show activation of the mesencephalon, demonstrating a fundamental anatomic difference from cluster and migraine headaches. Indomethacin is usually administered at doses of 75–150 mg/day. The disorder is typically unremitting; therefore, indomethacin treatment may be life-long, although doses can often be reduced over time.

May A. Headaches with (ipsilateral) autonomic symptoms. *J Neurol* 2002;11:1273–1278. [PMID: 0014648142]

Pareja J, et al. Dose, efficacy and tolerability of long-term indomethacin treatment of chronic paroxysmal hemicrania and hemicrania continua. *Cephalalgia* 2001;21:906–910. [PMID: 0011903285]

4. SUNCT Syndrome

 ESSENTIALS OF DIAGNOSIS

- ▶ At least 20 attacks
- ▶ Attacks of unilateral orbital, supraorbital, or temporal stabbing or pulsating pain lasting 5 seconds to 4 minutes
- ▶ Accompanied by ipsilateral conjunctival injection and lacrimation
- ▶ Attack frequency ranging from 3–200 per day

SUNCT (short-lasting unilateral neuralgiform attacks with conjunctival injection and tearing) is a rare syndrome. Sufferers, usually men, have multiple daily attacks lasting only seconds or a few minutes. Turning of the head or touching the face on the symptomatic side often triggers attacks. Pain is generally located in the eye, temple, and cheek, with prominent ipsilateral lacrimation, conjunctival injection, and lacrimation. Nausea and vomiting are not part of the syndrome. Most patients report being pain-free between attacks, although some report a dull discomfort. Tumors of the pituitary and posterior fossa may mimic SUNCT syndrome, and patients with this constellation of symptoms should undergo MRI scanning.

Therapy usually is only moderately effective at relieving patients' symptoms; however, successful treatment with lamotrigine, gabapentin, and topiramate has been reported.

Maharu MS, et al. Short-lasting unilateral neuralgiform headache with conjunctival injection and tearing syndrome: A review. *Curr Pain Headache Rep* 2003;7:308–318. [PMID: 0012828881]

▼ SECONDARY HEADACHES

Secondary headaches are caused by an acquired structural, metabolic, or infectious disorder. They are more common in people with a primary headache syndrome, who have a lowered threshold for the development of head pain, often on a hereditary basis. In primary care practice, 94% of periodic recurring headaches are migraine or migrainous; however, secondary headaches must always be considered.

MENINGITIS

The head pain experienced by patients with meningitis tends to be generalized, pulsatile in quality, and associated with photophobia and nausea. There is often posterior radiation. In these ways, it is similar to migraine, but meningitis produces a nonrecurring pain that tends to escalate rapidly. Nuchal rigidity becomes prominent as the headache progresses and, because migraine can also be associated with neck pain, early in the course it may be difficult to distinguish the two headache types. However, the nuchal rigidity of meningitis is most prominent with flexion. In addition, fever is not a feature of migraine and, if present in this setting, lumbar puncture becomes mandatory. Migraine is associated with neurogenic dural inflammation that can cause a modest pleocytosis; therefore, even this test might not always be diagnostic of meningitis.

▶ SINUS HEADACHE

So-called *sinus headache* is frequently diagnosed but usually with little supporting evidence. Most patients with episodic head pain and "sinus" symptoms are actually experiencing migraines. Many migraineurs experience a worsening of their pain when they lean forward and have facial discomfort, rhinorrhea, nasal stuffiness, and lacrimation. Acute sinusitis can cause pain in the head, face, or teeth, but objective evidence of acute sinusitis with purulent nasal discharge or abnormal imaging studies is necessary to make this diagnosis. Chronic sinus disease rarely causes headache and does not imitate paroxysmal headache syndromes such as migraine. An isolated sphenoid sinusitis can imitate a chronic tension-type headache with unremitting vertex pain. Some individuals with chronic headache who have identifiable septal contact points which, when topical anesthesia to these regions relieves the pain, may benefit from local resection.

Blumenthal H. Headaches and sinus disease. *Headache* 2001;41:883–888. [PMID: 0011703475] (A comprehensive review of the relationship between headache and sinusitis.)

Mohebbi A, Memari F, Mobehhi S. Endonasal endoscopic management of contact point headache and diagnostic criteria. *Headache* 2010;50:242–248. [PMID: 19804393]

OCULAR CAUSES OF HEADACHE

Ocular causes of eye pain, including acute glaucoma, are associated with a "red eye," characterized by conjunctival and scleral injection, corneal clouding, and visual disturbance. Refractive errors of the eye rarely cause headache. When they do, the headache is clearly related in time to the use of new glasses and is absent upon awakening.

HYPERTENSION

Hypertension rarely contributes to headaches. There is no correlation between the degree of hypertension and the burden of headache except in patients with extreme blood pressure elevations.

Spierings E. Acute and chronic hypertensive headache and hypertensive encephalopathy. *Cephalalgia* 2002;22:313–316. [PMID: 0012100095]

SUBARACHNOID HEMORRHAGE

The hallmark of headache resulting from subarachnoid hemorrhage is the apoplectic onset of intense head pain, referred to as a "thunderclap" headache. The headache of an aneurysmal rupture is most commonly unilateral and accompanied by nausea, vomiting, photophobia, nuchal rigidity, and varying degrees of encephalopathy. Because low-volume subarachnoid hemorrhages precede catastrophic bleeding in 50% of patients, it is essential to consider the diagnosis of subarachnoid hemorrhage even if the headache resolves spontaneously or with medication.

Patient characterization of the headache as "the worst headache of my life" generally signifies the worst *migraine*, because migraine is a far more prevalent condition than subarachnoid hemorrhage. It is the rate of onset of pain, rather than the absolute pain intensity, that usually distinguishes the two. The response to a medication, particularly a triptan, is in no way diagnostic of migraine. Patients with apoplectic headaches who respond to treatment still require a complete evaluation. Subarachnoid hemorrhage is discussed in detail in Chapter 11.

Landtblom AM, et al. Sudden onset headache: A prospective study of features, incidence and causes. *Cephalalgia* 2002;22:354–360. [PMID: 0012110111]

BRAIN TUMOR

Headache is seen at the time of presentation in 50% of patients with intracranial neoplasms and even more frequently in those with intraventricular tumors or tumors of the posterior fossa. The widely held view that headaches associated with brain tumors awaken an individual out of sleep and improve as the day progresses is inaccurate in most cases. Migraine and cluster headaches are far more likely than a cerebral neoplasm to cause headaches that awaken the sufferer from sleep.

Headache in association with brain tumors is seen more commonly in patients with a preexisting primary headache syndrome, and in these patients tends to develop as a worsening in the pattern of the preexisting headache type. Invariably brain tumor–associated headaches are progressive over time. The location of the headache does not usually localize the tumor because, as noted in the introduction to this chapter, most pain-sensitive structures within the head are innervated by the first division of the trigeminal nerve and therefore refer pain to the eye or temple. The degree of headache correlates best with the degree of cerebral edema rather than the size of the mass. Other mass lesions causing increased intracranial pressure (eg, brain abscess, subdural hematoma) will cause headache of the same type. Brain tumors are discussed in detail in Chapter 12.

IDIOPATHIC INTRACRANIAL HYPERTENSION

In this condition, also known as *pseudotumor cerebri*, the pain is intermittent, generalized, throbbing, and associated with nausea. The often-cited "typical" patient profile of an obese woman with menstrual abnormalities is overstated. The neurologic examination of patients with idiopathic intracranial hypertension is nonfocal and generally reveals papilledema. Cranial bruits or noises in the head are commonly noted. Because root sleeves may be dilated, radicular pains are common. Disorders associated with intracranial hypertension and its management are discussed in Chapter 25.

Binder BD, Horton JC, Lawton MT. Idiopathic intracranial hypertension. *Neurosurgery* 2004;54:538–551. [PMID: 0015028127]

Friedman DI, Rausch EA. Headache diagnoses in patients with treated idiopathic intracranial hypertension. *Neurology* 2002;58:1551–1553. [PMID: 0012034799]

Loh Y, Labutta RJ, Urban ES. Idiopathic intracranial hypertension and postlumbar puncture headache. *Headache* 2004;44:170–173. [PMID: 0014756857] (Reviews headaches of the opposite end of the spectrum: low and high intracranial pressure.)

INTRACRANIAL HYPOTENSION

The most common cause of low-pressure headache is a lumbar puncture that creates a tear in the dura, leading to reduction in cerebrospinal fluid volume. Dural tears can also develop with vigorous exercise, surgery of the spine, erosive skull or sinus lesions, and head trauma. Other causes of intracranial hypotension are severe dehydration and uremia. Pain is generalized and diffuse and either dull or throbbing in quality. It is typically triggered by standing and rapidly resolves with bed rest. After a short time, the postural nature may subside, and the headache becomes more reminiscent of meningitis, with nuchal rigidity, photophobia, nausea, vomiting, and tinnitus. The management of intracranial hypotension is discussed in Chapter 25. POTS (postural orthostatic tachycardia syndrome) can be associated with headaches and symptoms of cerebral hypoperfusion, and if suspected, a tilt table test should be performed.

GIANT CELL ARTERITIS

Giant cell arteritis rarely occurs in patients younger than 55 years of age. Symptoms include generalized allodynic pain and tenderness of the scalp. Headache is never the sole symptom of giant cell arteritis, and patients often have polymyalgia rheumatica, fatigue, dysphoria, a low-grade fever, and weight loss. This condition is systemic, sometimes affecting medium-sized arteries throughout the body, with an attendant risk for myocardial infarctions, limb gangrene, and visceral infarctions. Obstructions of the mandibular and temporal arteries can lead to jaw claudication, and narrowing of the lingual artery can lead to tongue claudication or tongue necrosis. The response to corticosteroids tends to be immediate and dramatic. Management of giant cell arteritis is discussed in Chapter 32.

Nordborg E, Nordborg C. Giant cell arteritis: Strategies in diagnosis and treatment. *Curr Opin Rheumatol* 2004;16:25–30. [PMID: 0014673385] (Reviews the current diagnostic criteria and management of giant cell arteritis.)

EXERTIONAL HEADACHE

Headaches that occur with exertion, other than as a symptom of angina, can be apoplectic in onset, and any headache of abrupt onset always raises the possibility of subarachnoid hemorrhage. Exercises performed against a closed glottis (eg, those occurring with a Valsalva maneuver) are most likely to trigger such a headache. Exertional headaches often occur with weight lifting, coughing, or sneezing, or are associated with orgasm. Such attacks are often self-limited and nonrecurrent, after lasting several days. Although most cases are benign, lesions of the posterior fossa (eg, neoplasm and decompensated Chiari malformations) must be considered in patients with exertional head pain.

SEXUALLY INDUCED HEADACHE

The most common headache to occur with orgasm is pain with an explosive onset, likely related to the other causes of benign exertional headaches. Aside from the apoplectic headache associated with orgasm, a low-pressure headache can also occur. Like all forms of low-pressure headache, there is postural pain initially, followed by symptoms suggestive of meningitis, with nuchal rigidity, generalized headache, and photophobia. A generalized pressure-like headache of gradual onset and resolution can also occur with sexual activity.

Frese A, et al. Headache associated with sexual activity: Demography, clinical features, and comorbidity. *Neurology* 2003;61:796–800. [PMID: 0014504323]

CARDIAC HEADACHE

Periodic head pain can be a symptom of angina. The forehead and jaw are the most common locations, but angina can refer pain to any location above the umbilicus. Headache, when a symptom of angina, tends to occur more frequently with vigorous exercise and to resolve with rest. Such headaches often respond to nitroglycerin.

Martinez HR, et al. Cardiac headache: Hemicranial cephalalgia as the sole manifestation of coronary ischemia. *Headache* 2002;42:1029–1032. [PMID: 0012453035]

CAROTID OR VERTEBRAL ARTERY DISSECTION & CAROTIDYNIA

Carotid artery dissection can follow major or minor trauma to the neck. **Vertebral dissection** can follow hyperextension of the neck or cervical manipulation but has occurred even after nose blowing. Some cases follow infection, usually of the upper respiratory tract. With dissection, increasing neck pain occurs, often associated with a hemicranial headache of abrupt onset. After a delay of hours to days, this pain may be complicated by ischemic symptoms of the ipsilateral cerebral hemisphere, the brainstem, or the cerebellum. Horner syndrome is often seen on the side of the carotid dissection. The management of carotid and vertebral dissections is discussed in Chapter 14.

Carotidynia is an inflammatory, although idiopathic, condition of the carotid artery. An increase in the erythrocyte sedimentation rate is common. Local carotid tenderness occurs, and the pain is often provoked by swallowing, coughing, sneezing, or yawning. The associated head pain can be throbbing, dull, or continuous. Treatment with corticosteroids generally leads to dramatic improvement. Recurring bouts of carotidynia are sometimes referred to as "facial migraine." Attacks are similar to those of migraine, including chronic migraine, but with superimposed paroxysms of throbbing and sharp pain, and are associated with significant tenderness of the carotid artery.

Buetow MP, Delano MC. Carotidynia. *AJR Am J Roentgenol* 2001;177:947. [PMID: 0011566713]

Evans RW, Mokri B. Headache in cervical artery dissections. *Headache* 2002;42:1061–1063. [PMID: 0012453042]

COLD STIMULUS HEADACHE

This type of headache has most commonly been associated with the ingestion of ice cream but can be triggered by any cooling of the mouth, for example, during outdoor activities in the cold. The pain is typically experienced in the temples or forehead but can also be referred to the ears or throat. As with other forms of secondary headache, this pain is most commonly experienced in migraineurs and often referred to the same location as their migraines.

Jankelowitz SK, Zagami AS. Cold-stimulus headache. *Cephalalgia* 2001;21:1002. [PMID: 0011843876]

Mattson P. Headache caused by drinking cold water is common and related to active migraine. *Cephalalgia* 2001;21:230–235. [PMID: 0011442559]

MEDICATION OVERUSE HEADACHE

Any medication that can provide acute relief of headache is capable, if overused, of transforming episodic pain into a chronic headache. The most common culprits are opioids and agents containing butalbital or caffeine, but the overuse of ergotamines, triptans, and other agents can also result in chronic daily headaches. In such cases, sufferers note that the episodic headache is superimposed on a more pervasive, generalized pain. Medications used for symptomatic relief become ineffective or their effect is short-lived. Prophylactic agents tend not to be helpful in this setting. The type of medication that is overused can provide some hints regarding possible underlying psychopathology that might be unmasked during the withdrawal process. For example, individuals who are depressed or who have an underlying sleep disorder often use excessive caffeine. Butalbital-containing drugs are often used to self-treat anxiety disorders. Dysphoric individuals might overuse opioids.

Although medication overuse is not the only cause of chronic headaches, it accounts for the majority of cases. Thus, when questioned, patients with secondary headaches who were previously taking a drug as needed may state that their requirement for the drug increased and that they are responding to the increased need.

Significant improvement in headache after withdrawal of the offending agent is common but not necessary for diagnosis of medication overuse headache. In triptan-induced medication overuse headache, the pain can be unilateral, pulsatile, and severe. With other agents, it is more commonly generalized, nonpulsatile, and mild or moderate in severity. The patient is generally weaned off the overused medication and preventive antimigraine agents begun, but the process of reduction is dependent on the offending agent, the quantities used, and comorbid conditions. Improvement in headache usually occurs after 22 months, but the time varies with the offending drug and amounts used.

Lipton R, Bigal M. Chronic daily headache. Is analgesic overuse a cause or consequence? *Neurology* 2003;61:154–155. [PMID: 0012874389]

Pini LA, Cicero A, Sandrini M. Long-term follow-up of patients treated for chronic headache with analgesic overuse. *Cephalalgia* 2001;21:878–883. [PMID: 0011903281]

Zwart J, et al. Analgesic overuse among subjects with headache, neck, and low-back pain. *Neurology* 2004;62:1540–1544. [PMID: 0015136678]

NEW DAILY PERSISTENT HEADACHE

 ESSENTIALS OF DIAGNOSIS

▶ Headache lasting more than 3 months
▶ Daily and unremitting headache pain from onset
▶ At least two of the following pain characteristics:
  · Bilateral location
  · Pressing or tightening quality
  · Mild to moderate intensity
  · Not aggravated by routine physical activity
▶ If present, only mild photophobia, phonophobia, or nausea

This form of chronic daily headache begins de novo and continues without remission. The cause is unknown and likely to be heterogenous. Headaches may follow a flulike illness. Patients typically recall the exact moment when the headache began. Because such headaches can have features of migraine or tension-type headache, a previous history of these syndromes needs to be evaluated and secondary causes of chronic headache excluded. These causes include medication overuse, low-pressure headache, trauma, and infection.

Goadsby PJ, Boes C. New daily persistent headache. *J Neurol Neurosurg Psychiatry* 2002;72(Suppl 2):ii6–ii9. [PMID: 0012122194]

Li D, Rozen T. The clinical characteristics of new daily persistent headache. *Cephalalgia* 2002;22:66–69. [PMID: 0011993616]

HEADACHES ASSOCIATED WITH SLEEP

1. Hypnic Headache

Hypnic headaches primarily affect the elderly, with the first event occurring after the age of 50. Individuals awaken from sleep nearly nightly with a generalized, often throbbing headache that persists upon awakening. No significant autonomic symptoms accompany the pain, but nausea is common. Giant-cell arteritis and other forms of secondary headache, in particular those causing increased intracranial pressure, need to be excluded. Treatment with lithium carbonate or caffeine at bedtime is generally satisfactory.

Dodick DW, et al. Clinical, anatomical, and physiologic relationship between sleep and headache. *Headache* 2003;43:282–292. [PMID: 0012603650] (Reviews the relationship between sleep and various headache syndromes, including hypnic headaches, cluster headaches, and migraine.)

Evers S, Goadsby PJ. Hypnic headache: Clinical features, pathophysiology, and treatment. *Neurology* 2003;60:905–909. [PMID: 0012654950]

2. Headache Associated With Sleep Apnea

Sleep apnea can be associated with morning headaches, possibly triggered by carbon dioxide accumulation, hypoxia, or sleep deprivation. Pain is generally bilateral, nonpulsatile, and not associated with autonomic symptoms. Other sleep disorders, such as periodic leg movements of sleep, can also trigger headaches upon awaking due to disturbance of sleep. Patients who awaken frequently with headaches should undergo polysomnography.

Neau JP, et al. Relationship between sleep apnoea syndrome, snoring and headaches. *Cephalalgia* 2002;22:333–339. [PMID: 0012110108]

Sand T, Hagen K, Schrader H. Sleep apnea and chronic headaches. *Cephalalgia* 2002;23:90–95. [PMID: 0012603364]

3. Turtling

People who sleep under blankets with their faces covered might accumulate carbon dioxide and awaken with headache. Most headache sufferers instinctively prefer sleeping in cool, well-aerated environments.

4. Exploding Head Syndrome

This is actually not a headache syndrome, but a parasomnia. Sufferers are awakened out of sleep by a nonpainful sound in the head that simulates a severe explosion. It can be associated with other forms of sensory sleep starts. Treatment with clomipramine is generally satisfactory.

Green M. The exploding head syndrome. *Curr Pain Headache Rep* 2001;5:279–280. [PMID: 0011309216]

PAIN IN THE FACE, PHARYNX, JOINT, & EAR

TRIGEMINAL NEURALGIA

ESSENTIALS OF DIAGNOSIS

► Paroxysmal attacks of severe facial pain, lasting seconds

► Sudden, sharp, superficial, stabbing, or burning in quality

► Distribution along one of more trigeminal distributions

► Precipitated by touching or moving trigger regions (eg, while eating, speaking, or brushing teeth)

► Absence of symptoms between attacks

▶ General Considerations

Trigeminal neuralgia is the most common cause of neuralgic pain in the face, with an incidence of 3 cases per 100,000 people. Patients are usually older than 40 years of age.

▶ Clinical Findings

A. Symptoms and Signs

The pain is usually unilateral and typically involves the second, third, or both of these trigeminal nerve distributions. Involvement of the first division is exceedingly rare. Movement of the face or light touch on the face typically triggers the pain. Onset of pain is instantaneous, pain is severe but brief, and often paroxysms are multiple. Facial pain between these paroxysms should not occur. Trigger zones are generally, but not invariably, in the same distribution as the pain. Attacks are usually experienced daily for weeks to months. Spontaneous remissions are common.

B. Imaging Studies

All patients with trigeminal neuralgia require MRI scans, with special attention directed to the pons and trigeminal nerve root entry zone.

▶ Differential Diagnosis

Most cases are associated with pathologic processes located at the trigeminal root entry zone, the junction of central and peripheral myelin. Most commonly, an ectatic vascular loop, often of the superior cerebellar artery, compresses and demyelinates the trigeminal nerve. Because ectatic loops occur rarely in young patients, cases involving patients younger than 40 years are unusual. Should a younger person develop trigeminal neuralgia, multiple sclerosis or a neoplasm is a common cause.

▶ Treatment

A. Pharmacotherapy

Pharmacotherapy includes a variety of antiepileptic agents, which attenuate polysynaptic reflexes. Phenytoin, carbamazepine or oxcarbazepine, and divalproex are the most commonly employed. Clonazepam, gabapentin, lamotrigine, and topiramate can also provide relief. Tizanidine or baclofen, although marketed as centrally acting muscle relaxants, can also be effective in trigeminal neuralgia. Because spontaneous remissions are common, medication is reduced or discontinued after significant asymptomatic periods.

B. Neurosurgical Treatment

In cases refractory to medical management, surgical intervention should be considered. One approach involves a selective injury of the appropriate trigeminal root, accomplished with a gamma knife, balloon compression, radiofrequency probe, or glycerol. These procedures always cause some degree of numbness and carry the risk of anesthesia dolorosa. Microvascular decompression of the trigeminal nerve has higher attendant serious risks, but the results are often more satisfactory because there is no numbness and less risk of developing dysesthetic facial pain. In rare cases involving V1 where the development of corneal anesthesia with these blocking procedures would be problematic, microvascular decompression is always favored in those refractory to medical therapy,

Merrison AF, Fuller G. Treatment options for trigeminal neuralgia. *BMJ* 2003;327:1360–1361. [PMID: 0014670852]

Rozen T. Antiepileptic drugs in the management of cluster headache and trigeminal neuralgia. *Neurology* 2001;41:25–33. [PMID: 0011903537] (Reviews the medications that are effective in the management of trigeminal neuralgia.)

GLOSSOPHARYNGEAL NEURALGIA

Glossopharyngeal neuralgia is far less common than trigeminal neuralgia, with a prevalence of 0.5 cases per 100,000 people. Similar to trigeminal neuralgia, it is more prevalent in the elderly; however, it is less likely to have a benign origin. Sharp, repetitive pains are experienced in the throat, tongue, ear, and tonsillar fossa. Swallowing commonly triggers these severe paroxysms of pain. Syncope and even sudden death have been reported. Evaluation of the brain by MRI scan is essential to identify the presence of a vascular loop or neoplasm cross-compressing the glossopharyngeal nerve, evidence of multiple sclerosis, or a malignancy or infection

of the peritonsillar region. Glossopharyngeal neuralgia is more refractory to treatment than trigeminal neuralgia, although the same medications are employed, and surgical procedures include a microvascular decompression of the ninth cranial nerve.

Bruyn GW. Glossopharyngeal neuralgia. *Cephalalgia* 1983;3:143–157. [PMID: 6313200] (A classic description of the syndrome.)

YAWNING HEADACHE

Yawning can trigger head pain in subjects with temporomandibular joint dysfunction and with trigeminal or glossopharyngeal neuralgia. In such secondary cases, pain is referred to the regions of the affected nerve or joint. Primary yawning headache consists of retroauricular, submandibular, or facial pain felt exclusively upon yawning. The pain is sharp and shooting but not triggered by other facial movements or cutaneous stimulation. Yawning headache is a benign and self-limiting condition.

Jacome DE. Primary yawning headache. *Cephalalgia* 2001;21:697–699. [PMID: 0011531903]

EAGLE SYNDROME

The pain of Eagle syndrome is experienced in the pharynx and, similar to glossopharyngeal neuralgia, radiates to the ear. Some individuals complain of a foreign body sensation in the throat. The cause is an elongation of the styloid process or calcification of the stylohyoid ligament. Radiographs of the skull can assist in diagnosing this syndrome, which may be confused with glossopharyngeal neuralgia.

Restrepo S, Palacios E, Rojas R. Eagle's syndromes. *Ear Nose Throat J* 2002;81:700–701. [PMID: 0012405087]

RED EAR SYNDROME

Patients with red ear syndrome, often migraineurs, have recurrent attacks of unilateral pain in the ear, which becomes red and burns. Attacks tend to be triggered by chewing, drinking, sneezing, or exposure to heat or cold. Because they are associated with migraine and are unilateral, it is likely that a mechanism is shared by the two syndromes, perhaps mediated through the convergence of trigeminal and upper cervical neurons in the trigeminal nucleus caudalis, with subsequent activation of the auriculotemporal nerve, a branch of the mandibular nerve. The treatment is uncertain, but attacks can respond to other migraine therapies.

Donnet A, Valade D. The red ear syndrome. *J Neurol Neurosurg Psychiatry* 2004;75:1077. [PMID: 0015201382]

Kumar N, Swanson JW. The 'red ear syndrome' revisited: Two cases and a review of literature. *Cephalalgia* 2004;24:305–308. [PMID: 0015030541]

Raieli V, et al. Red ear syndrome and migraine: Report of eight cases. *Headache* 2002;42:147–151. [PMID: 0012005292]

TEMPOROMANDIBULAR JOINT DISORDER

This is a common disorder but is often overdiagnosed to explain more severe headaches. The syndrome frequently accompanies chronic tension-type headache. Pain may reflect either spasm of the temporalis and masseter muscles or primary pathology of the temporomandibular joint, such as rheumatoid arthritis. In patients with temporomandibular joint disorder, chewing triggers pain, clicking and pain are experienced over the joints during jaw movement, and reduced or uneven movements occur upon opening the jaw. Frequently a self-limited attack follows chewing or overopening of the mouth. Muscle relaxants and NSAIDs can be helpful. If the syndrome becomes chronic, a dental evaluation is indicated. Reports of improvement after injection of botulinum neurotoxin A into the masticatory muscles are promising.

Graf-Radford SB, Newman AC. The role of temporomandibular disorders and cervical dysfunction in tension-type headache. *Curr Pain Headache Rep* 2002;6:387–391. [PMID: 00122007852] (Addresses the interactions and distinctions between tension-type headache and temporomandibular disorder.)

Uyanik JM, Murphy E. Evaluation and management of TMDs, Part 1. History, epidemiology, classification, anatomy, and patient evaluation. *Dent Today* 2003;22:140–150. [PMID: 0015011535]

PRIMARY STABBING HEADACHE

Primary stabbing headaches (also referred to as *jabs-and-jolts syndrome, needle-in-the-eye syndrome,* or *ice-pick headache*) are not actually neuralgias. Patients experience a sharp pain in the eye or temple that frequently changes locations. Idiopathic stabbing headache often occurs in migraineurs, primarily women, and sometimes interictally to their migraine attacks. The pain differs from that of trigeminal neuralgia because it usually involves the first division of the trigeminal nerve (rare in trigeminal neuralgia) and is not triggered by cutaneous stimuli. Primary stabbing headaches also often accompany other primary headache syndromes, such as hemicrania continua, SUNCT syndrome, and cluster headache. Other than reassurance, treatment is usually not warranted. Periodic attacks are frequent and troublesome. In that setting, indomethacin or aspirin may be effective.

Fusco C, Pisani F, Faienza C. Idiopathic stabbing headache: Clinical characteristics of children and adolescents. *Brain Dev* 2002;25:237–240. [PMID: 0012767453]

NUMMULAR HEADACHE

Nummular headache is a focal dysesthetic pain in the head, of mild-moderate severity, either continuous or intermittent. Most cases are idiopathic, although intracranial, meningeal, bony, and scalp lesions need to be excluded. Treatment is difficult, with some reported cases responding to onabotulinum toxin A or gabapentin.

Grosberg B, Solomon S, Lipton R. Nummular headache. *Curr Pain Headache Rep* 2007;11:310–312. [PMID: 17686396]

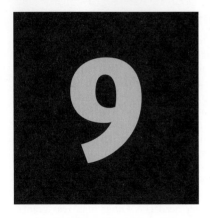

Dementia & Memory Loss

Karen Marder, MD, MPH (editor)

Among the most important dementing disorders are Alzheimer disease (AD), which affects over 5 million people in the United States; vascular-related dementia, the second most common dementia; the spectrum of parkinsonian-related dementias, including dementia associated with Parkinson disease and dementia with Lewy bodies; frontotemporal dementia and related "tauopathies," including corticobasal degeneration and progressive supranuclear palsy (PSP); and normal pressure hydrocephalus (NPH). Two other conditions that merit discussion in this context are mild cognitive impairment, a state that may precede AD, and transient global amnesia.

Dementias have traditionally been divided into cortical and subcortical dementias, with AD being the prototypical cortical dementia and PSP the prototypical subcortical dementia. In reality, features of both cortical and subcortical dementia often coexist, although cortical or subcortical features may be more prominent (Table 9–1).

▼ ALZHEIMER DISEASE

Karen L. Bell, MD, Jennifer L. Williamson, MS, & Sarah C. Janicki, MD, MPH

ESSENTIALS OF DIAGNOSIS

▶ Insidious onset and gradual progression of memory loss

▶ Impairment of one or more other cognitive domains, including aphasia, apraxia, agnosia, or executive functioning

▶ General Considerations

Alzheimer disease (AD) is the most common form of dementia. The prevalence of AD rises from 5% of those older

than 60 years to almost 50% of those older than 85 years. The pathologic hallmarks of AD are neurofibrillary tangles and neuritic (amyloid) plaques. The cause of the disease is unknown but involves abnormal cleavage of a neuronal membrane protein called *amyloid precursor protein* (APP) and abnormal accumulation of a fragment called *β-amyloid*, which is deposited in plaques.

▶ Pathogenesis

A. Genetic Influences

AD is a genetically heterogeneous disorder. Four AD genes have been identified that are clinically available for genetic testing (Table 9–2), and additional chromosomal regions and genes are being investigated. Three of the four genes are causative genes in which mutations result in autosomal-dominant, early-onset AD (EOAD), typically defined as onset before 60 years of age. Mutations in these genes, *PSEN1*, *PSEN2*, and *APP*, account for fewer than 5% of all cases of Alzheimer disease. Not all families with autosomal-dominant EOAD have identifiable mutations in *PSEN1*, *PSEN2*, or *APP*; therefore, there may be additional genes involved in EOAD. Predictive testing for asymptomatic individuals with a known family history of EOAD is most informative when a mutation has been confirmed in a symptomatic family member. Mutations in *PSEN1* and *APP* are associated with complete penetrance, meaning that all individuals who have a mutation will develop AD if they live a normal lifespan. However, mutations in *PSEN2* show 95% penetrance, meaning that not everyone with a *PSEN2* mutation will develop AD. Additionally, mutations in *PSEN2* have been identified in only a few families worldwide. In most patients, the cause of AD is believed to be complex; the result of susceptibility genes interacting with each other as well as with environmental factors. The fourth gene, *APOE*, is a known susceptibility gene for AD and is distinct from the causative genes because it is not sufficient or necessary to cause AD. *APOE* has three isoforms, *E2*, *E3*, and *E4*. The *E4* variant of

Table 9–1. Features of Cortical and Subcortical Dementias

Function Affected	Subcortical Dementia[a]	Cortical Dementia[b]
Cognition		
Attention and concentration	Impaired	Intact
Speed of mental processing	Slow	Normal
Language skills	Relatively intact, including naming	Impaired
Orientation to time and place	Often preserved	Often impaired
Memory (short-term recall)	Impaired retrieval	Impaired storage
Movement		
Speed of movement	Slow	Normal
Gait	Slow	Normal
Sense of equilibrium	Imbalanced	Normal
Posture	Stooped	Normal

[a]Primarily subcortical dementias include progressive supranuclear palsy, Parkinson disease–associated dementia, Huntington disease dementia, and normal pressure hydrocephalus.
[b]Primarily cortical dementias include Alzheimer disease and frontotemporal dementia.

APOE is associated with an increased risk for AD. Risk figures associated with *APOE E4* vary between studies, suggesting a two- to threefold increased risk for E4 heterozygotes and a two to 10-fold increased risk for E4 homozygotes, and are not clinically useful for individual risk assessment. Family history of AD may be just as useful as *APOE* genotype for risk assessment. First-degree relatives of an affected individual in sporadic or familial cases are estimated to have a two- to fourfold increased risk for AD compared with that of the general population.

Genetic testing for diagnostic and predictive purposes is available for early-onset autosomal-dominant AD, and genetic counseling is strongly recommended. For individuals who present with late-onset dementia, *APOE* genotyping may be part of the diagnostic workup, but *APOE* genotyping alone is not warranted because it lacks sufficient sensitivity and specificity to make a diagnosis. Currently, predictive testing for both causative and susceptibility genes for AD is limited, but family members will benefit from genetic counseling which includes information about the genetic influences of AD, a risk assessment via pedigree analysis, and current information about ongoing genetic research studies.

B. Risk Factors

Various environmental, systemic, and behavioral risk factors for AD have been investigated (Table 9–3). An increasing number of reports point toward an association between vascular disease, vascular risk factors, and risk of AD. Postmenopausal estrogen use has been associated with risk reductions of about 50% in several observational studies, but clinical trials of hormone replacement in women already diagnosed with AD have failed to show benefit. The Women's Health Initiative Memory Study showed that the combination of estrogen and progesterone as well as estrogen alone increased risk of dementia nearly twofold among women aged 65 years and older, potentially through a vascular mechanism.

▶ Clinical Findings

A. Symptoms and Signs

AD is characterized by a gradual, progressive decline in intellectual function, coupled with impairment of memory, judgment and problem solving, language, and perception. The symptoms can be divided into cognitive and noncognitive.

The typical cognitive symptoms include:

- Memory: misplacing things, missing appointments
- Impaired judgment: hiding money or possessions
- Impaired abstract reasoning
- Impaired language: word-finding difficulty or anomia
- Poor orientation to time of place
- Difficulty performing familiar tasks
- Decreased attention

Table 9–2. Genes Associated With Alzheimer Disease Available for Clinical Testing

Gene	AD Type	Associated Risk
Presenilin 1 (*PSEN1*)	Early-onset autosomal dominant	100% if mutation present
Presenilin 2 (*PSEN2*)	Early-onset autosomal dominant	95% if mutation present
Amyloid precursor protein (*APP*)	Early-onset autosomal dominant	100% if mutation present
Apolipoprotein E {e}4 (*APOE* {e}4)	Late-onset familial and sporadic	Risk increased by factor of ~3 for each copy of {e}4

AD = Alzheimer disease.

Table 9–3. Potential Risk Modifiers in Alzheimer Disease

Adverse Factor	Beneficial Factor
Stroke	Moderate alcohol consumption
Hypertension	Education
Diabetes mellitus	Intellectual leisure activity
Smoking	Physical exercise
Hyperlipidemia	Consumption of fish and
Systemic vascular disease	polyunsaturated fat
Postmenopausal estrogen ± progesterone	
Elevated caloric and fat intake	
Head injury	
Elevated homocysteine level	
Low vitamin B_{12} level	

The noncognitive manifestations include:

- Changes in personality and mood, such as apathy, withdrawal, and depression
- Changes in behavior, such as suspiciousness, paranoia, delusions, anger, aggression, restlessness, agitation, wandering, sundowning, sleep disturbance, hallucinations, and illusions

B. Stages

Standardized instruments are available for the staging of AD, such as the Clinical Dementia Rating scale (CDR) and the Global Deterioration Scale (GDS). Staging is useful for following progression of disease and also has some value for family counseling and patient management. The CDR divides AD into broad categories of mild, moderate, and severe based on review of performance in six categories (memory, orientation, judgment and problem solving, community affairs, home and hobbies, and personal care).

Mild AD is characterized by impairment of work or social activities but patients maintain the capacity for independent living, with adequate judgment and adequate personal hygiene. Patients may exhibit forgetfulness, word-finding problems, and difficulty with complex tasks, such as following directions, managing their finances, taking medications according to a schedule, planning meals and following recipes, shopping, driving, maintaining hobbies, and problem solving. Behavioral changes seen in mild AD include apathy, withdrawal, and depression.

Moderate AD is distinguished by the need for some supervision, with impaired recent memory, orientation, and insight. Patients require help with instrumental activities of daily living (ADLs) and may need help with the sequence and selection of clothing/dressing. The behavioral manifestations at the moderate stage include wandering, getting lost, agitation, and delusions. Sleep disturbance may become apparent.

Severe AD is characterized by significant impairment of ADLs, resulting in the need for constant supervision and personal care. Patients have very limited language and are unable to manage their basic ADLs, such as eating, dressing, bathing, and continence, and require assistance with walking. In the final stages of AD, patients can be bedridden with flexion deformities, mute, and unable to swallow. Weight loss is common.

C. Diagnostic Criteria

In 1984, the National Institute of Communicative Disorders and Stroke and the Alzheimer's Disease and Related Disorders Association (NINCDS-ADRDA) extended criteria to enable clinicians to have a range of certainty in the diagnosis of AD: probable, possible, and definite. By using these criteria, the clinician can achieve 85% accuracy in the diagnosis of AD.

1. Probable AD—Patients can be between the ages of 40 and 90 years and have intellectual decline that can be documented by neuropsychological tests. Memory and at least one of the following higher brain functions must be defective: judgment, language, perception, or cognition. Systemic diseases or other brain disorders that might cause dementia or altered consciousness must be absent. The diagnosis is supported by lack of ability to be independent in ADLs and associated symptoms such as depression, insomnia, incontinence, delusions, hallucinations, illusions, and outbursts of irrational verbal, emotional, or physical behavior in patients whose laboratory studies are generally normal. Conditions that can cause cognitive impairment and mimic AD, such as Parkinson disease, depression, multi-infarct or vascular dementia, and drug intoxication, are excluded. Thyroid disease, pernicious anemia, syphilitic brain disease or other chronic infections of the nervous system, occult hydrocephalus, Creutzfeldt-Jakob disease (CJD), subdural hematomas, and brain tumors are also excluded.

2. Possible AD—This category is used when a second condition that might contribute to the dementia is present but is not considered to be the causal factor. The clinical diagnosis of possible AD may also be used if the presentation or course is atypical.

3. Definite AD—This classification is reserved for patients who meet the clinical criteria and have autopsy or brain biopsy confirmation (neurofibrillary tangles and senile plaques).

D. Dementia Evaluation

The Quality Standards Subcommittee of the American Academy of Neurology (AAN) revised the guidelines on the evaluation of dementia in 2001. The evaluation usually consists of neurologic, neuropsychological, and psychiatric assessments and neuroimaging and blood evaluations. Although all of these tests may not be necessary in patients with clear histories and advanced symptoms, those individuals with subtle complaints may require the full set of tests to discriminate the earliest symptoms of MCI from early AD.

Thyroid disease, neurosyphilis, fungal infections, vitamin deficiencies, and structural brain lesions such as tumors, subdural hematomas, and hydrocephalus are treatable disorders that may be identified in a small percentage (<13%) of patients with cognitive impairment and dementia.

1. Mental status assessment—One structured mental status test is the Mini Mental State Exam (MMSE), which is an 11-item test used to measure memory, language, attention, calculations, fund of knowledge, and orientation. The scores range from 0–30, with lower scores indicating increasing impairment (ie, mild dementia, 20–26; moderate dementia, 10–19; and severe dementia, 0–9). This test may be administered serially to measure disease progression.

2. Laboratory studies—Routine blood tests are performed as screens to eliminate metabolic derangements or other conditions associated with cognitive impairment. The standard workup consists of blood count, electrolytes, blood urea nitrogen/creatinine, liver function tests, thyroid function tests, and serum vitamin B_{12} level. Optional studies include syphilis testing, serum folate, erythrocyte sedimentation rate, and human immunodeficiency virus testing.

3. Lumbar puncture—Lumbar puncture is useful in patients with cancer, suspicion of central nervous system (CNS) infection, reactive serum syphilis serology, rapidly progressive dementia, immunosuppression, suspicion of CNS vasculitis in patients with connective tissue disease, and in patients under age 55. Biochemical markers are abnormal in AD. Cerebrospinal fluid (CSF) tau levels are elevated and CSF β-amyloid levels are reduced in patients with AD. Lumbar puncture has the potential to become a useful screening tool to ascertain the level of these biomarkers for diagnosis of AD and possibly for prediction of disease in mild cognitive impairment (MCI).

4. Neuroimaging studies—Structural neuroimaging is recommended. Brain imaging with computed tomography (CT) demonstrates that individuals with AD have greater general brain atrophy; however, this finding is not specific to people with AD, limiting its diagnostic value. Magnetic resonance imaging (MRI) has greater resolution than CT and generates coronal and sagittal views to better visualize the hippocampus. Additionally, the atrophy rates of the medial temporal lobe and hippocampus as assessed by MRI are correlated with cognitive decline in individuals with AD. Both CT and MRI allow clinicians to rule out other pathology that could be contributing to cognitive complaints, including tumors, stroke, and other focal destructive and mass lesions, but their use in diagnosing neurodegenerative diseases has been more challenging.

Molecular brain imaging, including positron emission tomography (PET) and single-photon emission tomography (SPECT), was developed parallel to structural imaging and has demonstrated technical improvements over time. Although PET provides better functional information with higher resolution and greater sensitivity than SPECT, there are more SPECT scanners than PET imaging devices installed for routine clinical imaging, which provides one advantage of using SPECT imaging agents.

PET enables imaging of biological activity and therefore can identify abnormal biological activity in AD. Regional differences in brain glucose metabolism using PET have been explored in dementia, and 18F 2-fluoro-2-deoxy-D-glucose (FDG-PET) has become the most widely investigated radioligand. Glucose hypometabolism identified in FDG-PET is thought to represent both local decreases in synaptic activity in neurons affected by typical Alzheimer pathologic changes as well as decreased synaptic activity in regions receiving projections from these diseased neurons. Thus abnormalities in regional cerebral metabolism found on FDG-PET are thought to reflect the pattern of neuropathologic development of AD with early prominent AD changes in the medial temporal cortex as well as the temporoparietal association cortices. This typical pattern of AD change has been demonstrated to have a diagnostic sensitivity of 86–94% and specificity of 73–99% relative to neuropathologic diagnosis in people with AD. The capability of FDG-PET to differentiate AD from other types of dementia is more variable, with sensitivity values as high as 93–94% but as low as 44% and specificity values ranging from 63–80%. These studies have demonstrated that FDG-PET is a useful supplement to current surveillance techniques.

The presence of Aβ plaques in the brain of individuals with dementia is being studied as a possible biomarker for AD. PET tracers have been developed for in vivo imaging of Alzeimer disease pathology. Six amyloid PET ligands, including 18F-FDDNP, 11C-PIB, 11C-SB13, 11C-BF-227, 18F-BAY94-9172, and AZD2184, have so far been tested in PET studies in individuals with AD. The most comprehensively studied compounds so far have been 18F-FDDNP, developed in 2002 as the first amyloid ligand studied in patients, and 11C-Pittsburgh compound B (PIB). 11C-PIB was designed to measure the amount of amyloid plaque deposits, whereas 18F-FDDNP has been reported to label not only amyloid, but also other proteins, including neurofibrillary tangles. Individuals with AD show higher PIB retention in the frontal, temporal, parietal, and occipital cortices and the striatum compared with healthy controls. Correlations between PIB imaging and the β-amyloid deposits in the brain seen either at postmortem or in vivo by biopsy demonstrate good agreement on measures of β-amyloid deposition.

Data regarding the specificity of PIB-PET in the clinical diagnosis of AD is somewhat limited but so far has shown relatively low specificity (high false positives for AD) in some subjects. The reason for this is unclear but could be related to several possibilities. First, the detection of presymptomatic individuals could lead to false-positive findings: autopsied brains of cognitively normal elderly demonstrate some type of amyloid deposition in 25–67% of subjects. Therefore, it may not be amyloid deposition itself but the secondary downstream alterations in brain structure and function that cause the cognitive changes seen in clinical AD. Second, PIB amyloid binding is found in other cerebral amyloidoses, including cerebral amyloid angiopathy and Lewy body dementia. Additionally, once detected, PIB imaging may not provide useful information on clinical dementia staging or progression. Serial imaging evaluations of Alzheimer individuals with both PIB and FDG imaging demonstrate that there is no significant change in PIB retention over time compared with baseline, although a decline in cerebral glucose metabolism is observed. The unchanged PIB retention suggests that there are different time courses for the amyloid load compared with changes in functional activity in brain, and it is possible that maximal amyloid load in the brain is reached already in early AD. It seems likely that amyloid imaging will be useful for differentiating dementias associated with β-amyloid from those that are not, but the utility of this approach will depend on the availability of effective β-amyloid–directed treatments.

Acetylcholinesterase, nicotine, and their receptors have also been mapped by PET. Lower acetylcholinesterase activity has been measured in cortical brain regions of patients with MCI who later convert to AD.

Other processes that may play an important role in AD pathology include tau formation, oxidative stress, inflammatory reactions, and microglial activations. Imaging modalities that explore and elucidate these processes may warrant further exploration in the future. It will also be important to study these non-neuronal cell processes after amyloid immunization therapies.

5. Neuropsychological testing—Neuropsychological testing is considered optional. Tests that assess orientation, memory (recall and recognition), language skills, praxis (constructional ability), attention, visual perception, and problem-solving skills are performed and can yield information about the pattern of impairment. Neuropsychological testing may be valuable in diagnosing early dementia and can be used to assess progression of disease. It may also useful to distinguish depression from dementia.

▶ Differential Diagnosis

Acute or subacute onset of cognitive and functional impairment with focal symptoms raises the possibility of a dementia other than AD. If deterioration is rapid and accompanied by fluctuating levels of alertness and inattention, then the patient is likely to have delirium (acute confusional state). Delirium must be evaluated and treated before the diagnosis of dementia can be considered. Infections, dehydration, medications, and cerebral hypoperfusion are common causes of delirium in the elderly. If the dementia course is subacute (over weeks to months), then expanding mass lesions, CJD, and hydrocephalus are possible diagnoses. An acute (over

days to weeks) deterioration of function and cognition is more typically secondary to infection, strokes, or toxic/metabolic conditions. Using the standard recommended workup and criteria, thyroid disease, neurosyphilis, fungal infections, vitamin deficiencies, and structural brain lesions such as tumors, subdural hematomas, and hydrocephalus are treatable disorders that may be identified in a small percentage (<13%) of cognitive impairment and dementia cases. The other types of dementia, including dementia with Lewy bodies, vascular dementia, normal pressure hydrocephalus, and frontotemporal dementia, are discussed later in this chapter.

▶ Treatment

Drugs approved by the US Food and Drug Administration (FDA) for the treatment of AD are shown in Table 9–4.

A. Cholinesterase Inhibitors

Cholinesterase inhibitors are used to enhance cholinergic function by blocking the breakdown of acetylcholine. Four cholinesterase inhibitors have been approved by the FDA for the treatment of mild-to-moderate AD; three of these agents (donepezil, rivastigmine, and galantamine) are commonly used to treat AD. **Donepezil** is a reversible, highly specific inhibitor of acetylcholinesterase with minimal effect on peripheral butyrylcholinesterase. Donepezil is a piperidine-based molecule and has none of the hepatotoxicity associated with the acridine-based cholinesterase inhibitors. Donepezil has linear pharmacokinetics, a slow clearance, and a long half-life and therefore can be administered once a day. Donepezil has been approved by the FDA to treat mild, moderate, and severe AD. In the pivotal double-blind, placebo-controlled trials, donepezil demonstrated a significant benefit over placebo in terms of cognitive measures and clinical global scales. Both 5 mg/day and 10 mg/day were efficacious doses in the pivotal clinical trials. The dose can be raised to 23 mg/day in patients with moderate-to-severe AD who have been on 10 mg/day for at least 3 months. The most frequent side effects are nausea, diarrhea, abdominal discomfort, headache insomnia, fatigue, and nightmares. The medication can be administered at bedtime or in the morning. If sleep disturbance side effects occur, they may be lessened by morning administration.

Rivastigmine is a selective pseudo-irreversible inhibitor of both acetylcholinesterase and butyrylcholinesterase. In a 26-week double-blind, placebo-controlled, multicenter trial, rivastigmine 6–12 mg/day and rivastigmine 1–4 mg/day showed significant benefit over placebo in terms of cognitive measures. The 6–12-mg/day group showed greater benefit than the low-dose group. The most common side effects associated with rivastigmine treatment were nausea, vomiting, dizziness, diarrhea, headache, and weight loss. Rivastigmine treatment with a slower titration and the option of temporary decrease in dose if side effects occur yields a smaller percentage of side effects. Oral rivastigmine

Table 9–4. Medications Commonly Used in the Treatment of Alzheimer Disease

Drug	Class	AD Stage Indication		Dosing	Range	Target Daily Dose	Side Effects
Donepezil	Cholinesterase inhibitor	Mild to moderate	Oral	QD	Begin 5 mg, increase to 10 mg Q day after 4 weeks if necessary	5–10 mg	N, V, diarrhea, abdominal discomfort, insomnia, dreams
		Moderate to severe	Oral		Increase to 23-mg tablet after 3 months if necessary	5–23 mg	N, V, diarrhea, weight loss
Rivastigmine	Cholinesterase inhibitor	Mild to moderate	Oral	BID with food	Begin 1.5 mg BID, increase by 1.5 mg BID at 4-week intervals	6–12 mg	N, V, dizziness, diarrhea, headache, weight loss, anorexia
			Transdermal patch	QD	Apply 4.6 mg/24 h patch to skin QD, increase to 9.5 mg/24 h patch QD after 4 weeks if necessary		
Galantamine	Cholinesterase inhibitor	Mild to moderate	Oral	BID with food	Begin 4 mg BID, increase by 4 mg BID at 4-week intervals	16–24 mg	N, V, diarrhea, weight loss, anorexia
Galantamine-ER				QD	Begin 8 mg QD, increase to 16 mg after 4 weeks, then to 24 mg QD if necessary	16–24 mg	N, V, diarrhea, weight loss, anorexia
Memantine	NMDA-receptor antagonist	Moderate to severe	Oral	BID	5 mg q AM for 1 week, then increased to 5 mg BID for 1 week, then 10 mg Q AM and 5 mg Q PM for 1 week, with 10 mg BID	20 mg	Dizziness, headache, constipation, confusion Diarrhea
Memantine XR				QD	7 mg QD, increase gradually in increments of 7 mg, more often than once a week, to maximum dose of 28 mg	28 mg	Diarrhea, dizziness, headache

BID = twice a day; ER = extended release; N = nausea; NMDA = *N*-methyl-D-aspartate; Q = every; QD = every day; V = vomiting; XR = extended release.

treatment begins with 1.5 mg twice a day (BID), and titration upward to the therapeutically effective dose (6–12 mg/day administered as two equally divided doses) should occur at intervals of no less than 2–4 weeks. Oral rivastigmine is taken with food to decrease the risk of side effects. Rivastigmine is also available in a transdermal patch formulation. The initial strength is 4.6 mg/24 h for 4 weeks, which is then increased to 9.5 mg/24 h dose. The patch formulation was shown in its pivotal trials to cause fewer gastrointestinal side effects than the oral formulation.

Galantamine is a selective, competitive, acetylcholinesterase inhibitor and also potentiates cholinergic nicotinic neurotransmission by possible modulation of nicotinic receptors. The target dose based on the pivotal clinical studies is 16–24 mg/day.

Oral galantamine treatment begins with 4 mg BID and is increased to 8 mg BID and 12 mg BID as tolerated at 4-week intervals. Absorption is slowed and side effects minimized by administration during a meal. Side effects include nausea, vomiting, anorexia, weight loss, and diarrhea. Galantamine is also available as an extended-release oral formulation designed to reduce potential gastrointestinal side effects. The initial dose of galantamine extended release is 8 mg every day (QD), followed by 16 mg QD and then 24 mg QD.

B. NMDA Receptor Antagonists

The *N*-methyl-D-aspartate (NMDA) receptor is a glutamate receptor that may be relevant in the production of pathologic changes in AD. Glutamate receptor blockade may protect against excitatory amino acid–mediated toxicity, which has been noted to lead to cell death.

Memantine is a noncompetitive, low-to-moderate affinity NMDA-receptor antagonist that may selectively block the excitotoxic effects associated with abnormal transmission of glutamate, while allowing for the physiologic transmission associated with normal cell functioning. Memantine was approved by the FDA for the treatment of moderate-to-severe AD. In double-blind, placebo-controlled trials in patients with moderate-to-severe AD, treatment indicated slowed rate of cognitive and functional decline, and a similarly designed trial demonstrated benefit of memantine/donepezil combination therapy compared with donepezil alone. Oral administration of memantine follows a 4-week titration schedule beginning with 5 mg every morning for 1 week, then increased to 5 mg BID for 1 week, then 10 mg every morning and 5 mg every evening for 1 week, then to 10 mg BID as the maintenance dose. The most frequent side effects of the immediate release formulation are dizziness, headache, constipation, and confusion. Namenda XR 28 mg/day, a once-a-day extended-release formulation of memantine, is also available. The most common side effects of the extended-release formulation were headache, diarrhea, and dizziness.

C. Vitamins/Supplements

The antioxidant α-tocopherol (vitamin E), at a dose of 1000 IU twice daily, was shown in one study to prolong the time needed to reach predetermined end points correlated with severe disease when given to patients with moderate AD in a randomized placebo-controlled study. Vitamin E therapy did not improve cognition. Vitamin E also has failed to show any benefit in a large study of mild cognitive impairment in which half the subjects developed AD. Two studies noted increased mortality and cardiac adverse events associated with high-dose vitamin E use, but no such adverse effects were noted in either of the two vitamin E treatment trials using cognitively impaired (MCI or AD) populations. Thus there is considerable variance of opinion on whether vitamin E should be prescribed for patients with AD, and if so, at what dose.

A combination of homocysteine-lowering agents (vitamin B_6, vitamin B_{12}, and folic acid) failed to demonstrate any beneficial effect on slowing the progression of AD in randomized clinical trial.

Although animal studies have shown docosahexaenoic acid (DHA) supplementation reduces Alzheimer-type pathology in the brain, and epidemiologic studies have suggested that DHA consumption, usually in the form of a fish-rich diet, is negatively associated with AD risk, a double-blind placebo-controlled phase III trial of DHA supplementation in mild-to-moderate AD failed to demonstrate benefit.

D. Anti-Inflammatory Agents

Low-dose prednisone, standard nonsteroidal anti-inflammatory drugs (NSAIDS), and the cyclooxygenase-2 (COX-2) inhibitors have been studied in randomized controlled trials as treatment for AD and to prevent progression of MCI, but these studies have failed to demonstrate positive results.

E. Estrogen

Although cohort studies suggested that hormone-replacement therapy in postmenopausal women reduced the risk of AD, none of the prospective controlled clinical trials using HRT demonstrated any improvement in cognitive function in women with AD. There is no evidence to support the use of estrogen as a treatment for AD.

F. Cholesterol-Lowering Agents

There have been conflicting reports in the literature about the role of statins in AD. Although a single-site double-blind trial of a statin suggested possible benefit on cognition in AD, a phase III randomized trial of simvastatin to slow progression of AD failed to demonstrate any benefit after 18 months of treatment. There is no evidence to support the administration of statins as treatment for AD.

▶ Prognosis

Although the disease duration in AD may range from 3–20 years, the usual duration is 7–10 years, with slow progression. Longitudinal studies from the pretreatment era suggest that patients remain in the early stage for 1–2 years, the middle stage for 2–12 years, and the late stage for 1–2 years, depending on the type of care they receive.

The 30-item MMSE generally declines 2–4 points each year. Longitudinal studies suggest that rigidity and the presence of hallucinations and delusions predict a more rapid cognitive and functional decline. Patients with AD are susceptible to unintentional injuries and infections, and death is most likely to occur from pneumonia, malnutrition, dehydration, and sepsis resulting from pressure ulcers or urinary tract infections.

Cummings JL. Drug therapy: Alzheimer's disease. *N Engl J Med* 2004;351:56–67. [PMID: 15229308] (Excellent discussion of available medication to treat AD.)

Cummings JL, et al. Disease-modifying therapies for Alzheimer's disease. *Neurology* 2007;69:1622–1634. [PMID: 17938373]

Doody RS, et al. Practice parameter: Management of dementia (an evidence-based review): Report of the Quality Standards Subcommittee of the American Academy of Neurology. *Neurology* 2001;56:1154–1166. [PMID: 11342679]

Knopman DS, et al. Practice parameter: Diagnosis of dementia (an evidence-based review): Report of the Quality Standards Subcommittee of the American Academy of Neurology. *Neurology* 2001;56:1143–1153. [PMID: 11342678] (Useful report outlining the basic workup for dementia.)

Mayeux R. Early Alzheimer's disease. *N Engl J Med* 2010;362:2194–2201. [PMID:20558370]

Rocchi A, et al. Causative and susceptibility genes for Alzheimer's disease: A review. *Brain Res Bull* 2003;61:1. [PMID: 12788204]

MILD COGNITIVE IMPAIRMENT

Karen L. Bell, MD

ESSENTIALS OF DIAGNOSIS

- ▶ Subjective memory complaints
- ▶ Objective evidence of memory impairment
- ▶ Normal function in activities of daily living
- ▶ Preserved general cognitive function

▶ General Considerations

Mild cognitive impairment (MCI) is a syndrome, not a disease, but is considered to be a transitional state between normal cognitive function and Alzheimer disease (AD). Researchers have defined MCI in different ways, but one widely used set of criteria focuses on the amnestic subtype, which has been shown in longitudinal studies to exhibit high conversion rate to AD (10–15% per year).

▶ Clinical Findings

A. Symptoms and Signs

The criteria for amnestic MCI are memory complaints, normal ability to perform activities of daily living, no deficits in general cognitive function, and abnormal memory for age and education when compared with normally functioning individuals. If a clinician sees a patient with impaired delayed recall performance or difficulty benefiting from semantic cues during learning or recall in the setting of relatively preserved general cognition, then the diagnosis of MCI should be entertained.

B. Special Tests

1. Neuropsychological testing—Formal cognitive testing can help identify category naming and verbal memory problems, which may predict the future development of dementia. Some studies have shown that deficits in delayed recall were predictive of conversion to AD in non-demented subjects.

2. Lumbar puncture—Potential cerebrospinal fluid (CSF) AD biomarkers, such as CSF β–amyloid protein$^{1-42}$ and phosphorylated tau protein, are being studied to determine whether concentrations can predict conversion of MCI to AD.

3. Neuroimaging studies—Individuals with MCI typically demonstrate no clinically significant findings on computed tomography or magnetic resonance imaging. The utility of 18F 2-fluoro-2-deoxy-D-glucose positron emission tomography (FDG-PET) as a prognostic indicator in individuals with MCI is still unclear. Although there are few existing longitudinal FDG-PET studies in AD and MCI, there is some

evidence that FDG-PET accurately predicts subsequent decline and conversion to AD. However, these studies have relatively small sample sizes and have not established strong evidence for longitudinal associations between existing cognitive measures and FDG-PET. Detection of amyloid deposition with 11C-Pittsburgh compound B (PIB) PET in individuals with mild cognitive impairment may provide useful prognostic information. PIB-positive individuals with MCI are significantly more likely to convert to AD than PIB-negative individuals, with faster converters having higher PIB retention levels at baseline than slower converters.

▶ Treatment

There are no FDA-approved treatments for MCI. The studies of cyclooxygensase-2 inhibitors as prevention of conversion from MCI to AD failed to demonstrate efficacy.

▶ Prognosis

Patients with MCI have a conversion rate of 10–15% per year to AD (compared with a rate of 1–2% in the general population).

Farlow MR. Treatment of mild cognitive impairment (MCI). *Curr Alzheimer Res* 2009;6:362–367. [PMID: 19689235] (Discussion of therapeutic issues in MCI.)

Peterson RC. Early diagnosis of Alzheimer's disease: Is MCI too late? *Curr Alzheimer Res* 2009;6:324–330. [PMID: 19689230] (Discussion of therapeutic issues in MCI.)

VASCULAR COGNITIVE DEMENTIA

Lawrence Honig, MD, PhD

ESSENTIALS OF DIAGNOSIS

- ▶ Dementia or cognitive change that has a subcortical pattern
- ▶ Clinical strokes with radiologic evidence of cerebral infarcts
- ▶ Evidence of relationship between the dementia and stroke(s)
- ▶ Motor dysfunction, sometimes including gait disorder
- ▶ Urinary dyscontrol, typically incontinence or frequency

▶ General Considerations

Vascular dementia may be defined as a decline in cognition that results in functional impairment and is caused by cerebrovascular disease. Vascular insults may include ischemic or hemorrhagic strokes, ischemic white matter disease, or sequelae of hypotension or hypoxia. Diagnosis of vascular dementia has been controversial. During much of the 20th century, it was assumed that most dementia of the elderly was usually vascular in origin, but modern autopsy studies and neuroimaging have shown that most cases of dementia among the elderly in Europe and North America are rather the result of Alzheimer disease (AD). Pure vascular dementia is rare. However, many individuals do have some cognitive impairment due to stroke; for this reason, the term *vascular cognitive impairment* is increasingly in use. For example, in individuals presenting with cataclysmic aphasia or cortical blindness, there would be no tendency to confuse these deficits (usually of acute onset, then static with some improvement) with the steady progressive cognitive decline usually associated with the term *dementia*. However, many elderly people with progressive cognitive decline have concomitant pathologic vascular and AD-related changes causing dementia. In these individuals with mixed vascular and AD pathology, it is often difficult during life (or even after autopsy) to determine the principal cause of the dementia.

Various categories of cerebrovascular disease can cause dementia; these include:

1. Multiple large-vessel infarcts
2. Strategic "single" infarcts (eg, occlusions of the posterior cerebral artery causing bilateral thalamic infarction, or anterior cerebral artery syndromes causing bilateral frontal infarction)
3. Small vessel ischemic disease (eg, multiple lacunae in the basal ganglia or in subcortical or periventricular white matter)
4. Hypoperfusion (eg, global, due to cardiac arrest or hypotension)
5. Hemorrhagic cerebrovascular disease (eg, intracerebral or subdural hematomas or subarachnoid hemorrhage)
6. Other mechanisms (eg, combinations of those previously listed)

The first three listed mechanisms are often respectively termed *multi-infarct dementia, strategic-infarct dementia,* and *Binswanger disease*. Rare genetic syndromes also may produce vascular dementia (Table 9–5).

Because of the frequency of cerebrovascular disease in the elderly population, a diagnosis of vascular dementia requires the following criteria: (1) dementia; (2) stroke(s), evident clinically and radiologically; and (3) a temporal relationship between the dementia and the stroke(s). But even with such criteria, concomitant AD is common. For individuals who clearly fulfill clinical criteria for AD but who also have clinical or radiologic evidence of stroke, the appropriate diagnosis is AD with cerebrovascular disease.

▶ Clinical Findings

A. Symptoms and Signs

The symptoms and signs of vascular dementia may include memory loss, language impairment, visuospatial change, and

Table 9–5. Genetic Forms of Vascular Dementia

Disease	Chromosome	Gene
Cerebral autosomal-dominant arteriopathy with subcortical infarcts and leukoencephalopathy (CADASIL)	19	*Notch3*
Cerebral amyloid angiopathy (CAA)	21	*β-Amyloid precursor protein (βAPP)*
Mitochondrial encephalomyopathy with lactic acidosis and strokelike episodes (MELAS)	Mitochondrial (mtDNA)	*tRNA$^{Leu(UUR)}$*

lack of insight, similar to the symptoms of AD. Memory loss, a key feature in the dementia of AD, may be less prominent in cases of vascular dementia, particularly if the temporal lobe structures responsible for memory consolidation and retrieval are affected to a lesser degree. The cognitive symptoms of vascular dementia are often more subcortical; these include decreased concentration, forgetfulness, inertia, slowed thinking (bradyphrenia), apathy, and deficits in executive function (the ability to initiate, plan, and organize). In nearly all cases of vascular dementia, there are also motor symptoms and signs, including abnormal gait, focal weakness, or dyscoordination of one or more extremities. Bilateral cerebral dysfunction is generally required to cause dementia on a vascular basis, and this bihemispheric dysfunction may also result in emotional incontinence (so-called pseudobulbar affect), including inappropriate crying or laughing, and urinary frequency or incontinence due to bladder hyperreflexia.

Historic features that favor vascular dementia rather than AD include abrupt onset of dementia, stepwise deterioration, fluctuating course, nocturnal confusion, depression, somatic complaints, and emotional incontinence, as well as hypertension, prior strokes, and focal signs or symptoms.

Most vascular dementia is represented by one of the two of subcategories listed earlier: multi-infarct dementia and Binswanger disease. **Multi-infarct dementia** involves a history of multiple stepwise deteriorations in cognitive capacity. There are symptoms or signs of multiple cerebral infarcts, usually sudden motor or sensory changes, and radiologic studies confirm strokes. **Binswanger disease** may or may not include a history of multiple steps of deterioration. Dementia is accompanied by gait and urinary dysfunction, and extensive bilateral white matter abnormality is evident on radiologic studies.

B. Laboratory Findings and Neuropsychological Assessment

There are no radiologic or laboratory findings that specifically confirm vascular dementia. The diagnostic evaluation of stroke in general is discussed in Chapters 10 and 11.

Neuropsychological testing is also nonspecific for vascular dementia. However, typically patients may demonstrate deficits in frontal or executive function, including decreased speed of processing and difficulty with initiation. Memory deficits, when present, may be more subcortical, with a greater defect in free recall of recently learned information, than in recognition of this information, and improved recall with aural or written cues.

C. Diagnostic Criteria

The existing criteria for the diagnosis of vascular dementia suffer from poor apparent sensitivity and specificity. Even autopsy is not a gold standard for vascular dementia, because (1) it is not possible for the neuropathologist to state with certainty that pathologically evident cerebrovascular lesions caused the dementia, and (2) the white matter abnormalities visualized on MRI may be undetectable by standard neuropathologic examinations performed on autopsy. However, in the extreme case, absence of pathologic changes characteristic of AD or another neurodegenerative condition on autopsy, together with the presence of brain infarcts, provides reasonably strong evidence that vascular disease, rather than AD, was responsible for the dementia.

▶ Prevention & Treatment

Vascular dementia syndromes are caused by stroke. Thus prevention (primary treatment) or secondary treatment of stroke is key to preventing these varieties of cognitive impairment. Because of the relative rarity of pure vascular dementia, few studies have examined the efficacy of cholinesterase inhibitors and memantine in this condition, which are proven therapies for dementia due to AD. However, studies with each of these medications have shown efficacy in patients with mixed AD and stroke. It is reasonable, particularly given the lack of diagnostic accuracy, to offer such therapy to patients who have been diagnosed with vascular dementia. For agents and dosage, see Table 9–4.

▶ Prognosis

The prognosis in vascular dementia is more variable than that in AD. Deterioration may not be as relentlessly progressive, because stroke by nature is episodic. Some patients have a series of strokes and then are stroke-free for some years, particularly if they receive therapies to modify stroke risk factors.

Jellinger KA. The pathology of "vascular dementia": A critical update. *J Alzheimers Dis* 2008;14:107–123. [PMID: 18525132] (Reviews several clinical series, and an autopsy series of dementia cases, discussing prevalences and typologies of cases with pure vascular etiology.)

Menon U, Kelley RE. Subcortical ischemic cerebrovascular dementia. *Int Rev Neurobiol* 2009;84:21–33. [PMID: 19501711] (Review of Binswanger disease.)

Pendlebury ST, Rothwell PM. Prevalence, incidence, and factors associated with pre-stroke and post-stroke dementia: A systematic review and meta-analysis. *Lancet Neurol* 2009;8:1006–1018. [PMID: 19782001]. (Review of relationships between stroke and dementia.)

Roman GC. Vascular dementia prevention: A risk factor analysis. *Cerebrovasc Dis* 2005;20 (Suppl 2):91–100. [PMID: 16327258] (Reviews epidemiology and risk factors for vascular dementia, in comparison with Alzheimer's disease, and discusses overlap between these disorders.)

▼ FRONTOTEMPORAL DEMENTIAS

Nikolaos Scarmeas, MD, MS

ESSENTIALS OF DIAGNOSIS

▶ Prominent changes in personality and behavior (behavioral frontotemporal dementia)

▶ Primary progressive aphasia, which is subdivided into:
  • Progressive expressive nonfluent aphasia
  • Progressive receptive aphasia with loss of semantic knowledge for environmental objects (semantic dementia)

▶ Frontal and temporal dysfunction (personality, language, and memory impairment) with preservation of parietal lobe function (visual-spatial skills)

▶ Frontal and temporal circumscribed atrophy (MRI) or hypoperfusion-hypometabolism (SPECT or PET)

▶ Variety of underlying pathologic changes

▶ General Considerations

In 1892, Arnold Pick described cases of dementia with language and personality changes and pathologically evident severe and markedly circumscribed gross atrophy of the frontal and temporal lobes. The microscopic pathologic hallmarks were described several years later. Recent classifications use the term frontotemporal dementia (FTD) as an umbrella term, covering behavioral and language degenerative syndromes involving frontal/temporal lobes. The term *FTD* may be used for either the entire set of disorders or for behavioral frontotemporal dementia (bvFTD) itself. The language-predominant cases (primary progressive aphasia [PPA]) can be further divided into those with anterior, expressive, nonfluent aphasia (Progressive expressive nonfluent aphasia [PNFA]) and those with more posterior language deficits (semantic dementia [SD]).

Overall, FTD is less common than Alzheimer disease (AD) and Lewy body dementia, but it is a very common dementia cause for those with young onset (<~50–55 years of age). Neuropathologic studies, which benefit from diagnostic rigor but have the disadvantage of referral bias, report frequencies of FTD among dementia autopsies from 1–12%. Reviews of clinical records in the United Kingdom for demented subjects 45–64 years of age calculated a prevalence of FTD of 15 cases per 100,000 people (12–16% of the dementia population), with similar prevalences for AD in this younger age group. A study attempting complete ascertainment of FTD cases nationwide in the Netherlands resulted in an estimated FTD prevalence (per 100,000 people) of 2 for age 50–60 years and 4 for ages 60–80 years.

FTD is generally reported to occur at younger ages than AD, with mean ages of onset in the 50–65 years age range. There is no clear male or female predominance.

The relative distribution of different types of FTD varies in different reports. In one, 40% of patients were identified as having bvFTD, 20% were identified as having PNFA, and 40% were identified as having SD. In another report, 76% had bvFTD, 17% had PNFA, and 6% had SD.

▶ Pathogenesis

Several related histopathologic changes may underlie clinical FTD. Most cases of FTD (either bvFTD or PPA) can be broadly divided into (1) those with pathology involving tau, a protein that normally binds to neuronal microtubules; (2) those with pathology involving the transactive response DNA-binding protein 43 (TDP-43); and (3) those with pathology involving the "fused in sarcoma" (FUS) gene product. Tauopathies include among others tau (microtubule-associated protein tau [MAPT]) mutations, classic Pick disease (with Pick bodies), corticobasal degeneration (CBD), and progressive supranuclear palsy (PSP). TDP-43 proteinopathies include cases with and without mutations in the progranulin (PGRN) gene. FUS-proteinopathy appears to be associated with amyotrophic lateral sclerosis.

FTD has been reported to be familial (ie, present in at least one other first-degree relative) in 28–60% of cases. The two most commonly associated genes identified include MAPT (9–43% of familial cases and 5% of sporadic cases) and PGRN (13–20% of familial cases and 3–5% of sporadic cases). More rarely encountered genes include valosin-containing protein (VCP) and charged multivesicular body protein 2G (CHMP2B) (each seen in fewer than 1% of cases). There is substantial intra- and interfamilial variability in phenotype.

▶ Clinical Findings

A. Behavioral FTD

1. Symptoms and signs—The disorder is marked by progressive alterations in character and comportment in the setting of relative preservations of spatial skills and memory. Impaired insight usually includes both lack of awareness of an underlying disease process and lack of concern or distress regarding the personality changes. Symptoms include decline in social conduct, loss of social awareness, markedly increased or decreased sexual interests, impulsivity, disinhibition including tactlessness, inappropriate jocularity, and decline in personal hygiene and grooming. Utilization behavior may be seen, with unrestrained exploration of objects in the environment. Hyperorality, overeating, or changes in dietary habits, often with increased craving of sweets, is common. FTD patients may also manifest mental rigidity, inflexibility, fixed ideation, and perseverations encompassing simple or complex repetitive behavioral routines and stereotyped behaviors, including mannerisms or ritualistic preoccupations. Although emotional blunting, with unconcern, indifference, remoteness, and lack of empathy, is common, depression is infrequent.

The majority of patients with bvFTD do not have significant aphasia at initial presentation, but speech abnormalities may occur, including perseverative features such as echolalia or verbal stereotypies. There is lack of spontaneity, economy, and emptiness of speech, with progressive reduction of speech quantity.

Focal motor, sensory, or reflex neurologic signs are typically absent early in the disease, except for the nonspecific presence of primitive reflexes, such as a grasp reflex and a palmomental response. Extrapyramidal signs may be present in particular in FTD-parkinsonism linked to chromosome 17, CBD, and PSP. A subset of FTD patients have associated motor neuron disease symptoms and signs.

Despite these distinct symptoms, differentiation of FTD from AD or other dementing diseases may be difficult.

2. Behavioral assessment—Although impulsiveness, distractibility, and lack of cooperation tend to interfere with testing, patients may perform surprisingly well on neuropsychological assessment (including tests sensitive to frontal lobe function). Behavioral changes may occur before structural or functional brain imaging studies show discernible abnormalities. Behavioral inventories that focus more on unusual behaviors and personality changes rather than cognitive testing may be more sensitive and helpful for diagnosis in early stages.

3. Neuropsychological assessment—Performance of bvFTD patients may not always have true localizing value because it may be compromised by inattention, inefficient retrieval strategies, poor organization, lack of self-monitoring, and lack of effort or interest.

Cognitive changes are mostly indicative of frontal lobe dysfunction. Patients show attentional deficits, poor abstraction, difficulty shifting mental set, perseverative tendencies, and executive and planning dysfunction in tests such as the Wisconsin Card Sorting Test, the Stroop Test, and the Trail Making Test.

FTD patients usually remain oriented, often keep good track of recent personal events until late in the disease process, and are usually less impaired than those with AD on measures of anterograde memory. Performance on anterograde memory tests does vary, and patients often do poorly on tasks based on "free recall" as opposed to recognition. In more advanced disease, marked amnesia may develop, with severe loss of remote memory.

The most striking neuropsychological finding differentiating patients with FTD from those with AD is the preservation of visuospatial abilities early in the disease.

3. Imaging studies—Frontal and temporal atrophy is usually noted in CT and MRI. Abnormalities in functional imaging studies usually precede changes detected in structural imaging modalities: perfusion (hexamethylpropyleneamine [HMPAO] SPECT) and metabolism (FDG-PET) studies typically show decreased flow or metabolism in the frontal and temporal regions, usually of the right hemisphere.

B. Progressive Nonfluent Aphasia

1. Symptoms and signs—The clinical diagnosis of PNFA is made when language is the only area of salient and progressive dysfunction for at least the first 2 years of the disease. Patients present with anomia leading to speech simplification, circumlocution, substitution of words by fillers, paraphasias, and empty speech or logopenia (poverty of speech). Many PNFA patients develop gradually worsening anomia throughout most of their disease, whereas others develop agrammatism (inappropriate word order and misuse of small grammatical words). In the late stages of illness, patients become mute. As the disease progresses, PNFA patients may develop comprehension deficits, executive dysfunction, constructional deficits, and behavioral changes suggesting bvFTD. However, language dysfunction remains the most striking feature: in some, the principal symptoms and signs may be confined to the area of language for as many as 10–14 years.

2. Neuropsychological assessment—In addition to the above deficits, PNFA patients are impaired in phonemic fluency tests (the ability to generate words starting with a particular letter). Performance on visual-spatial function tests is well preserved.

3. Imaging studies—Left-sided perisylvian atrophy, usually anterior, on CT or MRI is the most common structural feature of PNFA. Functional imaging studies showing left-sided Sylvian hypoperfusion or hypometabolism may precede atrophy.

C. Semantic Dementia

1. Symptoms and signs—Semantic memory refers to knowledge of facts, concepts, and words. Patients with SD typically complain of loss of memory for words, and semantic paraphasias are noted. They usually have good day-to-day

(episodic) memory and orientation but show impaired recall of more distant life events. In other words, they show a reversal of the usual temporal gradient found in AD. Despite the profound loss of semantics, these patients often cope surprisingly well in activities of everyday life. Over time, other cognitive deficits and behavioral features such as those seen in bvFTD emerge.

2. Neuropsychological assessment—Patients with SD display profound deficits of picture naming and are impaired on single-word comprehension, as judged by tasks such as word–picture matching. They are also impaired in categorical fluency tests (ability to generate words belonging to a certain semantic category, such as animals). As in other types of FTD, SD subjects may have striking preservation of basic visual-spatial ability.

3. Imaging studies—In contrast to PNFA cases, atrophy (by CT or MRI) and hypoperfusion or hypometabolism in SD cases principally involves left posterior perisylvian regions.

▶ Prognosis

Average disease duration is estimated to be 3–17 years, with an average of 8–9 years. Patients with concomitant motor neuron disease have a poorer prognosis, with death usually occurring in 3–5 years.

▶ Treatment

There are no therapies known to affect the course of FTD. Anecdotal reports describe benefit from selegiline, selective serotonin reuptake inhibitors, memantine, and trazodone. There is no evidence regarding the efficacy of acetylcholinesterase inhibitors. The mainstay of treatment of FTD is for the psychiatric and behavioral symptoms, which often contribute more to caregiver burden than does cognitive impairment and are a frequent contributor to institutionalization. Acetylcholinesterase inhibitors, memantine, atypical neuroleptics, antidepressants, anxiolytics, and anticonvulsants (for mood control) are commonly prescribed.

Grossman M. Primary progressive aphasia: Clinicopathological correlations. *Nat Rev Neurol* 2010;6:88–97. [PMID: 20139998]

Josephs KA. Frontotemporal dementia and related disorders: Deciphering the enigma. Ann Neurol 2008;64:4–14. [PMID: 18668533]

Mackenzie IR, et al. Nomenclature and nosology for neuropathologic subtypes of frontotemporal lobar degeneration: An update. *Acta Neuropathol* 2010;119:1–4. [PMID: 19924424]

Rabinovici GD, Miller BL. Frontotemporal lobar degeneration: epidemiology, pathophysiology, diagnosis and management. *CNS Drugs* 2010;24:375–398. [PMID: 20369906]

Rogalski E, Mesulam, M. An update on primary progressive aphasia. *Curr Neurol Neurosci Rep* 2007;7:388–392. [PMID: 17764628]

▼ PROGRESSIVE SUPRANUCLEAR PALSY

Sarah C. Janicki, MD, MPH

ESSENTIALS OF DIAGNOSIS

▶ Dementia or cognitive impairment accompanied by axial rigidity and vertical supranuclear gaze palsy

▶ Preservation of memory recognition with deficits in encoding and retrieval

▶ Diagnosis is dependent upon clinical signs and symptoms rather than imaging findings

▶ General Considerations

Progressive supranuclear palsy (PSP) is categorized as an atypical parkinsonian syndrome or Parkinson-plus syndrome. Disease prevalence is estimated at 1.39 cases per 100,000 people. It occurs more frequently in men, and the mean age of onset is 65 years. PSP is a tauopathy. Neuropathologic findings include subcortical neuronal and glial loss with tau-positive neurofibrillary tangles and tufted astrocytes in the basal ganglia, brainstem nuclei, and frontal lobe.

A comparison of the pathologic and clinical features of frontotemporal dementia, PSP, and corticobasal degeneration is shown in Table 9–6.

▶ Clinical Findings

A. Symptoms and Signs

The history is notable for early onset of falls and parkinsonism with prominent axial rigidity, a wide-based gait, and an absence of postural responses. Typical eye findings include blepharospasm, ocular square wave jerks, and supranuclear ocular palsy, typically causing impairment of voluntary vertical downgaze with preserved ocular reflex movements.

Frontal executive impairments are early and pervasive. Although simple tests of attention and orientation are typically normal, more complex tasks of planning, task shifting, abstraction, and reasoning are significantly impaired, which contributes to patients' inability to formulate goal-directed behaviors. Memory complaints are usually mild and consist of impaired free recall with preserved recognition memory that is significantly improved by cued recall. Signs of cortical dementia, such as aphasia, apraxia, and agnosia, are absent.

Personality and behavior changes may appear before oculomotor and movement symptoms, most commonly as apathy and disinhibition. Patients may also occasionally demonstrate disinhibited behaviors typically seen in patients with frontotemporal dementia, such as obsessions, compulsions, stereotyped or ritualistic behavior, and extreme dietary preferences, including hyperphagia.

B. Imaging Studies

Structural imaging studies in patients with progressive nuclear palsy are often normal; however, MRI occasionally shows midbrain atrophy, particularly in the dorsal midbrain. Atrophy of the rostral and caudal midbrain tegmentum may create changes in the midbrain anatomy, which make its profile resemble a hummingbird on sagittal midline MRI sections. This is fittingly called the "hummingbird sign." However, these imaging findings tend to occur late in the disease course, and as a result, the diagnostic accuracy of PSP by conventional MRI is unsatisfactory, with a sensitivity of about 70%. Most functional imaging studies to date are based on relatively small numbers of cases with clinical diagnosis, which may not always be correct when compared with pathologic verification; however, some have demonstrated medial anterior thalamic or frontal lobe dysfunction. More work is required to better determine the diagnostic value of structural and functional imaging.

▶ Treatment

There is no treatment for cognitive changes associated with PSP. A treatment trial with donepezil demonstrated only mild benefit to memory function at the expense of decreased motor functions such as swallowing and gait, which led to the recommendation of avoiding its use in this patient population. Most patients demonstrate a limited response to treatment with levodopa, and many have only mild and short-lived improvement. Treatment with levadopa does not alter survival. Pallidotomy or deep brain stimulation is unhelpful. As a result, most current therapies are supportive, although none are of proven value. Common interventions include physical and occupational therapy, which may utilize weighted walkers for imbalance; speech therapy for dysarthria; and counseling and antidepressants for depression.

▶ Prognosis

Survival among patients with PSP is shorter than among with those with Parkinson disease, a median of 5–6 years with a range of 1–13 years. Early presentations of falls, dementia, dysphagia, or urinary incontinence are poor prognostic indicators of disability and death.

Dickson DW, Radamakers R, Hutton ML. Progressive supranuclear palsy: Pathology and genetics. *Brain Pathol* 2007;17:74–82. [PMID: 17493041] (A useful review of the pathology and genetics of progressive supranuclear palsy.)

Houghton DJ, Litvan I. Unraveling progressive supranuclear palsy: From the bedside back to the bench. *Parkinsonism Relat Disord* 2007;13:S341–S346. [PMID: 18267262] (Update regarding the clinical presentation of progressive supranuclear palsy, as well as the pathology and genetics.)

Magherini A, Litvan I. Cognitive and behavioral aspects of PSP since Steele, Richardson and Olszewski's description of PSP 40 years ago and Albert's delineation of the subcortical dementia 30 years ago. *Neurocase* 2005;11:250–262. [PMID: 16093225] (Reviews the cognitive and behavioral changes associated with progressive supranuclear palsy and related neurodegenerative disorders.)

Table 9–6. Pathologic and Clinical Features of Frontotemporal Dementia, Progressive Supranuclear Palsy, and Corticobasal Degeneration

Disease	Pathology	Clinical Presentation	Survival
Frontotemporal dementia	• Spectrum includes 3R tauopathies, 4R tauopathies, Pick bodies, and TDP-43 proteinopathies	• Behavioral variant marked by progressive alterations in personality and behavior with preservations of spatial skills and memory • Progressive nonfluent aphasia demonstrates isolated language dysfunction for at least the first 2 years of the disease • Semantic dementia manifests loss of memory for words and semantic paraphasias. In contrast to Alzheimer patients, orientation and recent episodic memory is preserved, whereas memory of distant events is impaired	• Average survival 8–9 years • Poor prognosis predicted by concomitant motor neuron disease
Corticobasal degeneration	• 4R tauopathy • Presence of H1 allele • Tau-positive astrocytic plaques and threads in both white and gray matter	• Asymmetric parkinsonism, rigidity, gait disturbances • Alien limb phenomenon • Depression more frequent than in PSP or FTD • Occasional agitation, aggression, and disinhibition • May have aphasia, first expressive and later receptive • Memory storage preserved with deficits in encoding and retrieval • Absence of psychosis and hallucinations	• Average survival 5–7 years • Poor prognosis predicted by severe or bilateral parkinsonism or prominent behavioral changes
Progressive supranuclear palsy	• 4R tauopathy • Presence of H1 allele • Tau-positive neurofibrillary tangles and tufted astrocytes in the basal ganglia, brainstem nuclei, and frontal lobe	• Symmetric motor signs and symptoms, including axial rigidity • Vertical supranuclear gaze palsy • Notable impairment in executive function • Mild memory complaints with preserved recognition • Absence of psychosis and hallucinations	• Average survival 5–6 years • Poor prognosis predicted by early falls, dementia, dysphagia, or urinary incontinence

3R tauopathy = 3 repeat tauopathy, 4R tauopathy = 4 repeat tauopathy.

CORTICOBASAL DEGENERATION

Sarah C. Janicki, MD, MPH

ESSENTIALS OF DIAGNOSIS

▶ Dementia or cognitive impairment associated with progressive, asymmetric cortical, and extrapyramidal signs

▶ Cognitive deficits including cortical deficits such as apraxia and aphasia accompanied by executive dysfunction including deficits in planning, task shifting, and memory encoding

▶ Absence of psychosis and severe memory impairment as an early manifestation

▶ General Considerations

Corticobasal degeneration is an atypical parkinsonian syndrome or Parkinson-plus syndrome. The mean age at onset is 60.9 years, with a range of 51–73 years, more than 10 years younger than that in Alzheimer disease. The current diagnostic accuracy of corticobasal degeneration is relatively poor. Despite a high specificity of clinical diagnosis, sensitivity is only about 35% at presentation, rising to about 48% at the last clinical visit. This may be due in part to clinical and pathologic heterogeneity. The evidence of this poor clinico-pathologic correlation has led to the use of the term *corticobasal syndrome* (CBS) in the case of a clinical diagnosis of corticobasal degeneration without pathologic verification.

▶ Pathogenesis

The clinical presentation of the corticobasal syndrome likely reflects the distribution of underlying pathology in cortical and subcortical regions rather than specific histopathology. As a result, a diagnosis of corticobasal degeneration requires pathologic diagnosis, and specific neuropathological criteria have been detailed. These validated pathologic diagnostic criteria do not require a specific clinical phenotype, as it has been demonstrated that a number of clinical phenotypes can occur as a result of similar pathologic changes. Core pathologic features include focal cortical neuronal loss in the parasagittal region, particularly in the peri-Rolandic gyri, with secondary changes in the associated corticospinal tracts, increased pallor of the substantia nigra due to neuronal loss, and cortical and striatal tau-positive neuronal and glial lesions, especially astrocytic plaques and threads, in both white and gray matter. Although ballooned achromatic neurons identical to Pick cells were initially believed to be the hallmark of the disorder, they are now considered only a supportive feature due to rare cases lacking this pathology but with otherwise typical findings.

▶ Clinical Findings

A. Symptoms and Signs

Classic corticobasal syndrome presents as a progressive and asymmetrical akinetic-rigid parkinsonism. Patients demonstrate axial rigidity associated with a gait disorder characterized by bradykinesia, postural instability, and falls. Asymmetric limb rigidity or dystonia is observed as the disease progresses and occurs more commonly in the arm than the leg, with rare involvement of the head, neck, or trunk. The "alien hand" phenomenon occurs in approximately 20–60% of cases. Cortical sensory deficits may present as agraphesthesia, astereognosia, or extinction to double simultaneous stimulation. The eye movement abnormality most strongly associated with corticobasal degeneration is difficulty and delay in initiating saccades. Additional eye movement abnormalities include ocular gaze apraxia or Balint syndrome. Eyelid movement disorders are also common, particularly apraxia of eyelid opening, closure, or both.

Although cognitive impairment was thought to be a rare or late-occurring manifestation of corticobasal syndrome, recently it has become apparent that cognitive decline is a common feature of the disorder. Furthermore, dementia may be the presenting feature, with extrapyramidal and motor features presenting later. Language dysfunction is the most commonly reported early cognitive complaint, and up to 44% of patients with pathologically confirmed corticobasal degeneration have some type of aphasia. Examination of patients reveals worsening expressive aphasia as the disease progresses; language comprehension is preserved for a longer period of time, but this too appears to worsen as the disease approaches an end stage. Additionally, many patients exhibit prominent executive difficulties at onset, including disinhibition, increased agitation, aggressiveness, hypersexuality, hyperorality, and obsessive compulsive disorder.

B. Imaging Studies

CT and MRI scans of the brain tend to be normal in early stages of the disease. Even as the disease progresses, the diagnostic accuracy of MRI abnormalities is poor. If present, MRI findings may include atrophy of the posterior frontal cortex, superior parietal cortex, and middle portion of the corpus callosum. Atrophy is worse in the parasagittal and peri-Rolandic areas contralateral to the clinically affected side, with dilatation of the lateral ventricle. Functional imaging studies may be of use in the differential diagnosis of patients with suspected corticobasal degeneration. The most notable findings in functional imaging studies are asymmetrical hypoperfusion on SPECT and asymmetrical hypometabolism on PET involving the frontoparietal cortex, basal ganglia, and thalamus.

▶ Treatment

There are no known treatments for cognitive impairment in corticobasal syndrome, and therapeutics are limited to treatment of depression with selective serotonin reuptake inhibitors, as well as treatment of early motor symptoms with physical and occupational therapy. There are no placebo-controlled studies of cholinesterase inhibitors in corticobasal syndrome. Although no formal studies have been performed, the neurosurgical procedures used in treatment of Parkinson disease have been uniformly ineffective as they are in most other levodopa-resistant Parkinson-plus syndromes.

▶ Prognosis

Disease duration is 5–7 years, with a range of 24–96 months. Poor survival is predicted by early presence of severe or bilateral parkinsonism or prominent behavioral changes. Falls and dysphagia are important causes of morbidity and mortality.

Dickson DW, et al. Office of rare diseases neuropathologic criteria for corticobasal degeneration. *J Neuropathol Exp Neurol* 2002; 61:935–46. [PMID: 12430710] (The Office of Rare Diseases of the National Institutes of Health [United States] developed neuropathology criteria for accurate diagnosis of corticobasal degeneration.)

Murray R, et al. Cognitive and motor assessment in autopsy-proven corticobasal degeneration. *Neurology* 2007;68;1274–1283. [PMID: 17438218] (Investigates the clinical features of cases of corticobasal degeneration with verified pathology.)

Wadia PM, Lang AE. The many faces of corticobasal degeneration. *Parkinsonism Relat Disord* 2007;13:S336–S340. [PMID: 18267261] (Updated review of the pathology, clinical presentation, and causes of the corticobasal syndrome.)

▼ PARKINSON DISEASE DEMENTIA

James M. Noble, MD

Parkinson disease dementia and dementia with Lewy bodies, along with Parkinson disease itself, arguably present a continuum of motor and cognitive disorders related to a common neuropathologic hallmark of α-synuclein, which is now considered the primary aggregated protein constituting Lewy bodies. Thus these diseases are collectively referred to as Lewy body disorders or α-synucleinopathies.

ESSENTIALS OF DIAGNOSIS

▶ Development of dementia or cognitive impairment in a patient with levodopa-responsive parkinsonism

▶ Cognitive deficits include impaired attention, executive function, and processing speed, with a relative preservation of memory

▶ General Considerations

Parkinson disease (PD) is characterized by the cardinal features of rigidity, bradykinesia, tremor, and postural instability. Cognitive impairment and subsequent dementia occurring in the context of PD (Parkinson disease dementia [PDD]) is common among PD patients. The prevalence of dementia in PD is between 20% and 40%, with 10–15% having dementia at the time of PD diagnosis. Among those surviving 20 years of PD, dementia is prevalent in >80%. In contrast to AD, potentially modifiable risk factors such as stroke and head injury have not been consistently associated with risk of PDD. In addition to increasing age, risk factors for the development of PDD may reflect severity of underlying parkinsonism, specifically postural instability–gait disorder predominant PD, speech and swallowing difficulty, and mesenteric or urologic autonomic dysfunction. A family history of dementia is associated with increased risk of PDD. A growing literature suggests a role of glucocerebrosidase (GBA) mutations in PDD. Carriers of GBA mutations have fourfold risk of PD; one study demonstrated 48% of PDD patients having a GBA mutation, and the importance of this mutation may be greater in younger patients.

▶ Pathogenesis

Disruption of dopaminergic, noradrenergic, cholinergic, and serotonergic neurotransmitter systems has been implicated in the pathogenesis of PDD. The clinicopathologic correlations of patients with PD and dementia suggest that patients fall into one of three categories: Lewy body pathology restricted to subcortical areas (typical of PD), concomitant PD and AD pathologies, or predominant cortical Lewy bodies. In general, patients with PDD have a greater burden of AD pathology compared with PD, with no or minimal cognitive impairment. Studies using α-synuclein immunohistochemical staining have emphasized the importance of cortical Lewy body pathology in PDD. Therefore, multiple underlying pathologic changes may account for the presence and degree of cognitive impairment in PD patients.

▶ Prevention

No randomized controlled trials have been performed with development of PDD as a primary end point, and one large prospective study of PD patients showed no benefit in cognitive test performance from selegiline, tocopherol, or a combination of the two. In a cross-sectional study, postmenopausal estrogen use was associated with a reduced risk of PDD. Although some studies have associated higher levels of baseline physical activity and favorable diet with decreased risk of developing PD, no studies have demonstrated diminished PDD risk.

▶ Clinical Findings

A. Symptoms and Signs

In PDD, cognitive impairment occurs at least 1 year after onset of PD symptoms. In general, the early and predominant symptoms of cognitive impairment associated with PD include impairments of frontal-executive functions (concept formation, problem solving, set shifting and maintenance, difficulties with internally cued behavior), attention and concentration, and processing speed. With disease progression, memory may also become affected.

Severity of executive function likely plays a significant role in the manifestation of memory impairment in some PDD patients. Speed of information processing has been shown to differentiate PDD from AD as well.

B. Laboratory Findings

Routine laboratory studies for reversible causes of dementia (covered earlier in this chapter) should be performed in patients with PD who develop dementia. No additional studies are routinely indicated for PDD.

C. Imaging Studies

Structural and functional imaging studies have been performed in patients with PDD. Results of these studies, although of interest, must be interpreted with caution, as few studies have included neuropathologic correlation. No clear pattern of abnormality has been consistently shown on structural imaging studies in PDD. The primary utility of structural imaging in PDD is to exclude an identifiable alternative cause, such as stroke and subdural or epidural hematoma. MRI findings can range from normal to atrophy patterns typical of AD. Functional imaging studies in PDD have shown patterns of either frontal or temporoparietal cortical dysfunction. Supporting pathologic considerations, research studies of amyloid imaging suggest low cortical amyloid burden in PDD patients.

D. Special Examinations

Formal neuropsychological testing is helpful in determining the extent of executive, attention and concentration, processing speed, verbal fluency, visuospatial, and memory impairment in PD patients with cognitive impairment.

Differential Diagnosis

Several diagnoses must be considered among PD patients with new cognitive symptoms, including mild cognitive impairment, depression, medication side effect (related to PD regimen or other medications), and delirium associated with metabolic or systemic disorders. Atypical features, including poor response to dopaminergic medications, should raise suspicion of related disorders such as dementia with Lewy bodies (DLB), multiple systems atrophy, or corticobasal degeneration (discussed elsewhere). Distinguishing PDD from DLB can be difficult, and these patients may be indistinguishable clinically and pathologically when identified in an advanced stage. The feature that distinguishes PDD from DLB is contemporaneous onset of cognitive and motor symptoms within 1 year of another in DLB. The possibility exists that PDD and DLB lie along a clinical and pathologic spectrum, with motor-onset and cognitive-onset presentations, respectively.

Treatment

Treatment with levodopa has been reported to be associated with both improvement and worsening of specific domains of cognitive function in PD, although no claims have been made of improved cognition in PDD. More recent studies have suggested that the cognitive effects of levodopa are subtle and largely limited to beneficial effects on arousal and mood. Concerns about adverse effects of long-term levodopa treatment on cognition in PD have not been substantiated. Because the cholinergic neurotransmitter system has been shown to be involved in PDD, and features of cognitive impairment (namely attention and concentration) that may be responsive to enhanced cholinergic tone are frequently present, cholinesterase inhibitors could be useful in symptomatic treatment of PDD. However, theoretically, this enhancement of cholinergic tone could also worsen extrapyramidal features of the disease. Rivastigmine has been approved for treatment of PDD given that it briefly slows cognitive decline, but it has been associated with a worsening motor symptoms (mainly tremor). One small randomized controlled study of memantine in PDD and DLB also suggested a modest benefit, particularly among the PDD subjects.

Prognosis

PD patients with dementia have higher mortality rates than PD patients without dementia, regardless of age or disease duration. PDD is associated with a decline in quality of life, nursing home placement, and increased caregiver burden.

Aarsland D. Memantine in patients with Parkinson's disease dementia or dementia with Lewy bodies: A double-blind, placebo-controlled, multicentre trial. *Lancet Neurol* 2009;8: 613–618. [PMID:19520613]

Aarsland D, Kurz MW. The epidemiology of dementia associated with Parkinson's disease. *Brain Pathol Sci* 2010;20:633–639. [PMID: 20522088]

Emre M, et al. Rivastigmine for dementia associated with Parkinson's disease. *N Engl J Med* 2004;351:2509–2518. [PMID: 15590953] (A randomized controlled trial warranting use of cholinesterase inhibitor in treatment of PDD.)

Hely MA, et al. The Sydney multicenter study of Parkinson's disease: The inevitability of dementia at 20 years. *Mov Disord* 2008;23: 837–844. [PMID: 18307261]

Lippa CF, et al. DLB/PDD Working Group. DLB and PDD boundary issues: Diagnosis, treatment, molecular pathology, and biomarkers. *Neurology* 2007;68:812–819. [PMID: 17353469]

Neumann J, et al. Glucocerebrosidase mutations in clinical and pathologically proven Parkinson's disease. *Brain* 2009;132(Pt 7): 1783–1794. [PMID: 19286695] (Along with Clark et al [see next section, DLB], one of two early articles identifying a surprisingly high frequency of GBA mutations among patients with Lewy body disorders.)

Uc EY, et al. Incidence of and risk factors for cognitive impairment in an early Parkinson disease clinical trial cohort. *Neurology* 2009;73:1469–1477. [PMID: 19884574]

▼ DEMENTIA WITH LEWY BODIES

James M. Noble, MD

ESSENTIALS OF DIAGNOSIS

► Dementia or cognitive impairment preceding or in temporal association with onset of parkinsonism

► Fluctuating levels of attention and alertness

► Recurrent visual hallucinations; auditory hallucinations and delusions

► History suggestive of sleep disruption, acting out dreams, nocturnal aggression or wandering

General Considerations

Dementia with Lewy bodies (DLB) is characterized by elements of psychosis (delusions, hallucinations), fluctuations in alertness and cognition, and sleep disturbance in addition to dementia and parkinsonism. The prevalence of DLB is unknown, but DLB comprises approximately 5% of dementia cases seen in memory disorders clinics. Less is known about the incidence or potential risk factors for DLB than for Parkinson disease dementia (PDD). The genetics of DLB is uncertain; however, recent studies suggest that glucocerebrosidase mutations play an important role, with GBA carriers having an approximate sevenfold risk of cortical Lewy bodies at autopsy.

Pathogenesis

Hypotheses about the pathophysiology of DLB center on the abnormal accumulation of α-synuclein protein (a normal synaptic protein implicated in vesicle production) into an insoluble form that is the major constituent of Lewy bodies. Lewy bodies and dystrophic Lewy neurites are found at autopsy involving pigmented nuclei of the brainstem as well as limbic and cortical areas. Many have noted a considerable clinical overlap between Parkinson disease (PD), DLB, and the pathologic burden of cortical Lewy bodies. The degree and duration of both diseases are not consistently correlated with pathology, and increasing evidence implicates Lewy neurites and neurotransmitter deficits as important in the etiology of the clinical syndrome. The nucleus basalis of Meynert, a critical element of the cholinergic system, is typically involved in DLB, and varying degrees of parkinsonism have been attributed to involvement of the dopaminergic system, as in other parkinsonian disorders.

Prevention

No controlled trials have been performed regarding prevention of DLB.

Clinical Findings

A. Symptoms and Signs

DLB characteristically presents contemporaneous onset of parkinsonism and cognitive impairment within the same year. Fluctuations in cognition, including distinct periods of depressed levels of alertness, are a core feature of the clinical diagnosis of DLB and involve varying dysfunction of level of attention and arousal. These fluctuations should be distinguished clinically from "sundowning" in Alzheimer disease (AD) or complex partial seizures, which also increase in frequency with advancing age and among dementia patients. As with PDD, DLB patients may have predominant impairments in domains of executive function, attention, and processing speed; visuospatial functioning may be particularly impaired. This profile of cognitive deficits, as well as less severe involvement of verbal memory, helps to differentiate DLB from AD.

Psychiatric symptoms are common in DLB, the most notable of which are elements of psychosis (delusions and hallucinations), and may be the presenting feature. Extrapyramidal signs are variably present at diagnosis of DLB, and most patients with DLB develop some parkinsonism during the natural history of the disease.

REM sleep behavior disorder, a parasomnia with vivid dreams and aberrant vocalizations and/or motor behavior, may precede the onset of dementia by many years. Autonomic dysfunction, including orthostatic hypotension, urinary incontinence, and constipation, is common in DLB patients.

B. Laboratory Findings

As with PDD, laboratory studies should be performed in patients presenting with the preceding symptoms to exclude identifiable systemic/metabolic, infectious, and inflammatory disorders. Currently there is no laboratory test in blood, urine, or cerebrospinal fluid specific for a diagnosis of DLB.

C. Imaging Studies

In addition to eliminating structural causes such as a mass lesion, stroke, or hydrocephalus, neuroimaging can be helpful in supporting a clinical diagnosis of DLB. The degree of cortical and hippocampal atrophy in DLB is often minimal and useful in differentiating DLB from AD. Functional neuroimaging in DLB has been characterized by parietal and occipital hypoperfusion/hypometabolism. Demonstration of occipital lobe dysfunction by SPECT and PET has been used to differentiate DLB from AD. Research studies of amyloid-labeled PET ligand Pittsburgh compound B suggest a greater degree of cortical amyloid in DLB than in PDD subjects.

D. Special Tests

Neuropsychological testing in DLB may demonstrate impairment in the domains of executive function, attention, and visuospatial functioning. This is similar to the profile seen in PDD but is useful in differentiating DLB from AD. Electroencephalography (EEG) may demonstrate significant slowing and variability in background rhythm and transient temporal slow-wave activity. Polysomnography may demonstrate loss of the normal electromyographic atonia during REM sleep in patients with REM sleep behavior disorder.

Differential Diagnosis

The main differential diagnostic considerations in DLB are AD, vascular dementia, and parkinson-plus disorders, such as multiple system atrophy, progressive supranuclear palsy, and corticobasal degeneration. Creutzfeldt-Jakob disease is a consideration in more rapidly progressive cases. Clinical differentiation from PDD is based mainly on the mode of presentation, as outlined previously.

Treatment

No treatments aimed at the underlying pathophysiologic process are currently available. Cholinesterase inhibitors have been shown to improve both cognition and the psychiatric manifestations of the disease and are considered by some to be first-line agents for treatment of DLB. A double-blind placebo-controlled study of the NMDA antagonist memantine in subjects with either PDD or DLB suggested benefit, although the findings may have been driven by the PDD patients.

Fluctuations in cognition and sleep disturbance also may be ameliorated by these cholinesterase inhibitors, but they may also exacerbate symptoms of autonomic dysfunction (eg, postural hypotension) seen in some patients with DLB. Similar to PDD, the hypothetical worsening of parkinsonism with cholinesterase inhibitors is infrequently seen in DLB.

Parkinsonism can be addressed with carbidopa/levodopa or dopamine agonists at the risk of exacerbating psychosis or autonomic dysfunction. In general, if antiparkinsonian medications are to be used, the lowest effective dose should be the goal of therapy.

Dopaminergic D2 receptor-blocking agents (both traditional and atypical neuroleptics) have been associated with severe (sometimes fatal) idiosyncratic reactions, including sudden cardiac arrhythmias and death. A recent "black box" warning by the FDA outlined the risks of sudden cardiac death associated with atypical antipsychotics. Thus any consideration of their use in low dose should be done with extreme caution and with full disclosure to the patients' care providers. Moreover, these agents may exacerbate parkinsonism and postural hypotension (in either DLB or PDD).

REM sleep behavior disorder may be managed with clonazepam, melatonin (or melatonin agonists), or atypical neuroleptics. Clonazepam should be used with caution, as low doses used for REM sleep behavior disorder can adversely affect cognition in DLB patients. One small study suggested that memantine may improve sleep patterns in patients with DLB or PDD.

▶ Prognosis

In general, the progression in cognitive decline seen in DLB is similar to that seen in AD. However, some patients with DLB exhibit a rapid clinical course. No significant difference has been consistently shown between DLB and AD in terms of survival time to death from symptom onset.

Clark LN, et al. Association of glucocerebrosidase mutations with dementia with Lewy bodies. *Arch Neurol* 2009;66:578–583. [PMID: 19433657]

Larsson V, et at. The effect of memantine of sleep behavior in dementia with Lewy bodies and Parkinson's disease dementia. *Int J Geriatric Psychiatry* 2010t;25:1030–1038. [PMID: 20872929]

McKeith IG, et al. Dementia with Lewy bodies. *Lancet Neurol* 2004;3:19–28. [PMID: 15261605]

McKeith IG, et al. Diagnosis and management of dementia with Lewy bodies: Third report of the DLB Consortium. *Neurology* 2005;65(12):1863–1872. [PMID: 16237129] (Reviews essential, sufficient, supportive, and suggestive clinical features to help the clinician best identify cases of DLB from mimickers such as PDD or AD with parkinsonism.)

Noe E, et al. Comparison of dementia with Lewy bodies to Alzheimer's disease and Parkinson's disease with dementia. *Mov Disord* 2004;19:60–67. [PMID: 14743362]

Salzman C, et al. Elderly patients with dementia-related symptoms of severe agitation and aggression: Consensus statement on treatment options, clinical trials methodology, and policy. *J Clin Psychiatry* 2008;69:889–898. [PMID: 18494535] (Reviews FDA "black box" warning of antipsychotics and the implication in clinical care of psychosis among dementia patients.)

▼ NORMAL PRESSURE HYDROCEPHALUS

Lawrence Honig, MD, PhD

ESSENTIALS OF DIAGNOSIS

▶ Gait disorder, typically wide-based "magnetic" gait, with short stride

▶ Urinary dyscontrol, typically incontinence or frequency and urgency

▶ Cognitive change or dementia, typically subcortical in nature

▶ Ventricular enlargement without commensurately enlarged sulci

▶ General Considerations

Hydrocephalus is defined as excessive fluid accumulation in the brain. Acute hydrocephalus is a medical emergency, usually caused by obstruction of cerebrospinal fluid (CSF) outflow from the lateral ventricles at the foramen of Munro, from the third ventricle at the aqueduct, or from the fourth ventricle at the foramina of Luschka and Magendie (so-called noncommunicating hydrocephalus). Typically, the intracranial fluid pressure is elevated. By contrast, chronic hydrocephalus is better compensated; pressure may be in the higher range of normal (eg, 12–20 cm H_2O), but not formally increased. Hence the term *normal pressure*. Most often there is no clear evidence of obstruction. Because ventricular enlargement is common in a variety of dementing disorders, and because urinary and gait abnormalities are also common in the elderly, diagnosis of hydrocephalus in the elderly is often difficult.

▶ Pathogenesis

Normal pressure hydrocephalus is often termed *communicating hydrocephalus* because, in most cases, and in contrast to so-called noncommunicating hydrocephalus, there is less evident obstruction of the normal pathway of CSF flow. However, communicating chronic hydrocephalus must involve either overproduction of CSF (rare) or, more commonly, inadequate resorption (which can be said to be obstructive). Chronic hydrocephalus is also often termed *idiopathic*, although in many cases, impediments to CSF flow may relate to prior subarachnoid hemorrhage from trauma or aneurysm, meningitis, tumor, or surgery and, perhaps in some cases, simply to aging. The exact mechanism by which ventricular enlargement at the expense of brain volume causes symptoms is also not well understood.

▶ Clinical Findings

A. Symptoms and Signs

The most frequent symptom of chronic hydrocephalus is gait disorder that worsens either subacutely or chronically over weeks, months, or years. The gait impairment is classically described as "magnetic" (with "freezing" and inability to lift the feet off the floor) and "apraxic" (as if the patient cannot figure out how to move the legs to initiate and continue walking). The gait has parkinsonian features, with slowness, shuffling, imbalance, and shortened stride length. In contrast to patients with Parkinson disease, patients with normal pressure hydrocephalus frequently adopt a position offering a wide base of support, often with external rotation of the legs.

Urinary symptoms are also nearly a sine qua nonfinding in patients with hydrocephalus. Patients may have minor symptoms, such as increased urinary urgency and frequency. Alternately, unsuppressed bladder contractions together with decreased voluntary ability to keep the outlet closed can result in incontinence. There may be incontinence *sans gêne*, in which the affected individual seems unconcerned about the incontinence.

Cognitive symptoms usually occur after the onset of gait and urinary dysfunction. Impaired cognition ranges from subtle to severe. Typically, dementia is of a subcortical type, involving forgetfulness, inertia, bradyphrenia, apathy, decreased processing speed, and impairment in decision making, set switching, and other aspects of executive function. Patients with memory impairment often demonstrate seemingly poor learning and impaired delayed recall of learned material, with better recognition of learned material with cues; this pattern suggests a primary retrieval deficit rather than defective encoding of learned material (see Table 9–1). In severe cases, bradyphrenia may progress to an akinetic mute state.

B. Laboratory Findings and Imaging Studies

Routine laboratory blood testing is noninformative in patients with chronic hydrocephalus. Imaging studies using CT, or preferably MRI, are a key component in diagnosis of the condition. Specifically, central, ventricular enlargement out of proportion to peripheral sulcal enlargement is mandatory for consideration of this disorder (Figure 9–1). Frequently, there is an impression of sulcal effacement, presumably due to compression of the gyri from the increased central ventricular volume. Radiologists may not agree on whether the ventricular enlargement is indicative of hydrocephalus or represents, instead, dilation secondary to brain atrophy (in which sulcal enlargement is usually commensurate with ventricular enlargement). In addition to disproportionate ventricular enlargement, evidence of abnormal periventricular white matter, with low attenuation by CT or increased T2-weighted or fluid-attenuated inversion recovery (FLAIR) signal by MRI imaging studies, is suggestive of transependymal fluid flow, consistent with hydrocephalus; however, periventricular white matter signal change can be nonspecific. Other less diagnostic structural changes include ballooning of the anterior ventricular horns, disproportionately dilated temporal horns, and bowing and apparent thinning of the corpus callosum. If multiple CT or MRI studies are available over time, progressive enlargement of ventricular volume, without concomitant increase in the subarachnoid, sulcal spaces, can be useful in identifying progressive hydrocephalus.

C. Special Tests

Special tests are useful both in determining the likelihood that hydrocephalus is present and in determining the likelihood of responsiveness of the syndrome to CSF shunting. The most common and convenient test is a single large-volume lumbar puncture accompanied by videotaped recording before and after the procedure. Typically, a defined 8–10 m walk is videotaped before the procedure. The procedure consists of a standard lumbar puncture, but including withdrawal of approximately 40 mL of CSF, with recording of both opening and closing pressures. The patient is videotaped again at intervals after the lumbar puncture. Higher pressures, even within the normal range (eg, 12–20 cm H$_2$O), are possibly supportive of a diagnosis of hydrocephalus, whereas lower pressures are nonsupportive. A positive test result consists of improvement of gait after CSF removal. Occasionally cognition or urination also improves, but most often the beneficial response observed 1–72 hours post-procedure involves gait. Typically improvement lasts less than 1 week. Lack of any beneficial response is considered a negative test result. Tests other than CSF removal, including radionuclide cisternography, brain SPECT, brain magnetic resonance spectroscopy, and intracranial pressure wave monitoring, have not been proven to be of utility.

Although a clear positive response has some specificity, it may lack sensitivity, and some clinicians prefer to perform sequential multiple lumbar punctures over 3–5 days to improve sensitivity, particularly in patients with chronic disease of longer duration. More invasive chronic attenuation of CSF volume is provided by insertion of a continuous lumbar CSF drain for a period of 3–5 days, but the presence of an external drain conveys significant risk of CNS infection. These procedures also require videotaped pre- and post-procedure testing. Serial neuropsychological testing may also be informative.

▶ Differential Diagnosis

Injury at a variety of other levels of the nervous system can cause gait disorder and incontinence, including multiple infarcts in the brain, white matter disease, spinal cord compression, and sometimes polyradicular disease. Elderly individuals may also have urologic (peripheral) causes of incontinence: prostatic enlargement in men and sphincter disturbances in women. Other causes of dementia, including Alzheimer disease, may also cause incontinence.

▶ Treatment

The principal treatment for hydrocephalus is shunting of CSF from the ventricle. Ventriculoperitoneal shunts are most commonly used, now nearly always with externally programmable valves. In some patients, depending on bodily

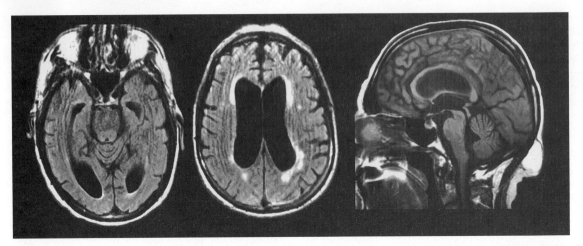

▲ **Figure 9–1.** MRI scans of the brain of a patient with dementia, gait disorder, and incontinence, who improved markedly post-shunting in all three domains. **Left and middle panels:** Axial FLAIR sequences showing markedly dilated ventricular system, including temporal horns (left panel) and prominent periventricular white matter signal hyperintensities (middle panel) consistent with transependymal flow from hydrocephalus. **Right panel:** Sagittal T1 sequence showing dilated ventricular system with marked bowing and thinning of corpus callosum.

habitus, ventriculoatrial or ventriculopleural shunts may be performed. Complications of shunting include "overshunting" with resultant headache, orthostatic symptoms, or development of subdural hematomas or hygromas; these problems can be obviated by checking the valve setting and changing the shunt-valve pressure. Shunt infections are rare, but may require removal of inserted hardware.

▶ **Prognosis**

Prognosis after shunting is most favorable in patients whose initial symptoms involve gait, in those with milder cognitive symptoms, in those with an identifiable secondary cause of hydrocephalus (eg, meningitis or subarachnoid hemorrhage), in those with positive spinal tap test, and possibly in those few patients who clearly have elevated intracranial pressure. Patients who first present with cognitive symptoms followed by gait and urinary involvement, as well as those with more severe cognitive symptoms or with marked sulcal atrophy, are less likely to have a favorable response to CSF shunting, possibly because their symptoms relate more to underlying Alzheimer disease. It is increasingly recognized that many persons with hydrocephalus may also be suffering from a neurodegenerative condition such as Alzheimer disease.

Eide PK, Sorteberg W. Diagnostic intracranial pressure monitoring and surgical management in idiopathic normal pressure hydrocephalus: A 6-year review of 214 patients. *Neurosurgery* 2010;66:80–91. [PMID: 20023540] (Review of the possible utility of intracranial pressure monitoring in predicting improvement after shunting.)

Finney GR. Normal pressure hydrocephalus. *Int Rev Neurobiol* 2009;84:263–281. [PMID: 19501723] (A review of imaging finding and prognostic variables predicting shunt responsiveness.)

Tarnaris A, Kitchen ND, Watkins LD. Noninvasive biomarkers in normal pressure hydrocephalus: Evidence for the role of neuroimaging. *J Neurosurg* 2009;110:837–851. [PMID: 18991499] (A review of studies of imaging and other biomarkers useful in selecting patients for shunting.)

▼ **TRANSIENT GLOBAL AMNESIA**

Clinton B. Wright, MD, MPH

 ESSENTIALS OF DIAGNOSIS

▶ Acute onset of anterograde amnesia (inability to form new short-term memories) lasting less than 24 hours

▶ Retrograde amnesia for events preceding the onset of symptoms of variable duration

▶ Diagnosis depends on eyewitness account

▶ No clouding of consciousness, loss of personal identity, or involvement of other cognitive domains

▶ No other focal neurologic symptoms or signs

▶ No recent seizures, active epilepsy, or recent head injury

General Considerations

During episodes of transient global amnesia, patients lose the ability to form new memories (termed *anterograde amnesia*), with a variable loss of episodic memory for events occurring before the attack (from minutes to decades in some cases; termed *retrograde amnesia*). About half of all attacks of transient global amnesia are temporally related to an emotionally stressful event or physical exertion. Many precipitants have been noted in the literature, including exercise, carrying heavy objects, driving, sexual intercourse, and immersion in hot or cold water. Transient global amnesia is relatively common, with an annual incidence between 3 and 10 per 100,000 people overall (higher in older age groups).

Pathogenesis

The cause of transient global amnesia is unknown. Neither an epileptic nor a vascular mechanism has been convincingly demonstrated, but epidemiologic evidence supports a greater prevalence among migraineurs. Dysfunction of the CA1 region of the hippocampus during attacks of transient global amnesia, and evidence that this region may be particularly vulnerable to various local stressors, suggests that this location may be in the critical path. The trigger for hippocampal dysfunction is not established, but numerous studies have documented a higher prevalence of internal jugular vein incompetence in those with transient global amnesia compared with controls. Venous congestion affecting the hippocampus in the setting of Valsalva is a postulated precipitant, but some studies support and others refute this hypothesis.

Clinical Findings

A. Symptoms and Signs

The typical patient with transient global amnesia is middle-aged or older (rarely under 40 years of age), and accurate diagnosis depends on having a witness to the attack to confirm the absence of seizure-like activity, recent head trauma, and any precipitating factors. During an attack, patients are alert and appear normal to casual inspection, except for anxiety about their loss of memory. Procedural memory remains intact during an episode, and patients are frequently able to carry out complex activities such as singing, driving, or playing an instrument during the acute phase. Patients often repeat the same question (eg, "How did we get here?" or "What are we doing?") and this feature should be sought from any witness. Memory for historical information preceding the onset of symptoms may be dramatically affected during an episode. For example, patients may be unable to remember that they are married, or that they have children. They may think they are still living at a prior address.

On examination, memory and orientation to place and time should be the only cognitive domains affected, and the neurologic examination should be otherwise normal. Short-term memory may be tested using delayed recall of words, figures, or the location of hidden objects. Attention should be normal. The patient's inability to recall his or her own identity suggests a psychogenic memory disturbance.

Attacks generally last about 4 hours but may persist as long as 24 hours. Once an attack has resolved and short-term recall has returned to normal, memory for events before the onset of the attack should return toward normal as time passes. However, patients usually remain amnestic for the episode itself and often for a brief period preceding the attack.

B. Diagnostic Studies

Current diagnostic studies cannot confirm the diagnosis of transient global amnesia, but they may be useful in ruling out other entities, such as stroke or epilepsy. Urine toxicology screening may help to exclude drug use, such as benzodiazepine intoxication. If there are vascular risk factors or if stroke is of particular concern in a given patient, an electrocardiogram should be obtained.

Brain imaging with MRI, or CT if the latter is unavailable, is recommended. Studies using MRI have found high signal on diffusion-weighted sequences in the medial temporal lobe(s) of subjects during and immediately after an attack, with normalization after symptoms resolve. Changes that persist or evolve on MRI or CT support an alternative diagnosis.

Differential Diagnosis

The presence of symptoms or signs suggestive of stroke, such as numbness, tingling, slurred speech, or weakness, especially those referable to the posterior circulation, should suggest stroke or transient ischemic attack. It is important to note that isolated infarction of the medial temporal lobe or thalamus can cause symptoms limited to an amnestic syndrome. Amnesia persisting beyond 24 hours should also suggest stroke, and brain imaging may confirm evolution of an infarct.

Amnesia during temporal lobe seizures is usually of much shorter duration than transient global amnesia and involves clouding of consciousness. Thus seizures can be mistaken for transient global amnesia if clouding of consciousness is missed, highlighting the necessity of a reliable informant that witnessed the attack. Multiple episodes in a short amount of time increase the likelihood of seizures, and serial electroencephalogram recordings may be necessary to rule out epilepsy in such cases. About 10% of patients experience headache during transient global amnesia, and an even larger number report a history of headache consistent with migraine. Given the potential for a common mechanism, patients without a prior diagnosis of migraine should be questioned further about the features and frequency of their headaches to allow for diagnosis and appropriate treatment.

Prognosis & Treatment

The prognosis after transient global amnesia appears to be excellent. When patients with transient global amnesia were compared with controls experiencing transient ischemic attacks in studies with long-term follow-up, a very low risk of subsequent transient ischemic attack and stroke, and other vascular outcomes comparable to those of normal controls, were demonstrated. Thus it is not necessary to begin antithrombotic therapy after a typical episode of transient global amnesia. A low risk of subsequent epilepsy has also been found in patients followed after a first episode, and treatment with antiepileptic drugs is not indicated. A brief hospital stay is warranted during the acute phase of the disorder to allow for an expeditious workup and brief observation to ensure resolution of symptoms, but a typical episode that has resolved by the time the patient is seen by a physician can be worked up in an ambulatory setting. Patients should be followed carefully; repeat imaging or electroencephalography can be obtained to ensure resolution of any abnormalities found on the initial examination. Recurrent episodes are uncommon (5–10% in some series), but a follow-up visit some weeks after the initial attack is recommended.

Bartsch T, Deuschl G. Transient global amnesia: Functional anatomy and clinical implications. *Lancet Neurol* 2010;9:205–214. [PMID: 20129169] (Review discussing refinement of the phenotype, updated imaging findings, and pathophysiology.)

Pantoni L, Lamassa M, Inzitari D. Transient global amnesia: A review emphasizing pathogenic aspects. *Acta Neurol Scand* 2000;102:275–283. [PMID: 11083503]

Quinette P, et al. Working memory and executive functions in transient global amnesia. *Brain* 2003;126(pt 9):1917–1934. [PMID: 12876141] (A small prospective study using detailed neuropsychological testing to examine working memory and executive function in relation to episodic memory in patients with transient global amnesia. Central executive function and working memory were not affected during attacks. The authors discuss transient global amnesia in relation to theories of memory.)

▼ HUNTINGTON DISEASE

Karen Marder, MD, MPH

▶ General Considerations

An autosomal-dominant neurodegenerative disorder characterized by motor, cognitive, and psychiatric deficits, Huntington disease (HD) is further discussed in Chapter 15. The gene associated with HD, the *HTT* gene, is located on chromosome 4 and contains a variably expanded trinucleotide repeat (CAG) sequence in exon 1. All individuals with 40 or more repeats will develop HD if they live long enough (full penetrance). CAG repeat length is inversely correlated with age of onset. Juvenile HD (before age 20 years) is associated with more than 60 repeats.

There are approximately 30,000 individuals with HD in the United States and 150,000 people who are at risk for the disease by virtue of having an affected parent. Among people of European ancestry, prevalence of HD is between 4 and 7 per 100,000 people; prevalence is lower among Chinese,

Japanese, and black Africans. Mean age of onset is 36–45 years of age; 6% of patients have juvenile onset.

HD includes impairments in motor, psychiatric, and cognitive function. The movement disorder is related to striatal pathology and consists of chorea, dystonia, parkinsonism, eye movement abnormalities, motor impersistence, and gait abnormalities. Psychiatric symptoms are common but variable and seem to cluster in some families and not in others. Cognitive impairment, secondary to dysfunction in frontostriatal pathways, is an invariable feature of this illness, although the onset of neuropsychological dysfunction is variable, as is its severity.

▶ Clinical Findings

Impairments in speed of processing, attention, verbal fluency, executive function, and visuospatial function have been described. Among individuals with symptomatic HD, deficits in executive function are prominent. Patients' ability to plan, organize, and monitor behavior is impaired. These domains of function have been closely associated with the frontal lobes and the frontostriatal circuits.

Patients with HD do not have a primary disorder of memory retention, but appear unable to acquire information efficiently or retrieve it consistently. in contrast to patients with Alzheimer disease (AD), patients with HD show marked improvement in response to cued recall, similar to that in other patients with frontal lobe disease. Unlike the cortical dementias, such as AD, HD does not prominently involve language until late in the illness.

Studies that have focused on carriers of an expanded CAG repeat (premanifest HD) who do not yet meet motor criteria for HD have documented clinical and biological changes associated with the disease up to 15 years before the predicted age at onset, with the most prominent cognitive impairments increasing during the decade before motor diagnosis. Compared with non-carriers, deficits in psychomotor speed (speeded finger tapping, self-paced tapping) may be the most sensitive cognitive measures to predict age at onset during the decade before diagnosis. Using traditional neuropsychological tests, 40% of premanifest individuals meet criteria for mild cognitive impairment (using cutoff scores 1.5 standard deviation [sd] below the mean of a comparison group). The prevalence of MCI increases as individuals get closer to their estimated age at onset of diagnosis. The majority have non-amnestic MCI (18%), followed by amnestic MCI (7.5%). Processing speed and impairment in episodic memory are the most commonly affected domains in premanifest HD. During the premanifest period, individuals may recognize subtle functional decline in capacity to perform their jobs and handle financial affairs.

▶ Differential Diagnosis

The differential diagnosis of HD dementia includes any dementing process that accompanies a hyperkinetic movement disorder, especially Creutzfeldt-Jakob disease, HIV dementia (in cases with chorea), and Wilson disease. Chorea and cognitive impairment may also occur with systemic lupus erythematosus or Graves disease. Because individuals with HD have a propensity for falls, the sudden onset of cognitive impairment or rapid worsening of cognition should suggest the possibility of subdural hematoma, and imaging should be performed immediately.

▶ Treatment

There is currently no effective treatment for HD dementia. A phase III multicenter trial of latrepirdine to assess performance on the MMSE and change in function is ongoing.

▶ Prognosis

Neuropsychological dysfunction worsens with the progression of the disease, but duration of illness is not a robust predictor of cognitive performance. Functional disability is strongly related to cognitive dysfunction, and neuropsychological dysfunction and depression are more important as predictors of overall function than motor impairment or chorea.

Duff K, et al. Mild cognitive impairment in prediagnosed Huntington disease. *Neurology* 2010;75:500–507. [PMID: 20610833] (First article to systematically use research criteria to define mild cognitive impairment in premanifest HD.)

Paulsen JS, et al. Neuropsychiatric aspects of Huntington's disease. *J Neurol Neurosurg Psychiatry* 2001;71:310–314. [PMID: 11511702]

Paulsen JS, et al. Detection of Huntington's disease decades before diagnosis: the Predict-HD study. *J Neurol Neurosurg Psychiatry* 2009;79:874–880. [PMID: 18096682] (This is the largest, most comprehensive study of individuals with premanifest HD.)

Sturrock A, Leavitt BR. The clinical and genetic features of Huntington disease. *J Geriatr Psychiatry Neurol* 2010;23:243–259. [PMID: 20923757] (Current review of neurobiology and clinical features of Huntington's disease.)

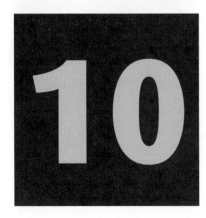

Cerebrovascular Disease: Ischemic Stroke

Brian-Fred M. Fitzsimmons, MD, & Marc Lazzaro, MD

ESSENTIALS OF DIAGNOSIS

▶ Sudden onset of focal neurologic deficits

▶ Initial computed tomographic (CT) scan of the head that excludes intracranial hemorrhage or mass lesion

▶ Follow-up brain imaging showing evidence of acute infarction

▶ Older age and other vascular risk factors (common)

▶ Rapid diagnosis is required to initiate thrombolytic therapy within 3 hours of onset

▶ General Considerations

Throughout the world, the public health burden of stroke is staggering. Stroke is one of the four leading causes of death in most countries, and the number one cause of severe neurologic disability in adults. In the United States alone, there are more than 4 million stroke survivors and more than 750,000 new strokes each year. The risk of stroke increases exponentially with age, with the highest incidence of stroke occurring in people older than 65 years. Men are affected more often than women (1.5:1), although women account for more than 60% of all stroke fatalities. In fact, more women die of stroke than of breast cancer in every decade of life. Blacks have more than twice the risk of stroke as compared with whites, whereas the risk for Hispanics is intermediate between the two.

The World Health Organization defines stroke clinically as "rapidly developing clinical signs of focal (at times global) disturbance of cerebral function, lasting for more than 24 hours or leading to death, with no apparent cause other than of vascular origin." Stroke, therefore, encompasses three major cerebrovascular disorders: ischemic stroke, primary intracerebral hemorrhage, and spontaneous subarachnoid hemorrhage. Ischemic stroke, or cerebral infarction, is the most common, accounting for approximately 70–80% of all strokes. Intracerebral hemorrhage and subarachnoid hemorrhage are classified as hemorrhagic strokes and are discussed in Chapter 11.

A transient ischemic attack (TIA) is an episode of focal brain ischemia in which all symptoms resolve within 24 hours. Most TIAs, however, usually resolve within 1–2 hours. TIAs that last longer than 3 hours may actually be "short-lived strokes," as more than 50% of these patients have evidence of brain infarction on magnetic resonance imaging (MRI). After a TIA, between 10% and 15% of patients suffer an ischemic stroke within 3 months, the majority of which occur in the first 48 hours. Therefore, both TIA and stroke are true medical emergencies and should be treated with the same urgency and level of medical resources as chest pain and acute myocardial infarction. Because TIAs are caused by the same pathogenic mechanisms as ischemic stroke (see Pathogenesis, later), they can be evaluated and managed in a similar fashion.

Johnston SC, et al. Short-term prognosis after emergency department diagnosis of TIA. *JAMA* 2000;284:2901–2906. [PMID: 11147987] (Large cohort study demonstrating a high incidence of stroke within 48 hours of a TIA.)

▶ Pathogenesis

As the name implies, ischemic stoke is caused by focal cerebral ischemia, a localized reduction in blood flow sufficient to disrupt neuronal metabolism and function. If ischemia is not reversed within a critical period, irreversible cellular injury ensues, resulting in cerebral infarction. Pathologically, cerebral infarction appears as focal pan-necrosis of neurons, glia, and blood vessels.

Although infarction by definition is ultimately the result of inadequate blood flow, several distinct mechanisms may disrupt cerebral blood flow to produce an ischemic stroke. The pathologic process responsible for the specific mechanism of infarction is then often used to categorize ischemic stroke into different etiologic subtypes, outlined next.

A. Cardioembolic Stroke

Emboli originating from the heart cause between 15% and 30% of ischemic strokes, depending on the population studied, and may be the most commonly identified cause overall. Cardiac emboli can travel into the cerebral circulation and obstruct cerebral blood flow by occluding an artery at the point where the lumen diameter equals the size of the embolic material. Common sources of cardioembolism include intracardiac and mural thrombi created by atrial fibrillation, a dilated cardiomyopathy with reduced ejection fraction, and wall motion abnormalities after myocardial infarction. Valvular heart disease is another common cause of cardiac thromboembolism, particularly rheumatic heart disease, severe mitral regurgitation or stenosis, prosthetic heart valves, and endocarditis (infectious and marantic). In patients with acute and subacute bacterial endocarditis, emboli may contain bacteria in addition to thrombus (septic emboli). A rare cause of cardiac embolism is atrial myxoma, in which emboli may be largely composed of neoplastic cells.

A paradoxic embolus refers to a thrombus in the venous circulation that travels to the heart and crosses into the arterial circulation through a cardiac defect, usually a patent foramen ovale. In addition to thrombus, other particulate matter may rarely enter the venous circulation and embolize through a cardiac defect. Examples include fat from a major bone fracture and air from trauma or surgical procedures involving the lungs, dural sinuses, or jugular veins. Nitrogen bubbles can also be created in the bloodstream after a rapid reduction in barometric pressure, such as in scuba divers surfacing too quickly, and may embolize to the cerebral circulation to produce an ischemic stroke.

Cardiac emboli produce both large and small branch occlusions of the major cerebral arteries, depending on the size of the embolic material. Cardioembolic occlusions usually recanalize, with up to 90% no longer visible on angiography after 48 hours. This tendency to recanalize may contribute to the high frequency of hemorrhagic transformation after cardioembolic stroke (see Management of Complications, later).

B. Atherosclerotic Stroke

Atherosclerotic infarctions account for approximately 14–25% of ischemic strokes and affect men more than twice as often as women. These strokes are associated with the accumulation of atherosclerotic plaque within the lumen of large or medium-sized arteries, usually at a bifurcation or curve in the blood vessel. Any artery from the aortic arch to the circle of Willis can be affected, but the most common sites of atherosclerosis related to stroke are the junction of the common and internal carotid artery, the origins of the middle and anterior cerebral arteries, and the origins of the

vertebral arteries. Overall, atherosclerotic infarctions are equally caused by intracranial and extracranial atherosclerotic disease, although extracranial atherosclerosis is more common in whites, and intracranial atherosclerosis is more common in blacks, Hispanics, and Asians.

Atherosclerotic strokes are immediately caused by one of three mechanisms. Embolic material can dislodge from a plaque and occlude a more distal cerebral artery. The atherosclerotic plaque may cause progressive stenosis of an artery that eventually leads to complete occlusion and infarction from local thrombosis. Finally, ischemia may develop distal to a severe atherosclerotic narrowing or occlusion as a result of progressive perfusion failure in the setting of inadequate collateral blood flow.

C. Lacunar Stroke

Lacunar infarctions, or small vessel strokes, account for 15–30% of ischemic strokes. These infarcts are usually less than 1 cm in diameter and are caused by the occlusion of a single small penetrating artery that supplies one of the deep structures in the brain, such as the internal capsule, basal ganglia, corona radiata, thalamus, and brainstem. The cause of the small vessel occlusion is generally considered to be endothelial damage from long-standing hypertension or diabetes, manifest as lipohyalinosis or microatheroma narrowing the penetrating artery to the point of occlusion through thrombosis. Rarely, small vessel occlusions may also be caused by atherosclerosis of the parent vessel from which they arise, or proximal microemboli. In up to 25% of patients with documented lacunar infarcts on neuroimaging, alternative stroke etiologies are also present, such as large artery atherosclerosis and cardiac sources of embolism.

D. Cryptogenic Stroke

In most series, between 20% and 40% of all strokes are of undetermined cause, or "cryptogenic." These infarcts often appear to have an embolic cause, but despite a complete diagnostic evaluation, no source of embolism can be found. Transesophageal echocardiography (TEE) suggests that patent foramen ovale and aortic arch atheroma may cause some of these strokes. Hypercoagulable states, such as the antiphospholipid antibody syndrome and factor V Leiden gene mutation, may also be responsible for some cryptogenic infarctions.

E. Other Causes of Ischemic Stroke

Other determined causes cumulatively account for less than 5% of ischemic stroke. Arterial dissections, particularly of the carotid and vertebral arteries, cause approximately 2% of all ischemic strokes, but approximately 20% of strokes in patients younger than 30 years of age. Arterial dissections may be spontaneous or traumatic and lead to cerebral infarction through artery-to-artery embolization, local thrombosis, or perfusion failure in approximately 50% of untreated

Table 10–1. Less Common Causes of Ischemic Stroke

Category	Disease
Vascular	Arterial dissection Fibromuscular dysplasia Moyamoya disease CADASIL syndrome (cerebral autosomal-dominant arteriopathy with subcortical infarcts and leukoencephalopathy)

Hematologic	Sickle cell disease
	Polycythemia vera
	Essential thrombocytosis
	Thrombotic thrombocytopenic purpura
	Waldenström macroglobulinemia
	Paroxysmal nocturnal hemoglobinuria
	Hypercoagulable states:
	  • Antiphospholipid antibody syndrome (lupus anticoagulant, anticardiolipin antibodies)
	  • Protein C, protein S, and antithrombin III deficiency
	  • Factor V Leiden and prothrombin gene mutations

Inflammatory	Primary central nervous system vasculitis
	Secondary vasculitis associated with systemic disorders:
	  • Polyarteritis nodosa, giant cell arteritis, Wegener granulomatosis, Churg-Strauss syndrome, Sjögren syndrome,
	    Behçet syndrome, lupus erythematosus, Takayasu arteritis, Sneddon syndrome

Drug-related	Cocaine/crack, amphetamines, heroin, PCP, LSD, marijuana Oral contraceptives, hormone-replacement therapy, tamoxifen Intravenous immunoglobulin
Infectious	Endocarditis Meningitis (bacterial, tuberculosis, fungal, amebic) Meningovascular syphilis, neuroborreliosis Hepatitis C with cryoglobulinemia HIV
Malignant	Leukemia (leukostasis) Angiocentric lymphomatosis Hypercoagulability associated with malignancy (Trousseau syndrome)
Metabolic	Homocystinuria Fabry disease MELAS syndrome (mitochondrial encephalomyopathy, lactic acidosis, and strokelike episodes)
Other	Migraine

LSD = lysergic acid diethylamide; PCP = phencyclidine.

patients. Other less common conditions that also cause ischemic stroke are listed in Table 10–1.

Homma S, et al. Effect of medical treatment in stroke patients with patent foramen ovale: Patent Foramen Ovale in Cryptogenic Stroke Study. *Circulation* 2002;105:2625–2631. [PMID: 12045168] (Patent foramen ovale was present in 34% of stroke patients receiving TEE. There was no difference in the risk of recurrent stroke between patients treated with aspirin or warfarin.)

Kremmer C, et al. Carotid dissection with permanent and transient occlusion or severe stenosis: Long-term outcome. *Neurology* 2003;60:271–275. [PMID: 12552043] (This series reports a relatively small long-term risk [0.3–0.7% per year] of ischemic stroke ipsilateral to a carotid dissection).

▶ Clinical Findings

A. Symptoms and Signs

The clinical hallmark of ischemic stroke is the sudden onset of focal neurologic deficits. Typically, new symptoms develop over seconds to minutes, or they may be present on waking from sleep. Headache is reported in approximately 25% of patients with ischemic stroke but is more common in patients with intracerebral or subarachnoid hemorrhage. Nausea and vomiting occur, particularly with stroke involving the brainstem and cerebellum. Decreased level of consciousness is unusual in the first several hours after ischemic stroke, unless the brainstem reticular activating system is affected. Hypertension is present acutely in more than 70% of cases but often returns to baseline spontaneously over the next several days.

Further evolution of neurologic symptoms depends on the mechanism of ischemic stroke and the degree of collateral blood flow. All infarction subtypes, from embolic to lacunar, may have fluctuating symptoms after onset, likely representing varying degrees of collateral blood flow to the ischemic tissue. TIAs precede ischemic infarction in only 20% of cases, and although they are more likely to be associated with atherosclerotic disease, they may precede any ischemic stroke subtype. In approximately 10–30% of patients with acute ischemic stroke, neurologic deficits progressively worsen over the first 24–48 hours; such a course is called *stroke in evolution* or *progressing stroke.* Stroke progression is likely caused by multiple mechanisms, including ongoing ischemia, inflammation, and glutamate-induced excitotoxicity, and is almost as common in the setting of lacunar infarction as in large vessel occlusions. The so-called *spectacular shrinking deficit* can occur when an embolus first lodges in a large proximal vessel, producing a large hemispheric ischemic syndrome, but then breaks apart and migrates distally into a smaller arterial branch, resulting in a much smaller clinical syndrome.

The specific neurologic deficits caused by an ischemic stroke are completely determined by the region of brain rendered ischemic, which in turn is determined by the artery occluded, the degree of collateral blood flow, and the presence of any vascular anatomical variants. A complete discussion of cerebrovascular anatomy is beyond the scope of this chapter, but a comprehensive understanding of the clinical syndromes associated with specific arterial occlusions is essential to the diagnosis and treatment of acute ischemic stroke.

1. Middle cerebral artery syndromes—The first segment of the middle cerebral artery (MCA) is called the *MCA stem* (or *M1 segment*), from which numerous small lenticulostriate arteries arise to penetrate and supply the internal capsule and basal ganglia. The MCA stem usually ends in a bifurcation, which gives rise to the superior and inferior divisions of the MCA. The superior division of the MCA supplies the lateral frontal lobe, anterior lateral parietal lobe, and insula, whereas the inferior division supplies the posterior lateral parietal lobe and lateral temporal lobe.

Occlusion of the MCA stem produces a complete MCA infarction with contralateral hemiparesis, sensory loss, homonymous hemianopia, and conjugate gaze paresis. Infarction in the dominant hemisphere produces global aphasia as well; infarction in the nondominant hemisphere results in impaired spatial perception and contralateral neglect. The weakness from a complete MCA infarction is severe, usually complete paralysis, and affects the face, arm, and leg equally due to the involvement of the posterior limb of the internal capsule. Sensory loss may also be severe, but proprioceptive and discriminative modalities are generally more affected than pain and temperature sensation. Contralateral homonymous hemianopia results from disruption of the optic radiations in the parietal and temporal white matter. The precise origin of the paresis of contralateral conjugate gaze

(eyes deviated toward the side of the infarction) is more controversial but usually implies a large infarction. Gaze deviation commonly resolves within 1–2 weeks.

Infarction resulting from an occlusion of the superior division of the MCA produces a contralateral hemiparesis and sensory loss that affects the face and arm more than the leg, due to the sparing of the internal capsule and the topographic organization of the motor and sensory cortices (face and arm lateral, leg medial). The weakness and sensory loss also tend to be worse distally than proximally. Paresis of contralateral conjugate gaze is often present, but a homonymous hemianopia should not occur. For superior division infarcts in the dominant hemisphere, the involvement of the frontal operculum produces a predominantly motor aphasia (Broca aphasia) with nonfluent speech and impaired writing but relatively preserved comprehension. Nondominant superior division infarcts may also produce hemineglect and spatial disorders, usually less severe than with complete MCA infarctions.

Infarction in the territory of the inferior division of the MCA often produces a contralateral homonymous hemianopia or quadrantanopia but little or no weakness, sensory loss, or gaze paresis. Inferior division infarctions in the dominant hemisphere result in sensory aphasias (Wernicke type), with fluent, often nonsensical speech filled with perseveration and paraphasic errors, as well as severely impaired comprehension and reading. Nondominant hemisphere infarcts can produce prominent contralateral neglect, impairments in spatial perception, and occasionally dramatic behavioral disorders.

Hemineglect refers to varying degrees of inattention to visual, auditory, and tactile stimuli from one side of space (usually the left). Frequently accompanying severe neglect are anosognosia, the unawareness of illness or disability, and asomatognosia, the failure to recognize a body part as belonging to oneself. Problems with spatial perception include constructional and dressing apraxias and loss of topographic memory. Rarely, severe confusion and delirium follow infarction, involving the nondominant parietal-temporal region.

2. Anterior cerebral artery syndromes—The anterior cerebral artery (ACA) predominantly supplies the medial portion of the frontal lobes. Unilateral ACA infarction usually produces contralateral leg weakness and sensory loss, distally greater than proximally. With involvement of the supplementary motor area, patients may appear to have a complete hemiparesis involving the arm as well, but they more likely have a form of motor neglect (a disinclination to move the contralateral limbs) in the absence of true arm weakness. Unilateral ACA infarctions can also produce various speech disturbances, most typically involving impairments in the initiation of spontaneous speech, but sometimes suggesting aphasia. Urinary incontinence can occur with either unilateral or bilateral ACA infarction.

Bilateral ACA territory infarction, which can occur in the setting of an incomplete circle of Willis, produces severe behavioral abnormalities including abulia (lack of will), muteness, motor inertia, psychomotor retardation, incontinence, and diffusely increased muscle tone. Severely affected patients display akinetic mutism; although awake with their eyes open, they do not speak or move unless encouraged by noxious stimuli.

3. Internal carotid artery syndromes—Through artery-to-artery embolization, internal carotid artery disease can produce the typical syndromes of MCA and ACA infarction. Embolization to the central retinal artery branch of the ophthalmic artery produces ipsilateral monocular blindness. The monocular blindness usually lasts less than 15 minutes (transient monocular blindness [amaurosis fugax]), but can be permanent.

Internal carotid artery occlusion can be asymptomatic or produce holohemispheric infarction, depending on the extent of collateral blood flow through the circle of Willis. In the setting of limited collateral blood supply, high-grade carotid stenosis or occlusion may induce symptoms through hemodynamic perfusion failure in the border zone (or "watershed") regions between the middle, anterior, and posterior cerebral artery territories. Symptoms include varying degrees of contralateral weakness, sensory loss, homonymous hemianopia, and aphasia or hemineglect. With the location of the MCA-ACA border zone at the upper portion of frontal-parietal convexity, the weakness usually affects the proximal arm and leg, with sparing of the face. Given the hemodynamic mechanism of the ischemia, symptoms frequently resolve and recur in a stereotyped fashion, creating stereotyped TIAs before complete infarction.

4. Posterior cerebral artery syndromes—The most proximal segment of the posterior cerebral artery (PCA) gives rise to numerous small penetrating arteries to the midbrain and thalamus. The PCA then crosses over the medial edge of the tentorium and supplies the occipital lobe and the inferior medial temporal lobe. Occlusion of the PCA most often produces a contralateral homonymous hemianopia due to infarction of the visual cortex in the occipital lobe. A pattern of macular sparing may be seen (preservation of central vision) as a result of collateral blood supply from the MCA to the occipital pole. When infarction involves the dominant hemisphere, there may be inability to read without other signs of aphasia (alexia without agraphia).

Bilateral PCA infarction may produce complete cortical blindness, or true tunnel vision (funnel vision) if macular vision is spared. In some instances, patients may be completely unaware that they are cortically blind, and even deny it on direct questioning (Anton syndrome). If the primary visual cortex is spared, bilateral occipital lobe injury may result in a variety of visual agnosias or achromatopsia. Impaired memory may be a prominent feature of bilateral PCA infarction if the inferomedial temporal lobe or medial thalamus is affected. Rarely, large bilateral PCA infarcts can produce behavioral disturbance, including agitated delirium.

Proximal occlusions of the PCA result in thalamic infarction, with severe contralateral sensory loss, or mid-brain infarction, with contralateral hemiparesis and ipsilateral occulomotor nerve palsy (Weber syndrome). There may be contralateral ataxia from involvement of cerebellar projections, or contralateral hemiballism from infarction of the subthalamic nucleus.

5. Vertebrobasilar syndromes—The vertebral arteries and basilar artery supply the major structures of the posterior fossa (brainstem and cerebellum). Ischemia of the posterior fossa is suggested by symptoms of diplopia, vertigo, hearing loss, circumoral numbness, dysphagia, hiccups, nausea and vomiting, decreased level of consciousness, and bilateral symptoms. On examination, posterior fossa infarction is supported by the presence of dysconjugate gaze, Horner syndrome, nystagmus, unilateral pharyngeal weakness, prominent ataxia, and bilateral or crossed (ipsilateral face, contralateral arm and leg) motor and sensory deficits. Infarcts in the medulla, pons, and midbrain produce several characteristic clinical syndromes (Table 10–2).

Acute infarction restricted to the cerebellum can occur from an occlusion of a superior cerebellar artery (SCA), an anterior inferior cerebellar artery (AICA), or a posterior inferior cerebellar artery (PICA). SCA cerebellar infarctions often have prominent dysarthria, ipsilateral limb ataxia, truncal ataxia, and nystagmus (fast phase generally toward lesion), but commonly have a very good prognosis. AICA infarcts usually involve the lateral pons in addition to the anterolateral region of the cerebellum, but rarely can produce isolated ipsilateral hemiataxia from pure cerebellar infarction, or isolated vertigo from infarction of the vestibular nuclei or nerve. PICA infarcts are the most common cerebellar infarctions and usually produce truncal ataxia, ipsilateral limb ataxia, and acute vertigo with nystagmus (fast phase away from lesion). PICA infarcts are also most likely to develop life-threatening edema and mass effect leading to acute hydrocephalus (from compression of the fourth ventricle), brainstem compression, and tonsillar herniation. Severe headache, nausea and vomiting, and somnolence are all symptoms of cerebellar infarction that may signal increasing mass effect requiring emergent intervention (see Management of Complications, later).

Occlusion of the basilar artery can also have catastrophic consequences. Occlusion of the distal basilar artery is usually embolic in origin, and can produce the "top of the basilar" syndrome from bilateral infarction of the midbrain, thalamus, and occipital and medial temporal lobes. Impairment in level of consciousness is the rule, ranging from somnolence to coma. If coma is not present, all the symptoms previously described for PCA infarction may occur. Peduncular hallucinosis, another symptom of distal basilar ischemia, refers to vivid, well-formed, often colorful visual hallucinations. Pupillary and eye movement abnormalities are also typical of the "top of the basilar" syndrome. Pupils are generally midsized and unreactive (midbrain pupils) and may be

Table 10–2. Brainstem Stroke Syndromes

Syndrome	Occluded Artery	Clinical Findings	Structures Involved
Medullary			
Medial medulla	Anterior spinal branch of distal vertebral artery	Contralateral arm and leg weakness Ipsilateral tongue weakness Contralateral loss of sensation (light touch, proprioception, vibration) (Above symptoms may be bilateral)	Pyramidal tract Hypoglossal nerve fibers Medial lemniscus
Lateral medulla (Wallenberg syndrome)	Distal vertebral artery (± PICA) Rarely, PICA alone	Ipsilateral limb ataxia Loss of pain and temperature sensation on ipsilateral face and contralateral body Ipsilateral Horner syndrome Vertigo and nystagmus Nausea and vomiting Hoarseness, dysphagia, and hiccups	Inferior cerebellar peduncle (± cerebellum) Spinal tract and nucleus of trigeminal nerve and spinothalamic tract Descending sympathetic fibers Vestibular nuclei Vestibular nuclei or dorsal tegmentum Nucleus ambiguus and fibers of glossopharyngeal and vagus nerves
Pontine			
Medial pons	Paramedian pontine perforators from basilar artery	Contralateral arm and leg weakness Dysarthria Sometimes, contralateral ataxia *plus* <u>Inferior infarcts:</u> Ipsilateral facial weakness Ipsilateral abducens weakness (ventral lesion) *or* Paralysis of conjugate gaze to the side of infarction (dorsal lesion) <u>Superior infarcts:</u> Contralateral facial weakness Internuclear ophthalmoplegia	Pyramidal tract Corticobulbar tract Crossing fibers to middle cerebellar peduncle Facial nerve fibers Abducens nerve fibers Pontine gaze center Corticobulbar fibers to facial nucleus Medial longitudinal fasciculus
Lateral pons • Inferiorly	AICA	Ipsilateral limb ataxia Loss of sensation on ipsilateral face and contralateral body Vertigo and nystagmus Unilateral deafness and tinnitus Ipsilateral facial weakness Ipsilateral Horner syndrome	Middle cerebellar peduncle (± cerebellum) Spinal tract and nucleus of trigeminal nerve and spinothalamic tract Vestibular nucleus, flocculus Cochlear nucleus of inner ear Facial nerve fibers Descending sympathetic fibers
• Superiorly	SCA and long circumferential branches of basilar artery	Ipsilateral limb ataxia Dysarthria Contralateral loss of pain and temperature sensation of face, arm, and leg Ipsilateral Horner syndrome Occasionally, ipsilateral choreoathetosis Occasionally, hearing loss	Superior cerebellar peduncle Paravermian cerebellum Mesencephalic trigeminal tract and spinothalamic tract Descending sympathetic fibers Superior cerebellar peduncle (or dentate) Lateral lemniscus

(Continued)

Table 10–2. Brainstem Stroke Syndromes (*Continued*)

Syndrome	Occluded Artery	Clinical Findings	Structures Involved
Midbrain			
Midbrain peduncle (Weber syndrome)	Paramedian peduncular branches of proximal PCA	Weakness of contralateral face, arm, and leg Ipsilateral paresis of medial rectus and vertical gaze, with mydriasis	Corticospinal and corticobulbar tracts Oculomotor nerve fibers
Midbrain tegmentum	Paramedian tegmental branches of PCA	Ipsilateral paresis of medial rectus and vertical gaze, with mydriasis Contralateral limb ataxia Contralateral choreoathetosis and hemiballism	Oculomotor nerve fibers Superior cerebellar peduncle Red nucleus

AICA = Anterior inferior cerebellar artery; PCA = posterior cerebral artery; PICA = posterior inferior cerebral artery; SCA = Superior cerebellar artery; ±, with or without.

oval and eccentrically positioned (corectopia). Abnormalities of vertical gaze are the most common eye movement abnormality and may be accompanied by convergence nystagmus. The combination of impaired vertical gaze and loss of the pupillary light reflex defines the Parinaud syndrome. Bilateral ptosis and abnormal retraction of the upper lids (Collier sign) are also signs of tectal injury. Severe quadriparesis with decorticate or decerebrate posturing may result from bilateral infarction of the midbrain peduncles or upper pons.

Occlusion of the proximal basilar artery can result in the locked-in syndrome, caused by extensive bilateral infarction of the ventral pons, with sparing of the midbrain through collateral blood flow. Patients are quadriplegic but completely awake and alert due to an intact reticular activating system. Vertical eye movements are usually preserved (horizontal eye movements and blinking less often) and serve as the only means of interaction with the outside world. Patients can usually communicate using these limited movements, demonstrating complete awareness of their disabilities and their environment.

6. Lacunar syndromes—Occlusions of single small perforating arteries supplying deep structures in the brain result in the clinical spectrum of lacunar infarctions. The most common arteries involved are the lenticulostriate branches of the MCAs supplying the internal capsule, basal ganglia, and corona radiata; the thalamoperforate branches of the PCAs supplying the thalamus; and the paramedian penetrating branches of the basilar artery supplying the pons. Several distinct clinical syndromes are associated with lacunar ischemic disease.

The most common lacunar syndrome is pure motor hemiparesis, which most often results from infarction of the contralateral internal capsule but may also be seen with infarcts in the corona radiata or the pons. The syndrome is clinically diagnosed with greatest confidence when the face,

arm, and leg are equally affected and there is no evidence of sensory loss, homonymous hemianopia, aphasia, or hemineglect.

With another typical lacunar syndrome, the pure sensory stroke, infarction almost always involves the thalamus. Typically, sensory loss is present throughout the contralateral side, but various partial hemisensory syndromes can occur. Sensation is usually decreased for all sensory modalities, and no other neurologic deficits are present. Patients often complain of abnormal spontaneous sensations, such as "pins-and-needles" or skin tightness. The Dejerine-Roussy syndrome is a complication of thalamic infarction characterized by severe, intractable pain and allodynia (pain produced by tactile stimuli) on the affected side. The pain may develop within days to months after the stroke, but often appears as the sensory loss is improving. Relief has been reported with the use of tricyclic antidepressants or gabapentin.

Sensorimotor stroke, another lacunar syndrome, is characterized by the combination of contralateral weakness and sensory loss in the absence of any visual, language, or cognitive disturbance. Infarcts usually involve both the internal capsule and adjacent thalamus.

The syndrome of ataxic hemiparesis consists of contralateral weakness and limb ataxia. Weakness and ataxia are present on the same side, with the ataxia usually more severe than the weakness. Infarctions associated with this syndrome most commonly occur in the pons, the internal capsule, or the corona radiata.

Another lacunar syndrome, the dysarthria clumsy-hand syndrome, may be a variant of ataxic hemiparesis. It is characterized by prominent dysarthria and ataxia of the upper limb. Other symptoms, however, are frequently present as well, including facial weakness, dysphagia, and varying degrees of weakness in the arm and leg. The dysarthria clumsy-hand syndrome is associated with infarction in the internal capsule or the pons.

B. Laboratory Findings

Currently, there are no laboratory findings diagnostic of cerebral infarction. All patients, however, should be evaluated with a complete blood count (CBC), prothrombin time (PT) and partial thromboplastin time (PTT), basic metabolic panel (Chem-7), fingerstick blood glucose level, and cardiac enzymes.

1. Complete blood count—The CBC is useful to detect anemia, leukocytosis, and abnormal platelet number. Anemia might suggest the presence of occult gastrointestinal bleeding, which would increase the risk of thrombolysis, anticoagulation, and even antiplatelet therapy. Anemia may also be associated with occult malignancy, which can produce a hypercoagulable state, or produce neurologic symptoms as a result of metastatic or paraneoplastic disease. Inflammatory and collagen vascular disorders, which can cause anemia, are also rare causes of ischemic stroke. Leukocytosis might reflect systemic infection, including endocarditis, or perhaps aspiration pneumonia secondary to dysphagia or decreased level of consciousness. Profound elevations in leukocyte count, as seen in acute leukemia, can lead to leukostasis within the cerebral arteries and subsequent cerebral infarction. A platelet count of less than 100,000/mm^3 is an absolute contraindication to treatment with intravenous recombinant tissue plasminogen activator (IV rt-PA) and increases the risk of treatment with anticoagulants and antiplatelet agents. Thrombocytopenia may also be associated with chronic diseases, such as HIV and collagen vascular disorders, or may be secondary to thrombotic thrombocytopenic purpura, a syndrome associated with cerebral ischemia.

2. PT and PTT—Significant elevations in the PT (international normalized ratio [INR] > 1.5) or PTT are also absolute contraindications to IV rt-PA therapy. An elevated PT may also suggest chronic treatment with warfarin, the indication for which may be relevant to the etiology of acute stroke, or it may be the result of chronic liver disease. An elevated PTT suggests heparin use in hospitalized patients; it may also reflect the presence of antiphospholipid antibodies, particularly lupus anticoagulant.

3. Basic metabolic panel and fingerstick blood glucose level—The Chem-7 provides a measurement of the basic electrolytes, serum creatinine, and blood glucose. Elevations in serum creatinine may indicate chronic renal disease, particularly relevant in patients with diabetes and hypertension, which increases the risk of renal toxicity from contrast agents used with CT scanning and angiography. Sodium and glucose abnormalities are common causes of metabolic encephalopathy. Hypoglycemia is notorious for sometimes producing focal neurologic deficits in the absence of acute cerebral ischemia; for this reason, a fingerstick blood glucose level should be checked immediately in all patients with symptoms of acute stroke.

4. Cardiac enzymes—Cardiac enzymes, such as cardiac troponin and creatine kinase-MB fraction, are measured to exclude concomitant myocardial ischemia. Approximately 20–30% of patients with acute ischemic stroke have a history of symptomatic coronary artery disease, and another 20–40% likely have presymptomatic coronary artery disease. Ischemic stroke can occur secondary to an acute myocardial infarction, and, conversely, the surge of adrenergic hormones that frequently accompanies acute stroke can sometimes trigger myocardial ischemia. Early detection and treatment of acute myocardial ischemia significantly improves survival and outcome.

5. Other tests—Several other laboratory tests may also be useful in evaluating patients with ischemic stroke. Hepatic function tests screen for liver disease, particularly important in patients with an unexplained elevation in the PT or a predominantly cognitive syndrome that could be explained by hepatic encephalopathy. Baseline hepatic function tests are also required when starting potentially hepatotoxic statin therapy. Urine toxicology should be especially considered in younger patients to screen for the use of illicit drugs associated with cerebral infarction, including cocaine, amphetamines, heroin, LSD, PCP, and, rarely, marijuana. An elevated erythrocyte sedimentation rate (ESR) can reflect systemic inflammatory disease, including vasculitis, which should be considered in patients with prominent headaches, myalgias, rash, hematuria, anemia, oral and genital ulcers, or monocular blindness. An elevated ESR of more than 50 mm/h, combined with monocular blindness, headaches, jaw claudication, and scalp tenderness, is practically pathognomonic of giant cell arteritis.

In younger patients (<50 years) without vascular risk factors, or with infarctions that otherwise appear cryptogenic, serologic tests can identify hypercoagulable states associated with the presence of antiphospholipid antibodies (anticardiolipin antibodies and lupus anticoagulant), or with deficiencies in protein C, protein S, and antithrombin III. Factor V Leiden and prothrombin 20210A gene mutations are also potential risk factors for stroke in younger patients.

Although not required as part of the initial evaluation of ischemic stroke patients, a fasting lipid profile is an essential part of vascular risk factor assessment. Elevations in serum homocysteine levels also appear to be associated with an increased risk of coronary artery disease and stroke. Nutritional supplementation with folic acid, pyridoxine (vitamin B_6), and cyanocobalamin (vitamin B_{12}) can effectively reduce elevated homocysteine levels, but whether such intervention reduces the risk of future vascular events is uncertain. C-reactive protein (CRP) is a marker of systemic inflammation that has been associated with an increased risk of myocardial infarction and stroke. In the setting of acute stroke, elevations in CRP may also predict neurologic deterioration and worse functional outcome. Treatment with statins reduces CRP levels, but the initiation of statin therapy based on CRP alone is not yet recommended.

Bushnell CD, Goldstein LB. Diagnostic testing for coagulopathies in patients with ischemic stroke. *Stroke* 2000;31:3067–3078. [PMID: 11108774] (Excellent review of the diagnostic yield of coagulation tests in patients with ischemic stroke.)

Cao JJ, et al. C-reactive protein, carotid intima-media thickness, and incidence of ischemic stroke in the elderly: The Cardiovascular Health Study. *Circulation* 2003;108:166–170. [PMID: 12821545] (Elevated CRP was demonstrated to be a risk factor for stroke, independent of the degree of atherosclerosis.)

Toole JF, et al. Lowering homocysteine in patients with ischemic stroke to prevent recurrent stroke, myocardial infarction, and death: The Vitamin Intervention for Stroke Prevention (VISP) randomized controlled trial. *JAMA* 2004;291:565–575. [PMID: 14762035] (Reduction in homocysteine levels after stroke did not reduce the risk of recurrent stroke, cardiac ischemia, or death.)

C. Imaging Studies

Brain imaging studies provide the most critical diagnostic information in the evaluation and treatment of patients with acute stroke. Both CT and MRI techniques can provide definitive confirmation that an ischemic stroke has occurred, as well as exclude the presence of hemorrhage and nonvascular intracranial processes. Information can also be gained regarding the size and location of the infarct, which aids in the determination of stroke etiology and influences treatment decisions. Acute brain imaging is also essential for the selection of patients for thrombolytic therapy, with newer modalities offering the potential for increased patient eligibility and safety. Vascular and cardiac imagings are also key elements in the evaluation of stroke patients, providing vital information about stroke etiology that may dictate both acute and long-term treatments.

1. Computed tomography—Emergent, nonenhanced CT of the brain remains the recommended diagnostic test for the initial evaluation of acute stroke. CT reliably detects intracranial hemorrhage, and in the era of thrombolysis, an emergent CT scan of the brain is performed on all patients who might be candidates for such therapy. The administration of intravenous contrast provides little additional information in this setting and is therefore obtained only in selected patients, for example, those suspected of harboring an intracranial neoplasm or infection.

Although sensitive for detecting intracranial hemorrhage, CT scanning is relatively insensitive for detecting small or early infarcts, particularly in the posterior fossa. The earliest signs of infarction are usually subtle and include loss of gray-white differentiation at the cortical-subcortical junction and basal ganglia and sulcal effacement. These signs appear within 6 hours of onset in more than 80% of patients with MCA infarctions, but are often less obvious when infarcts affect other territories. Hypodensity (edema) and mass effect develop next and, if present in more than 50% of the MCA territory within 24 hours of onset, correlate with early neurologic deterioration and death. The hyperdense MCA sign, representing thrombus or embolism in the MCA stem, also correlates with final stroke severity.

2. Magnetic resonance imaging—Conventional MRI sequences, such as T1-weighted and T2-weighted imaging, are also relatively insensitive for detecting early signs of cerebral ischemia and within hours of onset will show changes in less than 50% of patients. Diffusion-weighted imaging, however, detects subtle changes in the diffusion of water molecules within ischemic tissue and can accurately identify areas of ischemia within minutes of onset. The sensitivity of diffusion-weighted imaging for acute ischemia is greater than 90%, and the specificity greater than 95%. MRI using gradient-recalled echo (GRE) sequences or echo-planar susceptibility-weighted MRI can also accurately detect intracerebral hemorrhage and appears to be as sensitive as CT for this purpose.

The use of MRI in acute stroke is limited by several factors. MRI is generally not as emergently available as CT, and it takes more time to perform, potentially delaying the initiation of acute stroke therapy. The time required to complete an MRI is also important, because monitoring patients while they are in the MRI scanner can be difficult. MRI is also more expensive than CT, and there are more patient contraindications, such as pacemakers, metal implants, and claustrophobia.

For the nonemergent evaluation of ischemic stroke, MRI is clearly superior to CT for several reasons. MRI is more sensitive and specific than CT for identifying infarct location, size, and age. MRI can readily detect small cortical and subcortical infarcts, as well as those in the brainstem and cerebellum. MRI also enables the evaluation of cervical and cerebral arteries using a sequence called magnetic resonance angiography (MRA), a noninvasive test that can be performed without contrast injection and provides detailed three-dimensional images of the vascular system. For the detection of significant carotid stenosis, the sensitivity of MRA compares favorably with conventional catheter-based angiography but avoids the 0.5–3% risk of catheter-related neurologic complications. Information obtained from these studies is very useful for identifying patients with atherosclerotic mechanisms of infarction who might be appropriate candidates for surgical or endovascular therapies. MRA occasionally overestimates the degree of arterial stenosis present due to artifacts caused by turbulent blood flow, so confirmation with another study is generally recommended before finalizing treatment decisions.

3. Diagnostic ultrasound—Duplex Doppler ultrasound of the carotid arteries is another useful noninvasive test for identifying atherosclerotic disease after acute stroke or TIA. The sensitivity of Doppler ultrasound for detecting carotid stenosis is comparable to MRA and conventional angiography, but Doppler is less expensive, requires no exposure to radiation or magnetic fields, and can be performed at the bedside. Doppler is not susceptible to the same turbulence artifacts as MRA and so tends not to overestimate the degree of stenosis. However, the accuracy of Doppler is more susceptible to operator variability. Doppler can be performed to confirm MRA results (and vice versa); when results of the two studies differ significantly, conventional angiography is usually recommended.

Using an ultrasound probe with greater tissue penetration, the intracranial arterial circulation can be assessed with transcranial Doppler (TCD) techniques. TCD can be used in the evaluation of patient with acute stroke to rapidly identify large arteries of the circle of Willis occluded by thrombus or embolism, and it can be used to monitor for a response to thrombolysis. Recent clinical research also suggests that continuous insonation of an occluded cerebral artery during thrombolytic therapy may actually increase the likelihood of acute recanalization. TCD also provides information about the presence of intracranial atherosclerotic disease, as well as the degree and pattern of collateral blood flow in the setting of extracranial stenosis or occlusion. TCD is particularly useful in patients with sickle cell disease, in whom elevations in TCD velocities significantly correlate with the risk of stroke and the possible need for prophylactic transfusion therapy.

Cardiac ultrasound is obtained after most ischemic strokes to evaluate for a source of cardioembolism. The most convincing evidence of a cardiac source is the identification of an intracardiac thrombus, usually in the left atrial appendage or adjacent to an akinetic myocardial segment (mural thrombus). However, actual thrombi are rarely seen, and most often the information obtained provides indirect evidence for the likelihood of cardiac emboli, including a dilated left ventricle, reduced ejection fraction, focal wall motion abnormalities, or significant valvular pathology. With the injection of agitated saline, an intracardiac shunt may be identified, most commonly secondary to a patent foramen ovale.

Transthoracic echocardiography is usually the initial test of choice given the noninvasive nature of the study, but the use of transesophageal echocardiography (TEE) may significantly increase the yield for identifying potential sources of cardioembolism. The use of TEE has identified several new abnormalities that are associated with an increased risk of stroke, including spontaneous echo contrast, a smokelike echogenic signal likely caused by aggregation of cellular blood components due to slow-flow or stasis, and valvular strands, thin filamentous material seen on the aortic and mitral valves. TEE can also quantify the degree of aortic arch atherosclerosis, a potential source of artery-to-artery embolism that currently cannot be well-evaluated with other diagnostic techniques. TEE is more invasive than transthoracic echocardiography and therefore carries some additional risks. Patients are required to swallow the ultrasound probe, which usually requires some sedation and local anesthesia for discomfort. Rarely, patients may aspirate during the procedure if they are already dysphagic from a recent

stroke, and they can develop significant hypotension or bradycardia from vagal stimulation.

Alexandrov AV, et al. Ultrasound-enhanced systemic thrombolysis for acute stroke. *N Engl J Med* 2004;351:2170–2178. [PMID: 15548777] (Reports that transcranial Doppler improved the rate of rt-PA–induced arterial recanalization.)

Lee LJ, et al. Impact on stroke subtype diagnosis of early diffusion-weighted magnetic resonance imaging and magnetic resonance angiography. *Stroke* 2000;31:1081–1089. [PMID: 10797169]

Nederkoorn PJ, van der Graaf Y, Hunink MG. Duplex ultrasound and magnetic resonance angiography compared with digital subtraction angiography in carotid stenosis: A systematic review. *Stroke* 2003;34:1324–1332. [PMID: 12690221]

Rodriguez C, Homma S, Di Tullio M. Transesophageal echocardiography in stroke. *Cardiol Rev* 2000;8:140–147. [PMID: 11174887] (Reviews the use of TEE in the diagnostic evaluation of ischemic stroke.)

D. Other Tests

All patients with acute stroke should have an emergent electrocardiogram performed to evaluate for atrial fibrillation or myocardial ischemia. In selected patients, a 24-hour Holter monitor or continuous cardiac telemetry can identify paroxysmal atrial fibrillation. An electroencephalogram (EEG) is seldom needed in the evaluation of ischemic stroke but is indicated if a seizure is suspected. Lumbar puncture may be necessary to exclude subarachnoid hemorrhage or to identify inflammation consistent with central nervous system vasculitis or infection. A lumbar puncture should be avoided, however, if intracranial mass effect or anticoagulation is present.

▶ Differential Diagnosis

In the age of thrombolytic therapy, the prompt and accurate diagnosis of ischemic stroke is more critical than ever. Within 3 hours of onset, the physician must confidently arrive at the diagnosis of ischemic stroke and consider administering rt-PA. In the acute setting, the diagnosis is usually made based on clinical history, examination, and CT scanning alone, which makes a comprehensive understanding of potential stroke "mimics" very important. One prospective study of more than 400 patients hospitalized with an initial diagnosis of stroke found that almost 20% were misdiagnosed. Causes of misdiagnosis included seizures, brain tumors, trauma, migraine, hypertensive encephalopathy, and toxic-metabolic encephalopathy.

A. Spontaneous Intracerebral Hemorrhage

The most important diagnosis to distinguish from ischemic stroke is spontaneous intracerebral hemorrhage (ICH). The suddenness of symptom onset in ICH is generally slightly slower than that in infarction, and patients with ICH are more likely to have headache, nausea, vomiting, and decreased level of consciousness. The neurologic syndromes are otherwise usually indistinguishable. ICH is easily distinguished from ischemic stroke by CT imaging, with the exception of hemorrhagic transformation of ischemic stroke (see Complications, later). In this instance, the volume of hemorrhage into the infarction may mimic a primary ICH, and differentiation based on CT imaging may not be reliable. MRI with diffusion-weighted imaging may be more useful than CT in this setting.

B. Seizures

Seizures also have a sudden onset, and focal seizures, with or without secondary generalization, can produce a significant focal neurologic deficit postictally, referred to as *Todd's phenomenon,* sometimes mimicking the symptoms of a large hemispheric stroke. Postictal deficits are transient, usually resolving within 24 hours. If the seizure was not witnessed, the postictal syndrome may be indistinguishable from stroke, except that decreased consciousness and amnesia are more frequently encountered postictally. Focal seizures in adults are generally symptomatic of underlying brain pathology, and therefore the diagnosis of seizure may be supported by CT or MRI findings consistent with neoplasm, infection, or trauma. Differentiating between seizure and stroke is further complicated, however, by the rare instances of seizures caused by stroke. In this setting, the clinical manifestations of the stroke-related deficits are exacerbated by the postictal state, which is the primary reason for excluding stroke patients with acute seizures from treatment with IV rt-PA. Brain MRI with diffusion-weighted imaging may be helpful in assessing the extent of ischemia and infarction in patients with seizures.

Epilepsy as a chronic aftermath of stroke occurs in 2–4% of patients. A seizure in this setting often produces a relapse of the prior stroke symptoms, which may be clinically indistinguishable from a recurrent stroke. Symptoms usually resolve back to the recent preseizure baseline over several days. An MRI with diffusion-weighted imaging may again be helpful to identify any new ischemia. An EEG sometimes helps to differentiate between the two diagnoses but is nondiagnostic in more than 50% of patients who actually had a seizure. Furthermore, stroke can occasionally produce intermittent, even periodic epileptiform discharges on EEG, which correlate with an increased risk of seizure, but do not prove that the patient had one.

C. Migraine

Migraine is an important mimic of TIA and acute stroke. The diagnosis may be especially difficult when migraine aura occurs without headache and when migraine begins in later life without any history of prior headaches. The most common focal symptoms associated with migraine are visual auras, which must be distinguished from transient monocular blindness or PCA infarction. Visual manifestations of migraine generally begin in the central portion of vision and then slowly build up or march across the field of vision toward the periphery over the course of 5–25 minutes. C-shaped paracentral scotomas and scintillating, wavering lines are common. The subsequent development of a pounding, unilateral headache nearly ensures the diagnosis of migraine, but it may not occur. Migraine only rarely produces signs of transient hemispheric dysfunction, such as weakness, sensory loss, or aphasia, and should therefore not be seriously considered as a cause of these symptoms unless other etiologies are excluded. In such cases, symptoms usually last 20–30 minutes and are followed by contralateral headache. The affected side may change with recurrent attacks. The diagnosis of "complicated" migraine is further supported by younger age, absence of vascular risk factors, a history of classic migraine with visual auras, and a family history of similar episodes.

Familial hemiplegic migraine is an autosomal-dominant syndrome linked to a mutation in a calcium channel gene on chromosome 19. Attacks of hemiplegia usually affect the same side and may last for days to weeks. Sensory loss usually accompanies the weakness, and aphasia may be present in up to 50% of patients.

D. Hypertensive Encephalopathy

Hypertensive encephalopathy is a medical emergency that requires rapid diagnosis and treatment. Symptoms may resemble acute stroke, although there are many distinguishing features. Hypertensive encephalopathy may occur at any age but most commonly affects patients younger than 50 years. The presence of acute hypertension is required for the diagnosis, with blood pressure often higher than 240/140 mm Hg, and although hypertension in the setting of acute stroke is common, it is usually not to this extreme degree. Severe hypertension is thought to "break through" the limits of normal cerebrovascular autoregulation, leading to cerebral hyperperfusion, increased vascular permeability, forced dilation of cerebral vessels, cerebral edema, and hemorrhage. Infarction is rarely observed. Symptoms generally develop more slowly than in acute stroke and initially are often nonspecific, with headache, nausea, and vomiting. Visual symptoms are common and include blurring, dimming, frank visual loss, and cortical blindness. As encephalopathy develops, patients may become agitated, anxious, drowsy, confused, and disoriented. Seizures are a frequent complication of hypertensive encephalopathy and may be focal or generalized. Generalized hyperreflexia is also common, and funduscopic examination usually reveals hemorrhages, exudates, and papilledema. Focal motor or sensory deficits are less common but may result from seizures, edema, hemorrhage, or rarely ischemia. CT scan of the head may reveal diffuse cerebral edema, usually greatest in the posterior white matter, although MRI is much more sensitive than CT for detecting these abnormalities. Intracerebral hemorrhage and trace subarachnoid hemorrhage over the cerebral convexities may also be seen. Neurologic symptoms and imaging findings resolve with appropriate treatment of hypertension.

E. Head Trauma

Head trauma is rarely confused with ischemic stroke if an adequate history is available or external signs of injury are present. Subdural, epidural, or intraparenchymal hematomas can cause significant focal deficits, but they can be easily differentiated from ischemic stroke with nonenhanced CT. Brain tumor or abscess may also mimic stroke, but symptom onset is generally slower, over days to weeks, and CT and MRI abnormalities should clarify these diagnoses. One interesting observation is that in the setting of acute ischemic stroke, the initial CT scan often reveals minimal abnormalities, despite the presence of significant neurologic deficits. In contrast, patients with brain tumors often have dramatic abnormalities on neuroimaging with relatively mild symptoms.

F. Toxic or Metabolic Encephalopathy

When altered mentation or decreased consciousness dominates the clinical picture, the diagnosis of a toxic or metabolic encephalopathy must be considered. Focal deficits secondary to toxic and metabolic disorders are rare but can occur, particularly in patients who develop symptomatic seizures or who have prior neurologic injuries that become "unmasked" by the physiologic derangement. Frequently, the focal deficits do not reverse immediately after correction of the metabolic abnormality, particularly if the abnormality was severe or prolonged. Hypoglycemia is probably the most common metabolic cause of focal neurologic deficits.

▶ Treatment

A. Thrombolysis

Thrombolysis with IV rt-PA was approved by the US Food and Drug Administration (FDA) in 1996 for the treatment for acute ischemic stroke within 3 hours of onset, and to this day remains the only FDA-approved treatment for acute stroke. The rationale for thrombolytic therapy in acute stroke is based on two key concepts. First, the vast majority of ischemic strokes are caused by thrombotic or thromboembolic arterial occlusions. Angiographic studies of patients with ischemic stroke performed within 6 hours of onset find arterial occlusions in up to 80% of cases. Second, the eventual size and severity of an infarct is directly related to the degree and duration of ischemia sustained by the brain. Therefore, early recanalization of a thrombosed artery by a thrombolytic agent may limit the size of the final infarct and improve functional outcome.

Thrombolytic therapy for acute ischemic stroke was first tested in large clinical trials beginning in the late 1980s. Early trials, however, failed to show any clinical benefit and raised concerns about unacceptable bleeding complications.

Learning from the failures of prior studies, the National Institute of Neurological Disorders and Stroke (NINDS) tested a smaller dose of rt-PA within a shorter time interval from symptom onset in patients with acute ischemic stroke and found a significant benefit with treatment on 3-month functional outcome. The results of this randomized, double-blind, placebo-controlled trial were first published in 1995 and were the basis for FDA approval of IV rt-PA for the treatment of acute ischemic stroke. In the NINDS rt-PA study, patients with ischemic stroke received IV rt-PA (0.9 mg/kg; maximum, 90 mg) or placebo within 3 hours of symptom onset. The primary outcome measures were degree of neurologic improvement at 24 hours and degree of disability at 3 months. Although there was no statistical difference in neurologic improvement at 24 hours between rt-PA and placebo, the primary end point of minimal or no disability at 3 months was highly in favor of treatment with rt-PA. Treated patients were 30% more likely to have minimal or no disability at 3 months, corresponding to an absolute increase of 11–13% in excellent outcomes with rt-PA. Given this efficacy, only eight patients need to be treated with rt-PA to achieve one additional patient with minimal or no disability. Symptomatic intracranial hemorrhage occurred in 6% of rt-PA–treated patients versus only 0.6% of placebo-treated patients, but this did not adversely affect 90-day mortality (17% for rt-PA versus 21% for placebo).

Subsequent analysis of the NINDS rt-PA trial confirmed that all patients with acute ischemic stroke within 3 hours of symptom onset benefited from treatment with IV rt-PA, regardless of age, stroke severity, early ischemic changes on CT, or stroke subtype. Advanced age, severe neurologic deficits, and signs of early infarction on CT were all associated with an increased risk of intracranial hemorrhage following thrombolysis, but patients with these characteristics were still more likely to have minimal or no disability at 3 months when treated with rt-PA. Therefore, advanced age, severe stroke, and early infarct signs on CT should not absolutely exclude the administration of rt-PA in this population. In addition, patients with lacunar stroke were just as likely to benefit from treatment with rt-PA as patients with other stroke subtypes, so the use of rt-PA for lacunar stroke should be equally encouraged.

In 2004, published results of a pooled analysis of four separate stroke trials suggested that treatment with IV rt-PA might benefit stroke patients up to 4.5 hours from onset as well. The European Cooperative Acute Stroke Study (ECASS) III trial was then performed, and the results published in 2008 supported this conclusion. ECASS III trial was a randomized, double-blind, placebo-controlled trial that demonstrated a less robust, but still significant, benefit for IV rt-PA in the 3- to 4.5-hour window. The study was designed similarly to the NINDS trial, including treatment dose and primary outcome of 90-day disability. Patients treated with IV rt-PA between 3 and 4.5 hours from symptom onset were 16% more likely to have a favorable outcome at 90 days as compared with patients treated with placebo. This translates to an absolute increase of 7.2% in 90-day favorable outcome in the rt-PA group ($P = 0.04$), and a number needed to treat of 14 patients to achieve one additional patient with minimal or no disability. Symptomatic hemorrhage was higher in the alteplase group compared with the placebo group (2.4% versus 0.3% as defined in this study; $P = 0.008$); however, mortality did not differ (7.7% versus 8.4%, respectively; $P = 0.68$). Exclusion criteria differed slightly from the NINDS trial, selecting for patients with less severe strokes than in previous trials, and are reflected in Table 10–3. The results of the ECASS III trial provided the necessary evidence to demonstrate a benefit for IV thrombolysis up to 4.5 hours from onset increasing the potential to effectively treat more acute ischemic stroke patients than ever before.

Therefore, IV rt-PA is now the standard of care for treatment of acute ischemic stroke within 3 hours of onset and is rapidly being adopted for the extended time window of 3–4.5 hours. Eligibility criteria for treatment have been adopted from the NINDS study for administration within 3 hours and from the ECASS III trial for administration in the extended time window and are summarized in Table 10–3. Guidelines include a recommendation that a member of the stroke team be present at the bedside within 15 minutes, CT scan of the head be performed within 25 minutes, and IV rt-PA be administered within 60 minutes of presentation to the hospital. Even within the 4.5-hour time window, the sooner patients receive rt-PA, the greater the likelihood of achieving an excellent functional outcome. The dose of IV rt-PA for acute ischemic stroke is 0.9 mg/kg (maximum, 90 mg) initiated within 4.5 hours of symptom onset, with 10% of the dose given as an intravenous bolus, and the remaining 90% given as an infusion over 1 hour (Table 10–4).

Within the first 24 hours after IV rt-PA administration, patients should be monitored closely, with vital sign assessment and brief neurologic examinations performed every 15 minutes for the first 2 hours, every 30 minutes for the next 4 hours, and then every hour for the next 18 hours. Blood pressure must be tightly controlled to a level less than 180/105 mm Hg (Table 10–5). Intravenous antihypertensive agents such as labetalol and nicardipine are generally used for this purpose because they can be carefully and continuously titrated to the desired effect. Nitroprusside is reserved as a last resort, because the associated venous dilation may raise intracranial pressure and impair cerebral perfusion. An emergent CT scan of the head should be obtained for any neurologic deterioration and any remaining rt-PA discontinued until the possibility of an intracranial hemorrhage is excluded (Table 10–6). Arterial and central venous punctures should be avoided, particularly at noncompressible sites, as should Foley catheters and nasogastric tubes, unless they can be placed before IV rt-PA administration without delaying the initiation of treatment. Heparin, aspirin, and other antithrombotic medications should not be given for at least 24 hours after rt-PA dosing. A CT scan of the head should be routinely performed 24 hours after rt-PA to exclude the presence of asymptomatic intracerebral

Table 10–3. Criteria for Treatment With Intravenous Recombinant Tissue Plasminogen Activator (IV Rt-PA)

Inclusion criteria
- Age ≥ 18 y
- Clinical diagnosis of acute ischemic stroke
- Defined onset within 3 h (or 4.5 h) of starting treatment
- CT scan of head consistent with acute ischemic stroke (negative or minor early ischemic changes)

Exclusion criteria for patients within 3 h of onset
- CT scan with intracranial hemorrhage or significant mass effect
- Rapidly improving or minor symptoms (eg, pure sensory loss, isolated dysarthria, isolated facial weakness, isolated ataxia)
- Seizure at onset of stroke
- Any history of intracranial hemorrhage, subarachnoid hemorrhage, intracranial aneurysm, arteriovenous malformation, or tumor
- Stroke or serious head trauma within preceding 3 mo
- Gastrointestinal or urinary tract hemorrhage within preceding 21 d
- Major surgery or serious trauma within preceding 14 d
- Lumbar puncture within preceding 7 d
- Arterial puncture at noncompressible site within preceding 7 d
- SBP >185 or DBP >110 at time of treatment
- Coagulopathy: INR >1.5, aPTT >1.5 times normal, or platelet count <100,000
- Recent use of anticoagulants:
- Warfarin (unless INR <1.5)
- Heparin within past 48 h (unless aPTT <1.5 times normal)
- Glucose <50 or >400 (may use fingerstick value)
- Subacute bacterial endocarditis
- Pregnancy
- Symptoms of post-myocardial infarction (MI) pericarditis or known ventricular aneurysm

Additional exclusion criteria for patients within 3 to 4.5 h of onset
- Age >80 y
- History of prior stroke *and* diabetes
- Any anticoagulant use prior to treatment, regardless of INR level
- NIHSS >25
- CT or MRI with signs of acute ischemia in >one third of MCA territory

Warnings
- Recent MI or known left heart thrombus
- Diabetic hemorrhagic retinopathy or other hemorrhagic ophthalmic condition
- Any recent trauma

aPTT = activated partial thromboplastin time; CT = computed tomography; DBP = diastolic blood pressure; INR = international normalized ratio; MCA = middle cerebral artery; MRI = magnetic resonance imaging; NIHSS = National Institutes of Health Stroke Scale; SBP = systolic blood pressure.

hemorrhage that could influence decisions for subsequent antithrombotic therapy, blood pressure management, and neurologic monitoring.

With these guidelines for treatment, IV rt-PA can be administered in routine clinical practice with comparable efficacy and complication rates as that seen in the NINDS

Table 10–4. Protocol for IV Rt-PA Administration in Patients With Acute Ischemic Stroke

1. Review inclusion and exclusion criteria for IV rt-PA (see Table 10–3).

2. Discuss treatment with patient and family.
   a. Explain that IV rt-PA is the only FDA-approved treatment for acute stroke in patients who meet certain inclusion and exclusion criteria.
   b. Discuss benefits and risks.
   Benefits—
   • Recipients treated within 3 h are 30% more likely to have minimal or no disability at 3 mo.
   • Recipients treated between 3 to 4.5 h are 16% more likely to have minimal or no disability at 3 mo.
   Risks—
   • Increased risk of ICH
   • Increased risk of bleeding from other sites.
   • No increase in risk of death

3. If possible, have patient or a family member sign informed consent. However, *do not withhold treatment* from an eligible patient because he or she cannot sign (eg, aphasic) and family is not available.

4. Administer IV rt-PA (Alteplase, Activase): 0.9 mg/kg (maximum, 90 mg).
   a. Reconstitute appropriate amount of rt-PA in sterile water to achieve final concentration of 1 mg/mL.
   b. Start IV dose within 3 h of symptom onset, or within 4.5 h if appropriate.
   c. Administer 10% of total dose as an IV bolus over 1 min.
   d. Administer remaining 90% as an IV infusion over 1 h.

5. Perform neurologic examinations and obtain vital signs every 15 min for 2 h, every 30 min for 4 h, and then every hour for 18 h.

6. Maintain tight BP control for 24 h—
   SBP <180, DBP <105 (see BP management protocol, Table 10–5).

7. Do not administer anticoagulation or antiplatelet agents for 24 h.

8. Avoid central lines, arterial lines, nasogastric tubes, and Foley catheters for 24 h, unless medically necessary.

9. Admit to a monitored bed (stroke unit, ICU) as appropriate based on predicted medical and neurologic stability, and need for IV medications for BP control.

10. Repeat CT scan of head in 24 h, or STAT for any neurologic deterioration.

BP = blood pressure; CT = computed tomography; DBP = diastolic blood pressure; FDA = Food and Drug Administration; ICH = intracranial hemorrhage; ICU = intensive care unit; IV rt-PA = intravenous recombinant tissue plasminogen activator; SBP = systolic blood pressure; STAT = immediately.

and ECASS III trials. However, deviations from the treatment protocols outlined in the clinical trials are associated with significant increases in complication rates. One group reported a fivefold increase in the rate of symptomatic intracranial hemorrhage when 50% of treated patients had deviations from the treatment protocol, an increase that was subsequently corrected when strict adherence to NINDS guidelines was achieved.

Despite the proven benefit of IV rt-PA in the treatment of acute ischemic stroke, widespread adoption of systemic thrombolysis has been limited by the narrow time window and numerous contraindications. Furthermore, systemic thrombolysis may have limited efficacy against large vessel occlusions. This has led to growing enthusiasm for endovascular revascularization therapies. One randomized trial of intra-arterial (IA) prourokinase, Prolyse in Acute Cerebral Thromboembolism (PROACT) II, and several meta analyses combining additional, smaller randomized trial of using intra-arterial lytics (PROACT I, AUST, and MELT) both suggest of clinical benefit from the in intra-arterial administration of a thrombolytic agent up to 6 hours from stroke onset. With this limited randomized data, the FDA has not granted approval for IA thrombolytic therapy. However, these compelling findings have led most large stroke centers to adopt the use of endovascular revascularization therapy for select patients (Figures 10–1 and 10–2).

In addition to IA thrombolysis, mechanical thrombectomy devices are emerging with the hope of increasing the speed and efficacy of endovascular therapy. Two devices, the Merci Retriever (Concentric Medical, Mountain View, California) and the Penumbra System (Penumbra, Alameda, California), have received FDA approval for mechanical thrombectomy based on small prospective studies demonstrating their safety and efficacy for opening large artery occlusions in patients with acute ischemic stroke presenting within 8 hours of onset. Other devices based on a retrievable stent design, such as the Solitaire FR (ev3 Endovascular, Irvine, California) and the Trevo Stentriever (Concentric Medical, Mountain View, California) are in development, with clinical trials showing promise for rapid recanalization.

Table 10–5. Blood Pressure Management in the First 24 Hours After IV Rt-PA Administration[a]

Strict Goal: BP <180/105 mm Hg	
For SBP 180–230 mm Hg or DBP 105–120 mm Hg	• Give IV labetalol, 10 mg, over 1–2 min. Repeat or double as necessary every 10 min up to total dose of 150 mg (hold for heart rate <60). • Alternatively, consider starting continuous IV labetalol infusion at 20 mg/h and titrate upward to maximum dose of 150 mg/h. • Monitor BP every 5 min during treatment and observe for development of hypotension and bradycardia. • If labetalol is contraindicated due to bradycardia or bronchospasm, start IV nicardipine as a continuous infusion of 5 mg/h and titrate upward to maximum of 15 mg/h.
For SBP >230 mm Hg or DBP 121–140 mm Hg	• Give IV labetalol, 20 mg, over 1–2 min *and* start continuous IV labetalol infusion at 40 mg/h and titrate upward to maximum dose of 150 mg/h. • May give additional IV boluses of 20–40 mg over 1–2 min during infusion every 10–15 min as needed. • Monitor BP every 5 min during treatment and observe for development of hypotension and bradycardia. • If response is inadequate, *add* IV nicardipine as continuous infusion of 5 mg/h and titrate upward to maximum of 15 mg/h.
For DBP >140 mm Hg	• Start sodium nitroprusside (with thiosulfate buffer) at 0.5 μg/kg/min IV, and titrate to maximum of 5 μg/kg/min (doses up to 10 μg/kg/min may be used for brief periods <30 min). • Monitor BP every 3–5 min during treatment and observe for development of hypotension. • Try to wean patient to labetalol or nicardipine IV drip within 24 h to avoid cyanide-thiocyanate toxicity and to minimize risk of increasing intracranial pressure.

BP = blood pressure; DBP = diastolic blood pressure; IV = intravenous; rt-PA = recombinant tissue plasminogen activator; SBP = systolic blood pressure.
[a]An arterial line is recommended to monitor BP during prolonged labetalol and nicardipine infusions and is necessary during prolonged nitroprusside infusions. Risk of bleeding secondary to arterial puncture must be weighed against the possibility of missing dramatic changes in pressure during the infusion.

Table 10–6. Management of IV Rt-PA Treatment–Related Bleeding Complications[a]

Intracranial Hemorrhage (ICH)

If ICH is suspected[b]
• Discontinue IV rt-PA if still infusing.
• Obtain STAT CT scan of head.
• Send STAT CBC, PT, PTT, fibrinogen, type and crossmatch.
• STAT crossmatch 10 units of cryoprecipitate and 6 units of FFP.

If ICH is *not* present
• Do not restart rt-PA.
• Continue standard post-treatment protocol.

If ICH is present
• Administer epsilon aminocaproic acid (Amicar): 4 g IV × 1 (given over 1 h), then 0.5 g/h IV for 24 h.
• Request emergent neurosurgical consultation.
• Evaluate laboratory results, consider hematology consultation, consider transfusion of cryoprecipitate and FFP.
• Repeat CT scan of head in 6 h to assess for change.

Extracranial Bleeding

• Consider severity in determining need to discontinue rt-PA infusion.
• Consider mechanical measures to limit bleeding (eg, compression of an arterial or venous puncture site).

If more than mild bleeding is present
• Discontinue IV rt-PA if still infusing.
• Send STAT CBC, PT, PTT, fibrinogen, type and crossmatch.
• STAT crossmatch 4 units of packed red cells, 6 units of FFP, 10 units of cryoprecipitate, and 6 units of platelets.
• Obtain hematology consultation.
• Evaluate laboratory results and consider transfusion of blood products and administration of epsilon aminocaproic acid.

CBC = complete blood count; CT = computed tomography; FFP = fresh frozen plasma; IV = intravenous; rt-PA = recombinant tissue plasminogen activator; STAT = immediately.
[a]Consider occult internal bleeding in all patients with unexplained hypotension after rt-PA administration.
[b]Suspect ICH in patients with neurologic deterioration, new headache, acute hypertension, and vomiting.

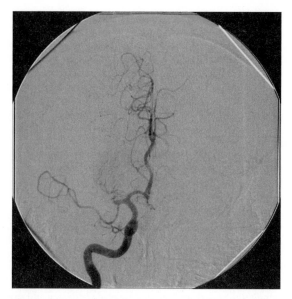

▲ **Figure 10–1.** Right internal carotid angiogram demonstrating a thromboembolic occlusion of the proximal right middle cerebral artery in a patient presenting with left-sided paralysis and left hemineglect.

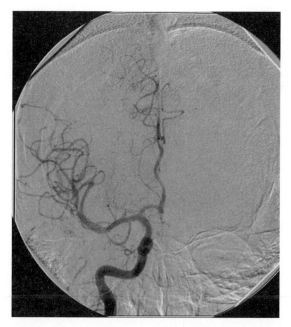

▲ **Figure 10–2.** Right internal carotid angiogram of the same patient in Figure 10–1 after endovascular treatment with intra-arterial rt-PA. Within 24 hours, the patient made a near-complete neurologic recovery.

Several larger ongoing randomized trials are intended to further clarify the role for endovascular therapy in acute ischemic stroke. The Interventional Management of Stroke Trial III (IMS III) is a phase 3, multicenter, randomized trial designed to compare the safety and efficacy of a combined IV/IA approach to an IV rt-PA approach alone. The Intra-Arterial Versus Intravenous Thrombolysis In Acute Ischemic Stroke (SYNTHESIS EXPANSION) trial is an Italian-based, multicenter, randomized trial designed to compare systemic administration of alteplase to endovascular revascularization using local IA alteplase, mechanical recanalization, or a combination of the two. MR and Recanalization of Stroke Clots Using Embolectomy (MR RESCUE) is an ongoing randomized trial investigating whether diffusion-perfusion MRI can identify patients who will benefit most from mechanical thrombectomy with the Merci clot retrieval device up to 8 hours from symptom onset.

At this time, the role of endovascular revascularization therapy in acute ischemic stroke remains unsettled, with questions surrounding patient selection using time and imaging parameters and the method of recanalization. Further study is needed, and ongoing randomized clinical trials will hopefully provide definitive evidence of benefit from endovascular revascularization therapies in the future.

Hacke W, et al. Association of outcome with early stroke treatment: Pooled analysis of ATLANTIS, ECASS, and NINDS rt-PA stroke trials. *Lancet* 2004;363:768–774. [PMID: 15016487] (Demonstrated better outcomes with earlier treatment, particularly within 90 minutes from onset.)

Hacke W, et al. Thrombolysis with Alteplase 3 to 4.5 hours after acute ischemic stroke. *N Engl J Med* 2008;359:1317–1329. [PMID: 18815396] (The ECASS III study that extended the time window for treatment with IV rt-PA up to 4.5 hours from onset in select patients.)

Lee M, Hong KS, Saver JL. Efficacy of intra-arterial fibrinolysis for acute ischemic stroke: Meta-analysis of randomized controlled trials. *Stroke* 2010;41(5):932–7. [PMID: 20360549] (Supports the use of intra-arterial thrombolysis for acute stroke treatment, with improved clinical outcomes and no increase in mortality.)

Wechsler LR. Intravenous thrombolytic therapy for acute ischemic stroke. *N Engl J Med* 2011;364(22):2138–46. [PMID: 21631326] (Recent review of IV rt-PA for acute stroke treatment, including a brief clinical vignette.)

B. Aspirin and Other Antiplatelet Agents

Aspirin (ASA) is the only treatment proven to reduce mortality after acute ischemic stroke when initiated within 48 hours of onset. Aspirin therapy also modestly reduces the risk of early stroke recurrence and long-term disability. All patients should be initially treated with aspirin after acute ischemic stroke unless they are being treated with thrombolytic therapy. In these instances, aspirin should be withheld for at least 24 hours and can then be started if no major bleeding complications are present. Minor hemorrhagic transformation of an ischemic infarct in the absence of a focal cerebral hematoma with mass effect is probably not a contraindication to aspirin therapy. Although newer antiplatelet agents (clopidogrel, dipyridamole) may be indicated as long-term therapies for reducing the risk of recurrent stroke, none of these agents have been evaluated in the acute treatment of ischemic stroke, so their relative efficacy compared with aspirin in this setting is unknown. ASA therapy, 160–325 mg/day, initiated within 48 hours of stroke onset results in 11 fewer in-hospital strokes or deaths, and 14 fewer patients dead or dependent at 6 months, per 1000 patients treated.

Although the efficacy of aspirin for reducing disability after ischemic stroke pales in comparison with the efficacy of rt-PA, aspirin remains the only other therapy for acute stroke shown to improve outcome for these patients, and it is the only such therapy that reduces mortality. Furthermore, the magnitude of these benefits is not trivial from a public health perspective. Because several million people each year are treated for acute ischemic stroke worldwide, the routine use of aspirin in this population could enable an additional 10,000 people to survive independently for every million treated.

Beyond the initial treatment period after ischemic stroke, most patients should be maintained on antiplatelet therapy to reduce the long-term risk of recurrent stroke and vascular death (Table 10–7). The one exception to long-term antiplatelet therapy after ischemic stroke is cardioembolic stroke due to atrial fibrillation, intracardiac thrombi, or prosthetic heart valves, for which long-term anticoagulation with warfarin is superior to antiplatelet therapy for secondary stroke prevention. For noncardioembolic stroke, aspirin 50–325 mg/day reduces the risk of recurrent stroke by approximately 18% overall; it is inexpensive, convenient (once-daily dosing), and generally well tolerated.

Two other leading antiplatelet therapies are clopidogrel (Plavix) and the combination of aspirin and extended-release dipyridamole (Aggrenox). The combination of aspirin (25 mg) and extended-release dipyridamole (200 mg) appears to be slightly more effective than aspirin alone for secondary stroke prevention, with the results of multiple clinical trials (European Stroke Prevention Study 2[ESPS-2], and European/Australasian Stroke Prevention in Reversible Ischemia Trial [ESPRIT]) demonstrating a relative risk reduction of approximately 23%. However, this combined formulation (Aggrenox) requires twice-daily dosing and may cause severe headaches in nearly one third of patients. Alternatively, clopidogrel appears to be as effective as the combination of aspirin plus extended-release dipyridamole for preventing recurrent stroke and is better tolerated with less headaches and the ease of once daily dosing. Both

Table 10–7. Antiplatelet Drugs for Secondary Stroke Prevention

Drug	Standard Dose	Mechanism	Comment
ASA	50–325 mg PO once daily	Inhibits platelet cyclooxygenase	18% reduction in recurrent ischemic stroke Inexpensive, easy once-daily dosing Contraindications-ASA allergy, severe peptic ulcer disease
ASA 25 mg plus extended-release dipyridamole, 200 mg (Aggrenox)	1 tab PO twice daily	Dipyridamole inhibits phosphodiesterase and increases prostacyclin-related platelet inhibition	23% relative reduction in recurrent stroke compared with ASA alone Severe headaches are frequently reported, diarrhea less often, which limit tolerability and compliance
Clopidogrel	75 mg PO once daily	Inhibits ADP-induced platelet aggregation	Equivalent to Aggrenox for secondary stroke prevention Alternative for patients who cannot tolerate ASA Rare cases of TTP reported, 4 cases per 1 million patients Avoid lumbar puncture and epidural anesthesia in patients receiving clopidogrel due to increased risk of epidural hematoma
Cilostazol	100 mg PO twice daily	Inhibits phosphodiesterase, increases cAMP, increases nitric oxide, inhibits vascular smooth muscle proliferation	Appears equivalent to ASA for secondary stroke prevention with fewer hemorrhagic events More side effects than ASA including headache, diarrhea, palpitation, dizziness, and tachycardia

ADP = adenosine diphosphate; ASA = aspirin; cAMP = cyclic adenosine monophosphate; PO = orally; tab = tablet; TTP = thrombotic thrombocytopenia purpura.

clopidogrel and Aggrenox are considerably more expensive than aspirin and therefore are often reserved for high-risk patients, or for those who cannot tolerate aspirin due to allergy or peptic ulcer disease (clopidogrel only).

More recently, cilostazol (Pletal), a phosphodiesterase inhibitor, was also shown to be effective for secondary stroke prevention. In a large clinical trial, Cilostazol Stroke Prevention Study 2 (CSPS 2), patients treated with cilostazol had a slight reduction in recurrent stroke compared with patients treated with aspirin and were significantly less likely to have an intracranial hemorrhage. Minor adverse events were worse in the cilostazol group and included headache, diarrhea, palpitations, and dizziness. Although cost and side effects may limit use, cilostazol may play an important role in the future, as an additional alternative agent for those patients unable to tolerate aspirin, or for those with a higher risk of intracranial hemorrhage.

Ticlopidine, an older thienopyridine derivative related to clopidogrel, is no longer recommended for stroke prevention given the risk of agranulocytosis and thrombotic thrombocytopenic purpura associated with its use.

Chen ZM, et al. Indications for early aspirin use in acute ischemic stroke: A combined analysis of 40 000 randomized patients from the Chinese Acute Stroke Trial and the International Stroke Trial. *Stroke* 2000;31:1240–1249. [PMID: 10835439]

ESPRIT Study Group. Aspirin plus dipyridamole versus aspirin alone after cerebral ischemia of arterial origin (ESPRIT): Randomized controlled trial. *Lancet* 2006;367:1665–1673. [PMID: 16714187]

Sacco RL, et al. Aspirin and extended-release dipyridamole versus clopidogrel for recurrent stroke. *N Engl J Med* 2008;359:1238–1251. [PMID: 18753638] (The PRoFESS study demonstrating equal efficacy of Aggrenox and clopidogrel for stroke prevention.)

Shinohara Y, et al. Cilostazol for prevention of secondary stroke (CSPS 2): An aspirin-controlled, double-blind, randomised non-inferiority trial. *Lancet Neurol* 2010;9(10):959–68. [PMID: 20833591]

C. Heparin and Other Anticoagulants

Many physicians prescribe intravenous heparin in the setting of acute ischemic stroke despite the lack of clinical evidence supporting its efficacy. Low-molecular-weight heparins (LMWHs) and heparinoids are alternative therapies for achieving therapeutic anticoagulation with simpler administration, more consistent hematologic effects, and less risk of thrombocytopenia. The goal of anticoagulation in acute ischemic stroke is to prevent early recurrent cerebral embolism, neurologic deterioration from propagation of intracranial thrombus, and systemic venous thromboembolic complications. Although anticoagulation may be effective at achieving some of these goals, the benefits are largely outweighed by an increased risk of intracranial and systemic

hemorrhage, and no improvement in death or disability has been demonstrated in clinical trials, even in patients with cardioembolic stroke. Current treatment guidelines do not recommend the routine use of full-dose anticoagulation in unselected patients with acute ischemic stroke. Although supportive data are limited, one possible exception is ischemic stroke caused by cervical artery dissection.

Low-dose anticoagulation, however, is recommended after acute stroke for the prevention of deep venous thrombosis (DVT) and pulmonary embolism. Both LMWH and unfractionated heparins can be used for this purpose. Low-dose enoxaparin (a LMWH) 40 mg daily was shown to be more effective than unfractionated heparin for the prevention of venous thromboembolism in acute ischemic stroke patients, with no increase in intracranial hemorrhage but a slightly higher rate of major extracranial bleeding. These findings, in addition to the convenience of once-daily administration, have made LMWHs a preferred choice for DVT prophylaxis in acute stroke patients. Subcutaneous heparin, 5000 units twice daily, is also effective and safe for prevention of venous thromboembolism and should be considered as an alternative therapy for all patients with ischemic stroke, particularly those with a contraindication to LMWH, such as renal insufficiency. Interestingly, low-dose anticoagulation may also achieve some of the elusive goals of full-dose anticoagulation but with a superior safety profile. In the International Stroke Trial (IST), the use of low-dose heparin (5000 units subcutaneously, twice daily) produced a modest reduction in the combined end point of death or recurrent stroke at 14 days (10.8% versus 12.0%) with no increase in major hemorrhagic complications and was even more effective when combined with aspirin.

Coull BM, et al. Anticoagulants and antiplatelet agents in acute ischemic stroke: Report of the Joint Stroke Guideline Development Committee of the American Academy of Neurology and the American Stroke Association. *Stroke* 2002;33:1934–1942. [PMID: 12105379]

Sherman DG, et al. The efficacy and safety of enoxaparin versus unfractionated heparin for the prevention of venous thromboembolism after acute ischaemic stroke (PREVAIL Study): An open-label randomised comparison. *Lancet* 2007;369:1347-55. [PMID: 17448820]

D. Antihypertensive Therapy

Significant blood pressure elevations are frequently seen after acute stroke, although the appropriate management of hypertension in this setting remains controversial. Arguments for aggressive treatment suggest that hypertension increases the risk of hemorrhagic transformation and cerebral edema. Arguments against aggressive treatment raise the concern that reductions in blood pressure may exacerbate ongoing cerebral ischemia and increase infarct size. Because data are lacking to support either point of view, current guidelines generally recommend avoiding antihypertensive therapy in the setting of acute stroke for the first 72 hours. In fact, blood pressure usually declines without treatment over the first several hours or days in the majority of patients.

Of course, extreme elevations of blood pressure cause end-organ damage; therefore, antihypertensive therapy should be initiated rapidly if systolic blood pressure is higher than 220 mm Hg or diastolic pressure is higher than 120 mm Hg. Parenteral agents such as intravenous labetalol or nicardipine are usually preferred, because they can be carefully titrated and produce no significant cerebral vasodilation. Intravenous nitroprusside may be required in refractory cases of extreme hypertension, but it is not a first-line therapy given the risk of increased intracranial pressure. Oral agents are less desirable, because they do not allow minute-by-minute dosage titrations. Sublingual use of calcium antagonists, such as nifedipine, should also be strictly avoided, given the risk of a precipitous drop in blood pressure due to rapid absorption. As noted previously, hypertension must also be treated aggressively in patients who are candidates for thrombolytic therapy, as hypertension in this setting is associated with an increased risk of intracranial hemorrhage.

E. General Management

All patients with acute stroke should have frequent assessments of their neurologic status and vital signs for at least 24 hours. Early mobilization should begin as soon as possible to lessen the risk of pneumonia, venous thrombosis, and pressure ulcers. Frequent turning and the use of alternating pressure mattresses help to prevent pressure ulcers in the immobile patient. Patients with severe weakness are at risk for developing contractures, so passive range-of-motion exercises should be started within 48 hours of stroke. Alternating pressure stockings and low-dose subcutaneous anticoagulants (heparin, LMWH, or heparinoids) are given for the prevention of deep venous thrombosis and pulmonary embolism (Table 10–8). Indwelling Foley catheters increase the risk of urinary tract infections and should be avoided unless medically necessary.

Providing adequate nutrition safely after acute stroke is also very important. Swallowing impairment is associated with aspiration pneumonia and increased mortality, and malnutrition may actually impair neurologic recovery. Physicians should assess all stroke patients for swallowing impairments before prescribing a diet. Patients with decreased level of consciousness, multiple infarcts, brainstem infarcts, or large infarcts are at the greatest risk for aspiration, and an abnormal gag reflex, impaired voluntary cough, dysphonia, or cranial nerve palsies should raise concern for potential swallowing impairments. A water-swallowing test can be performed at the bedside, with the presence of coughing, choking, or a wet voice after drinking suggesting aspiration. A formal swallowing evaluation by a trained speech and language pathologist or ear, nose, and throat physician is often indicated, and a fluoroscopic modified barium swallow, or a

Table 10–8. Pharmacologic Agents for Prophylaxis in Deep Venous Thrombosis

Drug	Dose	Comment
Dalteparin	5000 IU SQ every 24 h	LMWH HIT is less likely than with UH Contraindicated in patients with renal insufficiency
Danaparoid sodium	750 anti-Xa units SQ every 12 h	Heparinoid Preferred drug for prophylaxis of deep venous thrombosis in patients with known HIT
Enoxaparin	30 mg SQ every 12 h *or* 40 mg SQ every 24 h	LMWH HIT less likely than with UH Contraindicated in patients with renal insufficiency
Heparin	5000 units SQ every 12 h	UH Relatively inexpensive Watch for HIT

HIT = heparin-induced thrombocytopenia; IU = international unit; LMWH = low-molecular-weight heparin; SQ = subcutaneous; UH = unfractionated heparin

flexible endoscopic evaluation of swallowing with sensory testing (FEESST), may be obtained to definitively assess the effectiveness and safety of swallowing. If swallowing is impaired, a nasogastric or nasoduodenal tube should be placed to provide adequate nutrition and expedite the delivery of medications. If prolonged swallowing impairment is anticipated, the percutaneous placement of an endogastric tube is superior to a nasogastric feeding tube with regards to safety, reliability, and patient comfort.

Adams HP, et al. Guidelines for the early management of adults with ischemic stroke: A guideline from the American Heart Association/American Stroke Association Stroke Council. *Stroke* 2007;38(5):1655–711. [PMID: 17431204] (An excellent, comprehensive, evidence-based practice guideline for the evaluation and treatment of acute ischemic stroke.)

F. Management of Complications

1. Hemorrhagic transformation—Hemorrhage into an area of acute infarction is a common phenomenon referred to as *hemorrhagic transformation*. Most significant hemorrhages are believed to result from the reperfusion of infarcted tissue due to the delayed reopening of the occluded artery. This view is consistent with the observation that hemorrhagic transformation occurs most frequently after cardioembolic stroke, in which occlusions are most likely to recanalize. Hemorrhage can also occur distal to occlusions that have not recanalized, but in these instances it is usually less severe (petechial hemorrhages). Overall, some hemorrhagic transformation occurs in approximately 40% of all ischemic strokes and in more than 70% of strokes caused by embolism. However, symptomatic hemorrhagic transformation with significant bleeding and mass effect likely occurs in fewer than 5% of patients. Hemorrhagic transformation usually occurs within the first 2 weeks after stroke, but can be detected as early as hours and as late as 1 month. Additional risk factors for hemorrhage include large infarct size, arterial hypertension, and the use of anticoagulants and thrombolytics. The early use of aspirin after ischemic stroke does not significantly increase the rate of hemorrhagic transformation.

Serious hemorrhagic transformation is the most dreaded complication of thrombolytic therapy. As noted, symptomatic intracranial hemorrhage occurs in approximately 6% of patients treated with IV rt-PA for stroke. Signs of hemorrhage include severe headache, vomiting, sudden increase in blood pressure, and neurologic deterioration. If these signs develop, patients should be evaluated with an emergent CT scan of the head, and any remaining rt-PA infusion should be discontinued. Significant rt-PA related hemorrhage should be treated with an infusion of epsilon-aminocaproic acid (Amicar) for 24 hours, and transfusions of fresh frozen plasma, cryoprecipitate, and platelets based on the results of coagulation studies and a CBC. Emergent neurosurgical consultation should be obtained for consideration of surgical decompression, although neurosurgical interventions may not be feasible within the first several hours after rt-PA administration due to the presence of severe coagulopathy.

2. Brain edema—Clinically significant brain edema requiring treatment develops in 10–20% of patients with ischemic stroke, but it is responsible for 80% of the mortality after large MCA infarctions. Brain edema usually reaches its maximum between 3 and 5 days after stroke but can become symptomatic anytime from 1–10 days. Symptoms related to brain edema are primarily caused by mass effect, resulting in tissue shifts and compression of surrounding brain structures. Although elevated intracranial pressure may develop, it usually occurs after other signs of brainstem compression are present.

Symptoms of brain edema secondary to large supratentorial infarctions include progressive obtundation, worsening of neurologic deficits, nausea and vomiting, respiratory failure, and hypertension. The development of additional pyramidal signs ipsilateral to the side of infarction, such as hyperreflexia, spasticity, and Babinski sign, may be an early sign of impending transtentorial herniation. As edema worsens, signs of transtentorial herniation, such as an ipsilateral third nerve palsy and decerebrate posturing, may develop rapidly.

Brain edema secondary to cerebellar infarction can be particularly dangerous, because symptoms do not follow a predictable progression as is often seen with herniation due to supratentorial infarctions. Patients with cerebellar edema frequently present with nothing but headache, nausea, and vomiting before suddenly becoming comatose with bilateral decerebrate posturing. Other signs of brainstem compression may be present, including pupillary abnormalities (small pontine or midposition fixed midbrain pupils), loss of the oculocephalic reflex, abnormal respiratory patterns, hypertension, and bradycardia. Edema related to cerebellar infarction can also produce acute hydrocephalus secondary to compression of the fourth ventricle and cerebral aqueduct, leading to obtundation and bilateral pyramidal signs before the development of more severe brainstem compression.

In patients with brain edema, hypotonic fluids should be strictly avoided. Factors that raise intracranial pressure should be treated aggressively, such as hypoxia, hypercapnia, acidosis, and hyperthermia. Elevation of the head of the bed by 30 degrees may also reduce intracranial pressure by increasing venous drainage.

Hyperosmolar therapy with mannitol and hypertonic saline is effective at temporarily reducing brain edema and intracranial pressure and reversing the clinical signs of herniation. However, their efficacy in decreasing mortality and improving long-term outcome in this setting is unproven. These agents produce an osmolar gradient across the blood–brain barrier that draws excess water from the interstitial and intracellular spaces into the vasculature for redistribution and elimination through the kidney. Mannitol is given as a bolus, usually 0.5–1 g/kg every 4–6 hours as needed, with close monitoring of serum osmolarity. Mannitol is a strong osmotic diuretic, so dehydration and renal failure are the main side effects, both of which can be avoided by aggressively maintaining euvolemia with isotonic fluid replacement and by limiting the mannitol dose if serum osmolality is above 320 mOsm/L. Hypertonic saline may also be given as a bolus or as a standing infusion in various concentrations. Hypertonic saline may be slightly more potent than mannitol, but it is contraindicated in the setting of ongoing cerebral ischemia, because the resultant hypernatremia may increase the final size of brain infarction. After 24 hours from stroke onset, however, hypertonic saline is an acceptable alternative to mannitol. Serum chemistries should be monitored every 6 hours. The hypertonic saline solution should be buffered with acetate to prevent the development of a hyperchloremic metabolic acidosis, and the dose should be limited to maintain a serum sodium level less than 160 mEq/L. Severe fluid overload with congestive heart failure is a common complication of prolonged treatment with hypertonic saline, but it generally responds to diuresis.

There is currently no indication for the use of corticosteroids to treat brain edema after ischemic stroke. Numerous large clinical trials have tested both conventional and large doses of corticosteroids in this setting, but no beneficial effect was found. However, these studies did find an increase in infections, gastrointestinal bleeding, and hyperglycemia with corticosteroid use. Furosemide is another therapy sometimes used to treat brain edema, and although it may potentiate the effects of mannitol and hypertonic saline, used alone it is unlikely to be effective. Furthermore, the dehydration associated with repeated furosemide use can impair cerebral perfusion, leading to increased intracranial pressure, and can increase the risk of mannitol-induced renal toxicity.

Hyperventilation can rapidly reduce intracranial pressure by causing cerebral vasoconstriction through hypocapnia and should be tried in all patients with signs of herniation and brainstem compression. However, hyperventilation is less effective at reversing the mass effect seen with brain edema after infarction, so the prolonged efficacy of hyperventilation in this setting is limited. Extreme hyperventilation ($Pco_2 < 28$ mm Hg) might also worsen brain ischemia through severe vasoconstriction.

The ultimate treatment for relieving the mass effect created by brain edema after ischemic stroke is surgical decompression. Suboccipital decompression of large cerebellar strokes can reverse signs of brainstem compression and reduce mortality. Decompression should be considered with the earliest signs of decreasing consciousness or brainstem dysfunction. When obstructive hydrocephalus is present, an external ventricular drain should be placed. Decompression of large MCA infarctions can be accomplished by a generous hemicraniectomy with a relaxing durotomy, but its use in this setting is controversial. Hemicraniectomy reduces mortality after life-threatening MCA infarction—10–30% mortality after hemicraniectomy in most surgical series versus 80% mortality for historical controls treated with medical therapy alone—but the functional outcome and quality of life of most survivors is poor. Younger patients (<50 years old) have the best chance of achieving a good outcome after hemicraniectomy, so early decompression in this subgroup should be considered.

3. Seizures—The incidence of early seizures within the first 7 days after acute stroke is between 4% and 6%, with most occurring within the first 24 hours. Seizures are usually of focal onset, with or without secondary generalization, and are much more likely to occur after cortical infarction (6%) than deep infarction (0.6%). Early seizures do not appear to affect stroke mortality or functional outcome. However, approximately 25% of early seizures progress to status epilepticus, a life-threatening complication that should be treated aggressively, as outlined in Chapter 7.

The incidence of late seizures (usually within 12 months of the original stroke) is slightly greater than early seizures. Patients with late seizures are also more likely to have a recurrence (approximately 50%) than those with early seizures (approximately 30%). An EEG may help risk-stratify these patients; highly epileptiform EEGs correlate with higher risk of recurrence and normal EEGs with lower risk. Although only 2–4% of patients after stroke develop epilepsy, stroke remains the leading cause of epilepsy in the elderly.

Because of the relatively low incidence of seizure after stroke, routine seizure prophylaxis with antiepileptic medications is not recommended. An acute seizure should be treated according to established guidelines based on the clinical situation. After a first seizure, long-term antiepileptic therapy may not be necessary or advisable, because the risk for a second seizure is low, and traditional antiepileptic medications (eg, phenytoin and phenobarbital) can significantly impair neurologic recovery after stroke. Insufficient information is available about the effects of newer antiepileptic medications on stroke recovery. Recurrent seizures, however, require long-term antiepileptic therapy, and drug selection should be tailored to maximize patient safety, tolerability, and compliance.

4. Medical complications—More than 50% of stroke mortality overall is attributable to medical complications. The most common is infection, with pneumonia and urosepsis each occurring with a frequency of about 5%. Oropharyngeal weakness, decreased level of consciousness, and immobility all increase the risk of aspiration pneumonia after stroke, and indwelling bladder catheters increase the risk of urinary tract infections. Fever after stroke should prompt a thorough evaluation of potential sources of infection, including a chest x-ray and sputum culture to evaluate for pneumonia, urinalysis with microscopic examination and culture to evaluate for urinary tract infection, and blood cultures to exclude bacteremia. Venous and arterial catheters should be inspected for signs of infection. Potential sources of infection in patients with prolonged hospitalizations include *Clostridium difficile* diarrhea and decubitus ulcers. When infection is present, antibiotics should be tailored to treat the specific site of infection or the organism if known. Fever should also be treated aggressively with antipyretics and cooling blankets if needed, because hyperthermia worsens neurologic outcome after stroke. If no infectious source of fever can be identified, alternative explanations should be considered, such as a drug reaction or venous thrombosis.

Deep venous thrombosis (DVT) and pulmonary embolism are also important complications after stroke. Without prophylaxis, DVT develops in up to 50% of patients with severe stroke. Risk factors for DVT include advanced age, immobility, paralysis (particularly of the legs), atrial fibrillation, and hormone replacement therapy. Pulmonary embolism develops in about 1% of all stroke patients, but accounts for 10% of stroke-related deaths. Prophylactic use of low-dose subcutaneous heparin, LMWHs, and heparinoids is effective in preventing DVT and pulmonary embolism and should be administered to all patients without an absolute contraindication. Alternating pressure stockings may also be effective, but regular support stockings are not.

Hyperglycemia frequently develops after acute stroke, even in patients not previously diagnosed with diabetes. A surge in endogenous glucocorticoids and adrenergic hormones may explain some cases. Hyperglycemia in patients with acute stroke appears to increase infarct size and worsen neurologic outcome. If even mild hyperglycemia is detected, it should be monitored and treated aggressively with insulin as appropriate to maintain euglycemia. Clinical trials are ongoing to determine whether aggressive glucose control after stroke improves long-term outcome.

Baird TA, et al. Persistent poststroke hyperglycemia is independently associated with infarct expansion and worse clinical outcome. *Stroke* 2003;34:2208–2214. [PMID: 12893952]

Berger C, et al: Hemorrhagic transformation of ischemic brain tissue: Asymptomatic or symptomatic? *Stroke* 2001;32:1330–1335. [PMID: 11387495] (This study concludes that the majority of hemorrhagic transformation is clinically asymptomatic.)

Gupta R, et al. Hemicraniectomy for massive middle cerebral artery territory infarction: A systematic review. *Stroke* 2004;35:539–543. [PMID: 14707232] (Age > 50 years was associated with poor functional outcome after hemicraniectomy.)

Labovitz DL, Hauser WA, Sacco RL. Prevalence and predictors of early seizure and status epilepticus after first stroke. *Neurology* 2001;57:200–206. [PMID: 11468303] (Early seizures were more likely after lobar infarcts or hemorrhages than deep infarcts or hemorrhages.)

Qizilbash N, Lewington SL, Lopez-Arrieta JM. Corticosteroids for acute ischaemic stroke. *Cochrane Database Syst Rev* 2002;(2):CD000064. [PMID: 12076379]

Schwarz S, et al. Effects of hypertonic (10%) saline in patients with raised intracranial pressure after stroke. *Stroke* 2002;33:136–140. [PMID: 11779902] (Hypertonic saline was effective in treating raised intracranial pressure in stroke patients not responding to mannitol therapy.)

▶ Prevention

Whether the goal is to prevent first stroke or recurrent stroke, the identification and treatment of all modifiable stroke risk factors are the cornerstones of effective stroke prevention.

A. Hypertension

Hypertension is the most common and powerful risk factor for stroke after advanced age. Hypertension accelerates the progression of atherosclerosis and contributes to the development of small vessel disease. For every 10-mm Hg increase in systolic blood pressure, the relative risk of stroke rises by 1.7–1.9, even after controlling for all other risk factors. In patents with hypertension, reducing the systolic blood pressure to less than 140 mm Hg reduces the risk of first stroke by 40%. The strongest evidence for a reduction in stroke risk with antihypertensive therapy comes from studies using diuretics, β-blockers, and angiotensin-converting enzyme (ACE) inhibitors. Regular screening for hypertension is recommended in adults at least every 2 years, with antihypertensive treatment indicated to keep the blood pressure below 140/90 (or <130/80, if diabetic).

For patients with a history of prior stroke or cardiovascular disease, treatment with antihypertensive medications, particularly ACE inhibitors (ACE-Is), may be beneficial even in the absence of clear hypertension. In the Perindopril Protection Against Recurrent Stroke Study (PROGRESS), normotensive patients receiving perindopril (ACE-I) with or without indapamide (diuretic) had a 28% reduction in recurrent stroke compared with those receiving placebo. Stroke reduction, however, was greater with larger reductions in blood pressure. In the Heart Outcomes Prevention Evaluation (HOPE) Trial, patients received either ramipril (ACE-I) or placebo, and despite a very modest reduction in blood pressure with ramipril (3/2 mm Hg), there was a 30% reduction in stroke with this treatment. Alternative explanations for benefits of ACE-Is in addition to the blood pressure–lowering effects include modulation of angiotensin II–induced intimal and vascular smooth muscle proliferation, and atherosclerotic plaque stabilization. The Losartan Intervention For Endpoint reduction in hypertension (LIFE) study also supported a similar non–blood-pressure–mediated benefit for the angiotensin-receptor blocker losartan.

B. Cardiac Disease

Cardiac disease is another major risk factor for ischemic stroke, particularly atrial fibrillation, valvular heart disease, coronary artery disease, and congestive heart failure. Stroke risk is doubled for patients with coronary artery disease and four times greater for patients with congestive heart failure. Patients with these conditions should be treated according to established guidelines, many of which recommend interventions (antiplatelet therapy, lipid-lowering agents, ACE-Is, exercise) that may have robust secondary benefits for stroke prevention as well.

Atrial fibrillation is likely responsible for at least 50% of embolic strokes. The risk of developing atrial fibrillation increases with age, as does the risk of stroke associated with atrial fibrillation. The average risk of stroke in unselected patients is 4–5% per year, but it is 1.5% for patients younger than 60 years and 23.5% for patients older than 80. Concomitant factors that increase the risk of stroke attributable to atrial fibrillation include hypertension, impaired left ventricular function, diabetes, and prior stroke or TIA.

Anticoagulation with warfarin is the preferred treatment for most patients with atrial fibrillation to reduce the risk of cardioembolic complications. The intensity of warfarin therapy must be closely monitored, with frequent serologic measurements of the PT and INR, and the dose of warfarin adjusted to achieve an INR of 2.0–3.0. Five large, randomized, placebo-controlled trials, including the Atrial fibrillation Aspirin and Anticoagulation (AFASAK) Trial and the Stroke Prevention in Atrial Fibrillation I (SPAF I) trial, demonstrate that warfarin reduces the risk of first stroke by 68% in high-risk patients. The combined results of AFASAK and SPAF I also demonstrate a 21% reduction in the risk of first stroke due to atrial fibrillation in patients taking aspirin. In low-risk groups, generally patients younger than 65 years with no other risk factors, aspirin therapy is an acceptable alternative to warfarin for primary stroke prevention. For secondary prevention, however, aspirin has not been shown to reduce the risk of recurrent stroke due to atrial fibrillation. Warfarin should therefore be the treatment of choice in the high-risk population, unless an increased risk of bleeding complications prohibits its use.

A recent addition to the available treatment options for secondary prevention of ischemic stroke in patients with nonvalvular atrial fibrillation is the oral agent dabigatran (Pradaxa), a direct thrombin inhibitor. The Randomized Evaluation of Long-Term Anticoagulant Therapy (RE-LY) study demonstrated superiority of dabigatran 150 mg twice daily in comparison to adjusted-dose warfarin for the prevention of stroke or systemic emboli, with a similar major hemorrhage profile. Routine INR monitoring is not needed, and few food and drug interactions exist. Dabigatran will likely play a large role in secondary stroke prevention for patients with atrial fibrillation in the future, due to the favorable efficacy, safety, and convenience.

C. Diabetes

Diabetes is also associated with an increased risk of stroke, with relative risks ranging between 1.5 and 6.0, depending on the population studied and the type and severity of diabetes. Interestingly, tight glycemic control has not been proven to reduce the risk of stroke in diabetic patients, although aggressive control of hyperglycemia does reduce other microvascular complications, such as diabetic nephropathy, retinopathy, and peripheral neuropathy. Patients with diabetes often develop other medical comorbidities that further increase stroke risk, such as hypertension and cardiac disease. Hypertension is present in 40–60% of adults with type 2 diabetes, and several trials have shown a substantial reduction in cardiovascular complications and stroke with aggressive blood pressure reduction in these patients. The UK Prospective Diabetes Study Group found a 44% reduction in both fatal and nonfatal stroke with an aggressive antihypertensive regimen (mean blood pressure achieved = 144/82 mm Hg) compared with a less-aggressive regimen (mean blood pressure achieved = 154/87 mm Hg). In the HOPE study, diabetic patients at high risk for vascular events showed a 33% reduction in stroke with ramipril versus placebo, even after controlling for the minor difference in blood pressure between the two groups. These and other data have encouraged the recommendation of particularly aggressive blood pressure reduction in patients with diabetes (goal blood pressure <130/80) and the use of ACE-Is, such as ramipril, in high-risk diabetic patients to reduce the risk of stroke and other vascular complications.

D. Hyperlipidemia

Abnormalities of serum lipids are strongly associated with an increased risk of coronary artery disease, but less so with an increased risk of stroke. Early cohort studies considered ischemic and hemorrhagic stroke together and found no correlation between total cholesterol levels and stroke incidence; some studies actually found an inverse relationship between total cholesterol levels and hemorrhagic stroke. Subsequent studies found a more consistent association between lipid abnormalities and ischemic stroke specifically. The Honolulu Heart Program found a continuous increase in the risk of coronary artery disease and thromboembolic stoke with increasing total cholesterol levels, and the Northern Manhattan Stoke Study found an increased stroke risk with lower high-density lipoprotein levels. Other studies found correlations between lipid levels and the severity of carotid atherosclerosis.

Perhaps more compelling than the correlations between cholesterol levels and stroke risk, several randomized clinical trials—including the Scandinavian Simvastatin Survival Study (4S), the Cholesterol and Recurrent Events study (CARE), the Long-Term Intervention With Pravastatin in Ischemic Disease study (LIPID), and the Heart Protection Study (HPS)—demonstrated decreased stroke rates with the use of cholesterol-lowering medications (eg, HMG-CoA reductase inhibitors [statins]; see Table 10–9). In fact, the results of some trials indicate that in patients with coronary artery disease, treatment with statins reduces the risk of first stroke or TIA regardless of pretreatment cholesterol levels. To explain the benefit of statins regardless of pretreatment cholesterol levels, potential nonlipid effects include the ability to stabilize atherosclerotic plaques, enhance endothelial function and microvascular blood flow, and act as anti-inflammatory, antithrombotic, and neuroprotective agents.

In patients with a history of prior stroke, statin therapy has now been shown to reduce the risk of recurrent stroke as well. The Stroke Prevention by Aggressive Reduction in Cholesterol Levels (SPARCL) trial was the first study to demonstrate the effectiveness of cholesterol lowering with statin therapy to reduce the risk of recurrent ischemic stroke. This study investigated the effect of statin therapy in patients with prior stroke or TIA but no known cardiovascular disease. Patients treated with atorvastatin 80 mg/day had a significant 16% reduction in the risk of stroke over a follow-up period of 5 years. Post-hoc analysis demonstrated that low-density lipoprotein lowering of greater than or equal to 50% was associated with a greater reduction in the risk of stroke and major coronary events, suggesting that a significant benefit of statin therapy is in fact related to cholesterol-lowering properties. The recommendation for cholesterol management in secondary stroke prevention is the use of statin therapy, with a goal low-density lipoprotein below 100 mg/dL and below 70 mg/dL in high-risk patients with atherosclerotic disease.

E. Smoking

Cigarette smoking is a major risk factor for stroke. The biological effects of smoking include increased platelet aggregation, decreased vascular distensibility and compliance, and decreased high-density lipoprotein levels. Current smokers are at a 1.8-fold increased risk of stroke compared with nonsmokers, and between 12% and 18% of all strokes are

Table 10–9. Clinical Trials of Statin Therapy and Risk of Stroke

Trial	Study Population	Treatment	Result
Cholesterol and Recurrent Events (CARE)	4159 subjects with recent MI and average cholesterol levels	Pravastatin, 40 mg once daily, versus placebo for 5 y	32% relative risk reduction in stroke from all causes
Long-Term Intervention With Pravastatin in Ischemic Disease (LIPID)	9014 subjects with prior MI or unstable angina and average cholesterol levels	Pravastatin, 40 mg once daily, versus placebo for 6 y	19% relative risk reduction in stroke from all causes
Heart Protection Study (HPS)	20,536 subjects with history of CAD, stroke/TIA, peripheral vascular disease, or diabetes mellitus, or men ≥65 y with hypertension Overall average cholesterol levels	Simvastatin, 40 mg once daily, versus placebo for 5 y	30% relative risk reduction in ischemic stroke 21% relative risk reduction in any major vascular event in subjects with prior stroke/TIA and no CAD
Scandinavian Simvastatin Survival Study (4S)	4444 subjects with history of CAD and elevated cholesterol levels	Simvastatin, 20–40 mg once daily, versus placebo for 5 y	51% relative risk reduction in nonembolic stroke
Stroke Prevention by Aggressive Reduction in Cholesterol Levels (SPARCL) investigators	4731 subjects with history of stroke or TIA within 1–6 mo of study entry, with no history of CAD. LDL levels 100–190 mg/dL	Atorvastatin 80 mg once daily, versus placebo for 5 y	16–18% relative risk reduction in fatal and nonfatal stroke

CAD = coronary artery disease; LDL = lactate dehydrogenase; MI = myocardial infarction; TIA = transient ischemic attack.

attributable to current cigarette use. Prior cigarette smoking may also be associated with a relative risk of stroke of approximately 1.3. However, the risk of stroke dramatically declines with time from cessation. The Framingham Heart Study found a 50% reduction in stroke risk at 1 year after smoking cessation, and at 5 years the risk of stroke was comparable to that of nonsmokers.

A relative risk of stroke between 1.2 and 1.8 is estimated for nonsmokers exposed to environmental tobacco smoke. One study found that 90% of the nonsmoking population had detectable blood levels of chemicals indicating significant exposure to tobacco smoke, leading to the conclusion that approximately 12% of all strokes may be attributable to second-hand smoke. If so, the proportion of strokes attributable to tobacco use (current, previous, and second-hand) is nearly one third. To effectively modify the risk of stroke, any patient who smokes should quit completely (switching to a pipe or cigar is not beneficial), as should all close family members and household contacts.

F. Carotid Artery Stenosis

Atherosclerotic carotid artery stenosis of more than 50% is present in up to 10% of men and 7% of women older than 65 years. The risk of developing a stroke ipsilateral to an asymptomatic carotid stenosis of this degree ranges from 1–3% per year. Risk of stroke is likely higher in patients with greater degrees of stenosis, with a stenosis that is worsening over time, with contralateral carotid occlusion, and with poor collateral circulation. However, it is important to realize that up to 45% of strokes ipsilateral to a carotid stenosis may

actually be due to small vessel disease or cardioembolism, stressing the need for complete evaluation of all patients with ischemic stroke regardless of the presence of carotid disease.

The Asymptomatic Carotid Atherosclerosis Study (ACAS) was a large randomized trial designed to test the effectiveness of carotid endarterectomy for reducing the risk of first stroke in patients with asymptomatic carotid stenosis of more than 60%. Patients were randomized to endarterectomy plus aspirin versus aspirin alone. The trial was positive in favor of surgery, with a 5-year rate of ipsilateral stroke (plus perioperative stroke or death) of 5% for surgery versus 11% for aspirin (53% relative risk reduction, 1% absolute risk reduction per year). This means that to prevent one stroke in the next 5 years from asymptomatic carotid stenosis, one would need to treat 17 patients with carotid endarterectomy.

One unexpected result of the ACAS study was that the benefit for surgery over aspirin in women was not statistically significant, largely due to an increase in perioperative complications. This highlights a fundamental aspect of the ACAS results: The benefit of endarterectomy for any patient with asymptomatic carotid stenosis critically depends on perioperative morbidity and mortality. In ACAS, the incidence of perioperative stroke or death was only 1.5% (2.3% if complications of cerebral angiography are added), but the perioperative complication rate nationwide may be significantly higher (between 5% and 11% for all endarterectomies performed based on Medicare claims data in 1991). Before recommending endarterectomy for patients with asymptomatic carotid stenosis of more than 60%, physicians need to be aware of the endarterectomy complication rates among the potential local surgeons. Complication rates exceeding 3%

will negate the benefits of surgery for unselected patients and should encourage the alternative treatment options, including endovascular stent implantation or medical therapy with aspirin and aggressive risk-factor modification.

For patients with symptomatic carotid stenosis (ie, patients who have had a stroke or TIA presumed secondary to carotid disease), the benefit of endarterectomy for stroke prevention is much more robust. The North American Symptomatic Carotid Endarterectomy Trial (NASCET) randomized patients with carotid stenosis and a recent ipsilateral, nondisabling stroke or TIA to carotid endarterectomy plus aspirin versus aspirin alone. In patients with carotid stenosis of 70–99%, endarterectomy significantly reduced the rate of recurrent ipsilateral stroke at 2 years from 26% with aspirin alone to 9% with surgery, an absolute risk reduction of 17%. For patients with a carotid stenosis of 50–69%, the benefit of endarterectomy remained but was less significant, with a 5-year risk of ipsilateral stroke of 22.2% in medically treated patients versus 15.7% in surgically treated patients. This means that one needs to surgically treat six patients with symptomatic stenosis of more than 70% to prevent one stroke within 2 years, or 16 patients with symptomatic stenosis of 50–69% to prevent one stroke within 5 years. For patients with a stenosis of less than 50%, no benefit for endarterectomy could be demonstrated. The 30-day risk of perioperative stroke or death was 6.7%, but this did not negate the benefit of endarterectomy in this high-risk population. Clearly, in patients who have suffered a stroke or TIA secondary to a high-grade (>70%) carotid stenosis, endarterectomy significantly reduces the risk of subsequent stroke and should be considered in all patients.

Carotid artery angioplasty and stent implantation has become an alternative therapeutic option for extracranial carotid artery atherosclerotic disease. With advances in stent and balloon design, technique, and the emergence of embolic protection devices over the past three decades, carotid stenting has demonstrated comparable success and complication rates to carotid endarterectomy. Several large, randomized trials have investigated endovascular therapy for carotid stenosis. The Carotid and Vertebral Artery Transluminal Angioplasty Study (CAVATAS) randomized symptomatic patients to stenting or surgery and showed comparable 30-day rates of stroke or death, 10% in both groups. In the SAPPHIRE trial (Stenting and Angioplasty With Protection in Patients at High Risk for Endarterectomy), carotid artery stenting with an embolic protection device was compared with endarterectomy in high-risk patients and demonstrated 30-day perioperative combined stroke, death, and myocardial infarction (MI) rates of 9.9% versus 4.4% for surgery versus stenting, respectively, demonstrating a noninferiority of stenting to endarterectomy in high-risk patients. Two subsequent studies (EVA-3S and SPACE) compared carotid stenting with endarterectomy in a broader patient population, but both were stopped early due to higher 30-day stroke and death in the stenting groups. These early poor outcomes were inconsistent with other trials and were attributed to inadequate interventionalist experience and training. Most recently, the Carotid Revascularization Endarterectomy Versus Stent Trial (CREST) compared the efficacy of stenting with endarterectomy in both symptomatic and asymptomatic patients and found no significant difference in the composite primary outcome of 30-day stroke, death, MI, and 4-year ipsilateral stroke (7.2% versus 6.8% respectively, $P = 0.51$). The rate of stroke in the first 30 days was higher in the stenting group, whereas the rate of MI was lower. Additionally, for patients younger than 70 years of age, stenting showed greater efficacy, whereas in patients older than 70 years, endarterectomy appeared better. Overall, carotid angioplasty and stenting has proven to be a comparable alternative to carotid endarterectomy and is the preferred treatment for patients at high-risk for endarterectomy, expanding the available treatment options for carotid stenosis.

Adler AI, et al. Association of systolic blood pressure with macrovascular and microvascular complications of type 2 diabetes (UKPDS 36): A prospective observational study. *BMJ* 2000;321: 412–419. [PMID: 10938049]

Bosch J, et al. Use of ramipril in preventing stroke: Double blind randomised trial. *BMJ* 2002;324:699–702. [PMID: 11909785]

Chapman N, et al. Effects of a perindopril-based blood pressure-lowering regimen on the risk of recurrent stroke according to stroke subtype and medical history: The PROGRESS Trial. *Stroke* 2004;35:116–121. [PMID: 14671247]

CREST investigators. Stenting versus endarterectomy for treatment of carotid-artery stenosis. *N Engl J Med* 2010;363:11–23. [PMID: 20505173]

Furie KL, et al. Guidelines for the prevention of stroke in patients with stroke or transient ischemic attack: A guideline for healthcare professionals from the american heart association/american stroke association. *Stroke* 2011;42(1):227–76. [PMID: 20966421] (Recent evidence-based guidelines for secondary stroke prevention.)

Goldstein LB, et al. Primary prevention of ischemic stroke: A guideline from the American Heart Association/American Stroke Association Stroke Council. *Stroke* 2006;37:1583–1633. [PMID: 16675728]

Heart Protection Study Collaborative Group. Effects of cholesterol-lowering with simvastatin on stroke and other major vascular events in 20536 people with cerebrovascular disease or other high-risk conditions. *Lancet* 2004;363:757–767. [PMID: 15016485]

The SPARCL Investigators. Stroke Prevention by Aggressive Reduction in Cholesterol Levels (SPARCL) Investigators. High-dose atorvastatin after stroke or transient ischemic attack. *N Engl J Med* 2006;355:549–559. [PMID: 16899775]

Yadav JS, et al. Protected carotid-artery stenting versus endarterectomy in high-risk patients. *N Engl J Med* 2004;351:1493–1501. [PMID: 15470212] (The SAPPHIRE trial.)

▶ Prognosis & Rehabilitation

The risk of death after stroke is greatest in the first month and is less for ischemic than for hemorrhagic stroke. Thirty-day mortality after ischemic stroke is approximately 20%.

Death is more likely to occur from medical complications than neurologic complications and in patients with severe neurologic deficits, advanced age, cardiovascular disease, and hyperglycemia. Among patients surviving this initial period, the risk of death remains three to five times higher than that of age-matched controls, with estimated annual mortality rates ranging from 5–8%.

Recurrent stroke is a major cause of long-term morbidity and mortality. The risk is highest immediately after stroke, with estimates ranging from 3–10% within the first 30 days. Recurrence rates appear highest for patients with atherosclerotic infarction and lowest for patients with lacunar infarction. Long-term stroke rates range from 2–20% per year, depending on stroke etiology and other patient characteristics. Reducing the risk of recurrent stroke is one of the major goals of long-term stroke treatment (see Prevention, earlier).

Rehabilitation and recovery are additional goals critical to the long-term management of stroke patients. Stroke is the leading cause of long-term disability in most industrialized countries, and more than 70% of stroke survivors have some detectable neurologic deficit. The majority of neurologic recovery occurs within the first 3–6 months after stroke, but cognitive and language deficits may continue to improve dramatically for up to 2 years. However, even if deficits persist, rehabilitation services can teach patients effective adaptive techniques that increase function and independence.

Treatment in a comprehensive rehabilitation program appears to improve functional outcome and increases the likelihood of patients eventually returning home. Because the rate of recovery is most dramatic in the first 3 months, it is in this period that patients may benefit the most from aggressive rehabilitative therapy. Physical therapy is generally performed to maximize mobility, with a focus on strengthening of the legs and trunk, stretching and bracing to minimize spasticity and contractures, and retraining of gait and balance. Occupational therapy frequently addresses disabilities associated with hand and arm weakness and focuses on improving the performance of activities of daily living, such as feeding, dressing, toileting, washing, and grooming. Speech and language therapists specialize in the evaluation and treatment of both communication and swallowing disorders. Formal neuropsychological testing may also be useful to identify specific cognitive contributing to overall disability and subsequently to plan an appropriate program of cognitive rehabilitation. Depression, which develops in 30–60% of patients after stroke, should be identified and treated aggressively. Depression is associated with worse long-term functional outcome after stroke, but treatment with selective serotonin reuptake inhibitors, such as citalopram, has been shown to improve both depression and functional outcomes.

Regardless of the severity of the initial neurologic deficit, patients and physicians should be encouraged to pursue early, aggressive rehabilitation after stroke with hope and optimism. Within 3–6 months, more than 85% of stroke survivors walk independently, two thirds are independent with their activities of daily living, and more than one third have minimal or no disability. With an increased use of rt-PA and the development of new interventional and neuroprotective strategies, the number of patients with an excellent functional outcome after acute ischemic stroke should only increase in the future.

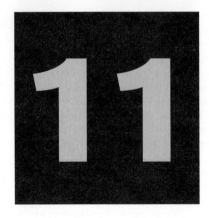

Cerebrovascular Disease: Hemorrhagic Stroke

Richard A. Bernstein, MD, PhD

Spontaneous intracranial hemorrhage accounts for about 20% of all strokes, but they are often devastating, accounting for a disproportionately large proportion of morbidity and mortality among stroke patients. There are two types of hemorrhagic stroke. Intraparenchymal hemorrhage (IPH) is characterized by bleeding within the brain itself, whereas subarachnoid hemorrhage (SAH) is characterized by vessel rupture in the cerebrospinal fluid (CSF)–filled subarachnoid space surrounding the brain. IPH and SAH have distinct clinical presentations, radiologic findings, etiologies, and treatment modalities.

▼ INTRAPARENCHYMAL HEMORRHAGE

ESSENTIALS OF DIAGNOSIS

► Sudden-onset focal deficit, with worsening over seconds to minutes; headache, nausea, vomiting, and coma are common

► Etiologies include hypertension, vascular malformations, vasculopathies, coagulopathies, and others

► Computed tomography (CT) and magnetic resonance imaging (MRI) are exquisitely sensitive to acute IPH

► Treatment and prevention of recurrence are based on etiology; there are no treatments for IPH that are known to improve outcome

▶ General Considerations

A. Incidence

Intraparenchymal hemorrhage (IPH) accounts for 10–15% of all strokes. Incidence worldwide is 10–20 cases per 100,000 persons and increases with age. It is more common in men, blacks, and people of Asian descent. The high incidence in blacks may reflect the prevalence of hypertension in that population, as well as inadequate access to primary prevention services. In the United States, approximately 45,000 people per year have an IPH, of whom 38–50% die. Most survivors are left with major neurologic deficits. The incidence is expected to double over the next 50 years due to aging of the population and changing racial demographics.

B. Risk Factors

The most prevalent modifiable risk factor for IPH is hypertension. IPH is a particular risk in hypertensive patients younger than 55 years, smokers, and patients who are noncompliant with antihypertensive regimens. Patients with IPH are usually hypertensive on presentation, in some cases probably due to the IPH itself. The presence of left ventricular hypertrophy or renal insufficiency may provide evidence of long-standing hypertension. Antihypertensive treatment lowers the risk of IPH by about 50%.

Other modifiable risk factors for IPH include smoking and heavy alcohol use. Chronic alcoholism may increase the risk of IPH by causing cirrhosis, thrombocytopenia, or both. Low serum cholesterol is associated with an increased risk of IPH, especially among patients with severe hypertension. High-intensity statin therapy may increase the risk of IPH in patients with a history of stroke.

There are genetic risk factors for IPH, as shown by a familial tendency in about 10% of patients. Important genes include the apolipoprotein E ε2 and ε4 alleles, which predispose to lobar hemorrhage by increasing the vasculopathic effects of amyloid deposition in cortical blood vessels. In patients with lobar hemorrhage, the presence of these alleles triples the risk of recurrent hemorrhage. As yet, screening of patients with IPH for genetic risk factors is not indicated in routine clinical practice.

▶ Pathogenesis

IPH can occur anywhere in the brain. The most common locations are shown in Figure 11–1. The hematoma spreads

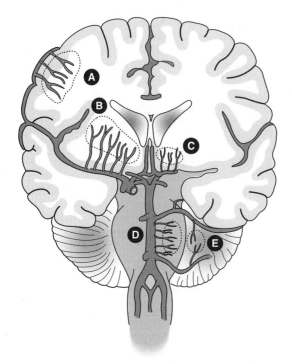

▲ **Figure 11–1.** Common locations of intraparenchymal hemorrhage. **A:** Lobar hemorrhage often due to cerebral amyloid angiopathy. **B:** Hemorrhage of basal ganglia and internal capsule. **C:** Thalamic hemorrhage. **D:** Pontine hemorrhage. **E:** Cerebellar hemorrhage. B–E are often due to hypertension. Hemorrhage due to tumor, arteriovenous malformation, and other etiologies may occur anywhere. (Reproduced with permission from Quereshi AI, et al. Spontaneous intracerebral hemorrhage. *N Engl J Med* 2001;344:1450–1460.)

Once the hematoma forms, cerebral edema develops around the clot as osmotically active serum proteins are released from the hematoma; thrombin also acts as a neurotoxin and contributes to edema. Edema peaks at about 48 hours and usually resolves by 5 days, but it may persist longer. Edema contributes to neurologic deterioration by causing tissue shifts, raised intracranial pressure, and transtentorial herniation (see later discussion). As the hematoma is absorbed and edema resolves, a slit-like hematoma cavity containing hemosiderin remains, with surrounding brain atrophy.

Whether brain tissue surrounding the hematoma is ischemic due to compression of vascular structures is controversial. Studies of cerebral blood flow and metabolism in regions immediately surrounding the hematoma favor a functional suppression of brain activity (diaschisis) rather than ischemia. The therapeutic implication of these observations is that acutely lowering blood pressure after IPH will not cause secondary brain injury by exacerbating ischemia. This is consistent with recent observations that acute blood pressure reduction in the setting of IPH is safe.

A. Deep Hemorrhages

Hypertension damages the small penetrating arteries of the brain, including those that supply deep structures such as the basal ganglia, internal capsule, pons, thalamus, and deep cerebellar nuclei (see Figure 11–1). Hypertension may contribute to lobar hemorrhages in conjunction with cerebral amyloid angiopathy (discussed next). Patients with hypertensive brain hemorrhage face a 2% yearly risk of recurrent hemorrhage.

B. Lobar Hemorrhages

In contrast to deep hemorrhages, hemorrhages occurring in the white matter immediately subjacent to the cortex (so-called *lobar hemorrhages*) are often due to cerebral amyloid angiopathy (CAA). CAA occurs in elderly, usually nonhypertensive patients. It is characterized by deposition of amyloid in the walls of leptomeningeal and cortical arteries. Amyloid hemorrhages tend to occur most frequently in the parietal and occipital lobes. For obscure reasons, CAA occasionally causes multiple, simultaneous hemorrhages in widely separated brain regions. Definitive diagnosis of CAA requires pathologic demonstration of apple-green birefringence under polarized light microscopy of cortical vessels. The diagnosis is suggested by the presence of one or more lobar hemorrhages in an elderly, often demented patient without hypertension and is also suggested by the presence of the ApoE2 or E4 alleles. Gradient-echo MRI may reveal multiple deposits of hemosiderin in the cortex and immediately subjacent white matter, probably reflecting ongoing, subclinical microhemorrhage formation; the number of lobar microhemorrhages is highly predictive of the risk of recurrent hemorrhage, which may be as high as 15% per year. Consistent with the idea that CAA is a generalized brain vasculopathy,

between white matter tracts, resulting in islands of viable brain tissue within the hematoma itself. In hypertensive brain hemorrhage, blood originates from the bifurcations of small, penetrating arteries that have sustained scarring and medial degeneration as a result of hypertension. Lobar hemorrhages may originate in leptomeningeal or cortical blood vessels that have become brittle due to deposition of amyloid (so-called *cerebral amyloid angiopathy*). The origin of bleeding in hemorrhage due to underlying brain lesions is specific to each particular etiology.

Bleeding usually stops shortly after the initial ictus, but in a substantial minority of patients the hematoma continues to expand, usually within the first hour after presentation; expansion beyond 24 hours is unusual except in the setting of an uncorrected coagulopathy. Severe hypertension may contribute to hematoma expansion. Early hematoma expansion portends a worse outcome.

patients with this disorder also often have severe chronic white matter ischemic changes and deep microhemorrhages on MRI. Blood pressure control may help prevent recurrent amyloid-related lobar hemorrhage.

C. Vascular Malformations

IPH may be caused by vascular malformations and anomalies, including arteriovenous malformation (AVM), arteriovenous fistula (AVF), and small vascular malformations such as cavernous angioma and so-called *micro-AVM*. The latter two are invisible by angiography but may be visible by MRI. Hemorrhages may be either lobar or deep and are unrelated to hypertension.

D. Sympathomimetic Agents

Sympathomimetic drug use has been associated with IPH, including amphetamine, methamphetamine, and cocaine. According to one large case-control study, use of appetite suppressants containing the sympathomimetic drug phenylpropanolamine (PPA, no longer available in the United States) increases the relative risk of IPH, although the absolute risk per dose is extremely low. Sympathomimetic agents probably cause IPH by producing reversible vasoconstriction with reperfusion hemorrhage, inflammatory vasculitis, or severe, acute hypertension. They may cause preexisting vascular malformations to rupture during hypertensive surges.

E. Neoplasms

Both primary and metastatic brain neoplasms may bleed, and in about half of such cases the hemorrhage is the first clinical manifestation of the brain tumor. High-grade primary brain tumors such as glioblastoma multiforme are the most likely to bleed. Among cerebral metastatic tumors, melanoma, bronchogenic carcinoma, renal cell carcinoma, and choriocarcinoma most commonly bleed. Diagnosis of an underlying neoplasm at the time of acute hemorrhage may be difficult. A history of subacute neurologic decline before the acute presentation, ring-enhancement on gadolinium MRI within the first 48 hours, and unusual location such as the corpus callosum all suggest underlying neoplasm. Biopsy of the suspect area, or repeat MRI after 6 weeks, may disclose the presence of a neoplasm in such cases.

F. Anticoagulation Therapy

The most common iatrogenic cause of IPH is anticoagulation with oral or parenteral agents. Long-term warfarin use accounts for about 10% of all spontaneous IPH and carries a risk of IPH between 0.5% and 1% per year. Warfarin-induced brain hemorrhage is disabling or fatal in 80% of cases, usually due to early catastrophic hematoma expansion. Risk factors for IPH in patients receiving warfarin include advanced age, cerebral leukoaraiosis, hypertension, an international normalized ratio greater than 2, and concomitant aspirin use. Cerebral amyloid angiopathy (CAA) is a major risk factor, and patients with known hemorrhage from CAA should never be placed on warfarin. Occasional patients have diffuse microhemorrhages but have never had a clinically detectable hemorrhagic stroke. The safety of anticoagulation in those patients is unknown. Whether patients with prior brain hemorrhage due to other causes can safely take warfarin if their risk factors are controlled is unknown. Acute anticoagulation with heparin or heparinoids in the setting of ischemic stroke also predisposes to IPH, especially in patients with large infarcts and uncontrolled hypertension.

Thrombolytic agents are also associated with a high risk of IPH, about 1% in patients given tissue-type plasminogen activator (tPA) for acute myocardial infarction and 6–10% in patients given thrombolytic agents for acute ischemic stroke. Predisposing factors for thrombolytic-associated brain hemorrhage include advanced age, severe stroke, deviations from accepted tPA protocol, and hyperglycemia. Underlying CAA may also increase the risk of tPA-induced hemorrhage.

G. Cerebrovenous Occlusion

An important, albeit rare, cause of IPH is cerebrovenous occlusive disease. In patients with saggital sinus thrombosis, especially when the thrombosis extends to cortical veins, lobar hemorrhagic infarction is common. This may initially be difficult to distinguish from primary IPH, and high clinical suspicion is required. This diagnosis should be considered in patients with high-convexity parietal lobar hemorrhage who are at high risk for thrombotic events, including pregnancy and puerperium, disseminated cancer, and collagen-vascular or other diseases predisposing to hypercoagulability. Brain magnetic resonance venography or catheter angiogram may be required to reveal underlying venous thrombosis.

H. Hyperperfusion Syndrome

Patients who have undergone cerebral revascularization by carotid endarterectomy or angioplasty may develop a syndrome of headache, confusion, focal deficits, cerebral edema, and IPH. This so-called *hyperperfusion syndrome* probably results from suddenly increased cerebral blood flow into a formerly ischemic, maximally dilated vascular bed. A similar syndrome occasionally complicates hypertensive encephalopathy, eclampsia, or so-called *cyclosporine encephalopathy*.

I. Other, Rare Causes

Other causes of IPH are relatively rare. Septic brain embolism from bacterial endocarditis may lead to IPH, SAH, or both due to infected (mycotic) aneurysm rupture, pyogenic arteritis, or brain abscess formation. IPH may result from any coagulopathy or severe thrombocytopenia. Cerebral vasculitis and syndromes of reversible cerebral vasoconstriction (eg, Call-Fleming syndrome) are associated with both IPH and ischemic stroke. The brittle dilated lenticulostriate arteries found in moyamoya syndrome may rupture, leading to

IPH. Finally, although not strictly a hemorrhagic stroke, head trauma may lead to brain contusion accompanied by minor or massive IPH.

▶ Clinical Findings

A. Symptoms and Signs

There is no single clinical finding that reliably differentiates IPH from ischemic stroke. The particular focal findings in IPH reflect the location of the hematoma and its effects on adjacent structures (see Differential Diagnosis). However, some general clinical patterns may be discerned. Patients with IPH develop a focal deficit that worsens over minutes, usually accompanied by acute hypertension. Onset during sleep is uncommon. Headache occurs in just under half of patients with IPH. Nausea, vomiting, and an early decline in level of consciousness result from large hematomas, which cause raised intracranial pressure and intracranial tissue shifts. Patients with acute IPH are at high risk of worsening due to ongoing or recurrent bleeding and therefore require careful monitoring.

B. History

History-taking in patients with the acute onset of central nervous system symptoms should focus on three areas: (1) determining whether the deficit is due to stroke, and if so, the type of stroke, (2) determining the location of the lesion, and (3) evaluating stroke risk factors and the likely mechanism of the stroke. In acute ICH, patients or families usually report the sudden onset of a focal deficit, which then progresses, sometimes to coma, over minutes. Headache, nausea, and vomiting are neither specific nor sensitive for differentiating ICH from ischemic stroke. Although transient symptoms are a rare manifestation of brain hemorrhage, some patients do have onset similar to that of transient ischemic attack.

Because hypertension is the most common cause of IPH, a history of hypertension, treated or untreated, must be assiduously sought. Often patients with known hypertension have discontinued antihypertensive medication. Patients may have a history of coronary artery disease, renal dysfunction, prior stroke, or retinal disease, all suggestive of hypertension. Causes of acute hypertension, such as the use of sympathomimetic drugs, should be considered.

In nonhypertensive elderly patients with ICH, a history of dementia or prior lobar IPH suggests the presence of CAA. The administration of systemic anticoagulants or thrombolytics is usually obvious by history. Review of systems should include hepatic and hematologic disorders and CNS or systemic neoplasm. A history of seizures or a pulse synchronous cranial bruit may suggest an underlying vascular malformation.

C. Examination

The examination of a patient with an acute stroke begins with an assessment of vital signs and general medical status. Acute, often very severe, hypertension is common in IPH. Management of elevated BP is controversial. Respiratory status should be assessed and arterial oxygen saturation measured, as aspiration pneumonia or pneumonitis may occur at any time. Careful evaluation of cardiac function, heart sounds, skin, and electrocardiogram may reveal cardiac ischemia or disclose murmurs suggesting endocarditis. Atrial fibrillation raises the possibility that the IPH is due to anticoagulants. Cutaneous bruising, petechiae, or an enlarged liver suggest hepatic failure or coagulopathy. Finally, it is important to address the effects of falling in patients found on the floor, including compartment syndromes, unstable cervical fractures, muscle necrosis, and pressure sores.

Neurologic examination should elicit signs that aid in localization (see Differential Diagnosis), including those that reflect signs of cerebral transtentorial herniation. These signs must be accurately recorded, especially the level of consciousness, so that a subsequent examiner can determine whether there has been worsening. Quantitation of limb strength is also important. Serial recording by nursing staff of the Glasgow coma scale and the National Institutes of Health stroke scale helps to determine response to treatment or neurologic deterioration.

▶ Differential Diagnosis

A. Syndromes Usually Due to Hypertension

1. Putamen hemorrhage—The hallmark of putamen hemorrhage is contralateral hemiparesis, hemisensory loss, or both, due to involvement of the adjacent internal capsule (Figure 11–2). Smaller putamen hemorrhages may mimic the deficits seen with lacunar infarction, including pure motor hemiparesis, pure hemisensory sensory stroke, and ataxic hemiparesis. Rarely, a movement disorder (eg, hemiballism) follows hemorrhage limited to the putamen itself. Larger putaminal hemorrhage often causes cortical signs in addition to contralateral hemiplegia, including aphasia (language-dominant hemisphere), contralateral hemineglect (either hemisphere), visual field disturbances, and ipsilateral gaze preference. Massive putamen hematoma can cause coma.

2. Caudate hemorrhage—Because the caudate nucleus abuts the frontal ventricular horn, bleeding into the caudate often extends into the ventricular system, causing severe headache, nuchal rigidity, nausea, and vomiting. There may be decreased verbal fluency or aphasia, but persistent language disturbance is uncommon. Many patients are apathetic or abulic. Hemiparesis, when present (about 30%), is usually mild. Ventricular extension of blood may cause acute hydrocephalus, with coma and oculomotor palsies. Many cases of so-called *primary intraventricular hemorrhage* are likely caudate hemorrhages, in which the intraparenchymal component is minimal compared with the intraventricular extension. Prognosis in isolated caudate hemorrhage is usually favorable, although subtle neuropsychiatric abnormalities often persist.

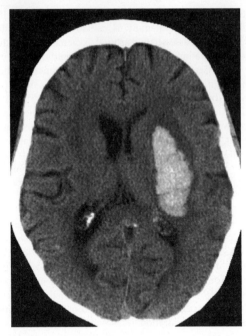

▲ **Figure 11–2.** Unenhanced cranial CT scan showing left putaminal hemorrhage in a 75-year-old right-handed woman with untreated hypertension and alcoholism. She presented with global aphasia, left gaze preference, and right hemiplegia. She survived, but the deficits did not improve.

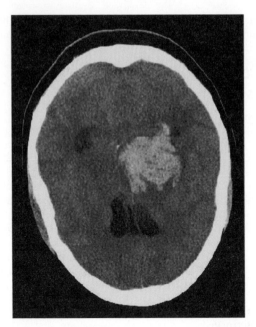

▲ **Figure 11–3.** Unenhanced cranial CT scan showing a massive right thalamic hemorrhage in a 33-year-old woman with untreated severe hypertension. She presented with left hemiparesis followed within minutes by deep coma. The patient failed to respond to medical therapy and placement of a ventricular catheter, and care was withdrawn at the family's request.

3. Thalamic hemorrhage—Most patients with thalamic hemorrhage have a rapid onset of contralateral weakness and hemisensory loss to all modalities (Figure 11–3). A minority experience initial hemisensory symptoms with subsequent appearance of hemiparesis. Receptive aphasia or hemineglect may be present. Small anterior or medial thalamic hemorrhages can cause amnesia or abulia with preserved motor and sensory function. Small lateral thalamic hemorrhages rarely mimic the thalamic lacunar syndrome of so-called *pure sensory stroke*. Massive thalamic hemorrhages cause a rapid descent into coma, either due to acute hydrocephalus from intraventricular extension or due to hematoma dissection into the midbrain reticular activating system.

Thalamic hemorrhage may be recognized at the bedside by characteristic and specific ocular findings. These include tonic downward gaze deviation with upgaze palsy; horizontal gaze deviations to either the ipsilateral or contralateral side; mid-position, unreactive pupils; and retractory nystagmus upon attempted upgaze. These ocular signs are probably the result of damage to the oculomotor complex in the midbrain tectum or acute obstructive hydrocephalus.

Patients with thalamic hemorrhages have a poor prognosis, with 25–50% mortality. Survivors occasionally develop a severe, medically refractory, contralateral thalamic pain syndrome.

4. Pontine hemorrhage—Ninety percent of pontine hemorrhages are due to hypertension. Massive pontine hemorrhage is due to rupture of pontine perforating arteries that arise directly from the basilar artery (see Figure 11–1). Eighty percent of patients have rapid descent into coma, accompanied by quadriplegia, stiffening of the limbs, extensor posturing, pinpoint reactive pupils, facial diplegia, absence of gag and swallowing reflexes, loss of spontaneous and reflexic horizontal eye movements, and loss of corneal reflexes. Other eye movement abnormalities include ocular bobbing (rapid conjugate downward saccade with slow return to neutral position). Rare patients have predicate symptoms of headache, deafness, numbness, or nausea, usually lasting a few minutes and followed by coma. Autonomic symptoms include high fevers and respiratory abnormalities. Mortality from large pontine hemorrhage is nearly 100%.

Occasional patients have small unilateral pontine hemorrhages, most often due to AVM rupture or bleeding from cavernous malformations. Such patients have syndromes that mimic lacunar infarction in the pons, such as pure motor stroke, ataxic hemiparesis, or isolated cranial neuropathies.

Treatment of massive pontine hemorrhage is supportive but usually futile. Survival with good function once coma has developed is extremely rare. Some patients with small pontine hemorrhages do survive, and good recovery has been reported after surgical removal of pontine AVMs or cavernous malformations that have bled.

5. Cerebellar hemorrhage—Cerebellar hemorrhages account for about 10% of all intraparenchymal hemorrhages. Hypertension is the most common etiology, but AVMs and tumors also occur. The most common symptom is the inability to stand or walk independently, with a "drunk" or unstable feeling. Vomiting, headache, and neck pain and stiffness are also common. Neurologic examination usually discloses nystagmus, dysarthria, occasional ipsilateral peripheral facial and gaze palsy (from compression of the ipsilateral pons), and ipsilateral appendicular incoordination. Frank weakness of the extremities is uncommon and, if present, suggests brainstem compression.

The level of consciousness may range from normal to coma and is a crucial clinical variable. Patients who remain alert have a good natural history with medical management. However, a decline in consciousness, which may occur abruptly in the first several days, portends a dismal prognosis in the absence of surgical evacuation. Hematomas greater than 3 cm in diameter are most often associated with neurologic decline. Because it is difficult to predict from either clinical or radiologic variables which patients will decline, all patients with cerebellar hemorrhage should be carefully monitored, and a neurosurgical team should be available if needed.

B. Syndromes Usually Not Associated With Hypertension

As noted, lobar hemorrhage in nonhypertensives is most often associated with CAA, AVM, neoplasm, or coagulopathy. About 20%, however, are of unknown cause (so-called *cryptogenic*). Neurologic deficits mimic those caused by cortical ischemic stroke and reflect the tendency of lobar hemorrhage to occur in the parietal and occipital lobes. Signs include contralateral hemiparesis, aphasia or hemi-neglect, and visual field disturbance. Because of their location near the cerebral cortex, seizures are more common in lobar than in deep hemorrhage. Coma is considerably less common. Outcome is generally better than with deep hemorrhage. In nonelderly patients with lobar hemorrhage, an extensive search for a treatable lesion is mandatory.

▶ Treatment

- Urgent neuroimaging is the key to diagnosis.
- Selected patients require vascular imaging with noninvasive or invasive angiography.
- Neurologic management focuses on stopping the bleeding, preventing secondary brain injury, and preventing rebleeding.
- Systemic management includes anticipating, preventing, and detecting the consequences of immobility and acute illness, such as infection, pulmonary embolism, and metabolic abnormalities.

There is no medical or surgical treatment that has been shown to improve outcome in IPH, and recommendations are based on anecdotal reports and small studies. Secondary prevention is a different matter, however, and treatments to prevent recurrent hypertensive hemorrhage are available.

A. Diagnostic Evaluation

The key to diagnosis of acute intraparenchymal hemorrhage is emergent neuroimaging with cranial CT or MRI. Both modalities are extremely sensitive. CT is considerably easier in acutely ill patients who may be neurologically and hemodynamically unstable, intubated, or confused. It is available in most emergency rooms and hospitals around the clock, and a head CT takes about 1 minute. For these reasons, head CT is usually the modality of choice. A negative head CT rules out acute IPH (see Figures 11–2 and 11–3).

The location of the epicenter of the hematoma aids in determination of the cause, as described previously. CT scans should be scrutinized for the presence of coexisting subdural, subarachnoid, and intraventricular hemorrhage, all of which would change treatment and the risk for specific secondary complications. The presence of mass effect, tissue shifts, and surrounding brain edema (which is hypodense on CT) should be evaluated.

Despite logistical disadvantages, MRI with appropriate scanning sequences (susceptibility-weighted or gradient echo imaging) is more sensitive than CT for detecting certain aspects of IPH, including subacute or temporally remote brain hemorrhage, in which hemosiderin staining of the brain may persist indefinitely (Figure 11–4). MRI can also detect the presence of abnormal blood vessels surrounding an acute hemorrhage, suggesting the presence of a vascular malformation (Figure 11–5). Gadolinium enhancement within the first 48 hours suggests an underlying neoplasm or abscess. Repeating the MRI after 6–12 weeks increases the yield for detecting a neoplasm.

Important laboratory tests include coagulation studies (prothrombin time, activated partial thromboplastin time, and possibly platelet function testing), complete blood count with platelets, liver function tests, urine toxicology in selected patients, electrocardiogram, chest X-ray, and, in obtunded patients, measurement of arterial blood gases.

Patients younger than 50 with unexplained hemorrhages should undergo catheter angiography, including views of the external carotid circulation, to rule out vascular anomalies (Figure 11–6). In cases where brain imaging suggests hemorrhagic infarction in the territory of a major dural sinus or vein, catheter venography or magnetic resonance venography should be performed to rule out venous thrombosis.

Acute therapy has the dual goals of minimizing brain injury and limiting systemic complications of the brain injury. The neurologic goals are to (1) stop the bleeding, (2) prevent further neurologic deterioration, and (3) prevent recurrence. Systemic goals are to anticipate, prevent, and quickly treat such complications as myocardial ischemia,

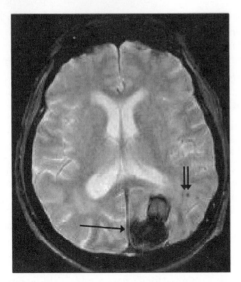

▲ **Figure 11-4.** Gradient-echo MRI scan showing a left occipital hemorrhage (*single arrow*) and an adjacent lobar hemosiderin deposit (*double arrow*), presumably due to cerebral amyloid angiopathy, in a 70-year-old non-hypertensive woman with mild dementia. She presented with a right homonymous hemianopia. The visual disturbance largely resolved, but she remained unable to read.

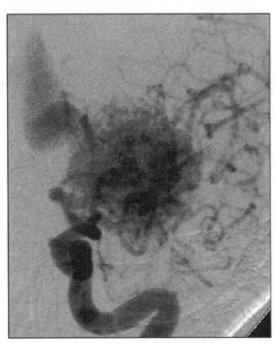

▲ **Figure 11-6.** Catheter angiogram, left internal carotid injection, showing the left temporal lobe arteriovenous malformation described in Figure 11-5. A dilated draining vein is seen in the upper left corner of the figure.

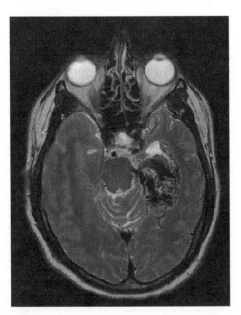

▲ **Figure 11-5.** T2-weighted MRI scan of the brain showing a left temporal arteriovenous malformation in a 35-year-old man with progressive memory loss and severe headache.

respiratory compromise, infections, deep venous thromboses, and decubitus ulcers.

B. Initial Management

Airway, breathing, and circulation should be the initial focus. Patients unable to protect the airway due to either diminished consciousness or bulbar dysfunction, or those with respiratory insufficiency due to aspiration pneumonia, should undergo endotracheal intubation. Precautions to avoid reflex arrhythmias or increases in blood pressure are essential. In unstable patients, intubation before CT scanning may be indicated. The patient should be evaluated for signs of trauma, especially if "found down." All patients found unconscious anywhere but in bed should be presumed to have an unstable cervical spine until proven otherwise, and spinal precautions should be instituted. Such patients should also be evaluated for pressure sores and compartment syndromes. In general, the head of the bed should remain at 30 degrees to optimize intracranial pressure and cerebral perfusion. Hypotonic fluids and lactated Ringers solution should be avoided; normal saline is appropriate. Urgent neurologic and neurosurgical consultation should be sought. Because of the high risk of neurologic deterioration in the first 48 hours, admission to a dedicated intensive care unit is important. American Heart Association consensus guidelines

Table 11–1. Medical Management of Intraparenchymal Hemorrhage: Summary of AHA Guidelines

1. **Initial management** should be focused on airway, breathing, circulation, and neurologic deficits.
2. **Intubation** is indicated for insufficient ventilation (Po_2 <60 mm Hg or Pco_2 >50 mm Hg) or obvious risk of aspiration.
3. **Systolic blood pressure** >200 mm Hg or mean arterial pressure >150 mm Hg should prompt consideration of aggressive reduction with continuous intravenous infusion of antihypertensive agents. If there is no suspicion of raised intracranial pressure, a target of 160/90 is reasonable as long as the neurologic examination does not worsen with a lower BP.
4. **Intracranial pressure (ICP) monitors** should be placed in patients with Glasgow coma scale score <9, and patients who are deteriorating due to presumed high ICP (Level of Evidence C, Grade C Recommendation). ICP should be maintained <20 mm Hg, with cerebral perfusion pressure (CPP) >70 mm Hg.
5. **Raised ICP** may be treated with hyperosmolar therapy (intravenous mannitol or hypertonic saline), hyperventilation, or neuromuscular paralysis. Steroids should be avoided.
6. **Ventricular drains** should be used in patients with or at risk for hydrocephalus.
7. **Fluid management:** Patients should be kept euvolemic, with central venous pressure between 5 and 12 mm Hg.
8. **Prophylactic anticonvulsant administration** in patients with lobar hemorrhage may reduce the risk of early seizures. (Class IIb, Level of Evidence C).
9. **Body temperature** should be maintained at normal levels, with cooling blankets or devices or acetaminophen as needed.
10. **Deep venous thrombosis** prevention with subcutaneous low-dose heparin or heparinoid should be initiated if the patient is neurologically stable after 3 or 4 days from onset (Class IIb, Level of Evidence B).

Based on information in Broderick J, et al. Guidelines for the management of spontaneous intracerebral hemorrhage in adults, 2007 update. *Circulation* 2007;116:e391–413.

for medical management of acute brain hemorrhage are summarized in Table 11–1.

C. Neurologic Management

1. Stopping the bleeding—Hematoma expansion in the first 24 hours after IPH, occurring in up to 40% of patients, is the most common cause of neurologic decline in the first 24 hours and portends a poor outcome (Figure 11–7). Why hematomas expand is unclear. Some studies suggest an association between severely elevated blood pressure and continued hematoma growth, but whether hypertension is a cause or an effect of hematoma expansion is unknown. An elevated blood pressure may reflect underlying hypertension, a nonspecific response to acute illness or pain, or even a protective response to raised intracranial pressure (ICP) and compromised cerebral perfusion (the Cushing-Kocher response).

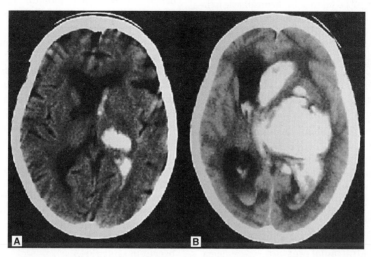

▲ **Figure 11–7.** Rapid expansion of thalamic hemorrhage. **A:** Initial CT scan, depicting moderate-sized left thalamic hemorrhage with extension into the left lateral ventricle. **B:** CT scan obtained 6 hours later, after neurologic deterioration. Dramatic expansion of the hematoma occurred, with diffuse cerebral edema, massive intraventricular hemorrhage, and hydrocephalus. (Reproduced with permission from Quereshi AI, et al. Spontaneous intracerebral hemorrhage. *N Engl J Med* 2001:344:1450–1460.)

Hemostatic therapy with recombinant activated factor VII and aggressive blood pressure lowering have both been shown to reduce hematoma expansion. However, neither measure has been shown to improve outcome in IPH.

Patients with warfarin-associated IPH should have their drug-induced coagulopathy corrected as soon as possible. Although the optimal agent for this is unknown, it is known that fresh-frozen plasma is not a feasible treatment. Better options probably include recombinant activated factor 7 or prothrombin complex concentrate. Both of the latter agents can be infused rapidly, require only minutes to prepare, and reverse warfarin-induced coagulopathy instantaneously. Some authors suggest platelet transfusion in the setting of IPH in users of antiplatelet agents or patients with abnormal platelet function test results, but the efficacy and safety of this approach are unknown.

A decrease in systolic blood pressure of 20% over the first 24 hours, or to less than 160 mm Hg, whichever is higher, is probably safe. It is essential to use intravenous, rapidly titratable agents such as labetalol or nicardipine. Nitroprusside, which can cause cerebral vasodilation and increased intracranial pressure, is a second-line agent and should only be used with an intracranial pressure monitor, if at all.

Neurosurgical hematoma evacuation should be considered in patients with imminent transtentorial herniation due to a large cerebral hematoma, in whom a reasonable prognosis for meaningful recovery exists. The latter consideration probably excludes those with coma and unreactive pupils for more than a few hours. Evacuation of deep, dominant hemisphere hematomas may worsen functional outcome by damaging cortical structures important for language.

Decompressive hemicraniectomy prevents death and may improve outcome in patients with massive hemispheric ischemic stroke; some clinicians use this surgical therapy, with or without hematoma evacuation, in patients with massive IPH, although reliable data on its effectiveness are not available. A large randomized trial comparing medical management with surgical hematoma evacuation in patients in whom the surgeon was "in equipoise" did not suggest any benefit of surgery. Therefore, a general policy of surgical hematoma evacuation is unwarranted.

Large cerebellar hemorrhages should be surgically evacuated regardless of the patient's level of consciousness. Endoventricular drainage is a consideration in patients with IPH and hydrocephalus due to aqueductal compression or intraventricular blood. A summary of the American Heart Association consensus guidelines on surgical evacuation of intracerebral hemorrhage is shown in Table 11–2.

2. Preventing secondary brain injury from mass effect, cerebral edema, and intracranial pressure—Large hematomas compress or distort adjacent brain regions. Cerebral edema develops more slowly, usually within the first 48 hours. In occasional patients, cerebral edema may occur as late as 2 weeks after a hemorrhage. Both mass effect and cerebral edema contribute to neurologic decline by compressing

Table 11–2. Surgical Treatment of Intracerebral Hemorrhage: Summary of AHA Guidelines

Surgical candidates:
1. Patients with cerebellar hemorrhage >3 cm who are neurologically deteriorating or who have clinical or radiographic evidence of symptomatic brainstem compression or hydrocephalus from ventricular obstruction (Levels of Evidence III–V, Grade C Recommendation).
2. Intracerebral hemorrhage associated with aneurysm, arteriovenous malformation, or cavernous malformation, if the patient has a chance for good outcome and the lesion is surgically accessible (Levels of Evidence III–V, Grade C Recommendation).
3. Young patients with moderate or large lobar hemorrhage who are clinically deteriorating (Levels of Evidence II–V, Grade B Recommendation).

Nonsurgical candidates:
1. Patients with small hemorrhages or minimal neurologic deficits (Levels of Evidence II–V, Grade B Recommendation).
2. Patients with a Glasgow coma scale score <5, except for those with cerebellar hemorrhages with brainstem compression (Levels of Evidence II–V, Grade B Recommendation).

Best therapy unclear:
    All other patients.

Based on information in Broderick J, et al. Guidelines for the management of spontaneous intracerebral hemorrhage in adults, 2007 update. *Circulation* 2007;116:e391–413.

otherwise uninvolved brain regions and in some cases progressing to transtentorial herniation. Patients with large hematomas or a rapidly declining level of consciousness may benefit from an ICP monitor. Intraventricular catheters allow withdrawal of ventricular fluid to lower ICP. Serial CT scanning twice per day over the first 48 hours may also aid in the monitoring of hematoma expansion, mass effect, and cerebral edema.

Interventions to decrease brain swelling should be reserved for patients with neurologic decline or CT-scan evidence of impending herniation and should not be used prophylactically. Mannitol is administered in 0.25–1.0 g/kg boluses to a target serum osmolality of 320 mOsm/L, although higher osmolalities may sometimes be used and are probably safe. Hyperventilation to a $PaCO_2$ of 30–35 mm Hg may also lower ICP, but the effect is transient, and this should be viewed as an emergent temporizing measure before more definitive therapy (eg, surgery). Rebound increased ICP may occur when either mannitol or hyperventilation are withdrawn, so withdrawal should be done slowly. Corticosteroids increase the risk of infection and are of no benefit in acute IPH.

Anticonvulsants are indicated in patients who have a seizure in the setting of acute IPH. Prophylactic administration of anticonvulsants is controversial. Because seizures may worsen cerebral edema and ICP, patients whose intracranial dynamics seem tenuous can be treated prophylactically for

2–4 weeks. Patients with lobar hemorrhage are more likely to have seizures.

3. Preventing recurrence—Long-term control of blood pressure significantly reduces the risk of recurrent hypertensive hemorrhage. Thiazide diuretics and angiotensin-converting enzyme (ACE) inhibitors in combination cut the risk of recurrence in half, regardless of blood pressure level. Oral antihypertensive therapy can be started as soon as the patient is stable, usually within a few days.

Patients with cerebral amyloid angiopathy should avoid all antithrombotic therapies, including aspirin. The risk of recurrent hemorrhage increases with the number of hemosiderin deposits seen on gradient-echo MRI. Patients with five or more areas of hemosiderin deposition have a risk of recurrent brain hemorrhage exceeding 10% per year. Blood pressure reduction has been shown to prevent recurrent lobar hemorrhage in patients with CAA.

The management of patients with vascular malformations is discussed later.

D. Systemic Management

The systemic complications of acute IPH, similar to those occurring in other unstable, immobilized patients, are cardiovascular, pulmonary, infectious, metabolic, and mechanical.

Many patients with IPH experience electrocardiogram changes and subendocardial ischemia. Antithrombotic therapy for prevention of coronary ischemia is avoided for the first several weeks after IPH. Low-dose β-blockers can be given during this period; short-acting agents that can be discontinued rapidly in the case of neurologic decline are preferred.

Aspiration of gastric contents may occur before hospital arrival, during intubation, during seizures, or at other times. Careful nursing attention to pulmonary toilet, prompt initiation of antibiotics, surveillance chest X-rays, and sputum cultures are important in management, especially in intubated patients. Deep venous thrombosis and pulmonary embolism are risks in immobilized patients. Prevention of deep venous thrombosis (DVT) includes compression stockings and pneumatic boots. Low-dose heparin or heparinoids to prevent DVT can be used safely in stable patients 3 days from the onset of hemorrhage.

Metabolic derangements in patients with IPH include hyponatremia due to syndrome of inappropriate antidiuretic hormone (SIADH), other electrolyte abnormalities, and the consequences of malnutrition. Hyponatremia is especially important to recognize and correct, as the accumulation of free water in the injured brain can worsen cerebral edema. Isotonic crystalloids should be used, and euvolemia (central venous pressure of 5–12 mm Hg) should be maintained.

IPH patients are at risk for pulmonary, urinary tract, skin, and intravenous site infections, calling for frequent surveillance and prompt treatment. Any metabolic or infectious derangement in patients with IPH may result in neurologic decline, including exacerbation of focal signs, decline in consciousness, or delirium.

▶ Prognosis

Prognostication in patients with IPH encompasses both the likelihood of survival and the potential for neurologic improvement. Accurate prediction of mortality might allow early withdrawal of futile care in devastated patients. Accurate prediction of neurologic recovery in patients who survive might allow families to weigh the relative risks and benefits of aggressive treatment. Unfortunately, neither mortality nor neurologic outcome can be precisely estimated. About 30–50% of patients survive acute intracerebral hemorrhage. Death may be due to catastrophic hematoma expansion, untreatable cerebral edema with herniation, or systemic complications such as pneumonia. Clinical predictors of mortality include age, level of consciousness, size of the hematoma seen on CT scan, and location of the hematoma. Extension of blood into the ventricles also portends a poor outcome. The "ICH score" (Table 11–3) is a useful, easily calculated scale that allows a rough estimate of 30-day mortality, but its use in bedside prognostication is controversial.

Table 11–3. The ICH Score

Component	ICH Score Points
Glasgow Coma Scale Score	
3–4	2
5–12	1
13–15	0
ICH Volume	
≥30 mL	1
<30 mL	0
Intraventricular Hemorrhage	
Yes	1
No	0
Infratentorial Origin	
Yes	1
No	0
Age ≥80 y	
Yes	1
No	0
Total ICH Score	0–6

Score	30-d Mortality (%)
0	0
1	3
2	26
3	72
4	97
5	100

Modified and reproduced with permission from Hemphill JC, et al. The ICH Score. A simple, reliable grading scale for intracerebral hemorrhage. *Stroke* 2001;32:891–897.

Patients who survive sometimes achieve a surprisingly good recovery. In one series of 120 patients with IPH who required mechanical ventilation, in-hospital mortality was 48%. Among the 62 survivors, 24 died, with death occurring an average of 6 months from hospital discharge. Patients were more likely to die after hospital discharge if they had reduced level of consciousness or if they were older than 65 years. In the 36 long-term survivors, 15 (42%) had slight or no disability. Patients who remain in coma after weaning from mechanical ventilation never achieve independent function, although some improve.

Prognostication in IPH must be done with great humility. Families must be appraised of the uncertainty with which prognosis is offered. Decisions about withdrawal of care, organ donation, code status, or aggressive interventions should be made with utmost respect for the family and patient wishes.

Anderson CS, et al. Effects of early intensive blood pressure-lowering on the growth of hematoma and perihematomal edema in acute intracerebral hemorrhage: The Intensive Blood Pressure Reduction in Acute Cerebral Haemorrhage Trial (INTERACT). *Stroke* 2010;41:307–312. [PMID: 20044534]

Broderick J, et al. Guidelines for the management of spontaneous intracerebral hemorrhage in adults: 2007 update. *Circulation* 2007;116:e391–413. [PMID: 17938297]

Brott T, et al. Early hemorrhage growth in patients with intracerebral hemorrhage. *Stroke* 1997;28:1. [PMID: 8996478] (Emphasizes the critical role of early hematoma expansion as a cause of neurologic deterioration in patients with acute intraparenchymal hemorrhage. It also demonstrates that acute brain hemorrhage is a dynamic, unstable process.)

Hemphill JC, et al. The ICH Score. A simple, reliable grading scale for intracerebral hemorrhage. *Stroke* 2001;32:891. [PMID: 11283388] (Describes an easily applied predictor of 30-day survival among patients with acute IPH.)

Mayer SA, et al. Efficacy and safety of recombinant activated factor VII in acute intracerebral hemorrhage. *N Engl J Med* 2008;358:2127–2137. [PMID: 18480205]

Nyquist P. Management of acute intracranial and intraventricular hemorrhage. *Crit Care Med* 2010;38:946–953. [PMID: 20068459]

Roch A, et al. Long-term outcome in intensive care unit survivors after mechanical ventilation for intracerebral hemorrhage. *Crit Care Med* 2003;31:2651. [PMID: 14605538] (Discusses survival and neurologic outcome among the most devastated patients with intracerebral hemorrhage, those requiring mechanical ventilation. Among long-term survivors, nearly half achieve good neurologic recovery.)

SUBARACHNOID HEMORRHAGE

Bleeding into the subarachnoid space surrounding the brain, subarachnoid hemorrhage (SAH), represents 5–10% of all strokes. About 80% of spontaneous (nontraumatic) SAHs are due to the rupture of an intracranial saccular aneurysm. The remaining 20% result from vascular malformations, infected (mycotic) aneurysms, and a few other generally benign conditions (see Table 11–1). Aneurysmal SAH differs from nonaneurysmal SAH in presentation, management, and prognosis and is the focus of this chapter.

ANEURYSMAL SUBARACHNOID HEMORRHAGE

 ESSENTIALS OF DIAGNOSIS

► Sudden onset of excruciating headache, sometimes accompanied by focal neurologic symptoms and signs or sudden coma

► May cause sudden death due to massive brain injury, raised intracranial pressure, or malignant cardiac arrhythmia

► Diagnosis requires emergent brain imaging with CT or MRI; lumbar puncture if imaging is negative

► General Considerations

Rupture of an intracranial saccular aneurysm leading to SAH is a neurologic emergency. There are more than 30,000 cases per year in the United States, likely including many cases of sudden death in which SAH goes undiagnosed. Although SAH represents only 5% of all strokes, it strikes younger patients than ischemic stroke or intracerebral hemorrhage and accounts for 25% of stroke-related years of potential life lost.

Overall mortality in SAH is very high, with a case-fatality rate between 25% and 50%. Ten percent of patients with SAH die before receiving medical attention, and some studies suggest that up to 25% of patients are at risk of death in the first 24 hours. Among patients who survive long enough for transfer to a major medical center, another 25% die over the following 3 months from the initial or recurrent hemorrhage, secondary brain injury, or medical complications. The causes of death and complications at each stage of the disease are relatively limited and often predictable. Nevertheless, SAH patients test the limits of technology in neurosurgery, interventional neuroradiology, and neurologic intensive care. Despite the grim statistics, advances in interdisciplinary management have improved the outlook for patients with SAH. Prompt diagnosis and treatment can result in good outcomes for many patients, including some who appear devastated at initial presentation. Patients have better outcomes when they are cared for in centers that treat large numbers of patients with SAH.

► Pathogenesis

Aneurysms are focal distortions of the normal blood vessel wall, possibly occurring as the result of a developmental abnormality. Most are thought to develop over time and not to be congenital. SAH is usually the result of the rupture of a saccular or berry aneurysm, in which there is a distinct neck and dome arising off the branch point of a major intracranial vessel on the circle of Willis. Less commonly, the artery itself dilates and the wall becomes thin and weak, forming a fusiform aneurysm. Eighty-five percent of saccular aneurysms occur in the anterior circulation. The most common sites for aneurysm formation are the anterior communicating artery/anterior cerebral artery junction, the junction of the posterior communicating and internal carotid arteries, the middle cerebral artery bifurcation, and the basilar artery apex.

About 5% of the healthy adult population harbors an intracranial aneurysm, although the vast majority of these remain unruptured and asymptomatic throughout life. Risk factors for rupture include aneurysmal size, hypertension, prior aneurysmal SAH, smoking, female sex, oral contraceptive use, psychostimulant use, and positive family history. Polycystic kidney syndrome, Marfan syndrome, and Ehlers-Danlos syndrome also predispose patients to formation of intracranial aneurysms.

▶ Clinical Findings

Symptoms and Signs

Patients with SAH typically have a sudden-onset headache, often described as "thunderclap headache," "the worst headache of my life," or "as if I was hit on the head with a baseball bat." The onset is almost always sudden, and patients may transiently lose consciousness or collapse at onset. Although onset may occur during physical exertion, sexual activity, or sympathomimetic drug use, two thirds of patients have onset during sleep or ordinary daily activities.

Some authorities believe that 10–50% of patients experience a so-called *sentinel hemorrhage* days to weeks before the major rupture. These are characterized by sudden-onset severe headache that reaches maximum intensity in seconds and lasts for days to a week. The headache is usually so severe that the patient cannot carry out normal activities. It is crucial not to misdiagnose a sentinel hemorrhage as a migraine, tension headache, or other benign headache. Sentinel hemorrhages generally come on much more rapidly than migraines, last longer, and are qualitatively different than benign headaches. Even with those caveats, it may be hard to clinically distinguish an especially severe migraine from a sentinel hemorrhage. Also, some patients with sentinel hemorrhage or frank SAH do not conform to the patterns just described. One should always err on the side of CT and lumbar puncture when in doubt, because the consequences of aneurysmal re-rupture may be catastrophic.

Examination may reveal meningeal signs such as nuchal rigidity, but this is variable. Examination of the optic fundi may reveal subhyaloid, vitreous, or flame-shaped hemorrhages, which likely result from retinal venous congestion due to raised intracranial pressure. Neurologic signs include focal findings such as cranial neuropathies (described later) or hemiparesis. A decline in level of consciousness is common, and many patients have sudden-onset coma. Severe SAH may cause transtentorial herniation, with coma, enlarged unreactive pupils, and motor posturing, similar to

Table 11–4. Hunt and Hess Grading Scale for Acute Subarachnoid Hemorrhage

Grade	Characteristic
1	Headache
2	Meningeal signs, severe headache, cranial neuropathy
3	Lethargy; inattentiveness, requiring repeated stimulation to remain alert; hemiparesis
4	Stupor; brief arousal only to painful stimulus
5	Coma: no arousal to any stimulus

the presentation of large intraparenchymal hemorrhage. In other patients, coma may be due to the rupture of an aneurysm abutting the brainstem, leading to parenchymal injury. In such cases, recovery is extremely unlikely.

In general, more severe declines in consciousness portend worse outcomes. The most widely used clinical grading scale for patients with aneurysmal SAH is the Hunt and Hess scale, shown in Table 11–4.

Clinical localization of the site of aneurysmal rupture is often impossible, but a few distinct topographic vascular syndromes are discernible. The sudden development of severe headache accompanied by pupil-involving third nerve palsy is highly suspect for a ruptured, thrombosed, or enlarging posterior communicating aneurysm. Aneurysms at the junction formed by the superior cerebellar or posterior cerebral arteries with the basilar artery may also cause painful third nerve palsy. Rare cases of painful third nerve palsies due to aneurysms with partial or even absent pupil involvement have been described.

Anterior communicating artery aneurysms may bleed into the anteromedial frontal lobes, causing leg weakness, abulia, and confusion. Middle cerebral artery aneurysms that rupture into the sylvian fissure may cause aphasia, hemiparesis, or contralateral neglect. Ophthalmic artery aneurysms may cause monocular visual disturbances and pain, including pain with eye movement, which can mimic optic neuritis. Giant aneurysms in any location may cause focal signs by compressing adjacent cranial nerves or brain structures, even in the absence of rupture. The sudden occurrence of symptoms due to an aneurysm, even in the absence of SAH, may indicate rapid enlargement or thrombosis of the aneurysm, both portending imminent rupture. This situation should be treated as urgently as aneurysmal SAH. Rarely, giant aneurysms may contain thrombus that then embolizes distally, leading to acute ischemic stroke.

B. Diagnostic Studies

1. Initial diagnosis—If subarachnoid hemorrhage is clinically suspected, its poor short-term natural history makes definitive diagnosis or exclusion essential. Unenhanced brain

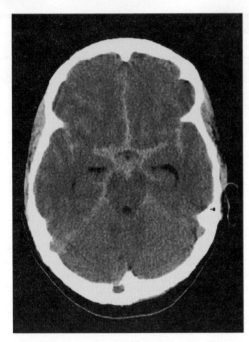

▲ **Figure 11–8.** Unenhanced cranial CT scan showing diffuse subarachnoid hemorrhage in the basal cisterns, interhemispheric cistern, and bilateral sylvian fissures. The bilateral temporal ventricular horns are abnormally dilated, suggesting the presence of hydrocephalus.

CT is an ideal first test (Figure 11–8). CT scans may show blood surrounding the circle of Willis at the base of the brain, over the convexity, or in the interhemispheric or sylvian fissures. The location of the highest density of blood may offer a clue to the location of the aneurysm, but this is not always reliable and is especially unreliable when imaging is performed more than 24 hours after symptom onset. CT may also disclose coexisting hydrocephalus or intraventricular hemorrhage, uncal transtentorial herniation, or mass effect from a large intra- or extra-axial hematoma. In some cases, aneurysmal rupture results in both SAH and intra-parenchymal hemorrhage. For example, a "jet" of blood in the medial orbitofrontal cortex is highly suggestive of a ruptured anterior communicating artery aneurysm.

The sensitivity of CT scanning is about 95% and is highest within the first 12 hours. Patients who are alert may not come to attention until after 12 hours, and so these patients may present a greater diagnostic challenge than patients who present promptly with an obvious neurologic catastrophe. Patients with SAH causing coma, hemiparesis, or other major focal findings due to SAH (Hunt and Hess grade III–V) almost never have a negative CT scan. A CT scan showing SAH makes lumbar puncture unnecessary.

Lumbar puncture (LP) must be performed in patients suspected of having SAH when the CT scan is negative, ambiguous, or technically inadequate. CSF analysis will show high numbers of red blood cells in SAH; if the red blood cell (RBC) count is zero, SAH is ruled out. It is important to distinguish a "traumatic" LP, in which the LP itself caused bleeding into the CSF, from an LP showing subarachnoid hemorrhage. There is no reliable way for the person doing the LP to determine whether it was traumatic or not. Clearing of red blood cells from the first to the fourth tube is an unreliable indicator of a traumatic LP.

The most reliable method for diagnosing SAH from spinal fluid is to measure the concentration of pigmented hemoglobin breakdown products (xanthochromia) by spectrophotometry. Xanthochromia develops in 100% of patients with SAH by 12 hours from aneurysmal rupture and lasts 2 weeks. Although delaying LP for 12 hours from headache onset would increase the sensitivity and specificity of CSF examination for ruling SAH in or out, most experts do not recommend such a delay. Waiting 12 hours from rupture causes logistical problems in ERs and delays definitive management; an aneurysm can re-rupture during the delay. Patients whose clinical presentation is suggestive of SAH and who have bloody spinal fluid before 12 hours from onset should be presumed to have a ruptured aneurysm. The appearance of xanthochromia may also be caused by elevated spinal fluid protein (usually > 150 mg/dL) in the absence of bleeding.

Causes of misdiagnosis of SAH include failure to appreciate the clinical spectrum of presentations of SAH, failure to understand the limits of CT scanning, and failure to perform LP and correctly interpret the results. Misdiagnosis occurs in 12% of patients, predominantly in patients with small hemorrhages and normal mental status. Patients who are initially misdiagnosed tend to have worse outcomes than patients who are correctly diagnosed at their first medical encounter.

2. Identifying the source of hemorrhage—Once the diagnosis of SAH is ascertained, the source must be found urgently. Catheter angiography has been the gold standard for many years for diagnosing the presence of an aneurysm after SAH, and may be required for planning surgical or endovascular treatment (Figure 11–9). Catheter angiograms reveal an aneurysm in 80% of cases; in 20%, patients are found to harbor more than one aneurysm, often in analogous locations on both sides of the circle of Willis (so-called *mirror aneurysm*). In about 1–2% of patients with negative initial angiograms, an aneurysm is disclosed by repeat angiography. It is unclear whether the low yield of repeat angiography is worth the cost and potential morbidity of the procedure, and noninvasive vascular imaging with computed tomographic angiography (CTA) may be a better option for a second study. It is important that catheter angiograms include detailed views of the anterior communicating artery region and both posterior inferior cerebellar artery origins; these sites are often poorly visualized on angiograms performed by operators without experience with SAH.

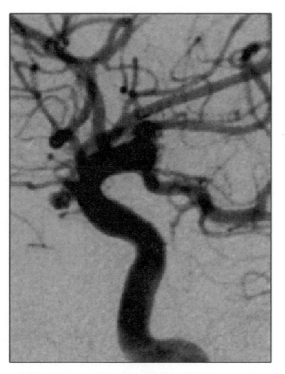

▲ **Figure 11–9.** Digital subtraction angiogram (carotid injection) showing aneurysm at the level of the ophthalmic artery.

In some centers, CTA is replacing catheter angiography because of its safety, rapidity, convenience, and high sensitivity for detecting aneurysms (Figure 11–10). In some cases, high-resolution CTA has identified aneurysms that were missed by catheter angiography. CTA also can disclose three-dimensional aspects of aneurysm morphology that can assist in surgical or endovascular planning. With CTA availability, patients with clinical presentations suggestive of SAH may undergo screening for intracranial aneurysms within minutes of arrival in the emergency department; patients with negative CTAs should still undergo a complete evaluation, including catheter angiography (see Differential Diagnosis, later), but their risk of harboring an aneurysm is quite low. Magnetic resonance angiography is not sufficiently sensitive to detect small, ruptured aneurysms but can play an important role in excluding other conditions that cause SAH (see next section).

▶ Differential Diagnosis

In addition to saccular aneurysmal rupture, the differential diagnosis of SAH includes head trauma with traumatic subarachnoid hemorrhage (usually over the brain convexity and not in the basal cisterns); spontaneous SAH due to bleeding diathesis; rupture of an infected (mycotic) aneurysm, cerebral sinus, or cortical vein thrombosis; ruptured cranial dural arteriovenous fistula (see Vascular Anomalies, later in this chapter); intracranial arterial dissection; cervical vertebral artery dissection with leakage of blood into the cervical

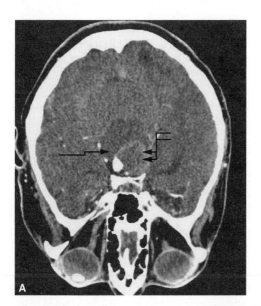

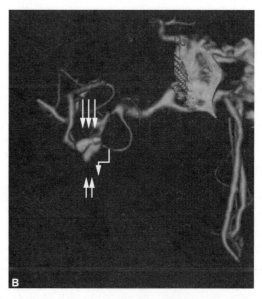

▲ **Figure 11–10.** **A:** CTA axial images of giant thrombosed basilar aneurysm with brainstem compression: basilar artery and aneurysm lumen (*single arrow*); thrombosed portion of aneurysm compressing pons (*double arrow*). **B:** CTA-3D reconstruction of middle cerebral artery (MCA) stenosis and multiple aneurysms: severe R (right). MCA stenosis (*single arrow*); 3-mm MCA aneurysm (*double arrow*); 7-mm multilobulated MCA aneurysm (*triple arrow*).

subarachnoid space; rupture of a cortical arteriovenous malformation; vasculitis or vasculopathy involving intracranial arteries; Call-Fleming syndrome of reversible cerebral vasoconstriction; or rupture of a spinal arteriovenous malformation or spinal dural fistula. Evaluation should include cranial MRI, magnetic resonance venography, catheter angiography of the head and neck including injection of the external carotid circulation and veins (to rule out dural arteriovenous fistula), and in some patients, MRI of the cervical and thoracic spine. A careful laboratory evaluation for hemorrhagic diathesis should be completed. Despite a complete evaluation, some cases of SAH remain cryptogenic.

Some patients present with severe headache and CT scan showing subarachnoid blood limited to the space anterior to the midbrain and pons, with no intraventricular or sylvian fissure blood. These patients, with so-called *perimesencephalic hemorrhage*, tend to be younger than other patients with SAH, present in good clinical grade, and often do not have aneurysms. An initial catheter angiogram is required and, if negative, a follow-up CTA suffices. The risk of rebleeding or poor outcome is extremely low. The etiology of perimesencephalic hemorrhage is unknown; many such patients have anomalous intracranial venous anatomy, but the significance of this finding remains unclear.

▶ Treatment

The clinical course of a patient with aneurysmal SAH comprises two distinct phases. The initial acute phase comprises the first 24–48 hours after aneurysmal rupture, generally before definitive treatment of the ruptured aneurysm. The second phase, which begins by day 3, comprises a very distinct set of clinical challenges.

A. Initial Management of Acute Aneurysmal SAH

The goals of early management of SAH are to secure the ruptured aneurysm to prevent rebleeding (neurosurgical management), prevent secondary brain injury from the initial hemorrhage (neurologic management), and prevent medical complications in these critically ill patients (medical management).

B. Neurologic and Medical Management

Patients with acute SAH are critically ill and require intensive care unit monitoring by an experienced staff. The goals of initial therapy are to anticipate, prevent, and treat medical and neurologic complications and rapidly address reversible causes of neurologic dysfunction.

1. Intubation—Patients should be intubated if they cannot protect the airway. Most do not require mechanical ventilation, but some patients may have aspirated gastric contents at the ictus and have acute lung injury. Occasional patients have acute pulmonary edema or cardiac failure due to the SAH itself (neurogenic pulmonary edema, neurogenic stunned myocardium) and may require pressor support.

Patients may be found unconscious and should be presumed to have an unstable cervical spine fracture until radiographs prove otherwise. Intravenous access should be established, and 0.9% NaCl infused at 100–150 mL/h. Coagulopathies should be reversed as rapidly as possible. Patients should be put on forced bed rest and kept calm and comfortable, with sedation and analgesia as needed. The headache of SAH is intense and should be treated with morphine.

2. Blood pressure management—The management of elevated blood pressure after acute aneurysmal rupture is controversial. Most patients have elevated blood pressure at the time of acute presentation, but the blood pressure may decline after treatment of pain or anxiety, or with bed rest. Some clinicians advocate maintaining a systolic blood pressure lower than 130 mm Hg, whereas others cite the absence of any reliable data justifying this recommendation and do not advocate lowering the blood pressure if the mean arterial pressure is less than 120 or systolic blood pressure is less than 180. Conscious patients are unlikely to have raised intracranial pressure (ICP), and blood pressure lowering to mean arterial pressure less than 100 mm Hg is unlikely to impair cerebral perfusion. Patients with depressed level of consciousness may require placement of an intraventricular catheter (discussed next), which facilitates both measurement and manipulation of ICP, thereby allowing blood pressure titration to levels that will not impair cerebral perfusion. Based on this reasoning, it is reasonable to lower the mean arterial pressure to 100–110 in conscious patients in the first 24 hours after SAH. Preferred agents are those that do not cause cerebral vasodilation and worsen raised ICP, such as intravenous labetalol, enalapril, or nicardipine. Because nitroprusside may increase cerebral blood volume and thereby raise ICP, it should be avoided unless ICP is directly monitored. In general, agents that are quickly reversible in case of neurologic decline are preferred.

3. Intraventricular catheterization—Many patients with acute subarachnoid hemorrhage develop acute hydrocephalus, due to either intraventricular extension of the hemorrhage or obstruction of cerebrospinal fluid drainage by cisternal blood. Ruptured anterior communicating artery and basilar artery apex aneurysms are most likely to cause hydrocephalus; overall hydrocephalus develops in 10–20% of patients and contributes to poor neurologic status in many of these. Symptoms of acute hydrocephalus include rapid-onset stupor or coma that persists after the initial hemorrhage. It is difficult to determine clinically whether a depressed level of consciousness is due to enlarged ventricles (symptomatic hydrocephalus) or to primary brain injury from the hemorrhage itself. Therefore, some authorities recommend that any SAH patient with a depressed level of consciousness and enlarged ventricles should be presumed to have symptomatic hydrocephalus, and an intraventricular catheter should be placed immediately. The catheter should be left open to drain at 10 cm above the internal acoustic meatus.

4. Pharmacotherapy—In patients with persistent stupor or coma, other causes of poor neurologic status should be considered, including seizure activity, electrolyte or other metabolic abnormalities, and infection. The use of prophylactic anticonvulsants is controversial, but it is reasonable to give patients prophylactically a loading dose of intravenous phenytoin, as seizure activity increases blood pressure, and cerebral blood flow, and the risk of aneurysmal re-rupture. If no seizure activity occurs by the time of hospital discharge, the anticonvulsant may be discontinued.

All patients should be started on the oral calcium channel blocker nimodipine 60 mg every 4 hours, continued for 21 days. This regimen leads to a slight improvement in clinical outcome in the setting of vasospasm (discussed later), although the mechanism of this improvement is unclear and probably does not involve reduction of angiographically visible spasm. A direct neuroprotective effect is possible. The main adverse effect of nimodipine is hypotension, which can be troublesome during attempts to induce hypertension after the aneurysm is secured (see later discussion). If hypotension does occur, the dose can be split and given every 2 hours, or reduced.

C. Neurosurgical Management

1. Preventing recurrent hemorrhage—Aneurysmal rebleeding doubles the risk of death from SAH, and prevention of rebleeding is one major goal of early therapy. The risk is between 4% and 10% in the first 24 hours after an acute SAH, and rebleeding often occurs while patients are awaiting aneurysm surgery. At least half of patients who rebleed die from the second hemorrhage; the presentation of rebleeding often includes sudden coma and loss of brainstem reflexes. The cumulative risk of rebleeding in the first month after aneurysmal rupture is about 30%.

Because of the high risk of early rebleeding, early neurosurgical intervention has become standard treatment in most viable patients. The goal of treatment is to exclude the aneurysm from the intracranial circulation and thereby eliminate the risk of bleeding.

2. Treatment of ruptured cerebral aneurysms—There are two treatments for ruptured cerebral aneurysms: neurosurgical clipping and endovascular coiling. Each has theoretical advantages and disadvantages (Table 11–5). Choice of therapy is often dictated by local expertise, aneurysm morphology and location, and the patient's clinical grade. The International Subarachnoid Hemorrhage Trial (ISAT) demonstrated that coiling may be a safer and more effective therapy for acute aneurysmal SAH patients in whom coiling and clipping are both feasible. Other studies have also suggested that coiling is less expensive than clipping, has lower short-term mortality and morbidity, and results in shorter hospital stays. Many patients were excluded from the ISAT trial during screening, and most treated aneurysms were anterior circulation. The generalizability of the ISAT result to routine clinical practice has therefore been questioned.

Table 11–5. Neurosurgical Options for Treating Aneurysmal Subarachnoid Hemorrhage

	Endovascular Coiling	Neurosurgical Clipping
Method	Placement of one or more platinum coils into the aneurysm via an angiographic catheter	Open craniotomy with placement of one or more surgical clips on the aneurysm neck
Advantages	Combines diagnostic angiography with direct treatment; no craniotomy or brain retraction required; one large randomized study demonstrated superiority over open surgical clipping; less short-term morbidity and mortality	Definitive treatment; established history of efficacy; allows contemporaneous evacuation of hematoma
Disadvantages	Risk of vessel perforation or dissection; may require repeat angiography and coiling due to compaction of the coil mass; long-term efficacy not known; may interfere with later surgical clipping if aneurysm enlarges	Requires craniotomy and brain retraction; clip may damage surrounding neural or vascular structures; inferior to coiling in a single, large randomized study; higher short-term mortality and morbidity

C. Management of Complications

Once the ruptured aneurysm has been secured, the patient is at risk for multiple neurologic and medical complications. Patients benefit from vigilant care by an experienced neurologic intensive care unit staff, and many complications may be anticipated and treated early, before irreversible brain injury occurs.

1. Vasospasm—Cerebral vasospasm is characterized by narrowing of large capacitance vessels at the base of the brain after SAH. It consists of an inflammatory vasculopathy that results in prolonged vascular smooth muscle contraction and vessel stenosis, thereby decreasing blood flow in the distal territory of these arteries. Vasospasm causes stroke or death in 14–20% of patients with SAH and is especially likely in poor-grade patients, patients with thick clot in the basal cisterns by CT scan, and patients with hydrocephalus.

The course of vasospasm after aneurysmal SAH is predictable. Vasospasm is rare before day 4 and peaks by day 10–14, usually rapidly and spontaneously resolving over the next 7 days. The parent artery of the ruptured aneurysm, which is usually the location of the thickest cisternal blood clot, is the vessel most likely to develop spasm, but any artery of the circle of Willis may be involved.

Vasospasm usually presents with new focal deficits during the high-risk time period. Patients may develop altered mental status, usually with coexisting focal signs. Patients with spasm in the anterior cerebral arteries after anterior communicating artery aneurysm rupture become markedly abulic and passive, sometimes with lower extremity weakness. Middle cerebral artery spasm causes hemiparesis and cortical signs such as aphasia or neglect. Basilar artery spasm can cause brainstem signs, quadriparesis, and visual field deficits.

A. DIAGNOSTIC STUDIES—Diagnostic evaluation begins with a cranial CT scan to exclude structural lesions, aneurysmal rebleeding, or hydrocephalus. If vasospasm is still suspected, transcranial Doppler ultrasonography may be performed. This modality may disclose elevated velocities in spastic vessels, most reliably in the middle cerebral artery distribution. Cerebral angiography is definitive. The roles of CTA and magnetic resonance angiography in diagnosing vasospasm, as well as cerebral blood flow measurements such as positron emission tomography and single-photon emission computed tomography, are still being defined.

B. TREATMENT—The traditional treatment of vasospasm is "triple-H" therapy, denoting hypertension, hypervolemia, and hemodilution. In actual practice, surgery and diagnostic phlebotomy tend to reduce hematocrit to the desired level (31%, where blood rheology is optimized for cerebral flow), so the need for therapeutic phlebotomy is rare. Hypervolemia is difficult to achieve in patients with normal cardiac function and presents special hazards in patients with low ejection fraction; therefore, a reasonable goal is strict maintenance of euvolemia.

Hypertension may be induced with intravenous pressor agents and is titrated to resolution of focal signs or to a maximum systolic blood pressure of 220 mm Hg. Careful cardiac and pulmonary monitoring in patients with coronary artery disease or neurogenic cardiac dysfunction is mandatory, usually requiring invasive hemodynamic monitoring.

Vasospasm that is unresponsive to hypertensive therapy may be treated with percutaneous transluminal balloon angioplasty of the involved arteries. The optimum timing of angioplasty is not known. In experienced hands, angioplasty results in significant improvement in neurologic function in 60–80% of patients, with a risk of complications (vessel rupture) of less than 5%. Arteries treated with balloon angioplasty do not generally undergo recurrent spasm in the absence of new SAH. Intra-arterial instillation of nicardipine can reverse vasospasm, but in contrast to angioplasty, the effect may be short-lived.

2. Hyponatremia—Patients with SAH may develop mild or profound hyponatremia between days 3 and 7, not usually the result of inappropriate secretion of antidiuretic hormone (SIADH), but rather reflecting renal salt and volume wasting (cerebral salt wasting). The distinction is important, as the treatment for hyponatremia in SAH is vigorous salt and volume supplementation, *not* free water restriction. Patients

should be treated with high infusion volumes of normal saline and oral NaCl supplements up to 2–3 g three to four times per day. If this is insufficient, 3% saline may be infused at 10–50 mL/h and oral fludrocortisone may be used. Normal salt homeostasis is usually re-established by 21 days.

3. Neurogenic cardiac stunning—Patients with severe acute SAH may develop electrocardiogram changes, including diffuse inverted T waves and ST-segment elevation, along with low-grade elevations of serum creatine kinase and cardiac troponins. In addition, reduced ejection fraction, frank congestive heart failure, and hypotension may develop. Neurogenic cardiac dysfunction is often discovered when patients develop congestive heart failure during attempted induced hypertension for vasospasm.

Echocardiography discloses global or focal wall motion abnormalities, and pressor support with dopamine or dobutamine may be required to support cerebral perfusion. Neurogenic cardiac dysfunction is almost never due to coronary disease or myocardial ischemia. Rather, SAH induces a large catecholamine surge, which is directly toxic to the myocardium, likely due to decoupling of membrane-bound receptors from intracellular signaling mechanisms. The syndrome is usually self-limited but may lead to hypotension, which exacerbates brain ischemia in the setting of vasospasm. Myocardial function usually returns to baseline values over several weeks.

4. Subacute and chronic hydrocephalus—Insidious-onset drowsiness, stupor, and coma accompanied by upward gaze palsy and bilateral grasp reflexes may develop over the first several days after SAH due to hydrocephalus. CT scanning may show slightly increased ventricular size; remarkably, a 1-mm increase in ventricular span at the level of the frontal horns may be sufficient to cause a dramatic decline in consciousness. Many patients with this subacute form of hydrocephalus do not have increased intracranial pressure—rather, the ventriculomegaly itself is the cause of the altered mental status. This syndrome is especially common in elderly patients with high brain tissue compliance. Placement of an intraventricular catheter set at 5 cm above ear level is effective at reducing ventricular size and improving neurologic status.

Beyond 10 days from the hemorrhage, some patients develop progressive gait disturbance, urinary incontinence, and apathy. CT scanning may show increased ventricular size, consistent with hydrocephalus. Intracranial pressure is usually not increased. High-volume lumbar puncture shrinks the ventricles and effectively relieves symptoms, but permanent ventriculoperitoneal shunting is usually required for lasting improvement.

▶ Prognosis

Thirty-day mortality after SAH ranges from 25–50%. Predictors of early mortality include poor neurologic status at presentation, advanced age, a large aneurysm, coexisting intraparenchymal hematoma, alcohol use, and hypertension.

Of these, presenting neurologic status, as rated by the Hunt and Hess score, is most predictive. Patients with good grade scores (1 or 2) have a 30-day mortality of 30%; grade 3 patients have a 65% mortality, and patients who are in stupor or coma (grades 4 and 5, respectively) have 85% mortality.

Most studies have shown that patients who survive past the first month do not have a significantly decreased life expectancy. However, one large study showed that 1-year mortality is increased by twofold in SAH survivors, with 70% of deaths resulting from cardiovascular disease or recurrent SAH. This statistic underscores the importance of long-term vascular risk factor reduction. Survivors of aneurysmal SAH are also at risk for the de novo generation of new aneurysms, which may occur in 10% of patients over 10 years. SAH survivors should undergo CT angiography every year during the decade after SAH to detect new aneurysms.

Failure to return to prior levels of social and occupational function is common after SAH. Ten percent to 20% of survivors are functionally dependent. However, 50% of patients with good clinical grades suffer long-term psychomotor and cognitive difficulties, with inability to return to full employment. Deficits in memory, concentration, mood, attention, and other cognitive functions are common, and patients require long-term support and cognitive rehabilitation even in the setting of an apparently good neurologic outcome.

UNRUPTURED INTRACRANIAL ANEURYSMS

ESSENTIALS OF DIAGNOSIS

▶ Includes incidental aneurysms, symptomatic aneurysms in patients without a history of rupture, or unruptured ("mirror") aneurysms in patients with hemorrhage from another source

▶ Rupture after diagnosis is fatal in more than 50% of patients

▶ Overall 5-year risk of rupture is 3%, but risk is strongly influenced by location and size of aneurysm

▶ The risk of death or disability from treatment is nearly 10% for most patients

Unruptured intracranial saccular aneurysms may be discovered by brain or vascular imaging performed to evaluate nonhemorrhagic conditions such as migraine or ischemic cerebrovascular disease. In addition, about 20% of patients with a ruptured aneurysm harbor an unruptured aneurysm at a different site. Unruptured aneurysms may also cause headache or exert mass effect on brain or cranial nerve structures. The discovery of an unruptured aneurysm may produce considerable anxiety for the patient, and treatment recommendations must take the patient's emotional response to the diagnosis into account.

Management options for unruptured aneurysms include no treatment, open surgical clipping, or endovascular coiling. Prospective data provide some guidance on the risks of these three options. The overall 5-year risk of SAH from an unruptured aneurysm is 3%, and 65% of these hemorrhages are fatal. However, the risk of SAH is strongly dependent on both the size and location of the aneurysm. Small (<7 mm) anterior circulation aneurysms in patients with no history of SAH have a 5-year rupture risk of 0%, and therefore likely require no treatment. At the other extreme, large posterior circulation aneurysms have a 5-year risk between 15% and 50%, and treatment may be justified.

The risks of surgical intervention have also been clarified by prospective analysis. The risk of mortality or significant disability from surgical clipping is about 11% and is higher in patients older than 50 years, patients with larger aneurysms, patients with compressive symptoms from the aneurysm, and patients with a history of ischemic cerebrovascular disease. Endovascular therapy carries a risk of morbidity and mortality of about 9%, and the risk does not seem to be as dependent on patient age or other clinical variables. These data suggest that endovascular therapy appears to be as effective and safe as surgical clipping, although the long-term (>5 year) durability of endovascular therapy has yet to be accurately defined.

Screening asymptomatic patients for unruptured aneurysms with catheter angiography is controversial. Catheter angiography carries a risk of disabling stroke or death between 0.1% and 1%, and the risk of not diagnosing an aneurysm must be weighed against the considerable psychological and surgical morbidity of finding and treating a lesion that may remain asymptomatic for life. Most experts do not recommend screening with catheter angiography unless patients have two or more first- or second-degree relatives with known aneurysms, especially if at least one is a sibling.

INFECTED (MYCOTIC) ANEURYSMS

ESSENTIALS OF DIAGNOSIS

▶ Infected aneurysms are most often associated with septic embolism from endocarditis

▶ Patients with brain embolism and endocarditis should undergo magnetic resonance angiography, computed-tomography angiography, or catheter angiography to rule out infected aneurysms

▶ Management decisions require balancing the chance of resolution of the aneurysm with antibiotic treatment with the risk of rupture during such treatment

Infected aneurysms are usually the result of septic emboli arising from infective endocarditis, infective aortitis, or, rarely, other systemic infections. They are thought to be the result of impaction of infectious material in the vasa vasorum of intracranial vessels, resulting in destruction of the vessel wall, but may also result from infectious material lodging in the lumen of the parent vessel itself. Unlike saccular aneurysms, infected aneurysms tend to be located beyond the circle of Willis in peripheral branches overlying the cerebral convexity. Intraparenchymal or subarachnoid hemorrhage from mycotic aneurysm rupture carries a high mortality rate.

Infectious aneurysms may be sought by catheter angiography in any patient with proven bacterial endocarditis and unexplained central nervous system symptoms or signs. The sensitivity of magnetic resonance angiography (MRA) and computed tomography angiography (CTA) may be insufficient to detect small infected aneurysms, although in most cases the aneurysm may elicit parenchymal inflammation that is detectable by MRI. In some patients with endocarditis, diffusion-weighted MRI reveals asymptomatic cerebral infarction, presumably the result of embolization. It is unclear whether such patients require vascular imaging to rule out infectious aneurysms, but noninvasive imaging with CTA or MRA seems prudent.

Management of infected aneurysms is complex, and the natural history of these lesions has not been clearly defined. Antibiotic treatment may allow aneurysm regression, but catastrophic rupture during antibiotic treatment has been reported. Surgical resection before completion of antibiotic therapy also has risks, because many patients with infectious endocarditis are suboptimal surgical candidates. Anticoagulation and thrombolysis of patients with infective endocarditis is contraindicated, because such treatment increases the risk of aneurysm rupture. Resection of infected aneurysms should be performed before procedures that require anticoagulation, such as prosthetic heart valve implantation.

Edlow JA, Caplan LR. Avoiding pitfalls in the diagnosis of subarachnoid hemorrhage. *N Engl J Med* 2000;342:29–36. [PMID: 10620647] (Reviews common errors in the diagnosis of SAH, with strategies for avoiding same.)

International Study of Unruptured Intracranial Aneurysms Investigators. Unruptured intracranial aneurysms: Natural history, clinical outcome, and risks of surgical and endovascular treatment. *Lancet* 2003;362:103–110. [PMID: 12867109] (The largest prospective study of the natural history of unruptured aneurysms and the risks attendant with surgical and endovascular treatment.)

International Subarachnoid Hemorrhage Trial Collaborative Group. International Subarachnoid Aneurysm Trial (ISAT) of neurosurgical clipping versus coiling in 2143 patients with ruptured intracranial aneurysms: A randomized trial. *Lancet* 2002;26:1267–1274. [PMID: 12414200]. (The first direct prospective comparison of two methods of acute aneurysm treatment in SAH, showing a distinct safety advantage of endovascular coiling over surgical clipping.)

Kowalski RG, et al. Initial misdiagnosis and outcome after subarachnoid hemorrhage. *JAMA* 2004;291:866–869. [PMID: 14970066] (Demonstrates that failure to properly diagnose SAH at the first physician encounter has adverse consequences for patient outcome, especially in good-grade patients, whose outcome would otherwise have been expected to be excellent.)

Mayberg MR, et al. Guidelines for the management of aneurysmal subarachnoid hemorrhage: A statement for healthcare professionals from a special writing group of the stroke council, American Heart Association. *Stroke* 1994;90:2315–2328. [PMID: 7955232]

Sen J, et al. Triple-H therapy in the management of aneurysmal subarachnoid hemorrhage. *Lancet Neurol* 2003;2:614–621. [PMID: 14505583]

Watanabe A, et al. Perimesencephalic nonaneurysmal subarachnoid hemorrhage and variations in the veins. *Neuroradiology* 2002;44:319–325. [PMID: 11914808] (Sheds light on the origin of benign perimesencephalic hemorrhage by showing the high prevalence of anomalous intracranial venous anatomy in such patients.)

▼ VASCULAR ANOMALIES

Vascular anomalies include a wide range of abnormal arteries and veins found within the central nervous system. Although some present with catastrophic hemorrhage, many are minimally symptomatic or incidental.

ARTERIOVENOUS MALFORMATIONS

ESSENTIALS OF DIAGNOSIS

- ▶ Abnormal tangles of arteries and veins in brain or spinal cord
- ▶ May be asymptomatic, or cause focal deficits, seizures, headaches, intraparenchymal hemorrhage, or subarachnoid hemorrhage
- ▶ Treatment may involve a combination of endovascular, radiologic, or surgical therapies

▶ General Considerations

Arteriovenous malformations (AVMs) are complex tangles of arteries and veins, linked by direct connections without capillaries. They may occur anywhere in the brain or spinal cord. Brain tissue found between the vascular tangles is nonfunctioning, largely composed of gliosis (scar), with or without evidence of hemorrhage. It is unclear whether AVMs arise during embryogenesis; some AVMs evolve, regrow, or regress over time. Because of the direct arteriovenous shunting that takes place in the center (nidus) of the AVM, high flow can cause symptoms by diverting blood from normal arteries (so-called *cerebral steal*).

The prevalence of cerebral AVM is estimated at 10 per 100,000 persons. The mean age at time of diagnosis is 31 years, and men and women are affected about equally.

▶ Clinical Findings

About half of patients present with subarachnoid, intraventricular, or intraparenchymal hemorrhage. Other presentations include seizures, focal deficits (which may be progressive), or intractable headaches; some AVMs are found on brain imaging performed for unrelated symptoms.

Patients who present without stroke have a risk of hemorrhage between 1.3–4% per year. Patients with a brain hemorrhage at the time of diagnosis have a much higher short-term risk of hemorrhage. Estimates of the subsequent risk of re-hemorrhage range from 1–18% per year. Estimates of the clinical impact of AVM hemorrhage also vary widely, with risk of morbidity ranging from 16–80% and risk of mortality ranging from 10–17%. The high rates of mortality, morbidity, and re-hemorrhage favor definitive treatment for most AVMs.

▶ Treatment

The goal of AVM treatment is complete elimination of the lesion. Partially treated lesions may recur, and the risk of hemorrhage may increase. Treatment may involve endovascular embolization of feeding arteries with glue, coils, or other materials; external brain radiation; or open neurosurgery. For small lesions, radiation alone may suffice. Larger lesions may require surgery, with endovascular embolization to decrease the extent of the lesion immediately before surgery. Preoperative evaluation by functional MRI or superselective angiography may help predict postoperative deficits and help guide patients in decision making.

CAVERNOUS MALFORMATIONS

ESSENTIALS OF DIAGNOSIS

- ▶ Thin-walled dilated vascular spaces found in the brain or spinal cord
- ▶ Primary yearly risk of rupture is about 0.5%, but the risk of rebleeding is higher

▶ General Considerations

Cavernous malformations are characterized by sinusoidal, thin-walled, enlarged vascular cavities. Because arterial input and venous outflow from cavernous malformations are often below the level of resolution of cerebral angiography, they have been called angiographically occult vascular malformations or "cryptic" malformations. Present in about 0.5% of the population, they may be disclosed by CT or MRI. A familial tendency toward harboring cavernous malformations has been identified in Hispanics of Mexican descent,

with an autosomal-dominant pattern. Multiple cavernous malformations are found in more than 80% of familial cases and 33% of nonfamilial cases.

▶ Clinical Findings

Cavernous malformations may be found incidentally on brain imaging or may present with seizures, intraparenchymal hemorrhage, or intraventricular hemorrhage. Seizures, occurring in 25–55% of cases, are often medically refractory, especially when the malformation is located in the temporal lobe. Clinically manifest hemorrhage occurs in 10–35% of cases. However, many lesions that never caused clinically evident hemorrhage show evidence on MRI of multiple layers of hemosiderin, suggestive of subclinical hemorrhage.

Clinically silent, incidentally discovered cavernous malformations have an annual risk of hemorrhage of about 0.5%. Lesions that present with symptomatic hemorrhage have an estimated yearly rate of hemorrhage between 4.5% and 30%. Deep or brainstem location is associated with a higher risk of symptomatic hemorrhage, but the reason may be that such lesions are more likely to be symptomatic. About 70% of patients with a clinically manifest hemorrhage are left with a permanent deficit.

▶ Treatment

Not all cavernous malformations require treatment. Treatment options include open surgery or stereotactic radiation. Decisions should be guided by an estimate of the risk of future hemorrhage, the surgical accessibility of the lesion, and the size of the target if radiation is planned. In general, asymptomatic lesions are managed conservatively. High-risk symptomatic lesions may undergo surgical resection with acceptable morbidity if they abut the pial surface. Surgically inaccessible lesions may be considered for stereotactic radiation, but the benefit of this therapy over natural history remains unproven.

DURAL ARTERIOVENOUS FISTULAS

ESSENTIALS OF DIAGNOSIS

- ▶ Direct connection between a dural artery and the CNS venous system or intracranial sinuses
- ▶ May cause hemorrhage, focal deficits, or generalized cerebral edema and raised intracranial pressure
- ▶ Rare cause of painless myelopathy or dementia

▶ General Considerations

A dural arteriovenous fistula (DAVF) is an abnormal direct connection between a dural artery and a vein or dural sinus. A DAVF can produce increased pressure and blood flow in the normally low pressure CNS venous system, leading to venous congestion in brain parenchyma and congestive ischemia or frank hemorrhagic infarction. In addition, rupture of draining veins may lead to Intraparenchymal, subarachnoid, or subdural hemorrhage. Rarely a DAVF causes global cognitive decline without focal findings, likely a result of increased venous pressure in the entire brain. Patients with brain dural fistulas may report pulsatile bruits in one or both ears. These bruits may be auscultated over the mastoid process, eye, or occiput. In some cases, bed partners report hearing the bruit.

DAVFs also arise in the spinal cord, where venous hypertension leads to a chronic, progressive painless myelopathy, radiculopathy, or both. A minority of patients with a spinal DAVF have paroxysmal onset of paraplegia due to infarction or hemorrhage. Because spinal venous pressure increases with Valsalva or upright posture, some patients report worsening of myelopathy in the standing position or with exercise or singing (so-called *singing paraplegia*).

▶ Clinical Findings

Diagnosis requires a high index of suspicion. Any patient with a pulsatile bruit, or unexplained brain or spinal cord edema, hemorrhage, or abnormal flow voids on MRI should undergo catheter angiography to exclude DAVF. Cerebral angiograms should include injections of the external carotid arteries, which usually supplies arterial feeders to the lesion. Spinal angiography requires separate injection of each radicular artery, including sacral arteries. Symptom localization does not always predict fistula location. Because the venous system of the entire brain and spinal cord is interconnected without valves, spinal cord fistulae may cause cerebral symptoms, and sacral fistulae may cause myelopathy referable to the thoracic or even cervical spinal cord.

▶ Treatment

A DAVF causing major CNS symptoms should be treated by surgical extirpation or endovascular occlusion. Elimination of the fistula may allow reversal of even long-standing deficits, and it is not uncommon for patients with severe deficits to be cured after treatment. DAVFs that cause minor symptoms such as bruit or headache should be assessed based on their venous anatomy. Fistulae with prominent venous drainage into brain surface veins, as opposed to dural sinuses, are probably at high risk for hemorrhage and may merit treatment.

The **carotid-cavernous fistula** is a type of DAVF in which the internal carotid artery, or an external carotid artery branch, is in direct communication with the cavernous sinus. Increased venous pressure in the eye results in acute glaucoma and vision loss. There may also be cranial nerve deficits (cranial nerves III, IV, VI, and V-I and V-II). Patients note a pulsatile bruit behind the eye, and the eye appears swollen and injected, with corkscrew veins visible on the sclera. Pupils are usually mid-position and fixed, and the eye may be immobile, with a severely ptotic upper lid. Symptoms and signs may be bilateral, if raised sinus pressure in the fistula is transmitted to the contralateral cavernous sinus through the circular sinus. Rarely, carotid-cavernous fistula may result in brainstem hemorrhages or cerebral symptoms such as hemiparesis. Most fistulas result from either trauma or rupture of a cavernous carotid aneurysm. Treatment by endovascular occlusion of the fistula or parent carotid artery is usually indicated; open surgery is rarely performed.

VEIN OF GALEN ANEURYSM

In neonates, aneurysmal dilatation of the vein of Galen results from an arteriovenous fistula draining directly into that structure. This results in noncommunicating hydrocephalus due to compression of the adjacent cerebral aqueduct, high-output heart failure due to arteriovenous shunting through the lesion, and a loud pulsatile cranial bruit. In some patients, symptoms are not manifest until later in childhood, when lethargy and oculomotor difficulties result from hydrocephalus and brainstem compression. CT or MRI allow accurate diagnosis. The preferred treatment is endovascular embolization.

DEVELOPMENTAL VENOUS ANOMALIES

These lesions, also known as venous angiomas, probably represent anatomically abnormal but physiologically normal variants of cerebral venous drainage. Usually asymptomatic and incidental, they appear as finger-like enhancing lesions on MRI, and have a caput medusa appearance on angiography. Some cases are associated with cavernous malformations. Hemorrhage or mass effect from the associated cavernous malformation is usually the basis of any focal symptoms. The risk of hemorrhage from an isolated venous angioma is extremely low, and therapy of any kind is rarely needed.

CAPILLARY TELANGIECTASIAS

These uncommon lesions consist of clusters of capillary-size vessels, often multiple, and usually present in the brainstem and cerebellum. Most are asymptomatic, although they may rarely bleed. The absolute risk is not well defined but is probably extremely low. In general, no treatment is required.

Bederson JB, et al. Recommendations for the management of patients with unruptured intracranial aneurysms. A statement for healthcare professionals from the stroke council of the American Heart Association. *Stroke* 2000;102:2300–2308. [PMID: 11056108]

Fleetwood IG, Steinberg GK: Arteriovenous malformations. *Lancet* 2002;359:863–873. [PMID: 11897302]

Central Nervous System Neoplasms

12

Christopher E. Mandigo, MD, & Jeffrey N. Bruce, MD

Tumors of the nervous system comprise a diverse, heterogeneous group of neoplastic lesions that affect every age group and every element of the central and peripheral nervous systems. The cause of most adult and pediatric central nervous system (CNS) tumors is largely unknown. A few genetic syndromes play a clear and independent role in brain tumor development, including neurofibromatosis types 1 and 2, Li-Fraumeni syndrome, Gardner syndrome, Turcot syndrome, and von Hippel-Lindau disease (Table 12–1). Independent of these disorders, a family history of malignant brain tumors is a risk factor for developing brain tumors. Most CNS tumors are thought to be sporadic in origin, as familial and genetic associations play a role in only about 5% of all cases. Nonetheless, many sporadic tumors arise as a result of combined somatic mutations that activate oncogenes such as platelet-derived growth factor and inactivate tumor suppressor genes such as *p53*. The role of environmental factors—physical, chemical, or infectious—in causing such mutations or otherwise acting as risk factors is as yet unclear.

BRAIN TUMORS

ESSENTIALS OF DIAGNOSIS

► Primary or metastatic

► Typical presenting signs are headache, seizures, focal neurologic deficits, and nonspecific cognitive and personality changes that follow a subacute course

► Detailed neurologic examination can localize lesions within the CNS

► Imaging tests are essential to direct further diagnostic and management strategies

► Surgical biopsy is almost always required for conclusive diagnosis

PRIMARY BRAIN TUMORS

General Considerations

Primary brain tumors are neoplastic and nonneoplastic lesions that arise directly from the brain tissue and its linings. In the United States, approximately 25,000 primary brain tumors are diagnosed in adults each year, with an incidence rate of about 8 cases per 100,000 people. There has been a general increase in incidence over the past 20 years that is most likely associated with the increased availability of computed tomographic (CT) and magnetic resonance imaging (MRI) scanning and an aging population. Approximately 2200 individuals younger than 20 years of age are diagnosed with a brain tumor every year. Malignant brain tumors are the leading cause of cancer death among children and the second most common type of pediatric cancer after leukemia. Astrocytomas account for 52% of childhood brain tumors, primitive neuroectodermal tumors (eg, medulloblastoma) for 21%, ependymomas for 9%, other gliomas for 15%, and 3% other types of tumors.

These tumors can be divided into two main categories: glial and nonglial neoplasms. Primary brain tumors have traditionally been further subdivided into categories based on the specific cell type of origin (Table 12–2). Diagnosis of these lesions and the subsequent direction of further treatment are ultimately dependent on biopsy and pathologic investigation. However, a presumptive diagnosis of these lesions can be very accurately made in most circumstances from the clinical history, physical examination, and radiographic imaging. The location of the tumor plays an important role in diagnosis, because certain types commonly occur in specific areas of the CNS (Table 12–3).

Clinical Findings

A. Symptoms and Signs

Patients with brain tumors usually present with headache, seizures, focal neurologic deficits, and nonspecific cognitive

Table 12–1. Genetic Syndromes and Corresponding Tumor Types

	Mutation	Tumor	Inheritance Pattern
Gardner syndrome	*APC*	Colonic polyps, astrocytomas	—
Li-Fraumeni syndrome	*p53* mutation	Solid systemic cancers, astrocytomas	Autosomal recessive
Multiple endocrine neoplasia types (MEN) 1 and 2	Chromosome 11	Pituitary adenomas	—
Neurofibromatosis (NF) types 1 and 2	Chromosome 17 (NF1); chromosome 22 (NF2)	Neurofibromas, acoustic schwannomas, meningiomas, skin lesions	Autosomal dominant
Turcot syndrome	Chromosome 5	Colonic polyps, astrocytomas	Both autosomal dominant and recessive
von Hippel-Lindau syndrome	Chromosome 3	Infratentorial and spinal cord hemangioblastomas	Autosomal dominant

Table 12–2. Major Categories of Primary Brain Tumors

Cell Type of Origin	Tumor
Glial Tumor	
Astrocytoma	Benign astrocytoma Pilocytic astrocytoma Anaplastic astrocytoma Glioblastoma multiforme Oligodendroglioma
Ependymal tumor	Cellular ependymoma Anaplastic ependymoma Myxopapillary ependymoma
Choroid plexus tumor	Choroid plexus papilloma Choroid plexus carcinoma
Nonglial Tumor	
Neural progenitor origin	Neuroblastoma Primitive neuroectodermal tumor (PNET) Pineocytoma, blastoma Ganglioneuroma
Meningeal or mesenchymal tumor	Meningioma Hemangioblastoma Hemangiopericytoma
Pituitary adenoma	Microadenoma Macroadenoma
Other tissue type	Craniopharyngioma Hamartoma, teratoma Germ cell tumor Epidermoid or dermoid cyst Chordoma Colloid cyst of third ventricle Central nervous system lymphoma Hemangioblastoma, pericytoma Vascular malformation Cavernous malformation

Table 12–3. Common Primary Brain Tumors by Location

Location	Tumor
Cerebral (supratentorial) region	Astrocytoma Meningioma Oligodendroglioma Metastatic lesion Lymphoma
Cerebellar or brainstem (infratentorial) region	Schwannoma Meningioma Primitive neuroectodermal tumor (PNET)
Pineal region	Pineal cell tumor (pineocytoma, pineoblastoma) Germ cell tumor (germinoma, teratoma) Astrocytoma Meningioma Pineal cyst
Lateral ventricles	Astrocytoma Ependymoma Central neurocytoma
Third ventricle	Astrocytoma Colloid cyst Central neurocytoma
Fourth ventricle	Brainstem glioma PNET Ependymoma Hemangioblastoma
Cerebellopontine angle	Acoustic schwannoma Meningioma Epidermoid tumor
Sellar region	Microadenoma and macroadenoma Meningioma Craniopharyngioma Glioma (pilocytic optic nerve glioma) Aneurysm

and personality changes. Initially subtle, these findings gradually become more apparent as the disease progresses. It is important to pay attention to the details of these symptoms and signs, because tumors can be detected at early stages with increasingly sensitive diagnostic tests.

The symptoms and signs found with intracranial tumors relate to the destructive and compressive nature of the tumor on nervous tissue and to the secondary effects of the tumor, which include peritumoral edema, hydrocephalus, and mass effect. Headache, nausea and vomiting, seizures, and altered mental status are commonly seen with most types of brain tumors. Particular symptoms, such as focal neurologic deficits that are related to the site of the tumor, can localize the disease to a discrete area of the brain. These symptoms are typically the same across tumor types. The size and rate of growth of the tumor are also important factors in presentation, because the brain is confined within a limited volume. For example, a slowly growing tumor can be quite large when diagnosed, because the brain can accommodate to a decreasing volume over an extended period of time. In contrast, a fast-growing, small tumor with a significant amount of peritumoral edema may have a more dramatic presentation.

Headache, nausea, vomiting, and loss of consciousness are most often related to increased intracranial pressure. As more volume is added within the cranial vault, the volume of other compartments (eg, CSF and blood space) can compensate to a modest degree. When the capacity of these spaces is exhausted, intracranial pressure rises exponentially with increasing tumor volume. Increased intracranial pressure can also cause a variety of other brainstem symptoms, such as dizziness, hearing loss, or tinnitus. Very high intracranial pressure can lead to altered consciousness and the Cushing reflex of hypertension and bradycardia. Such symptoms are often associated with headache.

1. Headache—Headache is the presenting symptom in roughly one third of patients with brain tumors, and more than 70% of patients develop headache during the progression of their disease. There is no specific pattern that can lead to diagnosis of a brain tumor; most headaches in these patients are nonspecific and intermittent, progressively more intense, and longer in duration. Characteristics that raise suspicion of a brain tumor include headaches exacerbated by coughing, lying down, or sleep; headaches that wake the patient at night; new headaches that are different from prior patterns or are more severe; and headaches with associated nausea, vomiting, or neurologic deficits. The pain originates from pressure on the vasculature, dura, and some of the cranial nerves. Intense, episodic headaches occur when "spikes" of increased intracranial pressure are superimposed on already increased intracranial pressure.

2. Nausea and vomiting—Nausea and vomiting suggest increased intracranial pressure or, much less commonly, the direct effect of a tumor on the chemoreceptor trigger zone in the brainstem.

3. Altered mental status—Altered mental status is the presenting symptom in 10–20% of patients and ranges from subtle problems with behavior, memory, and concentration to depressed levels of consciousness. Changes in mental status can result from tumors that directly affect the cerebral cortex, especially the frontal lobes, or, more commonly, from increased intracranial pressure. If increased intracranial pressure is not treated, the patient may progress to stupor and coma. Elevated intracranial pressure can create shifts of brain tissue with disastrous consequences from herniation syndromes. Rapid onset of lethargy, coma, and herniation syndromes can result from intratumoral hemorrhages, as well.

4. Seizures—Seizures occur as the presenting symptom in approximately one third of patients with brain tumors, and 50–75% of patients develop seizures during the course of their illness. In half of patients seizures are generalized and in half they are partial. Seizures usually occur with tumors that affect the cerebral cortex, such as oligodendrogliomas and astrocytomas. The new onset of seizures in an adult strongly suggests the presence of a brain tumor and mandates an MRI scan of the brain.

5. Other findings—Higher cortical functions such as speech and praxis can be affected by tumors growing within various associative areas of the cerebrum. Disruption of cranial nerve function and facial pain occur when tumors impinge on these nerves as they exit the brainstem and skull base. For example, hearing loss and facial palsy are often found in patients with tumors of the cerebellopontine angle.

B. Physical Examination Findings

The clinical signs observed in patients with brain tumors are also encountered in other categories of neurologic disease. It is the time course for the development of these signs that helps determine the appropriate diagnosis. Signs used to determine the location of the tumor are listed in Tables 12–4 and 12–5. Table 12–6 identifies so-called *false localizing signs* that produce specific neurologic deficits from indirect effects of the tumor.

1. Astrocytoma

▶ General Considerations

Astrocytomas represent roughly half of all CNS tumors, with an incidence of approximately 3 cases per 100,000 people. The classification of these tumors is determined by histopathology, and they are graded from I (the most benign) to IV (glioblastoma multiforme [GBM], the most malignant). GBM represents about two thirds of all astrocytomas; the remainder of patients are almost evenly divided between anaplastic (grade III) and lower-grade (I and II) astrocytomas. The natural history of lower-grade astrocytomas is notable for heterogeneity. Some astrocytomas dedifferentiate into more malignant tumors over time, and others have a

Table 12–4. Physical Examination Findings Associated With Cerebral Tumors

Location	Clinical Signs
Frontal lobe	Personality changes (disinhibition, lack of judgment, abulia) Contralateral hemiparesis, apraxia Aphasia Gaze preference Primitive reflexes Seizures (generalized or partial)
Temporal lobe	Seizures (generalized or partial) Memory impairment Visual field deficits Aphasia
Parietal lobe	Contralateral sensory loss Aphasia Hemineglect or spatial disruption
Occipital lobe	Homonymous hemianopsia

Table 12–5. Physical Examination Findings Associated With Infratentorial Brain Tumors

Location	Clinical Signs
Brainstem	Cranial neuropathies Hemiplegia, paresis Sensory loss Vertigo, nausea, vomiting Hydrocephalus
Pineal region	Hydrocephalus Parinaud syndrome (paresis of upgaze and convergence, pupillary reflex disturbance)
Third ventricle	Hydrocephalus Hypothalamic dysfunction Impaired memory
Cerebellum	Occipital headaches Ataxia Hemiplegia, paresis Cranial nerve sign

stable pattern for many years. Low-grade astrocytomas are most commonly found in children and adults younger than 40 years of age. The more malignant anaplastic astrocytomas progress to GBM over a few years. These tumors can occur at any age but most typically affect 40- to 60-year-olds. GBM is usually found in patients older than 50 years.

Astrocytomas are thought to arise either from dedifferentiated glial cells or from neuroprogenitor stem cells of the glial lineage. The tumor cells have an invasive, infiltrative phenotype within the brain tissue. They rarely metastasize outside of the CNS, but they invade normal brain tissue and can seed throughout the cerebrospinal fluid (CSF) system. A tumor mass can be seen on imaging as a relatively discrete lesion, yet in higher-grade lesions, tumor cells are present up to centimeters away in the surrounding "normal" brain. Rarer cases present as multifocal lesions within the brain.

▶ **Clinical Findings**

A. Symptoms and Signs

Astrocytomas usually present with headache, seizures, and progressive neurologic deficits, depending on the location of the tumor. The majority of these tumors arise within the cerebrum, and the various symptoms relate directly to the location of the tumor. Symptoms of increased intracranial pressure, such as headache, nausea, vomiting, lethargy, coma, and false localizing signs, can also be seen in patients with advanced disease.

B. Diagnostic Studies

Low-grade gliomas are hypodense on CT scan and hypointense to isointense on MRI scan and usually do not enhance

Table 12–6. False Localizing Signs

Neurologic Sign	Mechanism	Clinical Findings
Sixth nerve palsy	Increased intracranial pressure	Manifests as unilateral or bilateral abducens palsy Ipsilateral, contralateral
Third nerve palsy	Uncal herniation	Pupillary reaction affected first, then extraocular movements
Hydrocephalus	Cerebrospinal fluid outflow obstruction	Ataxia that is difficult to differentiate from cerebellar ataxia Bitemporal hemianopsia and endocrine deficiency from dilation of anterior third ventricle and chiasmal compression
Parinaud syndrome	Rostral midbrain compression	Paralysis of convergence and upgaze
Ipsilateral hemiparesis	Uncal (transtentorial) herniation	Midbrain compression against tentorial edge

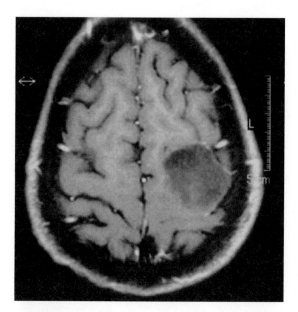

▲ **Figure 12–1.** Low-grade astrocytoma. Axial T1-weighted MRI scan after gadolinium contrast administration demonstrates a left-sided astrocytoma of the frontal lobe. There is no contrast enhancement, and the signal intensity is less than gray matter.

with contrast administration (Figure 12–1). They can appear as either well-circumscribed or diffusely infiltrating masses. Calcification occurs in 10–20%, and associated edema is uncommon. Higher-grade astrocytomas enhance with contrast and commonly have a central area of hypodensity that corresponds to necrosis (Figure 12–2A and 12–2B). These tumors are associated with peritumoral edema, best seen as hyperintensity on T2-weighted, fluid-attenuated inversion recovery (FLAIR) MRI sequences (Figure 12–2C). Definitive diagnosis relies on open or stereotaxic biopsy.

▶ Treatment & Prognosis

Malignant gliomas remain difficult to treat despite protocols that include surgery, radiotherapy, and systemically administered chemotherapy (Table 12–7). Aggressive surgical resection of the enhancing lesion is possible with current operative techniques and improves patient outcome. Whole-brain radiotherapy is the most effective therapy for this disease and can improve survival by 6–9 months in GBM. Adjuvant systemic chemotherapy with temozolomide is the current standard of care and has added months to the median survival time. There are a large number of experimental adjuvant treatment protocols for malignant glioma, which involve alternative chemotherapies, immune therapies, and direct infusion therapies. These are best directed by the treating neurosurgeon and neuro-oncologist. Treatment for lower-grade gliomas involves surgical resection when feasible with a decision

for radiation therapy made on an individual basis. Observation for tumor progression before surgical biopsy or resection is an option; radiation and chemotherapy generally have no role in the therapy of low-grade astrocytomas.

Patients with GBM, the most lethal form of astrocytoma, have a median survival of 1 year, with less than 2% of patients surviving beyond 5 years. Independent predictors of survival are patient age and functional status at diagnosis. For anaplastic astrocytoma, median survival is 2–3 years, as most of these tumors recur after therapy and progress to GBM. Lower-grade astrocytomas have a variable clinical course because this category comprises a mixed group of histologies. Some of these tumors eventually progress to more malignant forms. The 5-year survival rate for patients with most low-grade tumors is 50%; an exception is the childhood pilocytic astrocytomas, for which the 5-year survival rate after total resection may be 85%. A better prognosis in all of these tumor types is associated with age younger than 40 years, high functional status, greater extent of surgical resection, and lower histologic grade at the time of diagnosis.

2. Oligodendroglioma

▶ General Considerations

Oligodendrogliomas most often occur in middle-aged adults, with a predominance of women. They represent about 5% of all primary brain tumors and arise from the oligodendrocyte lineage, which represent glial cells responsible for the myelination of CNS axons. Their classification into low-grade or anaplastic oligodendrogliomas depends on histologic grade.

▶ Clinical Findings

A. Symptoms and Signs

Patients with oligodendrogliomas commonly present with seizures but can also present in a manner identical to those with astrocytomas.

B. Diagnostic Studies

Neuroimaging demonstrates cerebral hemisphere location, frequent intratumoral calcification, and characteristics similar to those of astrocytomas. Cysts are common, and necrosis is uncommon. Low-grade oligodendrogliomas are infiltrative, hypointense on T1-weighted MRI scans and hyperintense on T2-weighted FLAIR imaging (Figure 12–3). Higher-grade tumors share these findings and commonly enhance with contrast.

▶ Treatment & Prognosis

Treatment involves surgical biopsy and debulking followed by adjuvant radiation therapy and chemotherapy. A large subset of malignant oligodendrogliomas has shown long-term response to temozolomide or the PCV (procarbazine, lomustine, and vincristine) regimen of chemotherapy.

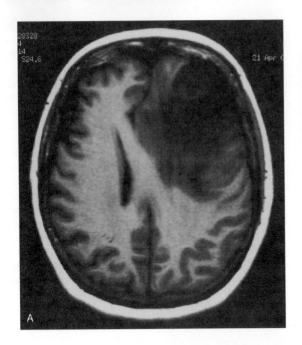

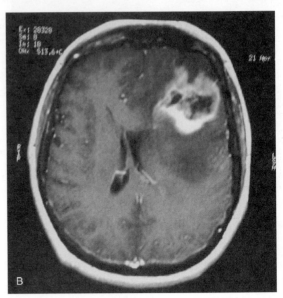

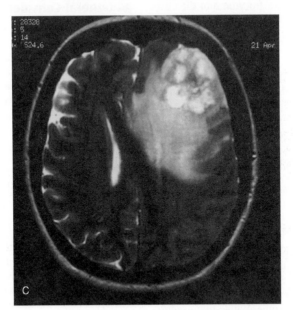

▲ **Figure 12–2.** Glioblastoma multiforme. **A, B:** Axial T1-weighted MRI demonstrates a large lesion of the left frontal lobe with rim enhancement after administration of contrast and extensive peritumoral edema. **C:** The axial T2-weighted MRI reveals the extent of the edema, seen as a hyperintense signal.

Genetic analysis has demonstrated a correlation between certain chromosomal aberrations and a response to chemotherapy, which makes genetic analysis of pathologic specimens essential. The prognosis is variable; some low-grade tumors grow slowly for many years, whereas more malignant forms can behave similarly to high-grade astrocytomas. The clinical course can be predicted by histopathologic grade, rate of tumor growth seen on serial imaging, and presence of contrast enhancement on CT or MRI. Patients with low-grade tumors have a 5-year survival rate of 75%.

Table 12–7. Chemotherapeutic Agents Commonly Used in the Treatment of Primary Brain Tumors

Drug	Tumor	Side Effects
Methotrexate	Lymphoma, primitive neuroectodermal tumor (PNET)	Myelosuppression, acute cerebellar syndrome
Nitrosourea (alkylating agent)	Malignant glioma	Myelosuppression, pulmonary fibrosis, renal damage
Platinum compounds (eg, cisplatin)	Malignant glioma, PNET, germ cell tumor	Peripheral neuropathy, ototoxicity, myelosuppression, nephrotoxicity
Podophyllotoxins (eg, etoposide)	Malignant glioma, PNET, germ cell tumor	Myelosuppression
Procarbazine (alkylating agent)	Malignant glioma, PNET	Myelosuppression, allergy, ataxia, hallucinations
Temozolomide (alkylating agent)	Malignant glioma	Myelosuppression
Vinca alkaloids (eg, vincristine)	Malignant glioma, PNET	Peripheral neuropathy

3. Ependymoma

▶ General Considerations

Ependymomas originate from ependymal cells lining the ventricles and central canal of the spinal cord. These tumors primarily affect children and young adults and are typically

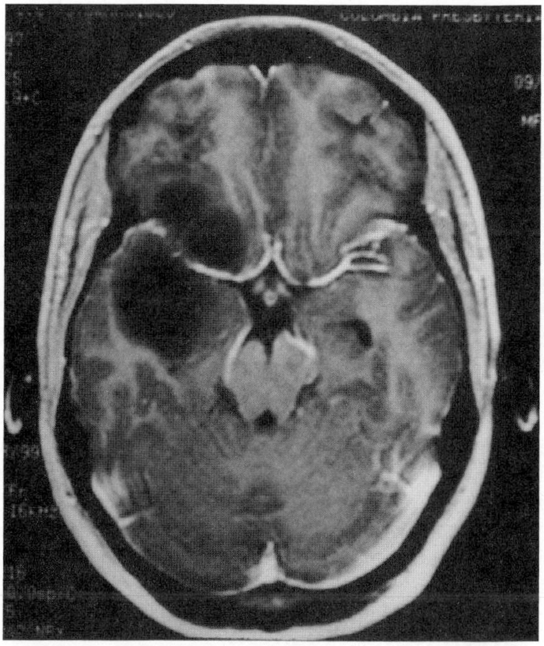

▲ **Figure 12–3.** Oligodendroglioma. Axial T1-weighted MRI scan after gadolinium contrast administration demonstrates a right frontotemporal hypointense lesion consistent with an oligodendroglioma.

found within or near ependymal surfaces; 70% are located within the fourth ventricle. Some arise from within the parenchyma, especially those in the cerebral hemispheres. Similar to astrocytomas, cellular ependymomas are graded according to their histology. They occur most often in children aged 1–5 years.

▶ Clinical Findings

A. Symptoms and Signs

Initial symptoms in patients with ependymomas usually relate to obstruction of CSF flow and resultant hydrocephalus. Depressed mental status is most common, and emergent management with CSF diversion may be necessary. Cranial nerve deficits can be seen as a result of local compressive or destructive effects.

B. Diagnostic Studies

These tumors can spread through the CSF to other sites in the CNS; therefore, it is necessary to evaluate the entire neuraxis with contrast-enhanced MRI. As with other types of gliomas, ependymomas usually have low intensity on T1-weighted MRI scans and high intensity on T2-weighted scans. Cysts, calcifications, and hemorrhages are often present, and the solid portion of the tumor usually enhances after contrast administration (Figure 12–4). Definitive diagnosis requires surgical biopsy.

▶ Treatment & Prognosis

Surgical excision is recommended, but it is frequently impossible to achieve because of the infiltrative nature of the tumor. Adjuvant radiotherapy is often used; chemotherapy is usually reserved for recurrent tumors. Intraparenchymal lesions and tumors in children younger than 5 years of age have a poor prognosis. In general these tumors have a 5-year survival rate of 45%, and tumor recurrence at the site of resection is common.

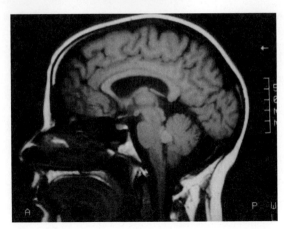

▲ **Figure 12–4.** Ependymoma. Sagittal T1-weighted MRI scan after gadolinium contrast administration demonstrates a tumor in the fourth ventricle consistent with an ependymoma.

4. Primitive Neuroectodermal Tumor and Medulloblastoma

▶ General Considerations

The term *primitive neuroectodermal tumor* (PNET) was originally used to describe a group of tumors, the prototype of which was considered to be medulloblastoma. Recent genetic analysis has differentiated the two into separate categories. Taken together, these are the second most common form of pediatric brain tumor after astrocytoma. Medulloblastomas are most often located in the posterior fossa in children, and PNETs are proportionally distributed throughout the brain and are found in children and adults.

▶ Clinical Findings

A. Symptoms and Signs

Headache, nausea, vomiting, and ataxia are the result of direct parenchymal damage and obstruction of CSF outflow, which can cause hydrocephalus in medulloblastoma. PNETs will cause symptoms similar to astrocytomas, which are usually related to the location of the tumor.

B. Diagnostic Studies

CT scans reveal a hyperdense, well-defined tumor of the cerebellar hemispheres or vermis that enhances after contrast administration. MRI signal characteristics are variable, but the tumor enhances with contrast and is usually hyperintense on T2-weighted imaging. MRI imaging with contrast of the entire neuraxis is necessary because this tumor commonly disseminates via CSF throughout the CNS.

▶ Treatment & Prognosis

Surgical resection is the first line of therapy, and survival is improved with gross total resection. All tumors should be treated with radiotherapy. Craniospinal irradiation is often indicated because of the high propensity for seeding. Chemotherapy is reserved for patients with high-grade lesions and a poor prognosis (see Table 12–7).

5. Meningioma

▶ General Considerations

Meningiomas are the most common benign brain tumor and represent approximately 20% of all primary brain tumors. They are more common in women than men (3:1 ratio), and incidence peaks in middle age. Thought to arise from the arachnoidal cap cells of the dura, meningiomas grow slowly, rarely invade brain tissue, and can become very large before they are symptomatic. Most (80–90%) are located supratentorially. These tumors can arise after exposure to high amounts of radiation and are a common form of secondary malignancy after adjuvant radiotherapy to the head and neck.

▶ Clinical Findings

A. Symptoms and Signs

Patients with meningiomas usually present with headache, seizures, and progressive neurologic deficits, depending on the location of the tumor. These tumors grow slowly and can be quite large at the time of diagnosis, especially when located over the frontal lobes.

B. Diagnostic Studies

CT and MRI findings are very specific for meningiomas. Most tumors are isodense or hyperdense on CT images, and they are well-defined smooth or lobulated masses that homogenously enhance after contrast administration. They can be calcified and appear to be attached to the meninges with dural tails. They also can create changes in the neighboring bone through erosion or hyperostosis. They are isointense to brain tissue on T1-weighted MRI scans and brightly and uniformly enhance with contrast (Figure 12–5). A CSF-filled space can often be seen between the tumor and nervous tissue. Sometimes, there is edema of the adjacent brain, which may signify invasion through the pia mater.

Conventional angiography is often used to assess the feasibility and safety of preoperative embolization, which can make resection easier and safer.

▶ Treatment & Prognosis

Total surgical resection is the goal of treatment (Figure 12–6). The location, size, and involvement of vascular and neural structures determine the difficulty of surgical resection. Stereotactic radiosurgery provides an alternative means of

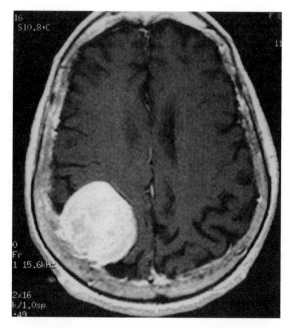

▲ **Figure 12–5.** Meningioma. Axial T1-weighted MRI scan after gadolinium contrast administration shows a right frontoparietal, well-circumscribed meningioma that enhances intensely and homogenously with contrast. This tumor grows from the meningeal covering of the brain and will typically compress but not invade into the brain tissue.

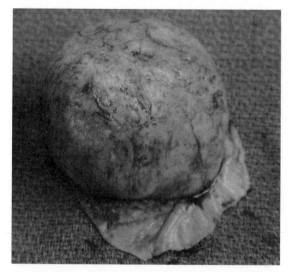

▲ **Figure 12–6.** Meningioma. Gross pathology of the convexity meningioma seen in Figure 12–5. The specimen was removed with the adjacent meningeal coverings.

therapy if the tumor is smaller than 3 cm and is not located near neural structures that are particularly radiosensitive, such as the optic nerves. Atypical and malignant forms of this tumor are characterized by invasion into normal brain, peritumoral edema, and faster growth patterns. Recurrence of the tumor after resection is related to the extent of resection; in general 7% recur within 5 years of total resection. Meningiomas are benign tumors, and surgical results are generally favorable.

6. Pituitary Adenoma

▶ General Considerations

Pituitary adenomas comprise up to 15% of all diagnosed primary brain tumors and are the third most common primary tumor. They become more common with age and have a female preponderance in younger patients. A genetic predisposition to development of these tumors has been identified: multiple endocrine neoplasia type 1 (MEN 1) syndrome. Pituitary adenomas can be categorized generally as secretory or nonsecretory tumors. Secretory tumors typically overproduce a single hormone, resulting in specific endocrine syndromes. Nonsecretory tumors cause symptoms from compression of local structures, including the normal pituitary, optic chiasm, hypothalamus, and third ventricle.

▶ Clinical Findings
A. Symptoms and Signs

The most common type of pituitary tumor is nonsecretory adenoma. Prolactinoma, the most common (40%) type of secretory pituitary adenoma, causes amenorrhea and galactorrhea in women and sexual dysfunction in men. Tumors that overproduce secretion of growth hormone are the next most common pituitary adenoma and cause acromegaly in adults and gigantism in children and adolescents. Tumors that secrete adrenocorticotropic hormone cause Cushing disease, which results in increased cortisol secretion from the adrenal glands. Adenomas that overproduce thyroid-stimulating hormone, luteinizing hormone, and follicle-stimulating hormone are much less common; symptoms usually result from mass effect and are similar to those occurring in patients with nonsecretory adenomas.

The central location of the pituitary gland results in a variety of neurologic symptoms from a growing pituitary tumor, including headache, visual loss, and hypopituitarism. Headaches are thought to result from compression of the diaphragma sella and the blood vessels. Compression of the optic chiasm results in progressive bitemporal visual field loss and decreased visual acuity. Unilateral visual loss can also occur if the tumor is asymmetric and compresses a single optic nerve. Hypopituitarism is caused by adenomas that compress and disrupt the normal secretory function of the anterior pituitary; there may be fatigue, weakness, hypothyroidism, and hypogonadism. Extraocular muscle palsies can follow invasion of the cavernous sinus. Hydrocephalus can occur from compression of the third ventricle. Compression of the hypothalamus can cause alterations in mood, sleep, and eating.

Extremely large tumors may produce the entire spectrum of symptoms encountered with meningiomas or astrocytomas. These tumors are also prone to spontaneous hemorrhage in up to 10% of cases. In 1–2% of cases, the dramatic clinical syndrome of pituitary apoplexy occurs after an acute hemorrhage. It is characterized by acute headache, meningismus, visual impairment, ophthalmoplegia, and alteration of consciousness. Without timely intervention and surgical decompression, patients can die of subarachnoid hemorrhage, acute hydrocephalus, or even hypopituitarism.

B. Laboratory Findings

Serum hormone testing for prolactin and growth hormone, thyroid function tests, and morning cortisol levels are used to determine the presence of a secretory adenoma and the functional status of the pituitary gland. Serum electrolytes can be altered from the disrupted regulation of cortisol and antidiuretic hormone and should be checked.

C. Imaging Studies

MRI scans can differentiate microadenomas (tumors smaller than 1 cm) from the normal gland on T1-weighted images after contrast administration; the adenoma is usually hypointense and the gland enhances. Macroadenomas (> 1 cm) are usually isointense on T1-weighted images and enhance homogenously with contrast (Figure 12–7). MRI

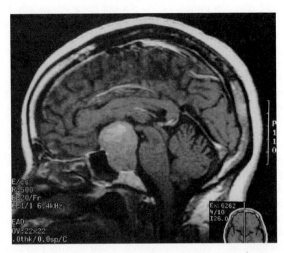

▲ **Figure 12–7.** Pituitary adenoma. Sagittal T1-weighted MRI scan after gadolinium contrast enhancement demonstrates a very large tumor arising from the sella.

can determine the relation of the tumor to nearby vital structures and is essential for surgical planning.

D. Other Tests

Even if visual loss is not detected on physical examination, a comprehensive neuro-ophthalmologic evaluation, including visual field testing, is indicated.

▶ Treatment & Prognosis

Treatment is directed at correcting any endocrine dysfunction and at tumor removal. Surgical resection, predominantly through trans-sphenoidal microsurgery, is the treatment of choice and can be curative. Pharmacologic therapy with dopamine agonists, typically bromocriptine, has been used with considerable success in prolactin-secreting tumors and should be considered as the first mode of treatment in patients with these tumors. Radiotherapy, especially stereotactic radiosurgery, is used primarily as an adjuvant to control recurrent or incompletely resected disease. Radiosurgery is sometimes used, but its role has not been completely defined and is often limited by the proximity of the optic nerves.

7. Central Nervous System Lymphoma

▶ General Considerations

There are two main categories of this disease: primary and secondary lymphomas of the CNS. Primary CNS lymphoma has become a more frequent diagnosis in adults, because of increasing instances of immunosuppressive states (eg, HIV infection, immunosuppressive therapy for organ transplantation), an aging population, and better diagnostic studies. Immunosuppressed patients have a lower age of presentation, and there is a male predominance in diagnosis, especially in cases associated with HIV and AIDS. (HIV-related primary CNS lymphoma is discussed in more detail in Chapter 28.)

▶ Clinical Findings

A. Symptoms and Signs

As with most primary tumors, the presenting symptoms relate to the location of the tumor within the CNS. The common frontal location of these tumors leads to personality change, cognitive dysfunction, and memory loss. Headache, motor or sensory loss, and depressed levels of consciousness are also noted. Lymphomas can occur in multiple locations, resulting in a constellation of seemingly unrelated neurologic signs and symptoms.

B. Diagnostic Studies

Neuroimaging may reveal single or multiple lesions that enhance with contrast and have associated edema (Figure 12–8).

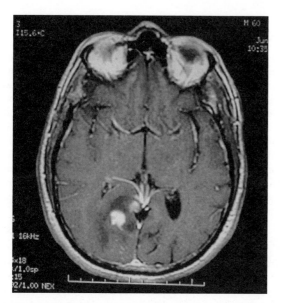

▲ **Figure 12–8.** Central nervous system lymphoma. Axial T1-weighted MRI scan after gadolinium contrast enhancement shows a tumor of the right occipital lobe that enhances intensely and has peritumoral edema.

▶ **Treatment & Prognosis**

Surgical resection has no role in treatment of these tumors. Stereotactic biopsy is often used for diagnosis and to direct subsequent chemotherapy treatment. Patients are usually treated with radiotherapy and methotrexate-based chemotherapy regimens (see Table 12–7). Despite aggressive therapy, the median survival for patients with primary CNS lymphoma is approximately 13 months. Survival for patients with metastatic lymphoma is dependent primarily on the status of the systemic disease.

8. Chordoma

▶ **General Considerations**

Chordoma is an embryonal tumor that develops from notochord remnants within the skull base and vertebrae. Accounting for less than 1% of all intracranial tumors, chordomas are most often located in the spheno-occipital and sacrococcygeal regions. They are slow growing and locally invasive and are characterized by continued recurrence after surgical resection. Men are nearly as likely as women to have a chordoma, which usually occurs in the second and third decades of life.

▶ **Diagnosis**

A. Symptoms and Signs

Headache and cranial nerve palsies are the most common presenting symptoms of skull base chordomas. Visual loss,

hemiparesis, and brainstem compression occur with disease progression.

B. Diagnostic Studies

CT and MRI scans are useful to delineate tumor margins and bony destruction. The tumor is well defined and enhances with contrast administration. The hyperintensity of the tumor as seen on T2-weighted images helps to define the tumor in relation to surrounding anatomy.

▶ **Treatment & Prognosis**

Complete surgical resection is the treatment that correlates with the best outcome. Treatment for recurrent tumor or residual tumor is surgical resection and radio-surgery or proton-beam therapy. Tumor-free survival at 5 years after complete resection ranges from 30–70%.

9. Schwannoma

▶ **General Considerations**

Schwannomas most often arise from the vestibular portion of the 8th cranial nerve and less commonly from the 5th, 9th, 10th, 11th, or 12th nerves. They account for 10% of all primary brain tumors. In 95% of cases tumors are unilateral; the 5% that are bilateral are associated with neurofibromatosis type 2.

▶ **Clinical Findings**

A. Symptoms and Signs

Hearing loss is present to some degree in nearly all patients with acoustic schwannomas but may not be the presenting symptom. Other early symptoms are vertigo, tinnitus, and facial weakness or numbness from compression of the eighth, seventh, or fifth cranial nerves. Large tumors cause brainstem and cerebellar compression, resulting in headache, hydrocephalus, hemiparesis, ataxia, and altered consciousness.

B. Diagnostic Studies

Tumors appear as hypointense lesions on T1-weighted MRI scans and are hyperintense on T2-weighted scans. They exhibit intense contrast enhancement (Figure 12–9). Audiograms demonstrate sensorineural hearing loss and decreased voice discrimination in almost all patients, and brainstem auditory evoked potentials can demonstrate auditory nerve compression.

▶ **Treatment & Prognosis**

Microsurgical resection is usually curative, with low morbidity and almost no mortality. Cranial nerve deficits are the most common complication of surgery. Facial nerve function after surgery depends on the size of the tumor; with tumors smaller than 2 cm, more than 95% of patients will

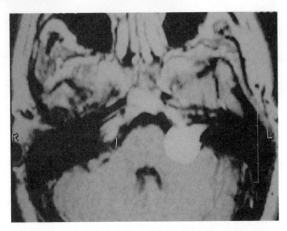

▲ **Figure 12–9.** Vestibular nerve schwannoma (acoustic neuroma). Axial T1-weighted MRI scan after contrast administration demonstrates an intensely enhancing, left-sided vestibular schwannoma at the cerebellopontine angle with some invasion into the internal auditory meatus.

have preserved function. Stereotaxic radiosurgery for lesions smaller than 2.5 cm is an alternative approach, especially in elderly patients.

10. Tumors of the Pineal Region

▶ General Considerations

Accounting for 1% of all brain tumors, primary tumors in this area arise from pineal parenchymal cells, producing either pineocytomas or pineoblastomas. Germ cell tumors occurring in the pineal region (and to a lesser extent in the suprasellar region) include germinomas, teratomas, yolk sac tumors, choriocarcinomas, and embryonal carcinomas. Other types of tumors found in this region include meningiomas, astrocytomas, ependymomas, gangliogliomas, epidermoid tumors, dermoid cysts, and pineal cysts.

▶ Clinical Findings

A. Symptoms and Signs

Pineal tumors commonly cause hydrocephalus and brainstem compression. Hydrocephalus leads to ataxia, depressed level of consciousness, and bladder dysfunction. Brainstem compression can cause Parinaud syndrome, various levels of coma, and ataxia.

B. Laboratory Findings

Serum levels of β-human chorionic gonadotropin or α-fetoprotein, or both, are pathognomonic for the presence of a malignant germ cell tumor and should be assayed in all patients with tumors in the pineal region.

C. Imaging Studies

CT and MRI scanning are very useful for diagnosis, because each type of pineal tumor demonstrates characteristic findings on neuroimaging. On CT scanning, pineal parenchymal tumors appear as lobulated hyperdense lesions that enhance with contrast and have areas of calcification. Germinomas are well-defined isodense to hyperdense lesions that enhance with contrast. Teratomas have a heterogeneous appearance that relates to their histologic structure of cystic, fatty, and solid tissues. MRI provides better anatomic definition of the tumor and its relation to neighboring structures and is essential for surgical planning. MRI scans of the entire brain and spinal cord should be performed, because many of these tumor types can seed along CSF pathways.

▶ Treatment & Prognosis

Treatment requires establishing a histologic diagnosis because of the variety of tumor types that can be found in this region. Open surgical biopsy is preferred, and intraoperative histopathology is helpful to determine whether aggressive resection is necessary. Nearly one third of these tumors are benign and can be cured by resection alone. Postoperative radiotherapy is given for all malignant pineal tumors, and chemotherapy is beneficial for germ cell tumors (see Table 12–7). The 5-year survival rate for patients with malignant pineal parenchymal tumors is 50%; for those with germinomas, 5-year survival is 80%, but other types of malignant germ cell tumor have a less favorable prognosis.

11. Craniopharyngioma

Accounting for about 2% of all primary brain tumors, craniopharyngiomas are most often diagnosed in children younger than 10 years of age, but they can occur in adults. They arise from remnant epithelial cells of the endoderm and undergo progressive growth. Classically located in the suprasellar region, they are histologically benign tumors, but they frequently recur after resection and can cause hypothalamic visual disturbances and hydrocephalus. Complete surgical resection is the treatment of choice, with radiation therapy indicated for residual or recurrent tumors.

12. Choroid Plexus Papilloma & Carcinoma

Choroid tumors are uncommon, and more than 90% of these tumors are papillomas. They most commonly affect children younger than 5 years of age and arise from the choroid plexus within the posterior lateral ventricles. When they occur in adults, they usually involve the fourth ventricle. Symptoms are the result of hydrocephalus and include headaches, ataxia, and altered mental status. Frondlike, occasionally calcified, masses within the ventricles are seen on imaging. Treatment is total surgical resection, and long-term survival is directly related to the pathologic grade. Resection of papillomas can be curative.

Behin A, et al. Primary brain tumours in adults. *Lancet* 2003;361:323–331. [PMID: 12559880] (Focuses primarily on the more common subsets of gliomas and CNS lymphomas, with an emphasis on the prognosis and treatment of these diseases.)

Ciric I. Long-term management and outcome for pituitary tumors. *Neurosurg Clin N Am* 2003;14:167–171. [PMID: 12690987] (Differential diagnosis and management of tumors arising near the pituitary region are reviewed with an in-depth discussion of the medical and surgical management of pituitary adenomas.)

Kleihues P, et al. The WHO classification of tumors of the central nervous system. *J Neuropathol Exp Neurol* 2002;61:215–225. [PMID: 11895036] (Provides an overview of the 2000 WHO classification of nervous system tumors, with an emphasis on genetic profiles of each tumor. This classification system is being used and implemented by neuro-oncology and biomedical research communities worldwide.)

Komotar et al. Surgical management of craniopharyngiomas. *J Neurooncol* 2009;92:283–296. [PMID: 19357956] (Provides a perspective on overall management of craniopharyngiomas.)

Rutka JT, et al. Pediatric surgical neurooncology: Current best care practices and strategies. *J Neurooncol* 2004;69:139–150. [PMID: 15527086] (Reviews the current treatment strategies of the three most common types of pediatric brain tumors—gliomas, medulloblastomas, and ependymomas—and discusses current and future diagnostic and therapeutic modalities.)

See SJ, et al. Anaplastic astrocytoma: Diagnosis, prognosis, and management. *Semin Oncol* 2004;31:618–634. [PMID: 15497115] (Summarizes the clinical diagnosis, prognosis, and treatment of anaplastic astrocytoma.)

Smith JS, et al. Role of extent of resection in the long-term outcome of low-grade hemispheric gliomas. *J Clin Oncol* 2008;26:1338–1345. [PMID: 18323558] (Extent of surgical resection in low-grade gliomas determines patient outcomes.)

Wen PY, et al. Malignant gliomas in adults. *N Engl J Med* 2008;359:492–507. [PMID:] (A comprehensive review of the current state of knowledge and treatment of malignant gliomas.)

Whittle IR, et al. Meningiomas. *Lancet* 2004;363:1535–1543. [PMID: 15135603] (Reviews the current rationale and the evidence basis for the different types of therapy used for meningiomas, as well as management controversies.)

METASTATIC BRAIN TUMORS

► General Considerations

Metastasis to the brain occurs in about 20–30% of all patients with systemic cancer. Therefore, approximately 50,000–100,000 patients per year in the United States develop these tumors. In 40% of symptomatic metastatic lesions, the primary site is the lung; in 20%, it is the breast. The next most frequent sources of metastatic brain lesions are melanoma, gastrointestinal cancers, and renal cancers. Most metastases (80%) are supratentorial; the cerebellum is the site of lesions in 10–15% of patients, and the brainstem in 3–5%. Half of metastatic lesions at presentation are single, and half are multiple. About 10% of patients have more than five lesions, and in these patients the most likely primary neoplasm is lung cancer or melanoma. Metastatic brain tumors are rare in children and are most often diagnosed in adults older than 40 years of age.

► Clinical Findings

The clinical pattern of metastatic brain tumors is very similar to that of primary brain tumors. The presence of neurologic symptoms and a lesion seen on MRI scan is almost diagnostic of a metastatic brain tumor in a patient with a known systemic neoplasm. In patients who present with a single lesion in the brain and no evidence of systemic cancer, there is a 15% chance that the lesion represents metastatic disease. Approximately one third of patients with metastatic brain lesions do not have a previous history of cancer. Patients with suspected or known metastatic brain lesions and no systemic diagnosis require a complete medical evaluation, including a CT scan of the chest and abdomen, stool guaiac test, and blood tests for various cancer markers.

A. Symptoms and Signs

Headache is the most common presenting symptom, followed by alteration in mental status and focal neurologic deficits. As with primary brain tumors, clinical signs are related to the location, size, and secondary effects of the lesion. The most common focal symptoms are hemiparesis, sensory disturbances, aphasia, and ataxia. Seizures occur in about 10% of patients and hemorrhage in about 15%, especially those with melanoma, choriocarcinoma, renal cell carcinoma, thyroid cancer, and lung cancer. The time from diagnosis of systemic cancer until the appearance of a metastatic lesion within the brain varies according to tumor type, but the median is usually 2–3 years. Lung cancer is an exception, producing widespread metastatic disease at 6–9 months.

B. Diagnostic Studies

MRI and CT scans typically reveal multiple lesions, often at the gray-white cortical junction. The lesions enhance with contrast (sometimes ring enhancing) and exhibit peritumoral edema, which is best seen on T2- or FLAIR-weighted MRI scans (Figure 12–10). Individual lesions appear similar to malignant gliomas, but the presence of multiple lesions suggests metastatic tumors. The differential diagnosis includes malignant glioma, primary CNS lymphoma, abscess, and radiation necrosis.

► Treatment & Prognosis

In general, patients with metastasis to the brain have a poor prognosis. The purpose of any intervention is to prolong survival and improve quality of life. Emergent situations, which usually involve a patient with a depressed level of consciousness or herniation syndrome from high intracranial pressure or tumoral hemorrhage, require high-dose corticosteroid, osmotic, and other therapies to lower intracranial

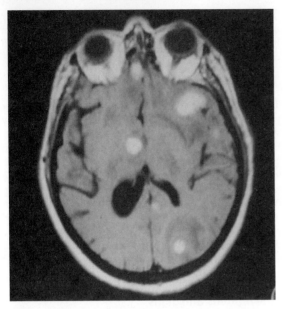

▲ **Figure 12–10.** Multiple metastatic lesions. Axial T1-weighted MRI scan after contrast administration shows four separate lesions throughout the cerebrum, consistent with metastatic systemic cancer.

pressure. Emergent surgical resection is often indicated. In most cases, a therapeutic decision is based on tumor type (if known), status of systemic disease, overall prognosis, and the number and location of lesions. Patients are stratified depending on whether the diagnosis of a systemic cancer is known.

Patients with probable metastatic lesions and no known primary neoplasm should have a complete medical evaluation followed by biopsy of either the brain or, if found, the systemic source. Surgical resection should be considered if there are only a few lesions that can be accessed easily, if the tumor is insensitive to chemotherapy or radiotherapy, and if the lesion is causing significant neurologic symptoms and can be removed without major morbidity. In situations where no systemic source is identified after a complete evaluation, stereotactic needle biopsy or open surgical resection should be performed. In patients with known or newly diagnosed systemic cancer, the first consideration is the possibility of a successful response to chemotherapy or radiotherapy. Certain types of cancer (eg, germ cell tumors and lymphomas) are treated effectively with chemotherapy and radiotherapy. Surgical resection improves survival and quality of life in patients with single metastatic lesions to the brain. Similar favorable results can follow removal of multiple metastatic lesions. Prognosis in these patients depends on the status of the systemic disease and the possibility of definitive therapy of the metastatic lesions.

Klos KJ, et al. Brain metastases. *Neurologist* 2004;10:31–46. [PMID: 14720313] (Summarizes the epidemiology, clinical features, pathophysiology, and diagnostic evaluation of brain metastases. A useful section presents the current therapeutic strategies from the perspective of the three most common primary tumor locations along with the treatment approach to other metastatic tumors.)

Soffietti R, et al. Management of brain metastases. *J Neurol* 2002;249:1357–1369. [PMID: 12382150] (Accurately describes the current algorithm generally used for determining the appropriate treatment modalities—surgery, radiotherapy, or chemotherapy—used for metastatic brain tumors.)

▼ TUMORS OF THE SKULL

Benign and malignant tumors of the skull create symptoms through compression and destruction of neural elements, the skull, and its supporting structures (Tables 12–8 and 12–9). Both CT and MRI are essential for diagnosis and for planning treatment. Surgical resection is the most common treatment measure.

Bulsara KR, et al. Skull base surgery for benign skull base tumors. *J Neurooncol* 2004;69:181–189. [PMID: 15527089] (Reviews the rationale for the use of surgery for the most common benign skull base tumors. The authors provide evidence that suggests that gross total resection of these lesions gives patients the best possible chance of a cure.)

DeMonte F. Evolving role of skullbase surgery for patients with low and high grade malignancies. *J Neurooncol* 2004;69:191–198. [PMID: 15527090] (Describes the multimodal approach to diagnosis and therapy for tumors of the skull and skull base from the perspective of surgical management.)

▼ SPINAL CORD TUMORS

 ESSENTIALS OF DIAGNOSIS

▶ Motor or sensory loss segmentally or below the level of the lesion

▶ Loss of bladder (or bowel) control

▶ Back pain

▶ Progressive course

▶ Abnormal findings on CT or MRI scan, indicative of tumor compression of the spinal cord or nerve roots

▶ General Considerations

These tumors, affecting primarily younger and middle-aged adults, are found throughout the spinal cord in a distribution that is in proportion to the length of each segment. The incidence of spinal cord tumors is approximately one quarter that of brain tumors. The most common extramedullary

Table 12–8. Benign Tumors of the Skull

Tumor	Description	Location	Clinical Findings	Treatment
Osteoma	Growth of dense cortical bone	Calvarium, paranasal sinuses, orbit	S&S—asymptomatic, sinusitis, proptosis Imaging—circumscribed lesion with density of bone	Surgery
Chondroma	Growth of cartilage	Skull base, paranasal sinuses	S&S—asymptomatic, cranial nerve palsies Imaging—lytic lesion with sharp margin, erodes into bone	Surgery
Hemangioma	Benign bone tumor, vascular channels	Vertebral column, calvarium	S&S—asymptomatic, headache Imaging—decreased density, "honeycomb" or trabeculated	Surgery
Dermoid or epidermoid cyst	Ectodermal remnants; most common lesion in children	Calvarium, sinuses, orbit, skull base	S&S—asymptomatic Imaging—rounded lytic lesions, sharp sclerotic margins	Rarely indicated, surgery

S&S = symptoms and signs.

tumors are metastatic tumors, meningiomas, neurofibromas, and schwannomas. The most common intramedullary tumors are ependymomas, astrocytomas, hemangioblastomas, and metastatic tumors (Table 12–10). The most common metastatic tumors, the majority of which are found in the vertebral body and epidural space, are lung, breast, prostate, and gastrointestinal cancers. Melanomas and lymphomas are found to a much lesser degree. Epidural spinal cord compression occurs in approximately 5–10% of cancer patients.

▶ **Clinical Findings**

Diagnosis of these lesions relies on findings from the clinical history, physical examination, and imaging studies. Extramedullary tumors cause symptoms through direct compression of nervous tissue, whereas intramedullary tumors affect the nervous tissue itself.

A. Symptoms and Signs

Extramedullary tumors typically affect a focal segment of the spinal cord and its associated nerve roots, producing symptoms referable to that level. Initial symptoms may be radicular pain and paresthesias and progressive numbness and weakness in the distribution of the affected nerve roots. With continued compression, descending and ascending pathways are compromised, resulting in spastic paresis and numbness below the lesion, hyperreflexia, and bowel or bladder dysfunction (Table 12–11).

Intramedullary tumors have a more variable presentation because they can involve only a few spinal segments or extend throughout the spinal cord. Symptoms depend on the specific areas of the spinal cord affected. If the lesions are restricted to only one or two segments, symptoms and signs resemble those of extramedullary tumors. Disassociated sensory loss suggesting syringomyelia can occur.

Table 12–9. Malignant Tumors of the Skull

Tumor	Description	Location	Clinical Findings	Treatment
Chondrosarcoma	Malignant cartilage tumor of men aged 30–40 y	Skull base	S&S—cranial nerve palsies, pain, sinusitis, proptosis Imaging—lytic lesion with sharp margin, erodes into bone	Surgery with wide margins; radiotherapy ineffective
Osteosarcoma	Malignant bone tumor, occurring in adolescence	Skull base, calvarium	S&S—asymptomatic, cranial nerve palsies, pain Imaging—lytic lesion with sharp margin, erodes into bone	Surgery with wide margins; radiotherapy ineffective
Fibrous sarcoma	Soft tissue tumor from associated connective tissue	Throughout skull	S&S—asymptomatic, headache Imaging—lytic lesion with sharp margin, erodes into bone	Surgery with wide margins; radiotherapy ineffective
Glomus jugulare	Paraganglia cell of jugular bulb	Skull base	S&S—tinnitus, cranial nerve palsies Imaging—contrast-enhancing lesion	Angiographic embolization, surgery

S&S = symptoms and signs.

Table 12–10. Categories of Spinal Cord Tumors

Location	Tumor[a]
Intramedullary	Ependymoma Astrocytoma Hemangioblastoma
Intradural, extramedullary	Meningioma Schwannoma Neurofibroma
Extradural	Metastatic cancer Primary bony lesions, including multiple myeloma

[a]Listed from most to least common.

B. Diagnostic Studies

The presence of a spinal tumor can be established with diagnostic imaging. MRI with intravenous gadolinium contrast can identify lesions and their relative compressive effects with high resolution. Plain radiographs demonstrate abnormalities in a small percentage of cases. CT scans will not show the same level of detail in the soft tissues as MRI. However, both imaging tests are useful for examining the structural elements of the spinal column and for determining the amount of bony destruction. Biopsy and surgical excision is the diagnostic end point for most cases of spinal cord tumors.

Table 12–11. Anatomic Localization of Symptom Patterns in Spinal Cord Tumors

Location	Symptoms
Cervical spine	Neck pain or paresthesias Radicular pattern of pain, numbness, or weakness in the upper extremity
Thoracic spine	Specific sensory level
Lumbar spine	Radicular pattern of pain, numbness, or weakness in the lower extremity
Conus or cauda equina	Back, rectal, or leg pain Saddle anesthesia Bowel or bladder dysfunction
Foramen magnum	Lower cranial nerve involvement (XII, XI, and sometimes IX and X)

▶ Treatment & Prognosis

A. Intramedullary Tumors

Intramedullary tumors are treated solely with surgical resection. There is no established role for postoperative adjuvant radiotherapy or chemotherapy in the treatment of these tumors. Ependymomas can be cured with total resection, and about half of all astrocytomas can be fully excised. Other, less common, types of intramedullary tumors (eg, hemangioblastomas, metastatic lesions, or dermoid cysts) should also be treated with surgical resection.

B. Intradural, Extramedullary Tumors

Intradural, extramedullary tumors are almost always benign tumors that cause symptoms through compression of the neural elements. Treatment should be total surgical resection. These tumors grow slowly and can take years to become symptomatic or recur.

C. Extradural Tumors

As previously discussed, extradural lesions that result in spinal cord compression are most often metastatic lesions from systemic cancer found in the vertebral bodies and epidural space. Management of patients with these lesions must be determined on an individual basis. Radiotherapy is usually the initial therapy of choice, but surgical resection may be warranted in cases of unknown diagnosis, good clinical condition, rapidly progressive neurologic deficits, spinal column instability, and radioresistant disease. In most cases, therapy will not extend survival but will improve quality of life, enabling patients to remain ambulatory and reducing their pain.

Gerszten PC, et al. Current surgical management of metastatic spinal disease. *Oncology* 2000;14:1013–1024; discussion 1024, 1029–1030, review. [PMID: 10929589] (Reviews the factors favoring an operative recommendation in patients with metastatic spinal disease in the context of the overall treatment options available. This article emphasizes the importance of an early surgical consultation as part of a multidisciplinary approach to their disease process.)

Parsa AT, et al. Spinal cord and intradural-extraparenchymal spinal tumors: Current best care practices and strategies. *J Neurooncol* 2004;69:291–318. [PMID: 15527097] (Describes the current best care practices and strategies for patients with the most common diagnoses of primary spinal cord tumors, with an emphasis on surgical management.)

Paraneoplastic Neurologic Syndromes

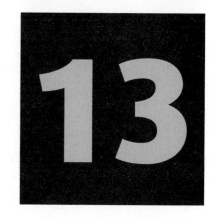

Lakshmi Nayak, MD, Alfredo D. Voloschin, MD, & Andrew B. Lassman, MD

ESSENTIALS OF DIAGNOSIS

▶ Acute or subacute onset (days to weeks)

▶ Up to 60% of cases precede the diagnosis of cancer

▶ Certain syndromes, along with specific markers, may herald the type and location of an occult cancer

▶ General Considerations

Immune-mediated paraneoplastic neurologic syndromes (PNSs) comprise a rare group of disorders in patients with cancer. They develop remotely and cause damage to neural structures, rather than as a direct effect of cancer or metastases. In general, patients present with neurologic symptoms, with cancer neither evident at onset nor previously diagnosed. Even when cancer is identified, it is often indolent and not widely metastatic although lymph node involvement is not unusual. PNSs can affect any part of the nervous system and mimic virtually any neurologic disorder; as a result, they are often diagnosed late when permanent damage has already occurred.

The reported incidence of 0.9–6% of patients is likely an underestimate because the lack of pathognomonic findings makes the diagnosis of PNSs challenging. Some patients also develop neurologic symptoms that are likely paraneoplastic in origin but without an identifiable antibody. For example, Lambert-Eaton myasthenic syndrome (LEMS) occurs in 3% of patients with small cell lung cancer (SCLC), but almost 50% of patients with SCLC develop muscle weakness that may be paraneoplastic.

▶ Pathogenesis

The PNSs are generally thought to occur because of abnormal autoimmunity, although the details remain unclear. The hypothesis is that the primary tumor expresses an onconeural antigen that is normally exclusive to the nervous system, or

testes in anti-Ma–related syndromes (Table 13–1), provoking an autoimmune response that leads to neurologic symptoms. This hypothesis is supported by the presence of serum and cerebrospinal fluid (CSF) autoantibodies and T cells that react against the nervous system and the associated cancer. The exact mechanism of damage to the nervous system by the autoimmune response is not known for most PNSs, except LEMS and myasthenia gravis (MG), which are primarily B-cell mediated with a T-cell component.

The observation that tumors of patients with PNSs are heavily infiltrated with inflammatory cells also supports the immune-mediated theory. In the nervous system, there is perivascular cuffing by lymphocytic infiltrates (T and B cells); T cells are also seen in the parenchyma. However, the pathologic findings may range from an entirely normal brain, as seen in some patients with paraneoplastic opsoclonus-myoclonus (POM), to marked neuronal cell (Purkinje cell) loss without any inflammation, as seen in severe cases of paraneoplastic cerebellar degeneration (PCD). From a clinicopathologic perspective, syndromes such as POM that often improve with treatment can be distinguished from those, such as PCD, that usually do not respond to therapy. Therefore, the importance of making an early, accurate diagnosis is twofold. First, the earlier the paraneoplastic syndrome is treated, the more likely that irreversible cellular damage might be prevented. Second, the earlier the syndrome is identified, the greater is the likelihood that the underlying malignancy will be localized and potentially treated.

▶ Clinical Findings
A. Symptoms and Signs

Most PNSs are of acute or subacute onset. They can affect any part of the nervous system and thus present with any neurologic symptom, including multifocal involvement. Up to 60% of patients present with neurologic symptoms without a known history of cancer. Even when the cancer is diagnosed, the neurologic symptoms typically overshadow

Table 13–1. Antibodies Associated With Paraneoplastic Syndromes and the Commonly Found Cancers

Antibody	Syndrome	Associated Cancer
Anti-Hu (ANNA-1)	PEM, including cortical, limbic, and brainstem encephalitis; PCD; myelitis; sensory neuronopathy; autonomic dysfunction	SCLC, other
Anti-Yo (PCA-1)	PCD	Gynecologic, breast
Anti-Ri (ANNA-2)	PCD, brainstem encephalitis, opsoclonus-myoclonus	Breast, gynecologic, SCLC
Anti-Tr	PCD	Hodgkin lymphoma
Anti-CRMP5(CV2)	PEM, PCD, chorea, peripheral neuropathy, uveitis	SCLC, thymoma, others
Anti-Ma proteins[a] (ANNA-3)	Limbic, hypothalamic, and brainstem encephalitis (infrequently PCD)	Germ cell tumors of testis, other solid tumors
Anti-amphiphysin	Stiff person syndrome, PEM	Breast
Anti-recoverin[b]	Cancer-associated retinopathy	SCLC
Anti-bipolar cells of retina	Melanoma-associated retinopathy	Melanoma
Anti-NMDA receptor	Encephalitis	Ovarian teratoma
Zic-4 antibodies	PCD	SCLC
Anti-mGluR1	PCD	Hodgkin lymphoma
SOX1 (anti-glial nuclear antibody)	LEMS, PCD	SCLC
Anti-gephyrin	Stiff person syndrome	Mediastinal tumor
Anti-spectrin	PMA	Breast
Antibodies That Occur With and Without Cancer Association		
Anti-VGCC(P/Q type)	LEMS, PCD	SCLC
Anti-AChR	Myasthenia gravis	Thymoma
Anti-VGKC	Peripheral nerve hyperexcitability (neuromyotonia), limbic encephalitis, Morvan syndrome	Thymoma, others
nAChR	Autonomic neuropathy	SCLC, others
Anti-GAD	PEM, PCD	Thymoma, solid tumors
Anti-GABA B receptor	Limbic encephalitis	SCLC
Anti-AMPA receptor	Limbic encephalitis	SCLC, breast
Aquaporin-4 (NMO) autoantibody	NMO	Breast, others
Anti-GM1	ALS, PMA	Lymphoma
Anti-MAG	ALS	Waldenström macroglobulinemia

AChR = acetylcholine receptor; ALS = amyotrophic lateral sclerosis; AMPA = alpha-amino-3-hydroxy-5-methyl-4-isoxazolepropionic acid; ANNA = antineuronal nuclear antibody; CRMP5 = collapsin response mediator protein 5; GABA B = gamma amino butyric acid type B; GAD = glutamic acid decarboxylase; GM1 = ganglioside; LEMS = Lambert-Eaton myasthenic syndrome; MAG = myelin-associated glycoprotein; mGluR1 = metabotropic glutamate receptor; nAChR = neuronal acetylcholine receptor; NMDA = N-methyl D-aspartate; NMO = neuromyelitis optica; PCA = Purkinje cell antibody; PCD = paraneoplastic cerebellar degeneration; PEM = paraneoplastic encephalitis; PMA = progressive muscular atrophy; SCLC = small cell lung cancer; VGCC = voltage-gated calcium channel; VGKC = voltage-gated potassium channel; Zic-4 = zinc finger gene of the cerebellum.
[a]Patients with antibodies to Ma2 are usually men with testicular cancer. Patients with additional antibodies to other Ma proteins are men or women with a variety of solid tumors.
[b]Other antibodies reported in a few or isolated cases include antibodies to tubby-like protein and the photoreceptor-specific nuclear receptor.

cancer symptoms. In many instances, the cancer does not lead to early death, but there is significant disability related to the neurologic manifestation.

B. Laboratory Findings

The CSF of patients with paraneoplastic neurologic syndromes of the CNS usually shows elevated protein concentration (most often, 50–100 mg/dL), mild lymphocytic pleocytosis (10–100 cells/mm^3), intrathecal synthesis of immunoglobulins, and/or the presence of oligoclonal bands. These findings are not diagnostic of PNSs, but rather reflect an inflammatory reaction. Specific antineuronal antibodies (discussed later for each syndrome) are found in higher concentration in the CSF than in serum, suggesting intrathecal synthesis.

Although identification of a PNS-associated antibody suggests the diagnosis of a PNS (and the presence of a malignancy), a negative test result does not exclude it. In other words, absence of proof is not proof of absence.

Depending on the site of neurologic involvement, magnetic resonance imaging (MRI) or electrodiagnostic tests may be helpful. These are suggestive of the neurologic involvement, but not diagnostic of the PNS. The suspicion of a PNS mandates a thorough evaluation for an occult tumor. The specific tumor may be predicted by the nature of the antibody (eg, the anti-Yo antibody suggests breast or ovarian cancer, the anti-Hu antibody suggests SCLC). Computed tomography (CT) of the chest, abdomen, and pelvis; 2-fluorodeoxy-D-glucose positron emission tomography (FDG-PET); mammogram; testicular ultrasound; and serum and CSF tumor markers may identify the underlying cancer. However, some paraneoplastic antibodies are not specific to a particular PNS. Conversely, some PNSs are associated with various cancers. Individual PNSs are described later.

C. Diagnostic Criteria

Specific diagnostic criteria have been established by Graus et al., which divide PNSs into definite and possible PNS. Definite PNS includes classic syndrome and cancer developing within 5 years, nonclassic syndrome that resolves with treatment of the cancer, nonclassic syndrome with onconeural antibodies and cancer developing within 5 years, or any neurologic syndrome associated with well-characterized onconeural antibodies without cancer. Possible PNS includes classic syndrome with neither onconeural antibodies nor cancer but high risk for an underlying cancer, nonclassic syndrome with development of cancer within 2 years, or any neurologic syndrome with no cancer but partially characterized onconeural antibodies.

D. Classification

Classification may be based on clinical syndromes, antibodies, or tumor type (Table 13–1). Although the association of some antibodies with specific syndromes and cancers is not absolute, recognizing the particular syndrome in association

with a specific antibody may lead to finding an occult cancer in certain organs. For example, one of the associations most commonly found is the anti-Yo antibody with PCD and ovarian cancer.

▶ Treatment & Prognosis

Therapy is targeted at the identified (or suspected) primary tumor. Occasionally, the autoimmunity that causes the PNS may also either control or obliterate the tumor. However, in most cases the underlying cancer remains active. Treating the primary tumor early in the course of the disease may prevent further neurologic deterioration and in some cases may lead to complete recovery. The inciting onconeural antigen is removed by treatment of the cancer, and further neurologic damage is averted. Immunosuppression in the form of corticosteroids, intravenous immunoglobulins, plasma exchange, tacrolimus, rituximab, and alemtuzumab has been employed to treat PNSs.

The prognosis varies with the nature of the syndrome. Some PNSs, such as LEMS and myasthenia, respond well to treatment of the underlying cancer or immunosuppression. Spontaneous resolution of symptoms has also been documented. However, in other syndromes, such as PCD that involves loss (degeneration) of neurons (Purkinje cells), the symptoms may stabilize, but usually do not improve. Patients with dysautonomia have a particularly poor prognosis and are likely to die from the PNS rather than tumor progression. Some studies suggest that survival in patients with PNS varies with the type of associated antibody and type of tumor.

Darnell R, Posner J. Paraneoplastic syndromes affecting the nervous system. *Semin Oncol* 2006;33:270–298. [PMID: 16769417]

DeAngelis LM, Posner JB. *Neurologic Complications of Cancer*, 2nd ed. Oxford University Press, 2009.

Giometto B, et al. Paraneoplastic neurologic syndrome in the PNS Euronetwork database: A European study from 20 centers. *Arch Neurol* 2010;67:330–335. [PMID: 20212230]

Graus F, et al. Recommended diagnostic criteria for paraneoplastic neurological syndromes. *J Neurol Neurosurg Psychiatry* 2004;75:1135–1140 [PMID: 15258215]

Honnorat J, et al. Onco-neural antibodies and tumour type determine survival and neurological symptoms in paraneoplastic neurological syndromes with Hu or CV2/CRMP5 antibodies. *J Neurol Neurosurg Psychiatry* 2009;80:412–416. [PMID: 18931014]

McKeon A, et al. Positron emission tomography-computed tomography in paraneoplastic neurologic disorders. *Arch Neurol* 2010;67:322–329. [PMID: 20065123]

Pittock SJ, Kryzer TJ, Lennon VA. Paraneoplastic antibodies coexist and predict cancer, not neurological syndrome. *Ann Neurol* 2004;56:715–719. [PMID: 15468074]

PARANEOPLASTIC CEREBELLAR DEGENERATION

▶ General Considerations

Cancers most commonly associated with PCD include SCLC, carcinomas of the breast and ovary, and Hodgkin lymphoma.

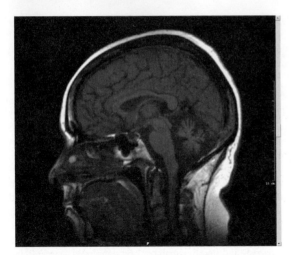

▲ **Figure 13–1.** Sagittal T1-weighted image of a 64-year-old woman with a history of breast carcinoma diagnosed 2 years before the onset of gait ataxia. She was found to have anti-Yo serum antibodies.

▶ Clinical Findings

A. Symptoms and Signs

Symptoms relate to loss of Purkinje cells in the cerebellum. These include gait imbalance, vertigo, nausea, vomiting, incoordination, and truncal ataxia. Other symptoms can include diplopia, oscillopsia, and blurred vision. On neurologic examination, nystagmus, dysmetria, dysarthria, and ataxia are commonly found. Whatever the presentation, there is a rapid onset and progression of the cerebellar syndrome which generally stabilizes; however, patients are often rendered severely and permanently disabled.

B. Imaging Studies

Initially, brain MRI may be normal. In advanced stages of PCD, however, there is usually significant cerebellar atrophy (Figure 13–1).

C. Special Tests

The anti-Yo antibody (also known as *anti–Purkinje cell antibody type 1* [PCA-1]) is commonly associated with breast and gynecologic cancers (mainly ovarian). The presence of anti-Yo antibodies in the setting of a cerebellar syndrome, without a history of cancer, warrants an aggressive search for an occult tumor, including laparoscopy and occasionally salpingo-oophorectomy.

Anti-Tr and anti-mGluR1 antibodies in a patient with PCD are associated with Hodgkin disease. Other antibodies associated with PCD are anti-CRMP5 (CV2), anti-Hu, anti-Ri, anti-Ma1, anti-ANNA3, anti-PCA2, and ZIC antibodies; patients with these antibodies often develop PCD along with involvement of other areas of the central nervous system.

PCD may occur in patients with LEMS; these patients usually have SCLC and voltage-gated calcium channel antibodies. A subgroup of patients with SCLC who develop PCD associated with voltage-gated calcium channel antibodies do not have symptoms of LEMS. Early in the course of the disease, CSF pleocytosis may be present with slightly elevated protein, but later the CSF becomes acellular.

▶ Differential Diagnosis

A subacute or acute cerebellar syndrome may be a presenting feature in patients with multiple sclerosis, cerebellar tumors, strokes, gluten ataxia, viral cerebellitis, and others. These causes of cerebellar dysfunction must be considered in addition to a PNS.

Cerebellar dysfunction is also associated with PNS other than PCD, such as paraneoplastic encephalomyelitis (PEM) and POM. However, the presence of limbic, focal, cortical, or diffuse encephalitis, myelitis, or peripheral neuropathy identifies PEM. Opsoclonus and myoclonus characterize POM.

▶ Treatment & Prognosis

PCD usually does not respond to therapy, reflecting the pathologic findings of severe and irreversible Purkinje cell loss. Although rare, case reports have described improvement with treatment of the underlying tumor, immunomodulation, corticosteroids, and immunosuppression with chemotherapy (cyclophosphamide, paclitaxel). However, PCD does not usually lead to death.

Brieva-Ruiz L, et al. Anti-Ri-associated paraneoplastic cerebellar degeneration and breast cancer: An autopsy case study. *Clin Neurol Neurosurg* 2008;110:1044–1046. [PMID: 18701208]

Nagayama S, et al. Case of anti P/Q type VGCC antibody positive small lung cell carcinoma that occurred with subacute cerebellar degeneration, Lambert-Eaton myasthenic syndrome, and brainstem encephalitis. *Brain Nerve* 2008;60:1470–1474. [PMID: 19110759]

Peterson K, et al. Paraneoplastic cerebellar degeneration. I. A clinical analysis of 55 anti-Yo antibody-positive patients. *Neurology* 1992;42:1931–1937. [PMID: 1407575]

Phuphanich S, Brock C. Neurologic improvement after high-dose intravenous immunoglobulin therapy in patients with paraneoplastic cerebellar degeneration associated with anti-Purkinje cell antibody. *J Neurooncol* 2007;81:67–69. [PMID: 16773214]

PARANEOPLASTIC ENCEPHALOMYELITIS

▶ General Considerations

The term *paraneoplastic encephalomyelitis* (PEM) refers to a complex of syndromes involving damage to more than one area of the nervous system (Table 13–1) that is often associated with the anti-Hu antibody (also known as *antineuronal nuclear autoantibody type 1* [ANNA-1]). Included is one or more of the following conditions: focal cortical encephalitis, limbic encephalitis, brainstem encephalitis, cerebellar dysfunction, myelitis, autonomic dysfunction and frequent peripheral nerve involvement.

▶ Clinical Findings

A. Symptoms and Signs

Typically, over days or weeks, patients develop confusion, lethargy, and seizures, with or without spinal cord involvement. Usually there is no significant past medical history, because symptoms precede the diagnosis of cancer. The subacute onset of severe memory deficits (mainly short-term memory) and change in mood or personality with or without temporal lobe seizures are characteristic of paraneoplastic limbic encephalitis. Hypothalamic dysfunction usually occurs in association with limbic or brainstem encephalitis. A diffuse cerebellar syndrome, including nystagmus, gait ataxia, and dysarthria, may be part of the pleomorphic and complex picture of PEM. Anti–NMDA receptor encephalitis presents typically in young women with psychiatric symptoms and memory problems that are followed by seizures, unresponsiveness, autonomic instability, hypoventilation, and dyskinesias. Psychiatric symptoms are often prominent and can lead to misdiagnosis of a primary psychiatric disorder.

Paraneoplastic brainstem encephalitis may develop as a component of PEM; lethargy and cranial nerve involvement are common features. Autonomic dysfunction may occur and cause orthostatic hypotension, hypertension, gastroparesis, abnormal sweating, and neurogenic bladder or impotence (which may also result from spinal cord involvement). Most importantly, a frequent cause of sudden death in this group of patients is acute cardiorespiratory or autonomic failure, often related to brainstem involvement. Occasionally, there is an associated peripheral nervous system syndrome. Rare cases of chorea have also been reported.

Usually, a localized SCLC lesion is found at the time of diagnosis. However, other types of cancer (thymoma, Hodgkin disease, non-Hodgkin lymphoma, germ cell tumors of the testis, ovarian teratoma, and others) are also associated with PEM.

B. Imaging Studies

In most patients with paraneoplastic limbic encephalitis, lesions are seen in the mesial temporal lobes, sometimes bilaterally, or on T2-weighted or fluid-attenuated inversion recovery (FLAIR) MRI studies, with or without enhancement on T1-weighted images. The lesions are not usually associated with mass effect, but mild edema may occur (Figure 13–2). It may be difficult to distinguish this lesion from a low-grade, infiltrative tumor. In some cases, brain biopsy may be necessary to make the correct diagnosis. Similar findings may be observed in other involved areas (cortical or brainstem), whereas cerebellar degeneration usually shows only atrophy.

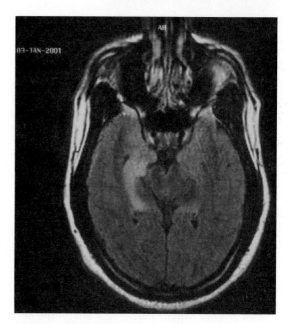

▲ **Figure 13–2.** FLAIR image of a 38-year-old man who presented with agitation and confusion. A diagnosis of limbic encephalitis was made. He was found to have malignant thymoma. Anti–glutamic acid decarboxylase (anti-GAD) antibodies and stiff person syndrome were also present. (From Ances BM, et al. Treatment-responsive limbic encephalitis identified by neuropil antibodies: MRI and PET correlates. *Brain* 2005;128:1764–1777; reproduced with permission of Oxford University Press.)

C. Special Tests

Most cases of PEM (and SCLC) are associated with anti-Hu (ANNA-1) antibodies. Other antibodies found in patients with PEM include anti-CRMP5(CV2), anti-VGCC, and anti-Ma antibodies, the last mainly associated with limbic-diencephalic-brainstem encephalitis. Younger male patients with this syndrome often harbor anti-Ma2 antibodies and have an underlying testicular tumor. Anti–NMDA receptor antibodies are seen in patients with limbic encephalitis with ovarian teratomas. Anti-amphiphysin antibodies may be seen in association with breast cancer and SCLC; these patients may also present with stiff person syndrome. Limbic encephalitis may present in a non-paraneoplastic form in association with anti-VGKC antibodies. Anti-GluR1/2 AMPAR antibodies are implicated in limbic encephalitis, which is reversible with treatment with intravenous immunoglobulins (IVIG).

In patients presenting with any of the symptoms and signs included in the PEM complex, an extensive search for an occult malignancy is often required. If the tumor is atypical for the antineuronal antibody encountered, analysis of the tumor for expression of the paraneoplastic antigen often clarifies whether it has triggered the immune response or whether another occult tumor should be suspected.

▶ Differential Diagnosis

The most common differential diagnoses include viral encephalitis, particularly herpes simplex encephalitis, low-grade glioma, multiple sclerosis, dementia, and other paraneoplastic syndromes. As above, cerebellar dysfunction may occur with other PNSs, such as POM and PCD. However, the presence of other associated clinical findings and specific antineuronal antibodies often helps the clinician to distinguish among these syndromes.

▶ Treatment & Prognosis

Treatment of the underlying malignancy is critical. This has been particularly effective in the management of certain syndromes, such as paraneoplastic limbic encephalitis. Other immunomodulating therapies, such as corticosteroids, IVIG, and plasmapheresis, as well as immunosuppression with cytotoxic agents, may be attempted. The efficacy of immunotherapies depends on early intervention and control of the underlying cancer. In general, encephalopathy, peripheral neuropathy, and cerebellar degeneration are less likely than limbic encephalitis to respond to treatment, and the prognosis is uncertain.

Dalmau J, et al. Anti-NMDA-receptor encephalitis: Case series and analysis of the effects of antibodies. *Lancet Neurol* 2008; 7:1091–1098. [PMID: 18851928]

Graus F, et al. Anti-Hu-associated paraneoplastic encephalomyelitis: Analysis of 200 patients. *Brain* 2001;124:1138–1148. [PMID: 11353730]

Graus F, Saiz A, Dalmau J. Antibodies and neuronal autoimmune disorders of the CNS. *J Neurol* 2010;257:509–517. [PMID: 20035430]

Gultekin SH, et al. Paraneoplastic limbic encephalitis: Neurological symptoms, immunological findings, and tumor association in 50 patients. *Brain* 2000;123:1481–1494. [PMID: 10869059]

Lai M, et al. AMPA receptor antibodies in limbic encephalitis alter synaptic receptor location. *Ann Neurol* 2009;65:424–434. [PMID: 19338055]

Lou E, et al. Paraneoplastic opsoclonus-myoclonus syndrome secondary to immature ovarian teratoma. *Gynecol Oncol* 2010; 117:382–384. [PMID: 20144470]

Nayak L, Rubin M. Amphiphysin autoimmunity in paraneoplastic neurologic disease. *Clin Adv Hematol Oncol* 2009;7:183–184. [PMID: 19398942]

Ohshita T, et al. Voltage-gated potassium channel antibodies associated limbic encephalitis in a patient with invasive thymoma. *J Neurol Sci* 2006;250:167–169. [PMID: 17028029]

Pittock SJ, et al. Amphiphysin autoimmunity: Paraneoplastic accompaniments. *Ann Neurol* 2005;58: 96–107. [PMID: 15984030].

Vincent A, et al. Potassium channel antibody-associated encephalopathy: A potentially immunotherapy- responsive form of limbic encephalitis. *Brain* 2004;127:701–712. [PMID: 14960497]

PARANEOPLASTIC OPSOCLONUS-MYOCLONUS

▶ General Considerations

Paraneoplastic opsoclonus-myoclonus (POM) is a potentially reversible disorder of the brainstem and cerebellum with an unclear pathophysiology. A more diffuse encephalopathy can also occur, varying in severity from mild confusion with depression and anxiety (in adults), to severe cases of stupor, coma, and death. Similar to PEM, POM can cause sudden death; possible mechanisms include acute brainstem or autonomic dysfunction. In adults, POM is associated with breast and ovarian cancers as well as SCLC. In children, it is most commonly associated with neuroblastoma.

▶ Clinical Findings

A. Symptoms and Signs

Patients with POM demonstrate spontaneous, arrhythmic conjugate saccades in all directions of gaze associated with shock-like muscle contractions. These contractions affect mainly the extremities, but in severe cases, the head and trunk may be involved. Gait ataxia is a frequent finding that may result from cerebellar dysfunction in addition to visual disturbance and myoclonus. Subacute in onset like most paraneoplastic syndromes, POM is often associated with fluctuations in severity, and spontaneous remissions have been reported.

Symptoms in adults include oscillopsia and mild to moderate "startle" myoclonus. The latter may be subtle and may initially be misinterpreted (by patients and physicians) as anxiety. In infants and young children, hypotonia, ataxia, and irritability precede opsoclonus and myoclonus and are the usual presenting signs.

B. Imaging Studies

Brain MRI scans in patients with POM may be completely normal. However, T2-weighted or FLAIR abnormalities without contrast enhancement may be visible in the brainstem and usually do not demonstrate mass effect or edema. Occasionally, complete radiologic resolution is observed with treatment (Figure 13–3A and 13–3B).

C. Special Tests

The large majority of children with neuroblastoma-related POM do not harbor a specific antineuronal antibody that could be used as a marker for the disease. The anti-Ri (ANNA-2) antibody has been found in serum and CSF of a few adult patients with POM; the most frequent associated cancers are breast, ovarian, and lung carcinomas. In rare instances, other antibodies (anti-Hu, anti-Yo, anti-Ma2) have been found in patients with POM and brainstem encephalitis.

▶ Differential Diagnosis

The most common differential diagnoses include multiple sclerosis, viral encephalitis, brainstem glioma, and toxic-metabolic

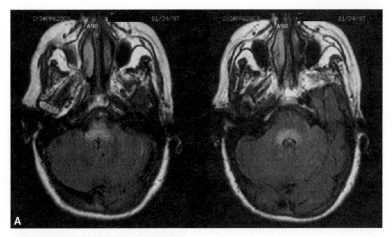

▲ **Figure 13–3A.** FLAIR images of a 62-year-old woman who presented with opsoclonus-myoclonus syndrome and was found to have a localized intraductal breast carcinoma. The lesion did not enhance after administration of gadolinium. Serum and cerebrospinal fluid tested positive for the presence of anti-Ri antibodies.

disturbances. Clinical findings (patient age, symptoms, and signs) and specific antibodies (when present) help make the correct diagnosis.

▶ Treatment & Prognosis

POM is one of the most treatment-responsive PNSs, especially when treated early. Occasionally, complete resolution of the syndrome is achieved with corticosteroids. Good results are also seen with IVIG, plasmapheresis, rituximab, and treatment of the underlying cancer. These clinical observations, along with the usual lack of neuronal loss on

postmortem examination, are the basis for the belief that POM (similar to paraneoplastic limbic encephalitis) may be a "reversible" syndrome and results from a transient inflammatory reaction rather than permanent neuronal death, as in PCD. Some patients, however, develop progressive neurologic deterioration and death, particularly if the underlying tumor is not treated.

POM in children may also respond to corticosteroids, adrenocorticotropic hormone, IVIG, rituximab, or chemotherapy. The ocular movement abnormalities and myoclonus often improve, but two-thirds of patients are left with psychomotor retardation and behavioral and sleep disorders.

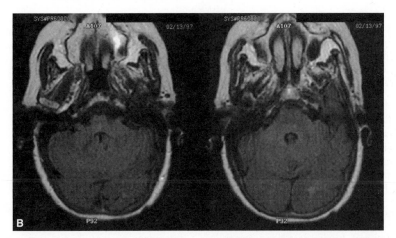

▲ **Figure 13–3B.** Cranial MRI scan of the same patient in Figure 13–3A shows complete resolution of the abnormalities seen on FLAIR imaging after 1 week of high-dose intravenous methylprednisolone administration.

Kirsten A, et al. New autoantibodies in pediatric opsoclonus myoclonus syndrome. *Ann N Y Acad Sci* 2007; 1110:256–260. [PMID: 17911440]

Ko M, Dalmau J, Galetta S. Neuro-ophthalmologic manifestations of paraneoplastic syndromes. *J Neuroophthalmol* 2008;28:58–68. [PMID: 18347462]

Luque FA, et al: Anti-Ri: An antibody associated with paraneoplastic opsoclonus and breast cancer. *Ann Neurol* 1991;29: 241–251. [PMID: 2042940]

PARANEOPLASTIC MYELOPATHIES

▶ General Considerations

Paraneoplastic myelopathy may occur by itself or as a part of PEM. Inflammatory myelitis usually occurs with PEM in association with the anti-Hu antibody and SCLC. Necrotizing myelopathy occurs with hematologic malignancies (leukemia, lymphoma, myeloma) and lung cancer. Devic disease or neuromyelitis optica (NMO) involves spinal cord and optic nerves and is seen with thymoma, lymphoma, lung, uterine, and breast cancers.

▶ Clinical Findings

A. Symptoms and Signs

Patients present with back pain followed by weakness of legs, paresthesias, sensory level, and loss of bladder and bowel function. Autonomic dysfunction and postural hypotension may occur. If present in association with PEM (as is usually the case in paraneoplastic inflammatory myelopathy), other neurologic symptoms develop. In necrotizing myelopathy, the course may be rapid and lead to respiratory failure and death. NMO is associated with optic neuritis and resembles multiple sclerosis.

B. Imaging Studies

Imaging studies may show spinal cord edema on T2 sequences and enhancement with gadolinium on T1 images. Evaluation of the CSF reveals an inflammatory reaction.

C. Specific Tests

Antibodies associated with paraneoplastic inflammatory myelopathy are anti-Hu, anti-amphiphysin, anti-GAD, anti-CRMP5(CV2), and anti-Ri (ANNA2) antibodies. Anti-CRMP5(CV2) antibodies have been found in a patient with Devic disease and thymoma. Autoantibodies to aquaporin-4 water channel may reflect a paraneoplastic process in a patient presenting with NMO.

▶ Differential Diagnosis

Transverse myelitis secondary to viral infections, especially herpes simplex type 2, and multiple sclerosis should be excluded.

▶ Treatment & Prognosis

The patient may benefit from immunosuppression or treatment of the underlying cancer. Patients with necrotizing myelopathy do poorly.

Dalmau J, et al. Anti-Hu-associated paraneoplastic encephalomyelitis/sensory neuronopathy. A clinical study of 71 patients. *Medicine* 1992;71:59–72. [PMID: 1312211]

Ducray F, et al. Devic's syndrome-like phenotype associated with thymoma and anti-CV2/CRMP5 antibodies. *J Neurol Neurosurg Psychiatry* 2007;78:325–327. [PMID: 17308295]

Pittock SJ, Lennon VA. Aquaporin-4 autoantibodies in a paraneoplastic context. *Arch Neurol* 2008;65:629–632. [PMID: 18474738]

PARANEOPLASTIC MOTOR NEURON DISEASE

▶ General Considerations

These syndromes include degeneration of upper and/or lower motor neurons. Amyotrophic lateral sclerosis (ALS) is the most common form. Other forms include primary lateral sclerosis, progressive spinal muscular atrophy (PMA), bulbar palsy, and pseudobulbar palsy. Whether paraneoplastic motor neuron disease (MND) occurs in patients with cancer by coincidence or as a paraneoplastic syndrome is debated, but the incidence of MND in patients with cancer does not appear to exceed the sporadic rate. The only hint of a relationship to underlying malignancy is improvement in neurologic symptoms with treatment of the tumor, as documented in isolated case reports. Cancers seen in association with MND are breast and ovarian cancers, lymphoma, plasma cell dyscrasias, and SCLC.

▶ Clinical Findings

A. Symptoms and Signs

The upper motor neuron syndrome is characterized by weakness, hyperreflexia, and spasticity. The lower motor neuron syndrome is characterized by weakness, atrophy, and fasciculations. Impairment of executive function and cognitive changes may be seen. The findings are no different from those of sporadic MND, but onset can be rapid.

B. Imaging Studies

Imaging studies are typically unremarkable, as in sporadic MND. Diffusion tensor imaging (DTI) may show damage to corticospinal tracts.

C. Specific Tests

The presence of paraneoplastic antibodies and neurologic recovery upon treatment of the cancer suggest that the MND is paraneoplastic. Antibodies seen in association with paraneoplastic MND are anti-Yo, anti-Hu, anti-Ma2, anti-CRMP5(CV2), anti-spectrin, anti-MAG, and anti-ganglioside

(GM1) antibodies. Electrodiagnostic studies demonstrate states of denervation and reinnervation.

Differential Diagnosis

The differential diagnosis is MND in the non-paraneoplastic context, which is more common, and mimickers such as structural disease in the cervical spine.

Treatment

Treatment of the underlying cancer is supportive management.

STIFF PERSON SYNDROME

General Considerations

Previously termed stiff man syndrome until it was well recognized that women are also affected, the stiff person syndrome (SPS) is a rare and unusual condition that may be paraneoplastic or non-paraneoplastic. SPS is associated with different types of cancer, including SCLC, breast carcinoma, Hodgkin disease, colon cancer, and thymomas.

Clinical Findings

A. Symptoms and Signs

Patients with SPS usually present with a subacute onset of painful muscle spasm involving mainly the paraspinal musculature and the lower extremities. The spasms, initially fluctuating and fairly localized, tend to increase in frequency and severity and occasionally lead to abnormal postures, incapacity, and bone fractures. Trigger factors for the spasms include tactile, auditory, or emotional stimuli. Clinical manifestations range from diffuse involvement of the trunk and four limbs to localized spasms in one limb (stiff limb syndrome). Typically, the spasms disappear with sleep and anesthesia.

B. Imaging Studies

MRI scans of the brain and spinal cord may show hyperintense signal on T2-FLAIR sequence and gadolinium enhancement or can be normal.

C. Special Tests

Antibodies against amphiphysin are associated with breast cancer and SPS. Anti–glutamic acid decarboxylase (anti-GAD) antibodies, which are also anti–pancreatic island cells, are found in patients with non-paraneoplastic SPS. The majority of these patients also have other autoimmune diseases such as type 1 diabetes mellitus. GAD and amphiphysin are enriched in the presynaptic terminals of spinal cord interneurons that secrete the inhibitory neurotransmitters γ-aminobutyric acid and glycine. Some patients with the paraneoplastic SPS have both anti-amphiphysin and anti-GAD antibodies. Other antibodies associated with SPS are anti-Ri and anti-gephyrin antibodies.

Characteristic electrophysiologic features include continuous activity of motor units in the stiffened muscles which typically improves with diazepam.

Differential Diagnosis

The main differential diagnosis is between paraneoplastic and non-paraneoplastic SPS. Although the latter condition is far more common, the former necessitates a search for an underlying cancer.

Treatment & Prognosis

Recent reports suggest that non-paraneoplastic SPS responds to immunotherapy, namely IVIG. Although this is not typically the case for paraneoplastic SPS, prompt therapy with corticosteroids and IVIG may help stabilize the neurologic syndrome. Benzodiazepines and muscle relaxants, such as baclofen, are useful for symptomatic management. As with most paraneoplastic syndromes, SPS may precede the diagnosis of an underlying malignancy, and prompt diagnosis and treatment may influence its clinical course.

Butler MH, et al. Autoimmunity to gephyrin in stiff man syndrome. *Neuron* 2000;26:307–312. [PMID: 10839351]

Dalakas MC, et al. High-dose intravenous immune globulin for stiff person syndrome. *N Engl J Med* 2001;345: 1870–1876. [PMID: 11756577]

Lockman J, Burns T. Stiff person syndrome. *Curr Treat Options Neurol* 2007;9:234–240. [PMID: 17445501]

Murinson BB, Guarnaccia JB. Stiff person syndrome with amphiphysin antibodies: Distinctive features of a rare disease. *Neurology* 2008;71:1955–1958. [PMID: 18971449]

Saiz A, et al. Spectrum of neurological syndromes associated with glutamic acid decarboxylase antibodies: Diagnostic clues for this association. *Brain* 2008;131:2553–2563. [PMID: 18687732]

PARANEOPLASTIC VISUAL SYNDROMES

General Considerations

Paraneoplastic visual syndromes, which are rare, may manifest as retinopathies or optic neuropathies. Two syndromes are well known: carcinoma-associated retinopathy (CAR) and melanoma-associated retinopathy (MAR). Less frequently, paraneoplastic retinitis or optic neuritis occurs. More common causes for visual disturbances in cancer patients should be excluded initially, including metastases to the optic nerves or leptomeninges and toxicity from chemotherapy or radiation therapy.

The tumor associated with MAR is melanoma. The most frequently involved malignancy in CAR is early-stage SCLC and occasionally gynecologic tumors.

Clinical Findings

A. Symptoms and Signs

Patients with CAR develop photosensitivity, progressive painless loss of vision and color perception, central or ring scotomas, and night blindness. Diagnosis of CAR should be considered in any patient who presents with these symptoms in the absence of a family history of retinitis pigmentosa. CAR affects rods and cones. Cones are rarely affected in isolation.

Patients with MAR present with the acute onset of night blindness and shimmering, flickering, or pulsating photopsias. Marked visual loss and central scotomata are uncommon. Patients with MAR have a known diagnosis of melanoma.

Paraneoplastic optic neuropathy is rare and manifests as subacute painless, bilateral visual loss. It usually occurs in combination with other neurologic symptoms, including cognitive changes, ataxia, and myelopathy. Afferent pupillary defects may occur with optic nerve involvement. Funduscopic examination may appear normal or show arteriolar narrowing; optic disc pallor may be present.

B. Imaging Studies

Imaging studies and evaluation of the CSF are not revealing.

C. Specific Tests

Serum antibodies that specifically react with retinal proteins include anti-recoverin, which is found in some patients with CAR. Anti-enolase antibodies are found in paraneoplastic and non-paraneoplastic retinopathies. Patients with MAR may have anti–bipolar cell antibodies. Some patients with paraneoplastic uveitis and optic neuritis have anti-CRMP5 (CV2) antibodies. Other antibodies associated with paraneoplastic optic neuropathy are anti-Hu, anti-amphiphysin, anti-GAD, and anti-VGCC antibodies.

In patients with CAR, the electroretinogram (ERG) shows attenuation of photopic and scotopic responses. The ERG of patients with MAR typically demonstrates reduction in B-wave amplitude with preservation of A-waves.

▶ Differential Diagnosis

As previously noted, the main differential diagnoses include other, more common causes of visual disturbances in cancer patients.

▶ Treatment & Prognosis

Paraneoplastic retinopathies usually do not respond to treatment. However, a few reports mention improvement with corticosteroids, immunomodulation (ie, IVIG, plasmapheresis, alemtuzumab), and treatment of the underlying cancer.

Adamus G, Ren G, Weleber RG. Autoantibodies against retinal proteins in paraneoplastic and autoimmune retinopathy. *BMC Ophthalmol* 2004;4:5. [PMID: 15180904]

Bazhin AV, et al. Recoverin as a cancer-retina antigen. *Cancer Immunol Immunother* 2007;56: 110–116. [PMID: 16444517]

Cross SA, et al. Paraneoplastic autoimmune optic neuritis with retinitis defined by CRMP-5-IgG. *Ann Neurol* 2003;54:38–50. [PMID: 12838519]

Keltner JL, Thirkill CE, Yip PT. Clinical and immunologic characteristics of melanoma-associated retinopathy syndrome: Eleven new cases and a review of 51 previously published cases. *J Neuroophthalmol* 2001;21:173–187. [PMID: 11725182]

Ko MW, Dalmau J, Galetta SL. Neuro-ophthalmologic manifestations of paraneoplastic syndromes. *J Neuroophthalmol* 2008;28: 58–68. [PMID: 18347462]

Myers DA, et al. Unusual aspects of melanoma. Case 3. Melanoma-associated retinopathy presenting with night blindness. *J Clin Oncol* 2004;22:746–748. [PMID: 14966102]

PERIPHERAL NERVE HYPEREXCITABILITY

▶ General Considerations

Peripheral nerve hyperexcitability encompasses a group of disorders known by different names, including *neuromyotonia, undulating myokymia, Isaacs syndrome,* and the *cramp-fasciculation syndrome.* Paraneoplastic peripheral nerve hyperexcitability has been associated with thymoma, SCLC, lymphoid malignancies, and other cancers.

▶ Clinical Findings

A. Symptoms and Signs

Patients usually present with muscle cramps, stiffness, weakness, and excessive sweating. The motor manifestations represent spontaneous and continuous muscle fiber activity of peripheral nerve origin and can be triggered by voluntary muscle contraction. On physical examination, the involved muscles may demonstrate undulating myokymia and hypertrophic changes. In some patients, central nervous system involvement in the form of memory loss, hallucinations, insomnia, mood and behavioral changes, and autonomic dysfunction may occur in addition to neuromyotonia (*Morvan syndrome*).

B. Imaging Studies

Imaging studies are noncontributory. PET scan in Morvan syndrome may show decreased metabolism in left inferior frontal and left temporal lobes.

C. Special Tests

Many patients have autoantibodies to voltage-gated potassium channels (VGKC) which, by increasing the release of acetylcholine, prolong the duration of the action potential, leading to nerve hyperexcitability. Electromyographic studies usually show fibrillations, fasciculations, and myokymic discharges. This abnormal activity continues during sleep and general anesthesia, is abolished by curare, and may be unaffected, reduced, or abolished by peripheral nerve block.

▶ Treatment

Symptomatic improvement is reported with phenytoin, carbamazepine, and immunomodulatory therapies such as plasmapheresis or IVIG, and agents such as azathioprine, cyclophosphamide, and rituximab.

Rueff L, et al. Voltage-gated potassium channel antibody-mediated syndromes: A spectrum of clinical manifestations. *Rev Neurol Dis* 2008;5:65–72. [PMID: 18660738]

PARANEOPLASTIC PERIPHERAL NEUROPATHY

▶ Clinical Findings

A. Symptoms and Signs

Patients with paraneoplastic sensory neuronopathy typically present with subacute and asymmetric onset of paresthesias that gradually progress to diffuse sensory loss. They may also have painful dysesthesias. Sensory gait ataxia can occur in advanced stages or as the only complaint. Rarely, patients develop sensorineural hearing loss. Paraneoplastic sensory neuronopathy should be suspected in patients with a subacute and asymmetric onset of sensory symptoms, even without a history of cancer, especially if thoracic and abdominal segments are involved.

Sensorimotor peripheral neuropathies may occur as primarily demyelinating or axonal degeneration. The demyelinating type, with clinical features that suggest chronic inflammatory demyelinating polyneuropathy, has a fluctuating course and better prognosis than the axonal type.

Commonly, paraneoplastic neuropathies develop as part of the PEM complex, but they can occur in isolation. Most paraneoplastic peripheral neuropathies precede the diagnosis of cancer, typically SCLC.

Brachial neuropathy, as well as an acute paraneoplastic polyradiculoneuropathy identical to the Guillain-Barré syndrome, may be associated with Hodgkin disease.

Pathologic findings in paraneoplastic sensory neuronopathy include degeneration of dorsal root ganglia, posterior nerve roots, and dorsal columns. In sensorimotor polyneuropathy, there may be demyelination or axonal degeneration with inflammatory lymphocytic infiltrates. Such changes are identified by peripheral nerve biopsy.

B. Imaging Studies

There are no relevant imaging findings other than those seen in PEM when neuropathies are part of that syndrome.

C. Specific Tests

The anti-Hu antibody is frequently detected in the serum and CSF of patients with SCLC who have paraneoplastic neuropathies associated with involvement of dorsal root ganglia. Anti-CRMP5(CV2) antibodies may be present in some patients with a predominantly axonal paraneoplastic sensorimotor neuropathy.

Electrophysiologic studies may help distinguish demyelinating from axonal neuropathies, providing information about management and prognosis.

▶ Differential Diagnosis

The main differential diagnoses include chemotherapy-induced neuropathy, metastases to plexus or peripheral nerves (usually as a component of leptomeningeal involvement), postradiation plexopathy (if applicable), Guillain-Barré syndrome, and chronic inflammatory demyelinating polyneuropathy.

▶ Treatment & Prognosis

In general, paraneoplastic neuropathies do not respond well to treatment. However, early therapy with high doses of corticosteroids, which are then tapered, may produce partial improvement in sensory deficits. As with chronic inflammatory demyelinating polyneuropathy, demyelinating paraneoplastic neuropathies may respond to immunomodulation with IVIG and plasmapheresis. Success in treatment of the underlying tumor is often a good predictor of prognosis, especially for neuropathies associated with SCLC and anti-Hu antibodies.

Antoine JC, Camdessanche JP. Peripheral nervous system involvement in patients with cancer. *Lancet Neurol* 2007;6:75–86. [PMID: 17166804]

Antoine JC, et al. Paraneoplastic anti-CV2 antibodies react with peripheral nerve and are associated with a mixed axonal and demyelinating peripheral neuropathy. *Ann Neurol* 2001;49: 214–221. [PMID: 11220741]

PARANEOPLASTIC SYNDROMES OF THE NEUROMUSCULAR JUNCTION

▶ General Considerations

Lambert-Eaton myasthenic syndrome (LEMS) and myasthenia gravis (MG) are discussed in detail in Chapter 22. The discussion that follows focuses on the clinical and diagnostic differences between these two neuromuscular disorders and highlights their association with specific cancers (Tables 13–1 and 13–2).

▶ Clinical Findings

A. Symptoms and Signs

Most patients with LEMS present with complaints of weakness or fatigue. Autonomic dysfunction is commonly present by the time of diagnosis. Dysphagia, dysphonia, ptosis, and diplopia are more frequent in MG than in LEMS.

Mild to moderate proximal weakness (legs worse than arms) and absent or depressed tendon reflexes are characteristics of LEMS. Proximal muscle weakness in MG usually affects all limbs and neck muscles, whereas deep tendon reflexes are normal. Strength improves after a few muscle contractions in patients with LEMS (facilitation), whereas it worsens in patients with MG. In 60% of patients with LEMS, the condition is paraneoplastic, usually associated with SCLC;

Table 13-2. Comparison of Lambert-Eaton Myasthenic Syndrome and Myasthenia Gravis

	Lambert-Eaton Myasthenic Syndrome	Myasthenia Gravis
Age at onset	Older (50s)	Younger (20s)
Proximal weakness	++	+++
Deep tendon reflexes	Often abolished	Normal
Autonomic symptoms	Present	Absent
Facilitation with exercise	Present (muscles become stronger)	Absent (muscles become weaker)
Anatomic level	Presynaptic	Postsynaptic
Mechanism	Release of acetylcholine is blocked by VGCC antibodies	Nicotinic receptor is blocked by AChR antibodies
Tumor association	SCLC	Thymoma (usually benign)
Specific treatment	3,4-diaminopyridine	Anticholinesterases

AChR = acetylcholine receptor; SCLC = small cell lung cancer; VGCC = voltage-gated calcium channel.

in contrast, 10–15% of patients with MG have an associated thymoma, most commonly benign.

B. Specific Tests

Antibodies against voltage-gated calcium channels (VGCC) are found in the serum of patients with LEMS. SOX1 antibodies are also seen in patients with SCLC and LEMS. Anti–acetylcholine receptor antibodies are found in 85–90% of patients with MG, but do not help to distinguish paraneoplastic from non-neoplastic MG. Patients who are seronegative for anti-acetylcholine antibodies may harbor muscle-specific kinase (MuSK) antibodies, but these antibodies are not usually associated with thymoma.

Fast repetitive stimulation (>20 Hz) on nerve conduction studies typically shows incremental change in amplitude (facilitation) of the compound muscle action potential in patients with LEMS. The opposite effect (amplitude decline of compound muscle action potential) is seen in patients with MG.

▶ Differential Diagnosis

The main differential diagnosis for paraneoplastic syndromes of the neuromuscular junction is between MG and LEMS (Table 13–2).

▶ Treatment & Prognosis

Symptoms of LEMS may improve with treatment of the underlying tumor. In some patients, 3,4-diaminopyridine may be beneficial. Immunomodulation with plasmapheresis and IVIG has shown only temporary benefits. Long-term immunosuppression with corticosteroids or azathioprine may be necessary.

For patients with MG associated with thymoma, resection of the tumor is an important intervention, along with anticholinesterase drugs and immunosuppression. Immunomodulation with IVIG and plasmapheresis can be helpful.

Sabater L, et al. SOX1 antibodies are markers of paraneoplastic Lambert-Eaton myasthenic syndrome. *Neurology* 2008;70:924–928. [PMID: 18032743]

Titulaer MJ, Verschuuren JJ. Lambert-Eaton myasthenic syndrome: Tumor versus nontumor forms. *Ann N Y Acad Sci* 2008;1132:129–134. [PMID: 18567862]

DERMATOMYOSITIS & POLYMYOSITIS

These two syndromes are discussed in more detail in Chapter 23. Both are autoimmune inflammatory diseases of muscle. The association between cancer and dermatomyositis, but not polymyositis, in adults is well documented.

Typically, patients present with a subacute onset of proximal muscle and neck flexor weakness. Other muscle groups may become involved, including pharyngeal and respiratory muscles. Tendon reflexes and sensation are normal. Serum creatine kinase concentrations are often elevated. The most common associated cancers are breast, lung, ovarian, and gastric malignancies.

Treatment is similar to that for patients without cancer, including corticosteroids, IVIG, and immunosuppressants such as mycophenolate and cyclosporine for refractory dermatomyositis.

ACKNOWLEDGMENTS

The authors thank Judith Lampron for her excellent assistance in the preparation of this chapter.

Trauma

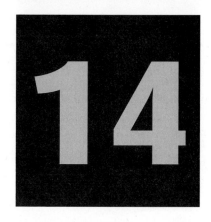

Katja E. Wartenberg, MD, PhD,
& Stephan A. Mayer, MD

HEAD TRAUMA

ESSENTIALS OF DIAGNOSIS

▶ History or clinical evidence of trauma

▶ Headache, altered mental status, seizure, focal neurologic deficit

▶ Signs of transtentorial herniation with progressive mass effect

▶ Computed tomography (CT) or magnetic resonance imaging (MRI) showing skull fractures; epidural, subdural, subarachnoid, or intraparenchymal hemorrhage; or cerebral edema

▶ General Considerations

Traumatic brain injury is a major cause of death and disability. The incidence is rising due to increasing motor vehicle accidents in low- and middle-income countries and falls of members of the aging population in high-income countries. Violence is reported to cause closed-head injury in about 7–10% of cases. Penetrating injuries are more common with the more frequent use of firearms, and a greater amount of blast injuries became the result of improved explosive devices used in terrorist and other attacks. More than 1.4 million patients with head injuries are treated annually in US emergency departments, and 21% of these patients are hospitalized. Almost 10% of all deaths in the United States are caused by injury, and about half of traumatic deaths involve the brain. In the United States, a head injury occurs every 7 seconds and a death due to traumatic brain injury every 5 minutes. The annual financial burden accounts to US $60 billion.

Brain injuries occur at all ages, but the peak is in young adults between the ages of 15 and 25 years. Head injury is the leading cause of death among people younger than 25 years. Men are affected three to four times as often as women.

Traumatic brain injury can be classified according to the mechanism of injury, clinical severity, structural damage on imaging, and prognosis (Table 14–1).

▶ Pathogenesis & Clinical Findings

A. Cerebral Concussion and Axonal Shearing Injury

Acceleration-deceleration movements of the head, especially with an angular-rotary component, cause stretching and shearing of axons that manifest clinically in loss of consciousness at the moment of impact. When the alteration of consciousness is brief (<6 hours), the term *concussion* is used. Patients may be completely unconscious or remain awake but dazed. Most recover within seconds to minutes (rather than hours) and have retrograde and anterograde amnesia surrounding the event.

The mechanism by which concussion leads to altered consciousness is believed to be transient functional disruption of the reticular activating system caused by rotational forces on the upper brainstem. Experimentally, violent head rotation can produce concussion without impact to the head. The computed tomography (CT) or magnetic resonance imaging (MRI) findings of the majority of patients are normal, because concussion is a result of physiologic, rather than structural, injury to the brain. Only 5% of patients who have sustained a concussion and are otherwise intact have intracranial hemorrhage on CT.

The term *diffuse axonal injury* defines traumatic coma lasting more than 6 hours caused by multiple small lesions in the white matter tracts. It is presumed that widespread microscopic and macroscopic axonal shearing injury has occurred in patients in whom CT or MRI cannot identify any other cause of coma. A comatose state lasting 6–24 hours is deemed mild diffuse axonal injury; coma lasting more than 24 hours is referred to as moderate or severe diffuse axonal injury, depending on the absence or presence of brainstem signs such as extensor posturing. Brainstem and hypothalamic

Table 14–1. Classification of Traumatic Brain Injury

Mechanism of injury
Closed, penetrating, crash, blast

Clinical severity: level of consciousness
(Glasgow Coma Scale, see Table 14–2)

Clinical severity: Injury Severity Score
Abbreviated injury score is obtained for six body regions:
- External (skin)
- Head/neck including the brain
- Thorax
- Abdomen and pelvis
- Spine
- Extremities

Scores:
0=none
1=minor
2=moderate
3=serious
4=severe
5=critical
6=virtually unsurvivable
The score (range 0–75) is the sum of the quadratic scores for each of the six body regions.

Radiographic damage on CT or MRI
Diffuse injury I: no visible pathology
Diffuse injury II: cisterns present, midline shift 0–5 mm and/or lesion densities present and no mass lesion >25 mL
Diffuse injury III: swelling, cisterns compressed or absent with midline shift 0.5 mm and no mass lesion >25 mL
Diffuse injury VI: shift, midline shift >5 mm, no mass lesion >25 mL
Evacuated mass lesion: any lesion surgically evacuated
Nonevacuated mass lesion: high or mixed-density lesion >25 mL, not surgically evacuated

Prognosis according to the CRASH or IMACT studies
Classification of the patient by expected outcome. Two examples can be found on the following websites:
http://www.crash2.lshtm.ac.uk
http://www.tbi-impact.org

Data from Marshall LF, Marshall SB, Klauber MR et al. A new classification of head injury based on computed tomography. *J Neurosurgery* 1991;75 (suppl):S14–20 and Baker SP, O'Neill BB, Haddon W Jr. et al. The Injury Severity Score: A method for describing patients with multiple injuries and evaluating emergency care. *J Trauma* 1974;14:187–196.

injury, reflected by autonomic dysfunction (eg, bradycardia or tachycardia, hypertension, hyperhidrosis, fever, or poikilothermia), is common in acute, severe diffuse axonal injury. Patients may remain unconscious for days, months, or years, and those who recover may have severe cognitive and motor impairment, including spasticity and ataxia. Diffuse axonal injury is considered the single most important cause of persistent disability after traumatic brain damage.

Axonal shearing injury tends to be most severe in specific brain regions that are anatomically predisposed to maximal stress from rotational forces. At the time of injury, diffuse microscopic damage occurs, seen as axonal retraction bulbs throughout the white matter of the cerebral hemispheres following microporation of membranes, leakage of ion channels, and stearic conformational changes of proteins. Macroscopic damage includes tissue tears, best visualized by MRI, specifically diffusion tensor imaging. They are most common in midline structures, including the dorsolateral midbrain and pons, posterior corpus callosum, parasagittal white matter, periventricular regions, and, occasionally, the internal capsule. Prolonged loss of consciousness from diffuse axonal injury tends to be associated with bilateral asymmetric focal lesions of the midbrain tegmentum, a region containing major parts of the reticular activating system. Small hemorrhages, known as *gliding contusions,* are sometimes associated with focal shearing lesions (Figure 14–1).

B. Skull Fracture

Skull fractures are important markers of potentially serious injury but are rarely the cause of problems by themselves. The severity of injury to the skull does not have a tremendous impact on prognosis. Skull fractures can be divided into linear, depressed, or comminuted types. If the scalp is lacerated over the fracture, it is considered an open or *compound fracture.*

Linear fractures comprise about 80% of fractures and occur most commonly in the temporoparietal region, where the skull is thinnest. Although detection of a linear fracture often raises the suspicion of serious brain injury, in most patients the CT scan does not show pathologic findings. Nondisplaced linear skull fractures generally do not require surgical intervention and can be managed conservatively.

In *depressed fractures* of the skull, one or more bone fragments are displaced inward, resulting in compression of the underlying brain. *Comminuted fractures* are defined as multiple shattered bone fragments, which may or may not be displaced. Eighty-five percent of depressed fractures are open (or compound) and at risk for infection or leak of cerebrospinal fluid (CSF). Even when closed, most depressed or comminuted fractures necessitate surgical exploration for debridement, elevation of bone fragments, and repair of dural lacerations (tearing of the meninges from sharp edges). In most patients, the adjacent cerebral tissue is injured. In some patients, depressed skull fractures are associated with tearing, compression, or thrombosis of underlying venous dural sinuses.

Basilar skull fractures are linear, depressed, or comminuted. They are frequently missed by plain skull radiographs and therefore best identified by CT with so-called *bone windows.* A cranial nerve injury or dural tear may be adjacent to the fracture site, which can lead to delayed meningitis. Suspicion of a fracture of the petrous portion of the temporal bone is high in the presence of signs such as hemotympanum or tympanic perforation, hearing loss, CSF otorrhea, peripheral facial nerve weakness, or ecchymosis of the scalp overlying the mastoid process (Battle sign). Anosmia, bilateral periorbital ecchymosis (raccoon

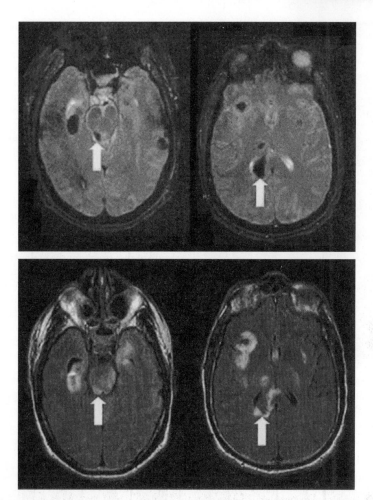

▲ **Figure 14-1.** Focal magnetic resonance findings characteristic of diffuse axonal shearing injury after trauma. **Top:** Gradient echo images demonstrate hemorrhagic lesions (gliding contusions, see *arrows*) of the right dorsolateral midbrain and splenium of the corpus callosum. **Bottom:** Fluid-attenuated inversion recovery (FLAIR) images show edema in the areas of hemorrhage (see *arrows*). (Reproduced with permission from Rowland LP, ed. *Merritt's Textbook of Neurology*, 11th ed. Lippincott Williams & Wilkins, 2005.)

eyes), and CSF rhinorrhea suggest possible fracture of the sphenoid, frontal, or ethmoid bones.

C. Cerebral Edema

Brain swelling after head injury is a poorly understood phenomenon that can result from several different mechanisms. It may be diffuse or focal, adjacent to a parenchymal or extradural hemorrhage. Post-traumatic brain swelling may result from masses (eg, hematoma), increased cerebral blood volume, or cerebral edema. Cerebral edema can be further classified into *cytotoxic* (cellular swelling), *vasogenic* (blood vessel leakage), and *interstitial* (extravasation through ventricular ependyma following ventricular dilation).

Brain swelling can follow any type of head injury. Curiously, the magnitude of edema does not always correlate with the severity of injury. In some cases, particularly in young adults, severe diffuse brain swelling, which may be fatal, occurs minutes to hours after a minor concussion. Abnormal dilation of the cerebral blood vessels is thought to result in increased cerebral blood volume, hyperperfusion, and increased vascular permeability, leading to secondary leakage of plasma and vasogenic cerebral edema. Cerebral blood flow studies indicate that hyperemia occurs to some degree in nearly all patients 1–3 days after severe head injury. This phenomenon might be related to a delayed inflammatory response or to dysfunction of cerebral vasomotor regulatory centers in the brainstem.

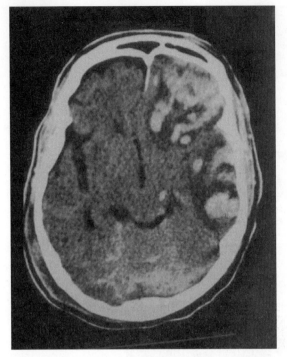

▲ **Figure 14–2.** Traumatic contusions. Axial noncontrast CT scan demonstrates areas of contusion with small focal hemorrhages involving the lower poles of the left frontal and temporal lobes adjacent to the rough cranial vault. (Used with permission from Dr Robert De La Paz.)

D. Cerebral Contusion and Hemorrhage

Cerebral *contusions* are focal parenchymal hemorrhages that result from "scraping" and "bruising" of the brain as it moves across the inner surface of the skull. They are the most common traumatic lesion, especially in the elderly. The most common sites of traumatic contusion are the inferior frontal and temporal lobes, where brain tissue comes in contact with irregular protuberances at the base of the skull (Figure 14–2). Contusions can be found at the site of a skull fracture, but they occur more often without a fracture and with the overlying pia and arachnoid intact. In most patients, contusions are small and multiple. With lateral forces, contusions occur at the site of the blow to the head (*coup lesions*) or at the opposite pole as the brain is shifted against the inner table of the skull (*contrecoup lesions*). Contusions frequently enlarge over 12–24 hours (10–25%), especially in the setting of coagulopathy. In some cases, contusions may appear one or more days after injury. Management is often conservative unless there is significant symptomatic mass effect, because contusions often consist of hemorrhagic or ecchymotic but potentially viable brain tissue. If diffuse axonal injury, brain swelling, or secondary hemorrhage is absent, recovery from one or more small contusions may be excellent. Healed

contusions are often found at autopsy in people with no clinical evidence of permanent brain damage.

Intracerebral *hemorrhage* results from tearing of a small- or medium-sized vessel within the parenchyma due to rotational forces. Hematomas are focal collections of blood clot that displace the brain, in contrast to contusions, which resemble bruised brain tissue. Most parenchymal hematomas are located in the deep white matter, whereas contusions tend to be cortical. Large parenchymal hematomas with mass effect may require surgical evacuation.

E. Subdural Hematoma

Subdural hematomas consist of blood within the potential space between the dural and arachnoid membranes. The most common cause is stretching and tearing of veins that drain from the surface of the brain to the dural sinuses as a result of movements of the brain within the skull. Less often, the source of the hematoma is a small pial artery.

Most subdural hematomas are located over the lateral cerebral convexities, but subdural blood can also collect between the tentorium and occipital lobe, between the temporal lobe and the base of the skull, or within the posterior fossa. CT usually reveals a high-density crescentic collection across the entire hemispheric convexity (Figure 14–3) or

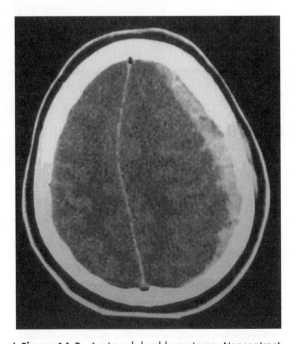

▲ **Figure 14–3.** Acute subdural hematoma. Noncontrast axial CT scan demonstrates a hyperdense, crescent-shaped, extra-axial collection showing mass effect (sulcal and ventricular effacement) and midline shift from left to right. (Used with permission from of Dr Robert De La Paz.)

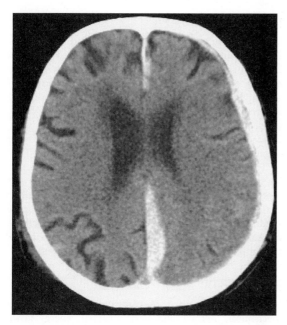

▲ Figure 14–4. Acute subdural hematoma. Noncontrast axial CT scan demonstrates a hyperdense, extra-axial collection along the anterior and posterior falx cerebri.

along the falx (Figure 14–4). Elderly or alcoholic patients with cerebral atrophy are particularly prone to subdural bleeding. Trivial impact or even pure acceleration-deceleration injuries such as whiplash can result in large hematomas in these patients.

Acute subdural hematoma, by definition, is symptomatic within 72 hours of injury, but most patients have neurologic symptoms from the moment of impact. These symptoms can occur after any type of head injury but seem to be more common after falls or assaults than after vehicular trauma. About half of patients with an acute subdural hematoma lose consciousness at the time of injury; one quarter are in a coma when they arrive at the hospital, and half of those who awaken lose consciousness for a second time after a lucid interval of minutes to hours, when the subdural hematoma grows in size. Hemiparesis and pupillary abnormalities are present in half to two thirds of patients, usually as ipsilateral pupillary dilation and contralateral hemiparesis. However, so-called *false localizing signs* (eg, abducens palsy, contralateral dilated pupil, or ipsilateral hemiparesis) are common with acute subdural hematoma, because uncal herniation can lead to compression of the contralateral midbrain or third cranial nerve against the tentorial edge (Kernohan notch phenomenon).

Chronic subdural hematomas become symptomatic 21 days after injury or later. They are more likely to occur in patients older than 50 years of age. There is no historical evidence of head trauma in 25–50% of patients. Nearly

50% of patients have a history of alcoholism or epilepsy, and the trauma may have been forgotten. In other cases the trauma may have been trivial with little or no brain compression because of coexisting cerebral atrophy. Other risk factors for chronic subdural hematoma include overdrainage of ventriculoperitoneal shunts and coagulopathies, including anticoagulant medication. One week after the initial event, fibroblasts on the inner surface of the dura form a thick outer membrane, and 2 weeks later a thin inner membrane develops, resulting in encapsulation of the clot, which begins to liquify. Enlargement of the hematoma may then be a consequence of recurrent bleeding (so-called *acute-on-chronic subdural hematoma*) or osmotic effects related to a high protein content of the fluid following serum exudation into the hematoma cavity. Symptoms may be restricted to altered mental status, which is sometimes mistaken for Alzheimer-type dementia. CT scanning typically shows an isodense or hypodense crescent- or lens-shaped mass that deforms the surface of the brain, and the membranes may enhance with intravenous contrast. Long-standing chronic subdural hematomas eventually liquify and form a *hygroma*, and, in some cases, the membranes may calcify.

F. Epidural Hematoma

Epidural hematomas are found in 5–15% of autopsies performed on patients with head injury. Bleeding into the epidural space is usually caused by a tear in the wall of one meningeal artery, especially the middle meningeal artery, but in 15% of patients the injury involves a dural sinus. Seventy-five percent of epidural hematomas are associated with a skull fracture. The dura is separated from the skull by the extravasated blood, and the size of the clot increases until the ruptured vessel is compressed or occluded by the hematoma.

Epidural blood has a "bulging" convex pattern on CT (Figure 14–5) because the collection is limited by firm attachments of the dura to the cranial sutures. Most epidural hematomas are located over the convexity of the hemisphere in the middle cranial fossa, but occasionally the hemorrhage may be confined to the anterior fossa, possibly as a result of tearing of an anterior meningeal artery. Extradural hemorrhage in the posterior fossa may arise when a venous sinus is torn. The hematoma is usually ipsilateral to the site of impact.

Epidural hematoma is primarily a problem of young adults. It is rarely seen in the elderly because the dura becomes increasingly adherent to the skull with advanced age. The clinical course in one third of patients proceeds from an immediate loss of consciousness due to concussion, to a lucid interval, and then to a relapse into coma as the hematoma expands. Contralateral hemiparesis develops, and the ipsilateral pupil may become dilated and eventually unreactive, signifying compression of the oculomotor nerve and impending transtentorial herniation. As with acute subdural

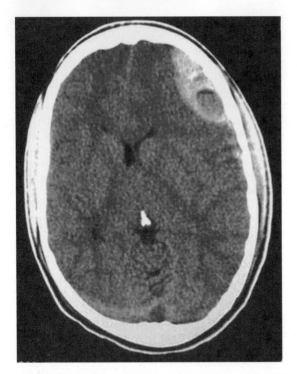

▲ **Figure 14–5.** Epidural hematoma is evident in the left frontal region on this CT scan. The convex bulging shape is highly characteristic and differentiates epidural from subdural hematoma. (Used with permission from Dr Robert De La Paz.)

hematoma, false localizing signs can be found. The presence of cerebellar signs, nuchal rigidity, and drowsiness associated with a fracture of the occipital bone suggests a hematoma in the posterior fossa. Progression to transtentorial or foramen magnum herniation and death can occur rapidly because the bleeding is arterial. The mortality rate approaches 100% in untreated patients.

G. Subarachnoid Hemorrhage

Extravasation of blood into the subarachnoid spaces can follow any head injury. In most cases, subarachnoid blood would be detected only by CSF examination and is of little clinical importance. In serious injuries, larger vessels traversing the subarachnoid space are torn, resulting in focal or diffuse subarachnoid hemorrhage detectable by CT. In these cases, blood is often distributed over the convexities, in contrast to aneurysmal bleeding, which results in collections of blood that are restricted to the basal cisterns. Although a large amount of subarachnoid blood is a poor prognostic sign, delayed complications of aneurysmal subarachnoid hemorrhage, such as hydrocephalus and ischemia from vasospasm, are uncommon after traumatic brain injury.

H. Penetrating Injury

Mortality from gunshot wounds to the head is more than 95%. The amount of tissue damage is dependent on the kinetic energy and velocity of the missile, angle of entrance, number of bony fragments, affected anatomic structures, and configuration of secondary bullet tracts due to ricochet. As a result of tissue destruction, perivascular edema, contusional or perivascular bleeding within the cerebral parenchyma, and hypoxic-ischemic brain injury may develop secondarily. These changes are detectable on MRI or CT.

The most common predictor of outcome after penetrating brain injury is the patient's level of consciousness after resuscitation. The chance of survival for patients with a Glasgow Coma Scale (GCS) score less than 4 is 20%. Subarachnoid, intraventricular, and subdural hemorrhage; vasospasm; proximity of the bullet to the brainstem; and bihemispheric injury are associated with higher mortality.

I. Blast Injury

Explosive missiles initiate overpressure waves that translate mechanical, thermal, and electromagnetic energy to the brain by spallation, implosion, and inertia directly through the cranium and indirectly through oscillating pressures in fluid containing large blood vessels. This primary injury pattern results in damage to the blood–brain barrier (high-frequency waves) and to the grey-white matter junction with de-afferentiation of the cortical columnar structure (low-frequency, high-amplitude waves) seen on MRI with diffusion tensor sequences. These patients suffer loss of consciousness and altered mental status even without a penetrating injury. About 30% of patients survive with long-term neurologic deficits; in 11%, post-traumatic stress disorder is diagnosed. Secondary blast injury is caused by debris physically displaced by blast overpressure or blast winds and results in penetrating and blunt trauma. Tertiary blast injury is defined as displacement of a person by the force of peak overpressure and blast winds or collapse of structures causing blunt trauma such as closed-head injury.

▶ Clinical Evaluation
A. Initial Assessment

Resuscitation, history taking, and examination should begin simultaneously once the patient arrives in the emergency department. Assessment and stabilization of airway, breathing, and circulation are the most important initial steps in management. Categorization of the severity of the head injury as low, moderate, or high risk; evaluation for fracture of the cervical spine; and identification of any extracranial injuries should follow immediately.

Because hypoxia and hypotension can have devastating effects in patients with a head injury, endotracheal intubation should be performed if the patient is unconscious,

Table 14–2. Glasgow Coma Scale

Response Category	Points
Eye Opening Response	
Spontaneous—open with blinking at baseline	4
To verbal stimuli, command speech	3
To pain only (not applied to face)	2
No response	1
Verbal Response	
Oriented	5
Confused conversation, but able to answer questions	4
Inappropriate words	3
Incomprehensible speech	2
No response	1
Motor Response	
Obeys commands for movement	6
Purposeful movement to painful stimulus	5
Withdraws in response to pain	4
Flexion in response to pain (decorticate)	3
Extension in response to pain (decerebrate)	2
No response	1

Adapted with permission from Teasdale G, Jennett B. Assessment of coma and impaired consciousness. A practical scale. *Lancet* 1974;2:81–84.

Table 14–3. Risk Stratification of Patients With Traumatic Brain Injury

Risk Category	Criteria
Low	Normal neurologic examination No concussion No drug or alcohol intoxication May complain of headache and dizziness May have scalp abrasion, laceration, or hematoma Absence of moderate or severe injury criteria
Moderate	Failure to reach GCS score of 15 within 2 h of injury Concussion Coagulopathy Anterograde amnesia >30 min Vomiting Seizure Signs of possible basilar or open skull fracture Dangerous mechanism of injury Alcohol or drug intoxication Unreliable historian or no history of injury Age <2 y or >65 y
High	GCS score of 3-8 (comatose) Progressive decline in level of consciousness ("talked and deteriorated") Focal neurologic signs Penetrating skull injury or palpable depressed skull fracture

GCS = Glasgow Coma Scale.
Adapted and reproduced with permission from Masters SJ, et al. Skull x-ray examinations after head trauma. Recommendation by a multidisciplinary panel and validation study. *N Engl J Med* 1987;316:87–91; and Stiell IG, et al. The Canadian CT Head Rule for patients with minor head injury. *Lancet* 2001;357:1391–1396.

unresponsive with a GCS (Table 14–2) score ≤8, unable to maintain an adequate airway, hypoxic (oxygen saturation <90%) despite supplemental oxygen, or in respiratory distress. Attention should be paid to immobilization of the spine, to avoid hyperventilation, hypotension, and stress in the setting of intracranial hypertensions, and to basilar skull fractures. A single episode of hypotension (systolic blood pressure <90 mm Hg) doubles the mortality rate. Hypotension should be corrected with intravenous boluses of isotonic fluids, blood transfusions, or vasopressors. Normal saline is preferred over lactated Ringer solution; fluids containing 5% dextrose or dextrane should be avoided. Hypertonic saline expands intravascular volume by 4- to 10-fold that of the volume infused. Albumin infusions have been associated with worse outcomes. Systolic blood pressure during the stabilization phase should be maintained above 90 mm Hg to ensure adequate cerebral blood flow. Potential causes of hypotension, such as bleeding into the abdomen, thorax, retroperitoneal space, or tissues surrounding a long bone fracture, should be treated. Hypotension may also reflect spinal shock related to a coexisting spinal cord injury (see the discussion of Spinal Trauma, later). Hypertension associated with a wide pulse pressure and bradycardia (Cushing reflex) may reflect increased intracranial pressure (ICP) or focal brainstem injury.

A baseline neurologic evaluation should be performed immediately, while airway, breathing, and circulation are assessed. Injuries can be ranked as low, moderate, or high risk based on risk factors, rapid initial neurologic assessment, and GCS score (Table 14–3). The GCS (Table 14–2) is based on eye opening and the patient's best verbal and motor responses. It is widely used as a semiquantitative clinical measure of the severity of brain injury and provides a guide to prognosis (see Table 14–7).

Patients who are comatose (GCS score ≤8) or who show clinical signs of herniation require emergency measures to reduce ICP, including head elevation, hyperventilation, and administration of intravenous mannitol, even before CT is performed (Table 14–4; see Treatment, later, for measures to manage increased ICP).

B. History and Physical Examination Findings

The circumstances of the accident and the clinical condition of the patient before admission to the emergency department should be ascertained from emergency medical services records, the patient (if possible), and eyewitnesses. It is important to determine the force and location of impact on the head as precisely as possible. Specific inquiries should be made regarding whether the patient suffered a concussion

Table 14–4. Emergency Measures to Reduce Intracranial Pressure in Unmonitored Patients With Clinical Signs of Herniation

- Head of bed elevated 15-30 degrees
- Normal saline (0.9%) at 80-100 mL/h (avoid hypotonic fluids)
- Intubation and hyperventilation (target $Pco_2 = 26$-30 mm Hg)
- Mannitol 20% solution, 1–1.5 g/kg via rapid IV infusion or 20–23.4% hypertonic saline 30 mL via central line over 20 min
- Foley catheter
- Neurosurgical consultation

Modified with permission from Rowland LP, ed. *Merritt's Textbook of Neurology,* 11th ed. Lippincott Williams & Wilkins, 2005.

with subsequent amnesia. Only an eyewitness can accurately gauge the duration of loss of consciousness.

Patients who have "talked and deteriorated" should be assumed to have an expanding intracranial hematoma until proven otherwise. Reports of headache, nausea, vomiting, confusion, or seizure activity must be noted. A medical history, including medications and drug and alcohol use, is crucial for management. Recent drug and alcohol use is common in trauma patients, and intoxication can confound assessments of mental status.

After the initial neurologic assessment, a more detailed physical and neurologic examination is performed. The skull should be inspected and palpated for fractures, hematomas, and lacerations. A "step off," or palpable bony shelf, represents a depressed skull fracture. A bloody discharge from the nose or ear may indicate leakage of CSF. Bloody CSF can be differentiated from blood by a positive halo test (a "halo" of CSF forms around the blood when dropped on a white cloth sheet). If there is no admixture of blood, CSF can be distinguished from nasal secretions because the CSF glucose concentration is 30 mg/dL or more, whereas lacrimal secretions and nasal mucus usually contain less than 5 mg/dL. The patient should be thoroughly examined for external signs of trauma to the neck, chest, back, abdomen, and limbs.

After determining the patient's level of consciousness (alert, lethargic, stuporous, or comatose) and GCS, a focused mental status examination should be performed if the patient is conversant. Particular attention should be paid to attention, concentration (counting backward from 20 to 1 or reciting the months in reverse), orientation, and memory, including assessment for retrograde and anterograde amnesia.

Eye movements and pupillary size, shape, and reactivity to light should be noted. A sluggishly reactive or dilated pupil suggests transtentorial herniation with compression of the third nerve. A midposition, poorly reactive, irregular pupil may result from injury to the oculomotor nucleus in the midbrain tegmentum. Nystagmus is common after concussion. In comatose patients, the oculocephalic and oculovestibular reflexes should be tested (see Chapter 4).

Motor examination should focus on identifying asymmetric weakness or posturing. Spontaneous movements should be assessed for preferential use of the limbs on one side. If the patient is not fully cooperative, lateralized weakness can be detected by an asymmetry in tone or tendon reflexes, or by the presence of an arm drift, asymmetric localizing response to sternal rub, or extensor plantar reflex. Noxious stimuli, such as pinching the medial arm or applying nail-bed pressure, may reveal subtle motor posturing in an extremity that moves purposefully otherwise. *Decorticate posturing* (flexion of arms, extension of legs) results from injury to the corticospinal pathways at the level of the diencephalon or upper midbrain. *Decerebrate posturing* (extension of legs and arms) implies injury to the motor pathways at the level of the lower midbrain, pons, or medulla.

Assessment of gait is particularly important in low-risk patients who are treated and released without a CT scan of the head. Balance and equilibrium, tested by tandem heel-to-toe walking, are frequently impaired after a concussion.

C. Imaging Studies

CT is the emergency imaging method of choice for head trauma, because it can be obtained quickly and provides important structural information. CT is superior to plain skull films in detecting skull fractures in the bone window setting and in three-dimensional reconstructions. In general, a CT scan of the head should be obtained in all patients with head injury, except those who are deemed low risk, that is, without concussion, with no neurologic abnormalities on examination, GCS <15, and with no evidence or suspicion of a skull fracture, alcohol or drug intoxication, or other moderate-risk criteria (see Table 14–3). The likelihood of detecting intracranial hemorrhage by CT in low-risk patients is only 1 in 10,000.

CT images should be assessed for the presence of epidural or subdural hematoma, subarachnoid or intraventricular blood, parenchymal contusions and hemorrhages, cerebral edema, and so-called *gliding contusions* related to diffuse axonal injury. With bone-window settings, fractures, sinus opacification, and pneumocephalus can be identified. CT evidence of mass effect and brain tissue displacement, compression or obliteration of the mesencephalic cisterns, or midline shift correlates with increased ICP and a decreased chance of survival.

MRI is more sensitive than CT in identifying subtle injury to the brain, particularly focal lesions related to diffuse axonal injury, hemorrhagic diffuse axonal injury, small contusions, and in penetrating injuries with wooden objects, but is generally not obtained in an emergency setting unless it is readily available. Acute axonal injury can be seen as bright lesions on diffusion-weighted sequences and dark regions on apparent diffusion coefficient (ADC) maps. The mean ADC value of the whole brain, fractionated anisotropy values obtained on diffusion tensor imaging that reflect disruption of axonal membranes and cytoskeletal network, correlates with poor outcome after traumatic brain injury. Microhemorrhages are detected on gradient-recalled echo and susceptibility-weighted imaging, which may explain impaired cognitive and memory function after relatively mild head trauma.

D. Management of Coagulopathy

Prehospital antiplatelet and anticoagulant therapy is associated with increased morbidity and possible mortality compared with patients with normal coagulation before trauma. Patients with abnormal coagulation require immediate reversal therapy. Treatment strategies for platelet dysfunction include transfusion of platelets, administration of intravenous or subcutaneous desmopressin (0.3 μg/kg), and intravenous recombinant factor VII. Patients on oral anticoagulation should receive fresh frozen plasma at 20 mL/kg or prothrombin complex concentrate at 30 U/kg along with vitamin K, 10 mg intravenously. Recombinant factor VII may aid to correct coagulopathies in the face of emergent craniotomy or other neurosurgical procedures. Protamin sulfate (0.25–1.5 mg of protamine for every 100 units of heparin given intravenously over 10 minutes) antagonizes heparin- and low-molecular-weight heparin–induced coagulopathies.

▶ Early Complications

A. Cranial Nerve Injury

Injury to the cranial nerves is a frequent complication of fractures at the base of the skull. The olfactory nerves and bulbs are most commonly affected (13%). Facial nerve dysfunction occurs in 0.3–5% of all head injuries, and every cranial nerve except IX–XII is at risk. Occasionally, dysfunction may not develop until several days after injury. Partial or complete recovery of function is the rule in traumatic injuries to cranial nerves, with the exception of the first or second nerves.

B. Cerebrospinal Fluid Fistula

CSF fistulae follow tearing of the dura and arachnoid membranes. They occur in 3% of patients with closed-head injury and in 5–10% of those with basilar skull fractures. There is usually a concomitant fracture of the ethmoid, sphenoid, or orbital plate of the frontal bone.

CSF leakage ceases after head elevation alone within a few days in 85% of patients. If it persists, a lumbar drain may lower CSF pressure, reduce flow through the fistula, and hasten spontaneous closure of the dural tear. Patients with dural leaks are at increased risk for meningitis. However, the use of prophylactic antibiotics is controversial. Persistent CSF otorrhea or rhinorrhea for more than 2 weeks is a clear indication for surgical repair, as is recurrent meningitis. If there is a CSF leak and the site of the fracture is not evident, metrizamide CT cisternography or

a combination of MR cisternography and plain high-resolution CT are the diagnostic studies of choice.

C. Pneumocephalus

Pneumocephalus—a collection of air in the intracranial cavity, usually in the subarachnoid space—commonly occurs as a complication of a fracture of the frontal sinus. The air may not appear for several days after injury and then only after the patient sneezes or blows his or her nose. The presence of intracranial air has the same implications as a CSF fistula. Most pneumoceles are asymptomatic, but headaches or cognitive symptoms may result from intracranial hypotension. The diagnosis is made by detection of air on CT, and the site of the dural defect can be identified by metrizamide CT cisternography. If spontaneous absorption of the air does not occur, the opening in the frontal sinus should be surgically repaired.

D. Carotid-Cavernous Fistula

A carotid-cavernous fistula is characterized by the clinical triad of pulsating exophthalmos, conjunctival chemosis, and orbital bruit. Most cases (80%) are the result of traumatic laceration of the internal carotid artery as it passes through the cavernous sinus. Other symptoms may include distended orbital and periorbital veins and paralysis of cranial nerves (III, IV, first and second divisions of V, and VI) that pass through or within the wall of the cavernous sinus. Traumatic carotid-cavernous fistulae may develop immediately or days after injury. Angiography confirms the diagnosis. Endovascular treatment with a balloon placed through the defect in the arterial wall into the venous side of the fistula can prevent permanent visual loss due to retinal venous infarction.

E. Vascular Injury and Thrombosis

Traumatic injuries can cause dissections of the extracranial or intracranial internal carotid or vertebral arteries, leading to thrombosis at the site of the intimal flap and infarction due to distal thromboembolism. The diagnosis is established by conventional CT angiography or MR imaging and angiography. Anticoagulation is recommended to prevent thrombosis and infarction, although such intervention may be contraindicated if there is coexisting coagulopathy and intracranial hemorrhage. Angioplasty and stenting may be a treatment alternative, but requires double inhibition of platelet aggregation.

Basilar skull fractures are sometimes associated with thrombosis of adjacent dural sinuses. *Dural sinus thrombosis* usually takes several days to develop; the sigmoid and transverse sinuses are most commonly affected. Symptoms are related to increased ICP or associated venous infarction and include headache, vomiting, seizures, depressed level of consciousness, and hemiparesis. Angiography or MR venography is the best diagnostic tool. Anticoagulation is the treatment of choice.

Cerebral infarction can occur as a complication of large epidural or subdural hematoma formation, when subfalcine or transtentorial herniation results in compression of the ipsilateral anterior cerebral artery against the falx or contralateral posterior cerebral artery against the tentorium. This complication is most commonly seen in patients with massive hematomas who do not undergo emergent clot evacuation. Border-zone ("watershed") pattern infarction can result from cerebral perfusion pressure (CPP) insufficiency in the setting of increased ICP, hypotension, or both.

F. Infection

Infection within the intracranial cavity after injury to the head may be extradural (osteomyelitis), subdural (empyema), subarachnoid (meningitis), or intracerebral (abscess) (see Chapter 26). *Extradural infection* is usually secondary to infection of the external wound or osteomyelitis of the skull. *Subdural empyema* is a closed-space infection between the dura and arachnoid. *Intracerebral abscess* may follow compound fractures of the skull or penetrating injuries to the brain. All these infections usually develop in the first few weeks after injury, but they can be delayed. Diagnosis is suggested by CT and MRI and confirmed by culture of the infected tissue. Treatment includes surgical debridement or drainage and administration of antibiotics.

Meningitis may follow any type of open fracture associated with a dural tear, including compound fractures, penetrating missiles, or linear fractures that extend into the nasal sinuses or the middle ear. Meningitis, described in up to 22% of patients with basilar skull fractures, commonly develops 2–8 days after injury but may be delayed for several months, particularly in patients with fractures through the mastoid or nasal sinuses. *Pneumococcus* or other gram-positive bacteria are the usual cause of meningitis occurring within a few days after injury, but any pathogenic organism may be present. Diagnosis depends on CSF examination. The principles of treatment are those recommended for meningitis in general. Persistent CSF fistula with rhinorrhea or otorrhea can cause recurrent meningitis. Treatment in such cases includes surgical closure of the fistula.

Antibiotics with gram-positive activity, such as oxacillin, are often used to reduce the risk of meningitis in patients with CSF otorrhea, rhinorrhea, or intracranial air; however, these agents may increase the risk of infection with more virulent or resistant organisms and are not recommended for routine use. Bacterial infections of the central nervous system are discussed in detail in Chapter 26.

▶ Late Complications

A. Postconcussion Syndrome

Approximately 40% of patients who have sustained minor or severe injuries to the brain complain of headache, dizziness, fatigue, insomnia or hypersomnia, blurred vision, tinnitus, irritability, restlessness, and inability to concentrate. Often, there is overlap with symptoms of anxiety and depression. This group of symptoms is known as *postconcussion syndrome.* It can be present for only a few weeks or persist for years (15%). Postconcussion syndrome is somewhat misleadingly named, because affected individuals do not need to have suffered loss of consciousness. There are no criteria that make it possible to define the role of either physiologic or psychological factors in the etiology. Patients may be severely disabled but have normal findings on neurologic examination and no evidence of brain injury on MR studies. The correlation between the severity of the original injury and the severity and duration of later symptoms is poor. For instance, the incidence of postconcussion syndrome does not correlate with the duration of retrograde amnesia, coma, or post-traumatic temporary anterograde amnesia. In some patients, symptoms may be related to brain damage seen on MRI. A worse outcome is associated with residual focal atrophy of a frontal or temporal lobe, resulting in executive dysfunction or personality change. Other proposed mechanisms are dysfunction of the hypothalamic-pituitary-adrenal axis, causing depression, and glucocorticoid-induced damage to dendrites within the hippocampus. In other patients, symptoms seem to be entirely psychogenic (eg, dissociative amnesia).

Post-traumatic symptoms are more likely to occur in patients with psychiatric symptoms before the injury. Social factors such as domestic or financial difficulties, unrewarding occupations, and the desire to obtain compensation, financial or otherwise, tend to produce and may prolong the symptoms once they have developed.

The prognosis for patients with postconcussion syndrome is uncertain. Generally, progressive improvement may be expected. Duration of symptoms is not related to the severity of the injury. In some patients with only mild injury, symptoms continue for a long period, whereas patients with severe injuries may have only mild or transient symptoms. Most often, 2–6 months elapse before headache, dizziness, or mental changes show much improvement. Treatment of postconcussion syndrome includes psychotherapy, cognitive and occupational therapy, vocational rehabilitation, and antidepressants or anxiolytics.

B. Seizures and Post-Traumatic Epilepsy

Post-traumatic seizures may be immediate (within 24 hours), early (within the first week), or late (post-traumatic epilepsy, after the first week). The incidence of seizures after head injury varies from 2.5–40% in the literature. As a rule, the more severe the injury, the greater is the likelihood that seizures will develop. The overall incidence of seizures is about 25% in those with brain contusion or hematoma and as high as 50% in those with penetrating head injury.

Immediate seizures, which are infrequent, are a risk factor for further early seizures but not for post-traumatic epilepsy. Early seizures occur in 3–14% of patients with head injury who are admitted to the hospital. Risk factors include depressed skull fracture, penetrating head injury, intracranial hemorrhage (epidural, subdural, or intraparenchymal), prolonged loss of consciousness (>24 hours), coma, and immediate seizures. The risk of early seizures in a patient with any of these risk factors is 20–30%. Children are more likely to develop early post-traumatic seizures than adults. Patients who experience early seizures remain at risk for late seizures and should be maintained on anticonvulsants after discharge from the hospital. The overall incidence of late seizures after closed-head injury is 5%, but the risk is as high as 30% among patients with intracranial hemorrhage or a depressed skull fracture and 50% among patients with early seizures. About 60% of patients experience their initial seizure during the first year, but an increased risk of seizures persists for up to 15 years after a severe head injury. Because 25% of patients with a late seizure do not have recurrent seizures, many practitioners begin anticonvulsant therapy only after a second seizure occurs.

C. Cognitive Impairment

Almost every patient with severe brain injury experiences cognitive changes after recovery of consciousness from prolonged coma; disorientation and agitation are particularly common. With time, there is usually considerable improvement, but permanent sequelae are common. Disabling cognitive problems include impaired memory, attention, and concentration; slowing of psychomotor speed and mental processing; and changes in personality. There may be loss of memory for the events that occurred in the immediate period after recovery of consciousness (post-traumatic amnesia) and a similar memory gap for the events immediately preceding the injury (pretraumatic amnesia). These periods of amnesia may encompass days, weeks, or years. Depression occurs in up to 40% of survivors of traumatic brain injury during the first year of recovery and is highly amenable to medical therapy. Post-traumatic stress disorder occurs in 10–30% of survivors of traumatic brain injury, especially after intensive care unit (ICU) admission, and needs to be recognized and treated.

D. Post-Traumatic Movement Disorders

Movement disorders are rare sequelae of head injury. Postural and intention tremor are most common, although their pathogenesis remains obscure. Cerebellar ataxia, rubral tremor, and palatal myoclonus are described in patients with focal shearing injuries of the cerebellum and brainstem. Parkinsonism and other basal ganglia syndromes have been reported after a single episode of head trauma.

▶ Treatment

A. Risk Stratification in the Emergency Department

The management of head trauma is stratified according to the level of risk of each individual patient.

Table 14–5. Criteria for Hospital Admission After Head Injury

- Intracranial blood or fracture identified on CT scan of head
- Confusion, agitation, or depressed level of consciousness
- Focal neurologic signs or symptoms
- Post-traumatic seizure
- Alcohol or drug intoxication
- Significant comorbid medical illness
- Lack of a reliable home environment for observation

CT = computed tomography.
Reproduced with permission from Rowland LP, ed. *Merritt's Textbook of Neurology,* 11th ed. Lippincott Williams & Wilkins, 2005.

1. Low-risk patients—Patients who meet all of the criteria for low risk outlined in Table 14–3 are generally discharged from the emergency department without undergoing CT imaging as long as they can be observed by a reliable person for the next 24 hours. Patients are given a checklist of symptoms such as headache, vomiting, and confusion and are instructed to return immediately to the emergency department if any occur.

2. Moderate-risk patients—Patients are at moderate risk, who have experienced a concussion but have a normal GCS score of 15 (alert, fully oriented, and following commands) and normal CT findings, do not need to be admitted to the hospital. Even in the presence of headache, nausea, vomiting, dizziness, or retrograde amnesia, these patients can be discharged to home for observation with a list of warning symptoms, because the risk of a significant intracranial lesion developing thereafter is minimal. Criteria for hospital admission for patients with head injury are listed in Table 14–5. Patients with mild-to-moderate neurologic deficits (generally corresponding to GCS scores of 9–14) and CT findings that do not require neurosurgical intervention should be admitted to an intermediate care unit or ICU for observation. A follow-up CT at 24 hours is often helpful to evaluate potential progression of bleeding or edema, or both, and required with clinical deterioration. New lesions develop in 16% of patients with diffuse injury, and 25–45% of cerebral contusions are shown to have grown significantly on follow-up CT.

3. High-risk patients—All patients with a serious head injury categorized as high risk are admitted to the hospital and require an early neurosurgical consultation. Once the patient has been stabilized and assessed and has undergone imaging, the immediate consideration is whether the patient needs to undergo an emergent surgical intervention. If necessary, surgery should proceed immediately, because delays can only increase the likelihood of further brain damage from increasing edema or hemorrhage. Medical management of severe injury requires an ICU setting. Although little can be done about brain damage that occurs on impact, ICU care can play a major role in reducing secondary brain injury that develops over hours to days.

B. Surgical Intervention

Simple wounds of the scalp should be thoroughly cleaned and sutured. Compound fractures of the skull have to be debrided completely. Operative treatment of compound fractures should be performed as soon as possible but may be delayed for 24 hours until the patient is transported to a hospital equipped for this purpose or until the patient is hemodynamically stable. Elevation of small depressed fractures does not require emergent surgical intervention, but the depressed fragments should be elevated before the patient is discharged from the hospital, particularly if the inner table of the skull is involved.

The treatment of choice for massive acute and chronic subdural, epidural, or parenchymal hematoma with mass effect is *craniotomy* and evacuation of the clot. Surgical evacuation of the thick, clotted blood that constitutes an acute subdural hematoma usually requires a large craniotomy. The source of bleeding should be identified and either ligated or clipped. Outcome after surgical evacuation depends primarily on the severity of the initial deficit, the degree of associated brain damage, and the interval from injury to surgery. Mortality ranges from 5–30% in surgically treated patients with epidural hematoma. Decreasing the interval between injury and surgical intervention results in improved survival. Underlying brain damage is less likely with epidural or chronic subdural hematoma than with acute subdural hematoma, and if the patient does not have parenchymal destruction, recovery after hematoma removal is remarkable, with disappearance of the hemiplegia or other focal neurologic signs. Reoperation for acute and chronic subdural hematoma is required in about 15% of patients.

Burr hole or *twist drill* evacuation is not sufficient for acute large subdural and epidural hematomas but is justified for liquified chronic subdural hematomas. Outcomes after burr hole or twist drill procedures are better than with craniotomy. A plastic catheter (Jackson-Pratt drain) is usually placed into the subdural space for several days until the drainage subsides.

Gunshot injuries require urgent surgical exploration and repair of major anatomic structures (arteries, internal organs, airway). Aggressive early debridement prevents osteomyelitis. Administration of intravenous cephalosporin antibiotics for 2 weeks is recommended in patients with high-velocity gunshot wounds, with the addition of intravenous gentamycin for soft tissue and cavitating lesions and penicillin for grossly contaminated wounds. Tetanus prophylaxis is mandatory.

Decompressive hemicraniectomy increases compliance, cerebral blood flow, and brain oxygenation and is used for treatment of cerebral edema and intracranial hypertension. Up to date, there are no randomized outcome studies proving a survival benefit, although an improvement of long-term disability could be demonstrated in large patient series. There is consensus that the craniectomy should be large enough (15 × 15 cm), done early (before clinical deterioration), and with duraplasty. Herniation through the craniectomy defect (up to 51%); subdural effusion (26–60%); the trephined syndrome of the sinking scalp flap presenting with headaches, seizures, mood swings, and behavioral disturbances due to cortical dysfunction caused by brain distortion under the scalp flap as the edema subsides); hydrocephalus (0.9–27%); seizures (7–20%); bone flap resorption (3–12%); and infection (1–10%) are more and more recognized complications of this procedure. Two randomized efficacy trials are currently ongoing: Randomised Evaluation of Surgery With Craniectomy for Uncontrollable Elevation of Intra-Cranial Pressure (RESCUEicp) in the United Kingdom and Early Decompressive Craniectomy in Patients With Severe Traumatic Brain Injury (DECRA) in Australia investigating the effect of an early hemicraniectomy on outcome.

C. Intensive Care Management

Head-injured patients at moderate and high risk are best managed in an ICU, preferably in a neurologic or neurosurgical ICU in experienced trauma centers. A time-coded flow sheet is helpful to allow for continuous updating of the patient's clinical, neurologic, and hemodynamic parameters. The patient should be examined repeatedly to evaluate level of consciousness and the presence or absence of signs of injury to the brain or cranial nerves. A change in level of consciousness, reflected by changes in the GCS score, or the appearance of focal neurologic signs should prompt a repeat CT scan.

1. Increased intracranial pressure—ICP should be monitored in all head-injured patients who are comatose (GCS score ≤8) after resuscitation, unless the prognosis is so poor that aggressive measures are not warranted. Intracranial hypertension occurs in more than 50% of comatose patients with CT evidence of mass effect from intracranial hemorrhage or cerebral edema and in 10–15% of patients with normal CT scans. Raised ICP is related to poor outcome. ICP monitoring devices such as ventricular catheters or fiberoptic parenchymal monitors can be placed into the lateral ventricle, the subdural or epidural space, or into the brain parenchyma in conjunction with a brain temperature and oxygen monitor. Ventriculostomy has the advantage of allowing CSF drainage to reduce ICP but carries a high risk of infection (~5%). The risk of infection or hemorrhage is substantially lower with parenchymal ICP monitors (~1%). Measurements of ICP utilizing subdural or epidural probes are less reliable.

Normal ICP is less than 15 mm Hg, or 20 cm H_2O. Cerebral perfusion pressure (CPP) is routinely monitored concurrently with ICP because it is the driving force of cerebral blood flow. CPP is defined as mean arterial blood pressure (MAP) minus ICP. The goal of ICP management after head injury is to maintain ICP less than 20 mm Hg and CPP greater than 60 mm Hg. The amount and duration of ICP and CPP derangements beyond these targets correlate with poor outcome.

Treatment of elevated ICP is most successful when a stepwise, preestablished protocol is followed. The Columbia University Medical Center management protocol for treatment of ICP elevations in monitored ICU patients is shown in Table 14–6.

If the ICP increases sharply, a repeat CT scan should be obtained to evaluate the need for a definitive neurosurgical procedure. If the patient is agitated or "fighting" the ventilator, a short-acting intravenous sedative agent such as propofol, fentanyl, or sodium thiopental should be given to attain a quiet motionless state. Thereafter, if CPP is less than 60 mm Hg, vasopressors such as dopamine, norepinephrine, or phenylephrine can lead to reduction of ICP by decreasing cerebral vasodilation that occurs in response to inadequate perfusion and can augment MAP, resulting in improved CPP. Alternately, if CPP exceeds 110 mm Hg, blood pressure reduction with intravenous labetalol, clevidipine, or nicardipine is sometimes followed by a parallel

Table 14–6. Stepwise Treatment Protocol for Elevated Intracranial Pressure in Monitored Patients[a]

1. Repeat CT scanning and surgical removal of an intracranial mass lesion, or ventricular drainage
2. IV sedation to attain a motionless, quiet state
3. Pressor infusion if CPP <70 mm Hg, or reduction of blood pressure if CPP remains >110 mm Hg
4. Mannitol, 0.25-1.0 g/kg IV every 2-6 h as needed or 7.5-23.4% hypertonic saline 0.5-2 mL/kg via central line over 20 min
5. Hyperventilate to Pco_2 level of 30-35 mm Hg
6. High-dose pentobarbital therapy (load with 5-20 mg/kg, maintain with 1-4 mg/kg/h)
7. Systemic hypothermia to 33°C (91.4°F)

CPP = cerebral perfusion pressure; CT = computed tomography; IV = intravenous.
[a]Defined as ICP >20 mm Hg for more than 10 minutes.
Reproduced with permission from Rowland LP, ed. *Merritt's Textbook of Neurology,* 11th ed. Lippincott Williams & Wilkins, 2005.

decrease in ICP. The relationship between extremes of CPP and ICP in states of reduced intracranial compliance is shown in Figure 14–6.

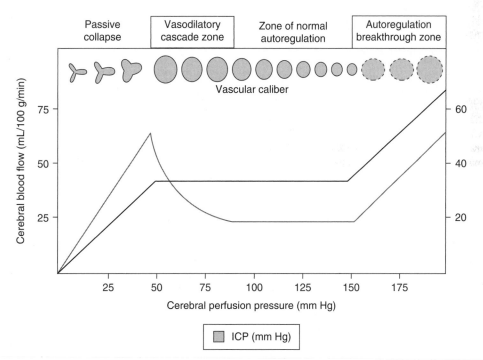

▲ **Figure 14–6.** Relationship between extremes of cerebral perfusion pressure (CPP) and intracranial pressure (ICP) in states of reduced intracranial compliance. In the vasodilatory cascade zone, CPP insufficiency and intact pressure autoregulation leads to reflex cerebral vasodilation and increased ICP; the treatment is to raise CPP. In the autoregulation breakthrough zone, pressure and volume overload, which overwhelms the capacity of the brain to autoregulate, leads to increased cerebral blood volume and ICP; the treatment is to lower CPP. (Reproduced with permission from Rose JA, Mayer SA. Optimizing blood pressure in neurological emergencies. *Neurocrit Care* 2004;1:287–299.)

Osmotherapy with mannitol or hyperosmolar sodium infusions and hyperventilation are the next steps if sedation and CPP management fail to normalize ICP. Mannitol, an osmotic diuretic, lowers ICP via reduction in brain water content through an osmotic gradient from interstitial and intracellular compartments to the intravascular space across the semipermeable blood–brain barrier. Additionally, it reduces blood viscosity, improves microvascular cerebral blood flow, and has free-radical scavenger properties. The initial dose of mannitol 20% solution is 1–1.5 g/kg, followed by doses of 0.25–1.0 g/kg as needed. Further doses should be administered on the basis of ICP measurements and serum osmolarity rather than on a standing basis. Rapid onset of action makes mannitol boluses very useful for reversal of acute herniation syndromes (ie, a dilated, unreactive pupil). The effect of mannitol is maximal when given rapidly; ICP reduction occurs within 10–20 minutes and can last for 2–6 hours. Serum osmolality should be monitored closely, with a secondary goal of attaining levels of 300–320 mOsm/L. Urinary losses should be replaced with normal saline to avoid secondary hypovolemia. Central venous pressure monitoring is generally recommended. Because of a potential rebound effect, resulting in rise of ICP, mannitol should not be used over prolonged periods and not abruptly withdrawn.

More recently, 7.5–23.4% hypertonic saline solution (0.5–2.0 mL/kg) has been used as an alternative to mannitol bolus therapy for the treatment of acute ICP elevations and herniation syndromes. Studies evaluating equiosmolar doses of mannitol and hypertonic saline indicate that in most cases hypertonic saline has a more profound and longer lasting effect on ICP reduction. Hypertonic saline solutions improve microvascular perfusion and CPP by rapidly expanding volume, increasing cardiac output and systemic blood pressure, decreasing production of CSF, modifying inflammatory responses, interacting with the neuroendocrine system, and expanding intracranial elastance. Hypertonic saline is generally preferable in patients who are hypotensive or hypovolemic, whereas mannitol is favored in patients who are relatively volume overloaded.

Hyperventilation lowers ICP by inducing cerebral alkalosis and reflex vasoconstriction, resulting in a concomitant reduction in cerebral blood volume. Hyperventilation to PCO_2 levels of 30–35 mm Hg can lower ICP within minutes, although the effect gradually diminishes over 1–3 hours as acid–base buffering mechanisms correct the alkalosis within the brain parenchyma. For every 1 mm Hg drop in PCO_2 there is a 3% decrease in CBF. Overly aggressive hyperventilation to PCO_2 levels less than 30 mm Hg may potentially exacerbate cerebral ischemia by producing severe vasoconstriction and should be avoided unless jugular venous oxygen saturation or brain tissue oxygen monitoring is available to ensure that cerebral hypoxia does not occur.

High-dose barbiturate therapy with pentobarbital given in doses equivalent to those used for general anesthesia (10–20 mg/kg as a loading dose, followed by 1–4 mg/kg/h) effectively lowers ICP in most patients who are refractory to the previously outlined steps. The effect of pentobarbital is multifactorial but probably involves reduction in cerebral metabolism, blood flow, and blood volume followed by reduction in edema formation. Barbiturates also have neuroprotective properties (free-radical scavenging). However, pentobarbital can cause profound hypotension and usually requires the use of vasopressors to maintain CPP of 60 mm Hg or higher. Further complications include pneumonia, sepsis, and hepatic dysfunction.

Mild-to-moderate systemic hypothermia (33°C [91.4°F]) can reduce ICP in patients who are refractory to pentobarbital. The application of hypothermia is complex and requires a management protocol that emphasizes the use of agents such as meperidine, fentanyl, or dexmedetomidine hydrochloride, and neuromuscular-blocking agents as well as skin counter-warming to control shivering, which increases cerebral and metabolic stress and consequently ICP. Routine application of mild-to-moderate hypothermia within 8 hours of traumatic brain injury does not improve outcome or mortality; its use should be limited to management of refractory intracranial hypertension and fever control. The Eurotherm3235 trial investigating the effect of hypothermia used for control of refractory intracranial hypertension in traumatic brain injury on ICP and long-term functional outcome is currently ongoing.

2. Additional neuromonitoring—More advanced techniques include monitoring of focal and global cerebral oxygenation, of cerebral metabolites, CBF measurements, and continuous EEG monitoring. Brain tissue oxygen tension ($PbrO_2$) is monitored focally by insertion of a Clark electrode (Licox) and represents the balance between oxygen delivery and consumption within a small brain tissue volume. $PbrO_2$ monitors can be used to titrate CPP by demonstrating a critical threshold below which $PbrO_2$ saturation falls. Therapy directed at normalization of CPP and $PbrO_2$ have indicated trends to better long-term outcome. The Brain Tissue Oxygen Monitoring in Traumatic Brain Injury (BOOST) trial investigating the efficacy of brain tissue oxygen monitoring in traumatic brain injury is being prepared. Normal values are 15–20 mm Hg. Global oxygenation can be determined by jugular venous oxymetry; in this study, a saturation below 55% indicated increased extraction or decreased supply. Focal measurements of CBF by thermal diffusion or laser Doppler methods demonstrated ischemia in a third of patients with severe traumatic brain injury. Microdialysis provides hourly measurements of brain glucose, lactate, pyruvate, glutamate, and glycerol as well as drug concentrations. Brain hypoglycemia and ischemia (high lactate/pyruvate ratio) can be detected. Continuous EEG monitoring with surface and depth electrodes identifies nonconvulsive seizures and status epilepticus as well as cortical spreading depression, which increase metabolic demand.

3. Airway and ventilation—Patients who are unable to protect the airway because of depressed level of consciousness should be intubated with an endotracheal tube and mechanically ventilated. In the absence of increased ICP, routine hyperventilation is not recommended. Ventilatory parameters should be set to maintain PCO_2 at 35–40 mm Hg and PO_2 at 90–100 mm Hg. Five percent to 30% of patients with traumatic brain injury develop acute lung injury and adult respiratory distress syndrome due to the catecholamine surge and systemic inflammatory reaction after trauma as well as inadequate ventilation strategies. This entity requires a compromise of ventilation strategies for ICP control (high positive end expiratory pressure [PEEP], high tidal volumes) and lung protection (low tidal volumes, permissive hypocapnia, high PEEP), which results in worse neurologic outcome, increased mortality, and longer ICU and hospital stays.

4. Blood pressure—If the patient shows signs of hemodynamic instability, a radial artery catheter should be placed to monitor blood pressure. Because cerebral blood flow autoregulation is frequently impaired in acute head injury, mean blood pressure (or CPP if ICP is being monitored) must be carefully regulated to avoid hypotension, which can lead to cerebral ischemia, or hypertension, which can exacerbate cerebral edema. Continuous infusion of short-acting vasopressors (eg, phenylephrine, dopamine, or norepinephrine) and antihypertensives (eg, labetalol, clevidipine, or nicardipine) are preferable because of their ability to stabilize blood pressure within a narrow therapeutic range. Sodium nitroprusside can cause vasodilation of the cerebral vasculature and raise ICP and should be avoided in patients with any brain injury.

5. Fluids—Only *isotonic fluids,* such as 0.9% (normal) saline, should be administered to patients with head injuries, because the extra free water in half-normal saline or D_5W can exacerbate cerebral edema. Hypertonic saline (3% sodium chloride/acetate solution) may be used as an alternative maintenance fluid in patients with significant brain edema or hypotension. The starting infusion rate is 1 mL/kg/h, adjusted to maintain serum osmolality between 300 and 320 mOsm/L. This strategy has been shown to reduce the frequency and amount of ICP elevations. Central venous pressure monitoring is helpful to guide fluid management in hypotensive or hypovolemic patients and is mandatory for patients treated with hypertonic saline solutions to prevent volume overload and congestive heart failure. A negative fluid balance is associated with poor outcome after traumatic brain injury.

6. Sedation—Patients may become agitated or delirious during their ICU course, putting them at risk for self-injury, removal of monitoring devices, systemic and cerebral hypermetabolism, and increased ICP. For agitated patients who are intubated, a continuous intravenous infusion of a rapidly acting analgesic and sedative agent such as propofol and

sufentanil or remifentanil should be given to attain a quiet, motionless state. Dexmedetomidine hydrochloride, a central α-antagonist, is an attractive alternative when the goal is attaining a calm and cooperative state, because it does not decrease level of consciousness as much as other anesthetic agents. Sedative infusions should be turned off at least once or twice a day to allow neurologic assessments; this strategy also minimizes oversedation and is associated with a shorter duration of mechanical ventilation. Nonintubated patients with delirium can be treated with haloperidol, 2–10 mg intramuscularly every 4 hours; ziprasidone, 10–20 mg intramuscularly or intravenously (maximum, 40 mg/day); or oral aripiprazole or quetiapine as needed.

7. Nutrition—Severe head injury is followed by a generalized hypermetabolic and catabolic response, with caloric requirements that are 50–100% higher than normal. Enteral feedings via nasogastric or nasoduodenal tubes should be instituted and titrated to goal as soon as possible (within 24–48 hours) with a daily goal of 30 kcal/kg. Early enteral feeding after injury is generally well tolerated and improves outcome in comparison with delayed feeding. Gastrokinetic agents (eg, metoclopramide) may help improve enteral tolerability. Total parenteral nutrition carries significant risks, such as infection and electrolyte derangement, and should be used only if enteral feeding cannot be tolerated.

8. Temperature—Fever (temperature >38.3°C [101.0°F]) is common after traumatic brain injury and may be the result of infection or impaired central temperature regulation. Because even small temperature elevations can exacerbate traumatic and ischemic brain injury, fever should be treated aggressively. Newer cooling devices using adhesive cooling pads or intravascular heat-exchange catheters are superior to standard water-circulating cooling blankets for maintaining normal central core temperature in comatose patients with brain injuries.

9. Normoglycemia—Severe head injury is predictably associated with a systemic stress response, which often includes significant levels of hyperglycemia. Continuous insulin infusion therapy to maintain blood glucose between 90 and 140 mg/dL in hyperglycemic patients reduces mortality in critically ill surgical patients. Caution must be exercised to avoid cerebral hypoglycemia, which has a detrimental impact on cerebral function and can be detected by cerebral microdialysis.

10. Corticosteroids—Although glucocorticoids have been used for many years in the treatment of cerebral edema, there is no scientific evidence that they favorably alter outcome or lower ICP in head-injured patients. Further, administration of these agents is complicated by increased risk of infection, hyperglycemia, psychosis, steroid myopathy, and other adverse effects and may increase mortality at 2 weeks. For these reasons, dexamethasone and other corticosteroids are not recommended for patients with head injury.

11. Deep venous thrombosis—Patients with head injury who are immobilized and have central intravenous catheters are at high risk for upper- and lower-extremity deep vein thrombosis and pulmonary thromboembolism. Pneumatic compression boots or antithrombotic stockings should be routinely used to protect against the risk of lower-extremity deep venous thrombosis. Subcutaneous heparin, 5000 IU every 8 hours, or low-molecular-weight heparin, can be added safely 48 hours after injury or surgery, even in the presence of intracranial hemorrhage.

12. Gastric stress ulcer prophylaxis—Patients receiving mechanical ventilation or with coagulopathy are at increased risk of gastric stress ulceration and should receive prophylaxis with either pantoprazole, 40 mg intravenously or orally daily; famotidine, 20 mg intravenously or orally every 12 hours; or sucralfate, 1 g orally every 6 hours.

13. Prophylaxis of vasospasm after subarachnoid hemorrhage—Nimodipine 60 mg orally every 6 hours improves outcome in head-injured patients with CT evidence of subarachnoid hemorrhage on admission. Nimodipine may increase neuronal ischemic tolerance at the cellular level or improve collateral blood flow. Hypotension is the most common adverse event.

14. Seizure prophylaxis—Routine seizure prophylaxis continues to be a debated topic. Administration of antiepileptic drugs is recommended in penetrating brain injury and the presence of a depressed skull fracture and a suspected dural lesion in patients with posttraumatic amnesia for more than 24 hours. Phenytoin or fosphenytoin (15–20 mg/kg loading dose, then 300 mg/day) reduces the frequency of early (ie, first week) post-traumatic seizures but does not prevent the development of later post-traumatic epilepsy. Intravenous valproic acid or levetiracetam is an acceptable alternative for patients with phenytoin allergies. If the patient has not experienced a seizure, prophylactic anticonvulsants should be discontinued after 7 days. Anticonvulsant levels should be monitored closely, because subtherapeutic levels frequently result from drug hypermetabolism or interaction, particularly in younger men. Nonconvulsive seizures or status epilepticus, diagnosable only with continuous electroencephalographic monitoring, occur in 15–18% of comatose patients with traumatic brain injury. These seizures are associated with poor outcome and warrant aggressive treatment with continuous infusion of midazolam, propofol, or similar agents.

▶ Prognosis

Outcome is usually evaluated after 6 months, and 85% of recovery occurs within that time period. GCS motor score, pupillary response, CT findings, and age are most predictive of long-term outcome after head trauma (Table 14–7). Also of prognostic importance are hypotension; hypoxemia on admission; eye and verbal components of the GCS; glucose,

Table 14–7. Estimated Mortality Based on Various Features of Head Injury

Clinical Finding	Mortality (%)[a]
Glasgow Coma Scale Score	
15	<1
11–14	3
8–10	15
6–7	20
4–5	50
3	80
Age[b]	
16–35 y	30
36–45 y	40
46–55 y	50
>56 y	60
CT Abnormalities[b]	
None	10
Intracranial pathology without diffuse swelling of midline shift	15
Intracranial pathology with diffuse swelling (cisterns compressed or absent	35
Intracranial pathology with midline shift (>5 mm)	55
Intracranial Pressure[b]	
<20 mm Hg	15
>20 mm Hg, reducible	45
>20 mm Hg, not reducible	90
Pathologic Entity	
Epidural hematoma	5–15
Gunshot wound	55
Acute subdural hematoma	
• Simple	20–25
• Complicated	40–75
• Bilateral	75–100

CT = computed tomography.
[a]Percentages are adapted from several sources and have been rounded.
[b]Among comatose patients.
Data are adapted from Greenberg J, Brawanshki A. Cranial trauma. In: Hacke W, ed. *Neurocritical Care.* Springer-Verlag, 1994:705; Vollmer DG, et al. *J Neurosurg* 1991;75(suppl 1):S37–S49; Marshall LF, et al. *J Neurosurg* 1991;75(suppl 1):S28–S36; Miller JD, et al. Significance of intracranial hyper-tension in severe head injury. *J Neurosurg* 1977;47:503–516. Reproduced with permission from Rowland LP, ed. *Merritt's Textbook of Neurology,* 11th ed. Lippincott Williams & Wilkins, 2005.

platelets, and hemoglobin on admission; coagulopathy; persistently elevated ICP; and critically reduced (<10 mm Hg) brain tissue oxygen levels. In the Traumatic Coma Data Bank (coma defined as GCS ≤8), an observational study of 746 patients, 33% died, 14% entered a vegetative state, 28% remained dependent with severe disability, 19% regained independence with moderate disability, and only 7% made a full or near-complete recovery.

As noted, the admission GCS score (see Table 14–2) has substantial prognostic value: Patients with a GCS score of 3 or 4 (deep coma) have an up to 80% chance of dying or remaining in a vegetative state. Such outcomes occur in only 5–10% of patients with a GCS score of 12 or higher. In general, elderly patients have a poor prognosis. In one series of comatose patients older than 65 years, only 10% survived and only 4% regained functional independence. Death may result from the direct effect of the injury or from complications. Attempts to predict a firm prognosis in patients with severe head injuries, especially in the early stages, are hazardous, however, because outcome depends on many variables.

Persistent vegetative state is a much-feared outcome of traumatic coma. In general, the prospects of recovery from prolonged traumatic coma are better than from prolonged coma of other causes. Functional MRI studies showed processing of external stimuli in the human cortex in patients with persistent vegetative state. Fifty percent of adults and 60% of children who are comatose for more than 30 days as a result of traumatic brain injury will recover consciousness within 1 year, compared with 15% of patients with prolonged coma from nontraumatic causes. Recovery of consciousness is operationally defined as the ability to follow commands convincingly and consistently.

Early cognitive, physical, and occupational therapy is an important part of optimizing recovery after traumatic brain injury. Physical therapy, including range-of-motion exercises to prevent limb contractures, can begin even while patients are still in the ICU. Once patients are stabilized, they should be transferred to a rehabilitation facility specializing in acute or subacute care. Whether cognitive rehabilitative measures truly improve neuropsychological outcome remains to be established.

In a study of patients with moderate or severe injuries, only 46% returned to work 2 years after initial injury, and most of those who did return to work did not go back to their positions held before traumatic brain injury. Only 18% were financially independent. Vocational training can play a key role in helping patients reintegrate into their workplace.

Individualizable outcome prediction models for patients with traumatic brain injury are available from the International Mission for Prognosis and Analysis of Clinical Trials in Traumatic Brain Injury (IMPACT) and Corticosteroid Randomisation After Significant Head Injury (CRASH) trial databases online (see Table 14–1).

Abdolvahabi RM, Dutcher SA, Wellwood JM, Michael DB. Craniovertebral missile injuries. *Neurol Res* 2001;23:210–218. (Review of gunshot injuries.)

Bell RB, Dierks EJ, Homer L, Potter BE. Management of cerebrospinal fluid leak associated with craniomaxillofacial trauma. *J Oral Maxillofacial Surg* 2004;62:676–684. [PMID: 15170277]

The Brain Trauma Foundation, American Association of Neurological Surgeons, Joint Section on Neurotrauma and Critical Care. Trauma systems: Guidelines for the Management of Severe Traumatic Brain Injury. 3rd Edition. *J Neurotrauma* 2007;24 (suppl 1):1–106 or www.braintrauma.org.

Clifton GL, et al. Lack of effect of induction of hypothermia after acute brain injury. *N Engl J Med* 2001;344:556–563. [PMID: 11207351] (Hypothermia with body temperature reaching 33°C [91.4°F] within 8 hours after injury assigned to 392 patients with head trauma in a randomized, controlled trial did not alter mortality and was associated with more frequent complications and prolonged hospital stay.)

Dennis LJ, Mayer SA. Diagnosis and management of increased intracranial pressure. *Neurol India* 2001;49(suppl 1):S37–50. [PMID: 11889475]

Glauser J. Head injury: Which patients need imaging? Which test is best? *Cleve Clin J Med* 2004;71:353–357.

Maas AIR, Stocchetti N, Bullock R. Moderate and severe traumatic brain injury in adults. *Lancet Neurol* 2008;7:728–741 [PMID: 18635021]

Mascia L. Acute lung injury in patients with severe brain injury: A double hit model. *Neurocrit Care* 2009;11:417–426. [PMID: 19548120]

Murray GD, et al. Multivariable prognostic analysis in traumatic brain injury: Results from the IMPACT Study. *J Neurotrauma* 2007;24:329–337. [PMID: 17375997]

Oertel M, et al. Progressive hemorrhage after head trauma: Predictors and consequences of the evolving injury. *J Neurosurg* 2002;96:109–116. [PMID: 11794591]

Roberts I, et al; CRASH Trial Collaborators. Effect of intravenous corticosteroids on death within 14 days in 10008 adults with clinically significant head injury (MRC CRASH Trial): Randomized placebo-controlled trial. *Lancet* 2004;364:1321–1328. [PMID: 15474134] (Randomized, placebo-controlled trial showing increase in mortality 2 weeks after head trauma with administration of methylprednisolone compared with placebo.)

Rohde V, Graf G, Hassler W. Complications of burr-hole craniostomy and closed-system drainage for chronic subdural hematomas: A retrospective analysis of 376 patients. *Neurosurg Rev* 2002;25:89–94. [PMID: 11954771]

Stiver SI, Manley GT. Prehospital management of traumatic brain injury. *Neurosurg Focus* 2008;25:E5. [PMID: 18828703]

Weigel R, Schmiedek P, Krauss JK. Outcome of contemporary surgery for chronic subdural haematoma: Evidence based review. *J Neurol Neurosurg Psychiatry* 2003;74:937–943. [PMID: 12810784]

SPINAL TRAUMA

ESSENTIALS OF DIAGNOSIS

▶ History or clinical evidence of trauma

▶ Spinal pain or tenderness

▶ Radicular signs at the level of injury; sensorimotor deficits and bladder and bowel dysfunction below the level of injury

▶ CT or MRI scan showing bone, joint, or disk abnormalities with root or cord compression

General Considerations

Between 8000 and 50,000 people suffer an acute spinal cord injury in North America each year. Multiple noncontinuous vertebral levels are involved in 20% of spinal cord injuries. Nearly 60% of those injured are children or young adults 30 years of age or younger. However, the mean age has increased steadily from 28.7 years in 1979 to 37.6 years in 2000; the proportion of persons older than 60 years at injury has also increased from 4.7% before 1980 to 10.9% after 2000. Men are affected four times more often than women. The aggregate cost for management of spinal cord injury is US $22.16 billion per year. The most common cause of spinal trauma is motor vehicle accidents, followed by gunshot wounds. In blunt polytrauma, the cervical spine is affected in approximately 2–12% of patients, and spinal trauma must be seriously considered in every unconscious victim. Missed or delayed recognition greatly increases the risk of permanent neurologic impairment.

Pathogenesis & Clinical Findings

The initial injury of the spinal cord occurs through four different mechanisms: (1) impact with persistent compression in burst fractures; (2) impact with only transient compression after hyperextension injuries; (3) distraction resulting in forcible stretching of the spinal column in the axial plane, with shearing of the spinal cord or its blood supply; or (4) laceration from missile injury, sharp bone fragment dislocation, or severe distraction, with or without transection.

The gray matter is primarily affected and irreversibly damaged within 1 hour of injury. There may be evidence of early hemorrhage within the spinal cord. The white matter may be spared initially but is irreversibly injured within 72 hours after initial insult as a result of hemorrhage, ischemia and reperfusion, excitotoxicity, calcium-mediated cellular dysfunction, fluid and electrolyte disturbances, immunologic mechanisms, or apoptosis. Neurogenic shock can ensue, with bradycardia and hypotension. Table 14–8 summarizes clinical findings and management of cervical and thoracolumbar spine injuries and cauda equina syndrome.

Clinical Evaluation

A. Transportation and Initial Assessment

Management of the patient with a potential spinal cord injury begins at the scene of the accident. Up to 25% of spinal cord injuries occur after the initial traumatic event as a result of inappropriate transportation or early intervention, and the outcome in these patients is poor. Complete immobilization of the spine is the crucial step in prehospital management of all trauma patients until spinal injury has been excluded. Hard backboards with occipital padding, a rigid cervical collar, lateral support devices, and straps and tapes to secure the patient to the collar, board, or lateral support are recommended. The spine should be in its normal anatomic position, defined as the position assumed while standing and looking ahead, with occiput elevation by 1.3–5.1 cm above ground in a supine position, which increases the spinal canal-to-spinal cord ratio at C5 and C6. Moving the patient onto the backboard should be done by experienced rescuers. Once the patient's spine is immobilized, he or she should be rapidly transported to a dedicated center with adequate resources and expertise.

In the emergency department, clearance of the airway, maintenance of oxygenation, and ventilation are complicated by the need for spinal immobilization. Pulmonary problems are expected in patients with injuries to the upper and midcervical spine (C3–C5, output to the phrenic nerve). Concurrent pulmonary and thoracic trauma, such as rib fracture, pulmonary contusion, pneumothorax, hemothorax, and aspiration, can also compromise pulmonary function. Intubation should be considered early in the course, and should be performed under fiberoptic guidance in a controlled environment. Any form of traction on the spine, neck hyperextension, and misalignment must be avoided. There is no benefit of nasotracheal over the orotracheal route. If intubation cannot be performed easily, alternatives such as laryngeal masks may be used until a surgical airway can be established.

Patients with spinal cord injury are extremely sensitive to hypoperfusion. Early hypotension is associated with increased mortality and decreased neurologic recovery. Autonomic instability with loss of sympathetic tone resulting in peripheral pooling of volume and bradycardia may complicate volume resuscitation. Hypotension can also be a symptom of spinal shock. The MAP (systolic plus 2 times diastolic pressure, divided by 3) should be maintained at 90–100 mm Hg by means of volume load or vasopressors for about 72 hours. α-Agonists (eg, phenylephrine) increase peripheral vascular resistance and counteract the loss of sympathetic tone. Dopamine or dobutamine are alternative vasoactive agents. Leg elevation and compression stockings or boots are helpful for volume distribution. A baseline electrocardiogram and cardiac enzymes should be obtained on admission in patients older than 40 years of age and those with a history of cardiac disease. Anticholinergic agents such as atropine, 0.5–1 mg intravenously, can reverse bradycardia. High-velocity chest injury with thoracic spine fracture can cause cardiac contusion and tamponade, diagnosed by echocardiogram.

Patients with spinal cord injury who arrive in the emergency department within 8 hours of initial injury should receive an intravenous methylprednisolone bolus of 30 mg/kg over 1 hour (see Treatment, later), followed by 5.4 mg/kg/h for the next 23 hours.

The spine must remain immobilized until it is specifically "cleared" by different neuroimaging techniques.

B. History and Physical Examination Findings

The time frame, circumstances of the accident, and previous condition of the patient should be obtained from witnesses,

Table 14–8. Spinal Injuries and Cauda Equina Syndrome: Clinical Findings and Management

Classification	Mechanism	Stability	Associated Injuries	Imaging Studies	Treatment
Upper Cervical Spine Injuries					
Atlanto-occipital dislocation	Traction and disruption of ligaments between skull, C1, and C2	Unstable	Usually none	Lateral radiograph–clivus–odontoid distance >5 mm	Surgical stabilization
C1/Atlas Fracture					
Bilateral posterior arch fracture	Compression and extension of cervical spine	Stable	Odontoid fracture	Odontoid-view radiograph through patient's open mouth CT scan through C1 arch	Orthosis
Lateral mass fracture	Fracture of ipsilateral anterior and posterior arches following compression with lateral bending	Stable if no lateral mass widening Unstable if lateral mass widening	Usually none	Same as above	Orthosis If intermass widening >6.9 mm or atlanto-dens interval >3 mm, traction and halo immobilization is required If atlanto-dens interval >5 mm, C1–C2 fusion is indicated
Jefferson fracture	Four-part C1 fractures from direct axial compression	Stable if no lateral mass widening Unstable if lateral mass widening	Retropharyngeal swelling	Same as above	Same as above
Hangman Fracture (Spondylolisthesis of Axis)					
I	Disruption of posterior arch; disk and posterior ligament intact	Stable	Usually none	Lateral radiograph	Orthosis
II	Anterior displacement of C2 on C3 through disk, with intact posterior ligament	Unstable	Usually none	Same as above	Traction and halo immobilization
III	Fracture of arch; facets of C2 attached to vertebral body	Unstable	Bilateral facet dislocation	Same as above	Surgical stabilization
Lower Cervical Spine Injuries (C3–C7)					
Unilateral or bilateral facet dislocation	Flexion with tension to facet capsule and interspinous ligaments; subluxation in 25% of patients	Unstable	Nerve root involvement	Lateral, anteroposterior, and oblique radiographs MRI to rule out disk herniation	Traction and fusion

(Continued)

Table 14–8. Spinal Injuries and Cauda Equina Syndrome: Clinical Findings and Management (*Continued*)

Classification	Mechanism	Stability	Associated Injuries	Imaging Studies	Treatment
Compression fracture	Flexion with 25% compression of middle column and intact posterior ligament	Stable or unstable	Usually none	Lateral flexion and extension radiographs MRI	Orthosis if posterior ligament is stable Fusion if posterior ligament is injured
Burst fracture	Compression and flexion	Stable or unstable	Cord and root compression	Lateral radiograph CT MRI	Halo immobilization if posterior ligament is intact and there is no neurologic deficit Posterior fusion and halo immobilization if posterior ligament is ruptured and there is no neurologic deficit Anterior corpectomy and fusion, posterior fusion, and halo immobilization if posterior ligament is unstable and neurologic deficit is present
Thoracolumbar Spine Injuries					
Compression fracture	Failure of anterior column with intact middle and posterior column	Stable	Usually none	Lateral radiograph	Hyperextension-type braces
Burst fracture	Axial load resulting in compression of anterior and middle columns and retropulsion of bone into canal	Unstable	Cord and root compression	Lateral radiograph—widening of interpedicle distance	Surgical stabilization Decompression and internal fixation if neurologic deficit is present
Chance fracture or seat belt injury	Flexion and distraction resulting in failure of middle and posterior columns with tension onto anterior column	Stable	Usually none	Lateral radiograph	Brace
Cauda Equina Syndrome	Traction and pelvic fractures following gunshot injuries, motor vehicle accidents, and falls from height	Unstable	Root compression resulting in paresthesias radiating down legs, leg weakness, sensory deficit in perineal area, and loss of bladder and bowel function	CT MRI	Surgical decompression, spinal nerve reconstruction, repair of ventral nerves and nerve transfer

CT = computed tomography; MRI = magnetic resonance imaging.

rescue service records, and family members. Patients should be questioned about neck pain, tenderness, neurologic deficits, and bladder or bowel incontinence.

Neurologic assessment of spinal cord injury should focus on strength testing of extremity muscle groups, muscle tone, sensation of touch, pain, vibration and proprioception according to dermatomes, identification of a sensory level, exaggeration or absence of deep tendon reflexes, and evaluation of rectal tone (see also Chapter 18).

If possible within the limits of immobilization, the spine should be inspected and palpated for open or closed fractures and hematomas. Chest, abdomen, and pelvis should be examined for fractures and internal organ injury. Stool and urine should be checked for presence of blood.

C. Imaging Studies: "Clearing" the Spine

Before a cervical collar and other measures of immobilization can be removed, spinal injury must be absolutely excluded ("cleared"). The preferred procedure for "clearing" the spine depends on the presence of pain and neurologic symptoms and on the mental status of the patient.

Patients who are awake, without other painful distracting injuries, and who do not complain of localized pain or tenderness of the cervical spine or neurologic symptoms do not require radiologic studies of the cervical spine after trauma. The negative predictive value of cervical spine radiographic assessment for significant cervical spine injury is virtually 100% in this population (Table 14–9).

The incidence of cervical spine injury in symptomatic patients is approximately 2–6%. Patients who complain of neck pain or spine tenderness, who have a neurologic deficit, who are unconscious, uncooperative, incoherent, or intoxicated, or who have associated traumatic injuries that can be confused with spinal cord injury require radiologic study of the cervical spine. In most patients, a lateral cervical radiograph will identify an unstable fracture. Many spinal injuries are detected by three-view cervical spine series (lateral,

anteroposterior, odontoid views); however, up to 60% of fractures are missed on radiographs compared with CT scans. Multislice CT through areas that are difficult to visualize and suspected of structural injury (eg, the upper three cervical vertebrae), with sagittal reconstruction in all and coronal reconstruction for craniocervical junction injuries, is now the standard imaging modality in acute cervical spine injury. The combination of CT and radiography represents the minimum in neuroimaging required for the symptomatic and unconscious patient and has a negative predictive value of 99–100%.

Dynamic flexion-extension radiographic views up to 30 degrees in each direction in the awake and symptomatic patient can be added to assess potentially unstable ligamentous or osteoligamentous injuries. They are most useful within 7–14 days after trauma. The negative predictive value of the combination of three-view and dynamic cervical spine radiography reaches more than 99%. Pain and spasm in alert patients with limited mobility often result in nondiagnostic flexion-extension radiographs. Those patients can be immobilized in a hard collar for 7–10 days to let muscle spasms subside before flexion-extension radiographs are repeated.

In obtunded and comatose patients, bedside flexion-extension radiographs under fluoroscopy are safe if performed by experienced staff trained in radiology or neurosurgery.

MRI is another option for spine "clearance" in obtunded patients. If performed within 48 hours, it is more sensitive than CT and radiography in identifying injury to neural tissue or ligaments. A negative finding on MRI within 48 hours after the incident is effective in eliminating significant ligamentous injury, but false-positive findings are common. If there is evidence of neurologic deficits or vascular injury, or if closed reduction of cervical spine is planned, an MRI evaluation should be obtained. Findings on MRT have been found to be a useful predictor of neurologic improvement after spinal cord injury.

▶ Treatment

Patients with acute spinal injury, especially in the context of multisystem trauma, are best managed in an ICU with continuous cardiovascular and pulmonary monitoring for the first 7–14 days after injury. They are at risk for hypotension, hypoxemia, pulmonary dysfunction, and cardiovascular instability, especially when there is concurrent neurologic dysfunction with dysautonomia.

A. Immobilization

Prolonged spinal immobilization on firm mattresses, spinal boards, and in cervical hard collars carries significant risks. It can lead to additional spinal pain and tenderness, pain in the cranial area, neurologic deficits, and respiratory compromise. Cutaneous pressure ulcers are present after 48–72 hours in up to 55% of patients with cervical spine injury and disturbed cutaneous vasoregulation. Skin grafts are required in many of

Table 14–9. NEXUS Low-Risk Criteria for Cervical Spine Injury

Neuroimaging is not needed in patients who meet the following criteria. All five criteria must be fulfilled:
1. No tenderness at midline of posterior cervical spine
2. No focal neurologic deficit
3. Normal level of alertness
4. No evidence of intoxication
5. No painful injury that might distract from pain of cervical spine injury

NEXUS = National Emergency X-Radiography Utilization Study. Reproduced with permission from Hendey GW, Wolson AB, Mower WR, Hoffman JR. National Emergency X-Radiography Utilization Study Group. Spinal cord injury without radiographic abnormality: Results of the National Emergency X-Radiography Utilization Study in blunt cervical trauma. *J Trauma* 2002;53:1–4.

Table 14–10. Complications of Prolonged Immobilization Following Spinal Trauma

- Infection of a skin ulcer or a spinal prosthesis after operative fixation, followed by septic shock
- Secondary ischemia and infarction of brain parenchyma resulting from elevated intracranial pressure through venous congestion
- Difficulty in performing intubation and percutaneous tracheostomy procedures, obtaining central venous access, and performing subsequent line care and oral-dental care
- Increased enteric nutrition intolerance and requirements for parenteral nutrition
- Bacterial translocation
- Gastrostasis, reflux, and aspiration risk
- Increased risk of ventilator-associated pneumonia because of restrictions in physical therapy regimens
- Increased incidence of cross-contamination because more staff is required for bedding and personal care

these patients. Additional complications are listed in Table 14–10. Consequently, "clearing" of the spine and discontinuation of immobilization should be made a priority. If there is evidence of an unstable spinal injury, reduction and surgical fixation should be undertaken as early as possible.

B. Surgical Intervention

Traumatic cervical spine fractures and cervical facet dislocation injuries compromising the spinal canal and its blood supply should be treated with closed reduction in awake patients by a trained specialist early in the course. Permanent neurologic deficits after this procedure occur in roughly 1% of patients. Transient neurologic complications are seen in 2–4%. Closed traction-reduction is safer than manipulation under anesthesia. Neurologic deterioration is usually related to inadequate immobilization, unrecognized head injury, loss of reduction, hemodynamic instability, or respiratory compromise. MRI obtained before reduction may demonstrate potentially hazardous cervical disk herniation that could lead to further neurologic deficits during the procedure, but it also delays fracture realignment and decompression of the cervical cord.

If closed reduction fails, patients should undergo detailed neuroimaging before open reduction is attempted. Disk herniation is a relative indication for anterior decompression, with or followed by a posterior procedure. MRI should be obtained in obtunded patients before any reduction procedure.

Early stabilization of the surgical spine is beneficial and safe in multitrauma patients with spinal injuries. However, the ideal timing of surgical intervention in patients with spinal trauma and neurologic deficits is controversial. Delay in admission, imaging, and availability of operating rooms are major hurdles in the timing of surgery. Increased functional improvement was observed in animal studies after early surgical decompression. The randomized, controlled, prospective Surgical Treatment for Acute Spinal Cord Injury

Study (STASCIS) demonstrated neurologic improvement in a greater proportion of patients at 1 year randomized to surgical decompression within 24 hours after injury compared with later surgery. In general, surgery as early as possible allows earlier mobilization and rehabilitation and reduces the incidence of postoperative infection, pulmonary disease, and thromboembolism.

C. Corticosteroids and Other Neuroprotection Strategies

Corticosteroids have the potential to stabilize membrane structures and maintain the blood–spinal cord barrier, resulting in decreased vasogenic edema, enhanced spinal cord blood flow, inhibition of endorphin release, scavenging of damaging free radicals, and reduced inflammation. Patients treated with methylprednisolone, given as an intravenous bolus of 30 mg/kg, followed by an infusion of 5.4 mg/kg/h for 23 hours, experienced significant improvement of motor function and sensation at 6 months and of right-sided motor function at 1 year if administered within 8 hours after injury. However, the use of methylprednisolone is associated with an increased incidence of wound infection, pneumonia, urinary tract infection, gastrointestinal bleeding, early hyperglycemia, glucosuria, and abnormal liver function tests, especially in older and diabetic patients, and it resulted in longer hospital stays, especially if administered for 48 hours. Moreover, improvement in functional recovery with the use of methylprednisolone appears not to be clinically important. Currently, the administration of intravenous methylprednisolone in conjunction with gastric protection is recommended for 23 hours if started within 8 hours of injury. Alternative pharmacotherapies of as-yet unproven benefit are shown in Table 14–11.

Table 14–11. Alternative Pharmacotherapies of Unproven Benefit in Spinal Cord Trauma

Drug	Proposed Mechanisms	Proposed Benefit
GM$_1$-ganglioside	Acceleration of neurite growth Stimulation of nerve regeneration and regrowth	Marked recovery earlier with GM1 administered within 8 h after injury compared with placebo
Tirilazad mesylate	Lipid peroxyl and hydroxyl radical scavenging mechanisms analogous to vitamin E	Similar efficacy compared with methylprednisolone
	Facilitation of endogenous vitamin E action	Lower rates of pneumonia and urinary tract infection
	Stabilization of membranes by decreasing membrane fluidity	

Systemic hypothermia slows neuronal metabolism and therefore reduces energy requirements. Whereas animal studies of hypothermia applied in acute spinal cord injury show controversial results, the prehospital cooling of Buffalo Bills player Kevin Everett followed by decompression and fusion of his cervical spine with a dramatic neurologic recovery at 4 months created enthusiasm to initiate a prospective trial of prehospital systemic hypothermia for acute spinal cord injury.

Other emerging treatment concepts include transplantation of olfactory ensheathing cells, which are specialized glia cells with the ability to facilitate the passage of new axons from the peripheral nervous system to a target neuron in the central nervous system, and human embryonic stem cell oligodendrocyte progenitor cells, which enhance remyelination into the injured spinal cord with the aim to improve paralysis.

D. Blood Pressure Management

In spinal cord–injured patients with hemodynamic instability as a consequence of autonomic dysfunction, an arterial line and a central venous catheter enable close monitoring of arterial blood pressure and fluid status. Hypotension can worsen the initial insult. The mean arterial blood pressure should be maintained at levels of 85–90 mm Hg to ensure adequate perfusion of the spinal cord for at least 7 days after injury. Vasopressors such as phenylephrine, dopamine, and norepinephrine and fluid boluses should be used as required, but weaned slowly.

E. General Care

Atelectasis and pneumonia result from difficulty clearing secretions and small spontaneous tidal volumes due to paralysis of respiratory muscles. Mucus plug formation can be life-threatening despite mechanical ventilation. Patients should be placed on kinetic therapy beds (RotoRest). Bronchodilator treatment, chest physiotherapy, and intermittent positive pressure breathing (recruitment maneuver) help reexpand lung volumes. In patients with mid- and high-level cervical injury, tracheostomy should be an early consideration.

Nonintubated patients should receive supplemental oxygen to maintain pulse oximetry saturation greater than 95%. The presence of pneumothorax in thoracic trauma necessitates thoracostomy tube placement and careful monitoring with concurrent use of positive pressure ventilation.

The risk of skin breakdown in immobilized patients is high and is increased further in those with decreased or absent sensation and autonomic failure. Early mobilization and early delivery of adequate enteral nutrition are the best preventive strategies. Orthoses should be well fitted. Frequent turning, use of air mattresses, daily bathing, lotion application, and careful skin inspection, especially of all contact areas, are crucial steps in managing these patients.

Deep venous thrombosis and subsequent pulmonary embolism are extremely common in patients with spinal cord injury, particularly in the context of leg and pelvic fractures. Administration of subcutaneous heparin at 5000 IU every 8 hours or low-molecular-weight heparin in conjunction with lower-extremity pneumatic compression devices, antithrombotic stockings, or electrical stimulation are recommended for at least 3 months after injury.

Patients with spinal cord injury frequently experience urinary retention caused by neurogenic bladder. An indwelling catheter is appropriate during the acute period in the ICU. After 1–2 weeks, once the patient is hemodynamically and neurologically stable, an intermittent sterile catheterization program every 4–6 hours should be instituted, and the indwelling catheter should be removed.

F. Nutritional Support

The hypermetabolic response seen after acute brain trauma seems to be blunted in spinal cord trauma because of muscle denervation. In the acute setting, protein catabolism leads to loss of lean body mass. Early enteral nutritional support should meet caloric and nitrogen requirements. Indirect calorimetry is recommended to assess energy expenditure in acute and chronic stages of spinal cord injury.

G. Management of Vertebral Artery Injuries

Vertebral artery injury occurs in approximately 11% of patients with nonpenetrating cervical spinal trauma. Most patients are asymptomatic, but complications from vertebral artery dissection, such as brainstem infarction, can be disabling and life-threatening. CT angiography, MRI and MR angiography, and duplex sonography can identify vertebral artery injury. When in doubt, cerebral angiography should be performed.

The optimal management of traumatic vertebral artery dissection is uncertain. Anticoagulation might prevent thromboembolic complications but carries a risk of bleeding complications as high as 14%. Therefore, whether to administer anticoagulant therapy to a patient with vertebral artery injury should be decided on an individual basis.

▶ Prognosis

Mortality after spinal cord injury ranges between 4% and 17%. Predisposing factors include advanced age, cord injury at a higher spinal level, pulmonary embolism, medical comorbidities, and suicide. Age greater than 20 years, male gender, severe systemic injuries (Injury Severity Score [ISS]≥15), comorbidities, poor neurologic status on admission, and level 1 trauma center admission have been identified as significant predictors of early mortality (before discharge).

Whether patients with spinal injury will return to previous occupations and lifestyles, as well as their subsequent care levels and ambulation potential, depends on several variables, which are outlined in Table 14–12.

Table 14–12. Predictive Factors for Recovery Potential in Patients With Traumatic Spinal Injury

- Neurologic level of injury, specifically motor level of injury
- Completeness of injury
- Patient age
- Energy expenditure
- Cardiopulmonary status
- Spasticity, contractures, and pain
- Associated injuries
- Motor power (pelvic control, hip flexors, knee extensors)

Patients with incomplete injury of the sensory pathways—even when loss of motor function is complete—have a better prognosis for regaining functional ambulation than tetraplegic patients with absent sensation below the level of injury. Recovery of distal muscles may not begin until 3 weeks or longer after injury. Patients with Brown-Séquard syndrome have the greatest potential for functional recovery; 75–90% can walk independently after discharge from rehabilitation, and 70% regain skills and activities of independent daily living. The recovery of lower-extremity strength in central cord syndrome is seen earlier than in other body regions and is followed by improved bladder function and proximal upper-extremity strength. The C7 segment is critical for triceps function and therefore for independent transfer, which contributes to bowel care, showering, and dressing. Patients aged 50 years or younger experience a faster and more successful recovery toward independence (97% versus 41% in older patients). Ambulation requires three to nine times more energy in paraplegic patients.

Most goals of rehabilitation, including ambulation, are not reached after the initial inpatient program, and a continuous interdisciplinary outpatient and inpatient process is obligatory. Several options in physical therapy might assist in decreasing the burden of neurologic injury and multisystemic complications. These include biofeedback, electrical and magnetic stimulation techniques, functional neuromuscular stimulation (to restore diaphragm function, bladder and bowel function, grasp and release, and upper-extremity control), tendon transfer, and rhizotomy of posterior sacral nerves (to minimize bladder reflex mechanisms).

Chesnut RM. Management of brain and spine injuries. *Crit Care Med* 2004;20:25–55. [PMID: 14979328]

Cohen WA, et al. Evidence-based approach to use MR imaging in acute spinal trauma. *Eur J Radiol* 2003;48:49–60. [PMID: 14511860]

Gittler MS, et al. Spinal cord injury medicine. 3. Rehabilitation outcomes. *Arch Phys Med Rehabil* 2002;83(suppl 1):S65–S71. [PMID: 11973699]

Kirshblum SC, et al. Spinal cord injury medicine. 1. Etiology, classification, and acute medical management. *Arch Phys Med Rehabil* 2002;83(suppl 1):S50–S57. [PMID: 11973697]

Morris CG, McCoy EP, Lavery GG. Spinal immobilization for unconscious patients with multiple injuries. *BMJ* 2004;329:495–499. [PMID: 15331475]

Morris CG, Mullan B. Clearing the cervical spine after polytrauma: Implementing unified management for unconscious victims in the intensive care unit. *Anaesthesia* 2004;59:755–761. [PMID: 15270965]

Patel RV, Delong W Jr, Vresilovic EJ. Evaluation and treatment of spinal injuries in the patient with polytrauma. *Clin Orthop Relat Res* 2004;422:43–54. [PMID: 15187832]

Varma A, et al. Predictors of early mortality after traumatic spinal cord injury. *Spine* 2010;35:778–783. [PMID: 20228715]

Movement Disorders

Amanda Deligtisch, MD, Blair Ford, MD, Howard Geyer, MD, & Susan B. Bressman, MD

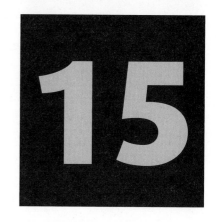

Movement disorders are conditions that produce inadequate or excessive movement. Neurologic disorders that result in a paucity or slowness of movement are termed *hypokinetic* disorders. The category of hypokinetic disorders is represented by Parkinson disease and other causes of parkinsonism. *Hyperkinetic* disorders are characterized by excessive, involuntary movements. Hyperkinetic disorders can usually be placed into one of five main categories of abnormal movement: dystonia, chorea, tremor, myoclonus, or tic.

Abnormal movements may be difficult to recognize or categorize because of their unusual appearance, complexity, subtlety, or variability. Movement disorder specialists tend to isolate or reduce abnormal movements to their unitary components, but often it is the pattern of the movement and its body part distribution that provides the important diagnostic clue. In addition, many diseases cause abnormal movements that can be fit into two or more categories or abnormal movement phenomenology. Table 15–1 provides descriptions of the main categories of movement disorders.

There are many other types of abnormal movements that do not fit cleanly into a simple classification of phenomenology. *Athetosis*, meaning "no fixed posture," was first coined in reference to postanoxic birth injury and characterized by a quivering "fibrillary" movement of the limbs and digits. In modern usage, the term describes a slow, continuous, writhing movement that bears similarities to both chorea and dystonia. *Ballism* refers to very large amplitude, random, flinging movements of the limbs and represents a proximal form of chorea. Unilateral ballism is termed *hemiballism* and is most often caused by an infarct of the contralateral subthalamic nucleus. *Akathisia*, meaning "inability to sit," describes inner restlessness and intolerance of remaining still, together with repetitive fidgeting, squirming, and pacing movements.

Many, but not all, movement disorders result from disordered function of the basal ganglia, a group of interconnected subcortical nuclei. The basal ganglia comprise the substantia nigra, putamen, caudate, globus pallidus, thalamus, and subthalamic nucleus, making up an extrapyramidal

motor control system with extensive, reciprocal connections to the cortex, brainstem, and cerebellum.

Very few movement disorders have specific treatment. Besides rare metabolic causes of parkinsonism or dystonia, most movement disorders are treated empirically, using agents that suppress or reduce unwanted symptoms but do not address the underlying pathophysiology. Nonetheless, movement disorders as a group of neurologic diseases represent a subspecialty that in recent decades has been driven by advances in therapeutics, pharmacologic and surgical. In the sections that follow, each of the major movement disorder syndromes are described, with an emphasis on clinical diagnosis and treatment.

PARKINSONISM & PARKINSON DISEASE

ESSENTIALS OF DIAGNOSIS

- ▶ Tremor at rest
- ▶ Bradykinesia
- ▶ Rigidity
- ▶ Loss of postural reflexes
- ▶ Flexed posture
- ▶ Freezing (motor blocks)

▶ General Considerations

The term *parkinsonism* may be used when a patient exhibits one or more of the following findings: tremor at rest, bradykinesia, rigidity, loss of postural reflexes, flexed posture, and freezing (motor blocks). Two of these findings, with at least one being tremor at rest or bradykinesia must be present to make a diagnosis of definite parkinsonism. Parkinson disease (PD), the most common form of parkinsonism,

Table 15-1. General Classification of Abnormal Movements

	Category of Movement	Description and Associated Clinical Features	Differential Diagnosis

Hypokinetic	Parkinsonism	Akinesia/bradykinesia, Rigidity
		Tremor at rest
		Postural instability
		Gait freezing
		Flexion posture
			Parkinson disease
			Diffuse Lewy body disease
			Atypical neurodegenerative Parkinson syndromes:
			    Progressive supranuclear palsy (PSP), multiple
			    systems atrophy (MSA), corticobasoganglionic
			    degeneration (CBGD)
			Hydrocephalus
			Vascular parkinsonism
			Neuroleptic-induced parkinsonism
			Wilson disease

Hyperkinetic	Dystonia	Torsional movements that are partially sustained and produce twisting postures	Idiopathic or primary dystonia Dopa-responsive dystonia Anoxic-hypoxic injury Trauma Post-encephalitic dystonia Tardive dystonia
	Chorea	Random, quick, unsustained, purposeless movements that have an unpredictable, flowing pattern	Huntington disease Neuroacanthocytosis Post-infectious chorea Drug-induced chorea Vascular chorea Autoimmune chorea Chorea gravidarum
	Tic	Stereotyped, automatic purposeless movements and vocalizations	Tourette syndrome Cerebral palsy/developmental delay syndromes Autism Huntington disease
	Myoclonus	Sudden, shock-like movements	Physiologic myoclonus Essential myoclonus Metabolic encephalopathy Postanoxic myoclonus Progressive myoclonic epilepsy
	Tremor	Repetitive oscillation of a body part	Essential tremor Physiologic tremor Parkinson tremor Cerebellar tremor

makes up 80% of cases of parkinsonism. PD has a prevalence of about 160 cases per 100,000 people and an incidence of about 20 cases per 100,000 people per year. Prevalence and incidence increase with age. Prevalence at age 70 is about 550 cases per 100,000 people, with an approximate incidence of 120 cases per 100,000 people per year. The mean age of symptom onset is 56 years in both sexes. However, the age range is wide, and young-onset PD (occurring in patients younger than 40 years) is not infrequent. PD is nearly twice as common in men as in similarly aged women. Family history of PD appears to be associated with an increased risk for development of PD, and mutations in identified PD genes account for 5–40% of cases depending on an individual's

ancestry. Most of the remainder of cases are thought to be etiologically complex, resulting from gene–environment and gene–gene interactions.

▶ Pathogenesis

The key motor symptoms of primary parkinsonism, PD, result from degeneration of dopamine-producing neurons within the pars compacta of the substantia nigra and the locus ceruleus in the brainstem. However, PD is a complex clinical disorder that includes impaired olfaction, autonomic dysfunction (eg, constipation, cardiac denervation), sleep disturbance (eg, rapid-eye movement [REM] behavior disorder), and alterations in mood and cognition. Underlying these clinical symptoms (many of which may precede overt motor signs) is pathology involving neurons outside the substantia nigra (eg, medullary and olfactory nuclei). The pathologic hallmark of PD is the presence of eosinophilic cytoplasmic inclusions, termed *Lewy bodies,* within many of the surviving neurons. When symptoms become clinically evident, 60% of dopaminergic neurons in the substantia nigra have been lost, and the basal ganglia (striatal) dopamine level has decreased by 80%. The precise cause of degeneration of dopaminergic cells within the substantia nigra is unknown, but recent advances in molecular genetics have clarified genetic influences that contribute to the development of neuronal toxicity and parkinsonism in highly penetrant, autosomal-dominant or autosomal-recessive familial PD. Mutations in six genes (SNCA, LRRK2, PRKN, DJ1, PINK1, and ATP13A2) have conclusively been shown to cause familial parkinsonism. In addition, common variation in three genes (MAPT, LRRK2, and SNCA) and loss-of-function mutations in GBA have been well-validated as susceptibility factors for PD. These genes encode proteins such as α-synuclein, Parkin, and DJ-1, which are involved in folding, trafficking, and clearance of intracellular proteins and in maintaining mitochondrial function. Gene mutations result in mishandling of intracellular proteins, increased oxidative stress, free-radical formation, and energy depletion within the cell, causing oxidative damage and cell death.

▶ Prevention

In PD, preventive strategies have focused on neuroprotection of healthy dopamine-producing cells. However, no drug or dietary supplement has been shown with certainty to have neuroprotective or restorative benefits. Some investigators believe that selegiline and rasagiline, selective, irreversible monoamine oxidase (MAO) B inhibitors, slow the progression of PD, and clinical data in support of rasagiline for neuroprotection are under consideration. Coenzyme Q10 is a supplement that may have neuroprotective properties and currently is under investigation.

▶ Clinical Findings

A. Symptoms and Signs

The cardinal motor findings of PD include resting tremor, bradykinesia, rigidity, loss of postural reflexes, flexed posture, and freezing. Onset of symptoms is insidious and usually unilateral. Progression is usually slow.

1. Resting tremor and bradykinesia—These are the most characteristic motor features of PD. Resting tremor, a tremor of four to six cycles per second that is present at rest, is the presenting symptom in 70% of patients. Classically, rest tremor remains in one limb or asymmetrically in the ipsilateral arm and leg for months or years and may over time generalize to all limbs. Although resting tremor usually

involves distal limbs, it may also affect the muscles of the lips, tongue, jaw, and trunk. Occasionally the tremor is felt as an inner tremor before it can be seen. Typically, the tremor disappears with action of the involved limb and reemerges with maintained posture. Stress, excitement, and walking can increase the tremor.

Bradykinesia manifests as a slowness in activities of daily living, production of movement, and reaction time and contributes to lack of automatic movement. Clinically, patients exhibit impaired fine motor movements, loss of facial expression, reduced arm swing when walking, and flexed (stooped) posture. Hypokinesia (reduced amplitude of movement) is most evident with repetitive movements such as finger and toe tapping. Hypomimia (decreased facial expression) results in decreased blink rate and loss of facial gestures. Other signs of bradykinesia include quiet voice (hypophonia), dysarthria, drooling, micrographia, and difficulty arising from a seated position.

2. Rigidity—Patients with PD have a sustained increased resistance to movement of a limb when that limb is passively extended, flexed, or rotated. Often cog-wheeling can be appreciated. Rigidity occurs proximally at the neck, shoulders, or hips or distally at the elbows, wrists, knees, and ankles. A painful, stiff shoulder is a frequent initial manifestation of PD and is often misdiagnosed as a rotator cuff injury, arthritis, or bursitis.

3. Loss of postural reflexes—A sign of advancing disease, loss of postural reflexes is evident by a patient's inability to maintain balance when pulled from behind. Preservation of postural reflexes occurs early in the course of disease.

4. Freezing—This symptom, which refers to the transient inability to perform active movement, can be one of the most disabling symptoms of PD. Also referred to as *motor blocks,* freezing occurs on initiation of walking, when turning, or walking through narrow passages, crossing streets, or approaching a destination. Patients experience a brief (seconds) inability to move their feet, as if glued to the ground. Freezing that occurs early or predominantly in the course of disease should raise suspicion of an alternate diagnosis such as an atypical parkinsonian syndrome. Festination can occur during walking; patients take faster and faster steps and step size becomes smaller. Freezing, festination, and loss of postural reflexes are important causes of falling in patients with PD.

5. Nonmotor symptoms—Nonmotor symptoms occur frequently in patients with PD and some (eg, impaired olfaction, constipation, REM behavior disorder) may precede overt motor signs by years. Cognitive changes are common and include slowed cognitive functioning, which manifests as prolonged time to verbalize thoughts (bradyphrenia). Dementia eventually occurs in 20–40% of patients with PD (for further discussion, see Chapter 9). Behavioral symptoms include personality changes, depression, reduced attention span, and visuospatial impairment. Sensory symptoms include pain, burning, and tingling. Autonomic disturbances include constipation, impotence, low blood pressure, and inadequate bladder emptying. Loss of motivation, depression, anxiety, sleep disturbances, constipation, loss of smell, and restless legs syndrome may occur in PD or predate the onset of classic motor symptoms. Most of the nonmotor symptoms can cause significant impairment, complicating the course of PD, and should be treated as necessary.

B. Laboratory Tests and Imaging Studies

To date, there is no blood or cerebrospinal fluid test that can diagnose PD. Similarly, there is no biological marker that can diagnose presymptomatic PD. Certain neuroimaging studies can be useful in confirming a diagnosis of PD. Routine magnetic resonance imaging (MRI) is typically normal in patients with PD. Positron emission tomography (PET) imaging of the brain using ^{18}F-fluorodopa shows significant decreases in fluorodopa uptake in the basal ganglia of patients with PD. However, a diagnosis can be made clinically without neuroimaging studies. When toxin-induced or metabolic causes of parkinsonism are suspected, appropriate laboratory studies should be performed.

▶ Differential Diagnosis

The diagnosis of PD is based on history, clinical examination, and the absence of incompatible clinical, laboratory, or radiologic abnormalities. No single feature absolutely confirms or excludes the diagnosis of PD. Initial response to levodopa, which is often dramatic, is expected in PD, but can also occur early in the course of atypical parkinsonian syndromes. Symptomatic improvement from levodopa helps to confirm a diagnosis of PD but is not foolproof.

Specific features that suggest the presence of an **atypical parkinsonian syndrome** rather than PD include symmetric onset of symptoms; absence of tremor; early gait abnormalities, including early falls and prominent freezing; early postural instability; dementia that precedes motor symptoms or occurs within the first year; corticospinal signs; cerebellar signs; abnormal eye movements other than restricted upward gaze; and symptomatic orthostatic hypotension.

Other major causes of parkinsonism are listed in Table 15–2. Drugs that block dopamine receptors (typical and atypical neuroleptics, certain antiemetics) or deplete striatal dopamine (reserpine, tetrabenazine) cause **drug-induced parkinsonism**; the symptoms usually improve slowly and hopefully resolve after the causative drug is stopped. Anticholinergic drugs can improve parkinsonism caused by antidopaminergic drugs.

Normal-pressure hydrocephalus causes a parkinsonian gait disorder notable for short, shuffling, or magnetic steps and loss of postural reflexes. These symptoms are accompanied by dementia and urinary incontinence that develop over time. Imaging of the brain reveals grossly enlarged ventricles. Diagnosis is confirmed by removal of CSF that results in

Table 15–2. Major Parkinsonian Syndromes

Primary Idiopathic Parkinsonism
Parkinson disease (sporadic and familial)

Secondary Parkinsonism
Drug-induced (dopamine antagonists and depletors)
Hydrocephalus (normal-pressure hydrocephalus)
Trauma
Tumor
Vascular (multi-infarct state)
Metabolic (hypoparathyroidism)
Toxin (mercury, manganese, carbon monoxide, cyanide, MPTP)
Infectious (postencephalitic)
Hypoxia

Atypical Parkinsonian Syndromes
Progressive supranuclear palsy
Corticobasal degeneration
Multiple system atrophy:
 • Shy-Drager syndrome
 • Striatal nigral degeneration
 • Olivopontocerebellar atrophy

Dementias
Diffuse Lewy body disease
Alzheimer disease

Inherited Degenerative Diseases
Wilson disease
Huntington disease
Neuroacanthocytosis
Hallervorden-Spatz disease

MPTP = methylphenyltetrahydropyridine.

significant improvement of gait, cognition, and urinary incontinence.

Lower-body parkinsonism may also be caused by vascular disease. **Vascular parkinsonism**, a slowly progressive gait disorder with freezing and loss of postural reflexes, results from multiple lacunar infarcts that are easily seen on MRI. Response to levodopa is not significant, and tremor is rare.

Parkinsonism also occurs in diffuse Lewy body disease, Alzheimer disease, Huntington disease, Wilson disease, and depression. Early, mild PD is commonly misdiagnosed as essential tremor.

▶ Treatment
A. Pharmacotherapy

PD is a progressive neurodegenerative disease. No medication has been proven definitively to stop, slow, reverse, or prevent the progression of disease, although several have been evaluated in clinical trials with debated disease-modifying effects. Therefore, current therapeutic strategies are directed at keeping the patient functioning independently for as long as possible with medications that improve symptoms, while considering evolving knowledge of potential neuroprotective

Table 15–3. Medications Used in the Treatment of Parkinson Disease

Class	Group	Drug
Dopaminergic agent	Dopamine precursor	Levodopa (with carbidopa)
	Dopamine agonist	Bromocriptine, pramipexole, ropinirole, amantadine, apomorphine
	COMT inhibitor	Entacapone, tolcapone
	MAO-B inhibitor	Selegiline, rasagiline
Nondopaminergic agent	Anticholinergic	Trihexyphenidyl, diphenhydramine, amitriptyline
	Antiglutaminergic	Amantadine
	GABAergic drug	Lorazepam or clonazepam
Atypical neuroleptic	Serotonin and dopamine antagonist	Quetiapine

COMT = catecholamine O-methyl transferase; GABA = γ-aminobutyric acid; MAO = monoamine oxidase.

benefit. Treatment must be individualized to the patient's symptoms and stage of disease. Deciding which drugs to use and when to use them remains one of the greatest challenges of treating PD patients. Medications and drug dosages change over the course of a patient's disease as new symptoms and adverse effects of drugs or loss of efficacy develop.

Because striatal (basal ganglia) dopamine deficiency causes the main motor symptoms of PD, replacement of dopamine with dopaminergic agents is the major medical therapy. Nondopaminergic agents such as anticholinergics, antiglutaminergics, and muscle relaxants are also used to treat motor symptoms (Table 15–3).

1. Levodopa—Levodopa is the most potent agent for the symptomatic treatment of PD. In early, mild PD, the cardinal motor symptoms are effectively ameliorated, leading to the notion that clinical response to levodopa is diagnostic. However, adverse effects, including the development of dyskinesias (involuntary movements) and motor fluctuations, can limit its usefulness. After 5 years of levodopa therapy, more than 50% of patients develop fluctuations, including wearing off and sudden offs, and dyskinesia; these complications of treatment are thought to represent both pre- and postsynaptic changes related to disease progression in the setting of levodopa exposure. Despite theoretical concerns, it remains unproven whether long-term levodopa use itself causes motor complications or is neurotoxic. Although levodopa has been prescribed for more than 30 years, its long-term effect on disease progression remains unknown.

There remains a lack of consensus about when treatment with levodopa should be started in patients with mild to moderate parkinsonism. Because of the probability of developing motor complications within the first 5 years of starting levodopa, many neurologists do not use levodopa as a first-line agent. Current practice includes using milder agents such as MAO-B inhibitors, amantadine, and dopamine agonists, often as monotherapy, in the mild stages of disease. Indications for starting levodopa include disabling symptoms and signs such postural instability and falling. Moderately severe PD (mild to moderate bilateral motor symptoms, some postural instability, physically independent) and a decline in the ability to carry out activities of daily living may also be indications for starting levodopa therapy. If patients are unable to tolerate dopamine agonists or do not obtain significant symptomatic benefit from a dopamine agonist in combination with nondopaminergic agents, initiation of levodopa therapy should be considered. Many patients older than 70 years of age and those with cognitive decline do not tolerate dopamine agonists or nondopaminergic agents, and early use of levodopa should be considered for these patients as well.

Levodopa, administered in combination with carbidopa (Sinemet), is converted to dopamine in the body. Carbidopa (Lodosyn), a peripheral dopamine decarboxylase inhibitor, inhibits the peripheral conversion of levodopa to dopamine and does not cross the blood–brain barrier. This increases the amount of levodopa that reaches the brain and is converted to dopamine and decreases peripheral dopamine-induced side effects such as anorexia, nausea, vomiting, hypotension, and cardiac irregularities. Carbidopa-levodopa is available in standard preparations that contain a fixed ratio of each drug, 10 mg carbidopa to 100 mg levodopa (10/100), 25 mg carbidopa to 100 mg levodopa (25/100), and 25 mg carbidopa to 250 mg levodopa (25/250). A controlled-release formulation is available in ratios of 25 mg carbidopa to 100 mg levodopa (25/100) or 50 mg carbidopa to 200 mg levodopa (50/200). Treatment is usually started by gradually increasing the dosage until one tablet of carbidopa-levodopa 25/100 is taken three times a day, preferably in the morning, early afternoon, and early evening for maximum benefit. Taking the medication with meals helps to prevent gastrointestinal upset, although protein intake may compete with levodopa transport across the duodenum. The dosage can be gradually titrated to symptomatic benefit. Long-acting controlled-release preparations of carbidopa-levodopa (Sinemet CR) provide a slower onset of effect, less bioavailability, and longer duration of effect than regular carbidopa-levodopa. Despite the theory that controlled-release levodopa formulations should provide a more constant level of bioavailable dopamine to the basal ganglia, thus reducing the frequency of motor complications, studies have failed to show that initial therapy with controlled-release formulations of levodopa decreased the development of motor fluctuations.

Adverse effects of levodopa therapy include anorexia, nausea, vomiting, confusion, drowsiness, hypersomnolence, vivid dreams, nightmares, hallucination, postural hypotension, and cardiac arrhythmias. The development of central nervous system adverse effects such as hallucinations is often dose-related and may require reduction in the dose of levodopa at the expense of worsening parkinsonian symptoms.

2. Dopamine agonists—After levodopa, the dopamine agonists are the most powerful antiparkinson medications. Dopamine agonists are synthetic compounds that stimulate striatal dopamine receptors. Although initially used as add-on therapy in patients receiving levodopa, the agonists are also commonly used as primary monotherapy in patients with mild PD. Many neurologists do not prescribe dopamine agonists for patients older than 70 years of age because these patients are more likely to develop confusion, sleepiness, and psychosis from antiparkinson medications. Because levodopa gives the greatest symptomatic benefit for the lowest risk of adverse effects compared with other agents, levodopa is often used as initial therapy in patients older than 70, especially those with preexisting cognitive decline. However, in patients with PD who are older than 70 but otherwise mentally and physically younger than this age, therapy with a dopamine agonist should be considered.

Studies of dopamine agonists as primary monotherapy in early PD show that drug-induced dyskinesias and motor fluctuations occur infrequently in these patients compared with those receiving levodopa monotherapy. In 70% of patients, however, monotherapy with a dopamine agonist is rarely sufficient for adequate symptomatic treatment after 3 years. Initial treatment of mild PD with dopamine agonists may give satisfactory reduction of PD symptoms while allowing for a delay in the initiation of levodopa therapy. Starting with a dopamine agonist also allows for a reduced dosages of levodopa used in combination with dopamine agonists when monotherapy with an agonist is no longer sufficient for symptomatic control and a lower risk of dyskinesias. These benefits need to be weighed against its relative lesser potency and greater risk of certain side effects compared with levodopa.

Dopamine agonists include the ergot agents pergolide and bromocriptine and the nonergot agents pramipexole and ropinirole. Reports of the development of idiosyncratic, irreversible pulmonary parenchymal fibrosis and cardiac valvular fibrosis from the ergot agonists have limited their use, and pergolide was withdrawn from the US market in 2007. The nonergot agonists pramipexole and ropinirole have been noted to cause sleep attacks (including when driving) and impulse control disorders such as gambling and shopping; other side effects include nausea, vomiting, sleepiness, peripheral edema, orthostatic hypotension, and psychotoxicity, including illusions, hallucinations, and mania. These symptoms stop when the drug is decreased or gradually stopped.

All dopamine agonists should be started at very low doses and increased gradually to reduce the risk of adverse affects. Drug selection is often made based on ease of titration and clinician experience. Patients respond individually to these medications, and if adverse effects develop from one agonist, another should be tried. If a sufficient therapeutic response is not attained with agonist therapy, other agents such as amantadine, selegiline, rasagiline, or trihexyphenidyl can be added. If none of these medications is tolerated or efficacious, treatment with levodopa may be required.

Apomorphine is a nonergot dopamine agonist that is available for subcutaneous injection to rapidly treat sudden, severe, disabling off periods. Dosing must be titrated slowly and under the supervision of a physician. Side effects include severe nausea, profound hypotension, dyskinesias, and hallucinations. Because severe nausea and vomiting occur at recommended doses of apomorphine, an antiemetic such as trimethobenzamide must be used in conjunction with this medication.

3. Other dopaminergic agents

A. SELEGILINE AND RASAGILINE—These drugs are both selective irreversible propargylamine MAO-B inhibitors that increase dopamine by impairing its metabolism via MAO-B. This mechanism of action gives selegiline and rasagiline their mild symptomatic effect. The propargyl chain also appears to have neuroprotective effects in both in vitro and in vivo models. In a large study, selegiline use was associated with an average 9-month delay in the need to initiate symptomatic treatment with levodopa; further, after 2 months of washout, patients treated with selegiline had milder PD compared with those given placebo. This could be consistent with a neuroprotective or disease-modifying effect. However, the reason for these results could be the known long-lasting symptomatic effects of the drug. Follow-up in this study showed that patients treated early with selegiline were less likely to develop freezing of gait but were still at risk for developing dyskinesias. Rasagiline has also been studied for potential neuroprotection in a delayed start design. At 1.0 mg/day, the results were consistent with neuroprotection; however, at 2.0 mg this effect was not observed, confounding interpretation.

Because selegiline and rasagiline have mild symptomatic benefit, may have neuroprotective effects, and are well tolerated, either can be used as initial therapy in patients with very mild symptoms or as add-on therapy, especially in patients with prominent gait difficulties such as freezing. The dosing of selegiline is 5–10 mg every day. Dosing should not exceed 10 mg/day because of risks associated with MAO enzyme inhibitors and ingestion of foods containing tyramine. Dosing of rasagiline is 0.5–1 mg once a day.

Current labeling advises against the coadministration with antidepressants because of the potential to develop a serotonin syndrome. This adverse interaction appears to be very uncommon but can occur. Because depression is so common in PD, cautious use of antidepressants with vigilance for symptoms of serotonin syndrome is advised. Other contraindicated drugs include meperidine, tramadol, methadone, propoxyphene, dextromethorphan, and St. John's wort. One of the metabolites of selegiline is an amphetamine, which may result in improved alertness but may also cause insomnia. Other side effects include dyskinesias, tremor, confusion, and psychosis.

B. **AMANTADINE**—This drug exerts its anti-PD effects by acting as a mild dopaminergic (augmenting release and possibly inhibiting uptake) and also has anticholinergic and antiglutaminergic properties. Amantadine is effective in both mild and advanced PD. In mild PD, amantadine can reduce symptoms of PD, especially tremor. In advanced PD, amantadine is a useful adjunct to therapy with levodopa and dopamine agonists. It is also effective in decreasing levodopa-induced dyskinesias. Side effects include peripheral edema, confusion, livedo reticularis, rash, and visual hallucinations. The usual dosage is 100 mg twice a day; doses up to 400 mg/day can be used.

C. **ENTACAPONE**—This drug is used in conjunction with levodopa to extend the "on time" (duration of action of each dose of levodopa) by inhibiting the enzymatic conversion of levodopa to its metabolite. This results in increased synaptic levels of dopamine. Side effects include diarrhea, dyskinesia, and orange discoloration of urine. Entacapone comes in a 200-mg tablet and is taken simultaneously with levodopa. A formulation that contains 25 mg carbidopa, 200 mg entacapone, and various dosages of levodopa (50 mg, 100 mg, 150 mg, 200 mg) in one tablet is now available as Stalevo.

D. **TOLCAPONE**—Tolcapone has the same mechanism of action and therapeutic effect as entacapone; however, tolcapone can cause fulminant hepatitis resulting in death, and explosive diarrhea. Although hepatitis is a rare adverse effect, patients require baseline and biweekly liver transaminase profiles to monitor transaminase activity. Tolcapone should not be used except when fluctuations are disabling and other drugs fail.

4. Nondopaminergic agents—Anticholinergic drugs such as trihexyphenidyl are mild anti-PD drugs used primarily as monotherapy or in conjunction with a dopaminergics in tremor-predominant PD. Bradykinesia and rigidity may also be minimally improved with anticholinergic therapy. Peripheral and central side effects can be prominent, including confusion, forgetfulness, blurred vision, constipation, dry mouth, urinary retention, hallucinations, and psychosis. Such side effects are especially problematic in older patients, and therefore anticholinergic drugs are generally avoided in this population. In such patients who might benefit from adjunctive therapy with an anticholinergic, a weaker anticholinergic such as diphenhydramine or amitriptyline can be used instead of trihexyphenidyl.

Benzodiazepines, such as lorazepam, with moderately long half-lives, used in small doses (0.5–1 mg twice a day), can be useful in treatment of anxiety that can result from and further complicate significant motor fluctuations.

Atypical neuroleptic agents are used frequently in PD therapy to treat hallucinations, a side effect of dopaminergic therapy. The safest approach for patients experiencing hallucinations and psychosis is to lower the dose of dopaminergic therapy, but many patients do not tolerate a reduction in dose. The most commonly used agent for treatment of mild to moderate hallucinations is quetiapine. If quetiapine is not tolerated or is ineffective, clozapine can be used. However, the risk of bone marrow suppression makes clozapine a difficult medicine to use. Low-dose quetiapine (12.5–25 mg at bedtime) may also be used to treat insomnia, which often occurs in patients with PD.

B. Surgery

Several neurosurgical procedures are used to improve the symptoms of PD. Since the 1950s, unilateral stereotactic lesioning of the pallidum (**pallidotomy**) or thalamus (**thalamotomy**) has been used to reduce the symptoms of PD, primarily tremor. The development of **deep brain stimulation** via electrodes implanted into specific sites in the basal ganglia has revolutionized the field of functional neurosurgery and the treatment of advanced PD. Electrodes may be placed into the subthalamic nucleus or the globus pallidus, and recent studies comparing these sites found both to be equally effective as measured by motor scores when stimulated and off medications. Each electrode lead is attached to a pulse generator that generates high-frequency electrical stimulation. Each pulse generator is surgically implanted subcutaneously below the clavicle. Stimulation parameters are easily adjusted and may change over time, allowing for flexibility and potential long-term symptom control. Surgical candidates are patients with idiopathic PD who are not demented or actively depressed and who have had symptoms for 5 years or more (to allow for atypical features to emerge and assess response to dopaminergics). Because surgery mimics that patient's optimal "on" from levodopa, there should be an excellent response to levodopa but also disabling fluctuations, dyskinesias, or other intolerable side effects despite medication optimization. Deep brain stimulation (DBS) can improve all of the cardinal signs of PD that have been levodopa responsive in a particular patient, especially tremor, bradykinesia, and rigidity. Medication dosages can often be lowered postsurgically, reducing dopamine-induced dyskinesias or other side effects. With deep brain stimulation, as opposed to stereotactic lesioning, stimulators are usually implanted bilaterally with the benefit of bilateral symptomatic improvement. DBS is reversible; pulse generators may be turned off or electrodes can be surgically removed without causing damage to brain tissue. Recent data have shown that DBS is better than best medical therapy in patients with moderately advanced symptoms. Proper patient selection by a neurologist with PD and DBS expertise is critical. Realistic expectations of the benefits of this surgical procedure are crucial for patients and families. Surgery is not curative and does not alter the progression of disease.

The major clinical trial of transplantation of human embryonic dopamine-producing neurons (**fetal cell transplantation**) for treatment of advanced PD was a partial success, demonstrating that fetal neurons could survive in vivo and produce dopamine, reversing parkinsonism, but the development of disabling dyskinesias prevents clinical use of this approach at this time.

Prognosis

PD is a neurodegenerative disorder that worsens slowly with time. The natural history of PD is influenced by the age of onset of disease, lifestyle, and medical therapy. Although there is no conclusive evidence that medical therapies slow the progression of disease, the mortality rate from PD has decreased 50% with the use of levodopa. In addition to prolonging survival time, functional capacity and quality of life are significantly improved by thoughtful treatment with available medications.

Follet K, et al. Pallidal versus subthalamic deep-brain Stimulation for Parkinson's disease. *N Engl J Med* 2010;362:2077–2091. [PMID: 20519680] (A randomized controlled trial comparing pallidal and subthalamic stimulation in DBS.)

Olanow W, et al. A double-blind, delayed start trial of rasagiline in Parkinson's disease. *N Engl J Med* 2009;361:1268–1278. [PMID: 19776408] (Discusses the trial results regarding possible disease modifying effects of two different doses of rasagiline.)

Weaver F, et al. Bilateral deep brain stimulation vs best medical therapy for patients with advanced Parkinson disease. *JAMA* 2009;301:63–73. [PMID: 19126811] (A randomized controlled trial comparing patients who received DBS vs best medical therapy.)

ATYPICAL PARKINSONIAN SYNDROMES

The atypical parkinsonian syndromes include progressive supranuclear palsy, corticobasal degeneration, and multiple system atrophy (Table 15–4). Many patients are initially misdiagnosed with idiopathic Parkinson disease (PD) early in the course of their disease. A lack of response to levodopa, early falls, early freezing (motor blocks), presence of cortical or corticospinal abnormalities on examination, and involvement of cranial nerve function distinguish these syndromes from PD. Notably, these syndromes progress rapidly and are difficult to treat.

PROGRESSIVE SUPRANUCLEAR PALSY

ESSENTIALS OF DIAGNOSIS

► Progressive parkinsonism
► Vertical supranuclear ocular palsy or slow vertical saccades
► Early onset of falling
► Axial rigidity

General Considerations

Progressive supranuclear palsy (PSP) is categorized as an atypical parkinsonian syndrome or Parkinson-plus syndrome. The prevalence of PSP is estimated at 1.39 cases per 100,000 people. Similar to PD, PSP occurs more frequently in men. The mean age of onset is 65 years.

Pathogenesis

The pathologic findings in PSP are distinctive for marked neuronal degeneration and neurofibrillary tangles and tau-positive astrocytes in basal ganglia and brainstem structures. The neurofibrillary tangles found in PSP, which contain the microtubule-associated protein tau, differ from those seen in

Table 15–4. Atypical Parkinsonian Syndromes

Syndrome	Parkinsonism Plus . . .	Neuroimaging Findings	
		PET	*MRI*
Progressive supranuclear palsy (PSP)	Impaired downgaze, neck and axial rigidity, early loss of postural reflexes	Hypometabolic basal ganglia and frontal cortex	Midbrain atrophy
Corticobasal degeneration (CBD)	Severe unilateral rigidity, alien limb phenomena, unilateral apraxia, unilateral cortical myoclonus, early dementia	Asymmetric cortical hypometabolism	Asymmetric parietal lobe atrophy
Multiple system atrophy (MSA)			
• Striatonigral degeneration	Laryngeal stridor, increased deep tendon reflexes, dysarthria, absence of tremor	Hypometabolic basal ganglia and frontal lobes (seen in all MSA syndromes)	Brainstem atrophy (in all MSA syndromes)
• Shy-Drager syndrome	Early, symptomatic orthostatic hypotension; urinary or fecal incontinence		
• Olivopontocerebellar atrophy	Cerebellar dysmetria and dysarthria		

MRI = magnetic resonance imaging; PET = positron emission tomography.

Alzheimer disease and other neurodegenerative disorders. Loss of striatal (basal ganglia) neurons and their postsynaptic dopamine receptors explains the poor symptomatic response to levodopa and dopamine agonists.

▶ Clinical Findings

A. Symptoms and Signs

The history is notable for early onset of falls, freezing, and parkinsonism. Common examination findings early in the course of disease include parkinsonism with prominent axial rigidity, dystonic retrocollis, and facial dystonia, giving patients an angry or surprised look. Typical eye findings include supranuclear ocular palsy, causing impairment of vertical gaze (more commonly downgaze), and ocular square wave jerks (small horizontal saccades alternately to the left and right). Patients may be unable to look downward voluntarily yet reflex ocular movements may be normal. Speech may be nasal, spastic, and slow. Gait is wide-based and postural reflexes are absent. As the disease progresses, dysarthria, dysphagia, and cognitive impairment occur. Cognitive impairment is notable for bradyphrenia, impaired verbal fluency, and difficulty with sequential tasks. Emotional lability, with inappropriate weeping or laughing, may occur. Some patients develop blepharospasm (inability to open their eyelids). Rest tremor is uncommon.

B. Imaging Studies

CT or MRI scans of patients with PSP may show brainstem atrophy, particularly in the midbrain, and generalized cerebral atrophy. PET scanning with ^{18}F-deoxyglucose shows hypometabolism in the frontal cortex brainstem, striatum, thalamus, and cerebellum. Further, specific patterns of hypometabolism involving the brainstem and medial frontal cortex may help distinguish PSP from other forms of parkinsonism.

▶ Differential Diagnosis

The major alternative diagnoses include PD, corticobasal degeneration, multisystem atrophy, cerebral multi-infarct disease, and diffuse Lewy body disease.

▶ Treatment

There is no specific treatment for PSP, and symptomatic improvement is difficult to obtain. Levodopa and other anti-PD medications should be tried but are rarely very effective. A recently approved combination of dextromethorphan/quinidine may help pseudobulbar affect (involuntary emotional expression disorder), and zolpidem has been reported to be beneficial for eye movements and motor function in two reports of PSP patients. Dystonia can be improved with botulinum toxin injections to affected muscles. Patients may choose to use enteric feeding if dysphagia becomes severe.

▶ Prognosis

Symptoms are steadily progressive, and death, often due to aspiration, usually occurs 5–10 years after onset of disease.

CORTICOBASAL DEGENERATION

ESSENTIALS OF DIAGNOSIS

▶ Parkinsonism
▶ Unilateral arm rigidity and dystonia
▶ Cortical sensory deficits

▶ Clinical Findings

A. Symptoms and Signs

Patients with corticobasal degeneration (also referred to as *cortical–basal ganglionic degeneration*) often describe unilateral hand clumsiness with corresponding limb rigidity and bradykinesia. The onset is usually insidious, involving asymmetric parkinsonism, focal rigidity, and dystonia involving one arm, and cortical sensory deficits. Cortical sensory loss, apraxia, myoclonus, and alien limb phenomena (unsuppressible, involuntary movements) occur in the affected limb. Patients may have coarse rest and action tremor. Speech becomes notably slurred and labored, causing disturbances in communication and language. Early features include falling and loss of postural reflexes. Other findings include hyperreflexia and the Babinski sign. Later in the course of the disease, both sides of the body are involved, disturbances of ocular motility occur, and dementia often develops.

B. Imaging Studies

CT and MRI scans may show asymmetric parietal lobe atrophy corresponding to the most affected side of the brain. Asymmetric frontoparietal atrophy helps to differentiate corticobasal degeneration from PSP. PET scans show reduced ^{18}F-fluorodopa uptake in the basal ganglia and asymmetric cortical hypometabolism.

▶ Differential Diagnosis

The main alternative diagnoses are PD and PSP.

▶ Treatment & Prognosis

No effective treatment exists. Levodopa and other dopaminergic drugs are rarely effective. Clonazepam may improve myoclonus. Dystonia and rigidity may improve with botulinum toxin injections. Corticobasal degeneration progresses more rapidly than PD. Mean survival is about 6 years after onset of symptoms.

MULTIPLE SYSTEM ATROPHY

▶ General Considerations

The term *multiple system atrophy* (MSA) encompasses distinct syndromes that have overlapping clinical and prognostic features. These include striatonigral degeneration, Shy-Drager syndrome, and olivopontocerebellar atrophy. Ten percent of patients with parkinsonism have MSA. In 100 patients with probable MSA (14 confirmed at autopsy) the median age of onset was 53 years, with a range of 33–76 years; 67 patients were men, and 33 were women.

▶ Clinical Findings

A. Symptoms and Signs

Patients with MSA present with parkinsonism and additional characteristic clinical features. **Striatonigral degeneration** is characterized by parkinsonism without tremor. Other features include dysarthria, dysphagia, laryngeal stridor, increased deep tendon reflexes, anterocollis, and early postural instability. Striatal neurons containing dopamine receptors are lost, resulting in a characteristically poor response to levodopa.

Shy-Drager syndrome is characterized by parkinsonism and symptomatic, autonomic dysfunction. Orthostatic hypotension may be severe, disabling, and difficult to treat. Other autonomic symptoms such as bladder and bowel dysfunction and impotence also occur. Brainstem, basal ganglia, preganglionic sympathetic neuronal, and cerebellar degeneration occurs in MSA. Occasionally, the basal ganglia are spared, accounting for unpredictable levodopa responsiveness.

Olivopontocerebellar atrophy (sporadic type) is characterized by parkinsonism and cerebellar symptoms. Degeneration of the pons, cerebellum, basal ganglia, and substantia nigra is present. If the basal ganglia are not severely degenerated, parkinsonism responds to levodopa therapy.

B. Imaging Studies

In MSA, T2-weighted MRI scans may show decreased signal intensity in the putamen as well as slit-hyperintensity in the lateral margin of the putamen. PET scan shows hypometabolism in the striatum and frontal lobes.

▶ Treatment

Treatment is based on the approach used in PD. Dopaminergic medications should be tried for symptomatic relief. A trial of levodopa (up to 2 g/day, as tolerated, with carbidopa) should be given to assess for levodopa responsiveness. Although patients with MSA may initially respond to levodopa because of preserved basal ganglia function, symptomatic benefits are rarely sustained, and moderate or high doses of levodopa may exacerbate preexisting orthostatic hypotension. In patients with Shy-Drager syndrome, several methods are used to treat symptomatic orthostatic hypotension. Initially, increasing salt intake and wearing support hose may be beneficial. Drugs such as midodrine or fludrocortisone may eventually be required if hypotension becomes disabling. Cerebellar symptoms in olivopontocerebellar atrophy may respond to amantadine, 100 mg, up to four times a day. Physical therapy with emphasis on balance, gait, and range of motion is critical for optimizing mobility. The symptoms of MSA respond poorly to deep brain stimulation.

▶ Prognosis

MSA (all three syndromes) progresses rapidly compared with Parkinson disease, and patients with prominent autonomic dysfunction have a worse prognosis. Many patients are wheelchair-bound or markedly disabled within 5 years of diagnosis. Mean survival rate in MSA is about 8–9 years after onset of symptoms.

ESSENTIAL TREMOR

▶ General Considerations

Essential tremor (ET) is the most common adult-onset movement disorder. More prevalent than Parkinson disease or Alzheimer disease, it has an estimated prevalence between 0.4% and 3.9% and up to 10% in those older than 65 years of age. Onset is most common in persons in their early twenties or in later adulthood, but ET may occur at any age. Both sexes are equally affected. Most patients never seek medical attention, because the tremor remains mild. Although ET is not a progressive neurodegenerative disease, tremor may be progressive, spreading to involve the head, vocal chords, and diaphragm, and becoming functionally disabling.

The etiology of ET is partly genetic. Many studies show that it is familial in 50–70% of patients, with autosomal-dominant transmission. Sporadic cases of ET suggest nongenetic or environmental risk factors causing or precipitating ET, perhaps explaining the variability in age of onset in familial cases.

▶ Clinical Findings

A. Symptoms and Signs

ET is characterized by a 4–10-Hz symmetric action tremor of the arms. Action tremor includes postural tremor (maintaining a posture against gravity) and kinetic tremor (tremor that occurs with voluntary movement of the affected limb). Ninety percent of patients have arm and hand tremor, 30–50% have head tremor, 20% have voice tremor, and approximately 12% have leg tremor. ET is described as a monosymptomatic syndrome, yet up to 50% of patients have very subtle cerebellar signs, such as impaired tandem gait or mild ataxia. In more that 50% of patients, tremor can be transiently diminished by ingestion of alcohol. Common tasks that are affected by kinetic arm tremor include writing, drinking out of a full cup, and eating soup with a spoon.

▶ Differential Diagnosis

ET is most frequently misdiagnosed as Parkinson disease (Table 15–5). Distinguishing features of ET include the absence of rest tremor, the symmetric onset of action tremor, and lack of parkinsonian features such as bradykinesia, rigidity, or loss of postural reflexes. In patients with ET, handwriting is large and tremulous rather than the tremulous micrographia seen in those with parkinsonism. It is often difficult to distinguish between mild ET and enhanced physiologic tremor. Cerebellar (intention) tremor can be differentiated from ET by the presence of cerebellar signs such

Table 15–5. Comparison of Essential Tremor and Parkinsonism Tremor

	Essential Tremor	Parkinsonian Tremor
Stimulus	Occurs with action	Occurs at rest
Family history of tremor	Yes	No
Body part involved	Hands, head, and voice	Hands, legs, rarely head or voice
Distribution at onset	Bilateral and symmetric	Unilateral or asymmetric
Sensitivity to alcohol	Yes	No
Course	Stable or slowly progressive	Progressive

Table 15–6. Treatment of Essential Tremor

Drug	Initial Adult Dose	Usual Effective Dose
Propranolol	20 mg/day	80–240 mg/day
Primidone	12.5–25 mg at bedtime	50–500 mg/day
Topiramate	12.5–25 mg/day	100–400 mg/day
Clonazepam	0.5 mg/day	2–4 mg/day
Gabapentin	100 mg	1200–1800 mg/day

as dysmetria and dysdiadochokinesis, and by marked exaggeration of the tremor with intention.

Various medications can cause symmetric action tremor similar to ET; these include lithium, valproate, selective serotonin reuptake inhibitors, tricyclic antidepressants, β-adrenergic agonists, ephedrine, theophylline, corticosteroids, cyclosporine, and neuroleptics. Hyperthyroidism can cause symmetric tremor that mimics ET.

▶ Treatment

Propranolol, a β-blocker, and primidone, an anticonvulsant, are the two most commonly used agents for treatment of ET (Table 15–6). Both reduce tremor amplitude when used as single agents or in combination. Either may be used as a first-line agent. If tremor reduction is unsatisfactory with one agent, the other may be added for further symptomatic benefit. Side effects may limit tolerability and necessitate switching to an alternate medication before tremor reduction is achieved. Topiramate, an anticonvulsant, can also reduce tremor. Clonazepam in small divided daily doses may be efficacious. The anticonvulsant gabapentin has been used as adjunct therapy in ET.

Chemodenervation using botulinum toxin improves limb tremor, head tremor, and voice tremor. Side effects include weakness at the site of injection and breathiness and weakened voice if used for vocal tremor. Success depends on correct selection of muscle sites, dose of toxin used, and overall skill and experience of the injector.

Thalamotomy, stereotactic lesioning of the ventral intermediate nucleus of the thalamus, can significantly improve tremor, with 80–90% of patients receiving moderate-to-complete resolution. Deep brain stimulation (described earlier, under treatment of Parkinson disease) is also used to treat severe ET. In patients with ET, the electrodes are placed into the ventral intermediate nucleus of the thalamus; the adjustable electrical stimulation allows for optimal, individualized tremor control. Deep brain stimulation has an advantage over thalamotomy because many of the side effects that are common to both procedures (eg, speech difficulty, hemiparesis, confusion, and weakness) can be resolved in patients who receive deep brain stimulation by adjustment of stimulation settings. Studies have shown tremor improvement of 60–90% after unilateral thalamic deep brain stimulation.

Louis ED. Essential tremor: Evolving clinicopathological concepts in an era of intensive post-mortem enquiry. *Lancet Neurol* 2010;6:613–622. [PMID: 20451458] (An overview of ongoing studies aimed at understanding the pathological basis of ET.)

Ondo WG, et al. Topiramate in essential tremor. *Neurology* 2006;66:672–677. [PMID: 16436648] (Double-blind, placebo controlled trial of topiramate for the treatment of ET.)

▼ DYSTONIA

ESSENTIALS OF DIAGNOSIS

▶ Sustained muscle contractions, often causing twisting movements or abnormal postures

▶ Varies in age of onset, anatomic distribution

▶ Can be primary, or can be a feature of an underlying neurologic disorder or exogenous insult

▶ When secondary, frequently accompanied by other abnormal movements or neurologic signs

Table 15–7. Classification of Dystonia

Distribution
Focal
  • Cervical dystonia
  • Blepharospasm
  • Spasmodic dysphonia
  • Oromandibular dystonia
  • Writer's cramp
Segmental
  • Meige syndrome
  • Craniocervical dystonia
Multifocal
Hemidystonia
Generalized

Age of onset
Early-onset (≤26 y)
Late-onset (>26 y)

Etiology
Primary dystonia
Secondary dystonia
  • Inherited
    —Dystonia-plus
    —Degenerative diseases
  • Complex/unknown etiology
    —Parkinson disease and other parkinsonisms
  • Symptomatic of an exogenous/environmental cause
Dystonic phenomenology in another movement disorder

▶ General Considerations

Dystonia is a movement disorder characterized by relatively sustained and directional muscle contractions that produce abnormal postures or twisting and repetitive movements. The movements are usually longer in duration than those seen in other movement disorders (eg, chorea or myoclonus), involve the co-contraction of agonist and antagonist muscles, and tend to be repetitive or patterned, consistently involving the same muscle groups. Dystonia is often aggravated by voluntary movement. In *action dystonia*, the dystonic movements are elicited only with voluntary movement. When dystonia is evinced only with particular actions, it is called *task-specific dystonia*; examples include writer's cramp and the embouchure dystonia of woodwind and brass musicians. Activation of dystonic movements by actions in remote parts of the body is called *overflow;* examples include leg dystonia while writing or axial dystonia with talking. Dystonia that is suppressed by voluntary activity is called *paradoxical dystonia;* for example, talking or chewing may suppress dystonia involving facial and oromandibular muscles (also known as *Meige syndrome*).

Factors that tend to exacerbate dystonia include fatigue and emotional stress, whereas the movements usually decrease with relaxation or sleep. Many patients discover a tactile or proprioceptive sensory trick (*geste antagoniste*) that minimizes the dystonia; for example, a patient with cervical dystonia may touch the chin. Severe dystonia is less likely to

respond to these maneuvers, and joint contractures can occur when dystonia is longstanding.

Dystonia is classified by *anatomic distribution,* by *age of onset,* and by *etiology* (Table 15–7). In *focal dystonia,* the abnormal movements involve a single body region, whereas *segmental dystonia* affects two or more contiguous body parts. When *multifocal,* two or more noncontiguous body areas are involved. *Hemidystonia* affects one side of the body and is suggestive of a secondary dystonia. *Generalized dystonia* involves the legs (or one leg and the trunk) plus at least one other area of the body.

Cervical dystonia is the most common of the focal dystonias. Various combinations of neck muscles may be involved to produce abnormal head positions, including horizontal turning (torticollis), tilting (laterocollis), flexion (anterocollis), or extension (retrocollis). Repetitive jerking of the head may resemble tremor, but can usually be distinguished by its directional preponderance. Approximately 75% of patients complain of neck pain. Less common than cervical dystonia are the focal dystonias that involve cranial muscles. *Blepharospasm* causes contraction of the orbicularis oculi; mild cases are characterized by increased blink rate with flurries of blinking, whereas more severely affected patients have visual impairment due to sustained forceful eye closure. *Spasmodic dysphonia* results from dystonia of the vocal cords; abnormal adduction, which causes a strained, strangled voice, is more common than abduction, in which the voice sounds whispering and breathy. In *oromandibular dystonia* there is abnormal activity in lower facial, tongue, jaw, and pharyngeal muscles that may interfere with speaking or swallowing. *Brachial dystonia* is a form of focal dystonia that may be primarily, or only, present with writing (*writer's cramp*); it is probably more common than is usually recognized. In about 15% of patients there is spread from the dominant to the contralateral arm, at which point it is considered segmental bibrachial dystonia. Other segmental dystonias involve the cranial muscles (eg, *Meige syndrome*), sometimes in combination with neck muscles (*cranial-cervical dystonia*).

Age at onset is an important prognostic consideration, as patients with onset of dystonia in childhood or adolescence are likely to progress to generalized or multifocal dystonia, especially when the dystonia initially involves the leg.

Classification of a patient's dystonia by etiology is useful for prognosis, for guiding therapy, and for genetic counseling. In *primary dystonia*, which may be familial or sporadic, no associated neurologic abnormalities (eg, dementia, ocular abnormalities, ataxia, spasticity, or paresis) are present. (An exception is tremor, which is common in patients with primary dystonia, especially cervical dystonia.) Primary dystonia is distinguished from the *secondary dystonias* by the absence of signs other than dystonia as well as by the absence of an identified exogenous cause or brain degeneration (Table 15–7). The secondary dystonias include (1) the inherited *dystonia-plus* syndromes, which are similar to primary dystonia in that there is no evidence of brain degeneration, but signs other than dystonia are present (specifically myoclonus and parkinsonism); (2) inherited neurologic conditions associated with neuronal degeneration (eg, Huntington disease, Wilson disease, the spinocerebellar ataxias); (3) dystonia associated with Parkinson disease and other parkinsonisms; and (4) dystonia due to environmental causes (eg, exposure to neuroleptics, stroke). Finally, dystonia may occur as a feature of other movement disorders, such as tic disorders and paroxysmal dyskinesias.

Most primary dystonias are focal or segmental in distribution, with onset in adulthood. About 10% of patients with primary dystonia have generalized dystonia, usually starting in childhood or adolescence (early-onset). DYT1, a major cause of early-onset primary dystonia, results from mutation of the gene *TOR1A* located on the long arm of chromosome 9 (9q34.1). *TOR1A* codes for torsinA, a heat-shock protein that binds ATP; in DYT1 dystonia, deletion of a GAG triplet from this gene results in loss of a glutamic acid residue from torsinA. This deletion is especially common in the Ashkenazi Jewish population, where its prevalence is 1 in 2000 persons. It is inherited in an autosomal-dominant fashion, with reduced penetrance of 30%. DYT1 dystonia (formerly called *Oppenheim dystonia* or *dystonia musculorum deformans*) has a mean age at onset of 12.5 years and in 94% of cases begins in a limb. It tends to progress to generalized dystonia; as mentioned earlier, the probability of generalization is related to age and site of onset. A less common early-onset inherited primary dystonia is DYT6 dystonia due to heterozygous mutations in the gene *THAP1*. *THAP1* is a member of a family of cellular factors that share a conserved THAP (thanatos-associated protein) DNA binding domain. Dystonia due to *THAP1* often involves the arms and axial muscles but differs from DYT1 in that speech is also frequently affected due to oromandibular or laryngeal involvement. It may, however, mimic DYT1. Other loci for primary dystonia include DYT7 (late-onset autosomal-dominant focal dystonia in a northwestern German family), DYT13 (autosomal-dominant cranio-cervico-brachial dystonia in an Italian family), and DYT17 (early-onset autosomal-recessive dystonia in a Lebanese sibship with segmental and generalized dystonia including dysphonia and dysarthria). Table 15–8 lists the hereditary forms of dystonia that have been identified.

The dystonia-plus syndromes include dopa-responsive dystonia, rapid-onset dystonia-parkinsonism, and myoclonus-dystonia. Perhaps the most important to recognize is *dopa-responsive dystonia* (DRD), or *Segawa disease*, as it is treated very effectively with levodopa. Typically, gait dysfunction (often appearing stiff-legged or spastic) begins in early or mid-childhood, and symptoms are worst late in the day and improve with sleep. Parkinsonism, including rigidity, bradykinesia, flexed posture, and loss of postural reflexes, may be prominent, making juvenile parkinsonism an important differential diagnosis. DRD has also been misdiagnosed as cerebral palsy. Girls are affected more often than boys. Onset in adulthood is uncommon, and may present as focal dystonia or parkinsonism. Most cases of DRD are caused by heterozygous mutations in the GTP-cyclohydrolase I (*GCH1*) gene located at 14q22.1 (DYT5); many different mutations have been identified, making genetic testing complex and expensive. The mutations impair the activity of GTP-cyclohydrolase I, which catalyzes the rate-limiting step in the synthesis of tetrahydrobiopterin, a necessary cofactor for tyrosine hydroxylase; tyrosine hydroxylase in turn converts tyrosine to levodopa. Inheritance is autosomal dominant with reduced penetrance that appears to be sex-influenced (ie, higher in girls). Although the dystonia may improve dramatically with anticholinergic medications such as trihexyphenidyl, a trial of oral levodopa therapy at low doses (usually no more than 300–400 mg daily) is useful for diagnosis as well as for treatment. Additional support for the diagnosis can be obtained from a phenylalanine-loading test, in which blood levels of phenylalanine remain elevated for a prolonged period, due to the role of tetrahydrobiopterin as a cofactor for phenylalanine hydroxylase as well as tyrosine hydroxylase. Measurement of biopterin metabolites in cerebrospinal fluid may also aid in diagnosis.

In addition to classic DRD due to heterozygous *GCH1* mutations, DRD may result from homozygous or compound heterozygous mutations in *GCH1*, in genes for other enzymes involved in pterin metabolism, and in genes encoding tyrosine hydroxylase. Patients with these defects are often more severely affected clinically, and features due to deficiency of norepinephrine and serotonin may predominate.

Table 15–8. Identified Hereditary Forms of Dystonia

Designation	Clinical Presentation	Inheritance	Gene Locus	Gene
DYT1	Early-onset generalized dystonia	AD	9q	TOR1A
DYT2	Autosomal-recessive dystonia	AR	—	—
DYT3	X-linked dystonia-parkinsonism (Lubag)	XR	Xq	TAF/DYT3 (gene transcription factor)
DYT4	Whispering dysphonia	AD	—	—
DYT5a/DYT14	Dopa-responsive dystonia	AD	14q	GCH1
DYT5b	Dopa-responsive dystonia	AR	11p	TH
DYT6	Adolescent-onset mixed dystonia	AD	8p	THAP1
DYT7	Adult-onset focal dystonia	AD	18p	—
DYT8	Paroxysmal nonkinesigenic dyskinesia	AD	2q	PNKD1/MR1
DYT9	Paroxysmal choreoathetosis with episodic ataxia and spasticity	AD	1p	—
DYT10	Paroxysmal kinesigenic choreoathetosis	AD	16p-q	—
DYT11	Myoclonus-dystonia	AD	7q	SGCE
DYT12	Rapid-onset dystonia-parkinsonism	AD	19q	ATP1A3
DYT13	Multifocal/segmental dystonia	AD	1p	—
DYT15	Myoclonus-dystonia	AD	18p	—
DYT16	Young-onset dystonia-parkinsonism	AR	2p	PRKRA (stress-response protein)
DYT17	Autosomal-recessive primary dystonia	AR	20p-q	—
DYT18	Paroxysmal exertion-induced dyskinesia 2	AD	1p	SLC2A1 (glucose transporter)
DYT19	Episodic kinesigenic dyskinesia 2	AD	16q	—
DYT20	Paroxysmal nonkinesigenic dyskinesia 2	AD	2q	—

AD = autosomal dominant; AR = autosomal recessive.

Myoclonus-dystonia (DYT11) is a dystonia-plus syndrome with prominent myoclonic jerks, usually affecting the arms and trunk more than the legs. Inheritance is autosomal dominant, and many patients have a mutation in the epsilon-sarcoglycan (*SGCE*) gene on chromosome 7q21. Onset is usually in childhood or adolescence. The symptoms characteristically respond to alcohol, and alcoholism (as well as other psychiatric disorders) is not uncommon.

Another rare dystonia-plus syndrome is *rapid-onset dystonia-parkinsonism* (DYT 12), in which dystonia and parkinsonism begin suddenly in adolescence or early adulthood and progress over hours to weeks, after which the symptoms usually stabilize. Inheritance is autosomal dominant and maps to 19q13. The responsible gene codes for the α3 catalytic subunit of the Na$^+$/K$^+$-ATPase pump.

Although the causes of secondary dystonia are numerous, patients with primary dystonia significantly outnumber the secondary cases. Nevertheless, it is important to identify patients with secondary dystonia, as treatment of the underlying condition may be warranted. Factors that raise the

likelihood that dystonia is secondary include history of a potentially causative insult (eg, perinatal injury, stroke, encephalitis, head trauma or peripheral trauma, brain tumor, exposure to neurotoxic agents); abnormalities in the neurologic examination (including hemidystonia), neuroimaging, or laboratory evaluation; onset of dystonia at rest rather than action; early onset of cranial dystonia or late onset of leg dystonia; and evidence that the dystonia is psychogenic.

One cause of secondary dystonia is exposure to drugs that block dopamine receptors; neuroleptic agents used in psychiatric practice and the antiemetics are most frequently responsible. Dystonia may occur soon after initiation of therapy (*acute dystonic reaction*) or after prolonged treatment (*tardive dystonia*). These are discussed in more detail in the section on drug-induced movement disorders. Exogenous causes also include injury to the central nervous system (especially the basal ganglia, cerebellum, and thalamus) or peripheral nervous system; dystonia can be a feature of complex regional pain syndrome. It is also relatively common for dystonia to emerge through psychogenic mechanisms; features that suggest a nonorganic etiology include movements that vary over time, disappearance with distraction, give-way weakness, and sensory findings that do not conform to a physiologically plausible pattern.

Inherited degenerative diseases that can cause dystonia include many autosomal-dominant and autosomal-recessive conditions, X-linked dominant and recessive conditions, and mitochondrial defects. As mentioned previously, these diseases usually do not cause pure dystonia. *Wilson disease* is an important consideration, because it requires early treatment. It results from mutations in the *ATP7B* gene on chromosome 13, which produce a defect in copper metabolism, leading to the insidious development of neurologic, psychiatric, or hepatic dysfunction. Inheritance is autosomal recessive; more than 200 different mutations have been reported, making genetic testing impractical. When onset is in childhood, Wilson disease usually presents with hepatic dysfunction, but neurologic presentation is most typical in adult-onset disease. Dystonia can be generalized, segmental, or multifocal, but cranial involvement is characteristic; Wilson's original 1912 monograph highlighted the typical "sardonic" smile. Other common neurologic abnormalities include tremor (classically "wing-beating"), dysarthria, dysphagia, drooling, ataxia, and dementia. In addition to brain and liver (cirrhosis, acute hepatitis) involvement, systemic findings can involve the eyes, heart, kidneys, bones, joints, glands, and muscles.

Rarer heredodegenerative causes of dystonia include other autosomal-recessive inborn errors of metabolism, such as Niemann-Pick type C, neuronal ceroid lipofuscinosis, GM1 and GM2 gangliosidoses, glutaric academia, and methylmalonic aciduria. Formerly called *Hallervorden-Spatz disease*, *pantothenate kinase–associated neurodegeneration* (PKAN) is an autosomal-recessive disease resulting in abnormal deposition of iron in the basal ganglia, producing childhood onset of dystonia, spasticity, seizures, and dementia. Other inherited causes of dystonia (often accompanied by parkinsonism and other neurologic signs) that are associated with neurodegeneration with brain iron accumulation include PLA2G6 (PARK14)-associated neurodegeneration, neuroferritinopathy, and Kufor-Rakeb disease (PARK9). *Lubag* (DYT3) is an X-linked recessive dystonia-parkinsonism affecting male Filipinos. Usual onset is in adulthood, with cranial or generalized dystonia; parkinsonism may co-occur or develop later. The course tends to be progressive. The *deafness-dystonia (Mohr-Tranebjaerg) syndrome* is an X-linked recessive condition with mutation in the *DDP1* gene. The spinocerebellar ataxias (especially SCA3 [*Machado-Joseph disease*], SCA2, and SCA17) can be associated with dystonia, as can *dentatorubropallidoluysian atrophy*.

Pathoanatomy

Many cases of secondary dystonia are associated with lesions of the basal ganglia (especially the putamen), or with their connections. Degenerative brain changes are not reported in primary dystonia, but relatively few brains have been studied.

One study described neuronal inclusions in the brainstem of DYT1 cases. Increased copper deposition in the basal ganglia of adult-onset focal dystonia has been described. Functional imaging of DYT1 patients with positron emission tomography (PET) demonstrates altered metabolism in neural circuits involving the cerebral cortex, basal ganglia, thalamus, and cerebellum.

Prevention

No intervention is known to prevent the development of dystonia. Genetic counseling is useful in educating patients about the likelihood of transmitting the condition to successive generations.

Clinical Findings

A. Laboratory Findings

Like most movement disorders, the diagnosis of dystonia is made on clinical grounds rather than on the basis of laboratory testing. Nevertheless, the cause of the dystonia sometimes can be elucidated through further investigations. The primary and dystonia-plus dystonias for which genetic testing is currently commercially available are DYT1, DYT6, DRD, and myoclonus-dystonia. A positive result obviates the need for further diagnostic testing. Genetic counseling must be available for patients undergoing this test.

Genetic testing for DYT1 dystonia is indicated for patients with onset of dystonia before 26 years of age, as well as for patients with later onset who have a relative with early-onset dystonia. Data to guide DYT6 testing are insufficient at present. Most patients with clinically typical DRD will have identified mutations in *GCH1* if comprehensive analysis is performed, including testing for deletions. There is genetic testing for myoclonus-dystonia, although many sporadic cases do not harbor *SGCE* mutations. Genetic testing is also available for many of the secondary dystonias, including SCAs and PKAN. An excellent resource for genetic counseling and testing information is www.genetests.org, a publicly funded resource.

If genetic testing is negative or is not indicated, much of the remaining work-up is directed toward identifying a secondary cause for the patient's dystonia. Treatable conditions that should always be considered in the differential diagnosis include DRD and Wilson disease. We offer a trial of carbidopa/levodopa to all non-DYT1 patients with early onset of symptoms as well as to late-onset patients with features suggesting DRD (ie, parkinsonism, diurnal variation). The dose is increased as tolerated over several weeks; although a daily dose of 600 mg levodopa is sometimes required, failure to respond to a dose of 300 mg/day usually excludes the diagnosis of DRD. Wilson disease should be excluded in patients with onset of dystonia before age 50. Diagnostic laboratory findings in patients with neurologic signs due to Wilson disease include MRI abnormalities involving the putamen, thalamus, and brainstem; reduced serum ceruloplasmin; increased 24-hour urinary copper excretion; and Kayser-Fleischer rings in the cornea due to deposition of copper in Descemet membrane. These are best seen with slit lamp examination. Although noninvasive studies are usually adequate for diagnosing neurologic Wilson disease, liver biopsy to assess copper content has high sensitivity and may be considered.

Evaluation of secondary dystonia is dictated by clues provided by the history and examination. Routine blood tests such as complete blood count, electrolytes, glucose, calcium, magnesium, coagulation profile, and kidney, liver, and thyroid function may be supplemented by sedimentation rate, antinuclear antibody screen, and syphilis screen. Specific clinical findings or laboratory abnormalities may dictate further investigations, including electrophysiologic studies, lumbar puncture, biopsy of various tissues, or metabolic studies of blood, urine, or cerebrospinal fluid. Testing for the human immunodeficiency virus should be considered in the appropriate setting.

B. Imaging Studies

All patients suspected of having a secondary form of dystonia should undergo MRI (or, if not possible, computed tomography) of the brain. In primary dystonia and in the dystonia-plus syndromes, brain MRI is normal. In secondary and heredodegenerative dystonias, MRI may show calcification, necrosis, or other abnormalities in the basal ganglia. In some cases, these changes are quite specific; for instance, T2-weighted MRI in PKAN often shows hypointensity in the globus pallidus with medial hyperintensity (the "eye-of-the-tiger sign"). PET scanning may be supportive of primary dystonia, but rarely is crucial in making the diagnosis.

▶ Differential Diagnosis

A variety of central and peripheral nervous systems disorders, as well as nonneurologic conditions, can be associated with abnormal postures that resemble torsion dystonia (sometimes called *pseudodystonia*). For example, tonic seizure activity can produce sustained twisting movements. Head tilt can reflect palsy of the trochlear nerve, vestibulopathy, pathology in the posterior fossa, or a retropharyngeal soft tissue mass. *Stiff person syndrome* causes contraction of axial and proximal limb muscles. Nerve and muscle abnormalities include *neuromyotonia (Isaac syndrome)*, the myotonic disorders, inflammatory myopathies, and glycogen storage diseases (eg, *Satoyoshi disease*). Carpopedal spasms of *tetany* can be the manifestation of hypocalcemia, hypomagnesemia, or alkalosis. Orthopedic and rheumatologic processes involving bones, ligaments, or joints can result in abnormal postures. In *Sandifer syndrome*, patients (typically young boys) with hiatal hernia develop head tilt in association with gastroesophageal reflux.

▶ Complications

Longstanding torsion dystonia can result in fixed contractures or scoliosis. Dystonic storm or status dystonicus is a rare but life-threatening disorder that may occur in primary or secondary dystonia, especially children or adolescents with underlying generalized dystonia. Severe repeated dystonic spasms may interfere with respirations and cause hyperpyrexia, dehydration, and acute renal failure secondary to rhabdomyolysis; it requires aggressive treatment that may include emergent deep brain stimulation.

▶ Treatment

When dystonia is secondary, treatment of the underlying condition may produce improvement in the dystonia. In patients with tardive dystonia or an acute dystonic reaction, dopamine receptor–blocking drugs should be eliminated or replaced whenever possible (as detailed in section on drug-induced movement disorders). Structural lesions may be amenable to surgical correction. Management of Wilson disease consists of copper chelation therapy (usually with penicillamine as a first-line agent) and oral zinc, which induces copper-binding metallothionein in enterocytes. Some of the inborn errors of metabolism may respond to dietary restriction or supplementation. Patients with DRD usually are maintained on low-dose carbidopa/levodopa therapy. Although currently there is no curative therapy for primary dystonia, several effective options for symptomatic treatment are available; these include oral pharmacologic agents, chemodenervation, and surgery. Of the various oral medications that have been studied, anticholinergic agents are the most efficacious (Table 15–9). Trihexyphenidyl is the best studied and probably the most widely used, although benztropine, diphenhydramine, and ethopropazine (which is not available in the United States) may be useful as well. Use is often limited by peripheral anticholinergic adverse effects, including blurred vision, dry

Table 15–9. Oral Medications Used in Management of Dystonia

	Usual Effective Dose (mg/day)
Anticholinergic agents	
Trihexyphenidyl	6–80
Benztropine	4–8
Ethopropazine[a]	100–400
Benzodiazepines	
Clonazepam	1–4
Diazepam	10–60
Lorazepam	1–6
Dopamine-depleting agents	
Tetrabenazine	50–200
Reserpine	1–3
GABA agonist	
Baclofen	30–80

GABA = γ-amino butyric acid.
[a]Not available in the United States.

mouth, urinary retention, sedation, and confusion, and doses should be titrated slowly. Pilocarpine eye drops or oral pyridostigmine, a peripherally acting anticholinesterase, may be effective in counteracting these unwanted effects. Anticholinergic medications can be used singly or in combination with other drugs, including baclofen, benzodiazepines, and muscle relaxants such as cyclobenzaprine. Dopamine-depleting agents and atypical antipsychotics may be helpful in the treatment of dystonia. Preliminary observations suggest that newer antiepileptic drugs (eg, zonisamide, topiramate, levetiracetam) may be useful in suppressing dystonic movements, but further study of their role is needed.

Chemodenervation of overactive muscles by injection of botulinum toxin is the treatment of choice for focal dystonia. The toxin produces muscle weakness by interfering with proteins in the presynaptic nerve terminal that are responsible for release of acetylcholine into the neuromuscular junction. This therapy is effective in the treatment of blepharospasm, cervical dystonia, spasmodic dysphonia, writer's cramp, and oromandibular dystonia. Side effects can arise from unintended weakness in nearby muscles due to diffusion of toxin. Antibodies to botulinum toxin can develop with repeated injections, resulting in loss of therapeutic effect.

Patients whose dystonia is disabling and refractory to oral medications and chemodenervation may be candidates for surgery of the peripheral or central nervous system (CNS). Thalamotomy, pioneered in the 1960s, is the oldest CNS surgical approach to dystonia. Based on the efficacy of pallidotomy for treating dyskinesias and dystonia in Parkinson disease and neurophysiologic studies that demonstrate an abnormal pattern of neuronal discharging from the globus pallidus in patients with generalized dystonia, current surgical interventions target this region of the basal ganglia. Although either pallidotomy or deep brain stimulation (DBS) can modulate the pallidal output, DBS has the advantages over ablative surgery of being reversible and having multiple stimulator parameters that can be adjusted noninvasively to optimize the outcome in a particular patient. DBS has been performed in patients with primary generalized dystonia, secondary generalized dystonia, cervical dystonia, blepharospasm, Meige syndrome, and tardive dystonia. In a 2006 meta-analysis of 24 studies including 137 patients who underwent DBS for dystonia, the greatest improvement was seen in patients with PKAN, DYT1 dystonia, and tardive dystonia. Surgical denervation procedures such as ramisectomy and rhizotomy as well as myectomy may be useful in selected cases of cervical dystonia.

Because patients with dystonia often have associated comorbidities, consultation with specialists including orthopedic surgeons, physiatrists, and psychiatrists can be useful. Many patients derive benefit from physical, occupational, and speech therapy. Various devices have been developed that provide sensory input via the affected body part, simulating a sensory trick. Alternative and complementary modalities such as acupuncture, biofeedback, massage, and relaxation techniques may be helpful.

Holloway KL, et al. Deep brain stimulation for dystonia: A meta-analysis. *Neuromodulation: Technology at the Neural Interface* 2006;9:253–261. doi: 10.1111/j.1525–1403 .2006.00067.x (A meta-analysis of reported cases of DBS for patients with dystonia.)

Jankovic J. Dystonia: Medical therapy and botulinum toxin. *Adv Neurol* 2004;94:275. [PMID: 14509685] (A review of nonsurgical treatment options in dystonia.)

Schwarz CS, Bressman SB. Genetics and treatment of dystonia. *Neurol Clin* 2009;27:697–718 [PMID: 19555827] (An overview of genetic causes and treatments of dystonia with a focus on DYT1.)

Wilson SAK. Progressive lenticular degeneration: A familial nervous disease associated with cirrhosis of the liver. *Brain* 1912;34:295. (Wilson's 1912 description of the disease that bears his name.)

▼ MYOCLONUS

ESSENTIALS OF DIAGNOSIS

► Brief, sudden, shock-like, involuntary muscle contractions

▶ General Considerations

Myoclonus means "a quick movement of muscle." Myoclonic jerks are shock-like, involuntary muscle contractions that may be rhythmic and repetitive or random and unpredictable. The jerks may be focal, segmental, or generalized. Myoclonic jerks are often stimulus-sensitive and induced by sudden noise or movement. Positive myoclonus, a sudden, brief muscle jerk, is caused by active muscle contraction. Negative myoclonus (eg, asterixis) is a sudden, brief, cessation of muscle contraction in actively contracting muscles that results in loss of posture followed by a compensatory contraction. Myoclonus may be difficult to distinguish from other hyperkinetic involuntary movements, especially tics and tremor. Unlike tics, myoclonus cannot be suppressed, and it does not wax and wane. In addition, myoclonus usually produces a faster movement than a tic. Tremor is usually slower than myoclonus and is rhythmic and oscillatory.

▶ Classification

Etiologic classification of myoclonus includes physiologic, essential, epileptic, and symptomatic forms. Normally occurring muscle jerks such as hiccups (myoclonus of the diaphragm) and hypnic jerks are termed *physiologic myoclonus.* *Essential myoclonus* is a rare disorder that may be hereditary (autosomal dominant), sporadic, or of unknown cause. An important inherited cause of myoclonus that usually starts in childhood and is commonly accompanied by dystonia is myoclonus-dystonia due to mutations in epsilon–sarcoglycan (DYT11); the syndrome is discussed earlier in the section on dystonia. Myoclonus that occurs in the setting of underlying epilepsy is termed *epileptic myoclonus*. Examples include epilepsia partialis continua and juvenile myoclonic epilepsy. Progressive myoclonic epilepsy includes a group of degenerative disorders characterized by epilepsy, myoclonus, and progressive neurologic deterioration. Examples of progressive myoclonic epilepsies include neuronal ceroid lipofuscinosis, Lafora body disease, Unverricht-Lundborg disease, MERFF (myoclonus with epilepsy and ragged-red fibers), and MELAS (mitochondrial encephalomyopathy, lactic acidosis, and strokelike episodes). *Symptomatic myoclonus* may occur in the setting of renal and liver failure, drug intoxication, anoxic brain injury (posthypoxic myoclonus), Creutzfeldt-Jakob disease, Huntington disease, Alzheimer disease, and parkinsonism.

Myoclonus may originate from the cerebral cortex, subcortical structures, brainstem, spinal cord, or peripheral nerves. Choice of antimyoclonic therapy is guided by the origin of the myoclonus. Definitive localization of the focus of myoclonus requires complex electrophysiologic studies that are not routinely available.

▶ Clinical Findings

A. Symptoms and Signs

Cortical myoclonus manifests as stimulus-sensitive, spontaneous, arrhythmic muscle jerks, often restricted to a body part such as the arm, leg, or face. Cortical myoclonic jerks originate within the sensorimotor cortex and may be manifestations of a focal cortical lesion (tumor, stroke, inflammation), focal epilepsy, or epilepsia partialis continua.

Subcortical myoclonus most often originates from the brainstem, resulting in stimulus-sensitive, generalized jerks. Subcortical myoclonus may occur in primary generalized epilepsy, multiple sclerosis, encephalitis, Creutzfeldt-Jakob disease, Alzheimer disease, degenerative disease, toxic states, and metabolic encephalopathies. Two types of myoclonus originate from the spinal cord. Spinal segmental myoclonus is typically rhythmic, stimulus-sensitive, and restricted to a few adjacent segments of the spinal cord. Propriospinal myoclonus causes slow, generalized truncal jerks that produce truncal flexion, and in a subset of patients the etiology is psychogenic. Myoclonus can result from a peripheral nerve lesion. Movements are limited to the involved motor unit, usually are not sensitive to stimuli, and are irregular. An example is hemifacial spasm caused by a lesion to the facial nerve.

B. Imaging Studies and Other Tests

Electroencephalography (EEG) may be useful to clarify an epileptic syndrome, but cortical myoclonus does not produce abnormalities on routine EEG. Definitive localization of a cortical myoclonic focus requires time-locked, back-averaged EEG, a highly specialized technique. In cortical myoclonus, somatosensory evoked potentials may show large-amplitude potentials. CT or MRI may reveal a focal, causal lesion.

▶ Treatment

Therapy of myoclonus is empiric, and for best results, antimyoclonic agents are used in combination (Table 15–10). Choice of therapeutic agents is based on diagnosis, origin of myoclonus, and side-effect profile. Standard antimyoclonic drugs include clonazepam, levetiracetam, piracetam,

Table 15–10. Treatment of Myoclonus

Drug	Initial Adult Dose	Usual Effective Dose	Indication
Clonazepam	0.5 mg/day	2 mg/day divided 3 times a day	Posthypoxic myoclonus Spinal myoclonus Progressive myoclonic epilepsy Essential myoclonus
Levetiracetam	250 mg/day	1000-1500 mg/day	Posthypoxic myoclonus Cortical myoclonus Spinal myoclonus
Piracetam	400 mg 3 times a day	1200-16,000 mg/day divided 3 times a day	Posthypoxic myoclonus Cortical myoclonus Progressive myoclonic epilepsy Essential myoclonus
Primidone[a]	25 mg/day	500-750 mg/day	Cortical myoclonus
Valproate	125 mg 2 times a day	750-1000 mg/day divided 2 times a day	Most forms of myoclonus

[a]Not approved by the Food and Drug Administration.

primidone, and valproic acid. Valproic acid is effective in both cortical and subcortical myoclonus. Levodopa-carbidopa and sodium oxybate have been reported to benefit myoclonus dystonia, and the latter also may help posthypoxic cortical myoclonus. Piracetam, available in Europe, is not approved by the US Food and Drug Administration (FDA), but tablets can be formulated by pharmacies.

Dijk JM, Tijssen MA. Management of patients with myoclonus: Available therapies and the need for an evidence-based approach. *Lancet Neurol* 2010;9:1028–1036. [PMID: 20864054]

TOURETTE SYNDROME & TIC DISORDERS

ESSENTIALS OF DIAGNOSIS

▶ Chronic disorder of motor and vocal tics, usually beginning before the age of 21
▶ Male predominance
▶ Frequently familial
▶ Frequently associated with attention-deficit/hyperactivity disorder and obsessive-compulsive disorder

General Considerations

Tic disorders are conditions that cause sudden, repetitive, stereotyped, purposeless brief actions, gestures, sounds, and words. The prototype tic disorder, Tourette syndrome (TS), was described in a seminal 1885 report by George Gilles de la Tourette, in which several cardinal observations were made: onset during childhood, the hereditary nature of the condition, male predominance, and association with psychiatric disease.

TS is worldwide in distribution, with a 3:1 male gender preponderance. Estimates of the prevalence of TS in the population vary markedly, ranging as high as 4.2%, depending on the methodology of the study. The prevalence of all types of tic disorders is considerably higher, in the range of 20%. Studies of schoolchildren with learning difficulties tend to show a higher prevalence of TS. Tic disorders may exist in pure form, but they are often associated with comorbid psychiatric symptoms, as described later.

Despite the overwhelming clinical evidence that most cases of tic disorder are familial, no gene for TS has been identified. The cause of tics is unknown, but the leading hypothesis postulates a heightened sensitivity of dopamine receptors in the caudate and putamen, termed the *dopamine hypersensitivity hypothesis*. This notion is supported by the clinical observation that tics occur in many disorders of the basal ganglia, including Parkinson disease and Huntington disease. In addition, dopamine receptor–blocking agents suppress tics.

▶ Clinical Findings

A. Tic Phenomenology

Tics are abrupt, purposeless, brief movements that occur suddenly out of a background of normal motor activity. Tics can be *simple* or *complex*. Simple motor tics are quick and short-lived: blinking, ocular deviation, facial grimacing, neck movements, and shoulder shrugging are examples of simple motor tics. Some simple motor tics are slower, sustained, tonic movements, such as limb muscle tensing or abdominal tightening. Other tics have a torsional, twisting aspect that is sustained at the peak of contraction, resembling dystonia.

Complex tics are coordinated, sequenced stereotyped acts, such as tapping or touching, or pantomiming an obscene gesture (copropraxia). Complex tics may have the appearance of compulsive acts, and indeed, the distinction is not always clear. Compulsions are driven by an irrational fear or anxiety that can be allayed by performing a specific sequence of gestures or actions, such as tapping a certain number of times.

The term *stereotypy* or *stereotyped movement* describes continuous and repetitive tic movement of restricted repertoire. Usage has linked stereotypy with developmental delay, autism, Asperger syndrome, mental retardation, and other neurobehavioral disorders—but in appearance, stereotypies resemble tics.

Simple vocal or phonic tics include throat-clearing noises, grunting, clicking, sniffing, barking, squeaking, and other purposeless sounds. Verbal tics, consisting of repetitive purposeless words and phrases, including obscenities (coprolalia), are example of complex vocal tics.

Most patients with tics report a premonitory sensation or urge, coincident with a build-up of inner tension that is relieved temporarily when the tic is released. Sometimes patients describe their prodromal feeling as a localized sensation, such as a tingling or burning, in the body part that participates in the tic. Many individuals can temporarily suppress their tics, especially during intense situations such as an interview or a visit to the physician, only to experience an amplified release of tics after the encounter. It is commonly observed that tics may decrease during times of intense concentration, such as when playing a videogame or participating in sports. Tics may also persist during sleep. Echo phenomena are common in TS: Some individuals can imitate with extraordinary speed and accuracy a sound (echolalia) or gesture (echopraxia). A related phenomenon is the tendency for some patients to repeat their own stereotyped phrases, words, and syllables, termed *palilalia*.

B. Clinical Features of Tic Disorders

Tic disorders usually begin in childhood. The mean age at onset is about 6 years, with increasing severity over the first several years. In 96% of patients, the tics present before age 11. The most common initial symptom is eye blinking, and during the course of the disorder, nearly all patients experience tics involving the face and neck. Vocalizations are reported as the initial symptom in about one third of patients, and the most common phonic tic is throat-clearing. Sniffing and coughing are frequent phonic tics that can be quite disruptive and trigger an initial medical evaluation for asthma or an otolaryngeal problem. Coprolalia, the most notorious and potentially disabling of tics, is present only in a small minority of patients with tic disorders, estimated at less than 3%.

About 50% of TS patients demonstrate symptoms of obsessive-compulsive disorder (OCD), such as compulsive checking, counting, obsessive orderliness, hoarding, and obsessive fears or worries. About half of patients with TS show evidence of attention-deficit/hyperactivity disorder (ADHD), manifested by inattention, distractibility, impulsivity, and hyperactivity, or pure attention deficit disorder without hyperactivity (ADD). Boys with TS are more likely to have ADHD symptoms, whereas girls with TS have OCD symptoms. In contrast to tics, ADHD and OCD symptoms are significantly associated with impaired emotional and social adjustment. A small number of individuals manifest self-injurious behavior. In addition to ADHD and OCD, the behavioral spectrum of TS includes conditions such as generalized anxiety disorder, panic attacks, phobias, and mood disorder. Overall, patients with TS have normal intelligence.

C. Classification of Tic Disorders

The spectrum of tic disorders ranges from mild, transient tics to multiple, chronic, disabling tics with associated psychopathology. For the purpose of diagnostic clarity, classification systems have evolved using standard clinical criteria. Primary tic disorders are "essential" idiopathic conditions in which the tics represent the only neurologic sign.

Secondary tic disorders are neurologic disorders in which tics are part of a larger neurologic syndrome that may include developmental delay, parkinsonism, dystonia, chorea, or a known genetic or acquired neurologic injury, including trauma, infection, or stroke. Secondary tic disorders almost always result from lesions of the basal ganglia. Among the many neurodegenerative causes of tic disorders are Huntington disease, neuroacanthocytosis, and Parkinson disease. The Pediatric Autoimmune Neuropsychiatric Disorders Associated With Streptococcal infections, or PANDAS, is a concept of some controversy suggesting that a large number of cases of tic disorders and obsessive-compulsive behaviors result from an immune-mediated cross-reaction between streptococcal infection and the basal ganglia. The strength of the association is weak, however, and does not justify the treatment of routine TS with antibiotics or immune-modulating therapy, such as plasmapheresis or intravenous immune globulin (IVIg).

The classification criteria for primary tic disorders, formulated by the Tourette Syndrome Classification Study Group in 1993, are listed in Table 15–11. The most common and mildest tic disorder is transient tic disorder (TTD), estimated to occur in up to 24% of schoolchildren. The disorder

Table 15–11. Primary Tic Disorders

Diagnosis	Criteria
Tourette syndrome	Presence of multiple motor and vocal tics Age at onset <21 y Tics must occur many times daily, nearly every day, over a period of >1 y Disturbance causes marked distress or significant impairment in daily functioning Condition cannot be ascribed to known neurologic disorder (symptomatic or secondary tic disorder)
Transient tic disorder	Duration of tic disorder <1 y
Chronic tic disorder	Chronic motor *or* chronic vocal tics (*but not both*) >1 y
Chronic single tic disorder	Chronic single motor *or* chronic single vocal tic
Adult-onset tic disorder	Tic disorder that begins after the age of 21 y Two temporal patterns: de novo adult-onset tics and *recurrent* childhood tics: a tic disorder that went into remission and recurred during adulthood

is characterized by tics that go into permanent remission within 1 year of onset, and so the diagnosis can only be made retrospectively. Chronic multiple tic disorder (CMTD) is a syndrome of multiple motor or vocal tics, but not both. Chronic single tic disorder (CSTD) is a condition in which patients experience only a single, recurrent motor or vocal tic. Such a classification is artificial, as all tic disorders represent variants that share a common underlying pathophysiology and genetic predisposition. The severity of a tic disorder is independent of the temporal profile, as a patient with a single, disruptive tic may be more disabled than an individual with multiple mild tics.

▶ Differential Diagnosis

Tics can usually be differentiated from other major types of hyperkinetic movements because they are uniquely stereotyped and usually preceded by a premonitory sensation. A blinking tic may have the appearance of blepharospasm, but the presence of tics at other body sites marks the condition as a tic disorder. Furthermore, although tics typically begin in childhood, blepharospasm is largely a disorder with onset in adult life. Complex motor tics may be difficult to differentiate from compulsions, and indeed many patients exhibit both types of behaviors. Tics occur automatically, with little premeditation, whereas compulsive motor acts are deliberately performed, purposeless actions often driven by an obsessive idea and may be repeated a specified number of times in a certain order.

▶ Treatment

A. General Approach

The first step in the management of TS is to determine whether treatment is even required. The goal of treatment is not to achieve complete tic suppression but to allow a patient to function and live normally. It is always important to consider the treatment of tics in the context of the associated psychopathology (ADHD, ADD, OCD, anxiety, depression, personality disorder), which, if present, can be more disabling than the tic disorder. Further, it is critically important to target the most distressing or disabling feature in the treatment plan. A comprehensive approach involves psychiatric evaluation and treatment, education of patients, family members, and school personnel, restructuring the school environment, and supportive counseling. In recent years, there has been increasing emphasis on behavioral modification techniques for controlling tics, although further study is needed.

B. Pharmacotherapy

Medication therapy should be considered only if the symptoms of TS are functionally disabling and not remediable by nonpharmacologic interventions. A number of therapeutic agents are available to treat the symptoms of TS, and each medication should be chosen on the basis of specific target symptoms and potential side effects. For example, tic suppression may be the most important goal for one patient, whereas treatment of OCD may take precedence in another.

The choice of medication depends on the severity of symptoms, side-effect profile, presence of comorbid psychopathology, and the physician's experience. For controlling tics, centrally acting α agonists, such as clonidine or guanfacine, are considered drugs of first choice because of a favorable side-effect profile. Clonazepam may be helpful in the treatment of tics and is well-tolerated in children. Medications that reduce or blunt dopaminergic transmission predictably suppress tics, but they carry a higher risk of adverse effects. The catecholamine-depleting agents tetrabenazine and reserpine are effective tic-suppressing agents, but may cause hypotension, depression, sedation, and reversible parkinsonism.

Neuroleptic drugs (haloperidol, risperidone, trifluoperazine, molindone, thiothixene, olanzapine, ziprasidone, pimozide, and most recently aripiprazole), which act as dopamine receptor antagonists, are the most predictably effective tic-suppressing medications but cause weight gain, depression, sedation, and also carry a small but definite risk of inducing permanent tardive dyskinesia. Risperidone has been shown in a number of studies to reduce tic frequency and intensity. Only haloperidol and pimozide have actually been approved by the FDA for the treatment of TS. The list of incompletely evaluated agents for treating tics is long and includes the dopamine agonist ropinirole and nicotine. Patients with focal tics restricted to a small body part, such as blinking tics or a stereotyped neck twitch, may be treated successfully using injections of botulinum toxin.

Table 15–12. Agents for Treating Tic Disorders

Drug	Usual Effective Dose (mg/day)	Potential Adverse Effects
Clonidine	0.05–0.5	Drowsiness, hypotension
Guanfacine	0.5–4	Drowsiness, hypotension
Clonazepam	0.25–2	Drowsiness, irritability
Tetrabenazine	12.5–100	Drowsiness, hypotension, depression, parkinsonism
Reserpine	0.25–3	Drowsiness, hypotension, depression, parkinsonism
Risperidone	0.5–12	Parkinsonism, weight gain, risk of tardive dyskinesias
Olanzapine	2.5–15	Parkinsonism, risk of tardive dyskinesias
Pimozide	0.5–10	Parkinsonism, risk of tardive dyskinesias, retinopathy, prolonged QT interval
Fluphenazine	1–5	Parkinsonism, risk of tardive dyskinesias
Haloperidol	0.5–20	Parkinsonism, risk of tardive dyskinesias

Patients with associated ADHD or OCD may require specific treatment, as drugs used for tic suppression do not help these behaviors. ADHD symptoms are treated using psychostimulants, and OCD symptoms are treated using serotonin reuptake inhibitors. Although many patients with tic disorders are followed by pediatricians or primary neurologists, a psychiatrist may be required to prescribe and supervise the required pharmacotherapy. The pharmacologic treatment of TS is summarized in Table 15–12. Many of the agents in common use are not approved for this indication, and caution must be exercised to avoid adverse effects and medication interactions. The dose ranges for each agent are provided, but it is important for clinicians to tailor treatment to the individual and seek the advice of specialists, including psychiatrists, in complex cases.

▶ Prognosis

The course of tic disorders is unpredictable, marked by tic patterns that evolve, wax, and wane, varying in severity and prevalence over time. The treatment of tic disorders is purely symptomatic, and there is no evidence that it has any effect on the long-term course of the condition. Approximately one half of patients experience a gradual and complete remission in tics by the end of adolescence. Tic severity during childhood does not appear to predict the long-term outcome. In general, the prognosis for normal occupational and social functioning depends more on the associated psychopathology than the tics.

Jankovic J. Treatment of hyperkinetic movement disorders. *Lancet Neurol* 2009;8:844–856. [PMID: 19679276] (Recent review article on the treatment of Tourette syndrome and related disorders.)

Piacentini J, et al. Behavior therapy for children with Tourette disorder: Randomized controlled trial. *JAMA* 2010;303:1929–1937. [PMID: 20483969] (A controlled trial of behavioral therapy shows improvements in tic severity using the Yale Global Tic Severity Scale.)

Schrag A, et al. Streptococcal infection, Tourette syndrome, and OCD: Is there a connection. *Neurology* 2009;73:1256–1253. [PMID: 19794128] (Case-control study that finds no association between Tourette syndrome, OCD, and antecedent streptococcal infection.)

Tourette Syndrome Classification Study Group. Definitions and classification of tic disorders. *Arch Neurol* 1993;50:1013–1016. [PMID: 8215958] (Clinical criteria for the classification of tic disorders.)

The Tourette's Syndrome Study Group. Treatment of ADHD in children with tics: A randomized controlled trial. *Neurology* 2002;58:527–536. [PMID: 11865128] (Clinical trial describing treatment of Tourette syndrome and ADHD concludes that methylphenidate can help behavioral symptoms without exacerbating tics.)

TARDIVE DYSKINESIA & OTHER DRUG-RELATED MOVEMENT DISORDERS

ESSENTIALS OF DIAGNOSIS

▶ Dopamine receptor–blocking agents (DRBAs) may cause acute, subacute, and chronic, persistent movement disorders

▶ Acute dystonia and akathisia are self-limited movement disorders that are triggered by exposure to high-potency DRBAs

▶ Tardive dyskinesias are a group of iatrogenic, persistent movement disorders induced by chronic exposure to DRBAs and include classic tardive dyskinesias, tardive dystonia, and tardive akathisia

▶ Tardive syndromes have a low spontaneous remission rate

▶ Drug-induced parkinsonism is a dose-dependent, reversible syndrome caused by DRBAs

▶ General Considerations

Many drugs cause abnormal movements. Of particular note are movement disorders resulting from exposure to neuroleptics and other agents that block dopamine receptors. These neurologic syndromes may be acute and self-limited or chronic and persistent. The range of abnormal movements caused by dopamine receptor–blocking agents

(DRBAs) varies widely, and it is important for clinicians to recognize these syndromes. Because drug-induced movement disorders are iatrogenic, and sometimes permanent, it is essential for clinicians to warn patients about their potential to occur in patients taking these medications.

The entire category of movement syndromes caused by DRBAs is sometimes lumped together as "extra-pyramidal symptoms" (EPS), but the term oversimplifies a complex group of disorders, each with its own distinct clinical features and treatment. The movement disorder tends to appear late in the course of treatment, hence the term *tardive*. DRBAs may also cause *acute* movement disorders, chiefly acute dystonia and akathisia. In addition, chronic exposure to DRBAs may produce reversible parkinsonism.

Most DRBAs are neuroleptics used for the treatment of psychosis, and although many newer agents are marketed as "atypical," such as risperidone, these drugs can also readily induce parkinsonism and tardive dyskinesias. In addition, many other agents used for depression (amoxapine), gastrointestinal ailments (metoclopramide), and cardiac disease (flunarizine) are DRBAs with the potential to cause tardive syndromes (Tables 15–13 and 15–14). The risk of developing a tardive syndrome is related to the intensity of D_2 receptor blockade but also presumably individual susceptibility factors that have not been elucidated. The only antipsychotic agents that appear to have no risk of inducing a tardive syndrome are clozapine and quetiapine, which have weak affinity for D_2 receptors, although the former drug carries a risk of inducing agranulocytosis.

MOVEMENT DISORDERS CAUSED BY DOPAMINE RECEPTOR–BLOCKING AGENTS

ACUTE SYNDROMES CAUSED BY NEUROLEPTICS

ESSENTIALS OF DIAGNOSIS

▶ Acute dystonia is a focal or segmental torsional muscle spasms that usually occurs within hours of treatment using a high-potency dopamine receptor–blocking drug

▶ Acute akathisia is a sensation of restlessness that occurs within hours of treatment using a high-potency dopamine receptor–blocking drug

1. Acute Dystonia

▶ Clinical Findings

The acute dystonic reaction is a sustained, torsional muscle contraction, usually confined to a body segment, occurring after initial treatment using a DRBA. The classic clinical scenario is

Table 15–13. Neurologic Adverse Effects of Dopamine Receptor Antagonists

Acute reactions
- Acute dystonia
- Acute (or subacute) akathisia

Drug-induced parkinsonism

Neuroleptic malignant syndrome

Tardive syndromes
- Classical tardive dyskinesia
- Tardive dystonia
- Tardive akathisia

that of a young patient who receives a high-potency neuroleptic in the emergency room and subsequently develops a sustained contraction of his neck muscles. All agents that block dopamine D_2 receptors can induce acute dystonic reactions, including risperidone and other so-called "atypical" agents. Serotonergic

Table 15–14. Dopamine Receptor–Blocking Agents

Class	Drug
Phenothiazines	
• Aliphatic	Chlorpromazine, triflupromazine
• Piperidine	Thioridazine, mesoridazine
• Piperazine	Trifluoperazine, prochlorperazine, perphenazine, fluphenazine
Thioxanthenes	
• Aliphatic	Chlorprothixene
• Piperazine	Thiothixene
Butyrophenones	Haloperidol, droperidol
Diphenylbutylpiperidine	Pimozide
Dibenzazepine	Loxapine
Dibenzodiazepine	Clozapine, quetiapine
Thienobenzodiazepine	Olanzapine
Substituted benzamide	Metoclopramide, tiapride, sulpiride, clebopride, remoxipride, veralipride
Indolone	Molindone
Pyrimidinone	Risperidone
Benzisothiazole	Ziprasidone
Benzisoxazole	Iloperidone
Quinolinone	Aripiprazole
Tricyclic	Amoxapine
Calcium channel blocker	Flunarizine, cinnarizine

Adapted with permission from Fahn S, Jankovic J, eds. *Principles and Practice of Movement Disorders.* Philadelphia: Churchill Livingstone/Elsevier, 2007.

agents have also been reported to induce acute dystonic reactions. The onset of symptoms ranges from immediately after the first dose to several days of treatment. In about half of the cases, the acute dystonic reaction occurs within 48 hours, and in 90% by 5 days after starting the therapy.

Acute dystonic reactions most often affect the ocular muscles (oculogyric crisis), face, jaw, tongue, neck and trunk, and less often limbs. A typical acute dystonic reaction may consist of head tilt backward or sideways with tongue protrusion and forced opening of the mouth, often with arching of trunk and ocular deviation upward or laterally. Rarely, the syndrome can recur with subsequent exposures to D_2 receptor–blocking agents.

▶ Treatment

In patients with acute dystonic reactions, symptoms can be relieved within minutes using parenteral anticholinergics or antihistaminics. Diphenhydramine 50 mg or benztropine mesylate 1 to 2 mg or biperiden 1 to 2 mg is given intravenously and can be repeated if the dystonia does not abate within 30 minutes. Intravenous diazepam is also effective and can be used as an alternative therapy. If untreated, the majority of cases resolve spontaneously within 12 to 48 hours after the last dose of the offending agent. DRBAs with high anticholinergic activity have a relatively low incidence rate of acute dystonic reactions, and therefore prophylactic use of anticholinergics (eg, benztropine) has been especially recommended in young patients beginning treatment with high-potency DRBAs.

2. Acute Akathisia

▶ Clinical Findings

Akathisia comprises two elements, one subjective and the other objective. The subjective symptom is extreme restlessness and intolerance of remaining still. Patients complain of a disturbing inner tension with vivid phrases like "I feel that I'm jumping out of my skin" or "I'm about to explode." The objective component, visible to an observer, are repetitive movements performed by the patient to relieve the inner restlessness, such as marching in place, shifting the limbs, writhing and rolling movements, or stereotypic caressing or rocking movements. Some patients moan as part of a generalized akathisic state. Most cases of akathisia occur within 1 month of drug exposure. Akathisia may occur in any condition of dopamine deficiency or blockade. It was first observed in patients with advanced parkinsonism but is now most frequently encountered as an acute side effect of neuroleptic drugs.

▶ Differential Diagnosis

The differential diagnosis of repetitive movements includes states of agitation due to encephalopathy, pain, or psychiatric disease such as agitated depression, psychosis, or obsessive-compulsive disorder. Hyperkinetic disorders, such as generalized chorea, tics or tremor, do not have the repetitive, driven, semipurposeful movements of akathisia, and the sufferers do not describe an inner state of restlessness. Unusual syndromes of inner vibrations and tremors are described in patients with parkinsonism, dementia, or tardive dyskinesia.

▶ Treatment

Acute akathisia is self-limited, disappearing on discontinuation of the offending neuroleptic. Acute akathisia can be controlled by anticholinergics when neuroleptics need to be continued; other agents that can reduce akathisia include β-blockers, clonidine, and mirtazapine.

NEUROLEPTIC-INDUCED PARKINSONISM

ESSENTIALS OF DIAGNOSIS

▶ Dose-dependent parkinsonism caused by dopamine receptor–blocking agents

▶ The syndrome may be clinically indistinguishable from classic Parkinson disease

▶ Parkinsonism gradually resolves if the offending agent is removed

Neuroleptic-induced parkinsonism is a dose-related side effect of DRBAs and may be indistinguishable in appearance from idiopathic Parkinson disease (PD), including typical rest tremor and asymmetric signs. It develops with use of either DRBAs or dopamine-depleting drugs such as reserpine and tetrabenazine. All neuroleptics can induce parkinsonism in proportion to their D_2 receptor affinity, the dosage, and duration of treatment, with the exception of clozapine. The incidence of drug-induced parkinsonism in patients taking DRBAs varies from 15% to 60%. Women are almost twice as frequently affected as men, a reverse of the ratio in idiopathic PD. Neuroleptic-induced parkinsonism also occurs increasingly with advanced age, in parallel with the incidence of idiopathic PD.

Drug-induced parkinsonism is typically reversible when the medication is reduced or discontinued, but sometimes the remission of symptoms takes many months. When parkinsonism develops in a patient receiving neuroleptics, the adverse effect should be weighed against the benefits of treatment. If a patient has strong need for DRBA therapy, some degree of parkinsonism may be tolerable. For patients at risk for falling due to drug-induced parkinsonism, a change in therapy should be considered, either reducing the dose of neuroleptic or replacing the DRBA with an atypical agent, such as quetiapine or clozapine. There is little evidence that dopamine agonists or levodopa ameliorate drug-induced parkinsonism in the presence of a DRBA. Some patients show persisting parkinsonism despite prolonged discontinuation of neuroleptics, probably reflecting the development of actual Parkinson disease; no pathologically proven case of tardive parkinsonism exists.

TARDIVE SYNDROMES

ESSENTIALS OF DIAGNOSIS

▶ Tardive dyskinesia is a syndrome of stereotyped, choreic movements involving the face and distal extremities caused by chronic exposure to dopamine receptor–blocking agents

▶ Tardive dystonia should be distinguished from classical tardive dyskinesias because it consists of sustained, torsional, often disabling muscle spasms that affect any part of the body

▶ Tardive akathisia is a syndrome of chronic restlessness resulting from exposure to dopamine receptor–blocking drugs

▶ Tardive syndromes have a low rate of spontaneous remission and often cause permanent disability

▶ General Considerations

Tardive syndromes are late, persistent abnormal movements induced by chronic exposure to dopamine receptor–blocking agents (DRBAs). The risk of developing a tardive syndrome is proportional to its dopamine D_2 receptor affinity and the duration of drug exposure, although some cases have appeared within weeks of the first doses. The three main tardive syndromes are classical tardive dyskinesia, tardive dystonia, and tardive akathisia. Tardive dyskinesias are hypothesized to result from permanent alterations in synaptic dopaminergic sensitivity induced by dopamine receptor blockade.

When a tardive syndrome develops, gradual withdrawal of the offending agent should be considered. Abrupt withdrawal of the inciting agent is associated with a more severe emergence of abnormal movements. General treatment guidelines for tardive syndromes are provided in Table 15–15. In patients with classical tardive dyskinesia, the remission rate is estimated at about one third over 2 years. The remission rates for tardive dystonia and tardive akathisia are 12% and 8%, respectively, underscoring the notion that for most patients, the likelihood of chronic, or even permanent, abnormal movements is high.

1. Classical Tardive Dyskinesia

▶ Clinical Findings

Dyskinesia is a general term simply meaning abnormal movements. Over the years, tardive dyskinesia has become synonymous with the first described complication of long-term dopamine receptor antagonist therapy: continuous, repetitive, rhythmical, stereotypic movements involving oral, buccal, and lingual areas. Prevalence estimates range from 0.5–65% in the literature, but is probably closer to 12%

Table 15–15. General Guidelines for Treating Tardive Syndromes

- Taper and slowly eliminate causative agents, if clinically possible. Avoid sudden cessation of these drugs, which may exacerbate symptoms.
- If it is necessary to treat the movements, the drugs of first choice are the dopamine-depleting drugs reserpine, tetrabenazine, and α-methylparatyrosine. It is important to monitor the development of depression, hypotension, sedation, and parkinsonism.
- If dopamine-depleting agents do not help, consider a trial of clozapine or quetiapine.
- Dopamine receptor-blocking agents may be used as medications of last resort for tardive syndromes, despite the risk of worsening the syndrome over the long term.
- Globus pallidus stimulation should be considered for disabling tardive dystonia if medication treatment fails.

in patients on chronic haloperidol treatment. Older age, female gender, cumulative drug exposure, and the presence of an affective disorder are associated with increased prevalence of classical tardive dyskinesia; African-Americans appear to have a higher risk than Caucasians. In the past decade, the incidence of tardive dyskinesias may be in slight decline due to the use of second-generation D_2 antagonists, which demonstrate less receptor blocking affinity. On the other hand, children are increasingly treated for psychiatric symptoms using "atypical" neuroleptics, so the long-term incidence of tardive dyskinesia in this population must be carefully tracked.

Classical tardive dyskinesia causes a pattern of repetitive, complex chewing motions, occasionally with lip-smacking and opening of the mouth, tongue protrusion, lip pursing, and sucking movements. The mouth movements in classical tardive dyskinesia are readily suppressed by patients when they are asked to do so, and they cease during talking or eating. Because tardive dyskinesias do not interfere with basic functions, patients are often unaware of their movements. The constant lingual movements may lead to tongue hypertrophy, and macroglossia is a common clinical sign. Tardive dyskinesias may also cause limb movements, usually distal, repetitive, patterned choreic movements of the toes and fingers, the latter sometimes termed piano-playing movements. Sometimes, there is rhythmic rocking of the trunk.

Differential Diagnosis

The differential diagnosis of choreic movements of the face includes Huntington disease, idiopathic dystonia of the face (primary oromandibular dystonia, or Meige syndrome), senile and edentulous chorea of the face, branchial myoclonus, facial tics, and myokymia. In tardive dyskinesias, the pattern of the movements is typically rhythmic, repetitive, and stereotypical, in contrast to the orofacial chorea seen in Huntington disease, which is random and unpredictable.

Treatment

The most effective agents for treating tardive dyskinesias are catecholamine depletors and, paradoxically, DRBAs. The rational for using dopamine-depleting drugs, such as reserpine and tetrabenazine, is that these agents effectively reduce dopaminergic synaptic activity, thereby reducing the TD symptoms, without exposing the brain to an offending DRBA. These agents are slowly titrated to the point of mild parkinsonism, usually reaching a dose range of reserpine 0.5–2 mg daily, or tetrabenazine 25–100 mg daily. Tardive dyskinesia can be temporarily suppressed using increasing doses of DRBAs, but continuing exposure to these agents may lead to worsening of the movements in the long term. α-methylparatyrosine is not very effective when used alone, but can be a potent antidopaminergic drug when combined with other presynaptically acting drugs, such as dopamine depletors. Clozapine and amantadine have reportedly been effective in suppressing tardive dyskinesia.

Tarsy D, Baldessarini RJ. Epidemiology of tardive dyskinesia: Is risk declining with modern antipsychotics? *Mov Disord* 2006;21:589-598. [PMID: 16532448] (Study of the decline in incidence of tardive dyskinesia in the era of second generation neuroleptics.)

2. Tardive Dystonia

Clinical Findings

Tardive dystonia differs from tardive dyskinesias in that the movements are sustained and interfere with normal motor function. Just as DRBAs may induce acute dystonia, persistent, sustained, disabling dystonic movements may result from chronic DRBA exposure. Tardive dystonia, which resembles idiopathic dystonia, is more disabling than classical tardive dyskinesia. The combination of retrocollis, trunk arching backward, internal rotation of the arms, and extension of the elbows and flexion of the wrists is a frequently observed pattern in severely disabled patients. The onset of tardive dystonia ranges from days to years after exposure to a DRBA. Severe tardive dystonia is more common in young men, whereas severe classical tardive dyskinesia is more common in older women.

Treatment

As with classical tardive dyskinesia, the most effective medications for tardive dystonia are antidopaminergic drugs, either dopamine depletors or DRBAs, but a smaller percentage of patients improves. As with classical tardive dyskinesia, increasing doses of DRBAs might temporarily help tardive dystonia, but continuing exposure may cause worse movements over time. In tardive dystonia, anticholinergics (eg, benztropine or trihexyphenidyl) are almost as effective as antidopaminergic drugs. The atypical antipsychotic, clozapine, is been helpful in some patients. For medically intractable tardive dystonia, bilateral globus pallidus stimulation using implantable electrodes can be effective.

3. Tardive Akathisia

 Clinical Findings

Tardive akathisia is a rare syndrome of restlessness and intolerance of remaining still, coupled with continuous, stereotyped, repetitive pacing and fidgeting movements. Tardive akathisia resembles acute akathisia in every way, except that it is persistent and may be permanent.

 Treatment

Tardive akathisia can be helped by reserpine and tetrabenazine. In this respect the clinical pharmacology more closely resembles that of classical tardive dyskinesia than acute akathisia. Opioids, such as codeine 15–60 mg daily, are reported to be beneficial in reducing the sensation of restlessness in chronic akathisia. Most of the patients develop tardive akathisia within the first 2 years of treatment.

Burke RE, et al. Tardive akathisia: An analysis of clinical features and response to open therapeutic trials. *Mov Disord* 1989;4:157–175. [PMID: 2567492] (Seminal article on the clinical features and treatment of tardive akathisia.)

Correll CU, Leucht S, Kane JM. Lower risk for tardive dyskinesia associated with second-generation antipsychotics: A systematic review of 1-year studies. *Am J Psychiatry* 2004;161:414–425. [PMID: 14992963] (Epidemiologic study on the risk of developing tardive dyskinesias in low potency "atypical" dopamine receptor blocking agents.)

Jeste DV. Tardive dyskinesia rates with atypical antipsychotics in older adults. *J Clin Psychiatry* 2004;65(Suppl 9):21–24. [PMID: 15189108] (Epidemiologic study on the incidence and prevalence of tardive dyskinesias.)

NEUROLEPTIC MALIGNANT SYNDROME

ESSENTIALS OF DIAGNOSIS

▶ Fever, rigidity, and changes in mental status, with elevated muscle enzymes, dehydration, and autonomic instability

▶ The syndrome usually develops on stable therapeutic doses of dopamine receptor–blocking agents

▶ Must be distinguished from serotonin syndrome, malignant hyperthermia, acute generalized parkinsonism or dystonia ("dystonic storm"), and other causes of metabolic encephalopathy

 Clinical Findings

Neuroleptic malignant syndrome (NMS) is an idiosyncratic, potentially life-threatening syndrome consisting of (1) hyperthermia, usually with other autonomic disturbances such as tachycardia, diaphoresis, and labile blood pressure; (2) extrapyramidal signs, usually muscle rigidity or dystonia, and often with elevated muscle enzymes; and (3) altered mental status, such as agitation, inattention, and confusion. The pathophysiologic mechanism of NMS and the individual susceptibility factors are not well understood.

NMS usually begins abruptly while the patient is on therapeutic, not toxic, dosages of medication. All the symptoms are fully manifest within 24 hours of onset and reach a maximum severity within 72 hours. There appears to be no relationship between the duration of therapy and the development of symptoms, as NMS can develop soon after the first dose or at any time after prolonged treatment. Recovery usually occurs within one to several weeks, but the syndrome is fatal in 20–30% of cases. Prolonged hyperthermia and generalized muscle contractions may cause rhabdomyolysis, with renal failure. Muscle biopsies show swelling, edema, and often vacuolar changes in muscle fibers. All agents that block dopamine D_2 receptors can induce NMS, including risperidone and other "atypical" neuroleptics. The differential diagnosis includes malignant hyperthermia, serotonin syndrome, and acute baclofen withdrawal, in addition to fever of any cause in the intensive care unit; the diagnosis depends on an accurate history of drug exposure and interactions.

 Treatment

Treatment of NMS consists of discontinuing the dopamine receptor–blocking agents and providing supportive measures. Rapid relief of symptoms usually follows administration of dantrolene, bromocriptine, or levodopa. Reexposure to dopamine receptor antagonists does not necessarily lead to recurrence of NMS. Residual catatonia lasting weeks to months has been reported after recovery from the acute syndrome, with some individuals responding to electroconvulsive therapy (ECT).

Trollor JN, Chen X, Sachdev PS. Neuroleptic malignant syndrome associated with atypical antipsychotic drugs. *CNS Drugs* 2009;23:477–492. [PMID: 19480467] (Recent review article on neuroleptic malignant syndrome.)

RESTLESS LEGS SYNDROME (RLS)

ESSENTIALS OF DIAGNOSIS

▶ A syndrome of restlessness and unpleasant sensations in the legs that is relieved by moving or walking

▶ RLS is associated with periodic limb movements of sleep

▶ Chronic, progressive course

▶ Responsive to dopamine agonists, opiates, and other agents

▶ General Considerations

Thomas Willis, 17th century English physician, first described a condition of leg restlessness ("unquietness") and involuntary movements that interfered with sleep and was relieved by walking. As fully delineated by Ekbom, restless legs syndrome (RLS) is a chronic condition that usually begins during middle age and worsens with time. The disorder is common, affecting 3–10% of individuals. Many cases are familial, inherited in an autosomal-dominant fashion. The cause of RLS is unknown, but the disorder is associated with iron-deficiency anemia, uremia, and peripheral neuropathy. RLS frequently responds to dopaminergic medication, implicating a role of central dopamine pathways in the pathophysiology of the disorder.

▶ Clinical Findings

A. Symptoms and Signs

The key diagnostic features of RLS include ill-defined discomfort or unusual sensations ("dysesthesias") in the legs, sometimes described as intolerable tingling, crawling, creeping, stretching, pulling, or prickling sensations (Table 15–16). Individuals with RLS usually do not describe their leg discomfort as painful muscular cramping or aching, a point of differentiation from nocturnal leg cramps. The legs are invariably involved, usually bilaterally, whereas the trunk and arms are rarely affected. RLS typically occurs during rest or sleep, or when patients are drowsy and attempting repose. The discomfort is associated with an urge to move the legs or walk about, which immediately relieves the unpleasant sensations. Symptoms typically begin intermittently and are mild but with time become more frequent and uncomfortable, impairing sleep and necessitating medical intervention. Some patients experience leg restlessness during the day or in wakeful situations that involve immobility, such as sitting in an audience or air travel.

Table 15–16. Clinical Features of Restless Legs Syndrome

Diagnostic Features
• Desire or need to move the limbs, usually associated with uncomfortable or unpleasant sensations
• Symptoms of motor restlessness
• Symptoms worse or exclusively present at rest, with at least partial or temporary relief by activity
• Symptoms maximal during evening and night

Typical Features
• Involuntary movements: periodic limb movements
• Sleep disturbance
• Normal neurologic examination
• Generally chronic course, often progressive
• Positive family history

RLS has long been linked to periodic limb movements (PLM), a movement disorder that occurs during sleep. The full cycle of these movements consists of brief jerks of either leg, dorsiflexion of the great toe and foot, and a briefly sustained tonic flexion spasm of the entire leg; the movement has the appearance of an exaggerated Babinski or flexor withdrawal reflex. The limb movements tend to recur every 20 seconds or so in trains that may last for hours. PLMs usually occur during periods of arousal in stage 1 and stage 2 sleep and decrease in deeper sleep stages. Present in more than 80% of patients with RLS, PLMs also occur in other sleep disorders, including narcolepsy and rapid-eye movement (REM) behavior disorder, a condition of acting out vivid dreams.

In recent years, a number of genetic risk factors for RLS have been identified, although a specific causative gene has not yet been found. In families with RLS, the disorder is transmitted as an autosomal-dominant trait. Several medical conditions are associated with an increased prevalence of RLS, including iron deficiency, uremia, peripheral neuropathy, diabetes, rheumatoid arthritis, pregnancy, gastric surgery, and the fibromyalgia syndrome. Patients with Parkinson disease (PD) experience leg restlessness, but the true prevalence of RLS in PD is uncertain.

B. Laboratory Findings

Laboratory testing in RLS is aimed at identifying secondary causes of the syndrome. Iron studies and ferritin levels are the most important tests. Additional testing includes routine serum chemistry. Electrodiagnostic testing should be performed in patients with symptoms or signs of peripheral nerve dysfunction. In selected cases, a routine sleep study, or polysomnography (PSG), will reveal an increased amount of nocturnal movement and wakeful periods, delayed sleep onset, and PLMS.

▶ Differential Diagnosis

It is important to distinguish RLS from akathisia, which may occur due to exposure to dopamine receptor–blocking agents or PD. In RLS, the sensory discomfort and urge to move are localized to the legs, unlike in akathisia, which causes generalized discomfort or restlessness. RLS can be distinguished from nocturnal leg cramps, which cause painful muscle contractions, tightness, and tenderness. RLS must further be differentiated from peripheral neuropathy, radiculopathy, reflex sympathetic dystrophy, and other localized sensory disturbances that can involve the legs; in these disorders, the symptoms do not show the nocturnal predilection of RLS, and neurologic evaluation reveals nerve or root dysfunction. The painful legs and moving toes syndrome is an unusual and rare disorder, sometimes associated with peripheral neuropathy, that causes cutaneous pain and writhing, choreic toe movements.

The differential diagnosis for PLMs comprises a wide variety of normal and abnormal movements in sleep, including hypnic jerks, normal postural shifts, nocturnal seizures, parasomnias such as sleep walking and pathologic arousals, and REM sleep behavior disorder.

Treatment

Several classes of medication are effective in RLS, including dopaminergic agents, opioids, benzodiazepines, and anticonvulsants, usually taken as a single dose before bed. The dopamine agonists bromocriptine and pramipexole are first-line drugs for RLS. Unfortunately, dopamine drug treatment is sometimes associated a gradual need to escalate the dosage, as well as the dopaminergic complications of pathologic gambling and other compulsive behaviors. Codeine and stronger opiates help RLS but carry a risk of dependence. Clonazepam, carbamazepine, baclofen, and clonidine have all been reported as successful treatments for RLS. Because RLS symptoms are chronic and progressive, it is important to treat using the lowest effective doses. Some patients, especially those treated using levodopa, develop dependence and rebound symptoms. In patients with iron deficiency and RLS, treatment with iron is curative. Any treatment approach for RLS must also include optimization of sleeping habits.

Prognosis

The prognosis for RLS is generally good. Although the disorder is lifelong, small doses of medication and the development of optimal sleep hygiene usually keep the symptoms under control.

Allen RP, et al; Restless Legs Syndrome Diagnosis and Epidemiology workshop at the National Institutes of Health; International Restless Legs Syndrome Study Group. Restless legs syndrome: Diagnostic criteria, special considerations, and epidemiology. *Sleep Med* 2003;4:101–119. [PMID: 14592341] (A report from the restless legs syndrome diagnosis and epidemiology workshop at the National Institutes of Health.)

Chesson AL, Jr, et al. Practice parameters for the treatment of restless legs syndrome and periodic limb movement disorder. Standards of Practice Committee of the American Academy of Sleep Medicine. *Sleep* 1999;22:961–968. [PMID: 10566915] (Diagnostic criteria for RLS and PLMs, with treatment recommendations.)

Trenkwalder C, et al. Treatment of restless legs syndrome: An evidence-based review and implications for clinical practice. *Mov Disord* 2008;23:2267–2302. [PMID: 18925578] (Recent review of restless legs syndrome treatment.)

Ataxia & Cerebellar Disease

16

Claire Henchcliffe, MD, DPhil

Ataxia (from the Greek "without order") denotes incoordination and imbalance, involving limbs, stance, and gait, as well as speech and ocular disturbances. In practice, the term is used when these symptoms arise from neurologic dysfunction involving the cerebellum and its connecting pathways. However, ataxia can also result from malfunction of sensory input from proprioceptive sensory pathways or the vestibular system into the cerebellum. Ataxia often results in significant loss of independence, and injuries from falls and other complications lead to considerable morbidity.

▼ APPROACH TO THE ATAXIC PATIENT

Once ataxic features of coordination or gait are recognized, cerebellar ataxia needs to be distinguished from so-called *sensory ataxia,* resulting from proprioceptive abnormalities, and from labyrinthine ataxia, seen with vestibular disorders. With proprioceptive ataxia, incoordination often increases dramatically when the patient's eyes are closed. Oculomotor symptoms such as nystagmus point away from sensory ataxia. Patients with labyrinthine ataxia also have impaired gait and balance, but speech is not affected and limb movements are coordinated. Myelopathy, basal ganglia disease, or bihemispheric disease can also cause incoordination and gait dysfunction. It is therefore important in assessing the patient with ataxia to ensure that the clumsiness observed is independent of isometric strength, muscle tone, reflex abnormalities, and problems with spatial planning. In practice, however, the clinical picture may be complicated by coexistence of these abnormalities with cerebellar disease.

Because ataxia may result from acquired disorders or be genetically inherited (Table 16–1), a careful family history is necessary. The time course of disease, age of onset, additional symptoms such as spasticity or cognitive dysfunction, and evidence of systemic disease help refine diagnostic possibilities.

▶ Clinical Findings & Their Relation to Cerebellar Anatomy

The close spatial and functional association of the cerebellum with the brainstem explains why cerebellar symptoms can originate in the brainstem itself. Additionally, space-occupying cerebellar lesions may rapidly lead to compression of the brainstem. The cerebellum can be functionally divided into three regions—anterior lobe and rostral vermis, flocculonodular and posterior lobes, and cerebellar hemispheres—corresponding to characteristic clinical syndromes (Table 16–2). Clinical signs of cerebellar disease are described in Table 16–3.

▶ Therapeutic Approaches in Cerebellar Disease

Particularly in patients with chronic ataxia, a multidisciplinary approach involving physicians, psychologists, therapists, nursing specialists, and social work services helps address diverse issues, including optimizing physical function, managing long-term disability, and social and psychological issues affecting both patient and caregivers. Genetic testing is best done in the context of rigorous and careful counseling. Some patients may wish to participate in trials offered at centers specializing in movement disorders. The National Ataxia Foundation is an excellent source of information and can be found at http://www.ataxia.org.

A. Physical and Occupational Therapy

Added weight can help decrease tremor and may also benefit limb ataxia, but at greater weight loads, performance tends to decline. Adaptive devices that incorporate damping mechanisms are available. Physical therapy is helpful for many patients who manifest generalized deconditioning, weakness, or spasticity.

Table 16–1. Causes of Ataxia: Categories of Diseases Affecting the Cerebellum and Time Course of Disease

Category	Disease	Time Course[a]		
		Acute	Subacute	Chronic
Developmental	Arnold-Chiari malformation, Dandy-Walker malformation, cerebellar hypoplasia	−	−	+
Hereditary	Autosomal-dominant spinocerebellar ataxias (see Tables 16-6 and 16-7)	−	−	+
	Autosomal-recessive spinocerebellar ataxias—Friedreich ataxia, others (see Table 16-9)	−	−	+
	Fragile X-associated tremor and ataxia syndrome	−	−	+
	Episodic ataxias (see Table 16-8)	+	−	(+)
	Mitochondrial disorders (see Table 16-10)	+	+	+
	Leukodystrophies, storage disorders	−	−	+
	Urea cycle disorders	+	+	+
Vascular	Ischemic cerebellar stroke (see Table 16-4), ataxic hemiparesis, lacunar stroke syndrome	+	−	−
	Cerebellar hemorrhage	+	−	−
	Arteriovenous malformations	+	+	+
	Cavernous malformations	+	−	−
Toxin-associated	Alcohol	+	+	+
	Metals (lead, thallium, mercury)	+	+	+
	Solvents	+	−	+
Medication-associated	Anticonvulsants (phenytoin, carbamazepine), amiodarone, cytotoxic drugs (methotrexate, cisplatin)	+	+	+
Neoplastic	Metastatic tumors (lung, breast, melanoma, renal, seminoma, teratoma)	−	+	+
	Medulloblastoma, glioma, oligodendroglioma, astrocytoma, meningioma, ependymomas, cerebellopontine tumors	−	+	+
	Cerebellar hemangioblastoma (von Hippel-Lindau syndrome)	−	+	+
Infectious	Abscess (bacterial, fungal)	−	+	+
	Acute viral cerebellitis (EBV, HHV-6, HSV-1, mumps)	+	−	−
	HIV encephalitis	−	(+)	+
	Prion disease	−	(+)	+
	Encephalitic bacterial infection, including listeriosis	+	(+)	−
Immune-associated	Multiple sclerosis	+	+	+
	Postinfectious cerebellitis	+	(+)	−
	Gluten ataxia	−	+	+
	Paraneoplastic (see Table 16-5)	−	+	+
Metabolic or nutritional	Hypothyroidism, hypoglycemia	−	(+)	+
	Deficiency in vitamins B_1, B_{12}, or E	−	−	+

EBV = Epstein-Barr virus; HHV-6 = human herpesvirus 6; HSV-1 = herpes simplex virus 1; +, present; −, absent.
[a]Parentheses signify a less likely, although possible, time course for that process.

B. Speech and Swallowing Therapy

Patients who have dysarthria often benefit from speech therapy. Many patients require formal swallowing evaluations, and exercises as well as dietary modification may help those with dysphagia, an important cause of morbidity. In advanced cases, feeding via a percutaneous endoscopic gastrostomy tube can reduce risk of aspiration.

C. Pharmacotherapy

There has been little success in treating ataxia with medications. Action tremor may respond to primidone, β-adrenergic blocking agents such as propranolol, and benzodiazepines. Appropriate medications may be given for associated symptoms such as spasticity, parkinsonism, dystonia, bladder dysfunction, and orthostatic hypotension.

Table 16-2. Cerebellar Syndromes: Functional Anatomy and Clinical Findings

Cerebellar Syndrome	Anatomic Location	Clinical Findings
Rostral vermis syndrome	Anterior lobe, rostral vermis	Wide-based stance and gait with proportionally less appendicular ataxia Infrequent presence of hypotonia, nystagmus, dysarthria
Caudal vermis syndrome	Flocculonodular and posterior lobes	Axial disequilibrium (trunk and head ataxia) but proportionally little or no appendicular ataxia Staggering gait Occasionally spontaneous nystagmus and rotated postures of head Vertigo Downbeat or gaze-evoked nystagmus, or both Impaired smooth pursuit
Cerebellar hemispheric syndrome	Cerebellar hemispheres	Ipsilateral appendicular (limb) ataxia with dysmetria, dysdiadochokinesia (arms > legs) Kinetic (intention) and statis tremors Dysarthria Muscle hypotonia (acute only) Excessive rebound Ocular dysmetria

D. Surgical Treatment

High-frequency electrical stimulation of the ventral intermediate nucleus of the thalamus, or surgical lesions, can reduce cerebellar tremor. There is, however, no effect on ataxia.

E. Gene and Stem Cell Therapy

Recent advances have enhanced our understanding of the genetic basis of many of the inherited ataxias, and the possibility of gene therapy is being studied in other neurodegenerative diseases. Currently there are no such therapies for ataxia.

Trujillo-Martin MM, et al. Effectiveness and safety of treatments for degenerative ataxias: A systematic review. *Mov Disord* 2009; 24:1111–1124. [PMID: 19412936]

Table 16-3. Clinical Signs of Cerebellar Disease

Sign	Definition
Truncal ataxia	Oscillations while sitting or standing; falling may occur toward the side of a unilateral lesion
Wide-based stance or gait	Feet placed widely apart; difficulty standing with feet together or walking tandem in heel-to-toe test
Dysdiadochokinesis	Impaired rapid alternating movements, tested by alternating supination-pronation of hands or by toe-tapping
Dysmetria	Errors in judging distance with body movements, tested by finger-to-nose test, which may result in underestimation (hypometria) or overestimation with transient overshoot (hypermetria)
Impaired check	Failure to arrest a limb movement, tested by flexing the arm at the elbow against resistance that is suddenly released
Past pointing	Termination of a movement, briefly, away from the target, tested by extending the arm in front, raising it, and attempting to return it to the identical position with eyes closed
Hypotonia	Decreased muscle tone
Dysarthria	Unclear pronunciation with normal language content and meaning
Scanning speech	Abnormally long pauses between words or syllables
Kinetic tremor	Tremor that occurs with voluntary movement, with worsening on target approach; also called *intention tremor*
Postural tremor	Tremor that persists once a target is reached, easily elicited by stretching arms out with palms facing down
Nystagmus	Inability to maintain gaze fixation, with slow phase followed by rapid saccadic correction, commonly gaze evoked but also in a primary position; may be downbeat, upbeat, or horizontal
Dysmetric saccades	Analogous to limb dysmetria, resulting in hypermetria or hypometria on saccade to a target presented by the examiner

ACQUIRED ATAXIAS

CEREBELLAR ISCHEMIC STROKE SYNDROMES

> ## ESSENTIALS OF DIAGNOSIS
>
> ▶ Acute onset of ataxia with other signs and symptoms
> ▶ Magnetic resonance imaging (MRI) of the brain, showing hyperintensity on diffusion-weighted images initially and on fluid-attenuated inversion recovery and T2-weighted sequences later

▶ General Considerations

Approximately 2% of all ischemic strokes and 10% of all intracerebral hemorrhages affect the cerebellum. Patients with cerebellar infarction often have brainstem signs because of common arterial supplies. The vessel most frequently implicated is the posterior inferior cerebellar artery, but infarctions also occur in the territories of the superior cerebellar artery and the anterior inferior cerebellar artery (see Chapter 10). Ataxia may also arise as a result of lacunar infarction, most commonly as the ataxichemiparesis syndrome.

▶ Clinical Findings

A. Symptoms and Signs

Symptoms and signs of cerebellar infarction are summarized in Table 16–4. Large cerebellar infarctions often cause headaches.

B. Laboratory Findings

There may be evidence of unrecognized risk factors such as diabetes or hypertension. Other tests for ischemic stroke are discussed in Chapter 10.

C. Imaging Studies

Computed tomography (CT) of the head is performed acutely to rule out hemorrhage. MRI of the brain with diffusion-weighted imaging can establish the clinical diagnosis acutely. Magnetic resonance angiography or vascular ultrasound can assess the extent of atherosclerotic disease in the basilar and vertebral arteries. In selected patients with recent whiplash or other trauma, vertebral artery dissection can be identified by MRI or cerebral angiography.

▶ Treatment & Complications

Therapy follows general recommendations for any patient with ischemic stroke (see Chapter 10). However, cerebellar infarctions that are more than 2.5 cm in diameter must be intensively monitored because of the risk of edema leading to

Table 16–4. Clinical Findings in Infarction of the Posterior Inferior, Superior, and Anterior Inferior Cerebellar Arteries

Symptom	PICA	SCA	AICA
Vertigo, nausea, vomiting	+	+	+
Nystagmus	+	+	+
Dysarthria	+	+	+
Ipsilateral Horner syndrome	+	+	+
Contralateral trochlear nerve palsy	−	+	−
Ipsilateral facial palsy	−	−	+
Ipsilateral facial hypalgesia and thermoanesthesia	+	−	+
Ipsilateral facial hypesthesia	−	−	+
Contralateral facial hypalgesia and thermoanesthesia	−	+	−
Ipsilateral hearing impairment or loss	−	+	+
Ipsilateral palatal, pharyngeal, and vocal cord paralysis	+	−	−
Contralateral trunk and limb hypalgesia and thermoanesthesia	+	+	+
Ipsilateral truncal lateropulsion	+	+	−
Ipsilateral appendicular ataxia	+	+	+

AICA = anterior inferior cerebellar artery; PICA = posterior inferior cerebellar artery; SCA = superior cerebellar artery; +, present; −, absent.

brainstem compression or obstructive hydrocephalus and coma 2–4 days after stroke onset. Surgical intervention may be required.

Jauss M, et al. Surgical and medical management of patients with massive cerebellar infarctions: Results of the German-Austrian Cerebellar Infarction Study. *J Neurol* 1999;246:257–264; erratum *J Neurol* 1999;246:628. [PMID: 10367693]

CEREBELLAR HEMORRHAGE

> ## ESSENTIALS OF DIAGNOSIS
>
> ▶ Sudden onset of ataxia, possible headache
> ▶ Hemorrhage detected by CT scan of the head

▶ General Considerations

The most frequent causes of cerebellar hemorrhage are hypertension and vascular malformations.

▶ Clinical Findings

A. Symptoms and Signs

Patients characteristically present with sudden onset of headache and inability to stand or walk. Ipsilateral limb ataxia is often present, and some patients have ipsilateral gaze or abducens paresis. Hemiparesis and long-tract sensory signs are usually conspicuously absent.

B. Laboratory and Imaging Findings

CT or MRI scan of the head demonstrates hemorrhage, and there may be surrounding signal abnormality as a result of edema. Evidence of herniation of the foramen magnum may be present. Laboratory tests should include coagulation studies.

C. Special Tests

MRI may identify an underlying vascular malformation, but if imaging findings are negative and such a lesion is suspected, cerebral angiography may be undertaken.

▶ Treatment

Cerebellar hemorrhages more than 3 cm in diameter require emergency surgical evacuation, even in patients who are seemingly stable with full alertness. Deterioration, when it occurs, can be abrupt and fatal. Medical treatment of smaller cerebellar hemorrhages follows the general recommendations for treatment of intracranial hemorrhage (see Chapter 11).

Rincon F Mayer SA. Clinical review. Critical care management of spontaneous intracerebral hemorrhage *Crit Care* 2008;12:237. [PMID: 19108704]

TOXINS & NUTRITIONAL DEFICIENCIES

1. Ethanol

Cerebellar ataxia in alcoholic individuals can be the result of acute intoxication, Wernicke-Korsakoff disease, or alcoholic cerebellar degeneration. These disorders are discussed in Chapter 33.

2. Solvents

ESSENTIALS OF DIAGNOSIS

- ▶ Usually sudden onset
- ▶ History of solvent abuse
- ▶ Associated findings include behavioral changes

Acutely, ataxia as well as other neurologic symptoms may accompany intoxication by inhalants (see Chapter 34). Most often, effects are short-lived and the ataxia needs no specific treatment, but other complications including cardiac arrhythmia can be fatal. Chronic toluene exposure has been linked to encephalopathy and ataxia, with brainstem and cerebellar white matter changes.

Uchino A, et al. Comparison between patient characteristics and cranial MR findings in chronic thinner intoxication. *Eur Radiol* 2002;12:1338–1341. [PMID: 12042936]

3. Medications Associated With Ataxia

Barbiturates, benzodiazepines, and many anticonvulsants, most notably phenytoin and carbamazepine, may all lead to dysarthria and ataxia. Chemotherapeutic agents, including 5-fluorouracil, methotrexate, cyclosporine, and cytosine arabinoside, are also associated with ataxia, as is lithium carbonate.

4. Heavy Metal Intoxication

Heavy metals, including mercury, lead, and thallium, may cause ataxia, in addition to other symptoms.

5. Nutritional Deficiencies

Deficiency in cobalamin (vitamin B_{12}), although typically recognized as a cause of dementia and myelopathy, may rarely give rise to isolated cerebellar ataxia. Deficiency of vitamin B_1, vitamin E, and possibly zinc can produce cerebellar signs and symptoms.

Morita S, et al. Cerebellar ataxia and leukoencephalopathy associated with cobalamin deficiency. *J Neurol Sci* 2003;216:183–184. [PMID: 14607321]

ENDOCRINE DISEASE & ATAXIA

Cerebellar dysfunction may be the result of hypothyroidism, hypoparathyroidism, or hypoglycemia. These disorders are discussed in Chapter 32.

CEREBELLAR NEOPLASMS

In children, tumors causing ataxic syndromes include medulloblastoma, cerebellar astrocytoma, and ependymoma. In adults, metastatic tumors and hemangioblastoma are the most common cerebellar neoplasms. For further discussion, see Chapter 12.

INFECTIOUS CAUSES OF ATAXIA

Several infectious agents produce cerebellar mass lesions such as abscess, tuberculoma, or toxoplasmoma. In children (and less often in adults) ataxia with explosive onset is the initial manifestation of encephalitis affecting predominantly the posterior fossa; agents include *Haemophilus influenzae*, rubella, and other viruses. Postinfectious ataxia may follow infection by varicella, although there is often only a vague viral prodrome. Postinfectious cerebellitis can be prolonged, and reports of improvement in isolated cases encourage the use of intravenous immunoglobulin (IVIG) when symptoms are protracted and debilitating. Ataxia is often a feature of sporadic Creutzfeldt-Jakob disease, which is characterized by rapidly progressive dementia and accompanied by myoclonus; 90% of affected patients die within 12 months. Ataxia has also been associated with other prion diseases, notably Gerstmann-Sträussler-Scheinker disease (see Chapter 29). Ataxia may result from cerebellar complications of HIV, usually from opportunistic infection, vasculitis, or malignancy (see Chapter 28). Rarely, cerebellar ataxia occurs in the absence of these processes, perhaps as a direct consequence of HIV infection.

Collins SJ, et al. Transmissible spongiform encephalopathies. *Lancet* 2004;363:51–61. [PMID: 14723996] (Reviews the clinical spectrum, epidemiology, and molecular biology of prion diseases in general, including those associated with cerebellar ataxia.)

Cooper SA, et al. Sporadic Creutzfeldt-Jakob disease with cerebellar ataxia at onset in the UK. *J Neurol Neurosurg Psychiatry* 2006;77:1273–1275. [PMID: 16835290]

De Brueker Y, et al. MRI findings in acute cerebellitis. *Eur Radiol* 2004;1478–1483. [PMID: 14968261]

Gruis KL, et al. Cerebellitis in an adult with abnormal magnetic resonance imaging findings prior to the onset of ataxia. *Arch Neurol* 2003;60:877–880. [PMID: 12810494]

Kwakwa HA, Ghobrial MW. Primary cerebellar degeneration and HIV. *Arch Intern Med* 2001;161:1555–1556. [PMID: 11427105]

Schmahmann JD. Plasmapheresis improves outcome in postinfectious cerebellitis induced by Epstein-Barr virus. *Neurology* 2004;62:1443. [PMID: 15111700]

Tagliati M, et al. Cerebellar degeneration associated with human immunodeficiency virus infection. *Neurology* 1998;50:244–251. [PMID: 9443487] (First report of primary cerebellar degeneration in association with HIV, in 10 patients presenting with gait ataxia and dysarthria.)

ATAXIA ASSOCIATED WITH INFLAMMATORY & AUTOIMMUNE DISEASE

Ataxia is a common manifestation of multiple sclerosis, occurring subacutely, chronically, or, less often, acutely (see Chapter 17). A few cases of cerebellar ataxia have been reported in patients with Hashimoto disease, in association with elevated titers of antithyroglobulin antibody and antithyroperoxidase antibody. Patients can develop ataxia in the euthyroid state. The significance of this association to Hashimoto encephalopathy is unclear. High titers of antiglutamic acid decarboxylase (GAD) antibodies have also been associated with some cases of cerebellar ataxia, and this may occur together with type 1 diabetes.

Bayreuther C, et al. Auto-immune cerebellar ataxia with anti-GAD antibodies accompanied by de novo late-onset type 1 diabetes. *Diabetes Metab* 2008;34:386–388. [PMID: 18583169]

Selim M, Drachman DA. Ataxia associated with Hashimoto's disease: Progressive non-familial adult onset cerebellar degeneration with autoimmune thyroiditis. *J Neurol Neurosurg Psychiatry* 2001;71:81–87. [PMID: 11413268]

GLUTEN ATAXIA

 ESSENTIALS OF DIAGNOSIS

▶ Chronic, progressive ataxia, sometimes with myoclonus

▶ Clinical features of celiac disease, including characteristic biopsy findings

▶ Associated antibodies—antigliadin immunoglobulins G (IgG) and A (IgA), antiendomysial, and antitransglutaminase antibodies

Celiac disease is an immune-mediated, gluten-sensitive enteropathy, with small bowel villous atrophy demonstrated on biopsy. Clinical improvement follows adherence to a gluten-free diet. The disease affects nearly 1% of the population. Neurologic syndromes, including ataxia, occur in 6–10% of such patients. Cerebellar atrophy and Purkinje cell loss have sometimes been observed at postmortem examination. The nature of this association, and the significance of serologic findings, including increased antigliadin antibody titers, is not yet fully understood.

Patients have progressive gait and limb ataxia, and sometimes dysarthria, abnormal eye movements, pyramidal signs, and memory decline. Some patients have myoclonus. Gastrointestinal complaints may or may not be present. Associated conditions sometimes include osteoporosis, dermatitis herpetiformis, autoimmune thyroiditis, and diabetes mellitus. Patients have an increased risk of lymphoma.

Antigliadin (IgA and IgG), antiendomysial (IgA), or antitransglutaminase (IgA) antibody titers are elevated. Antiglutamic acid decarboxylase autoantibodies and antiganglioside antibodies have also been detected. There may be vitamin deficiency, including folate, vitamin K, and vitamin D; iron-deficiency anemia; and elevated liver enzymes. MRI often shows cerebellar atrophy, sometimes limited to the vermis and sometimes pancerebellar.

Improvement sometimes follows implementation of a gluten-free diet, and intravenous immunoglobulin treatment has been reported to help in a small number of patients.

Hadjivassiliou M, et al. Gluten ataxia. *Cerebellum* 2008;7:494–498. [PMID: 18787912]

Souyah N, et al. Effect of intravenous immunoglobulin on cerebellar ataxia and neuropathic pain associated with celiac disease. *Eur J Neurol* 2008;15:1300–1303. [PMID: 19049545]

ATAXIA OF PARANEOPLASTIC ORIGIN

ESSENTIALS OF DIAGNOSIS

▶ Acute or subacute onset of ataxia

▶ Underlying neoplasm is often unrecognized

▶ Specific association of antibodies with some paraneoplastic syndromes

Paraneoplastic syndromes are discussed in Chapter 13. Syndromes that include cerebellar ataxia are summarized in Table 16–5.

MULTIPLE SYSTEM ATROPHY (TYPE C)

ESSENTIALS OF DIAGNOSIS

▶ Chronic, progressive ataxia with associated autonomic instability or parkinsonism

▶ Occurs in patients with no family history of the condition

▶ Olivopontocerebellar atrophy seen on MRI of the brain

▶ General Considerations

Multiple system atrophy (MSA) is a so-called *Parkinson-plus syndrome*, that is, one of a group of related movement disorders presenting with prominent parkinsonism, autonomic dysfunction, or cerebellar signs (see Chapters 15 and 21). These symptoms and signs may be present in any combination.

▶ Pathogenesis

Neurodegeneration occurs in multiple regions, including the substantia nigra, putamen, cerebellum, olivary nucleus, and pontine nuclei. Glial cytoplasmic inclusions form within the oligodendroglia. These inclusions contain α-synuclein, significant for its role in Parkinson disease pathogenesis.

▶ Clinical Findings

A. Symptoms and Signs

MSA is sporadic, presenting in patients without a positive family history. It is a progressive disease, with adult onset, and typically a faster course than Parkinson disease; in one series of 35 patients, median survival was 7.3 years. The diagnosis is suggested by a combination of cerebellar signs, including an unsteady wide-based gait, dysarthria, or scanning speech, along with bradykinesia and rigidity, although patients may present with isolated ataxia. Pyramidal signs occur in up to half of patients, and cognitive changes and autonomic dysfunction occur in some.

B. Imaging Studies

CT or MRI scan typically reveals pancerebellar and brainstem atrophy. The cross sign of hyperintensity in the pons on T2-weighted MRI scans arises from demyelination of transverse pontine fibers. Abnormal signals are often present in the putamen. Single-photon emission computed

Table 16–5. Paraneoplastic Syndromes Producing Ataxia and Cerebellar Degeneration

Antibody	Neurologic Findings	Associated Cancer	Commercial Test Available
Anti-Hu (ANNA-1)	PCD, sensory neuronopathy, encephalomyelitis	SCLC, prostate, neuroblastoma	+
Anti-Yo (PCA-1)	PCD	Breast, ovary, lung	+
Anti-Ri (ANNA-2)	PCD, opsoclonus-myoclonus	Breast, lung, gynecologic, bladder	+
Anti-Ma1	PCD, brainstem encephalitis	Lung, other	+
CV2	PCD, encephalomyelitis, neuropathy	SCLC, thymoma	+
Anti-metabotropic glutamate receptor R1	PCD	Hodgkin disease	–
Anti-Tr (atypical cytoplasmic antibody, PCA-Tr)	PCD	Hodgkin disease	–
Anti-PCA-2	PCD, encephalomyelitis, Lambert-Eaton syndrome	SCLC	
Anti-Zic4	PCD, encephalitis	SCLC	+

PCD = paraneoplastic cerebellar degeneration; SCLC = small cell lung carcinoma; +, available; –, not available.

tomography (SPECT) and positron emission tomography (PET) may be useful in some cases to differentiate MSA from Parkinson disease and other related disorders, but are not widely available.

C. Special Tests

Autonomic dysfunction may be investigated with tilt-table and other formal autonomic testing, neurogenic sphincter electromyography, and investigations of neurogenic bladder, as well as patterns of plasma levels of catecholamines and metabolites (see Chapter 21). However, these findings are not specific to MSA.

▶ Differential Diagnosis

Causes of acquired ataxias, including nutritional and associated systemic disease, need to be ruled out. Some patients with apparent sporadic ataxia turn out to have mutations in one of the *SCA* genes (see later discussion).

▶ Treatment

There is currently no disease-specific treatment for MSA. Parkinsonian symptoms improve in some patients treated with levodopa, although the response is rarely as marked as in idiopathic Parkinson disease. Standing blood pressures may be improved by increasing salt in the diet or with use of fludrocortisone or midodrine, but the risk of supine hypertension necessitates careful monitoring. Elastic stockings are beneficial for some patients. Unlike Parkinson disease, deep brain stimulation surgery does not appear to help MSA.

Brooks D, et al. Proposed neuroimaging criteria for the diagnosis of multiple system atrophy. *Mov Disord* 2009;24:949–964. [PMID: 19306362]

Colosimo C, et al. Management of multiple system atrophy: State of the art. *J Neural Transm* 2005;112:1695–1704. [PMID: 16284911]

Lee EA, et al. Comparison of magnetic resonance imaging in subtypes of multiple system atrophy. *Parkinsonism Relat Disord* 2004;10:363–468. [PMID: 15261878]

Stefanova N, et al. Multiple system atrophy: An update. *Lancet Neurol* 2009;8:1172–1178. [PMID: 19909915]

▼ HEREDITARY ATAXIAS

There exists a bewildering array of genetically inherited diseases in which ataxia may occur. Recent advances have focused attention on hereditary disorders in which ataxia is the most prominent feature. Despite limitations in treatment, it is important for the clinician to recognize these diseases in order to advise the patient and family appropriately. Ataxia may also occur in several hereditary disorders associated with other complaints, such as developmental delay or epilepsy; these disorders include inborn errors of metabolism, leukodystrophies, and storage disorders.

AUTOSOMAL-DOMINANT CEREBELLAR ATAXIAS

1. Spinocerebellar Ataxias

ESSENTIALS OF DIAGNOSIS

► Chronic, progressive cerebellar ataxia
► Family history of cerebellar ataxia (usually)
► Associated features that include oculomotor disturbance, hyperreflexia, macular degeneration (SCA7), dementia (SCA10)
► Genetic testing is available for a subset of these diseases

▶ General Considerations

Spinocerebellar ataxias (SCAs) are a set of genetically and clinically heterogeneous diseases that have in common progressive ataxia. SCAs are now classified genetically according to a specific mutation or mapped locus and also according to clinical findings (Table 16–6). In some cases, identification of the gene involved has clarified links to other disorders; for example, mutations in the calcium channel, voltage-dependent, P/Q type, α_{1A} subunit may lead to SCA6, to episodic-ataxia type 2 (see Table 16–8), or to familial hemiplegic migraine, and mutations in the inositol 1,4,5-triphosphate receptor type 1 gene lead to SCA15, SCA16, and SCA29. Dentatorubro-pallidoluysian atrophy (DRPLA) has not been assigned an SCA number, but is considered alongside the SCAs because of some similarities in presentation. In the older literature, a simpler clinical classification uses three major categories of autosomal-dominant cerebellar ataxia (ADCA), described along with their correspondence to SCAs in Table 16–7. To add to the confusion, many of these diseases have additional names in common use in the literature; for example SCA3 is also known as Machado-Joseph disease.

Prevalence of all dominantly inherited progressive ataxias is an estimated 0.9–1.3 cases per 100,000 people. Subtype prevalence depends on geographic location, but the most common ADCAs worldwide are SCA1 (6%), SCA2 (15%), SCA3 (21%), SCA5 (15%), SCA7 (5%), and SCA8 (3%). The pace of research in this field is rapid, and updated information may be obtained from the National Institutes of Health Web sites listed at the end of this discussion.

▶ Pathogenesis

The majority of known mutations involve expansion of a trinucleotide $(CAG)_n$ repeat within the coding region of the respective gene (see Table 16–6). This is translated into an abnormal polyglutamine tract in the corresponding protein, with formation of nuclear aggregates. The exact pathogenesis, however, is unknown.

Table 16–6. Autosomal-Dominant Spinocerebellar Ataxias

Type of Ataxia	Distinguishing Clinical Findings	Normal Alleles	Mutation and Alleles	Protein
SCA1	Pyramidal signs, executive dysfunction (rarely overt dementia), slow/absent saccades	CAG 6–39	CAG 41–83	Ataxin-1
SCA2	Slowed saccades, peripheral neuropathy, extrapyramidal signs (rare), myoclonus or action tremor, bulbar signs, dementia, rare pyramidal signs and may be hyporeflexia	CAG 14–30	CAG 33–77	Ataxin-2
SCA3	Gaze-evoked nystagmus, lid retraction, prominent spasticity, bulbar signs, peripheral neuropathy (variable), extrapyramidal signs including parkinsonism, dystonia	CAG 12–40	CAG 51–86	Ataxin-3 (MJD1)
SCA4	Cerebellar syndrome, sensory neuropathy (variable)	—	—	—
SCA5	Pure cerebellar syndrome, rare gaze palsy, facial myokymia	—	Missense mutations	Spectrin
SCA6	Pure cerebellar syndrome, often late onset (>50 y), pyramidal signs (variable)	CAG 4–18	CAG 20–31	Calcium channel, voltage-dependent, P/Q type, α_{1A} subunit,
SCA7	Progressive pigmentary retinopathy and macular degeneration with visual loss, hearing loss, slow saccades, pyramidal signs; childhood onset may be severe, with developmental delay, hypotonia, and sometimes cardiac failure, microcephaly, hemangiomas, hepatomegaly	CAG 4–27	CAG 37–>200	Ataxin-7
SCA8	Cerebellar syndrome, spasticity, sensory neuropathy in some, slow progression, congenital onset severe with epilepsy, static encephalopathy	CTG 15–37	CTG 80–300 (expanded repeats occasionally seen in healthy subjects, psychiatric disease)	Ataxin-8
SCA9	Ophthalmoplegia, some with optic atrophy, parkinsonism, pyramidal signs, weakness	—	—	—
SCA10	Cerebellar syndrome ± seizures	ATTCT 10–22	ATTCT 800–4500	Ataxin-10
SCA11	Pure cerebellar syndrome, hyperreflexia, nystagmus, slowly progressive	—	Stop/frameshift insertion/deletion	Tau tubulin kinase 2
SCA12	Early arm tremor, hyperreflexia in most, ± facial myokymia, peripheral neuropathy, dystonia in a few	CAG 7–32	CAG 55–93	Protein phosphatase 2, regulatory subunit B, β isoform
SCA13	Ataxia, ± mental retardation, early childhood onset	—	Missense mutations	Voltage-gated potassium channel, Shaw-related subfamily member 3 (KCNC3)
SCA14	Ataxia, myoclonus (with early onset), slow progression	—	Missense mutations	Protein kinase C, γ-polypeptide
SCA15	Pure cerebellar syndrome, slow progression, variants: SCA29, congential nonprogressive ataxia	—	Deletions	Inositol 1,4,5-triphosphate receptor type 1
SCA17	Dysphagia, intellectual deterioration to overt dementia, absence seizures, extrapyramidal signs (facial dyskinesia, limb dystonia, chorea, parkinsonism)	CAG/CAA 25–42	CAG/CAA 45–66	TATA box–binding protein
SCA18	Muscle atrophy, sensory loss with axonal neuropathy, slow progression	—	—	—

(Continued)

Table 16–6. Autosomal-Dominant Spinocerebellar Ataxias (*Continued*)

Type of Ataxia	Distinguishing Clinical Findings	Normal Alleles	Mutation and Alleles	Protein
SCA19	Mild cognitive impairment, myoclonus, slow irregular postural tremor, ± myoclonus	—	—	—
SCA20	Palatal tremor, dysphonia, dentate calcification on CT of brain	—	—	—
SCA21	Extrapyramidal features (akinesia, rigidity, tremor), cognitive impairment	—	—	—
SCA22	Pure cerebellar syndrome, slow progression, hyporeflexia	—	—	—
SCA23	Pyramidal signs, sensory loss	—	—	—
SCA25	Profound sensory neuropathy, severe cerebellar atrophy	—	—	—
SCA26	Pure cerebellar syndrome	—	—	—
SCA27	Ataxia, tremor, orofacial dyskinesias, cognitive decline, axonal peripheral neuropathy	—	Missense mutation	Fibroblast growth factor 14
SCA28	Ophthalmoparesis, pyramidal signs	—	Missense mutation	ATPase family gene 3-like 2
SCA30	Pure cerebellar syndrome, minor pyramidal signs	—	—	—
SCA31	Pure cerebellar syndrome, minor pyramidal signs	—	TGGAA repeat insertion mutation	Many (not all) PLEKHG, disease-causing mutation in pentanu-cleotide repeat insertion
DRPLA	Onset <age 20 y—ataxia, progressive intellectual deterioration, myoclonus, epilepsy	CAG < 26	CAG 49–88	Atrophin-1
DRPLA	Onset >age 20 y—cerebellar ataxia, choreoathetosis, dementia, psychiatric disturbances Spastic ataxia variant with spastic paraplegia	CAG < 26	CAG 49–88	Atrophin-1

CT = computed tomography; DRPLA = dentatorubropalliodoluysian atrophy; MJD = Machado-Joseph disease; PLEKHG = pleckstrin homology domain containing, family G; SCA = spinal cerebellar ataxia.

Table 16–7. Correspondence of ADCA Types I–III With SCA1–25[a]

ADCA Type	Clinical Findings	Corresponding SCA
ADCA I	Cerebellar ataxia *plus* • Spasticity (pyramidal signs) • Supranuclear ophthalmoplegia • Extrapyramidal signs • Peripheral neuropathy (sensory, motor, or both) • Cognitive deficit, dementia	SCA1, SCA2, SCA3, SCA9, SCA27, SCA28
ADCA II	Cerebellar ataxia *plus* • Pigmentary macular degeneration • Other CNS or PNS involvement, as in ADCA I	SCA7
ADCA III	Pure cerebellar ataxia *plus* • Mild spasticity (pyramidal signs)	SCA4, SCA5, SCA6, SCA10, SCA11, SCA30, SCA31

ADCA = autosomal-dominant cerebellar ataxia; CNS = central nervous system; DRPLA = dentatorubropallidoluysian atrophy; PNS = peripheral nervous system; SCA = spinocerebellar ataxia.
[a]The following ataxias have not been assigned to ADCA types I–III: SCA8, SCA12, SCA13, SCA14, SCA15, SCA17, SCA18, SCA19, SCA20, SCA21, SCA22, SCA23, SCA25, SCA26, and DRPLA.

Prevention

Genetic testing is available for a subset of SCAs and for DRPLA and can help obtain a molecular diagnosis to aid in counseling and to define options for participation in research. Some individuals from families with a history of ataxia request predictive and, occasionally, prenatal testing. Thorough and careful genetic counseling with a specialist trained in this area is mandated, both for diagnostic and predictive testing. There is no known intervention to delay symptom onset or to slow disease progression.

Clinical Findings

A. Symptoms and Signs

All SCAs produce a progressive cerebellar syndrome with gait and appendicular ataxia, dysarthria, and oculomotor disturbances. Patients may also have dysphagia, spasticity, brisk tendon reflexes with extensor plantar responses, noncerebellar oculomotor features, and signs of brainstem disease, such as facial atrophy and fasciculations. There is a tremendous heterogeneity within each type, as well as clinical overlap between types (see Table 16–6). Age of onset varies widely; typically onset is in the thirties for SCA1, SCA2, and SCA3, but later for SCA6, and may be inversely correlated with repeat expansion length. Additionally, the phenomenon of anticipation may be observed within a family, with an earlier age of onset and more severe phenotype in successive generations because of a tendency of expanded repeats to increase progressively from generation to generation. Because of clinical overlap, individual SCAs cannot be easily differentiated by clinical or imaging studies alone. Genetic testing is the only means to make a definitive diagnosis in a given patient.

B. Imaging Studies

There are no features specific for SCAs, but cerebellar or olivopontocerebellar atrophy is often revealed by MRI. Cortical atrophy may be observed in some patients with SCA2, SCA12, SCA17, and SCA19. Cerebral white matter abnormalities may be seen in DRPLA.

C. Special Tests

Genetic testing is commercially available for several SCAs and for DRPLA. A genetic cause may be assumed in patients with a clear family history. In sporadic cases, it is less clear when to test: in some patients, sporadic SCA1, SCA2, SCA3, or SCA6 mutations have been detected. In patients with a negative family history comprising three or more generations without ataxia, yield of testing for SCAs is low. However, testing may be considered if a patient with sporadic case has features very similar to one of the inherited ataxias. Erroneous assignment of paternity should also be kept in mind when recording family history. Despite careful evaluation and consideration of testing, some patients with clear evidence of autosomal-dominant inheritance do not obtain a clear molecular diagnosis because available tests do not cover all the known (and unknown) SCAs.

Treatment

There is no treatment to prevent neuronal cell death in ADCA, although patients may choose to participate in clinical trials of experimental treatments (an updated list is kept at the website www.clinicaltrials.gov). For symptomatic treatment, guidelines follow those for any ataxic patient. Parkinsonism may respond to levodopa or other dopaminergic medications. Seizures are treated with antiepileptic medications, and if myoclonus is debilitating, a trial of benzodiazepines, sodium valproate, or other medications is warranted. Spasticity is treated with baclofen, up to 20 mg four times daily; alternatives include benzodiazepines and tizanidine. Dystonia, if present, is treated as described in Chapter 15.

Prognosis

All SCAs are characterized by a progressive course, but there is tremendous variation in rate of progress and prognosis. Time from symptom onset to death typically ranges from one to three decades. However, progression is particularly slow in SCA5, SCA13, and SCA21, and patients with SCA8 and SCA11 typically have a normal life span.

Manto MU. The wide spectrum of spinocerebellar ataxias (SCAs). *Cerebellum* 2005;4:2–6. [PMID: 15895552]

Schols L, et al. Autosomal dominant cerebellar ataxias: Clinical features, genetics, and pathogenesis. *Lancet Neurol* 2004;3:291–304. [PMID: 15099544]

Web Sites
http://www.genetests.org, and http://www.neuro.wustl.edu/neuromuscular/. (These National Institutes of Health–funded sites provide up-to-date information on inherited ataxias.)

2. Episodic Ataxias

 ESSENTIALS OF DIAGNOSIS

▶ Episodes of ataxia and dysarthria lasting from seconds to minutes (type 1 disease) or hours to days (type 2)

▶ Provocation of episodes by startle and movement (type 1) or emotional stress and change of body position (type 2)

▶ Often associated with migraine (type 2)

▶ Interictal periorbital or hand muscle myokymia (type 1) or gaze-evoked or downbeat nystagmus (type 2)

▶ Autosomal-dominant inheritance

Eight different forms of episodic ataxia (EA) have been described to date: by far the most common are EA1 and EA2. Features of these rare disorders are summarized in Table 16–8.

Jen JC, et al. Primary episodic ataxias: diagnosis, pathogenesis and treatment. *Brain* 2007;130:2484–2493. [PMID: 17575281]

Tomlinson SE, et al. Clinical neurophysiology of the episodic ataxias: insights into ion channel dysfunction in vivo. *Clin Neurophysiol* 2009;120:1768–1776. [PMID: 19734086]

AUTOSOMAL-RECESSIVE CEREBELLAR ATAXIAS

Friedreich ataxia and ataxia-telangiectasia are the most common cerebellar ataxias inherited in an autosomal-recessive fashion. Table 16–9 lists other autosomal-recessive ataxias that, although extremely rare, should be recognized because of existing treatment options. Treatable ataxias include abetalipoproteinemia, ataxia with isolated vitamin E deficiency, hereditary motor and sensory neuropathy type IV, and cerebrotendinous xanthomatosis. Wilson disease, a treatable disorder resulting from copper accumulation and subsequent hepatic dysfunction, has variable presentations, but cerebellar symptoms may be present and tremor appears in up to 50% of patients. Wilson disease is discussed in Chapter 15.

1. Friedreich Ataxia

ESSENTIALS OF DIAGNOSIS

▶ Chronic, slowly progressive cerebellar ataxia
▶ Absent lower limb tendon reflexes (variants exist)
▶ Onset usually between ages 2 and 25 years
▶ Cardiomyopathy (common)
▶ Diabetes mellitus (up to 25% of patients)

▶ General Considerations

Friedreich ataxia (FRDA) is the most common of all hereditary ataxias in Caucasians, with a prevalence ranging from 2–4 cases per 100,000 person-years, but it is rare in populations of Asian or African descent. It is caused by a deficiency of the protein frataxin, encoded by the *FRDA1* gene. Approximately 98% of patients have a homozygous allele for an unstable expansion of GAA trinucleotide repeats. Approximately 2% of all FRDA patients have missense, nonsense, or splice mutations, making genetic testing more complex. A second genetic locus, *FRDA2*, has also been described.

▶ Clinical Findings

A. Symptoms and Signs

FRDA is characterized by slowly progressive gait and limb ataxia, absent lower limb reflexes, and reduction or loss of proprioception and vibration sense. Onset is typically between the ages of 2 and 25 years. The legs may be spastic, and extensor plantar responses may be present. Rarely, other movement disorders, including chorea, or spastic paraparesis may occur. Kyphoscoliosis is an early sign; pes cavus deformity occurs later. Hypertrophic cardiomyopathy is a prominent feature of classic FRDA and leads eventually to death. Diabetes mellitus occurs in later stages in up to 25% of patients and contributes significantly to morbidity and mortality.

Genetic testing has revealed a spectrum of milder cases with later onset and a less-debilitating course, as well as other movement disorders symptoms. Late-onset FRDA manifests in patients between 26 and 39 years of age, and very-late-onset FRDA, after age 40. These variants account for approximately 10–15% of known FRDA cases. Another variant is FRDA with retained reflexes, which also has a more benign course.

B. Imaging Studies and Special Tests

Commercial testing is available for trinucleotide repeat expansion in the *FRDA1* gene. MRI demonstrates atrophy of the cerebellum and often the cervical spinal cord. Electrocardiographic studies often show evidence of repolarization abnormalities, which may precede neurologic symptoms. Concentric hypertrophic cardiomyopathy, or other abnormalities, is revealed by echocardiogram in some patients. Electrophysiologic studies can demonstrate absent or reduced-amplitude sensory nerve action potentials.

▶ Treatment

Treatment of FRDA follows guidelines for ataxia in general; no curative treatment is as yet available. Monitoring for cardiomyopathy and diabetes is undertaken at least yearly. Idebenone, 5 mg/kg/day, reduces cardiac hypertrophy in most patients studied but does not halt progression of ataxia. However, it is well tolerated in high doses up to 55 mg/kg/day, and the possibility that these higher doses may improve neurologic function remains to be fully determined.

▶ Prognosis

Many patients are wheelchair-bound 10–20 years after symptom onset. The disease often leads to death in middle age, related to cardiomyopathy, diabetic complications, or pneumonia, although there are exceptions.

Pandolfo M. Friedreich ataxia. *Arch Neurol* 2008;65:1296–1303. [PMID: 18852343]

Schulz JB, et al. Clinical experience with high-dose idebenone in Friedreich ataxia. *J Neurol* 2009;256 (Suppl 1):42–45. [PMID: 19283350]

Table 16–8. Inherited Episodic Ataxias

Episodic Ataxia	Clinical Findings	Gene/Inheritance	Treatment
Type 1 (EA-1)	Onset childhood–2nd decade Episodes of ataxia and dysarthria lasting seconds to minutes Provoked by startle and movements Interictal periorbital or hand muscle myokymia but no interictal ataxia Neuromyotonia, seizure, and skeletal deformities in some Variants from this gene include: neuromyotonia and stiffness, chronic neuromyotonia with disappearance of ataxia, severe neuromyotonia and skeletal deformities, episodic ataxia plus paroxysmal dyspnea, fixed ataxia, hypomagnesemia	KCNA1—deficiency in voltage-gated potassium channel function	Phenytoin and carbamazepine Counseling to avoid sudden movements when possible
Type 2 (EA-2)	Onset childhood–teens Episodes of ataxia and dysarthria lasting 0.5–6 h, nausea, headache, dystonia and seizures in some, hemiplegia in 10% Provoked by emotional stress, physical exertion, heat, alcohol Interictal downbeat or gaze-evoked nystagmus Migraine may be present Interictal ataxia may slowly progress and become persistent, weakness may occur before or during spells MRI may demonstrate atrophy of cerebellar vermis	CACNA1A—subunit of P/Q-type calcium channel; different mutations in same gene lead to SCA6 and familial hemiplegic migraine (see Chapter 8)	Acetazolamide, up to 700 mg/day (effective in 75%) 4-aminopyridine 5 mg tid Phenytoin and carbamazepine may exacerbate symptoms
Type 3 (EA-3)	Periodic vestibulocerebellar ataxia with vertigo. Tinnitus, interictal myokymia Lasts 1 min–6 h Provoked by movement	Unknown Chromosome 1q42	Acetazolamide
Type 4 (EA-4)	Onset 3rd–6th decade Episodic ataxia, vertigo, diplopia, slowly progressive ataxia and defective smooth pursuit	Unknown	No response to acetazolamide
Type 5 (EA-5)	Onset 3rd–4th decade Episodic ataxia (typically hours), interictal ataxia with mild dysarthria and nystagmus (downbeat and gaze-evoked), also associated with JME, seizures	CACNB4 calcium channel	Acetazolamide
Type 6 (EA-6)	Onset in childhood Episodic ataxia with hypotonia lasting 2–4 days Delayed milestones Associated with migraine, alternating hemiplegia, hemianopia, seizures, coma Interictal mild truncal ataxia, increased tendon reflexes, mild static encephalopathy Provoked by fever MRI mild cerebellar atrophy, FLAIR hyperintensity during episodes; EEG seizure activity	EAAT1 glial glutamate transporter	
Type 7 (EA-7)	Onset < 20 y Paroxysmal ataxia with dysarthria, weakness, vertigo in some lasting hours to days Interictal mild truncal ataxia, increased tendon reflexes, mild static encephalopathy Associated with migraine, alternating hemiplegia, hemianopia, seizures, coma Provoked by exercise, excitement	Unknown Chromosome 19q13	

(Continued)

Table 16–8. Inherited Episodic Ataxias (*Continued*)

Episodic Ataxia	Clinical Findings	Gene/Inheritance	Treatment
EA + Choreoathetosis and spasticity (also named DYT9—see Chapter 15)	Onset 2–15 y EEG slowing Episodic ataxia lasting 20 minutes (2/d–2/y) with dystonia, headache, perioral and leg paresthesias Persistent spastic paraplegia Provoked by alcohol, fatigue, physical exercise	Unknown Chromosome 1p	Acetazolamide

CACNA1A = Cav2.1 P/Q voltage-dependent calcium channel; CACNB4 = voltage-dependent L-type calcium channel subunit β4; EAAT1 = excitatory amino acid transporter; DYT9 = dystonia gene 9; EMG = electromyography; JME = juvenile myoclonic epilepsy; KCNA1 = potassium voltage-gated channel subfamily A member 1; MRI = magnetic resonance imaging.

Table 16–9. Rare Autosomal-Recessive Cerebellar Ataxias

Disorder	Clinical Findings	Gene	Protein	Treatment
Abetalipoproteinemia, Bassen-Kornzweig syndrome	Neuronal—cerebellar ataxia, pigmentary degeneration of retina, progressive ataxic neuropathy (large fiber, demyelinating, sensory) Nonneuronal—defective intestinal lipid resorption, very low serum cholesterol levels, absent serum betalipoprotein, celiac syndrome, acanthocytosis	*MTP*	Microsomal triglyceride transfer protein	Vitamin E, 50–100 IU/kg/day
Hereditary motor and sensory neuropathy type IV (HMSM IV), Refsum disease	Neuronal—retinitis pigmentosa, chronic demyelinating polyneuropathy, cerebellar ataxia, nerve deafness, anosmia Nonneuronal—ichthyosis, cardiomyopathy with sudden cardiac death, skeletal deformities including short 4th metatarsal, epiphyseal dysplasia, syndactyly	*PHYH, PAHX, PEX1, PEX7*	Phytanoyl-CoA hydroxylase	Dietary restriction of phytanic acid; acute worsening by plasma exchange
Cerebrotendinous xanthomatosis	Neuronal—cerebellar ataxia, systemic spinal cord involvement, dementia, and later brainstem signs leading to death Nonneuronal—chronic diarrhea; premature atherosclerosis; widespread deposits of cholesterol and cholestanol, particularly in Achilles tendons, brain, and lungs; elevated cholestanol in serum; cataracts MRI—diffuse/cerebellar atrophy, bilateral focal cerebellar lesions	*CYP27A1, CTX*	Cytochrome P-450, subfamily XXVIIA, polypeptide 1 (sterol 27-hydroxylase)	Chenodeoxycholate, 750 mg/day
Ataxia with oculomotor apraxia	Neuronal—resembles ataxia-telangiectasia; progressive ataxia in early stages; progressive axonal motor neuropathy Nonneuronal—low albumin, high cholesterol, no immunodeficiency or increased risk for malignancies MRI—cerebellar atrophy	*APTX* (also leads to cerebellar ataxia with muscle Coenzyme Q10 deficiency), *SETX*	Aprataxin	—
Autosomal-recessive spastic ataxia of Charlevoix-Saguenay	Neuronal—ataxia, dysarthria, spasticity, extensor plantar reflexes, distal muscle wasting and sensory-motor neuropathy predominantly in legs, horizontal gaze nystagmus; in Quebec patients only, retinal streaks of hypermyelinated fibers seen in funduscopy Nonneuronal—none described MRI—cerebellar atrophy sparing pons	*Sacsin* (gene test available)	Sacsin	—

MRI = magnetic resonance imaging.

2. Ataxia-Telangiectasia

ESSENTIALS OF DIAGNOSIS

▸ Slowly progressive ataxia with onset usually in infancy

▸ Telangiectasias affecting conjunctivae and other structures

▸ Immunodeficiency (common)

▸ Malignancies (frequent, particularly in childhood)

▸ General Considerations

Ataxia-telangiectasia is a rare disease affecting the nervous, vascular, and immune systems, but it is the most common inherited progressive ataxia of childhood in most countries, with an incidence of 0.3 cases per 100,000 live births in the United States. It is caused by mutations of the *ATM* gene, one of the phosphatidylinositol-3 kinase family, involved in DNA repair and cell-cycle control. This deficiency is thought to be responsible for predisposition for malignancies and immune deficiency.

▸ Clinical Findings

A. Symptoms and Signs

Disease onset is typically in infancy, with truncal and later limb ataxia. Telangiectasias typically are found in the conjunctivae and earlobes. Immunodeficiency in 60–80% of patients often manifests as recurrent pulmonary and sinus infections. Nearly 40% of affected individuals develop malignancies during their lifetime, most before 20 years of age, and typically either lymphoma or leukemia. Older patients tend to develop solid tumors, including ovarian cancer, breast cancer, gastric cancer, malignant melanoma, leiomyoma, or sarcoma.

B. Laboratory Findings

Elevated α-fetoprotein level is found in more than 90% of patients. Serum levels of IgA, IgE, and IgG are decreased.

C. Special Tests

Western immunoblot analysis for the intranuclear serine-protein kinase ATM in lymphoid cell lysates demonstrates absent or very low levels of ATM protein. Given the diversity of mutations of the *ATM* gene that cause ataxia-telangiectasia, genetic testing is not used routinely.

▸ Treatment & Prognosis

Guidelines for managing neurologic symptoms follow those for other ataxias. Patients with ataxia-telangiectasia need to be closely monitored for malignancies. In those with tumors, dosages of radiation therapy need to be adjusted because of increased sensitivity to radiation.

The overall prognosis is grave. Most patients are wheelchair-bound by 10 years of age, and most die before age 30.

3. Ataxia With Isolated Vitamin E Deficiency

ESSENTIALS OF DIAGNOSIS

▸ Slowly progressive ataxia

▸ Depressed lower limb reflexes

▸ Onset typically before age 20 years

▸ Low serum α-tocopherol

▸ No abnormality of intestinal lipid absorption or other fat-soluble vitamins

▸ General Considerations

Ataxia with isolated vitamin E deficiency (AVED) is caused by mutations in the gene for α-tocopherol transfer protein, which is responsible in the liver for incorporating tocopherols into very-low-density lipoproteins for subsequent release into the circulation. In affected patients, therefore, vitamin E is rapidly eliminated, resulting in deficiency despite adequate enteric resorption. How this leads to neurodegeneration is unclear, but free-radical damage and mitochondrial dysfunction have been implicated.

▸ Clinical Findings

A. Symptoms and Signs

The diagnosis of AVED should be considered if a patient presents with clinical features suggestive of Friedreich ataxia, but molecular testing for the *FRDA* gene mutation is negative. Cardiomyopathy similar to the one in Friedreich ataxia is present in only 20% of affected patients.

B. Laboratory Findings

Serum vitamin E (α-tocopherol) is severely reduced or absent in affected patients. Levels of other lipid-soluble vitamins and betalipoprotein are normal.

▸ Treatment

Oral supplementation of vitamin E at a dose of 800–2000 IU daily or twice daily is the treatment of choice.

Cavalier L, et al. Ataxia with isolated vitamin E deficiency: Heterogeneity of mutations and phenotypic variability in a large number of families. *Am J Hum Genet* 1998;62:301–310. [PMID: 9463307]

4. Other Rare Autosomal-Recessive Ataxias

Table 16–9 summarizes neuronal and nonneuronal manifestations, clues for diagnosis, and underlying genetic defects of some of a subset of these heterogeneous disorders, but for a more comprehensive and up-to-date list, the reader is referred to http://neuromuscular.wustl.edu/ataxia. Abetalipoproteinemia, hereditary motor and sensory neuropathy type IV, and cerebrotendinous xanthomatosis are amenable to treatment. Other rare ataxias with childhood onset include childhood ataxia with central nervous system hypomyelination (also called *vanishing white matter disease*) and storage and metabolic disorders. Early-onset ataxias are also categorized by associated features, including retinal degeneration (Hallgren syndrome), hypogonadism (Holmes syndrome), cataracts and mental retardation (Marinesco-Sjögren syndrome), and myoclonus (Ramsay Hunt syndrome).

Bouchard JP, et al. Autosomal recessive spastic ataxia of Charlevoix-Saguenay. *Neuromuscul Disord* 1998;8:474–479. [PMID: 9829277]

Le Ber I, et al. Cerebellar ataxia with oculomotor apraxia type 1: Clinical and genetic studies. *Brain* 2003;126:2761–2772. [PMID: 14506070]

Le Ber I, et al. Frequency and phenotypic spectrum of ataxia with oculomotor apraxia 2: A clinical and genetic study in 18 patients. *Brain* 2004;127:759–767. [PMID: 14736755]

CEREBELLAR ATAXIA IN MITOCHONDRIAL DISORDERS

ESSENTIALS OF DIAGNOSIS

▸ Chronic, progressive multisystem disorders

▸ Common neurologic features—ptosis, external ophthalmoplegia, myopathy, exercise intolerance, sensorineural deafness, optic atrophy, pigmentary retinopathy, dementia or developmental delay, seizures, and mitochondrial myopathy, encephalopathy, lactic acidosis, and stroke-like episodes (MELAS)

▸ Common nonneuronal features—cardiomyopathy and diabetes mellitus

▸ Mostly maternal inheritance

Several of the clinically heterogeneous mitochondrial disorders may involve ataxia as part of their clinical course (Table 16–10). Family histories may be complex, with clinical heterogeneity resulting from organ mosaicism (heteroplasmy) and variable penetrance. These disorders are described fully in Chapter 24 and in the appropriate clinical context should be considered in the ataxic individual. There is, as yet, no treatment for these disorders, with the notable exception of hereditary coenzyme Q10 deficiency; for that reason, this disorder is described in more detail here.

DiMauro S, Schon EA. Mitochondrial disorders in he nervous system. *Annu Rev Neurol* 2008;31:91–123. [PMID: 18333761]

Familial Ataxia With Coenzyme Q10 Deficiency

ESSENTIALS OF DIAGNOSIS

▸ Ataxia and other features, including seizures, peripheral neuropathy, pyramidal signs, and developmental delay

▸ Low coenzyme Q10 (CoQ10) levels in muscle

▸ General Considerations

Despite its rarity, primary CoQ10 deficiency is important to recognize because it is a potentially treatable cause of progressive ataxia. CoQ10 is a component of the mitochondrial electron transport chain and is a potent antioxidant and membrane stabilizer. It is possible that increased oxidative damage therefore plays a role in progressive neurologic deterioration. Mode of inheritance and genetic basis are not yet well characterized.

▸ Clinical Findings

A. Symptoms and Signs

Ataxia can be prominent. Associated signs and symptoms include seizures, weakness, pyramidal signs, peripheral neuropathy, and developmental delay. The disorder can also occur in a myopathic form. Symptom onset is predominantly during infancy or childhood, but adult onset has been reported.

B. Laboratory Findings and Imaging Studies

Pyruvate and lactate levels are normal, and CoQ10 levels in serum may be normal or low. MRI of the brain characteristically reveals cerebellar atrophy, although individual cases may have other features.

C. Special Tests

Diagnosis depends on low CoQ10 levels in muscle. Ragged-red fibers are present in the rare, myopathic form but typically not in the ataxic form.

▸ Treatment & Prognosis

Some patients receiving CoQ10 supplementation (up to 3000 mg/day) show improvement in ataxia, strength, and seizures. Without treatment, symptoms progress. Weakness and wasting may lead to confinement to a wheelchair, and seizures can be difficult to control. Few cases have been

Table 16–10. Mitochondrial Disorders Producing Ataxia

Disorder	Clinical Findings	Diagnostic Clues
Autosomal-recessive mitochondrial ataxic syndrome	Onset often with migraine and epilepsy, with later sensory and cerebellar ataxia	MRI—abnormalities in cerebellum, olivary nucleus, occipital cortex, thalami Muscle biopsy—COX deficiency, depletion of mtDNA. Associated POLG mutations
Chronic progressive external ophthalmoplegia (CPEO)	Ataxia, extraocular muscle weakness, peripheral neuropathy, ataxia, tremor, depression, cataracts, pigmentary retinopathy, deafness, rhabdomyolysis, hypogonadism Can occur with sensory ataxic neuropathy dysarthria and ophthalmoplegia (SANDO) or mitochondrial recessive ataxia syndrome (MIRAS)	Muscle biopsy—variable POLG1 mutation
Familial coenzyme Q10 (CoQ10) deficiency	Variable age of onset Ataxia, generalized muscle weakness, pyramidal signs, neuropathy, developmental delay, seizures	Muscle biopsy—reduced levels of CoQ10 MRI—cerebellar atrophy
Infantile onset spinocerebellar ataxia (IOSCA)		Twinkle gene mutation
Kearns-Sayre syndrome (KSS)	Onset before age 20 y Ptosis and external ophthalmoplegia, retinopathy, ataxia, absent deep tendon reflexes, cardiomyopathy, short stature, hypogonadism, diabetes mellitus, hypoparathyroidism	Lactic acidosis in serum and CSF, CSF protein >100 mg/dL, Muscle biopsy—RRF MRI—sometimes shows leukoencephalopathy, often associated with cerebral or cerebellar atrophy or basal ganglia lesions
Maternally inherited Leigh syndrome (MILS)	Onset between 3 and 12 mo of age, often following viral infection Developmental delay, hypotonia, spasticity, chorea, ataxia, peripheral neuropathy, hypertrophic cardiomyopathy	Lactic acidosis in CSF > serum, elevated plasma alanine, hypocitrullinemia MRI—bilateral symmetric hyperintense signal abnormality in brainstem or basal ganglia on T2-weighted sequences
Maternally inherited diabetes, deafness, with cerebellar ataxia (MIDD)	Ataxia, deafness, diabetes	tRNA(Leu) 3243
Mitochondrial myopathy, encephalopathy, lactic acidosis, and stroke-like episodes (MELAS)	Onset usually between 4 and 15 y Episodic vomiting, seizures, and recurrent cerebral insults resembling strokes; myoclonic epilepsy; weakness; ataxia; deafness; retinitis pigmentosa; dementia	Lactic acidosis in serum and CSF, elevated CSF protein usually <100 mg/dL Muscle biopsy—RRF MRI—during stroke-like episodes T2-hyperintense lesions not conforming to distribution of major cerebral arteries
Myoclonic epilepsy with ragged-red fibers (MERRF)	Onset in childhood Myoclonic epilepsy, mental deterioration, weakness, truncal ataxia, dementia, spasticity, optic atrophy, peripheral neuropathy	Lactic acidosis in serum and CSF Muscle biopsy—RRF MRI—brain atrophy, basal ganglia calcifications
Neuropathy, ataxia, and retinitis pigmentosa (NARP)	Typical onset in young adults Developmental delay, retinitis pigmentosa, dementia, seizures, cerebellar ataxia, sensorimotor neuropathy	Lactic acidosis in CSF, hypocitrullinemia MRI—cerebral and cerebellar atrophy

COX = cytochrome oxidase; CSF = cerebrospinal fluid; MRI = magnetic resonance imaging; POLG1 = DNA polymerase γ subunit 1; RRF = ragged-red fibers.

characterized, and the true range in prognosis remains to be defined.

Musumeci O, et al. Familial cerebellar ataxia with muscle coenzyme Q10 deficiency. *Neurology* 2001;56:849–855. [PMID: 11294920]. (First description of six patients with ataxia and other symptoms, with response to CoQ10 supplementation.)

Quinzii CM, et al. CoQ10 deficiency diseases in adults. *Mitochondrion* 2007;7(Supp):S122–126. [PMID: 17485248]

X-LINKED ATAXIAS: FRAGILE X–ASSOCIATED TREMOR & ATAXIA SYNDROME

ESSENTIALS OF DIAGNOSIS

- ► Ataxia, tremor
- ► Cognitive decline (some patients)
- ► Occurs almost exclusively in males
- ► MRI of the brain may show atrophy and abnormal T2-weighted signal in the middle cerebellar peduncle

► General Considerations

Expansion of the triplet repeat CGG in the X-linked *FMR1* gene leads to mental retardation and other features of the fragile X syndrome. However, premutation expansions (55–200 repeats) have recently been identified as the cause of cerebellar tremor and ataxia in older male carriers without fragile X syndrome. Women, rarely affected, have less severe symptoms.

► Clinical Findings

A. Symptoms and Signs

Symptoms usually begin with progressive action tremor. Gait ataxia follows, and associated features include parkinsonism, peripheral neuropathy, autonomic dysfunction, and impaired memory and executive function. Depression and anxiety occur in some. Some patients present with isolated cerebellar ataxia.

B. Imaging Studies

MRI of the brain demonstrates generalized atrophy, including the cerebellum. Approximately 60% of male patients studied have increased signal intensity on T2-weighted images within the middle cerebellar peduncle.

C. Special Tests

Diagnosis is made by commercially available genetic testing for trinucleotide repeat expansion within the *FMR1* gene.

► Treatment

No disease-specific treatment is available, but symptom-targeted therapies are often employed. Action tremor sometimes responds to β-adrenergic blocking agents or primidone. Physical therapy for gait and balance, although not proven, should be tried.

Leehey MA. Fragile X-associated tremor/ataxia syndrome: Clinical phenotype, diagnosis, and treatment. *J Investig Med* 2009;57:830–836. [PMID: 19574929]

Multiple Sclerosis & Demyelinating Diseases

17

Bruce A.C. Cree, MD, PhD, MCR

 ESSENTIALS OF DIAGNOSIS

▶ Episodic or progressive multifocal symptoms and signs

▶ Onset most often in otherwise healthy young adults

▶ Abnormal findings on magnetic resonance imaging (MRI) of the brain (>95% of patients)

▶ General Considerations

Multiple sclerosis (MS) is the leading cause of neurologic disability in young adults. Although not generally a fatal disease, the social impact of disability caused by MS is substantial. MS results in loss of employment, causes dependency on care providers, and often leads to social isolation. MS affects approximately 300,000 Americans and more than 2.5 million individuals worldwide. The mean annual direct and indirect cost per patient in 2004 dollars was estimated to be $47,215 per patient, with an annual cost of MS in the United States of $14.2 billion.

There is no single test to diagnose multiple sclerosis, and its cause is unknown. The diagnosis relies on recognition of the clinical patterns of the disease. Waxing and waning neurologic deficits that localize to the central nervous system is the hallmark of the disease in most patients. The diagnosis can be supported by laboratory studies, including MRI of the brain and spinal cord, analysis of cerebrospinal fluid, and evoked potential studies of the visual and somatosensory pathways. Systemic or infectious etiologies with similar presentations should be excluded.

MS only affects the central nervous system, sparing the peripheral nervous system from injury. The pathologic hallmark of MS is focal demyelination within the brain and spinal cord. Myelin is a cellular layer formed by oligodendroglial cells that wraps around and electrically insulates axons, thereby allowing saltatory conduction of axon potentials. In MS, discrete areas of damaged myelin called plaques are embedded within normal-appearing tissue. Within each plaque, damaged myelin is associated with inflammatory infiltrates of lymphocytes and macrophages, antibody and complement deposition, activated microglia, and oligodendroglial cell loss. Because of this pathologic association with inflammation and demyelination, MS is considered an autoimmune disease. It is not known whether the immune response observed in MS plaques is a primary process or secondarily caused by other possibilities, such as infectious, toxic, or metabolic etiologies.

There is no cure for MS, and all currently available treatments are only partially effective in reducing MS relapses and disability. All MS therapies approved by the US Food and Drug Administration (FDA) alter immune function and reduce inflammation, adding support to the theory that MS is, at least in part, mediated by immune injury.

A. Epidemiology

MS affects women two to three times as often as men. MS is rare in the pediatric population, but its risk increases steadily from adolescence up to the age of 35 and then gradually decreases. MS is rarely diagnosed after the age of 65.

MS is uncommon in equatorial climates, and its prevalence increases with distance from the equator. Latitudinal gradients for MS susceptibility are observed in the United States, Europe, Japan, Australia, and New Zealand further suggesting an environmental risk factor associated with equatorial distance. Higher latitudes result in lower ultraviolet radiation exposure and consequently lower vitamin D levels. This observation in conjunction with the observation that MS patients consistently have lower levels of vitamin D than matched controls, and the observation that low levels of vitamin D were found associated with subsequent development of MS, led to the realization that vitamin D deficiency or insufficiency is an environmental risk factor for MS.

Additional evidence for an environmental risk factor, and possible infectious agent, in MS comes from the observations of clusters of MS cases and the observation that virtually all MS patients have been exposed to and develop high titer antibodies to the Epstein-Barr virus, the cause of infectious mononucleosis. Precisely how EBV infection and vitamin D deficiency contribute to MS pathogenesis, and what other environmental risk factors might also be involved, remains to be elucidated.

B. Genetic Susceptability

The risk of MS is much higher in populations of Northern European ancestry than in other ethnic groups residing at the same latitudes. This increased susceptibility might be due to genetic differences between ethnic groups. MS is much less common in both native Japanese and Japanese Americans (5 per 100,000) compared with Northern European populations (100 to 150 per 100,000). Similarly, MS is rare in Native Americans in both the United States and Canada.

The most compelling evidence for a genetic component to MS susceptibility comes from twin studies that demonstrate concordance rates of approximately 30% in monozygotic twins and 5% in dizygotic twins. The rate for fraternal twins is similar to that of first-degree relatives of MS patients. Linkage studies performed in multiple affected families in several populations show a consistent association of MS susceptibility with the major histocompatability complex (MHC) on chromosome 6p. This locus encodes the genes that present peptide antigens to T cells. Fine mapping studies indicate that the most likely contribution to MS susceptibility is a polymorphism, or group of polymorphisms, in the DR gene (the DRB1*15:01 allele). Recent studies have shown that the HLA-A*02:01 in the MHC class I region also contributes to MS susceptibility.

Genome-wide association screens have found additional minor contributions to MS susceptibility from a growing number of genes (Table 17–1). Currently more than 20 genes have been validated and nearly all are thought to be involved in immune regulation. The identification of many more genetic loci that contribute fractionally to MS susceptibility is expected. The individual contributions of these genes to MS risk is minor, and even their aggregate contribution to MS susceptibility appears to be have less influence than that of the MHC.

C. Pathologic and Immunologic Findings

The term multiple sclerosis comes from the disease's pathologic appearance. At autopsy, multiple discrete pink or gray areas that have a hard or rubbery texture are identified within the white matter of the brain and spinal cord. Although the lesions can occur at any site within the central nervous system, they have a predilection for involvement of the periventricular white matter, the corpus callosum, optic nerves, and the dorsal spinal cord. The lesions are composed of areas of myelin and oligodendrocyte loss accompanied by infiltrates of inflammatory cells, including lymphocytes and macrophages. The focal loss of normal myelin indicates a highly specific demyelinating process and helps distinguish MS from the leukodystrophies. The relative preservation of axons and neurons within these lesions helps distinguish MS from other destructive pathologic processes that are accompanied by focal inflammation. Although the relative sparing of axons in MS plaques is a defining feature of the disease, axonal transection occurs, is irreversible, and presumably leads to neuronal death by wallerian degeneration.

All active or acute MS plaques show evidence of a focal inflammatory process with infiltrates of T cells, plasma cells, and macrophages filled with myelin debris. As with chronic plaques, active plaques are characterized by demyelination with relative axonal sparing. Some plaques contain antibody and complement deposition, suggesting activation of the humoral immune system. Other plaques are characterized by prominent oligodendroglial cell loss. In progressive forms of MS, inflammatory active plaques are found less often; however, widespread microglial activation and cortical plaques are common. Whether these histopathologic features of progressive MS are secondary to earlier inflammatory injury or represent a distinct pathologic process remains to be determined.

Support for an autoimmune etiology for MS comes from animal studies. Experimental allergic encephalomyelitis (EAE) is an autoinflammatory response against the brain and spinal cord induced by inoculating animals with brain extracts or purified myelin proteins. Depending on the animal model used, causative roles for T cells or B cells have been implicated. However, the evidence that MS is caused by either T-cell or B-cell autoreactivity is limited. Challenging the idea that MS plaques are caused by inflammatory-mediated tissue injury is the observation that oligodendroglial cell loss can precede inflammatory infiltration and suggests that the inflammatory response is secondary to tissue injury of as yet an unknown etiology.

Ascherio A, Munger KL, Simon KC. Vitamin D and multiple sclerosis. Lancet Neurol 2010;9:599–612. [PMID: 20494325] (Reviews the evidence for a cause-effect relationship between vitamin D insufficiency and multiple sclerosis.)

Frischer JM, et al. The relation between inflammation and neurodegeneration in multiple sclerosis brains. Brain 2009;132(Pt 5): 1175–1189. [PMID: 19339255] (Finds that neurodegeneration and inflammation are pathologically linked and suggests that ongoing neuroinflammation, behind a closed blood–brain barrier, contributes to clinical decline in progressive MS.)

Henderson AP, Barnett MH, Parratt JDE, Prineas JW. Multiple sclerosis: Distribution of inflammatory cells in newly forming lesions. Ann Neurol 2009;66:739–753. [PMID: 20035511] (Suggests that inflammation in MS plaques is secondary to oligodendroglial injury.)

International Multiple Sclerosis Genetics Consortium (IMSGC). Risk alleles for multiple sclerosis identified by a genomewide study. N Engl J Med 2007;357:851–862. [PMID: 17660530] (Identifies the first two definitive, non-MHC genes involved in MS pathogenesis and paved the way for further large-scale studies of MS genetics.)

Table 17–1. MS Susceptibility Genes

Major Gene of Interest	Function	Other Disease Associations
HLA-DRB1*15:01	Presents antigens to T cells.	SLE
IL2RA[a]	Interleukin 2 receptor α subunit, expressed on activated and regulatory T cells, it regulates lymphocyte proliferation and differentiation.	Graves disease, RA, SLE, DM1
IL7R[a]	Interleukin 7 receptor promotes survival of CD4+ and CD8+ cells after positive selection and modulates peripheral memory cell homeostasis.	DM1
IL12A[b]	The α subunit of the interleukin 12 protein, secreted by monocytes and dendritic cells, is crucial for Th1 lymphocyte differentiation.	Celiac disease, primary biliary cirrhosis
CD6[b]	T-cell costimulatory molecule potentiates lymphocyte proliferation.	
IRF8[b]	A transcription factor that is induced by type I interferons.	
TNFRSF1A[b]	Tumor necrosis factor α receptor involved in apoptosis, inflammation and immunosuppression.	TRAPS
MPHOSPH9/CDK2AP1[b]	The function of MPHOSPH9 is unknown. CDK2AP1 encodes p12DOC-1, an inhibitor of DNA replication.	
RGS1[b]	It encodes a regulator of G-protein signaling, involved in lymphocyte migration and trafficking.	Celiac disease, DM1
CD58[b]	A ligand of CD2 signals this costimulatory molecule and enhances TCR signaling.	
CLEC16A[b]	C-type lectin family member expressed on B cells, dendritic cells, and NK cells. May signal for a decision between tolerance and immunity.	DM1
CD40[c]	TNFR superfamily member, a costimulatory molecule on B cells, dendritic cells, macrophages, and microglia.	Graves disease, RA
CYP27B1[c]	Encodes the enzyme 25-hydroxy-vitamin D-1 α hydroxylase. Hydroxylates 25-OH vitamin D to 1,25 (OH)$_2$ vitamin D.	DM1
EVI5 [c]	A common site of retroviral integration with unknown function.	
STAT3[d]	A transcription factor involved in multiple functions including the Jak-STAT signaling pathway, apoptosis, immune activation, neuronal guidance, and TH17 differentiation.	Crohn disease
TYK2[e]	A tyrosine kinase in the STAT signaling pathway that is important for type I interferon signaling and induction of Th1 T-cell differentiation.	SLE
KIF21B[f]	Kinesin super family motor protein involved in axonal transport.	
TMEM39A[f]	Unknown function.	
MMEL1[g]	A membrane metalloendopeptidase involved in neuropeptide degradation, also involved in degradation of β-amyloid.	RA, celiac disease, primary biliary cirrhosis
CBLB[h]	E3 ubiquitin ligase involved in regulation of self-tolerance.	

DM1 = type 1 diabetes mellitus; RA = rheumatoid arthritis; SLE = systemic lupus erythematosus; TCR = T-cell receptor; TNFR = tumor necrosis factor receptor; TRAPS = tumor necrosis factor receptor associated periodic syndrome, also known as familial Hibernian fever.

[a]International Multiple Sclerosis Genetics Consortium (IMSGC). Risk alleles for multiple sclerosis identified by a genomewide study. *N Engl J Med* 2007;357:851–862.

[b]De Jager PL, et al. Meta-analysis of genome scans and replication identify CD6, IRF8 and TNFRSF1A as new multiple sclerosis susceptibility loci. *Nat Genet* 2009;41:776–782.

[c]The Australia and New Zealand Multiple Sclerosis Genetics Consortium (ANZgene). Genome-wide association study identifies new multiple sclerosis susceptibility loci on chromosomes 12 and 20. *Nat Genet* 2009;41:824–828.

[d]Jakkula E, et al. Genome-wide association study in a high-risk isolate for multiple sclerosis reveals associated variants in STAT3 gene. *Am J Hum Genet* 2010;86:285–291.

[e]Ban M, et al. Replication analysis identifies TYK2 as a multiple sclerosis susceptibility factor. *Eur J Hum Genet* 2009;17:1309–1313.

[f]International Multiple Sclerosis Genetics Consortium (IMSGC). Comprehensive follow-up of the first genome-wide association study of multiple sclerosis identifies KIF21B and TMEM39A as susceptibility loci. *Hum Mol Genet* 2010;19:953–962.

[g]Ban M, et al. A non-synonymous SNP within membrane metalloendopeptidase-like 1 (MMEL) is associated with multiple sclerosis. *Genes Immun* 2010;11:660–664.

[h]Sanna S, et al. Variants within the immunoregulatory CBLB gene are associated with multiple sclerosis. *Nat Genet* 2010;42:495–497.

▶ Clinical Findings

A. Symptoms and Signs

1. Onset—The initial focal manifestation of disease that a patient recognizes may be acute or insidious and can vary in severity. Initial symptoms are often sensory disturbances, weakness, visual loss, abnormal gait, diminished dexterity, diplopia, ataxia, vertigo, or sphincter disturbances. Patients may recall nonspecific symptoms such as malaise, fatigue, or headache heralding the initial focal neurologic disturbance. From most to least common, Table 17–2 summarizes the presenting manifestations of MS, and Table 17–3 lists the most to least common clinical manifestations of MS over the entire course of the disease.

2. Sensory disturbance—The most common presenting manifestations of MS are paresthesias: tingling, pins and needles, dysesthesias (burning, gritty, sandy, electrical, or wet sensations), or hypoesthesia (loss of sensation or

Table 17–2. Frequency of Symptoms at Disease Onset Ranked in Order From Most to Least Common

Symptom	Percentage
Sensory disturbance	34
Weakness	22
Visual loss	13
Ataxia	11
Diplopia	8
Vertigo	4.3
Fatigue	2
Facial pain	2
Headache	2
Bladder dysfunction	1
Facial weakness	1
Dysarthria	0.6
Hearing loss	0.6
Cramps	0.6
Loss of consciousness	0.6
Psychiatric symptoms	0.3
Poor memory	0.3
Dysphagia	0.3
Loss of taste	0.3

Adapted with permission from Swingler RJ, Compston DA. The morbidity of multiple sclerosis. *Q J Med* 1992;83:325–337.

Table 17–3. Frequency of Symptoms During the Entire Disease Course in Order From Most to Least Common

Symptom	Percentage
Weakness	89
Sensory disturbance	87
Ataxia	82
Bladder	71
Fatigue	57
Cramps	52
Diplopia	51
Visual loss	49
Bowel dysfunction	42
Dysarthria	37
Vertigo	36
Facial pain	35
Memory dysfunction	32
Headache	30
Psychiatric symptoms	23
Hearing loss	17
Facial weakness	16
Dysphagia	13
Pressure sores	12
Loss of consciousness	11
Loss of taste	6

Adapted with permission from Swingler RJ, Compston DA. The morbidity of multiple sclerosis. *Q J Med* 1992;83:325–337.

procaine-like numbness). Some patients describe a swollen feeling or a squeezing sensation as if a limb or the trunk is tightly wrapped. These symptoms can be intermittent or constant and can spread from one location to adjoining areas. A common manifestation is unilateral numbness affecting one leg that spreads to involve the other leg and ascends to the pelvis, abdomen, or thorax. This pattern is indicative of spinal cord involvement, especially when a sensory level can be demonstrated on physical examination. Also useful is the Lhermitte symptom: upon neck flexion, an electrical or shock-like sensation travels down the spine and radiates into one or more limbs. The presence of a Lhermitte symptom localizes the pathologic process to the cervical spinal cord. Sensory disturbances associated with MS flares usually resolve but sometimes evolve into chronic neuropathic pain.

3. Motor symptoms—Motor symptoms are the second most common initial manifestation of MS and include limb weakness, loss of dexterity, and gait disturbance. Symptoms typically evolve over hours or days, but sometimes patients will awake with a motor deficit. Sometimes weakness becomes apparent only during exertion; fatigue after exercise is common. Weakness is often accompanied by spasticity, a velocity-dependent increase in tone. In addition to spasticity, hyperreflexia and pathologic reflexes such as the Babinski sign typically accompany weakness, indicating a central pathology. Sometimes deep tendon reflexes may be diminished or absent if MS plaques within the spinal cord impede transmission of afferent signals from stretch receptors to the lower motor neurons, thereby simulating peripheral nerve injury. Weakness can affect a single limb or cause hemiparesis or paraparesis. The hemiparesis of MS usually spares the face.

4. Optic neuritis—The third most common presenting manifestation of MS is optic neuritis, which is characterized by loss of vision affecting usually one eye evolving over hours or days. Bilateral optic neuritis is much less frequent. Multiple sclerosis is one of several disease states that cause monocular vision loss (Table 17–4). Loss of vision can be complete or partial; patients will often report a scotoma, an area of diminished or blurred vision in the monocular field. The size of the scotoma can vary. Loss of vision can be subtle and preferentially affects color vision. Red desaturation, the inability to distinguish shades of red, can be quantified using Ishihara color plates. Optic neuritis is often associated with periorbital pain during eye movements. Pathologically, optic neuritis is caused by inflammation and demyelination of the optic nerve. If myelin loss is close to the retina, relative pallor of the optic disc is seen on funduscopy. Additional funduscopic findings of optic neuritis include papillitis of the nerve head (mild swelling) and venous sheathing of retinal vessels, produced by transendothelial migration of lymphocytes.

5. Ataxia and tremor—Discoordinated movements of the limbs or gait are common in MS and can be caused by plaques affecting the cerebellar afferent or efferent pathways. Appendicular ataxia is often observed as dysmetria or tremor on finger-nose-finger and heel-knee-shin tests. Dysdiadochokinesia can be elicited by alternately clapping the palmar and dorsal surfaces of one hand on the opposite palm. Dysrhythmias can be demonstrated by finger or toe tapping. The Romberg sign, truncal swaying on standing with the feet together and eyes closed, can be caused by impaired proprioception from spinal cord dorsal column lesions. In a patient without leg weakness, proximal joint position of the legs can be assessed by the mirrored movement test. With the patient lying down with eyes closed, the examiner raises one leg of the patient into a position and asks the patient to mirror the position with the other leg. When proximal joint position sense is impaired, the movement mirrored by the patient will

Table 17–4. Diagnostic Considerations in Optic Neuritis

Demyelinating Diseases
　Multiple sclerosis
　Acute disseminated encephalomyelitis
　Neuromyelitis optica
　Idiopathic recurrent and nonrecurrent optic neuritis

Viral
　Varicella-zoster virus
　West Nile virus
　HIV

Mycobacterial and Bacterial
　Borrelia burgdorferi (Lyme disease)
　Treponema pallidum (syphilis)
　Brucella melitensis (brucellosis)
　Bartonella henselae (catscratch disease)

Parasitic
　Cryptococcosis
　Toxoplasmosis
　Histoplasmosis

Rheumatologic Diseases and Autoantibody Syndromes
　Collagen vascular diseases
　　• Sjögren syndrome
　　• Systemic lupus erythematosus
　　• Mixed connective-tissue disease
　　• Anticardiolipin autoantibodies
　　• Primary angiitis of the CNS
　　• Protoplasmic-staining antineutrophil cytoplasmic antibodies autoantibodies
　Temporal arteritis
　Sarcoidosis
　Behçet disease

Vascular
　Retinal artery occlusion
　Retinal vein occlusion
　Anterior ischemic optic neuropathy

Neoplastic and Paraneoplastic
　Lymphoma, leukemia, and other infiltrating tumors
　Carcinomatous meningitis
　Optic nerve glioma
　Meningioma of the optic nerve sheath
　Paraneoplastic
　　• Hodgkin lymphoma
　　• Other tumors (anti-AQP4, anti-CRMP5)

Glaucoma
　Acute angle-closure glaucoma
　Low-tension or normal-tension glaucoma

Nutritional
　Vitamin B_{12} deficiency

Toxic
　Methanol
　Ethambutol
　Halogenated hydroxyquinolines
　Amiodarone
　Chemotherapeutic drugs (eg, carmustine, cisplatin, cytosine arabinoside, fludarabine, and vincristine)

Hereditary
　Leber hereditary optic neuropathy

Trauma
　Retinal detachment

not match the leg positioned by the examiner. Tremors range in severity from subtle, manifested only by intention tremor on tests of limb coordination, to severe and disabling.

6. Diplopia—Double vision is common in MS and is caused by disconjugate eye movements. The deficits, which may be overt in primary gaze or elicited by vertical or horizontal eye movements, depend on which eye muscles are affected. Sometimes diplopia can be subtle and is manifested by blurred vision, similar to that of optic neuritis. To distinguish between these possibilities, blurred vision caused by diplopia resolves when either eye is covered, whereas blurred vision caused by optic neuritis resolves only when the affected eye is covered. The most common abnormal eye movement observed in MS is intranuclear ophthalmoplegia (INO). Demyelinating plaques affect the medial longitudinal fasciculus, a tract that yokes the sixth cranial nerve nucleus controlling abduction to the contralateral third nerve nucleus controlling adduction, enabling conjugate horizontal eye movement. Lesions in the MLF typically occur ipsilateral to the affected third nucleus and result in impaired adduction of the eye ipsilateral to the lesion when lateral gaze is attempted. Compensatory nystagmus of the abducting eye occurs. INO can be distinguished from isolated medial rectus palsy because INO does not impair convergence. MS is by far the most common cause of bilateral INO in young adults. Bilateral INO in MS can result in exotropia on primary gaze, so-called wall-eyed bilateral INO (WEBINO). MS lesions can also cause diplopia in the vertical plane or isolated impairments of the sixth, third, and fourth nerves.

7. Vertigo—Vertigo can be the initial manifestation of MS or can occur at any time during the course of the disease. Vertigo can be fleeting or last for days or even weeks. Vertigo caused by MS is sometimes associated with other signs or symptoms of brainstem pathology such as facial sensory loss or diplopia. Vertigo caused by labyrinthine pathology identified by the Dix-Hallpike maneuver is not due to MS. Although uncommon, unilateral hearing loss occurs in MS, sometimes with vertigo.

8. Fatigue—Over the course of the disease, fatigue is one of the most common MS symptoms and contends with cognitive impairment as the major cause of loss of vocation. Fatigue can occur as a consequence of exertion (the weakness associated with neuromuscular fatigue), as a manifestation of the vegetative symptoms of depression, as a consequence of insomnia (daytime drowsiness), or as a generalized lassitude. Fatigue can occur late in the afternoon or be present on awakening and persist throughout the day.

9. Facial pain—MS can present with trigeminal neuralgia, and the presentation of lancinating facial pain should always prompt the consideration of MS, followed by appropriate diagnostic imaging. The paroxysms of pain are lancinating and severe and can occur in clusters. Features that help distinguish trigeminal neuralgia associated with MS from its idiopathic counterpart are bilateral occurrence, constant duration, involvement of the first branch of the trigeminal nerve, and sensory loss detected by physical examination.

10. Bladder and bowel dysfunction—Patients often complain of urinary urgency, frequency, hesitancy, and incontinence. Although the symptoms of urgency and frequency imply a spastic bladder, whereas hesitancy is associated with a denervated bladder, it is difficult to determine the nature of bladder dysfunction by history alone. Incontinence can occur in the setting of a spastic bladder that is tonically contracted and incapable of filling completely and can also occur with a denervated bladder that fails to contract and overflows. The volume of postvoiding residual urine measured either by catheterization or by ultrasound is useful for distinguishing between a spastic and denervated bladder. Urodynamic studies may be helpful. Bladder dyssynergia, impairment of sphincter and detrusor coordination, is also a cause of hesitancy and incomplete voiding. Patients with urinary retention are susceptible to urinary tract infections. Urinary tract infections are thought to trigger MS flares by stimulating the immune system.

Bowel dysfunction is also common in MS and may be caused by spinal cord plaques. Chronic constipation can worsen appendicular spasticity. Incontinence occurs either as a consequence of sphincter dysfunction or from bowel spasticity and fecal urgency.

11. Facial weakness—Lower motor neuron facial weakness, similar to Bell palsy, can occur when MS plaques affect intraparenchymal emerging fibers of the 7th cranial nerve. Ipsilateral loss of taste, hyperacusis, retroauricular pain, and synkinesis are hallmarks of peripheral facial neuropathy and do not occur with central facial weakness.

12. Flexor spasms—One of the paroxysmal symptoms of MS, and a hallmark of the disease, is flexor spasms. Tonic spasms of a limb or the face are often preceded by paresthesias or dysesthesias. These can occur at night and in clusters and can be elicited by movements, hyperventilation, or other precipitating factors. Spasms usually are brief, can be painful, and are generally very distressing for the patient.

13. Neuropsychiatric dysfunction—Patients often report difficulties with short-term memory, attention, information processing, problem solving, multitasking, and language function. Cognitive deficits may not be detected by the Mini Mental Status Exam and often require more extensive neuropsychiatric testing. In many MS patients, cognitive deficits cause loss of vocation and impairment of activities of daily living. Emotional lability is common, and as many as 60% of MS patients suffer from depression. Some patients have a pseudobulbar affect with spontaneous and inappropriate laughter or tears. Later in the course of the disease, some patients develop "la belle indifférence," a seeming lack of concern for their severe disability, and some display striking euphoria.

14. Dysarthria—Impairments of speech are common in MS and can be caused by tongue weakness from lower brainstem dysfunction, spastic dysarthria from corticobulbar injury, or scanning dysarthria from cerebellar dysfunction.

15. Dysphagia—Impairment of swallowing occurs in MS, particularly later in the course of the disease. Choking on thin liquids such as water is consistent with neurologic injury as opposed to a pharyngeal structural abnormality that usually causes solid food dysphagia. Barium swallow and fiberscope endoscopic evaluation of swallowing are helpful in evaluating dysphagia and assessing aspiration risk.

16. Facial myokymia—Chronic flickering contractions of the orbicularis occuli or other muscles of facial expression occur and arise from injury to the facial nerve within the brainstem or to the corticobulbar tracts.

Other paroxysmal symptoms—Virtually all symptoms of MS, including the Lhermitte symptom, sensory disturbances, weakness, ataxia, and diplopia, can occur as transient paroxysms lasting for seconds to minutes, sometimes in clusters.

B. Disease Course

1. Relapsing remitting multiple sclerosis—Because there is no specific test for MS, diagnosis of the disease relies largely on the clinical history. Relapses, also known as flares or attacks, occur when patients develop symptoms caused by plaque formation. Patients become aware of an acute plaque in an area likely to cause symptoms such as the optic nerves, spinal cord, brainstem, and cerebellum. However, many plaques evolve in clinically silent areas, such as the corpus callosum and the periventricular white matter. Often patients gradually recover after resolution of the acute inflammation and possibly through myelin repair and plastic reorganization. These periods of recovery of neurologic function are termed remissions, and the episodic development of attacks and recoveries gives rise to the term *relapsing remitting multiple sclerosis* (RRMS). Approximately 90% of patients follow this disease course (Figure 17–1). Although complete recovery of neurologic function may follow acute attacks, patients may suffer sustained neurologic deficits as a consequence of irreversible axonal and myelin injury. In addition, plaque accumulation in clinically silent areas can eventually result in neurologic impairments.

2. Clinically isolated syndrome—Although the disease course of MS is characterized by multiple attacks affecting different regions of the central nervous system over time, many patients seek medical attention after the first attack. The first demyelinating event is called the clinically isolated syndrome, and such patients are considered at risk for developing MS. Some patients go on to develop RRMS and suffer from multiple attacks, whereas others have no further evidence of demyelinating disease. It is difficult to predict whether a given individual will develop MS after symptom

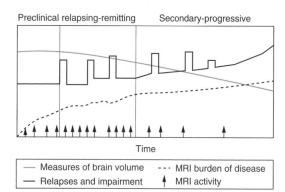

▲ **Figure 17–1.** The natural history of MS. Approximately 85% of MS patients follow a similar disease course. Brain MRI scans show that MS begins before the onset of the first focal neurologic deficit of which the patient is aware. Relapses then occur during the relapsing-remitting phase of the disease. Varying degrees of neurologic recovery follows each relapse. The secondary progressive phase of the disease is characterized by progressive neurologic deterioration independent of relapses. Relapses do occur during the secondary progressive phase of the disease but are less frequent and eventually stop. The MRI burden of disease increases and the extent of brain atrophy increases during the course of the disease. MRI activity, measured by new, contrast-enhancing lesions, decreases during the secondary progressive phase of MS.

onset; however, natural history studies show that the risk of having a second attack after 14 years of follow-up is 88% if there are any lesions present on the initial brain MRI and only 19% if the brain MRI is normal.

Brex PA, et al. A longitudinal study of abnormalities on MRI and disability from multiple sclerosis. *N Engl J Med* 2002;346: 158–164. [PMID: 11796849] (A 14-year natural history study of patients following the first demyelinating event shows that clinically silent brain MRI lesions predict development of MS.)

Comi G, et al; PreCISe Study Group. Effect of glatiramer acetate on conversion to clinically definite multiple sclerosis in patients with clinically isolated syndrome (PreCISe study): A randomized, double-blind, placebo-controlled trial. *Lancet* 2009;374:1503–1511. [PMID: 19815268] (These papers show that treatment with interferon beta-1a, interferon beta-1b, and glatiramer acetate delay the time between the first and second relapses in early MS.)

Jacobs LD, et al. Intramuscular interferon beta-1a therapy initiated during a first demyelinating event in multiple sclerosis. *N Engl J Med* 2000;343:898–904. [PMID: 11006365]

Kappos L, et al. Effect of early versus delayed interferon beta-1b treatment on disability after a first clinical event suggestive of multiple sclerosis: A 3-year follow-up analysis of the BENEFIT study. *Lancet* 2007;370:389–397. [PMID: 17679016]

3. Secondary progressive MS—Approximately 85–90% of subjects with RRMS eventually develop *secondary progressive* MS (SPMS), the insidiously progressive neurologic impairments that cause important ambulatory and cognitive disability. Relapses can still occur in SPMS; however, the frequency of relapses declines during SPMS. Eventually most patients stop experiencing attacks. Some patients with SPMS plateau with stable deficits for many years; however, in most patients neurologic disability relentlessly continues. Patients develop progressive ambulatory disability, eventually becoming bed bound, and finally succumbing to complications of immobility: pneumonia, pressure ulceration, and deep venous thromboses. Patients with RRMS initially have an average of less than one relapse per year, although the range is broad. The median time from diagnosis of RRMS to SPMS is 20 years, and the time from disease onset to requiring a cane to walk is 30 years.

4. Primary progressive multiple sclerosis—Although most central nervous system demyelinating disease follows the RRMS and SPMS clinical course, 10% of patients with MS have a disease course that is progressive from onset without relapses or remissions, termed *primary progressive* MS (PPMS). Patients with PPMS typically present with insidious onset of asymmetric leg weakness or gait disturbance; however, some present with sensory, brainstem/cerebellar, or sphincter dysfunction. In PPMS, visual loss at onset is rare, whereas it is common in RRMS. In contrast to patients with RRMS and SPMS, men are affected about as often as women, and the mean age of onset is older: 40 years for PPMS versus 30 years for RRMS. Natural history studies indicate that patients with PPMS develop ambulatory disability 50% faster than patients with RRMS; however, the rate of progression in PPMS is similar to that of the progressive phase of SPMS. The pathology of PPMS lesions is identical to that of RRMS and SPMS. PPMS can be distinguished from other progressive myelopathy by the presence of characteristic MS demyelinating plaques present on brain MRI. The number and total volume of plaques within the brain of patients with PPMS tend to be fewer than those observed in RRMS and SPMS. Furthermore, actively demyelinating plaques, which show uptake of gadolinium-diethylenetriamine pentaacetic acid (DPTA) contrast on brain MRI, are less common in PPMS. The reason for these differences is not known. Fewer than 5% of patients with MS have progressive symptoms from onset and will also have rare relapses. This disease course is termed *progressive-relapsing* MS.

C. Rating Scales and Diagnostic Criteria

The most commonly used measure of neurologic impairment in MS is the Expanded Disability Status Scale (EDSS, Figure 17–2). This scale ranges from 0 to 10. The EDSS quantifies components of the neurologic examination as functional scale scores and also takes into account the extent of ambulatory disability and limitations in self-care. The functional scales quantify vision, brainstem, corticospinal, sensory, cerebellar, cognitive, and bowel and bladder function. Many other

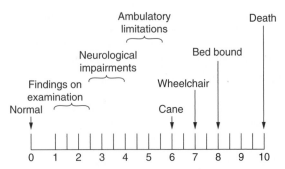

▲ **Figure 17–2.** The EDSS is a nonlinear rating scale with half-point intervals from 1 to 10. An EDSS score of 0 is normal. Scores of 1–2 reflect physical findings on examination. Scores of 2.5–3.5 correspond to impairments such as hemiparesis, paraparesis, cerebellar dystaxia, or substantial sensory loss. Scores from 4–5.5 usually reflect limitations in the distance a patient can walk without assistance. Scores of ≥6 are based on the extent of ambulatory disability and the ability to perform activities of daily living. A score of 10 is death due to MS. (Reproduced with permission from Kurtzke JF. *Neurology* 1983;33:1444–1452.)

tests have been used in MS clinical trials, including various measures of cognitive function by neuropsychiatric testing and tests of physical strength, dexterity, and vision.

D. Diagnostic Studies

Because MS is a disseminated disease that afflicts multiple areas of the central nervous system during an affected individual's disease course, it is said to evolve over space and time. An example would be a patient who develops optic neuritis and then several months later develops cerebellar ataxia. The recognition of this pattern of attacks accompanied by corresponding physical findings forms the basis of the diagnostic criteria used to define the disease (Table 17–5).

1. Magnetic resonance imaging—Although the diagnosis of MS relies on recognition of the clinical pattern of disease, several laboratory studies are useful in confirming the diagnosis. MRI is particularly helpful. The brain MRI is abnormal in 95–99% of cases of RRMS. Although sensitive, the brain MRI is not specific because several other disease states are associated with a similar pattern. Typically multiple areas of abnormal signal intensity are present on T2-weighted brain MRI imaging (T2, proton density, and fluid-attenuation inversion recovery sequences) that often have a round or ovoid appearance and are located within the corpus callosum and the periventricular and subcortical white matter (Table 17–6). On sagittal views, these plaques appear as linear or flame-like streaks oriented perpendicularly to the lateral ventricles. Perivenular plaques give rise to the distinct

Table 17–5. Proposed Multiple Sclerosis Diagnostic Criteria

Clinical Presentation	Additional Data Needed for Multiple Sclerosis Diagnosis
Two or more relapses[a]; objective clinical evidence of two or more lesions	None[b]
Two or more relapses[a]; objective clinical evidence of one lesion	Dissemination in space, demonstrated by: • MRI[c] *or* • Two or more MRI-detected lesions consistent with MS plus positive CSF[d] *or* • Await further clinical relapse[a] implicating a different site
One relapse[a]; objective clinical evidence of two or more lesions	Dissemination in time, demonstrated by: • MRI[e] *or* • Second clinical relapse[a]
One relapse[a]; objective clinical evidence of one lesion (monosymptomatic presentation; clinically isolated syndrome)	Dissemination in space, demonstrated by: • MRI[c] *or* • Two or more MRI-detected lesions consistent with MS plus positive CSF[d] *and* dissemination in time, demonstrated by: • MRI[e] *or* • Second clinical relapse[a]
Insidious neurologic progression suggestive of MS	One year of disease progression (retrospectively or prospectively determined) *and* two of the following: • Positive brain MRI (nine T2 lesions or four or more T2 lesions with positive visual-evoked potential)[f] • Positive spinal cord MRI (two focal T2 lesions) • Positive CSF[d]

Note: The 2005 International Panel Criteria revisions to the McDonald Diagnostic Criteria for Multiple Sclerosis allow establishment of a diagnosis of multiple sclerosis (MS) if one of five sets of criteria are fulfilled and that other etiologies be excluded. If criteria indicated are fulfilled and there is no better explanation for the clinical presentation, the diagnosis is MS; if suspicious, but the criteria are not completely met, the diagnosis is "possible MS"; if another diagnosis arises during the evaluation that better explains the entire clinical presentation, then the diagnosis is "not MS."

CSF = cerebrospinal fluid; MRI = magnetic resonance imaging; MS = multiple sclerosis.

[a]A relapse, or attack, is defined as an episode of neurologic disturbance for which causative lesions are likely to be inflammatory and demyelinating in nature. A subjective report (backed up by objective findings) or objective observation that the event lasts for at least 24 hours must occur.

[b]No additional tests are required; however, if tests (MRI, CSF) are undertaken and are negative, extreme caution needs to be taken before making a diagnosis of MS. Alternative diagnoses must be considered. No better explanation for the clinical picture is known, and some objective evidence supports a diagnosis of MS.

[c]MRI demonstration of space dissemination must fulfill the criteria derived from Barkhof and colleagues and Tintoré and colleagues, as presented in Table 17–6.

[d]Positive CSF determined by oligoclonal bands detected by established methods (isoelectric focusing) different from any such bands in serum, or by an increased IgG index.

[e]MRI demonstration of time dissemination must fulfill the criteria in Table 17–6.

[f]Abnormal visual-evoked potential of the type seen in MS.

Adapted with permission from McDonald WI, et al. Recommended diagnostic criteria for multiple sclerosis. *Ann Neurol* 2001;50:121–127.

appearance of these lesions, which are named Dawson fingers after the Scottish pathologist who described similar findings at autopsy. Their presence is strongly suggestive of MS. Other typically affected areas include the white matter of the brainstem and cerebellum. Less often, gray matter structures, such as the thalamus and basal ganglia, are affected. Although cortical plaques occur, they are not well visualized by MRI.

On T1-weighted imaging, areas of relative hypointensity can be identified that correspond to some of the areas of increased T2 signal. These areas, so-called T1 black holes, have been pathologically associated with chronic MS plaques and axonal loss. When gadolinium-DPTA contrast is administered intravenously, acute plaques show contrast uptake. Sometimes the pattern of enhancement is homogenous, and at other times it is associated with a ring or open ring pattern. Gadolinium enhancement typically persists for an average of 1–3 weeks and then subsides (Figure 17–3).

In patients with active disease who are otherwise asymptomatic, the brain MRI often shows evolution of new plaques

Table 17–6. MRI Criteria for Multiple Sclerosis

Dissemination in Space
Three of the following[a]:
- At least one gadolinium-enhancing lesion or nine T2 hyperintense lesions if no gadolinium-enhancing lesion is present
- At least one infratentorial lesion
- At least one juxtacortical lesion
- At least three periventricular lesions

Dissemination in Time
There are two ways to show dissemination in time using imaging:
1. Detection of gadolinium enhancement at least 3 months after the onset of the initial clinical event, if not at the site corresponding to the initial event
2. Detection of a *new* T2 lesion if it appears at any time compared with a reference scan done at least 30 days after the onset of the initial clinical event

[a]A spinal cord lesion can be considered equivalent to a brain infratentorial lesion: An enhancing spinal cord lesion is considered to be equivalent to an enhancing brain lesion, and individual spinal cord lesions can contribute together with individual brain lesions to reach the required number of T2 lesions.

over a several-month interval. Serial studies on the same patient show that the same plaque is susceptible to multiple rounds of recurrent inflammation. Detection of subclinical disease activity by MRI is helpful for diagnosing patients who have suffered only one clinical attack. In addition, the brain MRI is useful for evaluating a patient's response to treatment.

MRI of the spinal cord is also useful in MS. Although spinal cord imaging is not as sensitive as brain MRI, plaques within the parenchyma of the cord can be seen on T2-weighted imaging or on T1-weighted imaging after administration of gadolinium-DPTA. Typically these plaques are oriented longitudinally along the cord, often with a posterior (dorsal) location, spanning one or two vertebral cord segments. As with brain MRI plaques, acute spinal cord plaques may show areas of contrast enhancement in either a homogenous or ring pattern. Focal cord swelling may be present.

A recent prospective multicenter cohort study of patients presenting with clinically isolated syndromes was used to reevaluate the diagnostic criteria for dissemination in space and time. This study proposed use of new criteria for diagnosis of MS (Table 17–7). The primary advantage of these

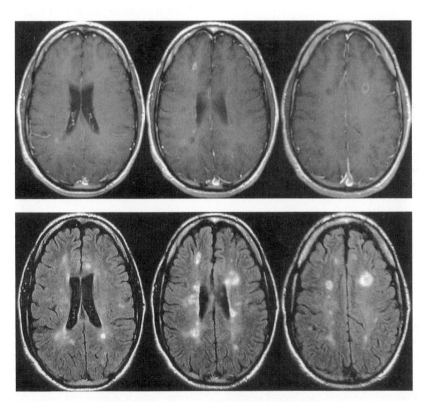

▲ **Figure 17–3.** Axial brain MRI. Contrast-enhanced T1-weighted images show several areas of contrast uptake in acute MS plaques and areas of T1 hypointensity (black holes). Multiple areas of increased signal intensity are present on T2-weighted FLAIR images, some of which correspond to the acute plaques seen on the contrast-enhanced T1-weighted images.

Table 17–7. Proposed MAGNIMS Criteria for Multiple Sclerosis[a]

Dissemination in Space

≥1 lesion in each of ≥2 characteristic locations:
- Periventricular
- Juxtacortical
- Posterior fossa
- Spinal cord

All lesions in symptomatic regions excluded in brainstem and spinal cord syndromes

Dissemination in Time

There are two ways to show dissemination in time using imaging:
1. Simultaneous presence of asymptomatic gadolinium-enhancing and nonenhancing lesions at any time
2. A new T2 and/or gadolinium-enhancing lesion on follow-up MRI irrespective of timing of baseline scan

[a]Cerebrospinal fluid was not systematically examined in the European Magnetic Resonance Network in MS (MAGNIMS) cohort and for this reason is not included in the proposed MAGNIMS criteria.

Adapted with permission from Montalban X, et al. MRI criteria for MS in patients with clinically isolated syndromes. *Neurology* 2010;74:427–434.

diagnostic criteria over those of the 2005 International Panel Criteria is that repeat brain MRI may not be needed in order to meet the dissemination in time criteria based on the premise that the simultaneous presence of an asymptomatic gadolinium-DPTA–enhancing lesion and other nonenhancing T2 lesions indicates dissemination in time. The sensitivity, specificity, and positive predictive value of these criteria compare favorably to that of the 2001 (McDonald criteria) and 2005 International Panel Criteria.

MRI is also used to investigate MS pathogenesis. Indices of brain volume loss (atrophy) correlate with progressive disability and underscore the neurodegenerative effects of MS. Magnetic resonance spectroscopy (MRS) can measure the ratio of *N*-acetylaspartate (NAA), an amino acid present within neurons, to creatine and has shown that in MS areas of normal-appearing white matter can have axonal injury. Changes in the magnetic transfer ratio (MTR), a measure of the association of water with protein, indicate that pathologic changes occur before the onset of contrast enhancement. Diffusion tensor imaging (DTI) measures the diffusion of water along white matter tracts and may become useful for anatomically demonstrating wallerian degeneration. Functional MRI (f-MRI) indicates that recovery after an acute exacerbation can be due to utilization of alternate neuronal circuitry in addition to myelin recovery. High-field strength MRI (7 Tesla) can reveal cortical plaques. These techniques are not yet being used in clinical practice but will likely become useful as surrogate measures of disease progression activity.

2. Cerebrospinal fluid analysis—In cases in which the MRI is normal or shows a pattern that is consistent with other disease processes such as microvascular ischemia or infection, cerebrospinal fluid (CSF) analysis is indicated. The CSF is abnormal in 85–90% of MS patients. Typically there is evidence of intrathecal synthesis of gammaglobulins as measured by elevated total immunoglobulin G (IgG), an elevated IgG ratio, an increased IgG synthesis rate, or the presence of two or more oligoclonal bands in the CSF that are not present in a simultaneously drawn serum sample. Intrathecal synthesis of gammaglobulins is not specific for MS and occurs in the setting of infections such as syphilis, subacute sclerosing panencephalitis, and Lyme disease. CSF can be further analyzed to help exclude potentially competing diagnoses using serologic or nucleic acid amplification techniques.

A lymphocytic pleocytosis with cell counts greater than 5 cell/μL is present in approximately 25% of MS patients. Cell counts are usually fewer than 20 cells/μL. The total protein is usually normal or mildly elevated. Cell counts greater than 50 cells/μL, the presence of polymorphonuclear cells, or protein elevation greater than 100mg/dL should raise suspicion for alternate diagnoses such as infection, collagen vascular diseases, or neoplasm.

3. Evoked potentials—Electrophysiologic studies of the visual pathways and spinal cord dorsal columns are sometimes useful in documenting involvement of these pathways when imaging studies or physical findings do not support the clinical impression. In up to 85% of MS patients, visual evoked potentials (VEP) are abnormal. The characteristic findings of the VEP that suggest demyelination include asymmetric delay of the P100 potential and conduction block (in the setting of acute optic neuritis). Delays or block of the N-20 potential of the median nerve, or the P37 potential of the tibial nerve, on somatosensory-evoked potential tests can also help in diagnosing MS when brain and spinal cord imagings do not meet criteria for dissemination in space. Evoked potential abnormalities are present in a broad range of diseases that affect the nervous system, therefore limiting their diagnostic utility.

Bourahoui A, et al. CSF isolectric focusing in a large cohort of MS and other neurological diseases. *Eur J Neurol* 2004;11:525–529. [PMID: 15272896] (Shows that the presence of 3 or more oligoclonal bands in cerebrospinal fluid has 85% sensitivity and specificity of 92% for the diagnosis of MS.)

Montalban X, et al. MRI criteria for MS in patients with clinically isolated syndromes. *Neurology* 2010;74:427–434. [PMID: 20054006] (Proposes new MS diagnostic criteria using dissemination in time criteria based on characteristics of a single MRI study in patients presenting with the first clinical relapse.)

Polman CH, et al. Diagnostic criteria for multiple sclerosis: 2005 revisions to the "McDonald Criteria." *Ann Neurol* 2005;58: 840–846. [PMID: 16283615] (Describes the current International Panel Criteria for MS diagnosis using both clinical and radiographic features.)

▶ Differential Diagnosis

Because MS can affect any function of the CNS, the differential diagnosis potentially can be broad (Table 17–8). Recognition of the clinical pattern of disease, typically waxing and waning focal neurologic symptoms in a young adult, should suggest the diagnosis. Signs and symptoms of systemic illness that should prompt consideration of alternate diagnoses include fever; concomitant systemic disease including cardiac, pulmonary, gastrointestinal, and renal disease; dermatologic involvement other than psoriasis; endocrinologic disease other than autoimmune thyroid disease; mucosal ulcerations; sicca; bone lesions; tendon xanthomas; hematologic manifestations; systemic thrombosis; recurrent spontaneous abortions; and symptom onset after the age of 50.

In addition, certain neurologic features warrant further diagnostic consideration and include peripheral neuropathy, myopathy, hearing loss, multiple cranial neuropathy, neuropsychiatric illness other than unipolar depression, prominent cognitive symptoms from the disease onset, cerebral venous sinus thrombosis, extrapyramidal signs and symptoms, amyotrophy, cortical and lacunar infarcts, meningismus, meningeal enhancement on brain MRI, unilateral lesions, isolated myelopathy normal brain MRI, retinopathy, CNS hemorrhage, and simultaneous enhancement of all lesions. The diagnosis of usually can be substantiated with imaging, CSF analysis, and in some cases, evoked-potential studies. However, several settings in which MS can be particularly difficult to distinguish from other disorders warrant further consideration.

A. Progressive Myelopathy

Although cerebellar and cognitive presentations may occur, PPMS typically presents as an asymmetric progressive myelopathy with insidious onset. The age of onset is usually older than that in RRMS, and men are equally affected as women. CSF analysis is essential in diagnosing PPMS; however, as with RRMS, 10–15% of PPMS cases will not have increased intrathecal gammaglobulin synthesis. Several other diagnoses must be scrutinized and include neoplasm, arteriovenous malformation (AVM), vitamin B_{12} deficiency, sarcoidosis, Sjögren syndrome, hereditary spastic paraplegia (HSP), adrenomyeloneuropathy (in women), syphilis, human immune virus, and human T-cell lymphotrophic virus I/II. MRI of the spinal cord is usually able to identify neoplasms and AVMs. Additional studies include blood tests for vitamin B_{12}, methylmalonic acid, homocysteine, angiotensin-converting enzyme, anti-SSA and anti-SSB, rheumatoid factor, antinuclear antibody, very long chain fatty acids, VDRL and FTA-ABS, HIV, and HTLV I/II serologies. In cases with minimal sensory involvement, normal bladder function, and relatively symmetric presentations of leg weakness and spasticity, primary lateral sclerosis and HSP are possibilities. DNA tests for HSP mutations are available.

Table 17–8. Differential Diagnosis for Multiple Sclerosis

Idiopathic CNS Demyelinating Diseases
  Multiple sclerosis
  Acute disseminated encephalomyelitis
  Neuromyelitis optica spectrum disorders
  Fulminant multiple sclerosis

Chronic Infections
  Borrelia burgdorferi (Lyme disease)
  Treponema pallidum (syphilis)
  Brucella melitensis (brucellosis)
  Bartonella henselae (catscratch disease)
  Mycoplasma pneumoniae
  Rickettsia conorii (Mediterranean spotted fever)
  HIV
  HTVL I/II
  HHV-6
  Hepatitis C
  JC virus (progressive multifocal leukoencephalopathy)
  Leptospira serovars (leptospirosis)
  Creutzfeldt-Jacob disease

Psychiatric Disease
  Somatization disorders
  Conversion disorder
  Malingering

Vascular Disease
  Stroke
  Spinal dural AVM
  Leukoaraiosis
  Primary CNS vasculitis
  Susac disease

Hereditary Diseases
  Adrenoleukodystrophy
  Metachromatic leukodystrophy
  Elongation factor 2a leukodystrophy
  Lamin B leukodystrophy
  Mitochondrial disorders
  CADASIL
  Fabry disease
  Cerebrotendinous xanthomatosis
  Neuronal ceroid lipofuscinosis
  Wilson disease
  Alexander disease
  GM2 gangliosidosis

Nutritional
  Vitamin B_{12} deficiency

Systemic Autoimmune Diseases
  Systemic lupus erythematosus
  Antiphospholipid antibody syndromes
  Sjögren syndrome
  Celiac sprue
  Sarcoidosis

Malignancies
  Primary CNS lymphoma
  Paraneoplastic syndromes

B. Progressive Cognitive Impairment With Symmetric White Matter Disease

Many leukodystrophies have adult-onset variations. In adults, the leukodystrophies often present with progressive cognitive impairment. White matter lesions similar to MS can be seen on brain MRI; however, several features suggest leukodystrophy. MRI changes in the leukodystrophies usually have a symmetric and confluent appearance in contrast to the focal plaques of MS. Widespread confluent white matter disease at disease onset should prompt diagnostic consideration of leukodystrophies. Differential diagnoses include adrenoleukodystrophy, metachromatic leukodystrophy, Krabbe disease, methylenetetrahydrofolate reductase deficiency, biotinidase deficiency, eukaryotic initiation factor mutations, cerebral autosomal dominant arteriopathy with subcortical infarcts and leukoencephalopathy, Lamin B mutations, and polyglucosan storage disease. Some leukodystrophies are associated with a peripheral neuropathy, and nerve conduction studies coupled with nerve biopsy can narrow the diagnostic considerations.

C. Cranial Neuropathies

MS can affect the optic nerves and eye movements and produce facial paresis. Many other conditions are capable of causing a solitary cranial neuropathy; however, the presence of more than one affected cranial nerve should raise suspicion for conditions other than MS. For example, Behçet

disease, Sjögren syndrome, and sarcoidosis can cause multiple cranial neuropathies. Behçet disease should be suspected in any patient with cranial neuropathies and oral ulceration (aphthous sores). Genital ulcerations, dermatographia, and an elevated erythrocyte sedimentation rate are other features of the disease. Sjögren syndrome is associated with xerostomia and xerophthalmia; the diagnosis is confirmed through biopsy of a minor salivary or lacrimal gland. Lyme disease and sarcoidosis may cause bilateral facial paresis. Sarcoidosis also causes optic neuropathy that may be poorly responsive to glucocorticoids.

Miller DH, et al. Differential diagnosis of suspected multiple sclerosis: a consensus approach. *Mult Scler* 2008;14:1157–1174. [PMID: 18805839] (Describes the differential diagnosis of multiple sclerosis including "red flags," clinical features that suggest alternate diagnoses.)

▶ Treatment

A. Disease-Modifying Therapies

Although there is no cure for MS, there are currently six FDA-approved drugs that alter the course of the disease (Table 17–9). Many additional drugs are commonly used in practice for disease refractory to standard therapies.

1. Interferons—Interferons (IFN) are cytokines secreted by immune cells that inhibit viral replication, and their use in

Table 17–9. Clinical Outcomes From Independent Registration Trials

Medication	Dose, Route, Frequency of Administration	% Reduction in Annualized Relapse Rate	% Reduction in Accumulation of Disability
Interferon β-1b (Betaseron Extavia)	8 MIU, SC, every other day	34	29 (NS)
Interferon β-1a (Avonex)	6 MIU, IM, once weekly	18	37
Interferon β-1a (Rebif)	12 MIU, SC, three times weekly	30	30
Glatiramer acetate (Copaxone)	20 mg, SC, daily	29	12 (NS)
Mitoxantrone (Novantrone)	12 mg/m², IV, once every 3 months	38	24
Natalizumab (Tysabri)	300 mg, IV, Q 4 weeks	68	42
Fingolimod (Gilenya)	0.5 mg, PO, daily	54	30

All comparisons are versus placebo within the same study. The relapse rate reductions are for 2-year data using the intention-to-treat method of analysis. Disability is measured by a confirmed, sustained change in the EDSS at 2 years. The patient populations for each study are different; therefore, direct comparisons between each medication should be interpreted with caution. IM = intramuscular; IV = intravenous; NS = nonsignificant *P*; value PO = orally; Q = every; SC = subcutaneous.

MS was initially proposed to act on the presumed, but unidentified, viral trigger for the disease. Not all IFNs are effective for MS treatment, and IFNγ actually worsens the disease; in contrast, IFNβ reduces disease activity. Although the precise mechanism of action of IFNβ in MS is not known, IFNβ has potent regulatory functions on the immune system, and its anti-inflammatory properties are presumably beneficial.

IFNβ 1-b (Betaseron) reduces the relapse rate by 32% and slows accumulation of new lesions on brain MR in RRMS. IFNβ 1-a (Avonex) reduces the annualized relapse rate by 18%, slows accumulation of neurologic impairment as measured by the EDSS by 37%, and reduces the number of new brain MRI lesions. Another preparation of IFNβ 1-a (Rebif) is available and reduces the annualized relapse rate by 30% and slows disability progression by 30% (Table 17–9 lists dosages and routes of administration of the IFNβ preparations). Patients treated with any of the IFNβ preparations are at risk for liver function abnormalities, leukopenia, thyroid disease, and depression. Monitoring of the liver functions (aspartate amino transferase and alanine amino transferase) and white blood cell count with differential is mandatory after initiation of treatment and periodically thereafter. Most patients do not experience significant transaminemia requiring treatment discontinuation. A flu-like reaction is common in patients treated with IFNβ 4–6 hours after the injection. The flulike symptoms are reduced by coadministration with acetaminophen or a nonsteroidal anti-inflammatory drug. With repeated treatments, the flulike reactions gradually subside over time. Erythematous skin site reactions can occur with the subcutaneously injected preparations. Long-term follow-up studies show that IFNβ is safe and in general well tolerated for at least 10 years.

2. Glatiramer acetate—Glatiramer acetate (GA, Copaxone) is a synthesized copolymer composed of L-glutamic acid, L-lysine, L-alanine, and L-tyrosine in random order injected 20 mg subcutaneously every day. In RRMS, GA reduces the annualized relapse rate by 29% and reduces the accumulation of contrast-enhanced lesions on brain MRI. GA resembles myelin basic protein and is thought to interact with the MHC class II molecule to alter T-cell immune function, inducing "bystander suppression," wherein GA-treated T cells reduce proinflammatory cytokines secreted by autoreactive T cells. Fourteen-year follow-up data demonstrate that many patients treated with GA are able to safely continue treatment. Unlike IFNβ, treatment with GA does not cause liver function abnormalities, leukopenia, or thyroid disease and is not associated with depression. The typical flulike reaction characteristic of IFNβ does not occur with GA; however, approximately 15% of GA-treated patients will experience a self-limited, post-injection systemic reaction characterized by chest tightness, flushing, anxiety, dyspnea, and palpitations that can be mistaken for cardiac ischemia. This reaction is unpredictable and can occur at any time during treatment.

Skin site reactions may occur. Laboratory studies do not need to be monitored in GA-treated patients.

When compared directly in head-to-head clinical trials, GA was found to have comparable clinical efficacy to that of thrice-weekly 44 µg IFNβ 1-a and IFNβ 1-b. Head-to-head clinical trials favored thrice-weekly IFNβ 1-a or IFNβ 1-b compared with once-weekly IFNβ 1-a. However, the more frequent occurrence of anti-interferon neutralizing antibodies may reduce this apparent benefit added over time.

3. Mitoxantrone—Mitoxantrone (Novantrone) is a chemotherapeutic agent that intercalates into DNA and inhibits topoisomerase II activity (Table 17–10 includes recommended dosage schedule). Because of its cytopathic effects on replicating cells, it is a potent immune suppressor. In a study of RRMS and SPMS patients with incomplete recovery after attacks, mitoxantrone reduced the accumulation of neurologic impairment and number of relapses compared with placebo. Mitoxantrone has cardiotoxic properties that limit its total lifetime cumulative dose to 140 mg/m^2 and systolic ejection fraction abnormalities occur in 12% of treated patients. Patients treated with mitoxantrone should undergo evaluation of left ventricular function at baseline and then before each subsequent treatment. Most patients are treated for 2 years, although some patients can be treated longer. In addition to cardiotoxicity, mitoxantrone causes leukemia in ~1 in 129 (0.8%) MS patients. Because of its toxicity, mitoxantrone is regarded as a second-line agent to be used in RRMS and SPMS patients who continue to have relapses and disease progression despite treatment with IFNβ or GA and is in practice only rarely used.

4. Natalizumab—Natalizumab (Tysabri) is a monoclonal antibody that binds α-4 integrin on the surface of lymphocytes, monocytes, basophils, and eosinophils. α-4 integrin binds vascular cell adhesion molecule-1 on the vascular endothelium, and this receptor–ligand interaction is important for lymphocyte adhesion. If lymphocytes cannot bind the vascular endothelium, they are unable to migrate into tissues and cause inflammation. Natalizumab was found to reduce the risk of relapses by 68%, accumulation of neurologic disability by 42%, and MRI markers of disease activity and progression by 83–92%. It is administered via intravenous infusion, 300 mg, once per month. Natalizumab was introduced to the market in 2004, but it was subsequently withdrawn from the market after two MS patients treated with natalizumab in a clinical trial succumbed to progressive multifocal leukoencephalopathy (PML). The drug was reintroduced in 2006 with a risk-monitoring plan called the TOUCH (Tysabri outreach unified commitment to health) program. The postmarketing experience found that the risk of PML is related to duration of exposure, with the risk during the first year of treatment being ~1 in 33,000. In the second year of treatment the risk increases to ~1 in 1800, and in the third year of treatment, it increases further to ~1 in 500. In addition to duration of exposure, prior treatment

Table 17–10. Diagnostic Considerations in Acute Transverse Myelitis

Demyelinating Diseases
  Multiple sclerosis
  Acute disseminated encephalomyelitis (postvaccination)
  Neuromyelitis optica

Viral
  Herpetoviridae
   • Varicella-zoster virus
   • Herpes simplex virus types 1 and 2
   • Epstein-Barr virus
   • Cytomegalovirus
  Group B arboviruses (West Nile and dengue)
  Exanthems
   • Measles
   • Mumps
   • Rubella
  Rare causes
   • Enteroviruses
    —Hepatitis A, B, and C
    —Lymphocytic choriomeningitis virus

Mycobacterial and Bacterial
  Mycobacterium tuberculosis
  Mycoplasma pneumoniae
  Chlamydia pneumoniae
  Borrelia burgdorferi (Lyme disease)
  Treponema pallidum (syphilis)
  Brucella melitensis (brucellosis)
  Bartonella henselae (catscratch disease)
  Bacterial meningitis
  Intraparenchymal abscess
  Epidural abscess

Parasitic
  Schistosoma haematobium
  Schistosoma mansonii
  Schistosoma japonicum
  Toxocara species

Rheumatologic Diseases and Autoantibody Syndromes
  Collagen vascular diseases
   • Sjögren syndrome
   • Systemic lupus erythematosus
   • Mixed connective-tissue disease
   • Anticardiolipin autoantibodies
   • Primary angiitis of the CNS
   • Protoplasmic-staining antineutrophil cytoplasmic antibodies
   • Hashimoto encephalopathy (myelopathy)
   • Linear scleroderma
  Sarcoidosis

Vascular
  Spinal dural arteriovenous malformation
  Stroke

Neoplastic and Paraneoplastic
  Lymphoma
  Leukemia
  Other infiltrating tumors
  Paraneoplastic
   • Hodgkin lymphoma
   • Other tumors

with immune-suppressive medications is an independent risk factor for developing PML in natalizumab-treated patients and increases the risk by approximately threefold. Because the overall risk of PML in the postmarketing experience is similar to the estimated risk based on the clinical trials, the medication continues to be available and is used primarily as a second-line treatment. Prior exposure to the JC virus as measured by the presence of anti-JCV antibodies appears to be useful for stratifying risk for individual patients. The prevalence of anti-JCV antibodies in the natalizuamb-treated population is approximately 50%. To date, all patients who developed PML with natalizumab treatment, for whom serum samples were available at least 6 months prior to the onset of PML symptoms, tested positive with this assay. Therefore, the negative predictive value is anticipated to be quite high: the risk of PML in patients who test negative for JCV is estimated to be less than 1:10,000 regardless of duration of exposure.

Plasmapheresis, or immune absorption, are commonly used to remove natalizumab in patients who develop PML, although the potential benefit of these treatments is not proven. An immune reconstitution inflammatory syndrome similar to that observed in AIDS patients treated with highly active antiretroviral therapy occurs in MS patients and itself is associated with substantial neurologic morbidity. Approximately one in five natalizumab-treated MS patients who develop PML die. Morbidity in the survivors is highly variable.

5. Fingolimod—Fingolimod (Gilenya) is a sphingosine 1-phosphate (S1P) modulator and is the first oral FDA-approved treatment for relapsing forms of MS. When fingolimod binds the S1P receptor on lymphocytes, the receptor is internalized, causing lymphocytes to become sequestered in lymphoid tissue. In a phase III, 2-year, placebo-controlled trial, fingolimod 0.5 mg/day taken orally reduced the risk of relapse by 54%, the accumulation of sustained neurologic disability by 30%, and brain MRI markers of disease activity by 75–82%. Fingolimod also slowed progression of brain volume loss. Fingolimod was also shown to be superior to once-weekly IFNβ 1-a in relapse rate reduction and accumulation of new MRI lesions. Fingolimod is currently under investigation in PPMS. Fingolimod reduces peripheral lymphocyte counts by approximately 73%, as expected from its mechanism of action. Adverse events include bradycardia after the first dose, elevation in hepatic transaminases, and macular edema. There were two deaths in the clinical trials associated with herpes virus infections: a case of herpes encephalitis and a case of de novo zoster resulting in fulminant hepatic failure. Herpes encephalitis is not considered to be an opportunistic infection, and therefore the relationship to fingolimod, if any, is not known. However, disseminated zoster is an opportunistic infection, and therefore fingolimod-treated patients who have not previously been exposed to herpes zoster should be vaccinated before treatment with fingolimod. Recommended safety studies include a baseline electrocardiogram, observation of the patient for 6 hours after the first dose, baseline ophthalmologic examination with repeat examination 3–4 months after starting fingolimod, and baseline herpes zoster IgG to determine prior exposure. Additional studies, including assessment of liver functions, may be indicated in symptomatic patients.

Benefits of early treatment—IFNβ 1-a, IFNβ 1-b, and GA are beneficial in treatment of clinically isolated syndromes (first attack) in patients with brain MRI studies consistent with MS. Administration of these drugs reduces the time between the first and second clinical or subclinical (as measured by brain MRI) attacks. Immediate treatment of clinically isolated syndromes appears to have a greater impact on the course of the disease than delaying treatment until after patients experience a second clinical attack.

B. Glucocorticoids

Glucocorticoids are the mainstay of therapy for treatment of acute MS relapses. Intravenously administered methylprednisolone dosed at 1 g/day or dexamethasone dosed at 2 mg/kg/day and administered over 3–5 days reduces the symptoms of flares and shortens the recovery time. One dose-comparative study found that patients treated with 2 g/day of methylprednisolone had significantly improved outcomes in terms of post-flare recovery compared with patients treated with 500 mg/day of methylprednisolone for 5 days. A rebound in disease activity sometimes occurs after glucocorticoid treatment, and for this reason, some clinicians follow intravenous treatment with an oral taper of prednisone. Because of the excellent oral bioavailability of oral glucocorticoids, some institutions use equivalent oral doses rather than intravenously administered glucocorticoids, although there are no comparative studies of route of administration in MS. Because of the possible long-term consequences of frequent exposure to glucocorticoids, clinicians usually withhold treatment with glucocorticoids for MS flares with purely sensory involvement. Biannual monitoring of bone densitometry is recommended for patients treated with frequent pulsed doses of glucocorticoids. Short-term risks of glucocorticoids include fluid retention, hypokalemia, flushing, acne, insomnia, psychiatric disturbance, dyspepsia, and increased appetite. Avascular necrosis of the femoral head, a serious complication of long-term glucocorticoid use, has been very rarely reported after short-term treatment. In patients with a history of gastroesophageal reflux disease or peptic ulcer disease, prophylaxis with a proton pump inhibitor during treatment with glucocorticoids is indicated. Lithium chloride is useful for treatment of patients who experience emotional lability on glucocorticoids. Patients with preexisting psychiatric illness may experience psychotic symptoms from glucocorticoids, and prophylaxis with an antipsychotic medication such as risperidone (Risperdal) may be necessary.

Although glucocorticoids are typically not considered disease-modifying therapies, one study showed that regularly dosed intravenous methylprednisolone reduced disability and MRI lesion burden compared with intravenous methylprednisolone administered for treatment of flares.

C. Treatments for SPMS

Two large studies of IFNβ 1-b in SPMS showed conflicting results. A European trial showed a highly significant reduction in relapse rate and disability, whereas a similar study in North America showed no benefit. Differences in the baseline characteristics of these populations might account for the discrepancy. The European population had a shorter disease duration and less disability and continued to have relapses, whereas the North American population had a longer disease duration and greater disability and was no longer experiencing relapses. Therefore, IFNβ 1-b appears to reduce the relapse rate and disability in patients who recently transitioned from RRMS into SPMS and are still experiencing relapses. IFNβ 1-b is probably of no benefit in SPMS patients who experience disease progression without relapses. Mitoxantrone is similarly indicated in SPMS patients who experience relapses.

D. Treatments for PPMS

There are no FDA-approved treatments for PPMS, and trials using IFNβ, GA, mitoxantrone, and rituximab (a B-cell–depleting monoclonal antibody used for treatment of non-Hodgkin lymphoma and rheumatoid arthritis) have not shown benefit.

E. Emerging MS Treatments

Many medications with immune-modulating or suppressing properties are being investigated in MS, either alone or in combination with FDA-approved treatments. It is likely that some of these drugs will find applications for treatment in MS.

1. Cladribine—Cladribine (Mylinax) is an adenosine deaminase- resistant purine nucleoside that is a relatively selective lymphocyte immunosuppressant. In a phase III clinical trial, an oral formulation of cladribine was shown to reduce the annualized relapse rate by 58%, slow accumulation of disability by 33%, and reduce MRI markers by of neuroinflammation by 77–88%. Cladribine is dosed at 3.5 mg/kg and is administered over a 2-week period once per year. By its mechanism of action, cladribine causes peripheral lymphopenia. Adverse events associated with cladribine include herpes zoster reactivation, myelosuppression, and possible associations with myelodysplastic syndromes and neoplasms. Because of FDA concerns about possible malignancies associated with cladribine treatment its development in MS has been halted and the medication was withdrawn from Russia and Australia where it previously had been approved.

2. Teriflunomide—Teriflunomide is a derivate of leflunomide (Arava), a broad-spectrum immunosuppressant used for treatment of rheumatoid arthritis. In phase II trials, teriflunomide, either alone or in combination with either IFNβ or GA, was found to reduce the accumulation of gadolinium-DPTA–enhancing lesions relative to placebo during a 36-week period in RRMS. A phase III clinical trial found that 14 mg teriflunomide reduced the annualized relapse rate by 31% and accumulation of neurologic disability by 30%. MRI markers of disease activity were reduced by 67–80%. Because teriflunomide is a known teratogen with an unusually long half-life, it will most likely be prescribed to patients who are not planning reproduction. Teriflunomide is currently under investigation in phase III clinical trials.

3. Dimethyl fumarate—Dimethyl fumarate is a combination of two fumaric acid esters and has been effectively used for treatment of psoriasis. In a phase II trial, 240 mg of dimethyl fumarate administered thrice daily reduced the accumulation of gadolinium-DPTA–enhancing lesions relative to placebo during a 24-week period in RRMS. The mechanism of action of dimethyl fumarate is not well understood, but it is thought to have immunomodulatory properties. A phase III clinical trial found that 240 mg of dimethyl fumarate administered twice daily reduced the annualized relapse rate by 53% and accumulation of neurologic disability by 38% relative to placebo. Dimethyl fumarate is currently under investigation in phase III clinical trials.

4. Laquinimod—Laquinimod is a quinoline-3-carboxamide derivative of linomide. The mechanism of action of laquinimod is not understood, but it may have immunomodulatory properties. In a phase II trial, 0.6 mg of laquinimod administered once daily reduced the accumulation of gadolinium-DPTA–enhancing lesions relative to placebo during a 36-week period in RRMS. A phase III clinical trial found that 0.6 mg of laquinimod administered once daily reduced the annualized relapse rate by 23% and accumulation of neurologic disability by 36% relative to placebo. Laquinimod is currently under investigation in phase III clinical trials.

5. Alemtuzumab—Alemtuzumab (Campath-1H) is a humanized monoclonal antibody directed against CD52, a lymphocyte surface antigen, which depletes lymphocytes and is indicated for treatment of fludarabine-resistant chronic lymphocytic leukemia. In a large phase II head-to-head trial, alemtuzumab compared with thrice-weekly IFNβ 1-a was found to significantly reduce the risk of relapse, the accumulation of disability, and MRI markers of disease progression. However, ~3% of treated patients developed immune thrombocytopenic purpura, and ~20% of patients developed autoimmune thyroid disease (both Hashimoto and Graves diseases). Other adverse events include Goodpasture disease (anti-glomerular basement antibody disease) and Burkitt lymphoma. Opportunistic infections are a recognized complication of alemtuzumab in leukemia treatment.

Alemtuzumab is currently under investigation in phase III clinical trials in RRMS.

6. Daclizumab—Daclizumab is a monoclonal antibody directed against the α subunit of the interleukin 2 receptor. Daclizumab is indicated for prevention of host-versus-graft disease in solid-organ transplantation. Daclizumab treatment causes expansion of NK56[bright] cells, a type of T-suppressor cell. Daclizumab was shown to reduce the risk of accumulation of active lesions on brain MRI when added to IFN-treated patients and is currently under investigation in a phase III clinical trial in RRMS.

7. Ocrelizumab and ofatumumab—Ocrelizumab and ofatumumab are monoclonal antibodies directed against CD20, a cell surface marker present on B lymphocytes. Both antibodies cause depletion of B cells but do not affect plasma cells. In phase II clinical trials in RRMS, both antibodies reduced the accumulation of new lesions on brain MRI. Phase III trials are in planning.

F. Off-Label Therapies

Several broad-spectrum immunosuppressants are still sometimes used in treatment-refractory MS. The use of these agents has declined sharply since the introduction of natalizumab.

1. Cyclophosphamide—Cyclophosphamide (Cytoxan) is a cytotoxic alkylating agent that may have benefit in younger SPMS patients who are still experiencing flares. An open-label study found benefit of combination treatment with IFNβ 1-a in RRMS patients who were experiencing disease progression despite treatment with IFNβ. Cyclophosphamide is usually administered using a protocol similar to the treatment for lupus nephritis and is dosed monthly at 800 mg/m^2 and titrated based on the preinfusion and 10-day postinfusion white blood cell counts.

2. Mycophenolate mofetil—Mycophenolate mofetil (CellCept) is an inhibitor of inosine 5′-monophosphate dehydrogenase type II and is a relatively selective immunosuppressant of activated lymphocytes. Several small series show that mycophenolate mofetil is well tolerated either alone or in combination with IFNβ and has been used in treatment of RRMS and SPMS patients who have ongoing disease activity despite treatment with FDA-approved therapies. Mycophenolate mofetil is administered orally at 500–1000 mg twice daily.

3. Azathioprine—Azathioprine (Imuran) is a nucleoside analogue of 6-mercaptopurine that impairs DNA and RNA synthesis. A meta-analysis of small studies showed that azathioprine reduces the relapse rate in RRMS and SPMS. Azathioprine is initially dosed at 50 mg/day and titrated to reduce the total white count to approximately 3.0 K/μL (usually 2–3 mg/kg/day).

4. Methotrexate—Methotrexate (Rheumatrex) is an inhibitor of dihydrofolate with potent anti-inflammatory properties; it also augments suppressor cell function. It has been used in treatment of SPMS, and a small trial showed a reduction in the T2 burden of disease on brain MRI and a test of arm and hand dexterity. Methotrexate is administered at 7.5 mg once weekly. Patients treated with methotrexate should be monitored for potential hepatotoxicity.

5. Rituximab—Rituximab (Rituxan) is a chimeric monoclonal antibody directed against CD20 and causes depletion of B cells. Rituximab is FDA approved for treatment of non-Hodgkin lymphoma and rheumatoid arthritis. A phase II study showed that rituximab reduced the frequency of relapses and accumulation of lesions on brain MRI in RRMS. A phase IIb/III trial in PPMS failed to meet its primary endpoint of disability reduction. Rituximab is sometimes used off-label in patients with progressive MS who have contrast-enhancing lesions on brain MRI, in cases of natalizumab-refractory MS, and in neuromyelitis optica.

6. Intravenous immunoglobulin—In small studies, monthly infusions of intravenous immunoglobulin, dosed at 0.15–0.20 g/kg, reduced the relapse rate in MS; the effects on disability are not known.

7. Plasma exchange—Small trials showed that plasma exchange may help resolve acute flares of severe demyelinating disease that are not responsive to glucocorticoids. Plasma exchange was shown not to be beneficial in treatment of SPMS.

Clifford DB, et al. Natalizumab-associated progressive multifocal leukoencephalopathy in patients with multiple sclerosis: Lessons from 28 cases. *Lancet Neurol* 2010;9:438–446. [PMID: 20298967] (Reviews the manifestations of PML in natalizumab-treated patients.)

Goodin DS, et al. Disease modifying therapies in multiple sclerosis: Report of the Therapeutics and Technology Assessment Subcommittee of the American Academy of Neurology and the MS Council for Clinical Practice Guidelines. *Neurology* 2002; 58:169–178. [PMID: 11805241]

Goodin DS, et al. The use of mitoxantrone (Novantrone) for the treatment of multiple sclerosis: Report of the Therapeutics and Technology Assessment Subcommittee of the American Academy of Neurology. *Neurology* 2003;61:1332–1338. [PMID: 14638950]

Goodin DS, et al; Therapeutics and Technology Assessment Subcommittee of the American Academy of Neurology. Assessment: The use of natalizumab (Tysabri) for the treatment of multiple sclerosis (an evidence-based review): Report of the Therapeutics and Technology Assessment Subcommittee of the American Academy of Neurology. *Neurology* 2008;71: 766–773. [PMID: 18765653] (Concise, evidence-based assessments of FDA-approved disease-modifying therapies in multiple sclerosis.)

Kappos L, et al; FREEDOMS Study Group. A placebo-controlled trial of oral fingolimod in relapsing multiple sclerosis. *N Engl J Med* 2010;362:387–401. [PMID: 20089952] (Randomized, placebo-controlled trial of fingolimod, the first FDA-approved MS disease-modifying therapy that is orally bioavailable.)

Keegan M, et al. Symptomatic Management Plasma exchange for severe attacks of CNS demyelination: Predictors of response. *Neurology* 2002;8;58:143–146.[PMID: 11781423] (Retrospective case series documenting response of severe demyelinating attacks to plasmapheresis.)

Zivadinov R, et al. Effects of IV methylprednisolone on brain atrophy in relapsing-remitting MS. *Neurology* 2001;57:1239–1247. [PMID: 11591843] (Phase II study showing benefit of pulsed intravenous methylprednisolone used as disease-modifying therapy for RRMS.)

G. Symptomatic Therapies

Because MS affects multiple functions of the nervous system, the symptomatic management of MS patients can be complex, especially for patients with SPMS and PPMS.

1. Spasticity—Spasticity is a velocity-dependent change in tone and occurs in MS as a consequence of damage to the motor pathways and subsequent reorganization within the spinal cord or higher centers. Spasticity typically co-occurs with weakness but may be isolated. Physical triggers of spasticity such as pain and constipation should be adequately treated before antispasmodic agents are prescribed. Baclofen (10 mg three times daily) and tizanidine (2 mg three times daily) are usually the first agents prescribed. The dosage of both agents can be gradually increased until symptomatic relief is attained. The recommended maximum dosage of baclofen is 80 mg/day; some clinicians prescribe doses up to 120 mg/day. Abrupt discontinuation can result in withdrawal symptoms and seizures. The maximum dosage of tizanidine is 36 mg/day. Drowsiness is often a limiting side effect of both baclofen and tizanidine. Liver function abnormalities and bradycardia can occur with tizanidine. Liver function should be monitored in patients treated with tizanidine, especially if there is preexisting hepatic disease. Gabapentin is also an effective antispasmodic agent. Patients should be started at 300 mg three times daily and rapidly escalated to 1800 mg/day. Further upward titrations may be necessary; doses of 3600 mg/day or higher are typical. Diazepam is also an effective antispasmodic agent and can be safely used in monotherapy or in combination with other therapies. Low starting doses (2 mg three times daily) can be titrated upward until symptomatic relief is obtained. As with the other agents, drowsiness may be limiting, and abrupt discontinuation may precipitate withdrawal symptoms, including seizures. In patients with spasticity who experience excessive side effects or limited relief with oral medications, an indwelling pump can administer intrathecal baclofen. Medical management is only part of spasticity therapy. Physical therapy and daily stretching exercises are essential to prevent contracture formation.

2. Fatigue—Before symptomatic management of fatigue is undertaken, the clinician must determine the type of fatigue. MS patients may experience neuromuscular fatigue (weakness), fatigue associated with depression, daytime drowsiness secondary to insomnia, and generalized lassitude.

Glucocorticoids may be helpful if a recent flare causes neuromuscular fatigue. Physical therapy and regular exercise are essential. For patients who experience neuromuscular fatigue associated with increases in body temperature, swimming is an excellent form of exercise. MS patients are at high risk for depression, which, if present, must be adequately treated. Sleep disturbance is also common in MS, and patients should be educated about sleep hygiene. Some patients may require treatment with hypnotics. The lassitude associated with MS may respond to amantadine 100 mg twice daily. Other stimulants used to treat excessive daytime drowsiness in MS include modafinil (Provigil) 100–200 mg twice a day, methylphenidate (Ritalin) 10–20 mg twice a day, and armodafinil (Nuvigil) 150 mg once per day. All CNS stimulants can cause insomnia that can further exacerbate fatigue, and caution must be exercised in patients who are treated with a hypnotic medication for insomnia and a stimulant for fatigue.

3. Pain—Acute or chronic neuropathic pain is a frequent complication of MS. Many patients describe chronic dysesthesias that are burning, lancinating, squeezing, or gritty as a consequence of spinal cord injury. The neuropathic pain of MS usually does not respond to treatment with nonsteroidal anti-inflammatory drugs. Gabapentin is often beneficial but usually requires doses of 1800 mg/day or higher. Carbamazepine (Tegretol), administered at 100 mg twice daily, or oxcarbazepine (Trileptal), administered at 300 mg twice daily, is particularly useful for the "squeezing" or "band-like" dysesthesias and for trigeminal neuralgia. Both these medications can be titrated upward until the patient's pain is relieved, up to a maximum of 1600 mg/day for carbamazepine and 2400 mg/day for oxcarbazepine. Hyponatremia can be a life-threatening consequence of these medications, and serum sodium concentrations should be monitored. Tramadol (Ultram) is also useful for neuropathic pain and is dosed at 50 mg three times daily and titrated up to 400 mg/day. Abrupt discontinuation can precipitate withdrawal symptoms, and the drug has been associated with serotonin syndrome. Therefore, it must be used with caution in patients treated with antidepressant medications. Topiramate (Topamax), lamotrigine (Lamictal), and zonisamide (Zonegran) are also useful in the treatment of neuropathic pain. Low-potency opiate analgesics such as codeine or hydrocodone may be used in combination with nonnarcotic analgesics. When monotherapy or combination therapy with nonnarcotic medications is unable to provide adequate pain relief, a continuous-release opiate preparation such as the fentanyl transdermal patch may be necessary.

4. Paroxysmal symptoms—The Lhermitte symptom and tonic spasms respond to treatment with carbamazepine, oxcarbazepine, gabapentin (as outlined earlier), and acetazolamide (Diamox) 125–250 mg two to three times daily. Acetazolamide and ondansetron (Zofran), 4–8 mg twice a day, can be useful for intermittent vertigo. Meclizine (Antevert) is rarely of benefit in central vertigo. Nocturnal flexor spasms respond well to antispasmodic agents such as baclofen or tizanidine.

5. Bladder dysfunction—Bladder spasticity is treated with anticholinergic agents such as oxybutynin (Ditropan) 5 mg three or four times daily or tolterodine (Detrol) 2 mg twice daily. Long-acting formulations and an oxybutynin transdermal patch applied twice weekly are available. The denervated bladder is treated by intermittent self-catheterization, and patients should be taught this technique as soon as urinary retention is diagnosed. Sphincter dyssynergia can be treated with terazosin (Hytrin) 1–5 mg at night in combination with an anticholinergic; in some cases, intermittent catheterization may be necessary.

6. Bowel dysfunction—Bowel dysfunction is common in MS and is often undertreated. Chronic constipation can be treated with a combination of fiber (Metamucil, 1 teaspoon three times a day with meals), stool softener (decussate sodium, 100 mg three times daily with meals), and a stimulant (senna, two tablets at night). Enemas, suppositories, and digital stimulation may be necessary. Urge incontinence can be treated with a bowel regimen to trigger voiding at a convenient time each day.

7. Sexual dysfunction—Male impotence can be treated with sildenafil (Viagra) 50–100 mg, vardenafil (Levitra) 5–20 mg, or tadalafil (Cialis) 5–20 mg before intercourse. Alprostadil (Edex) 2.5-40 micrograms injected intracavernously is used for nonresponders to oral preparations. Women experiencing vaginismus may be treated with antispasmodic medications. Diminished vaginal lubrication causes dyspareunia and can be treated with water-based lubrication.

8. Ambulatory impairment—Dalfampridine (4-amino pyridine, or Ampyra) was found to improve walking speed in patients with ambulatory impairment in phase III clinical trials and was recently FDA approved for this indication. Dalfampridine is administered as a 10-mg sustained release tablet and is taken twice per day. Approximately one of three treated patients experience improvement in ambulatory function. 4-Amino pyridine is a potassium channel blocker and improves electrical conduction along demyelinated axons. Seizures are a known complication of 4-amino pyridine.

Chou R, Peterson K, Helfand M. Comparative efficacy and safety of skeletal muscle relaxants for spasticity and musculoskeletal conditions: A systematic review. *J Pain Symptom Manage* 2004;28:140–175. [PMID: 15276195] (A comprehensive systematic review of antispasmodic medications.)

Goodman AD, et al; Fampridine MS-F203 Investigators. Sustained-release oral fampridine in multiple sclerosis: A randomized, double blind, controlled trial. *Lancet* 2009;373:732–738. [PMID: 19249634] (Phase III trial showing benefit of dalfampridine in a minority of treated patients.)

Rammohan KW, et al. Efficacy and safety of modafinil (Provigil) for the treatment of fatigue in multiple sclerosis: A two centre phase 2 study. *J Neurol Neurosurg Psychiatry* 2002;72:179183. [PMID: 11796766] (Phase II trial showing benefit of the wakeful-promoting agent modafinil in treatment of MS fatigue.)

▼ MS SUBTYPES

ACUTE TRANSVERSE MYELITIS

Acute transverse myelitis (ATM) is inflammation of the spinal cord that results in motor and sphincter impairment with a sensory level. ATM is usually bilateral and tends to cause more severe weakness than the typical attacks of partial myelitis characteristic of MS. Nevertheless, ATM occurs in many MS subjects at some point during the course of the disease and is the presenting manifestation in approximately 1–2% of cases. Other causes of ATM include infections (including herpes zoster and herpes simplex), collagen vascular diseases, sarcoidosis, and idiopathic inflammatory diseases (see Table 17–10). ATM can be a presenting manifestation of neuromyelitis optica. Recurrent ATM without cerebral or optic nerve involvement appears to be a rare and distinct syndrome. Because ATM is a manifestation of many disease processes, treatment depends on the underlying pathoetiology. Patients presenting with ATM should undergo spinal cord imaging to exclude compressive etiologies, tumors, and arteriovenous malformations. Brain imaging is also indicated to look for evidence of disseminated demyelination. CSF analysis is indicated to look for possible infectious etiologies, as are blood studies to look for evidence of systemic inflammation and infection. In severe or rapidly progressive cases, initial empiric treatment usually includes administration of high-dose glucocorticoids and intravenous acyclovir while definitive diagnostic tests are pending. In cases that are not responsive to pharmacotherapy, plasmapheresis is indicated (typically seven rounds of 1.5 volumes per exchange).

Occasionally, spinal cord inflammation can have the appearance at imaging of a tumor, and rarely, spinal cord biopsy may be necessary for diagnosis. Because of the risk of irreversible postsurgical injury, a comprehensive preoperative evaluation to exclude other possibilities, including neuromyelitis optica, MS, sarcoidosis, and vasculitis, is essential.

Infarcts of the anterior spinal artery and artery of Adamkiewicz may be distinguished from ATM by preserved dorsal column function in the setting of weakness and spinothalamic sensory loss. However, this pattern is not invariant. In addition, the appearance of a spinal cord infarct on MRI can be similar to that of ATM. CSF analysis is helpful because acute infarcts are not associated with leukocytosis or intrathecal synthesis of gammaglobulins.

NEUROMYELITIS OPTICA

Neuromyelitis optica (NMO or Devic disease) is a rare variant of central nervous system demyelinating disease. The co-occurrence of ATM with optic neuritis, a normal brain MRI study at onset, and spinal cord lesions spanning three or more vertebral segments of the cord are the hallmarks of the disease. Similarly to ATM, neuromyelitis optica is a syndrome with several etiologies (Table 17–11). The idiopathic form can be either monophasic or polyphasic. Although

Table 17–11. Diagnostic Considerations in Neuromyelitis Optica

Idiopathic Demyelinating Diseases
Neuromyelitis optica
Multiple sclerosis
Acute disseminated encephalomyelitis
Collagen Vascular Diseases and Autoantibody Syndromes
Systemic lupus erythematosus
Sjögren syndrome
Mixed connective tissue disease
p-ANCA autoantibodies
Anticardiolipin autoantibodies
Viral and Mycobacterial Infections
Varicella zoster virus
Epstein-Barr virus
HIV
Tuberculosis
Brucellosis

patients with the monophasic form recover less well than patients recovering from the first attack of the polyphasic form, patients with polyphasic disease are at high risk for mortality as a consequence of respiratory compromise from cervical cord lesions. Acute attacks are treated with a combination of glucocorticoids and plasma exchange.

Pathologic studies showed that NMO lesions are associated with antibody deposition and complement formation. An immunohistochemical assay was recently developed that identifies an autoantibody associated with the disease directed against aquaporin-4 (AQP4), a water channel expressed on astroglial cells. This autoantibody, although highly specific, has only 70% sensitivity. In animal models, the anti-AQP4 antibody can cause astroglial cell injury with histopathology that is similar to that seen in NMO patients. These observations suggested that the humoral immune system has a prominent role in pathogenesis. There are no proven treatments that alter the course of the disease; however, a small open-label study of azathioprine in combination with glucocorticoids, rituximab, and mycophenolate mofetil reported modest benefits. IFN and GA are considered to be ineffective.

ACUTE MS

Acute MS, or Marburg variant MS, is a rare fulminant disease that presents with acute or subacute neurological dysfunction. Brain MRI shows large edematous lesions that cause mass effect and enhance with contrast. The appearance of these lesions is similar to that of a brain tumor, and many patients undergo brain biopsy before diagnosis. Historically, acute MS was a fatal disease, with death occurring within a year of onset, often secondary to extensive brainstem demyelination. Because of its rarity, clinical trials have not been performed. Treatment recommendations, based on anecdotes, include plasma exchange (seven rounds) in conjunction with high-dose glucocorticoids (eg, 1–2 g/day of methylprednisolone for 10 days followed by a slow taper). Follow-up treatments include natalizumab, immunosuppression, and IFNβ or GA.

ACUTE DISSEMINATED ENCEPHALOMYELITIS

Acute disseminated encephalomyelitis (ADEM) is a monophasic illness characterized by multifocal inflammation and demyelination. It is more common in children than in adults. ADEM is associated with recent rabies or smallpox vaccination (postvaccination encephalomyelitis) and recent infection (postinfectious encephalomyelitis), usually childhood exanthemas such as measles and varicella (chickenpox). Other antecedent infections associated with ADEM include mononucleosis, influenza, parainfluenza, rubella, mumps, and *Mycoplasma pneumoniae*. An autoimmune response to myelin basic protein is observed in some patients with ADEM, suggesting that molecular mimicry underlies the pathogenesis. Acute hemorrhagic leukoencephalitis (Hurst disease) is a fulminant and devastating form of ADEM associated with microvascular hemorrhagic lesions. ADEM is usually distinguished from MS by history of antecedent vaccination or infection, a rapid onset, and multifocal symptomatic involvement of the cerebrum, brainstem, cerebellum, and spinal cord. Alterations in consciousness and seizures are common in ADEM and rare in MS. Brain MRI in ADEM shows multiple areas of abnormal signal change that are often contrast-enhancing, indicating that all lesions are acute. CSF analysis shows a lymphocytic pleocytosis, protein elevation, and intrathecal synthesis of gammaglobulins and is not clinically useful in distinguishing ADEM from MS. Treatment consists of high-dose glucocorticoids. Plasma exchange is used when patients do not respond to treatment with glucocorticoids. Epilepsy, learning disorders, and behavior disorders may be sequelae of this disease in children.

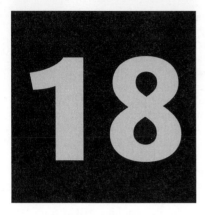

Nontraumatic Disorders of the Spinal Cord

Olajide Williams, MD, MSc,
& Michelle Stern, MD

▶ General Considerations

Anatomically, the spinal cord can be divided into four regions: cervical, containing 7 vertebrae and 8 spinal nerves; thoracic, containing 12 vertebrae and spinal nerves; lumbar, containing 5 vertebrae and spinal nerves; and sacral, containing 5 fused vertebrae and spinal nerves. In cross section, the spinal cord reveals butterfly-shaped gray matter surrounded by white matter. The gray matter contains the neuronal cell bodies; the white matter consists of nerve tracts (Figure 18–1).

The major clinically relevant tracts of the cord are the dorsal columns (ascending), which convey tactile discrimination, vibration, and joint position sense; the spinothalamic tracts (ascending), which convey pain, temperature, and crude touch; and the corticospinal tracts (descending), which convey fibers used for motor control. The spinal cord ends between the first and second lumbar vertebrae in adults. This distal area is called the *conus medullaris*, and its continuation as the filum terminale is composed of connective tissue that attaches to the coccyx. The cauda equina is a collection of nerve roots that begins at the end of the spinal cord and exits from the third lumbar vertebra to the fifth sacral vertebra. The spinal cord is protected from the bony canal by a layering of fatty connective tissue and by the meninges. The three meninges from inner to outer are pia, arachnoid, and dura. The subarachnoid space contains cerebrospinal fluid and separates the pia from the arachnoid.

Other structures that protect the spinal cord can be divided based on their location relative to the cord (Figure 18–2). The intervertebral foramen is the opening between the pedicles of adjacent vertebrae for the spinal nerve to pass through. Spinal nerves are composed of dorsal and ventral roots. The first seven pairs of cervical spinal nerves exit above the same-numbered vertebral bodies, whereas all the subsequent nerves exit below the same-numbered vertebral bodies because of the presence of eight cervical spinal cord nerves but only seven cervical

vertebrae. Intervertebral disks separate the vertebral bodies and act as shock absorbers. The avascular disk consists of an eccentrically located nucleus pulposus and the surrounding annulus fibrosus. The nucleus pulposus is a semigelatinous mass composed of 70–80% water. The water content declines with advancing age, and by the sixth or seventh decade of life, the nucleus has been transformed to fibrocartilage.

▶ Clinical Findings in Spinal Cord Disorders

A. Symptoms and Signs

Clinical findings in spinal cord disorders can be divided into sensory abnormalities, motor abnormalities, sphincter abnormalities, and sexual abnormalities (Table 18–1). Classic spinal cord syndromes are summarized in Table 18–2.

B. Diagnostic Studies

Magnetic resonance imaging (MRI) is the test of choice for the evaluation of spinal cord syndromes. Computed tomographic (CT) myelography may be used when MRI is unavailable or contraindicated. Somatosensory-evoked potentials are useful in the evaluation of conditions involving the dorsal columns (eg, multiple sclerosis). Electromyography and nerve conduction studies are useful for diagnosing amyotrophic lateral sclerosis and conditions with associated peripheral neuropathy. Transcranial magnetic stimulation (central motor conduction studies) can aid in the diagnosis of hysterical paraplegia.

Lumbar puncture is of limited value in most spinal cord syndromes. When cord compression is suspected, this procedure should not be performed until an MRI or CT myelogram has been performed to exclude a mass lesion. Infectious etiologies (eg, cytomegalovirus) may be diagnosed by polymerase chain reaction; cerebrospinal fluid cytology may reveal tumor cells; and, in suspected multiple sclerosis, the presence of oligoclonal bands in cerebrospinal fluid is supportive.

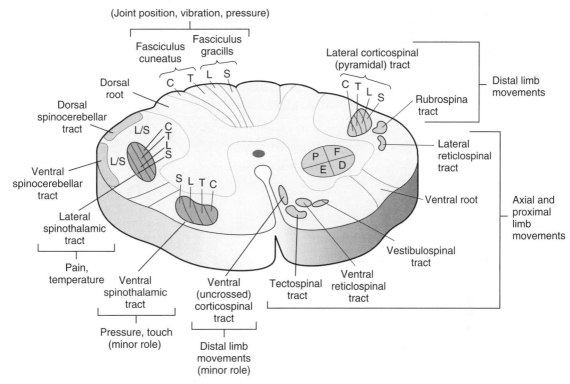

▲ **Figure 18–1.** Transverse section through the spinal cord, composite representation, illustrating the principal ascending (*left*) and descending (*right*) pathways. The lateral and ventral spinothalamic tracts ascend contralateral to the side of the body that is innervated. C = cervical; D = distal; E = extensors; F = flexors; L = lumbar; P = proximal; S = sacral; T = thoracic. (Reproduced with permission from Hauser S. Diseases of the spinal cord. In: Braunwald, ed. *Harrison's Principles of Internal Medicine Online*. McGraw-Hill, 2001.)

SPINAL CORD TUMORS

Spinal cord tumors are discussed in Chapter 12.

MYELITIS

ESSENTIALS OF DIAGNOSIS

▶ Poorly localized back pain or discomfort

▶ Fever (sometimes) with infectious etiologies

▶ Evolving paraparesis, tetraparesis, or a Brown-Séquard syndrome

▶ No evidence of a compressive lesion on MRI scan

▶ Frequently abnormal cerebrospinal fluid analysis (lymphocyte pleocytosis and elevated protein level)

▶ General Considerations

The term *myelitis* refers to infectious and noninfectious inflammatory processes of the spinal cord. *Leukomyelitis* involves the spinal cord white matter, and *poliomyelitis* involves the spinal cord gray matter. *Transverse myelitis* involves the entire cross-sectional area of the cord. Multiple or widespread lesions are classified as diffuse or disseminated, and *meningomyelitis* implies additional involvement of the meninges. In general, the term *acute* refers to rapid development of symptoms specified by hours or days, *subacute* refers to evolution of symptoms over a period of 2–6 weeks, and *chronic* refers to symptom evolution from onset to peak over 6 weeks. Myelitis can be caused by several conditions, as outlined in Table 18–3.

▶ Clinical Findings

A. Symptoms and Signs

The clinical picture of acute transverse myelitis is similar to acute cord transection from spinal trauma, tumor, or

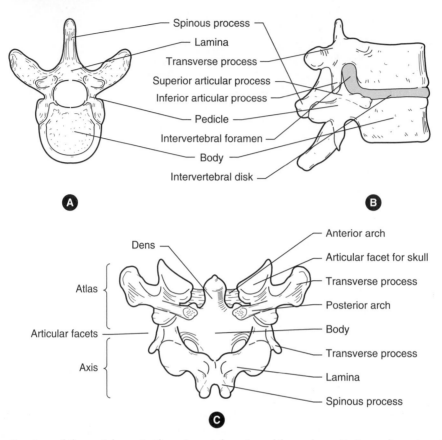

A: Thoracic vertebra viewed from above.

- Spinous process
- Lamina
- Transverse process
- Superior articular process
- Inferior articular process
- Pedicle
- Intervertebral foramen
- Body
- Intervertebral disk

- Dens
- Atlas
- Articular facets
- Axis
- Anterior arch
- Articular facet for skull
- Transverse process
- Posterior arch
- Body
- Transverse process
- Lamina
- Spinous process

▲ **Figure 18–2.** Structure of the vertebrae. **A:** Thoracic vertebra viewed from above. **B:** Two adjacent vertebrae, lateral view. **C:** structure of atlas (first cervical vertebrae) and axis (second cervical vertebrae) (Reproduced with permission from Jenkins DB. *Hollinshead's Functional Anatomy of the Limbs and Back,* 6th ed. Elsevier, 1991.)

infarction. Three groups are generally seen. The first is characterized by ascending sensory symptoms over 1–14 days, followed by good recovery. The second group, which has the poorest outcome, is characterized by almost instantaneous onset with rapid symptom evolution, back pain, and paraplegia. The third group is characterized by gradual onset and stuttering progression. In all three forms the midthoracic cord is usually involved, and a band of pain around the chest may mimic intrathoracic or cardiac disease. Incontinence of urine occurs, and fever may or may not be present.

B. Diagnostic Studies

Spinal fluid examination, which should be performed only after an MRI scan to exclude the presence of a compressive lesion, may be normal but often shows lymphocyte pleocytosis (greater in postinfectious and infectious causes) and elevated protein level. Spinal fluid analysis with polymerase chain reaction can detect infectious agents. Oligoclonal bands are often present, especially in patients with multiple

sclerosis. Multiple sclerosis is more likely in patients with partial, asymmetric syndromes. MRI may be normal or reveal cord edema with high signal lesions extending over several segments (Figure 18–3). Gadolinium enhancement may be present. In cases of suspected multiple sclerosis, MRI of the brain is also indicated.

▶ Treatment

Treatment is both supportive and disease specific. Acyclovir or ganciclovir therapy may be used for herpes zoster– or cytomegalovirus-related myelopathies, respectively. Specific antifungal, antiparasitic, or antibacterial medications, including antituberculous agents, may be used for other infectious myelopathies. Immunomodulating therapy (eg, corticosteroid) is used for autoimmune, postinfectious, and multiple sclerosis–related myelopathies. In tuberculous osteitis (Pott paraplegia) surgical intervention is usually indicated. The majority of children with transverse myelitis make a good recovery, but residual neurologic deficits may persist in adults.

Table 18–1. Clinical Findings in Spinal Cord Disorders

Sensory Abnormalities
Local pain
Radicular pain
Funicular pain (central-type, diffuse, aching, or burning pain
    with poor localizing value)
Dysesthesia
Hyperesthesia
Paresthesia
Lhermitte phenomenon (neck flexion elicits an electrical sensation
    down back and into arms)
Loss of joint position sense below level of lesion (sensory ataxia)
Loss of sensation at or below level of lesion

Motor Abnormalities
Weakness (often paraparesis or tetraparesis)
Upper motor neuron signs
    • Slow RAM out of proportion to weakness
    • Gait dysfunction out of proportion to weakness and not
      explained by proprioceptive loss
    • Mild atrophy in longstanding upper motor neuron dysfunction
    • Increased muscle tone
    • Hyperactive DTRs
Lower motor neuron signs
    • Slow RAM proportional to weakness
    • Prominent atrophy
    • Decreased muscle tone
    • Fasciculations
    • Hypoactive or absent DTRs

Sphincter Abnormalities
Nocturia (may be an early sign)
Urinary frequency
Incontinence

Sexual Abnormalities
Erectile dysfunction or ejaculatory dysfunction

DTR = deep tendon reflex; RAM = rapid alternating movement.

Defresne P, et al. Acute transverse myelitis in children: Clinical course and prognostic factors. *J Child Neurol* 2003;18:401–406. [PMID: 12886975]

Krishnan C, et al. Transverse myelitis: Pathogenesis, diagnosis and treatment. *Front Biosci* 2004;9:1483–1499. [PMID: 14977560] (Summarizes recent classification and diagnostic schemes that provide a framework for the management of patients with acute transverse myelitis and reviews current concepts of natural history, immunopathogenesis, and treatment strategies.)

SPINAL EPIDURAL ABSCESS

 ESSENTIALS OF DIAGNOSIS

▶ Fever

▶ Back pain

▶ Evolving paraparesis

 General Considerations

A spinal epidural abscess can occur from direct spread (vertebral osteomyelitis, local surgical or anesthetic procedures) or hematogenous spread from a distant infection (bacterial endocarditis, genitourinary infection). In some cases, no source of infection is found. Risk factors include immunosuppression and intravenous drug abuse. *Staphylococcus aureus* causes more than 50% of cases.

▶ **Clinical Findings**

A. Symptoms and Signs

Initial symptoms are usually local back pain and fever. Radicular pain soon develops, followed by rapidly evolving motor and sensory deficits below the level of the lesion and sphincter disturbances. In some patients neurologic evolution occurs over several weeks.

B. Laboratory Findings

Peripheral leukocytosis is usually present, but white blood cell count may be normal. Erythrocyte sedimentation rate is often elevated. Blood cultures should be performed. In the absence of abscess rupture, spinal fluid examination reveals an elevated white cell count (polymorphonuclear leukocytes or lymphocytes), increased protein level, and normal glucose level.

C. Imaging Studies

MRI is the imaging study of choice and reveals abnormal findings in 95% of patients. CT myelography is also useful.

▶ **Treatment**

Treatment consists of surgical decompression, drainage, and any necessary stabilization of the spine. Systemic antibiotics are given for up to 2 months. Prognosis is related to the clinical stage at which spinal cord compression is relieved. Patients who have paraplegia for more than 48 hours generally fail to improve.

MacKenzie AR, et al. Spinal epidural abscesses: The importance of early diagnosis and treatment. *J Neurol Neurosurg Psychiatry* 1998;65:209–212. [PMID: 9703173]

SYRINGOMYELIA

ESSENTIALS OF DIAGNOSIS

▶ Segmental loss of pain and temperature with intact proprioception

▶ Segmental lower motor neuron weakness

▶ Most often occurs in lower cervical and upper thoracic regions

Table 18-2. Spinal Cord Syndromes

Syndrome	Causes	Clinical Findings
Central cord	Hyperextension injuries, syringomyelia, intramedullary tumors	Often cervical Dissociated sensory deficits (loss of pain and temperature with preserved proprioception affecting dermatomes at level of lesion) As lesion enlarges, weakness, muscle wasting, absent DTRs in arms, and spastic paraparesis occur
Anterior cord	Anterior spinal artery territory ischemia (aortic dissection, aortic aneurysm surgery, atherosclerosis, vasculitis)	Sudden loss of pain and temperature below level of lesion, paraparesis and urinary incontinence, but preserved proprioception
Posterior cord	Multiple sclerosis or demyelination, cervical spondylitic myelopathy, spinal cord tumors, atlantoaxial subluxation, Friedreich ataxia, subacute combined degeneration	Sensory ataxia (proprioceptive loss), paresthesia, weakness, extensor plantar responses, urinary incontinence, and Lhermitte phenomenon
Lateral cord (Brown-Séquard)	Trauma, multiple sclerosis or demyelination, cord compression	Weakness paresthesia, and proprioceptive loss ipsilateral to lesion Loss of pain and temperature contralateral to lesion
Complete cord	Trauma, cord compression	Loss of sensory, motor, and autonomic function below level of lesion
Pure motor	Amyotrophic lateral sclerosis, primary lateral sclerosis, progressive muscular atrophy, poliomyelitis, HTLV-1 infection, hereditary spastic paraparesis	Spastic paraparesis or tetraparesis with hyperactive DTRs (UMN) Weakness (monoparesis, paraparesis, tetraparesis), atrophy, fasciculations (LMN)
Conus	Intramedullary tumors, dermoid tumors, lipomas, metastatic tumors	Rectal and urinary incontinence, loss of anal reflexes, impotence, saddle anesthesia (S3-5 dermatomes), little or no weakness
Cauda equina	Intervertebral disk herniation, tumors, infections, arachnoiditis	Areflexic and flaccid paraparesis with back pain that radiates down posterior aspect of both legs, sensory loss in distribution of involved roots, urinary and fecal incontinence

DTR = deep tendon reflex; HTLV-1 = human T-lymphotropic virus type 1; LMN = lower motor neuron; UMN = upper motor neuron.

► General Considerations

Syringomyelia is a disorder characterized by development of a fluid-filled gliosis-lined cavity within the spinal cord. The majority of lesions are between the C2 and T9–11 spinal levels, and they can extend into the brainstem (syringobulbia) or descend down the spinal cord. The cavity is usually irregular and disrupts the anterior horns of the gray matter and the gray matter ventral to the central canal.

Syrinxes are often associated with other spinal column or brainstem abnormalities, including scoliosis, Klippel-Feil syndrome, and Arnold-Chiari type I malformation. Symptoms usually appear in the third or fourth decade of life but sometimes begin in childhood or late adulthood. Syringomyelia has both congenital and acquired causes and is classified as communicating (in contact with the central canal) or noncommunicating (separated from the central canal).

Postinflammatory syringomyelia can occur after an infection (tuberculous, fungal, parasitic) or from chemical meningitis and is associated with arachnoidal scarring. Syringomyelia can also develop after resection of a spinal cord tumor. Spinal tumors most often associated with syringomyelia are ependymoma and hemangioblastoma.

Post-traumatic syringomyelia occurs in 1–3% of patients after spinal cord trauma. It is a progressive disorder in which initial spinal cord damage leads to altered cerebrospinal fluid hydrodynamics and arachnoiditis, resulting in progressive expansion and extension of the syrinx months or years after the initial spinal cord injury.

► Clinical Findings

A. Symptoms and Signs

The characteristic picture is segmental atrophy with areflexia and segmental loss of pain and temperature sensation with intact proprioception. As the disorder progresses, the long motor and sensory tracts become affected. Syringobulbia causes dysphagia, nystagmus, pharyngeal and palatal weakness, asymmetric weakness and atrophy of the tongue, and sensory loss in the distribution of the trigeminal nerve.

In post-traumatic syringomyelia, symptoms may be present above or below the level of the original neurologic injury, and the diagnosis should be suspected in spinal cord–injured patients who develop worsening pain or neurologic function.

Table 18–3. Causes of Myelitis

Infectious	Noninfectious
Viral	Multiple sclerosis and
Enteroviruses (poliomyelitis, coxsackievirus)	neuromyelitis optica (Devic disease)
HIV	Acute disseminated encephalomyelitis
Cytomegalovirus, herpes zoster, herpes simplex virus	Sarcoidosis
HTLV-1	
Hepatitis C	Other autoimmune and vasculitic diseases (eg, lupus erythematosus, systemic sclerosis)
	Postinfectious and postvaccinal myelitis
Bacterial	Paraneoplastic myelitis
Syphilis	Neoplastic myelitis
Lyme disease	Foix-Alajouanine myelopathy (vascular malformation)
Mycoplasma pneumoniae	Radiation
Tuberculous disease (Pott disease, meningomyelitis, tuberculoma)	Electric shock
	Idiopathic transverse myelitis
Mixed infections and pyogenic myelitis	
Cat-scratch disease (*Bartonella henselae*)	
Fungal	
Cryptococcus	
Nocardia	
Aspergillus	
Actinomyces, Blastomyces, Coccidioides	
Parasitic	
Schistosomiasis	

HTLV-1 = human T-lymphotropic virus type 1.

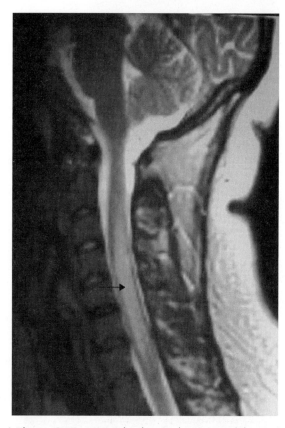

▲ **Figure 18–3.** T2-weighted sagittal MRI scan of the cervical spine showing a large plaque in the spinal cord characteristic of multiple sclerosis (*arrow*). (Used with permission from Alexander Flint, MD, PhD, and Alexander Khanji, MD.)

B. Imaging Studies

The imaging study of choice is MRI of the spine (Figure 18–4). If MRI is contraindicated, CT myelography can be used.

▶ Treatment

Patients with syringomyelia have two treatment options: conservative management and surgical decompression. Conservative treatment includes avoiding high-force isometric contractions and Valsalva expiration, head elevation at night, and maintenance of the neck in a neutral position.

Surgery, including decompression and shunt placement, is recommended for neurologic deterioration or intractable central pain. Pain and paraparesis show the best response; sensory loss, lower motor neuron signs, and brainstem findings are less likely to improve.

Syringomyelia resulting from an intramedullary spinal cord tumor is treated with tumor resection and radiation if complete excision is not possible. (Spinal cord tumors are discussed in Chapter 12.)

Grietz D. Unraveling the riddle of syringomyelia. *Neurosurg Rev* 2006;29:251–263. [PMID: 16752160]

Ushewokunze SO, et al. Surgical treatment of post-traumatic syringomyelia. *Spinal Cord* 2010;48:710–713. [PMID: 20309005]

SPINAL CORD ARTERIOVENOUS SHUNTS

 ESSENTIALS OF DIAGNOSIS

▶ Pain

▶ Leg weakness and sensory loss

▶ Slowly progressive myelopathy (most patients)

▶ Sudden onset of myelopathy (10% of patients)

▶ Most often affects lower thoracic cord and conus medullaris

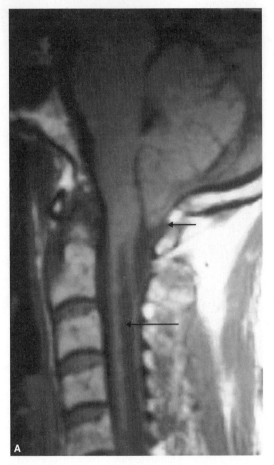

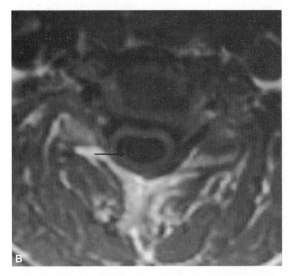

▲ **Figure 18–4. A:** T1-weighted sagittal MRI scan of the cervical spine showing a large syrinx (*long arrow*) and an Arnold-Chiari type I malformation (*short arrow*). **B:** T1-weighted MRI scan of the cervical spine showing a large syrinx (*arrow*). (Used with permission from Alexander Flint, MD, PhD, and Alexander Khanji, MD.)

▶ **General Considerations**

These rare lesions are categorized by their location within or adjacent to the spinal cord and the type of shunt involved (fistula or nidus). Arteriovenous fistulas have direct communications between arteries and veins without interposition of any pathologic network. In nidus-type lesions or arteriovenous malformations (AVMs), a vascular network is interposed between feeding arteries and draining veins. Lesions can be further categorized by location into four groups: paraspinal, epidural, dural, and intradural.

▶ **Clinical Findings**

A. Symptoms and Signs

The most common initial symptoms are radicular pain, sensory disturbance, leg weakness, and bladder dysfunction.

Seventy-five percent of patients have a slowly progressive myelopathy caused by cord compression from an AVM, and 10% have a sudden onset of cord compression due to hemorrhage or spinal cord infarction. Weakness and numbness may increase after ambulation. A pathognomonic bruit over the spinal cord is present in 25% of patients (usually with an intradural AVM). A cutaneous angioma may also overlie an AVM.

Foix-Alajouanine syndrome is a rapidly progressive myelopathy that develops because of venous thrombosis caused by venous stasis.

B. Imaging Studies

MRI and magnetic resonance angiography can identify the lesions, but angiography is the gold standard for analysis of the anatomic, morphologic, and architectural features necessary for therapeutic decisions.

Treatment

The goal of treatment should be complete closure of the shunt. Treatment options must be individualized for the patient and include: embolization (endovascular technique), surgery to ligate the feeding vessel and excise the abnormality, or a combination of these techniques. A complete cure by embolization can usually be achieved in patients with paraspinal lesions. Dural AVMs can be treated either with embolization or with surgery. If there are multiple feeders or tortuous vascular anatomy, surgery is usually the best option. Treatment may also consist of a combination of endovascular ablation followed by surgical excision. After treatment, most patients with spinal arteriovenous shunts show neurologic improvement.

Morgan MK. Outcome from treatment for spinal arteriovenous malformation. *Neurosurg Clin N Am* 1999;10:113–119. [PMID: 9855653]

Spetzler RF, et al. Modified classification of spinal cord vascular lesions. *J Neurosurg* 2002;96(2 Suppl): 145–156. [PMID: 12450276]

SPINAL CORD INFARCTION

ESSENTIALS OF DIAGNOSIS

- ► Sudden onset of symptoms
- ► Moderate to severe back pain at the site of cord infarction (most often in the thoracic region) followed within minutes by paraplegia
- ► Usually associated with paraparesis and loss of pain sensation below the level of the infarction bilaterally with intact proprioception and vibration
- ► Loss of bladder control
- ► Most common causes are severe hypotension, aortic dissection, and aortic surgery

General Considerations

Infarction of the spinal cord is uncommon. Arteries originating from the vertebral artery and the aorta supply the spinal cord. A single anterior spinal artery supplies the anterior two thirds of the cord, and the paired posterior arteries supply the dorsal one third. The anterior spinal artery is discontinuous and therefore requires multiple feeders. The region from T4 to T8, which contains few anastomoses, is considered to be at the greatest ischemic risk, especially in patients with systemic hypotension. An area at the boundary zones between the territories of the anterior and posterior spinal arteries is also at risk for ischemia. This may result in an acute progressive syndrome of weakness and spasticity, with little sensory

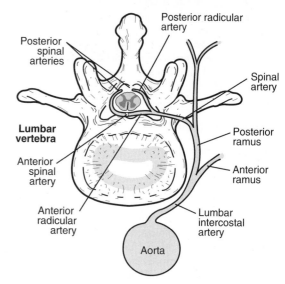

▲ **Figure 18–5.** Extrinsic arterial supply to the spinal cord. (Reproduced with permission of Lippincott Williams & Wilkins from Cheshire WP, Santos CC, Massey EW, Howard JF Jr. Spinal cord infarction: Etiology and outcome. *Neurology* 1996;47:321–330.)

change resembling amyotrophic lateral sclerosis. Infarction of the posterior third of the spinal cord is less likely because of the greater anastomosis of the posterior arteries (Figure 18–5).

Spinal cord infarction has many causes, including hypoxia and ischemia, cardiogenic thromboembolism, vasculitis, atherosclerosis, AVM, collagen and elastin disorders, sickle cell disease, polycythemia, hypercoagulability, paradoxical embolism via a patent foramen ovale, and cocaine use. Other causes include dissecting aortic aneurysm, hypotension, and surgical clipping of aortic aneurysms. Some cases are associated with pregnancy, acute back trauma, or exercise that, by an unknown mechanism, leads to embolism of nucleus pulposus material into spinal vessels. In a substantial number of cases, no cause can be found.

Spinal venous infarction is rare. It can be hemorrhagic or ischemic and is more likely to be subacute in onset, yielding variable deficits. Nitrogen bubbles may lodge in spinal veins in scuba divers with decompression sickness.

Clinical Findings
Symptoms and Signs

The usual presentation of the anterior spinal artery syndrome is characterized by sudden onset of paraplegia, loss of pain sensation, loss of bladder control, and pain at the site of infarction. Absent or hypoactive tendon reflexes may be present initially, later changing to hyperreflexia.

Spinal transient ischemic attacks typically manifest as painless paraparesis or quadriparesis that may be sporadic or associated with postural changes but without loss of consciousness or intracranial localizing features. They can occur in patients with foraminal stenosis during cervical or lumbar extension, which maximally compromises the intervertebral foramina through which the spinal radicular arteries pass.

B. Diagnostic Studies

Imaging studies such as MRI and CT are usually normal in the first 24 hours after acute spinal cord infarction and are initially performed to rule out other causes or paraplegia. A few days later, the MRI scan may reveal focal cord swelling, and if performed months or years later, focal cord atrophy is seen.

Lumbar puncture is indicated whenever the underlying cause has not been clarified. Laboratory studies are performed to detect infectious, inflammatory, hematologic, or cardiovascular disorders, including diseases of the aorta.

▶ Treatment

Therapy is directed at any predisposing condition. Standard drug therapy is aspirin, but no definitive study has been performed. Whether the acute effects of spinal infarction can be modified by high-dose corticosteroids, agents that increase blood flow, or anticoagulation is unknown.

▶ Prognosis

Young patients without total paralysis have the best prognosis. Patients with complete paralysis rarely show significant improvement.

Novy J, Carruzzo A, Maeder P, Bogousslavsky J. Spinal cord ischemia: Clinical and imaging patterns, pathogenesis, and outcomes in 27 patients. *Arch Neurol* 2006;63:1113–1120. [PMID: 16908737]

SPINAL EPIDURAL & SUBDURAL HEMATOMAS

ESSENTIALS OF DIAGNOSIS

▶ Sudden onset of pain at the site of hemorrhage (most often the upper thoracic region)

▶ Paresthesia and weakness occurring hours or days later below the level of the spinal pain

▶ Urinary retention

▶ General Considerations

Most spinal epidural and subdural hematomas occur in the upper thoracic region, although other levels can also be involved. Spinal epidural hematoma of the lower thoracic and lumbosacral spine most often affects patients younger than 40 years of age and can result from spinal surgery, inherited coagulopathy, therapeutic thrombolysis, anticoagulant therapy, lumbar puncture, epidural analgesia, spinal vascular malformation, hemangioma, Paget disease, and cocaine or amphetamine abuse. Spinal subdural hematoma is a rare entity associated with hemorrhagic disorders, anticoagulant therapy, lumbar puncture, spinal surgery, neoplasm, vascular malformation, and trauma.

▶ Clinical Findings

A. Symptoms and Signs

Spinal epidural and subdural hematomas are difficult to distinguish clinically. Onset in the thoracic region leads to acute progressive paraplegia. Typically, severe thoracic pain is followed by fast-spreading sensory and motor loss with sphincter dysfunction. Brown-Séquard syndrome can occur. Lesions in the upper part of the spine are often linked to vertebral or epidural dysplasia, whereas those in the lower spine are often related to mechanical or degenerative lesions.

B. Diagnostic Studies

Except in patients with preexisting vertebral lesions, plain radiographs are unremarkable. In patients with spinal epidural hematoma, CT shows a high-density, oblong mass that sometimes impinges on the lateral aspect of the spinal cord; MRI can reveal an epidural collection of blood. MRI is superior to CT in both diagnosis and follow-up of spinal subdural hematoma.

If no obvious source for the patient's neurologic symptoms is found, studies should include evaluation for a coagulopathy, including clotting factors, bleeding time, prothrombin time, partial thromboplastin time, and platelet count.

▶ Treatment

Surgical treatment involves evacuation of the hematoma. Conservative treatment of spinal subdural hematoma has been used in younger patients showing spontaneous neurologic recovery.

▶ Prognosis

For patients with spinal epidural hematoma, the prognosis depends not only on the degree of neurologic loss before surgery, but also on the time from symptom onset to surgical decompression. Surgery performed more than 12 hours after symptom onset is unlikely to be successful. About half of such patients who have complete motor and sensory loss at the time of surgery recover to some degree, and 10% recover completely. Patients with a modest already-improving neurologic deficit can be treated conservatively. For patients with spinal subdural hematoma, the worst outcomes occur when lesions are located at the cervical and thoracic levels.

SUBACUTE COMBINED DEGENERATION

ESSENTIALS OF DIAGNOSIS

▶ Paraparesis

▶ Sensory ataxia

▶ Areflexia

▶ Extensor plantar responses

▶ Low serum vitamin B_{12} level, or elevated homocysteine and methylmalonic acid levels in patients with borderline serum B_{12} levels

▶ Dementia and optic atrophy (less common features)

▶ General Considerations

Cyanocobalamin (vitamin B_{12}) deficiency can occur in pernicious anemia, Crohn disease, fish tapeworm (*Diphyllobothrium latum*) infestation, and blind loop syndrome; in strict vegetarians; and after total gastrectomy. Neurologic complications of vitamin B_{12} deficiency can occur in the absence of anemia or macrocytosis and include myelopathy, peripheral neuropathy, and dementia, alone or in various combinations. The myelopathy that occurs with vitamin B_{12} deficiency is similar to the vacuolar myelopathy seen in patients with AIDS and in patients with prolonged exposure to nitrous oxide. Most affected are the posterior and lateral columns of the spinal cord.

▶ Clinical Findings

Myelopathy plus peripheral neuropathy produce a combination of areflexia, sensory ataxia, paraparesis, and extensor plantar responses. Lhermitte phenomenon may be present. Dementia and optic atrophy are less common features. Elevated serum levels of homocysteine and methylmalonic acid are confirmatory tests in patients with borderline serum B_{12} levels. MRI scan of the spine may show normal findings or reveal abnormal signals or atrophy in the cord. Somatosensory-evoked potentials and motor-evoked potentials are usually abnormal. Nerve conduction studies may reveal peripheral neuropathy.

▶ Treatment

Dosages and routes used for cyanocobalamin replacement depend on the severity of neurologic deficits and the underlying etiology. For patients with severe deficits, 1 mg/day is given intramuscularly for 7–12 days, followed by 1 mg per week for 3 weeks, and then 1 mg every 1–3 months for life. An incomplete response is obtained in patients who have severe symptoms that have been present for more than 1 year.

Misra UK, Kalita J, Das A. Vitamin B12 deficiency neurological syndromes: A clinical, MRI and electrodiagnostic study. *Electromyogr Clin Neurophysiol* 2003;43:57–64. [PMID: 12613142]

AMYOTROPHIC LATERAL SCLEROSIS & OTHER MOTOR NEURON DISEASES

These disorders are discussed in Chapter 20.

SPINOCEREBELLAR DEGENERATION

This disorder is discussed in Chapter 16.

RADICULOPATHY

ESSENTIALS OF DIAGNOSIS

▶ Pain in a dermatomal distribution, sensory symptoms along the same dermatome, weakness in a corresponding myotomal distribution, and absent or depressed reflexes

▶ Frequency of incidence in order of occurrence—lumbar > cervical > thoracic (rare)

▶ Usually caused by a herniated disk or by spondylosis; other causes are infection, neoplasm, granuloma, cyst, and hematoma

▶ General Considerations

Many different terms are used to describe an abnormal disk, but a true disk herniation implies that annular fibers have been disrupted. A radiculopathy occurs when the disk herniates laterally; if the disk herniates more centrally, it causes cord compression in the cervical and thoracic spine and a cauda equina syndrome in the lumbar region.

A. Cervical Spine

In cervical radiculopathy, the C7 nerve root is most often affected (60%), followed by C6 (25%). Cervical disk herniation more commonly results from degeneration than from trauma. With the loss of the viscoelastic properties of the nucleus pulposus and annulus fibrosus, the disk loses height and bulges posteriorly into the canal. Osteophytes form around the disk margins and at the facet joints, leading to narrowing of the canal and radicular symptoms.

B. Lumbar Spine

Lumbosacral radiculopathy is usually caused by disk herniation or by spondylitic changes, especially at the facet joints or by calcification of the ligamentum flavum. When combined, these changes can result in stenosis of the lumbar canal.

Disk herniation occurs most frequently in middle-aged men, especially after physical activity. Other risk factors include any congenital condition that affects the size of the lumbar spinal canal.

In 90% of patients, herniated lumbar disks occur between L4–5 and L5–S1. L5 is the most commonly compressed nerve root, followed closely by S1. The disk commonly herniates posterolaterally and compresses the nerve root passing through the foramen below that disk. If the disk herniates far laterally into the foramen, it will compress the exiting nerve root.

Positions causing the highest intradiscal pressure and therefore the most discomfort are, in descending order, sitting while leaning forward, followed by sitting, standing, lying on the side, and finally supine. Bending forward, bending to the side, lifting, coughing, and sneezing also increase pain.

▶ Clinical Findings

A. Symptoms and Signs

1. Herniated cervical disk—Pain is present in the posterior neck, with spasms of the cervical paraspinal musculature and near or over the shoulder blades on the affected side. Pain, sensory disturbances, and arm weakness usually occur in a root-level distribution on the same side of the herniation (Figure 18–6, Table 18–4). Pain can be increased by coughing, straining, laughing, bending, or turning the neck to the side.

2. Herniated lumbosacral disk—Symptoms include severe low back pain and lumbar paraspinal spasms, with pain radiating to the buttocks, legs, and feet. Pain, sensory loss, and weakness typically occur in a radicular pattern, but weakness and atrophy are not usually early presenting features (see Figure 18–6 and Table 18–4). Maneuvers that increase the pain include coughing, straining, and laughing. Urinary symptoms, if present, require immediate attention.

Table 18–4. Radicular Pattern in Arms and Legs

Root Level	Sensory Changes	Motor Changes	Reflex Changes
Arms			
C5	Lateral proximal arm	Elbow flexion	Biceps, brachioradialis
C6	Thumb	Wrist extension	Brachioradialis and pronator teres
C7	Middle finger	Elbow extension	Triceps
C8	Little finger	Finger flexors	Finger flexors
T1	Medial proximal arm	Finger abduction	—
Legs			
L3	Medial thigh	Knee extensors	Knee jerk
L4	Medial calf	Ankle dorsiflexion	—
L5	Lateral calf or first toe	First toe extension, hamstring	Medial hamstring
S1	Lateral foot	Ankle plantarflexion	Ankle jerk

B. Diagnostic Studies

Plain radiographs using anteroposterior, lateral, and oblique views can reveal osteophytes encroaching in the intervertebral foramen but have limited utility in detecting a herniated nucleus pulposus.

MRI is the best imaging study to detect disk pathology, herniation of the nucleus pulposus, and nerve root impingement (Figure 18–7). MRI may also reveal disk abnormalities, such as a disk bulge or protrusion, in asymptomatic patients.

CT imaging is used to discern the bony architecture and can detect disk protrusion. CT with the addition of myelography can show foraminal and central stenosis as well as lateral disk protrusion that may be missed by MRI.

Electromyography (EMG) and nerve conduction studies (NCS) can be used to confirm the clinical impression, exclude other disorders in the differential diagnosis, and highlight findings that will alter clinical management. Denervation of muscle at one root level may indicate radiculopathy. EMG and NCS can also give information on acute or chronic changes and the severity of the neuronal deficit. These studies can help differentiate between radiculopathy and neuropathy, myopathy, or plexopathy. EMG and NCS are of limited value if symptoms are limited to the axial spine.

C. Special Tests

Spurling sign is useful to help diagnose a cervical radiculopathy. In this test, the patient's neck is extended while the head is rotated with a downward pressure on the head. A positive finding consists of pain radiating into the limb and the shoulder to the side at which the head is rotated and occurs as a result of maximal disk protrusion in the intervertebral foramen.

The **straight leg-raising test** is used to diagnose lumbosacral radiculopathy. With the patient supine, each leg is raised separately until pain occurs. Pain below the knee along the path of a nerve root (radicular pain) that occurs between 30 and 70 degrees of flexion, is a sign of nerve root irritation. Bending the knee while maintaining hip flexion should relieve pain, and pressure in the popliteal region should increase the pain. **Lasègue sign** is elicited by placing the knee in full extension during straight leg raising and then dorsiflexing the ankle; this maneuver increases the pain if a radiculopathy is present. A positive finding on the **crossed straight leg-raising test** occurs when the contralateral uninvolved leg is raised and pain is produced on the affected side.

The **femoral stretch test** is performed with the patient prone or in lateral decubitus position to help diagnose an L2–4 radiculopathy. The thigh is extended at the hip, and the knee is flexed; a positive finding is indicated by reproduction of the patient's pain. It may be falsely positive secondary to tight or injured muscles of the anterior thigh, and to osseous or joint pathology in and about the hip.

Other useful tests to help evaluate patients with back pain include Kernig sign, which is not only useful for meningitis. Have the patient supine, and flex the thigh to a 90-degree

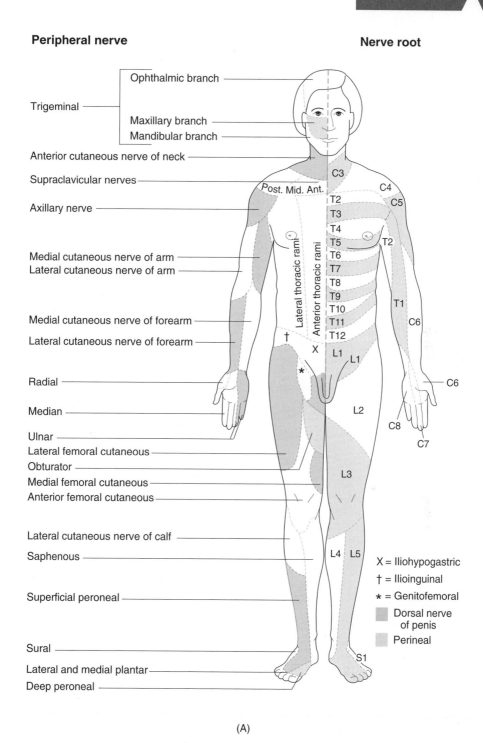

Peripheral nerve

Nerve root

(A)

▲ **Figure 18–6.** Cutaneous innervation. The segmental or radicular (root) distribution is shown on the left side of the body and the peripheral nerve distribution on the right. **A:** Anterior view. **B:** Posterior view. (Reproduced with permission from Simon RP, Aminoff MJ, Greenberg DA. *Clinical Neurology,* 4th ed. McGraw-Hill, 1999.)

Nerve root

Peripheral nerve

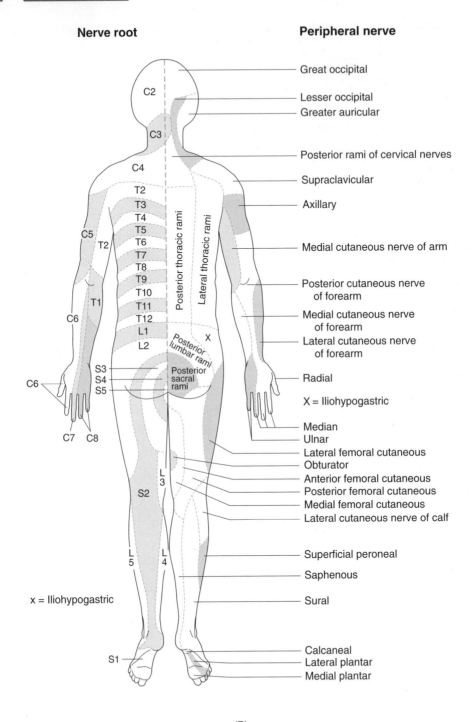

Great occipital

Lesser occipital
Greater auricular

Posterior rami of cervical nerves

Supraclavicular

Axillary

Medial cutaneous nerve of arm

Posterior cutaneous nerve
of forearm

Medial cutaneous nerve
of forearm
Lateral cutaneous nerve
of forearm

Radial

X = Iliohypogastric

Median
Ulnar
Lateral femoral cutaneous
Obturator
Anterior femoral cutaneous
Posterior femoral cutaneous
Medial femoral cutaneous
Lateral cutaneous nerve of calf

Superficial peroneal

Saphenous

Sural

Calcaneal
Lateral plantar
Medial plantar

(B)

▲ **Figure 18–6.** (*Continued*)

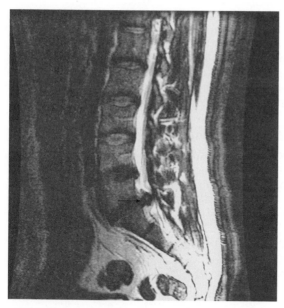

▲ **Figure 18–7.** T2-weighted sagittal MRI scan of the lumbosacral spine showing a large paracentral disk protrusion (*arrow*). (Used with permission from Alexander Khanji, MD.)

angle, keeping the leg extended. The test is positive if the patient is unable to completely extend the leg due to pain.

▶ Differential Diagnosis

Cervical radiculopathy must be differentiated from musculoskeletal disorders such as cervicalgia, shoulder pathology, elbow disorders, brachial plexus disorders, thoracic outlet syndrome, and peripheral nerve entrapment.

Lumbosacral radiculopathy must be differentiated from musculoskeletal disorders such as low back strain, hip and knee disorders, lumbosacral plexus disorders, and peripheral nerve entrapment.

▶ Treatment

The mainstay of treatment for a radiculopathy is a period of rest and anti-inflammatory medication. Most patients are managed well with conservative treatment. Bed rest for a maximum of 2 days is recommended; a longer course provides no additional benefit.

A. Pharmacotherapy

Nonsteroidal anti-inflammatory drugs are used for their anti-inflammatory and analgesic effects. These agents should be used with caution in patients with uncontrolled hypertension, in the elderly, and in those with a history of gastrointestinal symptoms. Adding misoprostol, an H_2 blocker, or a proton

pump inhibitor may offer added gastrointestinal protection. Acetaminophen can reduce pain without gastrointestinal toxicity but does not have any anti-inflammatory effect.

A short course of oral corticosteroids is useful in treating an acute herniated disk, especially in low-risk patients, but use of these agents is controversial. Muscle relaxants can be used, although most work at the central rather than the muscle level, and they may cause excessive drowsiness. Narcotics are reserved for control of severe pain. For neuropathic pain, useful medications (which are off label in the treatment of radicular pain) include gabapentin, pregabalin, duloxetine, 5% lidocaine patch, tramadol, and tricyclic antidepressants.

B. Nonpharmacologic Measures

Heat, ice, massage, stress reduction, activity limitation, postural modification, and the addition of a physical therapy program may provide additional relief. A soft cervical collar (for neck pain) and a lumbar corset (for back pain) may be useful. Once the acute pain has subsided, stretching exercises should be started to help restore range of motion. Exercises for the cervical region include neck rotation, bending and tilting, shoulder rolls, and upper back stretches. The McKenzie exercise program is widely used for low back pain and contains repetitive exercises (usually in passive extension) that "centralize" pain by moving it away from the extremities to the back. Traction can also be used.

C. Epidural Injection and Surgery

Epidural corticosteroid injection is gaining in popularity as a treatment for pain caused by herniated disks. They are usually more useful for leg pain as opposed to axial pain. Their use and timing is still controversial at this time, with limited studies regarding their long-term efficacy. The few absolute indications for surgery are (1) marked muscular weakness pertaining to a nerve root or roots; (2) progressive neurologic deficit; (3) cauda equina syndrome with urinary symptoms; and (4) pain that has existed for more than 4 months, has not responded to conservative treatment, and interferes with normal function.

Surgery for lumbosacral disk herniation usually involves laminectomy and disk excision and can be performed in an open procedure or by microdiscectomy. For cervical disk herniation, surgical treatment includes laminectomy and foraminotomy, using anterolateral or posterolateral approaches.

LUMBAR STENOSIS

 ESSENTIALS OF DIAGNOSIS

▶ Leg pain, numbness, and weakness exacerbated by standing or walking and relieved with lumbar flexion

▶ General Considerations

Spinal stenosis is narrowing of the spinal canal or neural foramina, which produces root compression, most commonly at L4–5 and L3–4. Stenosis may occur congenitally as a result of developmentally narrow spinal canal dimensions or bone dysplasias; however, degenerative disease is the most common cause.

Degenerative lumbar spinal stenosis usually affects patients older than 60 years. It may be localized to a single segment of the spine or may span multiple segments. Pathological hallmarks include, disk degeneration, facet joint osteoarthritis and hypertrophy of the pedicles, laminae, and supporting ligamentous structures. Other causes of lumbar stenosis include underlying spinal instability from spondylolisthesis, scoliosis, metabolic bone disorders, neoplastic or infectious processes, or post-traumatic degenerative changes. Precipitation of symptoms by walking is attributable to lumbar extension, which causes buckling of the ligamentum flavum, increases disk protrusion, decreases interlaminar distance, and narrows the spinal canal by as much as 60% when compared with lumbar flexion.

▶ Clinical Findings

Symptoms include insidious, poorly localized pain, paresthesias, and weakness during walking and lordosis that is relieved with flexion of the spine. The condition must be differentiated from vascular claudication (Table 18–5).

Special tests include those outlined above in the radiculopathy section. Patrick sign can help distinguish lumbar stenosis from hip joint pathology, which causes hip joint or groin pain during external rotation of the hip when the hip and knee are flexed (flexion, abduction, external rotation).

▶ Treatment

A. Pharmacotherapy and Nonoperative Measures

Medications are useful for pain control and muscle relaxation. Exercise regimens include therapeutic stretching of the lumbosacral spine, low back and abdominal muscle strengthening, and general aerobic conditioning. Use of a stationary bicycle or leaning forward while walking on a treadmill can help reduce symptoms. Walking on an upward incline tends to be more comfortable than flat or downhill walking. Physical modalities include heat, ice, or electrical stimulation. Lumbosacral corsets can help support the usually weak abdominal muscles during activities.

B. Surgical Management

Surgical referral is recommended for patients with severe and disabling pain, significant neurologic deficits, or bladder and bowel disturbance and poor response to at least 4 weeks of conservative treatment. The standard decompression procedure is laminectomy.

Andersson GB, et al. Consensus summary of the diagnosis and treatment of lumbar disc herniation. *Spine* 1996;21(Suppl): 75S–78S. [PMID: 9112328]

Clare HA, Adams R, Maher CG. A systematic review of efficacy of McKenzie therapy for spinal pain. *Aust J Physiother.* 2004; 50(4):209–16. [PMID: 15574109]

Peul WC, et al. Surgery versus Prolonged Conservative Treatment for Sciatica. *N Engl J Med* 2007;356:2245–2256. [PMID: 17538084]

Saal JA. Natural history and nonoperative treatment of lumbar disc herniation. *Spine* 1996;21(Suppl):2S–9S. [PMID: 9112320] (Ground-breaking articles describing the nonoperative management of lumbar herniated disks.)

Saal JS. General principles of diagnostic testing as related to painful lumbar spine disorders: A critical appraisal of current diagnostic techniques. *Spine* 2002;27:2538–2545. [PMID: 12435989]

Yamazaki S, Kokubun S, Ishii Y, Tanaka Y. Courses of cervical disc herniation causing myelopathy or radiculopathy: An analysis based on computed tomographic discograms. *Spine* 2003;28:1171–1175. [PMID: 12782988]

CERVICAL SPONDYLOTIC MYELOPATHY

ESSENTIALS OF DIAGNOSIS

▶ Most common in middle-aged and older adults

▶ Gradual onset of symptoms

▶ Radicular signs at the level of the lesion; upper motor neuron signs below the lesion

▶ Gait difficulties

▶ General Considerations

Cervical spondylotic myelopathy is the most common cause of acquired spastic paraparesis in middle and older adulthood. The patient may present with subtle findings of several

Table 18–5. Comparison of Key Characteristics in Vascular Claudication and Lumbar Stenosis

Characteristic	Vascular Claudication	Lumbar Stenosis
Location of pain	Distal-to-proximal calf pain	Proximal-to-distal pain, thigh pain
Response to activity or positioning		
• Walking uphill	Pain occurs early	Pain occurs later
• Bicycling	Evokes symptoms	Does not evoke symptoms
• Standing	Relieves symptoms	symptoms
• Sitting or bending		Relieves symptoms
• Lying flat	Relieves symptoms	May exacerbate symptoms

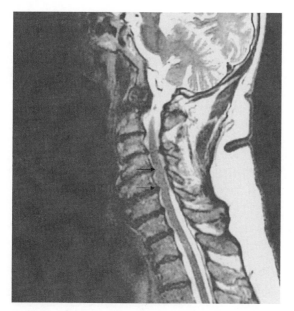

▲ **Figure 18–8.** Cervical MRI scan showing multilevel degenerative disk disease, disk osteophyte complexes, cord impingement, and spinal stenosis (*arrows*). (Used with permission from Alexander Khanji, MD.)

years' duration or with quadriparesis that developed over the course of a few hours. Myelopathic syndromes include *medial syndrome,* consisting primarily of long-tract symptoms; *lateral syndrome,* consisting primarily of radicular symptoms; *combined medial and lateral syndrome,* the most common clinical presentation; *anterior syndrome,* producing painless unilateral upper-extremity weakness; and *vascular syndrome,* producing a rapidly progressive myelopathy.

▶ **Clinical Findings**

Patients frequently have difficulties with balance, especially spasticity, and radicular symptoms. Bladder incontinence is uncommon, but urinary frequency is common when spasticity is present. On examination, lower motor neuron signs are present at the level of the lesion, and upper motor neuron signs are present below the lesion.

▶ **Diagnostic Studies**

MRI of the cervical spine is the imaging study of choice (Figure 18–8). CT can complement the MRI scan by providing additional bony detail. CT myelography can be used in patients who are unable to tolerate MRI.

▶ **Treatment**

Cervical myelopathy can be treated conservatively with the use of neck immobilization (cervical collar), physical therapy, and lifestyle modification. Pharmacotherapy can include

nonsteroidal anti-inflammatory drugs or other analgesics, as well as muscle relaxants.

If there has been rapid progression, decompressive surgery is recommended.

▶ **Prognosis**

Prognosis after surgery is better for younger patients and those with symptom duration of less than 1 year, fewer levels of involvement, and unilateral motor deficit.

Bednarik J, et al. Presymptomatic spondylotic cervical cord compression. *Spine* 2004;29:2260–2269. [PMID: 15480138]

Fouyas IP, Statham PF, Sandercock PA. Cochrane review on the role of surgery in cervical spondylotic radiculomyelopathy. *Spine* 2002;27:736–747. [PMID: 11923667] (Assesses the balance of risk and benefit from surgery; whether surgical treatment of cervical radiculopathy or myelopathy is associated with improved outcome, compared with conservative management; and whether timing of surgery [immediate or delayed on persistence or progression of relevant symptoms and signs] has an impact on outcome.)

Kadanka Z, et al. Approaches to spondylotic cervical myelopathy: Conservative versus surgical results in a 3-year follow-up study. *Spine* 2002;27:2205–2210. [PMID: 12394893]

Kadanka Z, et al. Predictive factors for spondylotic cervical myelopathy treated conservatively or surgically. *Eur J Neurol* 2005;12:55–63. [PMID: 15613148]

▼ ISSUES IN REHABILITATION OF SPINAL CORD–INJURED PATIENTS

BLADDER DYSFUNCTION

The bladder receives innervation from the following systems: sympathetic (T10–L2, hypogastric nerve), parasympathetic (S2–4, pelvic nerves), and somatic (S2–4 pudendal nerve). There are two micturition centers, the sacral and the pontine. Urodynamic studies can be used to evaluate bladder function.

Lower motor neuron lesions cause a flaccid bladder and urinary incontinence, with voiding by overflow and a large volume of residual urine. Voiding may be accomplished by increasing the intra-abdominal pressure, although excessive residual urine or intravesical pressure may result. Long-term bladder management ideally consists of intermittent, clean self-catheterization that is timed to regularly empty the bladder and prevent periods of overdistention.

Upper motor neuron lesion may cause a spastic bladder, which can present early as frequency, urgency, and nocturia. Patients with upper motor neuron lesions may have a local reflex of bladder contraction (reflex voiding), but this often occurs against high sphincter pressure (bladder-sphincter dyssynergia), which in turn results in high intravesical pressure. Detrusor-sphincter dyssynergia is common when lesions are located between the sacral and pontine micturition centers. Untreated, this dyssynergia can lead to urinary

Table 18–6. Pharmacotherapy for Bladder Dysfunction in Patients With Spinal Cord Lesions

Drug	Initial Dose	Maximum Dose	Common Side Effects
Anticholinergics			
Oxybutynin			Dry mouth, blurred vision, urinary retention, sedation, constipation
(Ditropan)	5 mg orally 2–3 times a day	5 mg orally 4 times a day	
(Ditropan XL)	5–15 mg orally once a day	30 mg orally once a day	
(Oxytrol transdermal patch)	3.9/day patch, 1 patch twice a week	—	
Tolterodine			Same as above
(Detrol)	1–2 mg orally 2 times a day	4 mg/day	
(Detrol LA)	2–4 mg orally once a day	4 mg/day	
Others			
Trospium	20 mg orally twice a day		
(Sanctura)			
Darifenacin	Initial dose is 7.5 mg orally once a day; after 2 weeks may increase to 15 mg daily		
(Enablex)			
Solifenacin succinate	Initial dose is 5 mg orally daily; may be increased to 10 mg daily		
(Vesicare)			
Adrenergic Blockers			
Doxazosin (Cardura)	1 mg orally once a day	16 mg orally once a day	Hypotension, sedation, headache
Prazosin (Minipress)	1 mg orally 2 times a day	5 mg orally 3 times a day	
Terazosin (Hytrin)	1 mg orally at bedtime	5 mg orally 2 times a day	
Tamsulosin (Flomax)	0.4 mg orally once a day	0.8 mg orally once a day	Causes less hypotension than other α-adrenergic antagonists

postvoiding residual, incontinence, vesicoureteral reflux, and hydronephrosis. Bladder hyperreflexia can be treated with anticholinergic agents such as oxybutynin and tolterodine (Table 18–6); however, intermittent catheterization may still be required. The addition of α-blockers such as tamsulosin and doxazosin to reduce resistance to outflow at the α-adrenergically innervated bladder neck and internal sphincter can also be useful (see Table 18–6). Transurethral and transperineal injections of botulinum A toxin have been used to treat dyssynergia by lowering resistance to urine outflow. Alternatively, outlet obstruction can be reduced by transurethral sphincterotomy or placement of a urethral stent. Bladder augmentation (a surgical procedure to increase bladder size by using a section of the bowel or stomach) is occasionally required, as well as the placement of an abdominal stoma to ease intermittent catheterization.

Another approach to the management of upper motor neuron bladder dysfunction is the use of electric stimulation such as the NeuroControl VOCARE Bladder System or the InterStim neuromodulation system.

Postvoiding residuals should ideally be maintained at less than 100 mL to confirm adequate emptying. If the patient is performing intermittent catheterization, target volumes should be 400–500 mL. Although intermittent catheterization is preferred, some patients may require the long-term use of an indwelling catheter (eg, Foley catheter or suprapubic tube). Foley catheters are associated with bladder stones, prostatitis, epididymitis, and urethral strictures. Indwelling catheters increase the risk of carcinoma of the bladder. Frequent urinary tract infections may plague patients with indwelling catheters, and they should be monitored appropriately for symptoms and signs of infection.

BOWEL DYSFUNCTION

Two patterns of bowel dysfunction are identified. In lesions located above the conus (upper motor neuron), a hyperreflexic bowel is present. Below this level (lower motor neuron), the patient develops an areflexic bowel. Most patients with an areflexic bowel experience constipation and fecal impaction. Developing a bowel program for these patients is essential. One such bowel management regimen consists of a stool softener, such as docusate sodium, one to three times a day, with a stimulant laxative given 6–8 hours before defecation and a suppository such as bisacodyl or rectal stimulation at the time of the desired bowel movement. Patients should also be instructed to ingest a high-fiber diet.

DECUBITUS ULCERS

The most common sites for decubiti are the ischium, sacrum, greater trochanter, and heels. It is much easier to prevent decubiti than to treat them. Therefore the use of special mattresses and wheelchair cushions that can provide support over a broad area, protecting bony prominences, is

Table 18–7. Pharmacotherapy for Spasticity in Patients With Spinal Cord Lesions

Drug	Initial Dose	Maximum Dose	Common Side Effects
Baclofen (Lioresal)	5 mg orally 3 times a day	80 mg/day	Sedation, fatigue, weakness, lower seizure threshold, hallucinations, and seizures if withdrawn abruptly
Tizanidine (Zanaflex)	2 mg orally at bedtime	36 mg/day	Hypotension, drowsiness, weakness, abnormal liver function tests
Diazepam (Valium)	2.5 mg orally 2 times a day	60 mg/day	Sedation, weakness, memory loss, dependence
Dantrolene (Dantrium)	25 mg orally once a day	400 mg/day	Weakness, sedation, hepatitis, abnormal liver function tests
Clonidine (Catapres) (Catapres TTS weekly patch)	0.1 mg orally 2 times a day 0.1 mg/patch	2.4 mg/day 0.3 mg/patch	Weakness, sedation, dry mouth, hypotension, withdrawal hypertension

recommended. Frequent changes in position, a shift of bed position every 2 hours or a shift of weight in the wheelchair (15 seconds for every 30 minutes) are crucial.

Full-thickness skin loss, with underlying osteomyelitis (which is difficult to diagnose), can preclude healing. Bone biopsy is needed for definitive diagnosis, but bone scans, CT, and MRI can be informative. Ulcers that involve bone or muscle require surgical treatment. Primary closure of an ulcer is not effective in most cases, and wide excision and coverage with a myocutaneous flap are often necessary.

SPASTICITY

Spasticity is defined as a velocity-dependent increase in tonic stretch reflexes. Spasticity occurs frequently in patients with lesions located above the conus medullaris. It is usually absent immediately after an acute injury but develops over subsequent weeks. Initial treatment includes a program of regular muscle stretching to reduce the spasticity and prevent contracture. Baclofen is the treatment of choice for spasticity caused by spinal cord disorders, but other useful medications include diazepam and dantrolene (Table 18–7). There is also a class of medications called the imidazolines that reduce spasticity through their action on the CNS. These drugs typically cause less muscle weakness than do the benzodiazepines and may be valuable when it is important for the patient to retain strength. Medications in this class include tizanidine and clonidine (which is also used as an antihypertensive agent, and low blood pressure may limit its use).

If orally administered medication is ineffective or if spasticity is localized, phenol nerve blocks or botulinum toxin can be used. An intrathecal baclofen pump can be used in patients whose symptoms are refractory. Destructive procedures such as rhizotomy or cordotomy are rarely performed today.

AUTONOMIC DYSFUNCTION

Autonomic dysreflexia, an exaggerated autonomic response to stimuli, can occur in patients with lesions located at or above T6. Symptoms include headache, flushing above the level of the lesion, piloerection, and hypertension. Any noxious stimuli below the level of injury can result in symptoms due to the loss of supraspinal inhibitory control of segmental sympathetic neurons. Common causes are bladder distention, bowel distention, and decubiti. Management consists of removing the precipitating stimulus.

CONTRACTURES

Muscles that cross multiple joints, such as the biceps, hamstrings, tensor fascia lata, and the gastrocnemius, are prone to contractures. Treatment options include range-of-motion programs, bracing (eg, ankle-foot orthosis), serial casting, and, if needed, surgical release of the contracted muscle(s).

SEXUAL DYSFUNCTION AFTER SPINAL CORD INJURY

The autonomic nervous system is essential to the initiation and maintenance of penile erection. Parasympathetic stimulation initiates the erectile response, and sympathetic stimulation is necessary for ejaculation. Treatment options for erectile dysfunction include surgical procedures, vacuum devices, and pharmacologic interventions. Oral medications that produce vasodilation of the penile vascular tissues (eg, sildenafil [25–100 mg], tadalafil [10–20 mg], and vardenafil [5–20 mg]) can be used in treatment of patients with erectile dysfunction. The intracorporeal injection of papaverine, phentolamine, and prostaglandin E$_1$ can also be used to achieve erection. Surgical treatment involves the implantation of penile prostheses.

DEEP VEIN THROMBOSIS

The three primary risk factors for deep vein thrombosis are venous stasis, hypercoagulability, and vessel injury. The risk appears greatest during the first 2 weeks after spinal injury, and fatal pulmonary embolus is rare more than 3 months after injury.

Recommendations for prevention include use of antiembolism stockings or pneumatic compression stockings for at least 2 weeks; 5000 units of unfractionated heparin in motor-incomplete patients for 8 weeks; and either heparin adjusted to high-normal activated partial thromboplastin time or low-molecular-weight heparin in motor-complete patients for 8–12 weeks.

Treatment for an acute deep vein thrombosis requires 3 months of dose-adjusted anticoagulation therapy. This can consist of intravenous heparin adjusted to maintain the activated partial thromboplastin time at 1.5–2.5 of normal until warfarin produces an international normalized ratio (INR) between 2 and 3 or, alternatively, use of a low-molecular-weight heparin at a dose based on the patient's weight. For patients in whom anticoagulation is contraindicated, an inferior vena cava filter can be used.

Peripheral Neuropathies

19

Clifton Gooch, MD, & Tanya Fatimi, MD

Neuropathy is defined as a disease or injury of the peripheral sensory, motor, or autonomic nerves. It is usually categorized separately from selective injury to the cell body of the axon (neuronopathy), injury to the nerve roots distal to their origin (radiculopathy), or injury to the brachial or lumbosacral plexus (plexopathy). Neuropathy may be pure motor, pure sensory, or mixed sensorimotor. It may occur symmetrically throughout the body (polyneuropathy), individually in single nerves (mononeuropathy), or in multiple, scattered nerves in an irregular distribution (multifocal neuropathy). Autonomic neuropathy may accompany a larger neuropathic process or occur independently. Disorders of the autonomic nervous system are discussed in Chapter 21.

▶ Epidemiology & Etiology

A. Mononeuropathy

Mononeuropathies, particularly those resulting from nerve entrapment, are among the most common diseases affecting the general population. They can be caused or significantly exacerbated by repetitive motion injury during manual tasks such as keyboard operation. Median nerve entrapment resulting from carpal tunnel syndrome is the most common mononeuropathy, with a symptomatic prevalence of 14% and a much higher lifetime incidence. The ulnar and peroneal nerves are also commonly injured (at the elbow and the knee, respectively).

Mononeuropathy can also result from multifocal demyelination (eg, multifocal motor neuropathy), from ischemic injury as a result of occlusion of the vascular supply to an individual nerve (eg, mononeuropathy multiplex), or from trauma (Table 19–1).

B. Polyneuropathy

Polyneuropathy has hundreds of potential etiologies, the most common of which are summarized in Table 19–2. Diabetes mellitus is the most common cause of polyneuropathy in the United States, as it is in most of the Western world, affecting at least 1–2% of the population. Leprosy remains the most common cause of neuropathy worldwide, affecting millions more. The total prevalence of chronic symmetric polyneuropathy is estimated to be approximately 3.5% in the outpatient elderly population.

▶ Pathogenesis & Classification

Peripheral nerves consist of an electrically active core, or *axon*, and an external fatty layer of electrical insulation known as *myelin*. Axonal integrity is critical to action potential propagation along the cellular membranes of either motor or sensory nerves. Injury to the axon at any point along its course may block transmission. Myelin is also critical to impulse transmission along the length of the axon and increases conduction velocity through saltatory conduction, in which an impulse leaps from node to node between myelin segments. Demyelination disrupts saltatory conduction, slowing nerve conduction velocity. In addition, focal demyelination can cause sufficient leakage of axonal current to halt action potential propagation at a specific point along the nerve, causing *conduction block*.

Pathologically, nerve injury can be divided into four major categories.

1. **Neuronal degeneration** results from damage to the motor or sensory nerve cell bodies, with subsequent degeneration of their contiguous peripheral axons.

2. **Wallerian degeneration** results from damage to the axon at a specific point below the cell body, with degeneration distal to the injury.

3. **Axonal degeneration** results from diffuse axonal damage. Because the distal portion of the axon is farthest from the cell body, it undergoes the earliest and most severe change during diffuse neuronal injury, accounting for initial symptoms in the feet and hands, followed by gradual proximal ascent with continued injury (the so-called *dying back phenomenon*).

4. Finally, **segmental demyelination** results from injury to the myelin sheath without injury to the axon.

Table 19–1. Common Compressive Mononeuropathies

Nerve	Site(s) of Entrapment	Cause of Compression
Median	Wrist Forearm	Carpal tunnel syndrome (common) Anterior interosseous syndrome (rare)
Ulnar	Across elbow Upper forearm Wrist	Tardy ulnar palsy (common) Cubital tunnel syndrome (rare) Guyon canal stenosis (rare)
Radial	Axilla Spiral groove Forearm Wrist	Crutch palsy Pressure of hard object (eg, back of chair) against inner upper arm Entrapment of posterior interosseous nerve upon forceful supination Superficial radial nerve (handcuff palsy)
Lateral femoral cutaneous (lumbosacral plexus)	Anterior superior iliac spine	Meralgia paresthetica; compression occurs with obesity, pregnancy, tight belts
Femoral	Anterior upper leg	Compression of femoral artery postcatheterization
Sciatic	Pelvis	Piriformis syndrome; entrapment under ischial tuberosity while sitting
Peroneal	Across knee At fibular head	Prolonged squatting (strawberry picker palsy) Sitting with crossed legs (captain chair palsy)
Tibial	Across knee Ankle	(Rare) Tarsal tunnel syndrome (rare)

Table 19–2. Causes of Polyneuropathy

Category	Specific Process
Infectious diseases	Leprosy HIV infection Borreliosis (Lyme disease)
Inflammatory diseases	Acute inflammatory demyelinating polyneuropathy (Guillain-Barré syndrome) Chronic inflammatory demyelinating polyneuropathy Multifocal motor neuropathy Collagen vascular disease (eg, rheumatoid arthritis, sarcoidosis, Sjögren syndrome) Vasculitis
Other systemic diseases	Diabetes mellitus Chronic renal failure Thyroid dysfunction Parathyroid dysfunction Paraneoplastic neuropathy Paraproteinemia Amyloidosis Vitamin deficiency (eg, vitamin B_{12}) Critical illness neuropathy Acute intermittent porphyria
Genetic disorders	Hereditary motor sensory neuropathies (Charcot-Marie-Tooth family of diseases) Hereditary sensory and autonomic neuropathies
Toxins	Therapeutic drugs (eg, chemotherapeutic agents, antivirals, statins) Drugs of abuse (eg, alcohol, aromatic hydrocarbons) Poisons (eg, arsenic, n-hexane)

Peripheral neuropathies are classified according to rate of onset (acute, subacute, chronic), type of symptoms or deficits (sensory, motor, autonomic, or mixed), and distribution (distal or proximal; symmetric, asymmetric, or multifocal). Electromyographic (EMG) and nerve conduction studies determine whether the injury is primarily axonal, demyelinating, or mixed, and identifies the distribution and degree of deficit.

▶ General Diagnostic Approach

Evaluation of someone with suspected neuropathy begins with a comprehensive history, general physical examination, and neurologic examination, focusing on the diagnostic possibilities listed in Tables 19–1 and 19–2. Several blood studies should be considered (Table 19–3). Other blood studies may also be indicated, including assays for antibodies directed against specific nerve or myelin components, some of which may be associated with specific clinical syndromes, such as anti-GM_1 antibody (acute motor axonal neuropathy), anti-GQ_{1b} (Miller Fisher variant of Guillain-Barré syndrome), anti-Hu antibody (carcinomatous paraneoplastic sensory neuronopathy), anti–myelin-associated glycoprotein (MAG) antibody (multiple myeloma), and anti-sulfatide antibody (symmetric polyneuropathy with prominent distal sensory loss). Searches for other infectious processes, particularly HIV and hepatitis, may also be indicated. More rarely, serum cryoglobulins and serum and urine heavy metal screening may be needed.

Table 19–3. Commonly Ordered Laboratory Tests for Evaluation of Neuropathy

Category	Test
General serologic testing	Standard electrolyte panel (sodium, potassium, bicarbonate) Glucose and glycosylated hemoglobin levels Magnesium, calcium, and phosphorus levels Renal and liver function tests Creatine kinase levels Vitamin B_{12} methylmalonic acid and homocysteine Complete blood count with differential Erythrocyte sedimentation rate Thyroid function testing
Immunologic screening	Antinuclear antibody Rheumatoid factor Serum protein electrophoresis Quantitative immunoglobulins
Infectious disease screening	Rapid plasma reagin Lyme titers

Lumbar puncture is especially important for the diagnosis of acute inflammatory demyelinating polyradiculopathy and chronic inflammatory demyelinating polyneuropathy, and may provide additional information regarding infectious and neoplastic diseases as well, but is not needed for most neuropathy evaluations. EMG and nerve conduction studies, the single most important diagnostic test for the evaluation of neuropathy, are described in Chapter 2.

The indications for nerve biopsy are highly limited, and it should be used sparingly, as harvesting of the sural nerve at the ankle (the most common procedure) carries a 10–15% risk of chronic neuropathic pain at the biopsy site. Biopsy can help to establish the diagnosis in suspected vasculitis, amyloidosis, sarcoidosis, giant axonal neuropathy, and leprosy. More refined diagnostic tools include quantitative sensory testing, autonomic studies, and skin biopsy with staining and quantitation of intraepidermal small sensory nerve fibers.

England JD, Asbury AK. Peripheral neuropathy. *Lancet* 2004;363:2151–2161. [PMID: 15220040] (Excellent review of the causes, diagnosis, and treatment of peripheral neuropathy, with a listing of Internet resources.)

Fuller G. Diagnosing and managing mononeuropathies. *Clin Med* 2004;4:113–117. [PMID: 15139726] (Brief, clinically relevant review of common mononeuropathies.)

Pascuzzi RM. Peripheral neuropathies in clinical practice. *Med Clin North Am* 2003;87:697–724. [PMID: 12812409] (Focused discussions, in case-based format, of common peripheral neuropathy presentations to the general practitioner.)

MONONEUROPATHIES

CRANIAL NERVE DISORDERS

Injury most often affects the peripheral cranial nerves individually, although they can be damaged in combination. This chapter addresses lesions of cranial nerves (CNs) III through VII, and IX through XII. Injury to CN VIII is addressed in Chapter 6.

OCULOMOTOR NERVE (CN III)

ESSENTIALS OF DIAGNOSIS

► Horizontal diplopia that is worse on lateral gaze
► Exotropic (abducted) and hypotropic (depressed) eye
► Dilated pupil (mydriasis) on the affected side in most cases
► Ptosis

► General Considerations

The oculomotor nerve innervates the medial rectus, superior rectus, inferior rectus, inferior oblique, and levator palpebrae muscles and supplies parasympathetic innervation to the pupil, facilitating constriction (Table 19–4).

► Clinical Findings

A. Symptoms and Signs

Patients typically complain of diplopia, which is worse in horizontal gaze with the affected eye adducted. With a complete lesion, examination reveals a fixed, dilated pupil and exotropia, with the affected eye in a "down-and-out" position, as well as ptosis. Because the parasympathetic fibers travel in the periphery of the nerve, they are typically the first affected with extrinsic compression, causing isolated mydriasis. However, with nerve ischemia, the parasympathetic fibers are usually unaffected, causing a "pupil-sparing" third nerve palsy (typical of diabetic injury to the third cranial nerve). Third nerve palsy can result from many causes, including trauma (fracture to the supraorbital fissure), compressive lesions (posterior communicating artery aneurysm, intracranial tumor, herniation of the uncus of the temporal lobe due to increased intracranial pressure), ischemia (secondary to diabetic occlusion of the vasa nervorum, producing a pupil-sparing palsy), meningitis, syphilis, herpes zoster, tumor, and demyelination.

B. Diagnostic Studies

An acute or subacute third nerve palsy is a neurologic emergency and is treated as an expanding posterior communicating artery

Table 19–4. Actions of the Oculomotor, Trochlear, and Abducens Nerves

Nerve	Innervation	Eye Function	Clinical Presentation
Oculomotor (CN III)	Superior rectus	Elevates in abduction; intorts in adduction	Eye looks "down and out"; associated with paralysis of other muscles innervated by CN III
	Medial rectus	Adducts	Primarily horizontal diplopia; associated with paralysis of other muscles innervated by CN III
	Inferior rectus	Depresses in abduction; extorts in adduction	Upward and outward deviation of affected eye; associated with paralysis of other muscles innervated by CN III
	Inferior oblique	Elevates in adduction; extorts in abduction	Incyclotorsion; head tilt to the side of the paretic inferior oblique; associated with paralysis of other muscles innervated by CN III
	Levator palpebrae	Elevates upper lid	Ptosis
	Pupil and ciliary muscles	Accommodation	Dilated pupil; unreactive to light; paralysis of accommodation
Trochlear (CN IV)	Superior oblique	Depresses in adduction; intorts in abduction	Extorsion of eye; head tilt away from affected eye; vertical diplopia on down gaze
Abducens (CN VI)	Lateral rectus	Abducts	Inability to abduct eye; horizontal diplopia

CN = cranial nerve.

aneurysm until proven otherwise. The clinical examination may suggest either a compressive lesion or infarction, but expeditious imaging studies, including magnetic resonance imaging (MRI) with gadolinium contrast, magnetic resonance angiography (MRA), and, in some cases, cerebral angiography must be performed. Lumbar puncture and blood studies to exclude infectious, autoimmune, and other disorders are often needed (Table 19–5). Chronic syndromes should also be addressed without delay, because aneurysmal expansion and tumor can produce a chronic course prior to catastrophic sudden decline.

▶ **Differential Diagnosis**

The differential diagnosis of third nerve palsy includes brainstem infarction, myasthenia gravis, orbital disease (eg, Graves ophthalmopathy), Horner syndrome (although the pupil on the affected side is miotic), congenital ptosis, and congenital anisocoria.

TROCHLEAR NERVE (CN IV)

 ESSENTIALS OF DIAGNOSIS

▶ Vertical diplopia that is worse with the affected eye adducted
▶ Head tilt away from the affected eye

The trochlear nerve innervates the superior oblique muscle, which intorts and depresses the eye (see Table 19–4). Fourth nerve palsy is the most common cause of vertical diplopia, which is most severe when the eye is adducted. Head tilt is to the side opposite the affected eye. In primary gaze, the affected eye is vertically higher (hypertropic). Most acquired fourth nerve palsies are isolated and caused by trauma. Bilateral palsies can occur from a blow to the vertex of the head with damage to the decussating trochlear fascicles. Injury can also occur from ischemia to the

Table 19–5. Laboratory and Neuroimaging Tests for Evaluation of Cranial Neuropathies

Category	Test
General serologic testing	Standard electrolyte panel Magnesium and calcium levels Glucose and glycosylated hemoglobin levels Creatine kinase levels Complete blood count with differential Erythrocyte sedimentation rate Angiotensin-converting enzyme
Immunologic screening	Antinuclear antibody Lumbar puncture for oligoclonal bands, IgG synthesis rate Acetylcholine receptor antibodies Rheumatoid factor
Infectious disease screening	Rapid plasma reagin Lyme titers Screening for tuberculosis—chest radiograph, PPD test, lumbar puncture for TB-PCR
Imaging studies	MRI of brain with and without gadolinium Cerebral angiography, in some cases

IgG = immunoglobulin G; MRI = magnetic resonance imaging; PPD = purified protein derivative; TB-PCR = tuberculosis by polymerase chain reaction.

nerve, especially in diabetic patients. In children, isolated superior oblique palsies are usually congenital or traumatic. Demyelinating disease, tumor, and lesions of the cavernous sinus are less common causes of fourth nerve injury.

Acute-onset fourth nerve palsy, similar to other acute cranial nerve lesions, should be expeditiously investigated. MRI with gadolinium contrast should be performed to rule out tumor, lesions of the cavernous sinus, and other potential emergent intracranial diseases. Lumbar puncture may be needed to assess for infection or inflammation, and blood studies should be performed to assess for inflammatory disease, diabetes mellitus, thyroid disease, and myasthenia gravis (see Table 19–5).

The differential diagnosis is limited mostly to intraorbital lesions that mechanically interfere with the movement of the eye, such as Graves ophthalmopathy or intraorbital tumor. Myasthenia gravis should also be considered.

TRIGEMINAL NERVE (CN V)

1. Trigeminal Neuralgia

Trigeminal neuralgia is discussed in Chapter 8.

2. Trigeminal Neuropathy

 ESSENTIALS OF DIAGNOSIS

► Unilateral loss of facial sensation
► Absent corneal reflex
► Weakness of muscles of mastication with deviation of the jaw to the weak side

The trigeminal nerve innervates the muscles of mastication and provides sensory innervation to the face. Sensory branches are divided into the ophthalmic division (V1), the maxillary division (V2), and the mandibular division (V3).

In trigeminal neuropathy, sensory loss is most prominent on one side of the face; however, patients may report loss of sensation of mucous membranes of the oral and nasal cavities. The corneal reflex may be absent or diminished. Paralysis of the muscles of mastication and deviation of the jaw to the weak side may occur, as well as deafness to low-pitched sounds from paralysis of the tensor tympani muscle. Tumor, demyelinating disease, syringobulbia, or vascular disease can involve the trigeminal nucleus. Infection, trauma, aneurysm, and malignancy can affect the nerve fascicle.

Blood studies and neuroimaging can be used to investigate trigeminal neuropathy (see Table 19–5). The differential diagnosis includes supranuclear lesions (eg, infarction of the sensory cortex).

ABDUCENS NERVE (CN VI)

 ESSENTIALS OF DIAGNOSIS

► Horizontal diplopia that is worse when looking toward the affected side
► Adduction of the affected eye in primary gaze

The sixth cranial nerve innervates the ipsilateral lateral rectus muscle (see Table 19–4). Patients complain of horizontal diplopia looking toward the affected side and when looking into the distance. At rest, the eye is deviated inward (adducted).

Sixth nerve palsy may result from meningitis; compression by an enlarged, ectatic basilar artery; hydrocephalus; demyelinating disease; tumor; and disease of the cavernous sinus. Ischemia of the nerve most commonly affects diabetic patients. Unilateral or bilateral abducens palsy can be the result of increased intracranial pressure even in the absence of direct compression by a mass lesion.

Acute-onset sixth nerve palsy, similar to other acute cranial nerve lesions, should be expeditiously investigated. Diagnostic workup is similar to that of oculomotor and trochlear palsy (see Table 19–5).

The differential diagnosis includes brainstem lesions (especially ischemic and demyelinating) and intraorbital lesions such as Graves ophthalmopathy or intraorbital tumor. Myasthenia gravis must also be considered.

SYNDROMES INVOLVING CRANIAL NERVES III, IV, & VI

1. Tolosa-Hunt Syndrome

Tolosa-Hunt syndrome is an inflammatory process of CNs III, IV, or VI alone or in combination. Patients are usually 30–50 years old, and both men and women are affected equally. Unilateral, steady, orbital pain develops over several weeks. Optic nerve involvement is rare, but the ophthalmic division of the trigeminal nerve can be affected. Diagnosis is made after excluding other space-occupying lesions in the superior orbital fissure and its neighboring structures. Tolosa-Hunt syndrome is responsive to corticosteroids. Spontaneous remissions can occur.

2. Cavernous Sinus Syndromes

The third, fourth, and sixth cranial nerves traverse the cavernous sinus with the carotid artery and the first and second divisions of the trigeminal nerve. Carotid dissection, carotid aneurysm, thrombophlebitis of the cavernous sinus, and fungal infections (*Mucor* or *Rhizopus* species) can cause dysfunction of any or all of the cranial nerves coursing through the cavernous sinus.

FACIAL NERVE (CN VII)

ESSENTIALS OF DIAGNOSIS

- ▶ Unilateral weakness of the upper and lower face
- ▶ Loss of taste on the anterior two thirds of the tongue
- ▶ Hyperacusis
- ▶ Loss of blink reflex on the affected side

▶ General Considerations

The facial nerve contains a *motor division*, which innervates the muscles of facial expression, and an *intermediate nerve*, which carries parasympathetic fibers to the lacrimal, parotid, submandibular, and sublingual glands, as well as taste fibers from the anterior two thirds of the tongue and

sensory fibers from the external auditory canal and pinna (Figure 19–1).

▶ Clinical Findings

A. Symptoms and Signs

Patients typically present with unilateral facial weakness and a facial droop that is most obvious around the mouth. On careful questioning, they may also complain of increased sensitivity to sound and eye irritation on the affected side (resulting from corneal dryness secondary to incomplete eyelid closure). Physical examination reveals unilateral upper and lower facial weakness that includes decreased forehead wrinkling and difficulty raising the eyebrows. (In contrast, a supranuclear lesion affecting the face causes only lower facial weakness and spares the forehead.) The corneal reflex is decreased or absent. Hyperacusis may be noted on tests of hearing, and there may be loss of taste over the anterior two thirds of the tongue.

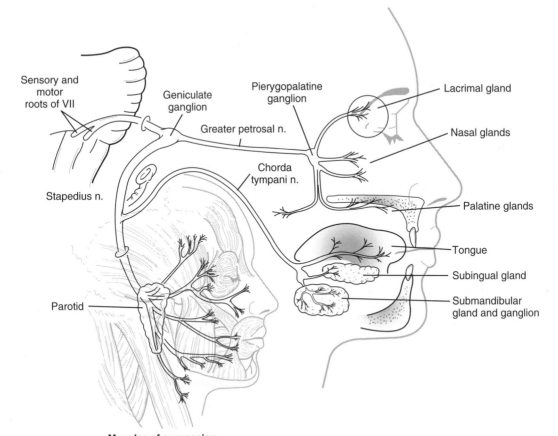

▲ Figure 19–1. Anatomy and histopathology of the facial nerve. (Reprinted from *Medical Clinics of North America,* 1999;83(1):179–195, Jackson CG, von Doersten PG, The facial nerve. Current trends in diagnosis, treatment, and rehabilitation. Copyright 1999, with permission from Elsevier.)

B. Diagnostic Studies

1. Electrophysiologic testing—Electrophysiologic studies are a critical part of the evaluation of seventh nerve injury, because they confirm its presence and define the type (axonal versus demyelinating), site, and severity of injury. As with other acute nerve injuries, abnormalities following proximal axonal injury may not be detectable for 72 hours or more, whereas purely demyelinating proximal injuries may have minimal effects on more distal nerve conductions.

2. Neuroimaging—Gadolinium-enhanced MRI is usually indicated, particularly if a parotid mass is found or clinical examination suggests a compressive lesion in the cerebellopontine angle or internal auditory canal. MRI can reveal enhancement of the geniculate ganglion in patients with Bell palsy. High-resolution computed tomography (CT) may be useful in patients with suspected temporal bone lesions and in patients in whom MRI is contraindicated.

3. Blood studies—Blood studies to investigate facial nerve weakness are similar to those employed for other cranial neuropathies (see Table 19–5).

► Differential Diagnosis

The differential diagnosis of seventh nerve palsy is summarized in Table 19–6. The most common cause of facial paralysis, by far, is the idiopathic syndrome of Bell palsy.

1. Bell Palsy

► General Considerations

Bell palsy is a clinical syndrome of idiopathic acute unilateral facial paralysis. The incidence of Bell palsy is approximately 1 case in 5000 people. It is more common during pregnancy and among the elderly.

Table 19–6. Causes of Facial Nerve Palsy

Category	Disease
Trauma	Temporal bone fracture
Infection and parainfection	Middle ear or mastoid infection Bacterial infections—Lyme disease, syphilis, diphtheria, leprosy Viral infections—herpes zoster (Ramsay Hunt syndrome), poliomyelitis, HIV, herpes simplex virus type 1 Tuberculous meningitis
Tumors	Parotid gland tumor Cerebellopontine angle tumor
Autoimmune disorders	Guillain-Barré syndrome Multiple sclerosis Neurosarcoidosis

► Clinical Findings

Patients may report that exposure to cold preceded their symptoms, and they may complain of facial numbness or stiffness without any objective sensory deficit. Some describe mild to moderate pain at the angle of the jaw. Decreased tearing and hyperacusis may appear or in some cases may precede weakness. Although not life threatening, Bell palsy may have severe functional, aesthetic, and psychological consequences.

True Bell palsy is idiopathic by definition. However, reactivation of herpes simplex virus type 1 may play an important role in some cases. Another proposed etiology is autoimmunity.

► Differential Diagnosis

The clinical features of seventh nerve infarction can be indistinguishable from those of Bell palsy. Infarction occurs either within the brainstem or along the course of the nerve and is usually associated with diabetes mellitus or hypertension.

► Treatment
A. Pharmacotherapy

Although not all studies concur, corticosteroids are safe and probably effective for improving functional outcome in patients with Bell palsy. Prednisone, 1 mg/kg/day for 1 week, can be given. Antiviral therapy is more controversial; studies suggest that acyclovir combined with prednisone is possibly effective in improving functional outcome. Dosing schedules vary, but acyclovir, 400 mg five times daily for 7–10 days, can be given if renal function is normal. Valacyclovir, 1 g three times daily, is commonly used because it requires less frequent dosing.

B. Surgical Therapy

Surgical decompression was suggested as acute therapy for Bell palsy based on the hypothesis that neuronal swelling within the temporal bone contributes to compressive nerve injury. However, prospective, randomized data are lacking in this area, and the treatment is highly invasive and risks permanent hearing loss.

C. Supportive Care

Although the great majority of patients with Bell palsy recover, temporary or permanent facial paralysis warrants attention to eye protection. Patients should receive artificial tears and ophthalmic ointments. Glasses or goggles are important to protect from light, wind, and dust. Protection of the eye at night with an eye patch is often necessary. Ophthalmologic consultation should be sought in patients with long-term disability.

► Prognosis

Bell palsy has a good prognosis; at least 70–90% of patients improve without treatment, and 90% achieve complete functional recovery with corticosteroid treatment. During the recovery period, patients may experience synkinesis, or involuntary activation of facial muscles in one region during voluntary activation in another (eg, uncontrolled, simultaneous blinking with chewing), as a result of aberrant reinnervation during recovery. Patients with incomplete recovery may have permanent deficits ranging from a cosmetic deformity to chronic corneal desiccation. Recurrence occurs in up to 10% of patients, either unilaterally or contralaterally.

2. Ramsay Hunt Syndrome

Ramsay Hunt syndrome is acute unilateral facial palsy caused by herpes zoster. Its clinical presentation differs from Bell palsy in that patients often complain of exquisite pain in the ear prior to the onset of facial weakness 1–3 days later. On examination they have eruption of vesicles in the external auditory meatus and over the mastoid process. Similar to Bell palsy, Ramsay Hunt syndrome is more prevalent during pregnancy, and it may involve other cranial nerves, especially the trigeminal nerve. Most patients regain full functional facial strength.

Treatment of Ramsay Hunt syndrome includes corticosteroids (1 mg/kg/day, tapering over 10 days) and early administration of acyclovir, 400 mg five times daily for 7–10 days.

3. Benign Hemifacial Spasm

Benign hemifacial spasm is characterized by continual facial twitching predominantly around the eye and mouth. It is usually caused by compressive irritation of the facial nerve by an anomalous arterial supply or by a tumor in the cerebellopontine angle. Treatment typically consists of botulinum toxin injections every 4–6 months. More definitive treatment involves tumor removal or microvascular decompression of the facial nerve.

VESTIBULOCOCHLEAR NERVE (CN VIII)

Disorders involving the eighth cranial nerve are discussed in Chapter 6.

GLOSSOPHARYNGEAL NERVE (CN IX)

ESSENTIALS OF DIAGNOSIS

- ▶ Loss of the gag reflex
- ▶ Loss of sensation in the pharynx, tonsils, and posterior tongue
- ▶ Loss of taste in the posterior one third of the tongue
- ▶ Hypersensitive carotid sinus reflex

▶ General Considerations

The glossopharyngeal nerve conveys taste from the posterior one third of the tongue, provides parasympathetic innervation to the parotid gland, controls swallowing in conjunction with CNs X and XII, and carries sensation from the pharyngeal wall. It also receives input from the carotid sinus, which has baroreceptors and mediates arterial blood pressure, and from the carotid body, which has chemoreceptors for carbon dioxide and oxygen levels in the blood.

▶ Clinical Findings
A. Symptoms and Signs

Ninth nerve injury may be accompanied by loss of the ipsilateral gag reflex, loss of taste on the posterior one third of the tongue, and diminished sensation in the posterior pharynx. Injury that involves other neighboring cranial nerves, such as mass lesions compressing CNs IX, X, and XI at the jugular foramen (jugular foramen syndrome), is more common.

Examination may reveal an asymmetric gag reflex, decreased pharyngeal sensation, or reduced taste sensation over the posterior tongue. Glossopharyngeal neuralgia is discussed in Chapter 8.

B. Diagnostic Studies

MRI can identify brainstem infarctions or other intraparenchymal lesions, as well as lesions along the course of the nerve.

▶ Differential Diagnosis

The differential diagnosis of glossopharyngeal nerve dysfunction includes disorders that cause focal bulbar motor injury, resulting in dysarthria, hoarseness, and dysphagia. These disorders include infarction, bulbar amyotrophic lateral sclerosis, and bulbar myasthenia gravis, as well as rare myopathic disorders (eg, oculopharyngeal dystrophy).

VAGUS NERVE (CN X)

ESSENTIALS OF DIAGNOSIS

- ▶ Ipsilateral weakness of the soft palate, pharynx, and larynx, causing hoarseness, dyspnea, dysarthria, and dysphagia
- ▶ Loss of the gag reflex
- ▶ Loss of the cough reflex

▶ General Considerations

The vagus nerve controls phonation, swallowing (along with CNs IX and XII), elevation of the palate, taste, and cutaneous sensation from the ear, along with motor innervation to the vocal cords. It also provides important parasympathetic innervation to the heart, lungs, stomach, upper intestine, and ureter.

► Clinical Findings

A. Symptoms and Signs

Lesions of the vagus nerve can cause hoarseness and dysphagia. Impaired palatal elevation may be seen ipsilateral to the lesion, and the uvula deviates away from the side of damage. Bilateral vagal nerve injury causes significant autonomic dysfunction. Aortic aneurysms and neck and thoracic surgery can damage the recurrent laryngeal nerve, resulting in hoarseness. Bilateral recurrent laryngeal nerve paralysis can cause stridor and death.

B. Diagnostic Studies

MRI studies can assess the integrity of the vagus nerve from the nucleus outward. Laryngoscopic examination by an otorhinolaryngologist may reveal unilateral vocal cord paralysis. If bilateral injury is suspected, autonomic testing may be informative (see Chapter 21).

► Differential Diagnosis

The differential diagnosis of vagus nerve dysfunction is the same as that of glossopharyngeal nerve dysfunction, described earlier.

► Treatment

Vagus nerve dysfunction may have serious implications and may cause upper airway respiratory compromise due to vocal cord paralysis, which may necessitate endotracheal intubation or more permanent tracheostomy. Severe swallowing difficulty may warrant the placement of an enteral feeding tube. Consultation with a therapist to evaluate speech and swallowing function, an otolaryngologist to assess the airway, and a gastroenterologist may be required.

SPINAL ACCESSORY NERVE (CN XI)

ESSENTIALS OF DIAGNOSIS

► Weakness on rotating the head away from the side of injury (sternocleidomastoid muscle)
► Weakness of neck extension and shoulder elevation (trapezius muscle)

► General Considerations

The spinal accessory nerve arises from motor neurons in the upper cervical spinal cord, ascends through the foramen magnum, and then exits through the jugular foramen to supply the sternocleidomastoid and trapezius muscles.

► Clinical Findings

A. Symptoms and Signs

Causes of spinal accessory nerve injury include iatrogenic damage (eg, lymph node dissection, placement of central venous catheters, other types of neck surgery), traumatic injuries such as indirect traction during blunt trauma and dislocations of the sternoclavicular and acromioclavicular joints, extended use of an arm sling with compression of the spinal accessory nerve, and basilar meningitis.

Injury to the spinal accessory nerve causes weakness of the trapezius muscle, along with shoulder droop and lateral scapular winging (rotation of the inferior border of the scapula laterally). The entire shoulder girdle loses strength and abduction, and forward flexion becomes impaired. Subacromial impingement, spasm of other periscapular muscles, additional weakness from traction on the brachial plexus, adhesive capsulitis, and thoracic outlet syndrome are potentially disabling secondary effects.

When the lesion is proximal to the branch to the sternocleidomastoid muscle, the patient has difficulty turning the head to the opposite side.

B. Diagnostic Studies

Plain radiographs, CT scan, or MRI of the head, cervical spine, and shoulder can be helpful. EMG and nerve conduction studies can identify the lesion, assist with prognosis, and help with decisions regarding nerve exploration or muscle transfer.

► Differential Diagnosis

Injury to the spinal accessory nerve must be differentiated from central ischemic lesions, anterior horn cell disease (eg, poliomyelitis or amyotrophic lateral sclerosis), or injury to peripheral nerves or the proximal brachial plexus, such as the long thoracic nerve (to the serratus anterior) or the branch to the rhomboid muscles, which also produce abnormalities of scapular function and scapular winging. Upper cervical radiculopathy affecting the third and fourth nerve roots can also cause trapezius weakness. Myasthenia gravis, polymyositis, and some hereditary myopathies can cause weakness of neck flexion and extension. Mechanical dysfunction secondary to musculoskeletal injury and disease, such as shoulder girdle injury, scapular injury, contracture formation, adhesive capsulitis, and glenohumeral instability, may also suggest trapezius injury.

► Treatment

Treatment depends on the type of injury, the degree of dysfunction, and the patient's needs. If a clearly reversible cause is identified (eg, mass lesion), appropriate therapy is obvious.

In patients with nerve laceration, microsurgical repair or grafting may restore function if performed acutely. If the injury cannot be repaired, the nerve may regenerate; the odds of spontaneous recovery can often be estimated from clinical and electrophysiologic data. If axonal injury is limited, the odds of some recovery are usually good. If functional improvement is poor after 1 year, surgery to provide compensatory function may be indicated. Transfer of the levator scapulae to provide the functions of the trapezius (elevation, retraction, and rotation of the scapula) is one surgical option.

HYPOGLOSSAL NERVE (CN XII)

ESSENTIALS OF DIAGNOSIS

▶ Dysarthria

▶ Tongue deviation on protrusion toward the side of the lesion

The hypoglossal nerve innervates the ipsilateral tongue. With nerve injury and ipsilateral tongue paralysis, the tongue deviates toward the side of the injury. With long-standing, severe hypoglossal damage, hemiatrophy and fasciculations of the tongue can be seen. Ischemia to the medial medulla can cause unilateral hypoglossal nerve palsy. Amyotrophic lateral sclerosis and poliomyelitis can affect the hypoglossal nucleus. Bilateral lesions of the hypoglossal nerve are rare. Multiple sclerosis, syringobulbia, and tumors can cause unilateral or bilateral hypoglossal damage because of the close proximity of the two hypoglossal nuclei.

Electrophysiologic testing can identify tongue denervation, but nerve conduction studies are not feasible. MRI can detect mass lesions and central ischemia and can sometimes reveal a pattern of unilateral genioglossus atrophy.

The differential diagnosis of hypoglossal nerve injury includes other disorders causing dysarthria and dysphagia, such as stroke and myasthenia gravis.

Apart from resection of mass lesions, few treatments are available for most of the causes of hypoglossal injury. Speech therapy may help patients by providing strategies for improving pronunciation and food handling, and by strengthening further the unaffected side of the tongue.

Friedman RA. The surgical management of Bell's palsy: A review. *Am J Otol* 2000;21:139–144. [PMID: 10651450] (Reviews literature on pathophysiology of Bell palsy and the history of facial nerve surgery for this disorder.)

Gilchrist JM. Seventh cranial neuropathy. *Semin Neurol* 2009;29:5–13. [PMID: 19214928]

Grogan PM, Gronseth GS. Practice parameter: Steroids, acyclovir, and surgery for Bell's palsy (an evidence-based review). *Neurology* 2001;56:830–836. [PMID: 11294918] (Evaluation of

literature on Bell palsy treatment, with American Academy of Neurology recommendations.)

Hazin R, Azizzadeh B, Bhatti MT. Medical and surgical management of facial nerve palsy. *Curr Opin Ophthalmol* 2009;20:440–450. [PMID: 19696671]

Holland NJ, Weiner GM. Recent developments in Bell's palsy. *BMJ* 2004;329:553–557. [PMID: 15345630]

Lee AG, Hayman LA, Brazis PW. The evaluation of isolated third nerve palsy revisited: An update on the evolving role of magnetic resonance, computed tomography and catheter angiography. *Surv Ophthalmol* 2002;47:137–157. [PMID: 11918895] (Reviews recent literature on the use of neuroimaging in patients with third nerve palsy.)

UPPER EXTREMITY NERVES

MEDIAN NERVE

The median nerve arises from the lateral (C6–C7) and the medial cords (C8–T1) of the brachial plexus. The nerve runs deep in the proximal arm, the medial antecubital fossa, and the ventral forearm before becoming more superficial as it approaches the wrist, enters the carpal tunnel, and passes into the palm. The median nerve supplies muscles in the forearm and hand as shown in Figure 19–2 and described in Table 19–7. It also provides cutaneous sensation to the palmar side of the first three-and-a-half digits, as well as their dorsal sides to the first interphalangeal joint.

1. Median Mononeuropathy at the Wrist (Carpal Tunnel Syndrome)

ESSENTIALS OF DIAGNOSIS

▶ Numbness and pain in the first three digits

▶ Exacerbation of symptoms by manual activity or during sleep

▶ Difficulty with fine manual tasks (eg, buttoning)

▶ Weakness of thumb abduction and opposition

▶ Atrophy of thenar muscles

▶ General Considerations

The carpal tunnel, located at the base of the palm, is formed by carpal bones on the median, dorsal, and lateral sides and is covered ventrally by the flexor retinaculum, a tough fibrous band. The median nerve is prone to compression at this location with repetitive flexion or extension (Figure 19–3). Consequently, carpal tunnel syndrome is one of the most common occupational diseases. Several medical conditions also increase the risk of carpal tunnel syndrome, including diabetes mellitus, hypothyroidism, pregnancy, rheumatoid arthritis, obesity, and, less commonly, amyloidosis and acromegaly.

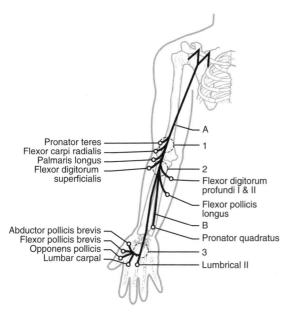

▲ **Figure 19–2.** Median nerve (A) with its branch, the anterior interosseous nerve (B), and the muscles they supply. The nerve may undergo compression at the elbow between the two heads of the pronator teres (1), or slightly distally (2), as in anterior interosseous syndrome, or at the palm (3), as in carpal tunnel syndrome. (Reproduced with permission from Kimura J. *Electrodiagnosis in Diseases of Nerve and Muscle: Principles and Practice,* 3rd ed. Oxford University Press, 2001, p. 14. Modified from *The Guarantors of Brain: Aids to the Examination of the Peripheral Nervous System,* 4th ed. Saunders, 2000.)

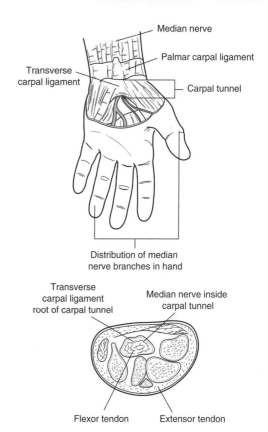

Distribution of median
nerve branches in hand

▲ **Figure 19–3.** Median nerve coursing through the carpal tunnel. (From Katz JN, Simmons BP. Carpal tunnel syndrome. *N Engl J Med* 2002;346:1807–1812, used with permission.)

Table 19–7. Motor Functions of the Median Nerve

Action	Muscle
Forearm pronation	Pronator teres, pronator quadratus
Wrist flexion, radial side	Flexor carpi radialis
Flexion of IP joint of thumb	Flexor pollicis longus
Flexion of proximal IP joint of digits 2–5	Flexor digitorum superficialis
Flexion of distal IP joints of digits 2 and 3	Flexor digitorum profundi I and II
Thumb abduction	Abductor pollicis brevis
Opposition of thumb and 5th digit	Opponens pollicis
Extension of finger at proximal IP joint with MCP joint fixed	Lumbricals to index and middle fingers

IP = interphalangeal; MCP = metacarpophalangeal.

▶ Clinical Findings

A. Symptoms and Signs

Patients with carpal tunnel syndrome complain of pain, paresthesias, or numbness in the first three digits. Symptoms are usually worse with repetitive or sustained wrist flexion or extension (eg, typing, driving) but are also often exacerbated during sleep due to unconscious sustained wrist flexion. In some patients, pain may radiate up the medial forearm. Numbness often is difficult for patients to localize and may involve only part of the dermatome (ie, the thumb). Symptoms are initially intermittent but can become constant if injury continues. Hand weakness, manifested by difficulties with fine manual coordination, particularly in tasks involving the thumb, is a feature of more severe, long-standing disease and may be accompanied by thenar flattening.

On examination, sensation may or may not be abnormal in the median territory at rest. Tinel sign is elicited by lightly percussing the median nerve at the wrist with a reflex hammer.

Phalen sign is performed by flexing and holding the wrist with some pressure at 90 degrees for 1 minute. With active nerve compression, paresthesias in the median nerve territory may be elicited with either maneuver. Detectible clinical weakness is usually limited to the abductor pollicis brevis, because the other muscles of the thumb (flexor pollicis brevis and adductor pollicis) receive dual innervation by both the ulnar and median nerves. Weakness of thumb opposition can appear as the disease advances. Thenar atrophy may be evident.

B. Diagnostic Studies

EMG and nerve conduction studies are critically important in the evaluation of carpal tunnel syndrome, not only for confirming the diagnosis but also to ensure that other nerve injuries are not also present.

The evaluation of motor and sensory conduction time through the carpal tunnel is a standard technique. Patients with mild nerve compression demonstrate only sensory slowing, whereas those with more severe compression demonstrate motor abnormalities. Loss of motor amplitudes is a worrisome sign because it heralds motor axonal injury, which might not improve with decompression, arguing for early surgical intervention.

Depending on the clinical setting, blood studies to assess for diabetes mellitus, thyroid dysfunction, rheumatoid arthritis, and other systemic diseases may be indicated. Although not needed in most patients, imaging studies, including MRI, may be used to screen for joint abnormalities and nerve compression.

▶ Differential Diagnosis

The differential diagnosis of numbness or weakness of the hand includes stroke, cervical radiculopathy, brachial plexopathy, more proximal median nerve injury, and ulnar nerve injury. Pain alone may be caused by joint or tissue injury or inflammation such as flexor tendonitis and arthritis of the wrist. These disorders, particularly cervical radiculopathy and arthritis of the wrist, may occur simultaneously with carpal tunnel syndrome. Traumatic injuries may also injure the median nerve.

▶ Treatment

Conservative therapy should be attempted first, except in patients with progressive motor injury, intractable and severe pain, or in those for whom median nerve–associated numbness is disabling (eg, diamond cutters, microsurgeons). Conservative therapy consists of wrist splinting in the neutral position at night and during activities that encourage wrist flexion and extension. Splinting can provide relief of pain and numbness within days in some patients. Concurrently, anti-inflammatory agents, vitamin B_6, or diuretics are sometimes used. Short courses of oral prednisone may also be useful for symptomatic improvement. Local corticosteroid injection, although increasingly popular, remains controversial. The effects of injection are transient in most patients, and there is a risk of worsening with inadvertent injection into the carpal tunnel.

Carpal tunnel release surgery is an option for patients who do not respond to more conservative management. The traditional or "open" approach involves transection of the transverse carpal ligament. The procedure has excellent success rates with few complications. Newer methods include endoscopic carpal tunnel release surgery, although the efficacy of this approach compared with more traditional methods is not yet clear.

2. Median Mononeuropathy at the Elbow

Entrapment of the median nerve can occur at or immediately below the elbow. In addition, the anterior interosseous branch can become compressed in the forearm. Each of these entrapments is far less common than carpal tunnel syndrome. Table 19–8 summarizes the modes of entrapment and their clinical presentations. Trauma, especially elbow fracture and dislocation, is another cause of median nerve injury at the elbow, as is penetrating injury of the antecubital fossa (eg, hypodermic injection). The differential diagnosis and diagnostic evaluation of these disorders is similar to that for carpal tunnel syndrome, and electrophysiologic testing and appropriate imaging studies are essential. Treatment depends on the specific cause, severity, and location of the injury. In general, the efficacy of surgical release in treating these disorders is less clear than in carpal tunnel syndrome.

High median nerve compression at the shoulder or proximal humerus is very rare. The majority of lesions are traumatic, with associated injury to the soft tissue and bones around the shoulder. Extrinsic compression caused by crutches can rarely occur but much more commonly causes radial nerve dysfunction. Vascular compression by an aneurysm of the brachial or axillary arteries can cause spontaneous median nerve injury. High median nerve compression results in significant loss of all median motor functions, especially in the wrist and the hand. Treatment is usually conservative. Early return of function usually predicts a complete recovery. Arteriography should be considered in patients with nontraumatic compression.

ULNAR NERVE

ESSENTIALS OF DIAGNOSIS

- ▶ Numbness and pain in the fourth and fifth digits
- ▶ Exacerbation of symptoms by prolonged elbow flexion
- ▶ Difficulty with fine manual tasks
- ▶ Weakness of finger abduction
- ▶ Claw-hand deformity

Table 19–8. Median Neuropathy Sites Above the Wrist

Location	Mechanism of Neuropathy	Clinical Findings
Above elbow	Entrapment by ligament of Struthers (fibrous band extending from humerus to medial epicondyle)	Rarely severe Pain above elbow Local tenderness near ligament of Struthers
At elbow	Entrapment by hypertrophied pronator teres Entrapment by tendinous band of pronator teres	Moderate aching pain in proximal forearm Hand clumsiness Paresthesias in median nerve distribution Worse with repetitive elbow motion
Forearm (anterior interosseous branch)	Entrapment by pronator teres tendon (deep head) Entrapment by flexor digitorum superficialis tendon Forearm fracture or inflammation	Acute pain in proximal forearm Recent trauma or muscle exertion Pinch weakness Absent flexion of distal IP joint (thumb) Absent flexion of the distal IP joint (2nd digit) Associated with neuralgic amyotrophy

IP = interphalangeal.

► General Considerations

The ulnar nerve, composed of fibers from the C8 and T1 nerve roots, travels medial to the brachial artery in the upper arm, across the elbow in the ulnar groove (where it may be stretched and compressed with elbow flexion), through the cubital tunnel just distal to the elbow (another potential entrapment site), and then through the canal of Guyon (yet another entrapment site) into the hand. The ulnar nerve innervates muscles in the forearm and hand (Figure 19–4, Table 19–9). Its sensory territory includes the hypothenar eminence, medial dorsum of the hand, and dorsal and palmar surfaces of the fifth finger and half of the fourth finger.

► Clinical Findings

A. Symptoms and Signs

As noted, the ulnar nerve is liable to damage at several points along its course. Compression at the elbow is very common, and second only to carpal tunnel syndrome as a cause of compressive mononeuropathy (Table 19–10). The ulnar nerve can also be damaged in the axilla, upper arm, forearm, wrist, and hand. Ulnar neuropathy can cause more prominent motor than sensory loss, leading to a debilitating impairment of the intrinsic hand muscles. Although most injuries result from compression, penetrating trauma and injury associated with elbow, forearm, and wrist fracture also occur.

Patients with mild ulnar nerve entrapment typically present with intermittent numbness and tingling along the medial aspect of the hand, which is often worsened by elbow flexion. More severe entrapment can result in constant paresthesias, cramping, and pain in the medial hand. Weakness of grasp or pinch and hand clumsiness may be the first motor findings. Atrophy of the intrinsic hand muscles can occur with prolonged ulnar nerve damage. On physical

examination, elbow range of motion and deformity should be evaluated. Worsening of symptoms with sustained elbow flexion or a positive Tinel sign at sites of compression lends

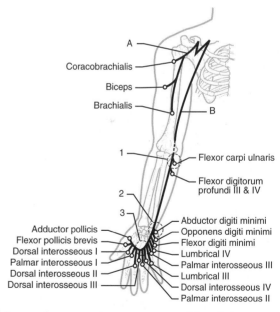

Figure 19–4. Musculocutaneous nerve (A) and ulnar nerve (B), and the muscles they supply. Common sites of lesion include the ulnar groove and cubital tunnel (1), Guyon canal (2), and mid-palm (3). (Reproduced with permission from Kimura J. *Electrodiagnosis in Diseases of Nerve and Muscle: Principles and Practice,* 3rd ed. Oxford University Press, 2001, p. 14. Modified from *The Guarantors of Brain: Aids to the Examination of the Peripheral Nervous System,* 4th ed. Saunders, 2000.)

Table 19–9. Motor Functions of the Ulnar Nerve

Action	Muscle
Wrist flexion, ulnar side	Flexor carpi ulnaris
Flexion at distal IP joint	Flexor digitorum profundus, digits 4 and 5
Touching 2nd digit to 4th digit; spreading fingers	Interossei
Extension of finger at proximal IP joint with the MCP joint fixed	Lumbricals to digits 4 and 5
Adduction of thumb at right angle to palm	Adductor pollicis
Flexion at MCP joint	Flexor digiti minimi
Abduction of 5th digit	Abductor digiti minimi
Pinch between thumb and 5th digit	Opponens digiti minimi

IP = interphalangeal; MCP = metacarpophalangeal.

support to the diagnosis. With sustained motor weakness, a claw-hand deformity of the fourth and fifth digits, and loss of sensation in these digits and the ulnar half of the hand may be found. Ulnar strength may be assessed using several maneuvers (see Table 19–9).

B. Diagnostic Studies

As with median neuropathy, EMG and nerve conduction studies are critically important in the evaluation of ulnar mononeuropathy. Blood studies and imaging can be informative in some cases.

▶ Differential Diagnosis

The differential diagnosis in patients with ulnar neuropathy includes the same disorders that can be confused with median neuropathy. Some of these disorders, particularly cervical radiculopathy and arthritis of the wrist, may occur simultaneously with ulnar mononeuropathy.

▶ Treatment

Patients without substantial motor axonal involvement, intractable pain, or disabling sensory loss (for certain professions) should be treated conservatively in most cases. Sustained elbow flexion and resting the elbow on hard surfaces such as desks are common precipitators of ulnar compression, and patients should avoid such activities or postures. Patients may wear simple elastic elbow bandages during sleep to prevent sustained elbow flexion. If these measures prove ineffective, a short course of oral corticosteroids followed by long-term nonsteroidal therapy may be useful.

If conservative therapy is ineffective within 4–8 weeks, ulnar decompression may be considered. Many techniques for decompression or transposition have been proposed, but the surgeon performing these procedures should be specifically trained in ulnar nerve decompression and transposition.

RADIAL NERVE

 ESSENTIALS OF DIAGNOSIS

▶ Wrist drop
▶ Weakness of finger and thumb extension
▶ Difficulty with manual tasks
▶ Numbness over the radial aspect of the dorsum of the hand (dorsolateral)

▶ General Considerations

The radial nerve begins in the axilla, courses down the upper arm in the spiral groove of the humerus, and in the forearm branches into a posterior interosseous branch, supplying forearm muscles (Figure 19–5, Table 19–11), and a sensory branch to the dorsolateral aspect of the hand. A proximal branch of the radial nerve provides sensation to the skin of the lateral arm and the dorsal forearm.

Table 19–10. Ulnar Nerve Compression Sites

Location	Mechanism of Entrapment	Clinical Findings
Elbow	Ulnar groove (compression or stretch) Cubital tunnel syndrome (anatomic)	Numbness in medial hand, worsened by elbow flexion Weakness of grasp or pinch Claw hand in severe, chronic compression
Wrist (Guyon canal)	Extrinsic compressive neuropathy Anatomic entrapment Wrist fracture	Pure motor (deep palmar branch), hypothenar weakness Pure sensory (superficial palmar branch), palm numbness Mixed motor and sensory (both)
Palm	Deep palmar branch (blunt trauma to palm) Superficial palmar branch (blunt trauma to palm)	Pure motor (deep palmar branch), hypothenar weakness Pure sensory (superficial palmar branch), palm numbness

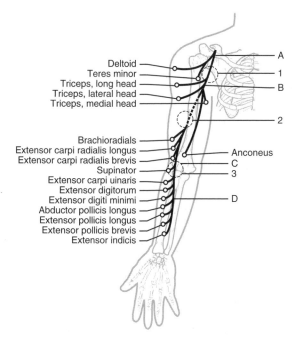

Deltoid — A
Teres minor — 1
Triceps, long head — B
Triceps, lateral head
Triceps, medial head — 2

Brachioradials
Extensor carpi radialis longus — Anconeus
Extensor carpi radialis brevis — C
Supinator — 3
Extensor carpi uinaris
Extensor digitorum — D
Extensor digiti minimi
Abductor pollicis longus
Extensor pollicis longus
Extensor pollicis brevis
Extensor indicis

▲ **Figure 19–5.** Axillary nerve (A) and radial nerve (B) with its main terminal branch, the posterior interosseous nerve (C), and the muscles they supply. Nerve injury may occur at the axilla (1), spiral groove (2), or elbow (3), as in posterior interosseous nerve syndrome. (Reproduced with permission from Kimura J. *Electrodiagnosis in Diseases of Nerve and Muscle: Principles and Practice,* 3rd ed. Oxford University Press, 2001, p. 14. Modified from *The Guarantors of Brain: Aids to the Examination of the Peripheral Nervous System,* 4th ed. Saunders, 2000.)

Table 19–11. Radial Nerve Injury Sites

Location	Mechanism of Entrapment	Clinical Findings
Axilla	Crutches	Wrist drop Triceps involved Sensory loss
Spiral groove	Extrinsic compression, fracture	Wrist drop Sensory loss
Posterior interosseous nerve	Entrapment at supinator muscle Occurs with rheumatoid arthritis, trauma, fracture, strenuous use of arm	Weakness of finger extensors Radial wrist deviation
Superficial sensory branch (cheiralgia paresthetica)	Handcuffs	Paresthesias on dorsum of hand

▶ **Clinical Findings**

A. Symptoms and Signs

The radial nerve is susceptible to injury in many different locations. Compression is the most common cause; other kinds of trauma, ischemia, and inflammation may also cause damage. Compression in the axilla, most commonly resulting from improperly fitted crutches, causes triceps weakness in addition to wrist drop, finger extensor weakness, and sensory loss. Humeral fracture or extrinsic compression of the nerve against the humerus, such as resting a head on the inside of the upper arm or propping the arm on a hard edge (so-called *Saturday night palsy*), causes weakness of wrist and finger extension but may spare the triceps. Sensation may be impaired, and the brachioradialis reflex may be lost. In the forearm, the posterior interosseous branch may be compressed by the supinator muscle during forceful supination, causing weakness of the finger extensors and partial weakness of the wrist extensors. Compression of the superficial sensory branch at the wrist from a tight watch, bracelet, or handcuffs causes paresthesias in the dorsum of the hand. Radial nerve injuries caused by compression usually improve within several weeks.

B. Diagnostic Studies

As with median and ulnar neuropathy, EMG and nerve conduction studies are critically important in the evaluation of radial mononeuropathy, particularly to differentiate radial injury from brachial plexopathy and cervical radiculopathy. Electrodiagnostic testing can gauge the type, precise location, and severity of the damage, and aid in prognostication. Imaging studies, including MRI, may be used to screen for shoulder, humerus, and joint injury and for nerve compression caused by mass lesions.

▶ **Differential Diagnosis**

The differential diagnosis of radial neuropathy includes the same disorders considered in patients with median and ulnar neuropathy. Pain alone, particularly in the forearm, may be caused by extensor tendonitis (so-called *tennis elbow*).

▶ **Treatment**

Therapy is directed at removing causes of compression. Rehabilitation, with passive range-of-motion and other exercises, as well as wrist splinting, may be indicated.

Gerritsen AAM, et al. Systematic review of randomized clinical trials of surgical treatment for carpal tunnel syndrome. *Br J Surg* 2001;88:1285–1295. [PMID: 11578281] (Quantitative meta-analysis and qualitative analysis of 14 studies evaluating open carpal tunnel release.)

Katze JN, Simmons BP. Carpal tunnel syndrome. *N Engl J Med* 2002;346:1807–1812. [PMID: 12050342] (Concise review of the diagnosis and treatment of carpal tunnel syndrome with excellent illustrations.)

LOWER EXTREMITY NERVES

FEMORAL NERVE

ESSENTIALS OF DIAGNOSIS

▶ Weakness of hip flexion and knee extension

▶ Atrophy of the quadriceps compartment

▶ Buckling of the knee with ambulation

▶ Loss of deep tendon reflex at the knee

▶ Loss of sensation over the anterior thigh and medial calf

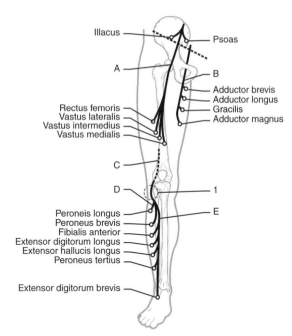

▲ **Figure 19–6.** Femoral nerve (A), obturator nerve (B), and common peroneal nerve (C), branching into superficial (D) and deep peroneal nerve (E), and the muscles they supply. Compression of the peroneal nerve commonly occurs at the fibular head (1). (Reproduced with permission from Kimura J. *Electrodiagnosis in Diseases of Nerve and Muscle: Principles and Practice,* 3rd ed. Oxford University Press, 2001, p. 14. Modified from *The Guarantors of Brain: Aids to the Examination of the Peripheral Nervous System,* 4th ed. Saunders, 2000.)

▶ General Considerations

The femoral nerve originates from the L2–L4 spinal roots and the lumbar plexus and then passes into the thigh, where it innervates the hip flexors and knee extensors (Figure 19–6) and gives off sensory branches to the anterior thigh and the medial calf. Diabetes mellitus can produce femoral neuropathy as a result of ischemic infarction of the nerve. Hip or pelvic fractures can cause local lacerations of the femoral nerve at the level of the inguinal ligament. Iatrogenic injury to the femoral nerve may occur during intrapelvic surgery or femoral artery catheterization in the femoral triangle (usually during compression of the artery after the procedure). Prolonged hip flexion (as in childbirth) or extension can stretch and injure the femoral nerve. Compression from retroperitoneal tumors and hematomas is a rare cause of injury.

▶ Clinical Findings

A. Symptoms and Signs

On examination, patients may have quadriceps weakness with sparing of the hip adductors (obturator nerve function) and knee flexors (sciatic nerve). Sensation is typically lost over the anterior thigh and medial calf. The patellar reflex is diminished or absent.

B. Diagnostic Studies

Electrodiagnostic testing can usually differentiate between lumbar radiculopathy, plexopathy, neuromuscular junction disease, myopathy, and femoral neuropathy. Although direct nerve conduction studies of the femoral nerve are technically challenging and often unreliable, needle EMG can clearly detect denervation isolated to the femoral myotome and can exclude the aforementioned mimics. As with other nerve injuries, electrophysiologic studies aid in localizing the site of injury along the nerve and in determining prognosis.

▶ Differential Diagnosis

Upper lumbar radiculopathy and lumbar plexopathy may closely mimic femoral mononeuropathy. Proximal leg weakness, especially when bilateral, has a host of causes, including neuromuscular junction disease (myasthenia gravis, Lambert-Eaton myasthenic syndrome) and most acquired myopathies. These entities do not cause sensory loss and are rarely strikingly asymmetric. Osteoarthritis of the hip and knee may limit hip flexion and knee extension mechanically or because of pain.

▶ Treatment

Treatment of femoral neuropathy is usually conservative and is aimed at eliminating any source of compression. Physical therapy and knee bracing to keep the leg extended during ambulation may be helpful.

SCIATIC NERVE

ESSENTIALS OF DIAGNOSIS

► Weakness of knee flexion and of dorsiflexion and plantar flexion of the ankles and toes
► Atrophy of the muscles below the knee
► Foot drop during ambulation
► Loss of the Achilles tendon reflex
► Loss of sensation over the entire foot (except the medial malleolus)

▶ General Considerations

The sciatic nerve, originating from L4, L5, S1, and S2, is composed of two distinct and functionally separate halves, which ultimately become the peroneal and the tibial nerves. The sciatic nerve passes underneath the piriformis muscle in the pelvis and exits through the sciatic notch to enter the posterior leg. In the distal thigh, it divides to form the peroneal and tibial nerves (Figures 19–6 and 19–7). The sciatic, posterior tibial, and peroneal nerves supply sensation to the anterolateral leg and the entire foot except for the medial malleolus.

▶ Clinical Findings
A. Symptoms and Signs

Although patients often use the term *sciatica* to describe pain radiating down the leg, actual damage to the sciatic nerve is rare. The most common cause of true sciatic nerve injury is hip surgery and hip fracture. Gunshot wounds and other types of external trauma can also damage the sciatic nerve. Compression to the nerve can occur in the pelvis from neoplasm or retroperitoneal hemorrhage. The peroneal division is much more likely to be injured during crush or stretch injury of the sciatic nerve, although the tibial division is more susceptible to misplaced injection injury in the buttocks. Rarely, the piriformis muscle can entrap the sciatic nerve trunk as it passes through or over the piriformis muscle (piriformis syndrome). In addition to trauma, ischemia (eg, diabetic mononeuropathy), inflammation, infection, and other processes may selectively damage the nerve.

When the sciatic nerve is damaged, weakness may be found in the hip extensors and the foot and toe dorsiflexors and extensors. In partial injury, foot dorsiflexion is more severely weakened than plantar flexion. Sensation can be lost over the anterolateral leg and entire foot (sparing the medial malleolus), and the ankle jerk may be diminished.

B. Diagnostic Studies

Electrophysiologic testing is useful to distinguish among anterior horn cell disease, radiculopathy, lumbar plexopathy, peroneal or tibial mononeuropathy, and true sciatic nerve

damage. Imaging studies of the lumbosacral spine, pelvis, thigh, and knee may also be needed.

▶ Differential Diagnosis

Sciatic nerve injury is most commonly mimicked by lower lumbosacral radiculopathy, although peroneal or tibial mononeuropathies can produce the deficits of sciatic nerve damage. Foot drop and distal leg weakness may also be seen in central disorders, such as stroke or mass lesion, and may be the presenting feature in patients with anterior horn cell disease.

▶ Treatment

Treatment is aimed at alleviating the underlying cause of compression or injury, if reversible. Physical therapy and orthotics, particularly ankle-foot orthoses, may help to compensate for permanent deficits.

PERONEAL NERVE

ESSENTIALS OF DIAGNOSIS

Common Peroneal Nerve
► Foot drop
► Weakness and atrophy of the anterior compartment muscles
► Sensory loss over the anterolateral leg and dorsum of the foot

▶ General Considerations

The common peroneal nerve originates as a branch of the sciatic nerve in the popliteal fossae and receives innervation from L4, L5, and S1 (see Figure 19–7). Passing through the knee and wrapping around the lateral aspect of the fibular head, it splits into the deep peroneal and superficial peroneal nerves. The deep peroneal nerve innervates ankle and toe dorsiflexors but not the ankle evertors, as well as a small patch of sensation to the web space between the first and second toes. The superficial peroneal nerve supplies the ankle evertors, as well as the anterolateral lower leg and dorsum of the foot.

▶ Clinical Findings
A. Symptoms and Signs

Injury to the common peroneal nerve is the most common mononeuropathy of the lower extremity. It is frequently caused by weight loss during prolonged illness and hospitalization, with extrinsic compression of the nerve between the fibular head and firm mattresses or side rails. Fracture of the fibular head and external blunt trauma, knee surgery, suspension of legs in straps, and positioning for lithotomy during gynecologic procedures can also cause compressive injury.

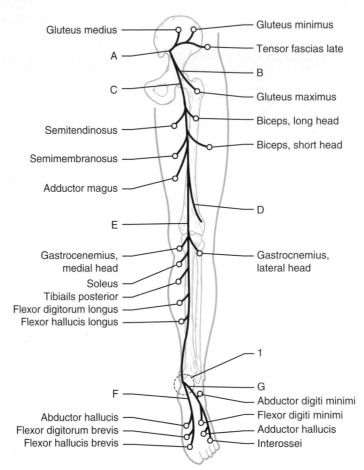

Gluteus medius — A

Gluteus minimus

Tensor fascias late

B

C

Gluteus maximus

Biceps, long head

Semitendinosus

Biceps, short head

Semimembranosus

Adductor magus

D

E

Gastrocenemius, medial head

Gastrocnemius, lateral head

Soleus

Tibiails posterior

Flexor digitorum longus

Flexor hallucis longus

1

G

F

Abductor digiti minimi

Abductor hallucis

Flexor digiti minimi

Flexor digitorum brevis

Adductor hallucis

Flexor hallucis brevis

Interossei

▲ **Figure 19–7.** Superior gluteal nerve (A), inferior gluteal nerve (B), and sciatic nerve trunk (C), and the muscles they supply. The sciatic nerve bifurcates to form the common peroneal nerve (D) and the tibial nerve (E). The tibial nerve in turn gives rise to the medial (F) and lateral plantar nerve (G). Compression of the tibial nerve may occur at the medial malleolus in the tarsal tunnel (1). (Reproduced with permission from Kimura J. *Electrodiagnosis in Diseases of Nerve and Muscle: Principles and Practice,* 3rd ed. Oxford University Press, 2001, p. 14. Modified from *The Guarantors of Brain: Aids to the Examination of the Peripheral Nervous System,* 4th ed. Saunders, 2000.)

Ankle trauma involving inversion and plantar flexion can result in sudden traction of the common peroneal nerve as it is anchored to the peroneus longus. Another very common cause of peroneal nerve injury is chronic crossing of the legs, as well as prolonged squatting or sitting with the feet folded under the buttocks. Trauma to the knee or mass lesions in the popliteal fossa (eg, tumor or hematoma) may involve the peroneal nerve.

Table 19–12 summarizes clinical findings in peroneal nerve compression. Lesions of the common peroneal nerve cause loss of ankle dorsiflexion with foot drop. Patients may lift the affected foot high off the ground by taking very high steps, resulting in a "steppage gait." Sensory loss over the anterolateral leg and dorsum of the foot may occur, but pain and paresthesias are rare and usually are not part of the presenting complaint.

Damage to the deep peroneal nerve causes similar weakness of dorsiflexion, but in contrast to common peroneal nerve injury, eversion is normal and sensory loss is restricted to the dorsal web space between the first two digits. With lesions at the anterior tarsal tunnel of the ankle, weakness of toe extensors occurs, with sparing of foot dorsiflexion. This syndrome can be painful, with aching at the ankle, and patients may plantar flex and medially deviate the foot to avoid pain.

Damage to the superficial peroneal nerve causes isolated weakness of eversion, with sensory loss over the anterolateral leg and dorsum of the foot. The superficial peroneal nerve is rarely injured near the fibular neck, but may become entrapped as it pierces the fascia in the mid-anterior leg.

Table 19–12. Peroneal Nerve Compression Sites

Location	Mechanism of Entrapment	Clinical Findings
Common peroneal nerve	Compression at fibular head	Impaired dorsiflexion and eversion of ankle Sensory loss to anterolateral leg and dorsum of foot
Deep peroneal nerve	Entrapment in anterior tarsal tunnel at ankle	Weakness of toe dorsiflexion Eversion spared Sensory loss in first dorsal web space
Superficial peroneal nerve	Entrapment at fascial exit on anterolateral leg	Weakness of eversion (proximal damage only) Dorsiflexion spared Sensory loss of anterolateral leg and dorsum of foot

Injury at the mid-leg or below causes a pure sensory mononeuropathy.

B. Diagnostic Studies

Electrophysiologic studies enable differentiation between peroneal mononeuropathy and anterior horn cell disease, lower lumbosacral radiculopathy, lumbosacral plexopathy, sciatic nerve injury, asymmetric polyneuropathy, and distal myopathy. They can also localize the site of the peroneal injury. Imaging studies of the pelvis, thigh, knee, or ankle may also be needed and should be guided by findings on electrodiagnostic testing. Other studies may be indicated if a more generalized polyneuropathy or myopathy is found.

▶ Differential Diagnosis

Peroneal nerve injury is often confused with L5–S1 radiculopathy. However, peroneal mononeuropathy does not affect the deep tendon reflex at the ankle or the strength of plantar flexion. Other processes that may present with prominent foot drop include stroke and motor neuron disease. Injury to the lumbosacral plexus and sciatic nerve must also be considered. Some distal myopathies (eg, myotonic dystrophy) and generalized polyneuropathies (eg, Charcot-Marie-Tooth family) may also produce foot drop, but these should be readily distinguished after careful history, physical examination, and electrophysiologic studies.

▶ Treatment

Conservative treatment with bracing may be needed in common peroneal nerve injuries at the knee. Patients should refrain from crossing their legs, squatting for prolonged periods, or sitting with their knees bent over the surface of a hard chair or bench. Surgical treatment with end-to-end anastomosis may be indicated in acute laceration injury. As with other mononeuropathies, the prognosis depends on the degree and chronicity of axonal injury, which can be assessed through historical, clinical, and electrophysiologic data.

POSTERIOR TIBIAL NERVE

ESSENTIALS OF DIAGNOSIS

▶ Weakness of plantar flexion of the ankle and toes

▶ Weakness and atrophy of calf muscles

▶ Sensory loss over the sole of the foot

The posterior tibial nerve branches off the sciatic nerve at the knee and provides innervation to the muscles that control plantar flexion and many of the intrinsic foot muscles, as well as sensation to the sole of the foot and the lateral heel. Posterior tibial nerve injury is much rarer than peroneal nerve injury but can occur in the popliteal fossa during trauma or surgery. Entrapment may occur as the tibial nerve passes through the posterior tarsal tunnel behind the medial malleolus, causing pain at the ankle and painful paresthesias of the sole, which is worse during standing or walking. Tinel sign may sometimes be elicited posterior to the medial malleolus. Foot and ankle fractures, diabetes mellitus, peripheral vascular disease, rheumatologic conditions, and tenosynovitis may contribute to tarsal tunnel syndrome.

Electrophysiologic studies enable differentiation between tibial mononeuropathy, lower lumbosacral radiculopathy, lumbosacral plexopathy, and sciatic nerve injury. Imaging studies of the pelvis, thigh, knee, or ankle may also be needed.

S1 radiculopathy and partial sciatic nerve injury most commonly mimic tibial nerve injury. Injury to the lumbosacral plexus is a much more rare cause.

In patients with mild posterior tarsal tunnel syndrome, anti-inflammatory agents and orthotics can be used. Corticosteroid injection and occasionally decompression of the tibial nerve in the ankle are sometimes performed, but the role of surgery in the management of these patients remains controversial.

LATERAL FEMORAL CUTANEOUS NERVE

ESSENTIALS OF DIAGNOSIS

▶ Numbness and pain over the lateral aspect of the thigh
▶ Absence of weakness, atrophy, or lower leg symptoms

The lateral femoral cutaneous nerve, a pure sensory nerve derived from the upper lumbar roots (L2–L3), supplies sensation to the lateral aspect of the thigh, passing underneath the inguinal ligament. The nerve is susceptible to compression as it courses from the pelvis to the leg underneath the inguinal ligament. Patients present with unilateral paresthesias, pain, or numbness in the outer and upper thigh without motor complaints (meralgia paresthetica). Tight clothing, heavy utility belts, obesity, and pregnancy all may precipitate this syndrome. Prolonged standing can worsen the symptoms.

Electrophysiologic studies are useful to exclude radiculopathy and femoral neuropathy. Direct conductions of the lateral femoral cutaneous nerve are technically difficult but can sometimes demonstrate a unilateral defect. Imaging studies of the lumbosacral spine or pelvis are sometimes needed.

The differential diagnosis includes femoral neuropathy and radiculopathy affecting the L2–L4 nerve roots. Unlike meralgia paresthetica, these disorders cause motor symptoms and loss of the patellar reflex.

Patients should be instructed to lose weight and avoid tight clothing and heavy utility belts. Meralgia paresthetica is usually self-limiting but may become chronic if the inciting factors are not addressed.

MULTIPLE MONONEUROPATHY SYNDROMES

Specific disease syndromes may involve a series of nerves, either regionally or in a multifocal pattern, mimicking focal or multifocal entrapment neuropathies.

IDIOPATHIC BRACHIAL PLEXITIS (NEURALGIC AMYOTROPHY)

ESSENTIALS OF DIAGNOSIS

▶ Acute shoulder pain
▶ Arm weakness and numbness within hours to days
▶ Monophasic course with recovery over months

Idiopathic brachial plexitis (neuralgic amyotrophy or Parsonage Turner syndrome) is an idiopathic, presumably inflammatory attack on the brachial plexus, often in a multifocal distribution. An autoimmune mechanism is likely.

Patients typically present with acute shoulder pain, followed within hours to days by numbness and weakness of the arm or hand. These symptoms rapidly plateau and are usually followed by gradual recovery over months. Most patients recover completely and recurrence is rare, although some patients may have permanent deficits.

Electrophysiologic studies are of critical importance, but nerve conduction abnormalities may not appear for up to several days after onset, and needle EMG may not become abnormal for 2–3 weeks. Imaging studies of the neck and shoulder may be indicated, and blood studies to assess for a broader autoimmune process may be needed.

The differential diagnosis includes stroke, acute radiculopathy, and traumatic injury to the shoulder or plexus, such as shoulder dislocation or rotator cuff injury.

Most patients recover without treatment. Physical therapy is helpful for aiding recovery and preventing complications. Within days of onset, a tapering course of corticosteroids may be given, although the efficacy of this intervention remains uncertain.

DIABETIC AMYOTROPHY

This disorder is discussed under Diabetic Neuropathies later in this chapter.

MONONEUROPATHY MULTIPLEX

ESSENTIALS OF DIAGNOSIS

▶ Multiple mononeuropathies appearing over hours to days
▶ Completely different and unrelated nerves affected in different areas
▶ Wrist drop, foot drop, and facial palsies (common)
▶ Usually occurs as part of a more generalized vasculitis or vasculopathy
▶ A neurologic emergency that may progress to respiratory compromise

▶ **General Considerations**

Mononeuropathy multiplex is the name given to several syndromes in which autoimmune attack on the vasculature of the peripheral nerves (the vasa nervorum) results in inflammation, occlusion, and ischemia in separate peripheral, cranial, and respiratory nerves throughout the body.

▶ **Clinical Findings**

A. Symptoms and Signs

Patients typically present with acute onset of motor weakness, which may be preceded by pain. Within hours to days, a second nerve, often in a different extremity, may be affected. In some instances, generalized vasculitic infarction of the peripheral nerves follows, which may include the nerves of the respiratory system, resulting in respiratory compromise. In other cases, peripheral nerve infarction precedes a rapidly progressive generalized vasculitis. Most cases of true mononeuropathy multiplex are not isolated to the peripheral nervous system but are instead part of a broader vasculitis.

Medical conditions associated with mononeuropathy multiplex include not only vasculitis, but also rheumatoid arthritis and other collagen vascular diseases (eg, sarcoidosis), viral infections (eg, HIV, hepatitis B and C), Lyme disease, leprosy, tumor infiltration, and lymphoid granulomatosis. Diabetes mellitus can cause multiple mononeuropathies but not typically as a rapidly progressive syndrome over days.

B. Diagnostic Studies

Electrophysiologic studies are of critical importance, but nerve conduction abnormalities may not appear for up to several days after the onset of the initial deficit, and needle EMG may not become abnormal for 2–3 weeks. If the deficits are restricted to a specific region (eg, leg), imaging studies of the back or extremity may be indicated. If embolic stroke is a consideration, MRI of the brain may be needed. Blood studies to assess for a broader autoimmune process may be indicated.

▶ Differential Diagnosis

The differential diagnosis includes multiple strokes, regional peripheral nerve syndromes (eg, brachial plexitis, diabetic amyotrophy), atypical polyneuropathy, and multiple compressive mononeuropathies. Multifocal motor neuropathy and hereditary neuropathy with liability to pressure palsies are part of the differential diagnosis of mononeuropathy multiplex. They are discussed later in this chapter.

▶ Treatment

Acute decompensation may require aggressive treatment with powerful immunosuppressive agents, such as intravenous cyclophosphamide, high-dose corticosteroids, or both, and patients may require observation in a critical care unit. If respiratory symptoms appear, mechanical ventilation may be needed. Specific autoimmune diseases should be treated in consultation with a rheumatologist after the initial episode of mononeuropathy multiplex has been adequately controlled.

▼ ACQUIRED POLYNEUROPATHIES

AUTOIMMUNE NEUROPATHIES

GUILLAIN-BARRÉ SYNDROME

ESSENTIALS OF DIAGNOSIS

- ▶ Rapidly progressive paralysis, often ascending
- ▶ Areflexia
- ▶ Increased cerebrospinal fluid (CSF) protein without increased cell count (albuminocytologic dissociation)
- ▶ Evidence of demyelination on nerve conduction studies (may be delayed)
- ▶ A neurologic emergency that may rapidly progress to respiratory compromise

▶ General Considerations

Guillain-Barré syndrome refers to a group of immune-mediated disorders targeting the peripheral nerves (Table 19–13).

Table 19–13. Guillain-Barré Syndrome: Subtypes and Clinical Findings

Guillain-Barré Subtype	Clinical Findings	Antibodies	EMG/NCS Findings
Acute inflammatory demyelinating polyneuropathy (AIDP)	Ascending paralysis Minor sensory symptoms	Nonspecific	Demyelination on NCS Absent F waves
Acute motor axonal neuropathy (AMAN)	Flaccid paralysis Often with *Campylobacter jejuni* infection	IgG anti-GM$_1$, IgG anti-GD$_{1a}$	Reduced motor amplitudes Normal sensory studies
Acute motor sensory axonal neuropathy (AMSAN)	Acute (< 1 wk) Profound quadriparesis Ventilation often required	IgG anti-GM$_1$	Reduced or absent motor amplitudes Reduced or absent sensory amplitudes Axonal injury by EMG
Miller Fisher syndrome	Ataxia Areflexia Ophthalmoplegia	IgG anti-GQ$_{1b}$	Decreased sensory nerve action potential Motor conductions often normal

EMG = electromyography; NCS = nerve conduction studies.

This syndrome has an annual incidence ranging from 1–2 cases per 100,000 people.

The most common form of Guillain-Barré syndrome, **acute inflammatory demyelinating polyradiculoneuropathy (AIDP)**, accounts for 85–90% of cases. It is characterized by progressive weakness of the extremities (more than one limb) and attenuation or loss of reflexes. The suspected target antigens are located on the myelin sheath, but the precise epitope has yet to be identified. Pathologically, demyelination begins in the proximal nerves then extends distally as the disease progresses.

Upper respiratory infection, gastrointestinal infection, or nonspecific febrile illness precedes neurologic symptoms in about 60% of patients. Although respiratory infections are most common, *Campylobacter jejuni* (a cause of gastroenteritis) is the most frequently identified organism. There is growing evidence that cross-reactivity of *C jejuni* epitopes and peripheral nerve gangliosides may play a role in the development of postinfectious AIDP. Cytomegalovirus, Epstein-Barr virus, *Mycoplasma* pneumonia, HIV, and hepatitis A and B infection have all been associated with AIDP. Several other antecedent events including surgery, cancer, pregnancy, autoimmune disease, and vaccinations (eg, the swine flu vaccine of 1976) have also been linked to AIDP.

Less common variants of Guillain-Barré syndrome include **acute motor axonal neuropathy (AMAN)**, also associated with *C jejuni*, and **acute motor sensory axonal neuropathy (AMSAN)**, which together account for approximately 10% of Guillain-Barré cases. **Miller Fisher syndrome**, which accounts for about 3–5% of Guillain-Barré cases, is characterized by ataxia, areflexia, and ophthalmoplegia; its antibodies are directed at the glycolipid GQ_{1b} found at nerve terminals, and it usually occurs in young men. Because of varying diagnostic criteria for these variants of Guillain-Barré syndrome, little clear epidemiologic data are available.

► Clinical Findings

A. Symptoms and Signs

AIDP often begins 1–3 weeks after an infection or inciting event such as surgery. Seventy percent of patients initially have paresthesias or vague numbness in their hands and feet. Symmetric weakness appears a few days later and progresses over days to a few weeks. Paralysis is maximal by about 2 weeks in more than 50% of patients and by 1 month in more than 90%. If the disease progresses longer, it is considered subacute or chronic inflammatory polyradiculoneuropathy. Ascending weakness beginning in the distal legs is typical, although descending paralysis with predominant proximal muscle weakness rarely appears. Facial weakness occurs in half of patients with AIDP and ophthalmoparesis and lower cranial neuropathies can cause dysarthria and dysphagia.

Life-threatening respiratory paralysis may rapidly appear as the disease progresses, necessitating intubation and mechanical ventilation, and all patients with AIDP must be identified as quickly as possible and carefully monitored until the disease has stabilized. One quarter of patients with AIDP require mechanical ventilation. Another very serious complication, more common in patients with severe quadriparesis and often difficult to control, is autonomic nervous system involvement, which can cause dangerous fluctuations in blood pressure or precipitate cardiac arrhythmia. Significant autonomic dysfunction in AIDP carries a high mortality.

On examination, weakness is symmetric and ranges from mild to severe flaccid quadriparesis. Sensation is usually normal despite sensory symptoms, although mild distal vibratory loss may be found. Reflexes are diminished or absent, but sphincter tone is normal. Bedside pulmonary function testing (forced vital capacity and negative inspiratory force) may reveal impending respiratory failure. Patients with autonomic involvement may demonstrate cardiac arrhythmia, fluctuations in blood pressure, flushing and sweating, and abnormalities of gastrointestinal motility.

B. Diagnostic Studies

Imaging studies of the spinal cord may be necessary to rule out myelopathic disease. All patients with acute to subacute onset of symmetric weakness and areflexia should have a lumbar puncture after spinal cord disease has been excluded. CSF protein concentration begins to rise a few days after onset of symptoms and peaks in 4–6 weeks. The cell count typically remains normal or shows only mild lymphocytic pleocytosis (more common in patients with HIV infection). Appropriate evaluations for infection should be performed, and electrocardiogram and chest radiographs should be obtained. Blood studies should be directed at possible underlying collagen vascular disease. Baseline electrolyte levels, blood counts, coagulation studies, and hepatic and renal function tests should be obtained in the event that critical care becomes necessary.

In AIDP, nerve conduction studies demonstrate demyelination with reduced motor conduction velocities and prolonged distal motor latencies within 3–5 days of symptom onset, but may be normal if performed within the first few days of onset. Studies assessing proximal demyelination (F-wave responses), an early feature of Guillain-Barré syndrome, may be diffusely abnormal at the time of clinical presentation. Sensory conduction studies are often normal at presentation but may be slowed. In early Guillain-Barré syndrome, needle EMG may show a reduction in motor unit recruitment. Evidence of axonal injury (denervation change with fibrillations and positive sharp waves), if present, usually does not appear on EMG for 2–3 weeks. Prominent axonal change on needle EMG supports significant axonal injury and suggests a worse prognosis for complete recovery (AMAN or AMSAN).

Differential Diagnosis

Guillain-Barré syndrome is most commonly mimicked by acute spinal cord disease (acute myelopathy, transverse myelitis), but brainstem ischemia may also mimic severe Guillain-Barré syndrome with cranial neuropathy (ie, locked-in syndrome). Acute disorders of the neuromuscular junction, such as myasthenia gravis and, particularly, botulinum intoxication, may have a similar time course and may also cause weakness of the extremities with bulbar muscle involvement. Although rare, other acute neuropathies, such as porphyric neuropathy, diphtheritic neuropathy, and mononeuropathy multiplex, must be considered, along with toxic neuropathy (eg, organophosphates, arsenic).

Treatment

Both intravenous immunoglobulin (IVIG; 0.4 g/kg/day for 5 days) and plasmapheresis (five to six exchanges over 1–2 weeks) appear equally effective when given within the first 2 weeks after onset. Combination therapy consisting of both does not seem to confer additional benefit. Plasmapheresis may be precluded in hemodynamically unstable patients. These measures generally increase the pace of recovery, although their effects on the severity of the disease, the risk of respiratory and autonomic dysfunction, and ultimate disability are less clear. Randomized trials of oral and intravenous corticosteroids (methylprednisolone and prednisolone) have failed to show benefit in Guillain-Barré syndrome.

Prognosis

Most patients with Guillain-Barré syndrome return to normal function. After disease progression stops, symptoms usually plateau for 2–4 weeks, followed by gradual recovery. About 20–25% of patients require mechanical ventilation, and 5% die, usually from the complications of respiratory failure or autonomic dysfunction. Residual motor weakness is present in 25% of patients after 1 year. Older age (60 years or older), ventilatory support, rapid progression (< 7 days), and low motor amplitudes (suggesting axonal injury) on early nerve conduction studies are poor prognostic factors associated with a less than 20% probability of walking independently at 6 months.

Govani V, Granieri E. Epidemiology of the Guillain-Barré syndrome. *Curr Opin Neurol* 2001;14:605–613. [PMID: 11562572] (Incidence, antecedent events, prognosis, prognostic indicators, and treatment of Guillain-Barré syndrome.)

Hartung HP, Willison HJ, Kieseier BC. Acute immunoinflammatory neuropathy: Update on Guillain-Barré syndrome. *Curr Opin Neurol* 2002;15:571–577. [PMID: 12352001] (Reviews the pathogenesis of Guillain-Barré syndrome.)

Pritchard J. Guillain-Barré syndrome. *Clin Med* 2010;10:399–401. [PMID: 20849020]

Vucic S, Kiernan MC, Cornblath DR. Guillain-Barré syndrome: An update. *J Clin Neurosci* 2009;16:733–741. [PMID: 19356935]

CHRONIC INFLAMMATORY DEMYELINATING POLYRADICULONEUROPATHY (CIDP)

 ESSENTIALS OF DIAGNOSIS

- ▶ Gradual, progressive weakness over at least 2 months
- ▶ Areflexia
- ▶ Increased CSF protein without increased cell count (albuminocytologic dissociation)
- ▶ Evidence of demyelination on nerve conduction studies

General Considerations

The precise cause of chronic demyelination in CIDP remains unclear, but there is growing evidence that both humoral and cell-mediated immune mechanisms may be involved. The prevalence of CIDP is estimated to range from 1.0–7.7 cases per 100,000 people. However, this is likely an underestimate related to differing diagnostic criteria and underreporting. CIDP disproportionately affects men and those older than 50 years of age.

Clinical Findings

A. Symptoms and Signs

CIDP can present in a stepwise progression with periods of plateau, a steadily declining course, or a course with recurrent episodes. Most patients initially have predominantly motor symptoms, although examination typically reveals both motor and sensory signs. Weakness may begin focally but usually becomes bilateral or multifocal within a few months of onset. Like Guillain-Barré syndrome, CIDP is usually symmetric, and both proximal and distal muscles are affected. Some degree of proximal hip flexor weakness on examination (often unnoticed by the patient at presentation) is considered by some authorities to be an essential feature. Cranial neuropathies and respiratory muscle weakness are rare.

B. Diagnostic Studies

Nerve conduction studies typically reveal significant demyelination with slowed conduction velocities, prolonged distal latencies, conduction block, and abnormal late responses (eg, F waves). Both motor and sensory nerves may be affected. In severe cases, evidence of secondary axonal injury may be seen. Lumbar puncture reveals an elevated protein concentration, but the cell count typically remains normal or shows only mild lymphocytic pleocytosis. Nerve biopsy, which carries a substantial risk of permanent focal neuralgia (10–15%), is no longer routinely recommended.

Differential Diagnosis

The differential diagnosis includes multifocal stroke, motor neuron disease, polyradiculopathy, inflammatory myopathy, neuromuscular junction disease (myasthenia gravis and Lambert-Eaton myasthenic syndrome), and other causes of progressive neuropathy, such as diabetes mellitus and vitamin B_{12} deficiency. After a demyelinating neuropathy has been confirmed electrically, diagnostic considerations include paraproteinemic neuropathy (especially IgM associated), anti-MAG antibody syndrome, and multifocal motor neuropathy.

Treatment

Most patients improve with immunomodulatory therapy, although individual responses to specific agents vary, and specific therapeutic regimens often must be devised through trial and error (Table 19–14). Long-term therapy is often required, and complete remission is rare.

Oral prednisone therapy is effective in most patients. Dosage is 1.0–1.5 mg/kg/day, titrated according to clinical response after several weeks. Alternate-day therapy (in equivalent weekly doses) may be instituted after 2–3 months in patients who improve, with subsequent taper by 5–10 mg every 2–4 weeks thereafter. The side effects of long-term corticosteroid administration may limit their use, particularly in older patients. Some patients respond incompletely to corticosteroids and require adjunctive therapy or a switch to an alternate modality.

IVIG and plasmapheresis are both effective but often must be continued indefinitely. Disease severity, long-term side effects, concurrent illness, cost of treatment, venous access, and age should all be taken into consideration when selecting therapy. The goals of treatment are to restore patients to a level of function sufficient to enable them to go about their daily activities while minimizing the adverse effects associated with therapy. Some patients have persistent symptoms despite aggressive combination therapy.

Other adjunctive immunosuppressive therapies, such as azathioprine or mycophenolate, are often considered in patients with persistent symptoms, although there is limited evidence of their benefit in CIDP. In patients with disease that is refractory to all other modalities, cyclophosphamide (oral or intravenous) may be of benefit.

Latov N. Diagnosis of CIDP. *Neurology* 2002;59(Suppl 6):S2–S6. [PMID: 12499464] (Reviews the diagnosis and prevalence of CIDP and discusses the difficulties of diagnosis in clinical practice due to strict research criteria.)

Nobile-Orazio E, et al. Chronic inflammatory demyelinating polyradiculoneuropathy and mutifocal motor neuropathy: Treatment update. *Curr Opin Neurol* 2010;23:519–523. [PMID: 20689427] (Reviews the treatment options and history of therapeutic trials for CIDP and MMN up to 2010.)

Pollard JD. Chronic inflammatory demyelinating polyradiculoneuropathy. *Curr Opin Neurol* 2002;15:279–283. [PMID: 12045725] (Clinical features, diagnostic studies, pathogenesis, and treatment of CIDP.)

Ropper AH. Current treatments for CIDP. *Neurology* 2002; 60(Suppl 3):S16–S22. [PMID: 12707418] (Reviews efficacy, tolerability, and limitations of therapies for CIDP.)

MULTIFOCAL MOTOR NEUROPATHY

 ESSENTIALS OF DIAGNOSIS

- ▶ Asymmetric distal weakness, especially of the hands
- ▶ Subacute to chronic progression (months)
- ▶ Proximal conduction block in motor nerves
- ▶ Elevated CSF protein concentration
- ▶ Elevated anti-GM_1 antibody titers (some patients)

General Considerations

Multifocal motor neuropathy is a chronic, immune-mediated motor neuropathy typified by asymmetric, slowly progressive weakness that most commonly begins in the hands. Age of

Table 19–14. Treatment Options in Chronic Inflammatory Demyelinating Polyradiculoneuropathy (CIDP)

Therapy	Dosage	Considerations
Prednisone	1.0–1.5 mg/kg/day initially After 2–3 months initiate alternate-day dosing in equivalent weekly doses Once alternate-day dosing is instituted, continue to taper by 5–10 mg every 2–4 weeks	Side effects may limit use
Intravenous immunoglobulin (IVIG)	2 g/kg total over 5 days	Effective, but may need to be continued indefinitely
Plasmapheresis	6 exchanges (250 mL/kg each) over 7–10 days	Same as for IVIG
Azathioprine	50 mg orally, 3 times a day	Used in refractory cases, but evidence of benefit is limited
Mycophenolate	1000 mg orally, 2 times a day	Same as for azathioprine

onset ranges from 20–75 years, but men in their fifties and sixties are most commonly affected.

Clinical Findings

A. Symptoms and Signs

Weakness usually begins in one hand and gradually worsens over several months, eventually spreading to the opposite hand. Atrophy and fasciculations may be present, mimicking motor neuron disease. Reflexes are usually normal or absent, but patients have been reported as having multifocal motor neuropathy that includes upper motor neuron signs. Cranial nerve involvement is extremely rare, and sensory symptoms and signs are usually minimal or absent.

B. Diagnostic Studies

Nerve conduction studies are the most important single test for this disorder. In contrast to most other polyneuropathies, the electrodiagnostic features of multifocal motor neuropathy are often elusive, especially if only routine nerve conduction studies are employed. Careful segmental conductions must be performed in the proximal motor segments in suspected cases, especially in the arms, because focal demyelination and conduction block may be restricted to these areas. Sensory conductions are usually normal, although distal amplitudes may be slightly decreased in some patients. EMG may demonstrate evidence of scattered but widespread denervation, suggesting possible motor neuron disease.

High titers of serum IgM anti-GM_1 antibodies are found in many patients, but a substantial minority is seronegative, limiting the sensitivity of this assay. Anti-GM_1 antibodies are also commonly present in patients with motor neuron disease, AIDP, and other neuropathies. CSF protein concentration may be increased.

Differential Diagnosis

A patient presenting with typical features of multifocal motor neuropathy should be considered to have motor neuron disease until proven otherwise, especially if upper motor neuron signs are present. Pure motor stroke, polyradiculopathy, idiopathic brachial plexopathy or plexus tumor, and other neuropathies such as CIDP, as well as focal nerve entrapments and inclusion body myositis, must also be considered.

Treatment

There is better category I evidence for the efficacy of high-dose IVIG in multifocal motor neuropathy than in any other neuropathy. IVIG therapy (2 g/kg given in divided doses over 2–5 days and repeated monthly) usually results in improvement in strength, often beginning within a few weeks after the first course. Benefit usually lasts for 3–6 weeks after a single treatment, and symptoms usually recur if therapy is discontinued.

Cyclophosphamide (1 g/m^2) is the only immunosuppressant with long-term benefit in this disorder, and a regimen of several monthly treatments may induce remission lasting for a few years, although ultimate recurrence remains the rule. The toxicity of cyclophosphamide makes this therapy a last resort for most patients. The benefits of other immunosuppressants in this disorder are less clear. Corticosteroid treatment is rarely beneficial in patients with multifocal motor neuropathy and may worsen weakness, and the role of azathioprine, mycophenolate, and other agents has yet to be clearly defined.

Meuth SG, Kleinschnitz C. Multifocal motor neuropathy: Update on clinical characteristics, pathophysiological concepts and therapeutic options. *Eur Neurol* 2010;63:193–204. [PMID: 20150737] (This is an up to date review on the clinical features of MMN and what is known about its underlying pathophysiology, as well as the available treatment options through 2010.)

Nobile-Orazio E, Gallia F, Tuccillo F, Terenghi F. Chronic inflammatory demyelinating polyradiculoneuropathy and multifocal motor neuropathy: Treatment update. *Curr Opin Neurol* 2010;23:519–523. [PMID: 20689427]

PARAPROTEINEMIC POLYNEUROPATHY

 ESSENTIALS OF DIAGNOSIS

▶ Usually predominantly sensory neuropathies

▶ Most often associated with IgM and IgG gammopathies

▶ May be the first manifestation of malignancy

▶ Also seen with monoclonal gammopathy of uncertain significance (MGUS)

▶ Specific anti-MAG antibody syndrome includes numbness, ataxia, tremor, and distal weakness

General Considerations

Abnormally elevated serum immunoglobulin levels can cause a **paraproteinemic neuropathy** in which many of the antibodies are targeted at myelin components. Paraproteinemias typically affect men older than 50 years of age, and paraproteinemic neuropathies are associated with lymphoma, amyloidosis, cryoglobulinemia, multiple myeloma, POEMS syndrome (polyneuropathy, organomegaly, endocrinopathy, M protein, and skin changes), and Waldenström macroglobulinemia.

In about two thirds of patients, no underlying neoplasm or other cause for the monoclonal spike is found (ie, **MGUS**). However, 20% of patients with MGUS ultimately develop a malignant plasma cell disorder. IgG is the most common paraprotein found in patients with MGUS, but IgM is the most common one in patients with neuropathy, followed by IgG and, rarely, IgA.

Clinical Findings

A. Symptoms and Signs

1. IgM gammopathy—Patients with IgM gammopathy often present with large-fiber sensory loss, prominent tremor, and sensory ataxia. Distal weakness and atrophy can occur as the disease progresses. IgM gammopathy is predominantly a demyelinating neuropathy, although axonal loss may occur.

2. Anti-MAG antibody syndrome—Fifty percent of patients with IgM neuropathy have antibodies to myelin-associated glycoprotein (MAG), a protein found in the periaxonal Schwann cell membranes. Anti-MAG antibodies are associated with a discrete clinical syndrome consisting of a slowly progressive, large-fiber neuropathy with late distal weakness.

3. IgG gammopathy—IgG gammopathy can be either axonal or demyelinating. Its clinical presentation is usually similar to that of IgM gammopathy.

B. Diagnostic Studies

On laboratory testing, immunofixation can detect small amounts of M protein. In many cases, anti-MAG, which binds to myelin, is found. Electrophysiologic testing usually demonstrates demyelination and axonal loss.

Differential Diagnosis

The differential diagnosis is broad and includes most of the neuropathic syndromes described in this chapter.

Treatment

More than one third of patients with MGUS neuropathy improve within days to weeks of IVIG therapy (0.4 g/kg/day for 5 days), plasmapheresis (220 mL/kg in four to five treatments), or oral corticosteroids, often in combination with other immunosuppressants. Patients with IgG or IgA monoclonal gammopathy–associated neuropathies respond better than those with IgM monoclonal gammopathy. However, neuropathy associated with multiple myeloma responds poorly to plasmapheresis. Primary systemic amyloid neuropathy (nonfamilial) responds poorly to melphalan and prednisone, despite improvement in survival with these medications. Half of patients with POEMS neuropathy improve with resection of solitary bone lesions, focused radiation, or chemotherapy with melphalan, cyclophosphamide, or prednisone.

Kwan JY. Paraproteinemic neuropathy. *Neurol Clin* 2007;25:47–69. [PMID: 17324720] (Provides an overview of the paraproteinemic neuropathies, including their clinical features, diagnostic approaches, and therapeutic options available.)

Nobile-Orazio E, Carpo M. Neuropathy and monoclonal gammopathy. *Curr Opin Neurol* 2001;14:615–620. [PMID: 11562573] (Literature review of the pathogenesis and treatment of neuropathy and monoclonal gammopathy of undetermined significance and other monoclonal gammopathies.)

PARANEOPLASTIC NEUROPATHY

ESSENTIALS OF DIAGNOSIS

▶ Most commonly a distal sensory neuropathy

▶ Numbness, pain, or both

▶ Subacute to chronic progression (months)

▶ May be the first manifestation of a malignancy

▶ May be worsened by neurotoxicity of chemotherapy and radiotherapy

▶ Multiple different paraneoplastic neuropathy syndromes may occur together

General Considerations

Paraneoplastic neuropathy may appear as the first manifestation of an occult neoplasm or may not appear until after a cancer is diagnosed. There are several different paraneoplastic neuropathy syndromes (Table 19–15); these are discussed in more detail in Chapter 13. Paraneoplastic sensory neuropathy is the most common and is often associated with anti-Hu antibodies (type 1 antineuronal nuclear autoantibodies, or ANNA-1). It is strongly associated with small cell lung cancer, but it is also seen in liver, bladder, lung, breast, and pancreatic cancers, as well as lymphoma and sarcoma. Anti-amphiphysin antibody may also be present in paraneoplastic sensory neuropathy, although it is not as specific as anti-Hu for a sensory neuropathy. Anti-amphiphysin antibodies are also associated with other, often overlapping paraneoplastic syndromes (eg, encephalomyelitis and sensory neuronopathy), Lambert-Eaton myasthenic syndrome, and stiff-person syndrome. Autonomic neuropathy is also sometimes seen with anti-Hu–associated sensory neuropathy and may cause gastroparesis, achalasia, dysphagia, and pseudo-obstruction. Other paraneoplastic syndromes include subacute sensory neuronopathy, demyelinating neuropathy (usually a feature of paraproteinemic malignancies; see preceding discussion), mononeuropathy multiplex, motor neuron disease, and motor neuropathy.

Clinical Findings

A. Symptoms and Signs

Paraneoplastic sensory neuropathy is characterized by numbness, painful paresthesias, and lancinating pain. It may begin in one limb and then spread to the remaining limbs, but it is usually generalized by the time of presentation. All sensory modalities are lost, and proprioception is most severely affected. Strength is normal or only minimally decreased, and tendon reflexes are reduced or absent. Frequently there is concurrent involvement of the myenteric plexus, autonomic ganglia, spinal cord, brainstem, cerebellum, or limbic cortex.

Table 19–15. Paraneoplastic Neuropathy Syndromes

Neuropathy	Antibody	Tumor
Sensorimotor neuropathy	—	Multiple
Sensory neuropathy	Anti-Hu[a]	Breast, SCLC
Subacute sensory neuropathy	Anti-Hu	SCLC
Autonomic neuropathy	Anti-Hu, neuronal nicotinic, AChR	SCLC
Vasculitic neuropathy	Anti-Hu	Lung adenocarcinoma
Demyelinating neuropathy	Anti-Hu, polyclonal immunoglobulin M antibodies	Melanoma, CML, gallbladder
Motor neuropathy	Anti-Hu Anti-Yo	SCLC Ovarian
Paraproteinemia	—	POEMS
Mononeuropathies and multiple cranial nerves	Anti-Hu	SCLC
Neuropathy plus (overlap syndromes)	Voltage-gated potassium channel Anti-amphiphysin	Malignant thymoma SCLC, Lambert-Eaton myasthenic syndrome, stiff-person syndrome

AChR = acetylcholine receptor; CML = chronic myeloid leukemia; POEMS = polyneuropathy, organomegaly, endocrinopathy, M protein, and skin changes; SCLC = small cell lung cancer.
[a]Also known as type 1 antineuronal nuclear autoantibodies (ANNA-1).

Subacute sensory neuronopathy (Denny-Brown syndrome or dorsal root ganglionitis) appears to be distinct from paraneoplastic sensory neuropathy; the dorsal root ganglion is the site of primary injury. Women are affected twice as often as men, and small cell lung cancer is, again, the most common underlying tumor. Breast carcinoma, ovarian cancer, and lymphoma are also frequently associated with this neuronopathy.

Paraneoplastic demyelinating neuropathy can mimic either Guillain-Barré syndrome (usually associated with Hodgkin disease) or a CIDP (non-Hodgkin lymphoma). Multiple myeloma is also associated with a demyelinating neuropathy and can be associated with POEMS syndrome.

Vasculitic neuropathy is associated with hematologic malignancy, and patients typically present with mononeuropathy multiplex. A form of motor neuron disease has been described as part of paraneoplastic encephalomyelitis and may respond to treatment of an underlying associated tumor; subacute motor neuropathy has also been associated with malignancy. Finally, subacute paraneoplastic autonomic neuropathy may be associated with neuronal nicotinic acetylcholine receptor antibodies (see Table 19–15).

B. Diagnostic Studies

Anti-Hu antibodies are often associated with paraneoplastic sensory neuropathy, but their absence does not rule it out. Nerve conduction studies show low-amplitude or absent sensory nerve action potentials with preserved motor amplitudes. Nerve biopsy is not usually needed unless amyloidosis is suspected and cannot otherwise be confirmed. CSF analysis may reveal elevated protein concentration and mild pleocytosis, especially in patients with associated lymphoma. Patients with subacute sensory neuropathy in whom no underlying cause is found should be screened for the presence of a malignancy. Neoplastic screening may be indicated as well, in other instances of "idiopathic" neuropathy, depending on the patient's age, history, and risk factors.

▶ Differential Diagnosis

True paraneoplastic neuropathies must be distinguished from other forms of nerve injury associated with cancer and its treatments, especially tumor invasion of the peripheral nerves and the toxic effects of chemotherapy and radiation.

▶ Treatment

Treatment of the underlying neoplasm is the mainstay of therapy and offers the best chance of improvement, although neuropathic symptoms may persist if the nerve injury is well established. Treatment with corticosteroids, immunosuppressants, and plasmapheresis is of questionable benefit, although IVIG has been reported to be effective in some patients.

Grisold W, Drlicek M. Paraneoplastic neuropathy. *Curr Opin Neurol* 1999;12:617–625. [PMID: 10590899] (Excellent review of paraneoplastic neuropathy and overlap syndromes.)

Pelosof LC, Gerber DE. Paraneoplastic syndromes: An approach to diagnosis and treatment. *Mayo Clin Proc* 2010;85:838–854. [PMID: 20810794] (Review of contemporary approaches to therapy and treatment of a variety of paraneoplastic syndromes through 2010.)

INFECTIOUS POLYNEUROPATHY

HIV-ASSOCIATED NEUROPATHIES

ESSENTIALS OF DIAGNOSIS

▶ Many different neuropathic syndromes are possible; sensory neuropathy is the most common

▶ Numbness, pain, or both

▶ May be worsened by antiretroviral neurotoxicity

▶ General Considerations

HIV-associated axonal sensory neuropathy (HIV-SN) may be the result of either direct HIV infection or anti-retroviral drug therapy. HIV-SN affects 7% of patients with CD4+ counts of less than 200 cells/μL and 2.8% of HIV patients regardless of CD4+ count. In addition to this large-fiber sensory neuropathy, a small-fiber–mediated symmetric distal sensory polyneuropathy may also occur as part of HIV-SN or as a separate entity, causing pain and numbness (for further discussion, see Chapter 28). Punch biopsies show reduced intraepidermal nerve fiber density similar to diabetic and amyloid neuropathy. Proinflammatory cytokines, rather than direct toxicity from the HIV retrovirus, are thought to be toxic to these small pain fibers.

The advent of combination antiretroviral therapy in the mid-1990s drastically reduced the incidence of CNS opportunistic infections in HIV patients. The nucleoside reverse transcriptase inhibitors (NRTIs), however, can cause a toxic peripheral neuropathy that is now the most prevalent neurologic complication in patients with HIV or AIDS. In clinical trials of zalcitabine (ddC), stavudine (d4T), and didanosine (ddI), peripheral neuropathy was the dose-limiting toxicity. Zalcitabine is the most neurotoxic, and neuropathy occurs more frequently when these agents are used in combination. The onset of neuropathic symptoms ranges from 1 week to 6 months after initiation of NRTI therapy. Risk factors for toxic neuropathy from antiretroviral drugs include preexisting neuropathy (eg, diabetes mellitus, vitamin B_{12} deficiency, or alcohol), old age, poor nutrition, and advanced HIV disease.

HIV is also associated with both AIDP and CIDP, as well as mononeuropathy multiplex (discussed earlier in this chapter). It can also cause a subacute lumbosacral polyradiculitis with lumbosacral pain, saddle anesthesia, urinary retention, and flaccid paraparesis, most commonly caused by cytomegalovirus infection in patients with end-stage AIDS. Motor neuron disease, reversible with antiretroviral therapy, also rarely occurs.

▶ Clinical Findings

A. Symptoms and Signs

HIV-SN is characterized by the gradual onset of bilateral burning or aching pain. It is most severe on the soles of the feet and usually is worse at night. Patients may have hyperalgesia and allodynia of the feet. The neuropathic pain starts distally and ascends proximally over several months. The fingertips may be involved when the dysesthesia reaches the level of the mid-thigh. Examination usually reveals losses to all sensory modalities in a stocking distribution, with more severe deficits in pinprick and temperature sensation. Weakness is rare. Tendon reflexes are usually diminished or absent. The other HIV-associated neuropathies (AIDP, CIDP, mononeuropathy multiplex, cytomegalovirus polyradiculitis, motor neuron disease) have the clinical features of those syndromes.

B. Diagnostic Studies

Other potential causes of distal symmetric sensory neuropathy, especially diabetes mellitus, must be carefully excluded through appropriate history and physical examination and serum studies. CSF analysis may also be needed.

Nerve conduction studies usually reveal an axonal sensory polyneuropathy. In some patients with disproportionate small-fiber involvement, nerve conduction studies may be normal, but quantitative sensory testing or epidermal nerve fiber density studies (via skin biopsy) reveal small-fiber loss.

▶ Differential Diagnosis

The differential diagnosis is broad and includes most of the neuropathic syndromes described in this chapter.

▶ Treatment

HIV-associated neuropathy may improve or worsen with effective antiretroviral therapy, which usually must be continued in spite of these symptoms (see Chapter 28). Treatment of neuropathic pain includes modalities employed for other neuropathic pain states; lamotrigine appears particularly efficacious in controlling the pain of HIV-SN.

Robinson-Papp J, Simpson DM. Neuromuscular diseases associated with HIV-1 infection. *Muscle Nerve* 2009;40:1043–1053. [PMID: 19771594] (Overview and update of the various neuromuscular complications of, and neuromuscular diseases associated with, HIV infection.)

NEUROPATHIES ASSOCIATED WITH LYME DISEASE

ESSENTIALS OF DIAGNOSIS

▶ Painful radiculoneuritis and cranial neuritis, most commonly with meningitis

▶ Diffuse polyneuropathy (more common chronically)

▶ Other neuropathic syndromes may also occur

General Considerations

Lyme disease, caused by the spirochete *Borrelia burgdorferi* and transmitted by the bite of the *Ixodes* tick, is discussed in Chapter 26. Lyme neuroborreliosis most commonly causes lymphocytic meningitis, cranial neuritis, painful radiculoneuritis, and diffuse polyneuropathy. Brachial and lumbosacral plexopathy, mononeuropathy multiplex, and carpal tunnel syndrome can also occur. Motor neuron disease resembling amyotrophic lateral sclerosis has also been described.

Clinical Findings

A. Symptoms and Signs

Focal cranial neuropathies and radiculoneuropathies are common, especially in patients with Lyme meningitis. These findings are usually acute and self-limited, and occur within the first 1–2 months of infection. Involvement of CNs II–XII has been reported. Optic neuritis in patients who test positive serologically for Lyme disease has been described, but causality has not been established. The facial nerve is most often affected (80% of patients with Lyme neuroborreliosis) followed by the third, fifth, sixth, and eighth cranial nerves. In about 20% of patients, multiple cranial nerves are involved. The facial nerve can be affected either within the subarachnoid space or external to it, and loss of taste and hyperacusis may be present. Most patients with cranial neuropathies have CSF lymphocytic pleocytosis.

Radiculopathy is common, but Lyme disease may not be recognized as the cause. Patients typically have severe radicular pain, with or without weakness and hyporeflexia. Radiculoneuritis associated with Lyme disease is more often diagnosed in Europe than in the United States, possibly as the result of underdiagnosis in the United States or variation in strains of *Borrelia*. Brachial and lumbosacral plexopathies and mononeuropathy multiplex rarely occur in Lyme disease. Nerve entrapment causing a carpal tunnel syndrome may occur from synovial thickening in the wrist secondary to Lyme arthritis.

The polyneuropathy in chronic neuroborreliosis usually presents as a typical indolent peripheral neuropathy with a stocking-glove pattern of sensory loss, distal weakness, and areflexia. A more severe acute polyneuropathy may mimic axonal Guillain-Barré syndrome.

B. Diagnostic Studies

The diagnosis is made from the history and physical findings, supported by serum studies. Demonstration of an immune response to *B burgdorferi* supports the diagnosis of Lyme disease, but, as discussed in Chapter 26, the interpretation of such results remains controversial. Facial nerve palsy in Lyme disease can occur very early in infection when serologic results are negative; in these patients, follow-up testing in 2–4 weeks can show high titers of antibody. In some patients, the antibody response is repeatedly negative despite persistent infection with *B burgdorferi* in the joints or the nervous

system. These patients may have been treated with noncurative doses of antibiotics during early infection.

Positive results may also be difficult to interpret. Patients can remain seropositive for an extended period, even after successful treatment, and false-positive results can occur in patients with syphilis, vasculitis, systemic lupus erythematosus, or bacterial endocarditis.

Culture of skin biopsy of an active erythema migrans lesion is frequently positive, although most patients with peripheral nerve injury seek treatment after the rash has resolved. Culture of blood, CSF, or other affected tissues has a lower yield.

Nerve conduction studies are important to confirm the presence and site of nerve injury.

Differential Diagnosis

The differential diagnosis is broad and includes most of the neuropathic syndromes described in this chapter.

Treatment

For treatment of Lyme disease, refer to Chapter 26.

LEPROSY

ESSENTIALS OF DIAGNOSIS

► Sensory or sensorimotor polyneuropathy
► Ulnar and tibial nerves disproportionately affected
► Tendon reflexes preserved (an unusual feature in neuropathy)
► Cutaneous manifestations are usually present

General Considerations

Although rare in the United States, leprosy remains the most common cause of peripheral neuropathy worldwide. Caused by *Mycobacterium leprae*, the disease occurs predominantly in tropical countries and in persons emigrating from these areas. Fourteen to 20% of patients with leprosy have neuropathy. Infected monocytes from broken skin and mucosal membranes carry *M leprae* into the nerves during normal macrophage transport. The bacteria attack Schwann cells, producing axonal damage by infiltrating inflammatory cells and granuloma formation.

Clinical Findings

A. Symptoms and Signs

The clinical manifestations of leprosy depend on the patient's immune status. Tuberculoid leprosy damages nerves earlier in the course of disease when host resistance is high, and such damage is often severe. Lepromatous leprosy occurs with low host resistance and is associated with less severe nerve damage, late in the course of disease. Associated skin nodules, papules, macules, and ulcers are often found. Palpation of nerves, especially ulnar and posterior tibial (the most frequently effected), may reveal hypertrophy. Primary neuritic leprosy manifests as either pure sensory or sensorimotor dysfunction. Loss of sensory modalities occurs distally, often with more prominent deficits and weakness in the ulnar and posterior tibial distributions. An unusual and therefore helpful diagnostic feature is the preservation of tendon reflexes, which are typically decreased or absent in other neuropathies.

B. Diagnostic Studies

Nerve conduction studies demonstrate axonal and demyelinating sensory or sensorimotor neuropathy. A skin punch biopsy is essential for diagnosis and should be taken from the active borders of skin lesions. Granulomatous inflammation is found in tuberculoid leprosy, whereas in lepromatous disease multiple acid-fast organisms are found in Schwann cells.

▶ Differential Diagnosis

The differential diagnosis includes the full range of sensory neuropathies, but the preservation of tendon reflexes, despite obvious neuropathy, is nearly strongly suggestive.

▶ Treatment

Adult patients with paucibacillary or multibacillary disease are prescribed rifampin, 600 mg orally once a month. For patients with multibacillary leprosy, an extra drug, clofazimine, is prescribed at a dose of 300 mg per month and 50 mg daily. Dapsone is also recommended for both paucibacillary and multibacillary adult patients at a dose of 100 mg daily.

DIPHTHERITIC POLYNEUROPATHY

ESSENTIALS OF DIAGNOSIS

▶ Localized febrile pharyngitis initially

▶ Diphtheritic membrane, which may cover posterior pharynx

▶ Purely demyelinating sensorimotor neuropathy

▶ General Considerations

Diphtheria is caused by the organism *Corynebacterium diphtheriae*, which produces localized, febrile pharyngitis and a characteristic gray membrane that adheres to the posterior pharynx and tonsils. The organism emits a protein exotoxin, which can cause cardiomyopathy and segmental demyelination of nerve roots or peripheral nerves. Acute demyelinating polyneuropathy is the most common severe complication of diphtheria infection. Respiratory compromise can ensue from either direct obstruction of the airway or neuropathic weakness of the respiratory muscles. The mortality rate is approximately 10%, and the disease is more severe in young children and older patients.

▶ Clinical Findings

A. Symptoms and Signs

About 20% of patients develop focal paralysis of the palate 4–30 days after the primary infection, followed by diphtheritic sensorimotor polyneuropathy, affecting the extremities.

B. Diagnostic Studies

Culture of *C diphtheriae* from the pharynx or a cutaneous ulcer confirms the diagnosis. CSF analysis can show elevated protein concentration. Nerve conduction studies reveal severe, demyelinating neuropathy.

▶ Differential Diagnosis

The differential diagnosis includes AIDP (discussed earlier), which may follow a similar time course with similar electrophysiologic features. Other causes of demyelinating sensorimotor neuropathy must also be considered.

▶ Treatment

Administration of antitoxin within 48 hours of the onset of primary infection reduces the incidence of neuropathy. Diphtheria is also treated with antibiotics. Intramuscular administration of procaine penicillin G (300,000 U/day for patients weighing 10 kg or less and 600,000 U/day for those weighing more than 10 kg) for 14 days, or oral or parenteral erythromycin (40 mg/kg/day; maximum, 2 g/day) for 14 days is the recommended regimen. Respiratory support may be necessary in patients with severe symptoms. Prevention through vaccination remains the mainstay of therapy.

Haimanot RT, Melaku Z. Leprosy. *Curr Opin Neurol* 2000;13: 317–322. [PMID: 10871258] (Epidemiology, pathogenesis, clinical findings, and treatment of leprosy.)

Keswani SC, et al. HIV-associated sensory neuropathies. *AIDS* 2002;16:2105–2117. [PMID: 12409731] (Reviews clinical features of neuropathy in HIV disease.)

TOXIC & METABOLIC NEUROPATHIES

ALCOHOLIC NEUROPATHY

ESSENTIALS OF DIAGNOSIS

▶ Gradual-onset, distal, symmetric sensory loss

▶ Weakness (late complication)

▶ Usually begins after months to years of alcohol abuse

▶ Diminished tendon reflexes

Peripheral neuropathy is the most frequent neurologic disease associated with chronic alcoholism and is caused by both direct alcohol toxicity and thiamine deficiency. (Alcoholism is discussed in detail in Chapter 33.)

Clinically, patients present with paresthesias and sometimes allodynia in the distal legs. A mixed sensory and motor neuropathy causes sensory loss in a symmetric stocking-glove distribution, as well as weakness and atrophy in distal muscles, and hyporeflexia. Nerve conduction studies typically show axonal neuropathy, with reduced sensory amplitudes and normal or mildly reduced conduction velocities.

The differential diagnosis includes most of the many causes of gradual, distal, symmetric sensorimotor neuropathy. Alcoholic neuropathy is a diagnosis of exclusion, and other causes such as diabetes mellitus and vitamin B_{12} deficiency must be appropriately investigated. A slowly progressive compressive myelopathy may mimic distal symmetric neuropathy, although tendon reflexes are usually increased with upper motor neuron dysfunction.

Treatment consists of abstinence from alcohol and vitamin supplementation. Recovery is slow and rarely complete.

VITAMIN B_{12} DEFICIENCY

ESSENTIALS OF DIAGNOSIS

► Gradual-onset, distal symmetric sensory loss
► Weakness (late complication)
► May occur with upper motor neuron signs (due to concurrent myelopathy)
► Borderline to low vitamin B_{12} levels with elevated levels of homocysteine and methylmalonic acid

► General Considerations

Vitamin B_{12} (cyanocobalamin) is found in most animal products. Deficiency can cause neuropathy, myelopathy (subacute combined degeneration of the corticospinal tracts and dorsal columns), dementia, and megaloblastic anemia, although each of these manifestations may occur alone or in any combination. (Subacute combined degeneration is discussed in Chapter 18.)

► Clinical Findings

A. Symptoms and Signs

The peripheral neuropathy of vitamin B_{12} deficiency typically presents with distal symmetric numbness and gait instability, and, if untreated for a long period, distal weakness. Examination usually reveals reduced proprioception and vibration sense, with distal weakness and muscular atrophy in more advanced cases. Because of the frequent simultaneous occurrence of subacute

combined degeneration of the spinal cord, patients may exhibit the unusual combination of diminished deep tendon reflexes at the ankle in the face of robust Babinski signs. The extent of neuropathic and myelopathic contributions to observed sensory deficits and weakness in a given patient may be difficult to judge by neurologic examination alone, but is somewhat academic once vitamin B_{12} deficiency is identified as the cause.

B. Diagnostic Studies

Nerve conduction studies typically show axonal or demyelinating neuropathy, with reduced sensory amplitudes and normal or mildly reduced conduction velocities. The diagnosis is confirmed by low serum vitamin B_{12} level and normal folate level. About 35% of patients with neurologic symptoms of vitamin B_{12} deficiency have a serum level in the borderline range (150–200 pg/mL), and in these patients megaloblastic anemia may not be apparent. In such patients, levels of methylmalonic acid and homocysteine are elevated. Because of the sensitivity, simplicity, and wide availability of these adjunctive tests, the Schilling test is now rarely performed. Intrinsic factor antibodies are found in 70% and anti–parietal cell antibodies in 90% of patients with pernicious anemia.

► Differential Diagnosis

The differential diagnosis includes most of the many causes of gradual, distal, symmetric sensorimotor neuropathy. A slowly progressive compressive myelopathy may also mimic vitamin B_{12} deficiency.

► Treatment

Treatment consists of vitamin B_{12} supplementation. A standard regimen is 1 mg of intramuscular cyanocobalamin given daily for 1 week, followed by weekly injections for 12 weeks. Improvement is often rapid and dramatic. Maintenance injections can be given once a month or every 3 months.

PYRIDOXINE (VITAMIN B_6) DEFICIENCY

ESSENTIALS OF DIAGNOSIS

► Associated with isoniazid, hydralazine, and penicillamine therapy
► Preventable with supplementation

Pyridoxine deficiency may occur during isoniazid, hydralazine, or, rarely, penicillamine therapy. These medications are structurally similar to pyridoxine and interfere with vitamin B_6 coenzyme activity. Peripheral neuropathy is characterized by slowly progressive, distal sensory and motor deficits. Consequently, patients receiving isoniazid should be given supplemental vitamin B_6 as prophylaxis.

TOXIC NEUROPATHIES

ESSENTIALS OF DIAGNOSIS

► Symptoms vary, depending on the specific toxin
► Distal sensory or sensorimotor neuropathy is common
► Often an adverse effect of potent pharmacotherapy
► Onset may be acute to subacute (with overdose) or chronic (with cumulative toxicity)

A wide range of toxins may cause neuropathies. Nerves can be injured by industrial and environmental toxins (Table 19–16) (eg, aromatic hydrocarbons), heavy metals (eg, lead, arsenic), and many pharmaceutical agents (Table 19–17). Antineoplastic drugs are common offenders, causing a length-dependent sensorimotor axonal neuropathy, pure sensory neuropathy, or ganglionopathy. A symmetric stocking-glove distribution neuropathy is most often found with distal weakness and hyporeflexia. Treatment consists of discontinuing the offending agent.

NEUROPATHIES ASSOCIATED WITH SYSTEMIC DISEASE

DIABETIC NEUROPATHIES

► **General Considerations & Clinical Findings**

Diabetes mellitus, the most common cause of neuropathy in the United States, is identified by objective testing in two thirds of diabetic patients. Diabetic nerve injury produces many clinical syndromes (Table 19–18). Distal symmetric sensorimotor neuropathy is most common and may appear in isolation as the first manifestation of diabetes. Different syndromes, however, can appear in virtually any combination.

A. Symptoms and Signs

1. Distal symmetric neuropathy—This disorder begins with numbness, paresthesias, or dysesthesias (alone or in combination) in the feet. Over months or years, symptoms ascend up the leg and eventually affect the upper extremities. Painful diabetic neuropathy may also develop at this early stage (see the discussion of small nerve fiber injury that follows). Loss of foot sensation in diabetic patients greatly increases the chance of unrecognized cutaneous ulceration, which, along with impaired cutaneous healing, can result in gangrene and limb amputation.

Loss of light touch, pain, and temperature typically occurs early, followed by loss of proprioception, which may cause gait ataxia. Distal weakness and atrophy follow, with gradual subsequent ascension.

Table 19–16. Environmental Neurotoxins Causing Peripheral Neuropathy

Category	Toxin
Heavy metal	Arsenic Lead Mercury Thallium
Drugs of abuse	Alcohol Glue inhalation Nitrous oxide
Industrial toxin	Acrylamide Allyl chloride Carbon disulfide Cyanide (chronic) Ethylene oxide Hexacarbon solvents (glue) Organophosphates Polychlorinated biphenyls Tetrachlorobiphenyl Trichloroethylene

2. Small-fiber and painful neuropathy—The small cutaneous nerve fibers that sense pain and temperature are often damaged in diabetic patients, resulting in the loss of distal pinprick and temperature sensation and the

Table 19–17. Therapeutic Drugs Associated With Polyneuropathy

Class	Drug
Antineoplastic	Cisplatin Suramin Taxoids (paclitaxel, docetaxel) Vincristine
Antimicrobial	Antiretroviral agents Chloroquine Dapsone Isoniazid Metronidazole Nitrofurantoin
Cardiovascular	Amiodarone Hydralazine Perhexiline
CNS	Nitrous oxide Thalidomide
Other	Colchicine Disulfiram Gold L-Tryptophan Phenytoin Pyridoxine

Table 19–18. Diabetic Neuropathic Syndromes

Syndrome	Clinical Findings
Distal Symmetric Neuropathy	
Large-fiber sensory neuropathy	Numbness, paresthesias, dysesthesias, hyperesthesias, ataxia
Sensorimotor neuropathy	Any of the above *plus* distal weakness
Small-Fiber Neuropathy	
"Pure" small-fiber neuropathy	Numbness, paresthesias, painful dysesthesias, hyperesthesias
Diabetic neuropathic cachexia	Subacute, severe neuropathic pain and rapid weight loss
Autonomic neuropathy	Erectile dysfunction, orthostasis, cardiac dysrhythmia, diarrhea, constipation
Ischemic Mononeuropathy	
Cranial (eg, CNs III, VI, VII)	Diplopia, pupil-sparing third nerve palsy, hemifacial weakness
Radicular (thoracic, lumbosacral)	Pain, followed by numbness or weakness in a radicular distribution
Peripheral (eg, femoral)	Pain, followed by numbness, weakness, or both in territory of a single nerve
Regional Neuropathic Syndromes	
Diabetic amyotrophy	Subacute weakness and atrophy of proximal leg muscles
Diabetic thoracoabdominal neuropathy	Subacute weakness, numbness, and atrophy in thorax and abdomen

CN = cranial nerve.

development of burning, electric, aching, stabbing, and pins-and-needles dysesthesias and pain, which can be incapacitating. Patients may have allodynia (the perception of a nonpainful stimulation as painful), especially at night, and foot contact with bedsheets may interfere with sleep. Painful neuropathy spontaneously improves over months to years in some patients but becomes a chronic symptom in others.

The syndrome of diabetic neuropathic cachexia consists of rapidly progressive severe neuropathic pain throughout the body and profound weight loss. It is often precipitated by efforts to tighten glucose control (eg, the first use of insulin, aggressive increases in dosing of oral hypoglycemic agents). This syndrome closely mimics paraneoplastic sensory neuropathy, necessitating a thorough medical evaluation for occult malignancy. In true diabetic neuropathic cachexia, pain resolves spontaneously within several months of onset, and weight is gradually regained.

3. Autonomic neuropathy—Autonomic neuropathy affects nearly 50% of diabetic patients, commonly causing genitourinary dysfunction (erectile dysfunction and neurogenic bladder), postural hypotension, and gastrointestinal dysmotility. Autonomic derangement can contribute to silent cardiac ischemia and cardiac arrhythmia, the most common causes of death in diabetic patients.

4. Mononeuropathy—Acute ischemia of a peripheral nerve resulting from occlusion of the vasa nervorum classically presents with sudden, aching pain lasting minutes to hours near the site of the lesion, accompanied by numbness and weakness in its associated dermatome and myotome. Cranial nerves, nerve roots, or peripheral nerves may be affected. The third cranial nerve is the most commonly injured cranial

nerve in patients with diabetes. Because the oculomotor fibers are located deep within the nerve and have poor collateral circulation, they are vulnerable to decreased perfusion. In contrast, the parasympathetic pupillary fibers are located on the surface of the nerve, where circulation is more redundant. Consequently, diabetic patients with third nerve ischemia classically present with a pupil-sparing oculomotor palsy (the so-called *diabetic third*). Injury resulting from an expanding posterior communicating aneurysm, neoplasm, or herniation must be ruled out, however, and MRI, MRA, and potentially cerebral angiography (see Table 19–5) should be considered in all patients with acute third nerve palsy. The sixth and seventh cranial nerves, as well as the spinal nerve roots, are also vulnerable to ischemic injury, and ischemic thoracic radiculopathy causing a dermatomal strip of numbness or pain may be confused with the prodrome of herpes zoster. Peripheral nerves, such as the femoral nerve, may also be affected.

The nerves of patients with diabetes are also much more susceptible to compressive injury, but complaints of hand numbness, pain, and weakness in these patients are often attributed to distal symmetric neuropathy instead of carpal tunnel syndrome. Conservative therapy is most effective when instituted early for treatment of nerve compression, so it is important to recognize carpal tunnel syndrome as early as possible. Compressive ulnar mononeuropathy at the elbow and peroneal mononeuropathy at the knee should also be considered as causes of diabetic symptoms.

5. Regional neuropathic syndromes—Diabetes can selectively damage a group of nerves in a specific region, as in diabetic amyotrophy. This syndrome presents with subacute proximal leg weakness that progresses in a stepwise manner over weeks to months, often accompanied by significant weight loss and, sometimes, by intermittent thigh pain. Weakness is usually most severe in the femoral and obturator distributions, with some involvement of the knee flexor compartment as well, but less severe weakness distally. In most patients, weakness plateaus over weeks to months and then slowly improves over 1–3 years. Diabetic thoracoabdominal neuropathy is another regional syndrome, in which damage to multiple thoracic nerve roots causes thoracic and abdominal pain, often accompanied by abdominal muscle weakness and outpouching. The initial pain of thoracoabdominal neuropathy may mimic cardiac ischemia, malignancy, gastric ulcer, or other diseases of visceral organs.

B. Diagnostic Studies

No single test can prove that the primary cause of nerve injury is diabetes. Careful history and physical examination may define patterns conforming to a single diabetic syndrome or some combination. Diabetic patients may develop neuropathy from a cause other than diabetes, and at least one careful evaluation for other potential causes is warranted. In patients who present with neuropathy but no prior history of diabetes, a 3-hour glucose tolerance test may be useful when fasting glucose measures or glycosylated hemoglobin are normal or borderline.

EMG and nerve conduction studies define the type of nerve injury and are also critical for identifying superimposed conditions such as carpal tunnel syndrome and lumbosacral radiculopathy. Distal symmetric diabetic neuropathy begins as an axonal disorder, with decreased sensory and motor amplitudes. Demyelinating change causing nerve conduction slowing often follows, and patients frequently have both axonal and demyelinative features at electrodiagnostic testing. Pure small-fiber neuropathy, which does not produce nerve conduction or EMG abnormalities, can be diagnosed through quantitative sensory testing and quantitation of small nerve fiber density via epidermal skin biopsies. When autonomic symptoms are present, specific tests of autonomic testing may be indicated (see Chapter 21). Cardiac symptoms require more detailed cardiologic evaluation.

▶ Differential Diagnosis

The differential diagnosis of the diabetic neuropathic syndromes encompasses not only all the potential causes of chronic sensorimotor neuropathy, but also the potential causes of small-fiber neuropathy, autonomic neuropathy, radiculopathy, plexopathy, mononeuropathy, and other causes of weakness, numbness, or both, such as myopathy, myelopathy, and stroke. Common and potentially treatable problems (eg, carpal tunnel syndrome and compressive cervical and lumbosacral radiculopathy) are too often attributed to diabetic neuropathy, resulting in unnecessary pain and permanent loss of sensory and motor function.

▶ Treatment

Optimal glucose control is the most effective method of preventing the development of diabetic neuropathy and of limiting its progression if it does develop. Intensive control is less likely to reverse existing neuropathy. Table 19–19 summarizes the efficacy of various therapies for painful polyneuropathy.

Diabetic foot care is of critical importance, and patients should undergo diabetic foot care education. If other foot abnormalities (eg, bony deformities, ingrown nails, corns) are present, referral to a podiatrist may be necessary. Autonomic dysfunction may necessitate assistance from the following specialists: urologist, gastroenterologist, and, especially, cardiologist. Physical therapy, gait training, occupational therapy, and orthotics are also very important and should be appropriately utilized.

Table 19–19. Efficacy of Medications for Painful Diabetic Neuropathy

Drug	Efficacy
Capsaicin cream	Effective in blinded, controlled trials; difficult to use
Carbamazepine	Effective in small, randomized trial
Citalopram	Effective in double-blind, controlled trial
Duloxetine	Effective in randomized double-blind, controlled trial
Fluoxetine	Not effective in double-blind, controlled trial
Gabapentin	Effective in double-blind, controlled trial
Isosorbide dinitrate spray	Effective in double-blind, controlled trial
Lamotrigine	Variably effective in different trials
Lidocaine patch	Effective in blinded, controlled trial of focal neuropathic pain
Narcotic analgesics	Possibly effective, difficult to use
Paroxetine	Effective in controlled trial
Phenytoin	Conflicting trial data
Pregabalin	Effective in randomized, double-blind controlled trial
Tramadol HCl	Effective in double-blind, controlled trial
Tricyclic antidepressants	Effective in double-blind, controlled trial
Venlafaxine	Effective in a small, randomized comparative trial
Zonisamide	Effective in open-label pilot trial

Dyck PJ, Windebank AJ. Diabetic and nondiabetic lumbosacral radiculoplexus neuropathies: New insights into pathophysiology and treatment. *Muscle Nerve* 2002;25:477–491. [PMID: 11932965] (Reviews pathogenesis, clinical findings, and therapeutics of diabetic lumbosacral radiculoplexus neuropathy [or diabetic amyotrophy].)

Novella SP, Inzucchi SE, Goldstein JM. The frequency of undiagnosed diabetes and impaired glucose tolerance in patients with idiopathic sensory neuropathy. *Muscle Nerve* 2001;24:1229–1231. [PMID: 11494278] (Patients with painful sensory neuropathy had a higher frequency of abnormal glucose metabolism compared with patients who did not have painful symptoms.)

Podwall D, Gooch C. Diabetic neuropathy: Clinical features, etiology and therapy. *Curr Neurol Neurosci Rep* 2004;4:55–61. [PMID: 14683630] (Reviews pathophysiology, clinical findings, diagnosis, and treatment of diabetic neuropathy.)

Sumner CJ, et al. The spectrum of neuropathy in diabetes and impaired glucose tolerance. *Neurology* 2003;60:108–111. [PMID: 12525727] (Evaluation of patients with neuropathy of unknown etiology who were subjected to oral glucose tolerance testing; patients with impaired glucose tolerance, rather than frank diabetes, had a milder neuropathy than patients with diabetes mellitus.)

THYROID DISEASE

1. Hypothyroidism

ESSENTIALS OF DIAGNOSIS

▶ Gradual onset of sensorimotor neuropathy

▶ Carpal tunnel syndrome (common)

▶ Diffuse muscle fatigue and cramping

▶ Myopathy may be superimposed

▶ "Hung up" deep tendon reflexes

Neuromuscular symptoms (eg, paresthesias, cramps, or weakness) can be the first manifestation of hypothyroidism and may precede the diagnosis by up to 1 year. Seventy-five percent of patients report at least some neuromuscular symptoms at the time of diagnosis. Carpal tunnel syndrome is the most common neuropathy in hypothyroidism, affecting up to one quarter of patients. Distal sensorimotor axonal neuropathy with stocking-glove sensory loss and weakness is found in one third. Diffuse muscle cramps and fatigue are even more common. The classic sign of the "hung up" deep tendon reflex (slow return of the limb to resting posture after activation of the reflex) is the result of slow relaxation of the muscle in hypothyroidism. Creatine kinase levels may be mildly elevated, most likely due to superimposed hypothyroid myopathy. Nerve conduction studies reveal axonal sensorimotor neuropathy, whereas needle EMG examination may reveal mild denervation, myopathy, or both. Thyroid replacement improves the neuropathy, but recovery may take more than 1 year.

2. Hyperthyroidism

ESSENTIALS OF DIAGNOSIS

▶ Subacute onset of sensorimotor neuropathy

▶ Carpal tunnel syndrome (less common than in hypothyroidism)

▶ Diffuse muscle fatigue

▶ Myopathy may be superimposed

▶ Rapid resolution with treatment

Neuromuscular symptoms (usually generalized muscular weakness and fatigue) may also be the first manifestation of hyperthyroidism. Reported by over 60% of patients, they usually precede the diagnosis by a shorter period, up to 4 months. About 20% of untreated hyperthyroid patients have a sensorimotor neuropathy diagnosed by EMG and nerve conduction studies; however, fewer patients actually have clinical symptoms from neuropathy. Ten percent of untreated hyperthyroid patients have a myopathy identified by electrodiagnostic studies. Carpal tunnel syndrome occurs in only 5% of patients, approaching the incidence in the general population, in contrast to patients with thyroid insufficiency. Examination often reveals proximal or distal weakness plus stocking-glove sensory loss. Nerve conduction studies and EMG may demonstrate a mild axonal sensorimotor neuropathy or mild myopathic change, or be normal. Symptoms resolve rapidly with treatment, usually within a few months.

Duyff RF, et al. Neuromuscular findings in thyroid dysfunction: A prospective clinical and electrodiagnostic study. *J Neurol Neurosurg Psychiatry* 2000;68:750–755. [PMID: 10811699] (Evaluation of clinical features and electrodiagnostic testing in patients with hypothyroidism and hyperthyroidism.)

COLLAGEN VASCULAR DISEASE & VASCULITIS

ESSENTIALS OF DIAGNOSIS

▶ Usually produces sensory or sensorimotor neuropathy or mononeuropathy multiplex

▶ Systemic disease has usually been diagnosed or is identifiable after workup

▶ Often responds to immunomodulatory therapy

1. Rheumatoid Arthritis

Neuropathy is a frequent feature of many of collagen vascular diseases. Rheumatoid arthritis frequently produces a distal, symmetric sensory or sensorimotor neuropathy that is usually mild and often less troubling to patients than their other symptoms. The incidence of carpal tunnel syndrome is increased in these patients. Atrophy of the intrinsic hand muscles may also occur as a direct result of rheumatoid arthritis, unrelated to a more systemic neuropathy. Less commonly, the disease produces a more severe mononeuropathy multiplex that requires aggressive immunosuppressive therapy.

2. Systemic Vasculitis & Other Collagen Vascular Diseases

Mononeuropathy multiplex occurs in up to 60% of patients with diseases causing systemic vasculitis, including polyarteritis nodosa, Churg-Strauss syndrome, and mixed connective tissue disease. It may present subacutely but more commonly evolves over several months to a year. As more and more nerves are affected, a diffuse symmetric pattern of polyneuropathy may emerge.

Isolated vasculitis, rare in the central nervous system, is extraordinarily rare in the peripheral nervous system, and all patients presenting with mononeuropathy multiplex should be aggressively evaluated for a more global vasculitic process. Virtually all patients demonstrate serum evidence of a systemic autoimmune disorder or involvement of other organ systems. Treatment may require aggressive immunosuppression with agents such as cyclophosphamide in patients with more rapidly progressive neurologic symptoms. More slowly progressive symptoms may respond to therapies directed at treating the underlying systemic disease process.

Systemic lupus erythematosus can also cause distal symmetric sensory or sensorimotor neuropathy (and, rarely, mononeuropathy multiplex), but more commonly affects the central nervous system, causing behavioral change and seizures. Sjögren syndrome causes a small-fiber or axonal sensory neuropathy as well as autonomic neuropathy.

SARCOIDOSIS

Sarcoidosis is a granulomatous, multiorgan disorder of unknown etiology that has many possible presentations. It can affect both the central and peripheral nervous systems and may cause diffuse sensorimotor neuropathy, myopathy, or both. More rarely, it may present with multiple mononeuropathies.

Chest radiographs may reveal mediastinal lymphadenopathy, and serum or CSF levels of angiotensin-converting enzyme may be elevated. Nerve conduction studies confirm neuropathy, and EMG may show myopathic change. If the diagnosis remains in doubt, nerve or muscle biopsy may show characteristic granulomas.

Corticosteroids are often beneficial, but side effects limit their use to severely affected patients.

CRITICAL ILLNESS POLYNEUROPATHY

ESSENTIALS OF DIAGNOSIS

► Most often occurs after weeks to months of critical illness
► Other causes of neuropathy (eg, acute inflammatory demyelinating polyradiculoneuropathy, drugs, diabetes) must be excluded
► Subacute form may occur with concurrent use of corticosteroids and depolarizing muscle relaxants
► Patients may have concurrent critical illness myopathy
► Associated with high mortality

▶ General Considerations

Critical illness polyneuropathy (CIP) is a subacute, symmetric polyneuropathy that occurs in patients who remain critically ill over weeks to months. A particular form of this disorder was first described in pediatric patients with severe exacerbations of reactive airways diseases treated concurrently with corticosteroids and neuromuscular blocking agents to assist ventilation. The patients developed prolonged, diffuse weakness caused by predominantly motor neuropathy. A much broader form of CIP afflicts patients of all ages with many different disorders.

The cause of CIP is thought to be multifactorial, because it often appears in patients with prolonged sepsis, multiorgan failure, severe trauma, advanced cancer, or other disorders. Typically patients have also been exposed to potentially neurotoxic drugs during intensive care, including total parenteral nutrition, aminoglycoside antibiotics, and vasopressor agents. Hypoalbuminemia and hyperglycemia are also possible risk factors, as are many other metabolic disturbances.

▶ Clinical Findings

A. Symptoms and Signs

Typically, the disorder begins with difficulty weaning patients from mechanical ventilation. On examination, they may have distal or even generalized weakness (sparing of cranial nerve muscles), distal sensory loss, and areflexia.

B. Diagnostic Studies

There are no specific laboratory tests for CIP. Nerve conduction studies usually reveal an axonal polyneuropathy. In some patients, there may be a purely motor neuropathy, but in others, sensory involvement is present. Motor unit assessment via needle EMG is usually limited, because patients are often unable to follow commands for volitional activation of the muscle. Nerve and muscle biopsy specimens may be difficult to interpret due to advanced atrophy and fibrotic change. Muscle sufficiently preserved to allow interpretation may show neurogenic, myopathic, or mixed change.

Differential Diagnosis

CIP remains a diagnosis of exclusion. It is often a challenging disorder to confirm, because patients are often afflicted with disorders that may also cause neuropathy (eg, diabetes, renal failure), including greater risk for the development of AIDP. Some patients may also develop a critical illness myopathy, either exclusively or in concert with CIP.

Treatment & Prognosis

There is no treatment for CIP other than treatment of the underlying illness and careful glucose control. Many of these patients die from their primary disease, and mortality is 2–3.5 times higher in those who develop CIP. Although it could contribute to mortality by prolonging ventilation, CIP may simply be a marker of more severe critical illness. Supportive care includes intensive physical therapy and prevention of both decubitus ulcers and deep vein thrombosis. In patients who survive, CIP improves over several months as the underlying illness is treated; about half of surviving patients recover completely.

Van Mook WN, Hulsewe-Evers RP. Critical illness polyneuropathy. *Curr Opin Crit Care* 2002;8:302–310. [PMID: 12386490] (Excellent review of the epidemiology, clinical features, diagnosis, and prognosis of patients with critical illness polyneuropathy.)

IDIOPATHIC POLYNEUROPATHY

The term *idiopathic polyneuropathy* is used to identify the disease process in the 25% of patients with distal polyneuropathy for whom no cause is identified after extensive diagnostic evaluation. Patients with idiopathic polyneuropathy are typically in their sixth decade and have a slow progression of symptoms over years. Distal sensory or sensorimotor symptoms and signs are most common, and legs are affected more significantly than hands. Electrophysiologic testing shows axonal polyneuropathy, and nerve biopsy reveals degeneration and regeneration of axons without inflammatory changes. Immunomodulatory treatment with corticosteroids, IVIG, or plasmapheresis has not shown clear benefit.

Vrancken AF, et al. Progressive idiopathic axonal neuropathy: A comparative clinical and histopathological study with vasculitic neuropathy. *J Neurol* 2004;251:269–278. [PMID: 15015005] (Study comparing vasculitic neuropathy and idiopathic neuropathy. Rarely, vasculitic changes may be found on biopsy examination in patients with idiopathic neuropathy.)

▼ HEREDITARY PERIPHERAL NEUROPATHIES

The hereditary peripheral neuropathies are the most common monogenetically inherited disease of the nervous system, with a prevalence ranging from 1–4 cases per 10,000 people. The hereditary neuropathies may be primary disorders, or they may appear as part of a broader hereditary metabolic disorder (eg, Fabry disease, lipoprotein deficiencies, abetalipoproteinemia, leukodystrophies, glycogen storage diseases). Genetic advances have clarified molecular diagnosis in these cases. At the same time, however, increasingly recognized phenotypic variability has forced modifications of previous clinical classifications. Although no definitive therapy is currently available for these disorders, a precise diagnosis assists with prognosis and genetic counseling.

GENERAL CLASSIFICATION

Prior to the genetic era, Charcot-Marie-Tooth neuropathy was divided into several different categories based on clinical and pathologic features. Today, hereditary peripheral neuropathies are divided into three major categories: (1) hereditary motor and sensory neuropathies (HMSNs), (2) hereditary motor neuropathies (HMNs), and (3) hereditary sensory and autonomic neuropathies (HSANs). The eponym *Charcot-Marie-Tooth* refers to the hereditary motor and sensory varieties. Many other hereditary disorders fall outside of this classification scheme, including familial amyloid polyneuropathy and hereditary neuropathies with a metabolic basis (eg, mitochondrial disease, the leukodystrophies, the glycogen storage diseases). The discovery of different genes has resulted in an ever-lengthening list of HMSN subtypes (Table 19–20).

HEREDITARY MOTOR & SENSORY NEUROPATHIES (HMSNs)

ESSENTIALS OF DIAGNOSIS

Charcot-Marie-Tooth (CMT) Types 1 and 2

- ▶ Gradually progressive distal weakness, atrophy, and sensory loss over many years
- ▶ Foot drop (common presenting feature)
- ▶ Frequent hammer toe and pes cavus deformities
- ▶ CMT type 1A is the most common variety (PMP22 mutation)

The HMSNs are the most common hereditary neuropathies. CMT type 1 (CMT-1 or HSMN 1) is the most common of the HMSNs, followed by CMT type 2 (CMT-2; HMSN 2); the remainder of the HMSN syndromes are much less common. Patients with CMT types 1 and 2 generally present with gradually progressive distal weakness, atrophy, and sensory loss over many years. Weakness beginning in small foot and peroneal muscles and progressing to hand and forearm muscles, distal symmetric sensory loss, and diminished or absent tendon reflexes are hallmarks of CMT types 1 and 2,

Table 19–20. Hereditary Motor and Sensory Neuropathies (HMSNs)[a]

HMSN	Inheritance/Subtype	Identified Gene	Clinical Findings
1	Autosomal dominant		Distal weakness and atrophy
	CMT-1A	PMP22	Demyelinating neuropathies
	CMT-1B	P_0	Slowed conduction velocities
	CMT-1C	LITAF	
	CMT-1D	EGR2	
2	Autosomal dominant		Distal weakness and atrophy
	CMT-2A	KIF1B, mitofusin-2	Axonal neuropathies
	CMT-2B	RAB7	Normal conduction velocities
	CMT-2C	None	Decreased motor and sensory amplitudes
	CMT-2D	GARS	
	CMT-2E	NEFL	
	CMT-2F	HSPB1	
	CMT-2G	None	
	CMT-2L	None	
	Autosomal recessive		
	AR CMT-2A	Lamin A/C	
	AR CMT-2B	None	
3	Autosomal dominant	PMP22	Dejerine-Sottas disease
	CMT-3	MP2	Severe demyelinating neuropathy
		EGR2	Many patients never walk
			Hypertrophic infantile neuropathy
4	Autosomal recessive		
	CMT-4A	GDAP1	Distal weakness and atrophy (most patients)
	CMT-4B	MTMR2	Demyelinating neuropathies
	CMT-4B2	MTMR13	Onset in infancy or childhood
	CMT-4C	KIAA1985	
	CMT-4D	NDRG1	
	CMT-4E	EGR2	
	CMT-4F	Periaxin	
Others	X linked	Connexin-32 (GJB1)	Distal weakness and atrophy (most patients)
	CMT-X		Demyelinating neuropathy
	Autosomal dominant	PMP22	Multiple compressive nerve injuries
	HNPP		Mild, generalized demyelinating neuropathy

CMT = Charcot-Marie-Tooth (disease); HNPP = hereditary neuropathy with predisposition to pressure palsy.
[a]Partial listing of causes of hereditary neuropathy.

but are usually more prominent in patients with CMT-1. Foot deformities such as pes cavus and hammer toe are frequently found. Patients complain primarily of weakness, but they may have sensory ataxia, which, along with foot drop, can interfere with gait. Most patients adapt to their gradually worsening condition and remain functional, with normal careers and life spans; however, more severe presentations also occur. In addition to careful history, physical examination, and family history, evaluation often includes electrophysiologic and genetic testing. Management is supportive and includes regular podiatric care, physical and occupational therapy, and appropriate orthotics (such as ankle-foot orthoses for foot drop). Drugs that cause peripheral neuropathy should be avoided. Genetic counseling is based on the inheritance pattern of the disease.

1. CMT Type 1 (HMSN 1)

CMT-1 is a group of autosomal-dominant, chronic demyelinating neuropathies. Symptoms often begin in early adulthood. The most common subtype, CMT-1A, results from a genetic defect in peripheral myelin protein 22 (PMP22) and accounts for 60% of all hereditary neuropathies. In CMT-1B, the affected gene is the myelin protein zero (MPZ) gene, whose product is the major protein component of compact myelin. CMT-1B is clinically similar to CMT-1A but may present earlier and become more severe. Enlarged, palpable peripheral nerves, especially the greater auricular nerve, may be seen, and nerve biopsy reveals an "onion-bulb" appearance of myelin, a consequence of chronic demyelination and remyelination. Although the clinical phenotypes may overlap,

CMT-1 is distinguished from CMT-2 by severely slowed nerve conduction velocities on electrophysiologic testing. Genetic testing provides confirmation.

2. CMT-X

X-linked dominant CMT presents similarly to CMT-1. Men are usually more severely affected. Women have milder neuropathy or may be asymptomatic. Nerve conduction velocities in men show significant slowing; in women the slowing is usually less severe.

3. CMT Type 2 (HMSN 2)

CMT-2 is a group of autosomal-dominant or autosomal-recessive, chronic axonal neuropathies, which usually present in the second decade. The clinical phenotype may be very similar to CMT-1. Electrophysiologic testing shows normal or mildly reduced nerve conduction velocities and reduced motor amplitudes. Nerve biopsy reveals neuronal loss without demyelination. Genetic testing, if positive, may provide confirmation of the diagnosis.

4. CMT Type 3 (Dejerine-Sottas Disease; HMSN 3)

Dejerine-Sottas disease is HMSN type 3 (or CMT-3), an autosomal-dominant or autosomal-recessive demyelinating neuropathy that often presents in infancy. The neuropathy is extremely severe and can be disabling. Electrophysiologic studies show severely reduced nerve conduction velocities with absent sensory responses. Nerve biopsy shows severe demyelination and "onion-bulb" formation. De novo mutations have been described.

5. CMT Type 4 (HMSN 4)

CMT-4 is a group of autosomal-recessive neuropathies that present in early childhood with weakness. Progressive loss of strength leaves many adolescents wheelchair bound. Nerve conduction velocities are slowed.

6. Hereditary Neuropathy With Predisposition to Pressure Palsy (HNPP)

ESSENTIALS OF DIAGNOSIS

▶ Multiple compressive nerve injuries (carpal tunnel, ulnar at elbow, peroneal at knee)

▶ Mild, generalized demyelinating neuropathy may be present

▶ Many patients have no family history (variable penetrance)

HNPP is an autosomal-dominant neuropathy that usually presents in patients between 20 and 40 years of age. Patients have multiple, painless, focal peripheral nerve lesions after minimal trauma or compression, which most often involve the median nerve at the carpal tunnel, the ulnar nerve at the elbow, or the peroneal nerve at the fibular head. Symptoms typically improve over days to months. Rarely, brachial plexopathy can be the initial presentation of HNPP. Some patients have a slowly progressive symmetric peripheral neuropathy that is clinically similar to CMT. Electrophysiologic studies confirm multiple focal mononeuropathies at common anatomic sites of compression, sometimes with a mild demyelinating neuropathy superimposed (with mild diffuse slowing of nerve conduction velocities). Sural nerve biopsy (no longer necessary for diagnosis) shows characteristic focal thickening of the myelin sheath. Therapy includes avoiding activities that place the nerve at risk for compression, with careful observance of ergonomic measures at all times, and the use of bracing, padding, and surgical release when needed. Genetic testing may confirm the diagnosis.

HEREDITARY MOTOR NEUROPATHIES (HMNs)

ESSENTIALS OF DIAGNOSIS

▶ Pure motor weakness with no sensory loss

▶ Distal onset

▶ Slowly progressive over years

▶ Usually autosomal-dominant inheritance

▶ Much less common than HMSNs

The HMNs are rare disorders characterized by very slowly progressive distal paresis and atrophy. Onset occurs between the ages of 20 and 40 years, and affected persons have a normal life expectancy. Nerve conductions reveal a pure motor, axonal neuropathy with normal velocities, reduced motor amplitudes, and normal sensory responses. Most cases show an autosomal-dominant inheritance.

HEREDITARY SENSORY & AUTONOMIC NEUROPATHIES (HSANs)

ESSENTIALS OF DIAGNOSIS

▶ Sensory loss or dysautonomia

▶ Specific features depend on subtype

▶ Usually autosomal-recessive inheritance but some types are autosomal dominant

▶ Much less common than HMSNs

HSANs present with sensory loss or autonomic dysfunction without motor symptoms (Table 19–21). Sensory loss makes patients susceptible to unnoticed trauma, ulcers, infections, osteomyelitis, and neuropathic Charcot joint deformities. Treatment is mainly supportive. Foot care is extremely important in patients with HSAN to prevent ulcers and stress fractures. When ulcers do develop, weight bearing should be stopped until the ulcers heal. Daily inspection and moisturization of feet should be encouraged.

1. HSAN Type 1

HSAN 1, the most common familial sensory neuropathy, is autosomal dominant. Symptoms start in the second or third decade, with sensory loss and lancinating pain in the feet. Foot calluses, stress fractures, neuropathic joints, and recurrent painless plantar ulcers are common as the disease progresses. On examination, pain and temperature sensation are affected more than proprioception and vibration. Electrophysiologic testing may reveal diminished sensory responses, and nerve biopsy shows severe loss of unmyelinated and small myelinated axons with milder loss of large myelinated fibers.

Table 19–21. Hereditary Sensory and Autonomic Neuropathies (HSANs)

HSAN	Inheritance/ Subtype	Identified Gene	Clinical Findings
1	Autosomal dominant	SPTLC1	Predominant pain and temperature sensory loss in feet Onset in 2nd or 3rd decade Most prevalent of HSANs Acromutilation
2	Autosomal recessive	HSN2	All sensory modalities lost in distal hands and feet Onset in infancy
3	Autosomal recessive	IKBKAP	Riley-Day syndrome (familial dysautonomia) Onset in infancy Poor temperature control Excessive sweating Blood pressure fluctuations Pain and temperature sensation deficits (late)
4	Autosomal recessive	TRKA/NGF receptor	All sensory modalities lost in distal hands and feet Onset in infancy
5	Autosomal recessive	None	Congenital insensitivity to pain Onset in infancy Poor temperature control Anhidrosis Mild mental retardation

2. HSAN Type 2

HSAN 2 is autosomal recessive and begins in infancy. All sensory modalities of the distal upper and lower limbs are affected. The hands, feet, lips, and tongue are at risk of injury because of sensory loss. Autonomic dysfunction may include bladder dysfunction and impotence. The course is slowly progressive, with evolving axonal loss and absent sensory responses on electrophysiologic testing. Nerve biopsy shows virtually complete absence of myelinated fibers and reduced unmyelinated fibers.

3. HSAN Type 3

HSAN 3 is the Riley-Day syndrome or familial dysautonomia. It is an autosomal-recessive disease affecting people of Ashkenazi Jewish descent. The disorder disproportionately affects peripheral autonomic and sensory neurons, but it also affects motor neurons. Neonates may have poor feeding and autonomic symptoms such as excessive sweating, poor tear secretion, fluctuations in blood pressure, and poor body temperature control. Pain and temperature deficits appear later. Electrophysiologic studies show mixed axonal and demyelinating changes with slowed conduction velocities and decreased motor amplitudes.

4. HSAN Type 4

HSAN 4 is a rare autosomal-recessive disorder that includes congenital insensitivity to pain, anhidrosis, poor temperature control, and mild mental retardation. There is disproportionate loss of unmyelinated axons and small myelinated fibers. Because large fibers are minimally affected, tendon reflexes are normal and nerve conduction studies (which assess large-fiber function) reveal normal sensory responses. However, autonomic sweat testing and quantitative small-fiber assessment via skin biopsy reveal the loss and dysfunction of small cutaneous nerve fibers.

5. HSAN Type 5

HSAN 5 is clinically similar to HSAN 4, but there is loss only of small myelinated, not small unmyelinated, fibers.

FAMILIAL AMYLOID POLYNEUROPATHY

ESSENTIALS OF DIAGNOSIS

▶ Predominantly sensory and autonomic neuropathy
▶ Frequent carpal tunnel syndrome
▶ Cardiovascular, gastrointestinal, or ocular symptoms
▶ Autosomal-dominant inheritance
▶ May present in adulthood

General Considerations

Familial amyloid polyneuropathy is an autosomal-dominant disorder that causes a life-threatening sensorimotor and autonomic neuropathy. Most commonly, it is the result of a mutation in the transthyretin (*TTR*) gene, producing the most severe form of the disorder. TTR is a protein that handles thyroxin and retinol transport and is primarily synthesized in the liver. Mutations in this gene can cause neuropathy and cardiomyopathy through the deposition of amyloid within affected organs.

Clinical Findings

A. Symptoms and Signs

Familial amyloid polyneuropathy causes a length-dependent sensorimotor and autonomic neuropathy and has a variable presentation, depending on which organs are affected first. The incidence of carpal tunnel syndrome is dramatically increased in these patients. Cardiovascular involvement is common, and gastrointestinal, renal, and ocular injury also occurs. Several different mutations in the *TTR* gene have been identified, with varying phenotypes in each genetic group. Some mutations are associated with central nervous system involvement, including seizures, dementia, depression, infarction, or leptomeningeal amyloidosis. Despite multiorgan involvement, neuropathy is often a major source of disability in these patients, who may survive for a decade or more after diagnosis.

B. Diagnostic Studies

Neurophysiologic testing shows a sensorimotor neuropathy with axonal features. Nerve biopsy examination shows characteristic amyloid deposits with staining for TTR antibodies. There is involvement of unmyelinated and small myelinated fibers. Molecular genetic testing can establish a definitive diagnosis, and presymptomatic and prenatal molecular genetic diagnosis can be offered to family members at risk.

Differential Diagnosis

This disorder must be distinguished from acquired systemic or paraneoplastic amyloidosis, which is often associated with much shorter survival. Neuropathy may also be the presenting feature of acquired amyloidosis. Biopsy of the most affected tissue typically demonstrates characteristic amyloid deposition.

Treatment & Prognosis

Liver transplantation has been used as a primary treatment of familial amyloidosis because the liver is the primary source of TTR. Patients who undergo liver transplantation may show improvement in their neurologic symptoms, but some have worsening of cardiac failure. Liver transplantation early in the course of disease seems to result in fewer complications.

HEREDITARY NEUROPATHIES WITH A METABOLIC BASIS

Most of these disorders are rare and present in childhood with characteristic clinical syndromes. They include Fabry disease, lipoprotein deficiencies (Tangier disease), abetalipoproteinemia (Bassen-Kornzweig disease), the leukodystrophies (adrenoleukodystrophy, adrenoleukoneuropathy, metachromatic leukodystrophy, Cockayne syndrome, Krabbe disease, Pelizaeus-Merzbacher disease), phytanic acid storage disease (Refsum disease), and some of the glycogen storage diseases (eg, glycogen storage disease type II). Many of these disorders are discussed in Chapter 36.

Kuhlenbaumer G, et al. Clinical features and molecular genetics of hereditary peripheral neuropathies. *J Neurol* 2002;249:1629–1650. [PMID: 12529785] (Summary of the clinical and molecular genetic features of inherited neuropathies.)

Plante-Bordeneuve V, Said G. Transthyretin related familial amyloid polyneuropathy. *Curr Opin Neurol* 2000;13:569–573. [PMID: 11073365] (Reviews the molecular genetics, clinical presentation, and treatment of familial amyloid polyneuropathy.)

Young P, Suter U. The causes of Charcot-Marie-Tooth disease. *Cell Mol Life Sci* 2003;60:2547–1560. [PMID: 14685682] (Reviews the classification and molecular genetics of CMT disease.)

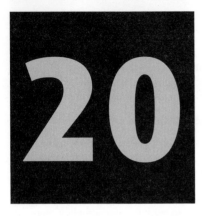

Motor Neuron Diseases

Michio Hirano, MD

▶ General Considerations

By convention, the term *motor neuron disease* encompasses disorders that predominantly or exclusively affect upper motor neurons, lower motor neurons, or both. By definition, sensory neurons are spared in these diseases. Motor neuron diseases can be acquired or inherited; however, the most common of these diseases in adults, amyotrophic lateral sclerosis (ALS), is typically sporadic and its cause is unknown (Tables 20–1 and 20–2).

Motor neuron diseases are clinically heterogeneous and occur worldwide, but several forms have been found in endemic foci. In the Western Pacific, ALS is particularly prevalent in Guam, Papua New Guinea, and the Kii Peninsula of Japan. In Guam, the prevalence of ALS was 50 times greater than that in other parts of the world, and it was often associated with parkinsonism and dementia. Curiously, since World War II, the incidence of ALS in Guam has declined markedly. There are controversial descriptions of clusters of ALS in veterans of the 1990–1991 Persian Gulf War, Italian soccer players, and other groups. In Southern India, a Madras motor neuron disease variant has been described.

▶ Pathogenesis

The pyramidal system comprises UMNs and LMNs and is responsible for the voluntary control of muscles. The cell bodies of UMNs reside in the motor cortex of the brain and project axons via corticospinal and corticobulbar tracts that descend through the cerebral white matter and the internal capsule. Corticobulbar tracts synapse on LMNs (motor cranial nuclei) in the brainstem. By contrast, corticospinal tracts pass through the cerebral peduncles of the midbrain and the anterior pons and, at the lower medullary pyramids, cross to the contralateral side before descending primarily through the lateral spinal cord to synapse predominantly on LMNs in the anterior horn of the spinal cord. The LMNs, in turn, project through the anterior spinal nerve roots and peripheral nerves to innervate muscle.

Motor neuron diseases can be divided into two broad etiologic categories, acquired and inherited. Both may be subclassified according to pattern of motor neuron dysfunction (see Tables 20–1 and 20–2). Acquired motor neuron diseases may have an infectious (eg, poliomyelitis), autoimmune (multifocal motor neuropathy with conduction block and motor neuropathy with paraproteinemia), or idiopathic cause (primary lateral sclerosis and sporadic ALS). Inherited motor neuron diseases are grouped according to the motor neuron involvement: hereditary spastic paraparesis when only UMNs are affected; spinal muscular atrophy when only LMNs are involved; and familial ALS when both UMNs and LMNs degenerate. To date, 12 genetically distinct forms of familial ALS and 41 types of hereditary spastic paraparesis have been delineated. In addition, syndromes of familial ALS plus other neurologic features have been described.

▶ Clinical Findings

A. Symptoms and Signs

Dysfunction of UMNs and LMNs produces characteristic symptoms and signs (Table 20–3).

1. Upper motor neuron dysfunction—UMN lesions manifest as spasticity, slowed rapid alternating movements, hyperactive tendon reflexes, and pathologic reflexes, including Babinski sign. **Spasticity** is a form of increased motor

Table 20–1. Acquired Motor Neuron Diseases

Presentation	Disease
Acute	
LMN only	Poliomyelitis
Chronic	
UMN and LMN	Amyotrophic lateral sclerosis
UMN only	Primary lateral sclerosis
LMN only	Progressive spinal muscular atrophy
	Fazio-Londe syndrome
	Monomelic muscular atrophy
	Madras motor neuron disease

LMN = lower motor neuron; UMN = upper motor neuron.

tone, which, in arms, usually affects flexor muscles to a greater extent than extensor muscles. Conversely, in the legs, extensor muscles of the legs are affected to a greater degree than flexors. Spasticity is more prominent at the initiation of passive movement and then diminishes, a sign described as *clasp-knife phenomenon.* Furthermore, the increased tone is velocity dependent and therefore becomes more evident as the speed of the passive movement is increased. Patients with severe spasticity often complain of muscle stiffness.

Hyperactive tendon stretch reflexes manifest as clonus (repetitive rhythmic muscle contractions) or spread (contractions of muscles not directly connected to the stretched tendon). Dysfunction of corticobulbar tracts causes dysphagia, dysarthria, and pseudobulbar affect, a tendency to laugh or cry spontaneously or with mild provocation. Frontal release signs indicate corticobulbar degeneration and include hyperactive jaw jerk and snout and suck reflexes.

Disorders of UMNs are described as spastic paraparesis when legs are weak or spastic paraplegia when legs are paralyzed.

2. Lower motor neuron dysfunction—LMN defects cause weakness and wasting of muscles. **Fasciculations** are spontaneous discharges of individual LMNs and are often visible as muscle twitches. Although often seen in healthy individuals, fasciculations in the setting of atrophic and weak muscles usually signify LMN disease. Hyporeflexia and areflexia are important signs of LMN defects.

B. History and Physical Examination Findings

The history of present illness can be helpful in defining the cause of a motor neuron disease. Subacute onset of weakness over days to weeks suggests an infectious or inflammatory process whereas a gradual onset of weakness over months to years is more typical of hereditary or degenerative diseases. Autosomal-recessive motor neuron diseases generally show juvenile onset, whereas autosomal-dominant forms usually begin in adulthood. The disease course in most motor neuron diseases is slow progression.

Patients with UMN dysfunction complain of stiffness and clumsiness, which often manifests as difficulty fastening buttons and tying shoelaces, and clumsy gait. By contrast, LMN defects cause weakness, atrophy, and twitching (fasciculations). Weight loss is common and is primarily due to loss of muscle mass. Decreased oral intake due to dysphagia may contribute to loss of weight.

The pattern of weakness in motor neuron diseases is variable and depends on the distribution and severity of UMNs and LMNs. When brainstem motor neurons (cranial nerves V, VII, IX, X, and XII) degenerate, muscles of the jaw, face, oropharynx, or tongue are weak, impairing speech and swallowing. Weakness of respiratory muscles is common. Absence of sensory changes distinguishes motor neuron disease from peripheral neuropathies; nevertheless, pure or predominantly motor neuropathies may manifest as weakness without sensory symptoms.

A thorough neuromuscular examination can usually distinguish motor neuron disease from myopathies or neuropathies. With ALS, the clinical diagnosis is based on medical history and physical findings and can be confirmed only at autopsy.

Inspection of muscle can reveal atrophy and fasciculations. Fasciculations may be elicited by lightly tapping the muscle or by transient contraction of the muscle.

Weakness is assessed semi-quantitatively by manual muscle testing; such testing is somewhat subjective and effort dependent. For example, a physician who applies full arm strength will be able to overcome normal small distal muscles such as finger extensor or interosseous muscles. For this reason, muscle strength must be tested judiciously. Sensory and coordination testing are important to exclude the involvement of sensory nerves and cerebellum. Tendon reflexes are variably abnormal. UMN defects cause hyperactivity, whereas LMN dysfunction causes hyporeflexia or areflexia. The Babinski sign indicates corticospinal tract pathology. It may be masked, however, by the severe weakness of toe extensors. Hoffmann sign, often seen in patients with UMN dysfunction, may also be present in normal individuals. Frontal release signs may be evident in the setting of UMN disease.

C. Diagnostic Studies

Laboratory and diagnostic studies are important to confirm the diagnosis of motor neuron disease and to exclude other possibilities (Table 20–4).

1. Electromyography and nerve conduction studies—Electrophysiologic studies can be essential in recognizing motor neuron diseases and are described in detail in Chapter 2. When LMNs are affected, nerve conduction studies show decreased amplitude of compound motor action potentials, with normal or mildly slowed motor nerve conduction velocities. In contrast, in demyelinating neuropathies, motor nerve conductions are severely slowed and there may be conduction blocks. In addition, abnormalities of

Table 20–2. Inherited Motor Neuron Diseases

Disease	Gene Locus	Gene Product (Gene Symbol)
Familial ALS		
Autosomal dominant		
ALS1	21q12	Superoxide dismutase (*SOD1*)
ALS3	18q21	Unknown
ALS4	9q34	Senataxin (*SETX*)
ALS6	16q12	FUS(*FUS*)
ALS7	20p13	Unknown
ALS8	20q13	Vesicle-associated membrane protein-associated protein B (*VAPB*)
ALS9	14q11	Angiogenin (*ANG*)
ALS10	1p36.22	TAR DNA-binding protein (*TARDBP*)
ALS11	6q21	Unknown
ALS12	10	Optineurin (*OPTN*)
Autosomal recessive		
ALS2	2q	*Alsin*
ALS5	15q	Unknown
ALS12	10	Optineurin (*OPTN*)
ALS-X	Xcen	Unknown
Maternally inherited	MtDNA	Subunit I of cytochrome c oxidase
Upper Motor Neuron		
Hereditary spastic paraparesis with known causative genes		
• Autosomal dominant		
SPG3A	14q11–q21	Atlastin (*ATL1*)
SPG4	2p22	Spastin (*SPAST*)
SPG6	15q11	Nonimprinted in Prader-Willi/Angelman syndrome region protein 1 (*NIPA1*)
SPG8	8q23–q24	Strumpellin (*KIAA0196*)
SPG12	19q13	Kinesin heavy chain (*KIF5A*)
SPG13	2q24–q34	Heat shock protein 60 (*HSPD1*)
SPG17	11q12–q14	Seipin (*BSCL2*)
SPG31	2p12	Receptor expression-enhancing protein 1 (*REEP1*)
SPG42	3q24.31	Acetyl-CoA transporter (*SCL33A1*)
• Autosomal recessive		
SPG5	8q21.3	Cytochrome P450, family 7, subfamily B, polypeptide 1 (*CYP7B1*)
SPG7	16q	Paraplegin (*SPG7*)
SPG11	15q	Spatacsin (*SPG11*)
SPG13	2q24–q34	Heat shock protein 60 (*HSPD1*)
SPG15	14q	Spastizin (*ZFYVE26*)
SPG20	13q	Spartin (*BSCL2*)
SPG21	15q21–q22	Maspardin (*SPG21*)
SPG39	19p13	Neuropathy target esterase (*PNPLA6*)
SPG44	1q42.13	Connexin 47 (*GJC2*)
• X-linked		
SPG1	Xq28	L1 cell adhesion molecule (*L1CAM*)
SPG2	Xq21	Proteolipid protein
SPG22	Xq13.2	Solute carrier family 16, member 2 (*SCL16A2*)
Adrenomyeloneuropathy	Xq21	Adrenoleukodystrophy protein
Lower Motor Neuron		
Spinal muscular atrophy (SMA)—infantile (Werdnig-Hoffmann disease), intermediate, childhood (Kugelberg-Welander disease), adult	5q11	Survival motor neuron protein

(Continued)

Table 20–2. Inherited Motor Neuron Diseases (*Continued*)

mtDNA depletion (SMA phenotype)	16q22	Thymidine kinase 2
X-linked spinobulbar muscular atrophy (Kennedy disease)	Xq	Androgen receptor
GM$_2$-gangliosidosis		
Adult Tay-Sachs disease	15q	Hexoaminidase A
Sandhoff disease	5q	Hexoaminidase B
AB variant	5q	GM$_2$ activator protein
Acid maltase deficiency—infantile (Pompe disease), childhood, adult	17q	Acid maltase
ALS-plus Diseases		
ALS with frontotemporal dementia and parkinsonism	17q	Tau protein
ALS with frontotemporal dementia	9q21–q22	Unknown
Adult polyglucosan body disease	3p12	Glycogen branching enzyme
Adult polyglucosan body disease	Unknown	Other causes

ALS = amyotrophic lateral sclerosis.

sensory nerve conductions should cast doubt on the diagnosis of motor neuron disease. In both motor neuron disease and peripheral neuropathies, electromyography will reveal fibrillations and positive sharp waves, which are caused by spontaneous discharges of denervated muscle fibers. In contrast, fasciculations are more specific to motor neuron disease.

Chronic peripheral neuropathies or LMN diseases lead to a reduction in motor axons with axonal sprouting from the remaining nerves providing compensatory reinnervation to larger-than-normal groups of muscle. As a consequence of denervation and reinnervation, fewer motor neurons are activated during muscle contractions, a phenomenon reflected in the electromyogram as reduced recruitment or, when the individual motor units are discernible, discrete activity (see Chapter 2).

2. Imaging studies—In patients with UMN degeneration, magnetic resonance imaging (MRI) of the brain may reveal abnormal hyperintensity of the corticospinal tract in the posterior limb of the internal capsule on T2-weighted images or fluid-attenuated inversion recovery (FLAIR) imaging. Magnetic resonance spectroscopy can detect the degeneration or dysfunction of UMNs within the motor cortex by demonstrating a decrease in the absolute level of *N*-acetylaspartate (NAA) or in the amount of NAA relative to creatine or choline. MRI scans of the brain and spine are often obtained to look for structural abnormalities that can produce weakness mimicking motor neuron disease. MRI of the cervical spine is particularly important to exclude structural lesions when the cranial nerves are spared.

3. Lumbar puncture—Lumbar puncture is useful to exclude inflammatory processes such as multiple sclerosis

Table 20–3. Symptoms and Signs of Upper and Lower Motor Neuron Dysfunction

	UMN Defects	LMN Defects
Muscle tone	Increased	Decreased
Rapid alternating movements	Slow out of proportion to weakness	Slow due to weakness
Fasciculation	Absent	Present
Weakness	+	++
Muscle wasting	±	++
Tendon reflexes	Hyperactive	Areflexia
Babinski sign	Present	Absent

LMN = lower motor neuron; UMN = upper motor neuron; + = positive; ++ = strongly positive; ± = may be positive or negative.

Table 20–4. Diagnostic Studies for Amyotrophic Lateral Sclerosis (ALS) and ALS-Like Disorders

Study	Diagnostic Utility
Nerve conduction studies/electromyography	Confirmation of LMN dysfunction in patients with ALS and LMN disorders Identification of focal conduction blocks in patients with multifocal motor neuropathy Detection of sensory nerve involvement in peripheral neuropathies
MRI of brain and spine	Detection of corticospinal tract abnormalities in ALS; however, lesions not always seen Identification of structural abnormalities affecting brain, spine, or both
Magnetic resonance spectroscopy	Detection or confirmation of UMN degeneration when UMN signs not clearly present
Lumbar puncture	Detection of inflammatory process Elevated CSF protein may indicate polyneuropathy, polyradiculopathy, or lymphoma
Metabolic studies • Routine blood chemistries • Fasting glucose level • Vitamin B_{12}, methylmalonic acid, and homocysteine levels • Lactic acid and pyruvate levels	 Detection of electrolyte abnormalities Screening for diabetes mellitus Screening for vitamin B_{12} deficiency Screening for mitochondrial dysfunction
Endocrinologic studies • Thyroid function tests • Calcium measurement	 Screening for hypothyroidism Screening for hyperparathyroidism
Serologic studies • Serum and urine protein electrophoresis, immunofix-ation electrophoresis, quantitative immunoglobulin, and cryoglobulins • In patients with possible myelopathies—HTLV-1 and HTLV-2, HIV, cytomegalovirus, herpes zoster, HSV-1 and HSV-2 screening	 Screening for monoclonal gammopathy Detection of viral causes of myelopathy
Hexosaminidase activity	Diagnosis of hexosaminidase A deficiency

CSF = cerebrospinal fluid; HIV = human immunodeficiency virus; HSV = herpes simplex virus; HTLV = human T-lymphotropic virus; LMN = lower motor neuron; MRI = magnetic resonance imaging; UMN = upper motor neuron.
Reproduced with permission from Brooks BR, Miller RG, Swash M, Munsat TL. El Escorial revisited: Revised criteria for the diagnosis of amyotrophic lateral sclerosis. *Amyotroph Lateral Scler Other Motor Neuron Disord* 2000;1:293–299.

that can cause weakness. Abnormally high white blood cell counts, the presence of oligoclonal bands, or elevated immunoglobulin G in cerebrospinal fluid (CSF) suggest inflammation rather than a primary degenerative or hereditary motor neuron disease. Elevated CSF protein concentration can be indicative of polyneuropathy, polyradiculopathy, or paraneoplastic diseases caused by lymphoma.

4. Other tests—Blood tests are important to identify causes of motor neuron diseases and motor neuron–like disorders, which include toxic-metabolic, endocrinologic, infectious, inflammatory, and genetic conditions (see Table 20–4). Indications for genetic testing are described in the context of each disease category (see later discussion and Table 20–2). No treatments exist for inherited motor neuron diseases. It is therefore generally considered unethical to perform genetic testing on asymptomatic minors at risk for inheriting these disorders. In contrast, once a patient develops a motor neuron disease that may be heritable, genetic testing can be confirmatory and will allow more accurate genetic counseling.

AMYOTROPHIC LATERAL SCLEROSIS

 ESSENTIALS OF DIAGNOSIS

▶ Subacute to chronic progressive weakness

▶ UMN symptoms and signs—stiffness, spasticity, clumsiness, hyperactive tendon reflexes, Babinski sign

▶ LMN dysfunction—weakness, wasting and fasciculations, areflexia or hyporeflexia

▶ Preservation of extraocular muscle movements

▶ Intact bladder and bowel functions

▶ Absence of cognitive and sensory changes

General Considerations

ALS, widely known as *Lou Gehrig disease*, is the most common motor neuron disease in adults. In 1874, Charcot described the disease as ALS because of the marked muscle atrophy (amyotrophy) and hardening of the lateral spinal cord (lateral sclerosis). These gross pathologic changes capture the essential features of the disease: UMN degeneration causing spasticity and clumsiness and LMN loss causing weakness and wasting.

The incidence of ALS is about 1–2 cases per 100,000 people, which translates to about 5000 new patients per year in the United States. Although ALS and multiple sclerosis have similar incidence rates, the prevalence of ALS is much lower, about 25,000 cases in the United States, because most patients die within 3–5 years of onset of symptoms.

Pathogenesis

About 5% of ALS patients have an inherited form of the disease, but the vast majority have a sporadic neurodegenerative disease of unknown cause. Autosomal-dominant, autosomal-recessive, and X-linked recessive forms of familial ALS have been delineated (see Table 20–2). Despite constituting a small minority of ALS, familial forms have stimulated new lines of research in the pathogenesis of ALS.

The first genetically defined form of familial ALS, ALS1, is an autosomal-dominant disease caused by mutations in the gene encoding SOD1, a superoxide dismutase that converts superoxide (O^{2-}) to hydrogen peroxide (H_2O_2). Mutations in SOD1 account for about 20% of familial ALS patients or about 1% of all ALS cases. Onset is typically after age 40, clinical manifestations may begin in bulbar or spinal innervated muscles, and survival ranges from 1–20 years.

Since the identification of SOD1 mutations, two genes responsible for juvenile forms of inherited ALS have been identified: *alsin*, which causes autosomal-recessive ALS2, and *senataxin*, responsible for autosomal-dominant ALS4. Five additional genes have been identified as causes of familial ALS that are predominantly autosomal dominant and mainly affect adults (see Table 20–2). Familial ALS has provided insights that may be applicable to sporadic ALS.

Intraneuronal inclusions are histologic hallmarks of sporadic and SOD1 mutant forms of ALS and may be pathogenic. Excitotoxic injury to motor neurons resulting from impaired removal of the excitatory neurotransmitter glutamate from synapses may play a role. Autoimmunity and environmental factors such as viruses and toxins have also been hypothesized to cause ALS. These pathogenic hypotheses are not mutually exclusive, and multiple mechanisms may contribute to the motor neuron degeneration seen in ALS.

Clinical Findings

The major clinical findings are UMN and LMN signs (see Table 20–3) that are typically asymmetric early in the course

of the disease. Extraocular muscles, cognitive, and sensory functions are usually spared.

Differential Diagnosis

In patients with clear UMN and LMN signs affecting bulbar and limb muscles, the diagnosis of ALS is relatively straightforward; early in the course, however, the disease can be difficult to distinguish from other disorders (Table 20–5). Furthermore, atypical patients with ALS may manifest only UMN or LMN signs or may show involvement of neurons outside the motor system. Because of these uncertainties,

Table 20–5. Differential Diagnosis of Amyotrophic Lateral Sclerosis

Disorders Associated With UMN and LMN Dysfunction
Structural lesions affecting the brainstem or cervical spinal cord:
• Parasagittal tumor
• Foramen magnum tumor
• Arnold-Chiari malformation
• Syringomyelia, syringobulbia
• Cervical spondylosis
• Intraspinal extramedullary tumor
• Brainstem or spinal cord arteriovenous malformation
• Brainstem or spinal cord tumor
Adrenomyeloneuropathy
Subacute combined degeneration (vitamin B_{12} deficiency)
Mitochondrial encephalomyopathies
UMN Disorders
Hereditary spastic paraparesis
Infectious myelopathies—HTLV-1, HTLV-2, HIV, herpes simplex, herpes zoster
Primary lateral sclerosis
LMN Disorders and Motor Neuropathies
Multifocal motor neuropathy with conduction block
Motor neuropathy with paraproteinemia
Spinal muscular atrophy
Hexoaminidase A deficiency
Kennedy disease
Monomelic amyotrophic lateral sclerosis
Polyradiculopathies and polyneuropathies—Lyme disease, CIDP, cytomegalovirus
Polio, postpolio syndrome
Paraneoplastic syndromes, including lymphoma
Myopathies
Inclusion body myositis
Acid maltase deficiency
Other Disorders
Hyperthyroidism
Hyperparathyroidism
Benign fasciculations
Cramp-fasciculation syndrome

CIDP = chronic inflammatory demyelinating polyneuropathy; HIV = human immunodeficiency virus; HTLV = human T-lymphotropic virus; LMN = lower motor neuron; UMN = upper motor neuron.

Table 20–6. Revised E1 Escorial Criteria for the Diagnosis of ALS[a]

	Criteria
Definite ALS	UMN and LMN signs in at least 3 body regions
Probable ALS	UMN and LMN signs in at least 2 body regions with some UMN signs rostral to LMN signs
Clinically probable laboratory-supported ALS	UMN signs with or without LMN signs in 1 region and electrophysiologic LMN signs in at least 2 regions, and neuroimaging and clinical laboratory studies to exclude other causes
Possible ALS	UMN and LMN in 1 region or UMN signs in at least 2 regions, or UMN signs caudal to LMN signs
Suspected ALS	Pure LMN signs

ALS = amyotrophic lateral sclerosis; LMN = lower motor neuron; UMN = upper motor neuron.
[a]Patients undergo clinical and electromyographic studies of four body regions—cranial, cervical, thoracic, and lumbosacral.
Reproduced with permission from Brooks BR, Miller RG, Swash M, Munsat TL. El Escorial revisited: Revised criteria for the diagnosis of amyotrophic lateral sclerosis. *Amyotroph Lateral Scler Other Motor Neuron Disord* 2000;1:293–299.

diagnostic criteria have been established for research studies (Table 20–6).

In patients suspected of having ALS, it is important to consider structural lesions such as arteriovenous malformation, tumor, or syrinx affecting the brainstem or cervical spinal cord (see Table 20–5). Cervical spondylosis can cause weakness, atrophy, and fasciculations in the arms with spasticity in the legs. Absence of cranial nerve signs and presence of sensory changes or bladder or bowel dysfunction may be clues that the patient has a restricted cervical cord lesion rather than ALS. Tumors of the foramen magnum or a syrinx can affect the 12th cranial nerve, causing tongue weakness and wasting. MRI scans of the brain and cervical spine can easily exclude these structural abnormalities.

A. Myelopathies

Myelopathies resulting from adrenomyeloneuropathy or infections (eg, human T-lymphotropic virus 1 or 2 [HTLV-1, HTLV-2] or HIV) can produce spastic paraparesis; however, sensory changes, lack of bulbar involvement, and sphincter complaints differentiate these disorders from ALS. Subacute combined degeneration (vitamin B_{12} deficiency) causes a myeloneuropathy that usually results in weakness and sensory

changes; however, in the absence of sensory abnormalities, this condition may resemble ALS. Hereditary spastic paraparesis (discussed later in this chapter) can be distinguished from ALS by family history, slow progression, sphincter involvement, and absence of bulbar and arm involvement, LMN symptoms, or respiratory dysfunction.

B. Lower Motor Neuron Disorders and Peripheral Neuropathies

Of the LMN disorders and peripheral neuropathies that resemble ALS, it is most important to recognize multifocal motor neuropathy with conduction block (MMNCB) and peripheral neuropathies caused by paraproteinemias because these conditions can respond to immunosuppressive therapies. Patients with MMNCB or paraproteinemic neuropathy often have abnormal serum antibodies. Although very rare, lead toxicity causes a motor neuropathy that characteristically produces wrist drop. Workup for motor neuron disease therefore includes nerve conduction studies and blood screening for anti-GM_1 antibodies and monoclonal antibody spikes by serum protein electrophoresis, immunofixation electrophoresis, and, if clinically indicated, lead level. These disorders are discussed in greater detail in Chapter 19.

C. Paraneoplastic Syndromes

In paraneoplastic syndromes, paraproteins can also cause motor neuron disease. In particular, lymphoma and myeloma may produce antibodies that are detectable in blood. Elevated CSF protein (> 75 mg/dL) may be a clue to the diagnosis of lymphoma. Bone marrow biopsies and imaging studies (eg, total body positron emission tomography scan, computed tomography [CT] or MRI of the chest and abdomen, and skeletal surveys) should be considered when malignancy is suspected (see Chapter 13).

D. Spinal Muscular Atrophy

Spinal muscular atrophy is an autosomal-recessive LMN disease that typically begins in infancy or childhood and rarely begins in adulthood (see later discussion). In patients with slowly progressive LMN dysfunction in proximal muscles without UMN signs, blood DNA should be tested for *survival motor neuron* (*SMN*) gene mutations. Kennedy disease is an X-linked spinobulbar motor neuron disease with endocrinopathy. The diagnosis is confirmed by genetic testing. Both disorders are discussed later in this chapter.

E. Polyradiculopathies and Polyradiculoneuropathies

Polyradiculopathies or polyradiculoneuropathies can resemble ALS but generally manifest sensory symptoms and signs. Nerve conduction studies will reveal sensory nerve involvement in radiculoneuropathies, but may not show abnormalities in pure polyradiculopathies. (Elevated CSF protein concentration is a sign of polyradiculopathy.) Serologies may support the diagnosis of an infectious polyradiculopathy.

F. Monomelic Amyotrophic Lateral Sclerosis

Monomelic ALS (discussed later in this chapter) can be difficult to distinguish from ALS in an early stage. The disease begins earlier in adulthood than typical sporadic ALS and does not affect upper or bulbar motor neurons. MRI of the cervical spine may reveal segmental asymmetric cord and ventral root atrophy in this disorder.

G. Inclusion Body Myositis and Adult-Onset Acid Maltase Deficiency

Although myopathies are relatively easy to distinguish from ALS, inclusion body myositis (IBM) and adult-onset acid maltase deficiency are often misdiagnosed as motor neuron disease. Similar to ALS, IBM is a late-onset, progressive disease with predominantly distal asymmetric weakness and normal or slightly elevated serum creatine kinase level. In IBM, electromyography may show spontaneous activity with subtle myogenic changes, resulting in the misdiagnosis of a neurogenic process. In most instances, however, IBM is recognizable clinically by disproportionate weakness of finger flexor and quadriceps muscles in the absence of UMN signs. Muscle biopsy reveals characteristic changes (see Chapter 23).

Adult-onset acid maltase deficiency typically begins after the second decade of life with axial and proximal limb weakness. Respiratory muscles are affected early in this disease. Electromyography typically reveals abundant spontaneous activity with myotonic or bizarre repetitive discharges, particularly in paraspinal muscles. The serum creatine kinase level is variably elevated. Muscle biopsy is usually diagnostic by revealing increased membrane-bound (intralysosomal) and free glycogen and reduced acid maltase activity.

H. Adult-Onset Hexosaminidase A Deficiency

Adult-onset hexosaminidase A deficiency is characterized by the progressive degeneration of UMN, LMN, and cerebellum, and is sometimes misdiagnosed as ALS. Cognitive dysfunction, including psychosis and depression, can be a manifestation of the disease. (An infantile-onset form of hexosaminidase A deficiency is well-known as *Tay-Sachs disease*.) Electromyography in this disorder reveals spontaneous activity, including unusually prominent complex repetitive discharges. The diagnosis is made by measuring hexosaminidase A activity in blood leukocytes.

▶ Treatment

Although ALS is a fatal disease, treatment is important. Once the diagnosis is made, it is important for the physician to inform the patient in an appropriate manner in a private setting with the patient's support network present. A discussion of the patient's understanding of his or her illness and of ALS in general, as well as the patient's desire to know the diagnosis, should precede informing the patient. The patient should be reassured that continuing medical care will be provided and that complications of ALS are treatable. Care of ALS is best provided through multidisciplinary clinics, which may extend survival and enhance quality of life.

A. Riluzole Therapy

Riluzole, 100 mg/day, is the only medication approved by the Food and Drug Administration (FDA) for the treatment of ALS. The drug is thought to block the presynaptic release of glutamate, an excitatory neurotransmitter that may contribute to motor neuron death. According to a 2007 Cochrane Review of four randomized clinical trials, riluzole probably prolongs the survival of ALS patients by about 2–3 months. The medication is very expensive (about $10,000 per year) and is rarely associated with elevated liver enzymes, nausea, and asthenia. Some ALS experts recommend a starting regimen of 50 mg riluzole at bedtime for 1–2 weeks to allow patients to adjust to the medication before beginning the full 50-mg twice-a-day dose.

B. Symptomatic Management

1. Pharmacotherapy—Symptom management includes pharmacologic treatment of sialorrhea, pseudobulbar affect, muscle cramps, spasticity, dyspnea, and depression (Table 20–7).

2. Swallowing—Dysphagia, often a major problem for ALS patients, can cause weight loss and aspiration. Swallowing issues should be addressed proactively. In patients who aspirate, barium swallow studies with video fluoroscopy are useful to guide which forms of food and food modifications may reduce aspiration, particularly when evaluated by an experienced speech therapist. However, barium swallow is not a sensitive screening test for aspiration. Aggressive nutritional care is essential. As the dysphagia worsens, percutaneous endoscopic gastrostomy (PEG) placement should be considered as a means to supplement or replace oral intake. PEG placement can stabilize weight and possibly prolong survival, but may not improve the quality of patients' lives. The PEG should be placed early to obtain maximal benefits and before the vital capacity falls below 50% of predicted value. Refractory sialorrhea may be treated with botulinum toxin B or low-dose radiation.

3. Respiratory care—As with dysphagia, physicians must address respiratory care issues proactively in ALS. Patients should be educated about the noninvasive and invasive forms of mechanical ventilation in order to make rational decisions about these potential treatments. Physicians should look for signs of respiratory insufficiency (dyspnea on exertion, orthopnea, disturbed sleep, and morning headaches).

Table 20–7. Pharmacologic Palliation for ALS and Related Disorders

Symptom	Pharmacotherapy	Common Side Effects
Sialorrhea	Glycopyrrolate, 1–2 mg 2–3 times a day	Anticholinergic effects
	Amitriptyline, 10–100 mg at bedtime	Anticholinergic effects
	Transdermal hyoscine (scopolamine), 0.1–0.2 mg SC or IM 3 times a day or 1.5-mg patch 4 times a day	Confusion, nausea, dizziness
	Trihexyphenidyl HCl, 6–10 mg daily divided 3 times a day	Anticholinergic effects
	Botulinum toxin injections to parotid glands, 5–10 units to each gland	Local muscle weakness and other complications at injection site
Pseudobulbar affect	Dextromethorphan 20 mg/quinine 10 mg once or twice daily	Hypersensitivity, cardiac effects (particularly QT interval prolongation), dizziness, drug interactions (increases desipramine, paroxetine, digoxin)
Muscle cramps	Carbamazepine, 200 mg 2 times a day	Lethargy, gastrointestinal upset, rash, cholestatic jaundice
Spasticity	Oral baclofen, 10–20 mg 3–4 times a day	Sedation, weakness, fatigue
	Tizanidine, 2–8 mg 3 times a day	Sedation and fatigue
	Dantrolene, 50–100 mg 4 times a day	Diarrhea, hepatotoxicity, increased weakness
Dyspnea	Lorazepam (for anxiety), 0.5–2 mg SL every 6–8 h	Sedation, agitation, dizziness
• Intermittent	Nebulized morphine in saline, 5 mg every 4–6 h	Sedation, respiratory depression, dizziness, wheezing, constipation, altered mood
	Midazolam (for severe dyspnea), 5–10 mg IV slowly	Respiratory depression
• Chronic	Morphine (PO, IV, SC, or TD), 2.5 mg every 4 h	Sedation, respiratory depression, dizziness, constipation, altered mood
	Other opiates with dosing equivalent to morphine	Sedation, respiratory depression, dizziness, constipation, altered mood
	Diazepam (for nocturnal symptoms), 2.5–5 mg at bedtime	Sedation, agitation, dizziness
	Continuous IV morphine for severe dyspnea, titrated dose	Sedation, respiratory depression, dizziness, constipation, altered mood, hypotension
• Chronic depression	Selective serotonin reuptake inhibitors	Insomnia, agitation

ALS = amyotrophic lateral sclerosis; IM = intramuscular; IV = intravenous; PO = by mouth (oral); SC = subcutaneous; SL = sublingual; TD = transdermal.

Vital capacity should be monitored regularly. Regardless of their advance directive plan, many ALS patients choose to use noninvasive positive-pressure ventilation (NIPPV) devices, which may prolong survival, slow the decline of forced vital capacity, and improve quality of life. NIPPV should be considered when patients experience orthopnea, have sniff nasal pressure (< 40 cm), have maximal inspiratory pressure (< 60 cm), have abnormal noctural oximetry (ie, noctural desaturatoin < 90% for 1 cumulative minute), or have functional vital capacity less than 50% of predicted. Only a small minority (5–10%) undergo tracheostomy and invasive ventilation. If patients decide not to have mechanical ventilation, then, in addition to NIPPV, pharmacologic palliation of dyspnea-associated anxiety should be considered (see Table 20–7).

4. Pseudobulbar affect—Because dextromethorphan with quinidine improves pseudobulbar affect, the FDA has approved this pharmacological combination. The recom-

mended starting dose is a single capsule containing dextromethorphan (20 mg)/quinidine (10 mg) once daily for 7 days, then one capsule every 12 hours. Side effects of this therapy include dizziness, nausea, and somnolence. The use of dextromethorphan/quinidine is contraindicated in patients with hypersensitivity to either or both components, or cardiac problems (eg, prolonged QT interval, heart block, or cardiac failure).

▶ **Prognosis**

The prognosis for patients with ALS varies widely. Rarely, patients die within several months of onset or survive more than 30 years. Most live from 3–5 years after onset. Younger patients generally have a longer duration of illness, and survival is also longer in patients with limb-onset rather than bulbar-onset ALS. Early respiratory dysfunction and low serum chloride level are associated with a worse prognosis.

Brooks BR, Miller RG, Swash M, Munsat TL. El Escorial revisited: Revised criteria for the diagnosis of amyotrophic lateral sclerosis. *Amyotroph Lateral Scler Other Motor Neuron Disord* 2000;1:293–299. [PMID: 11464847] (Provides diagnostic criteria for ALS that are widely applied to clinical trials.)

Dion PA, Daoud H, Rouleau GA. Genetics of motor neuron disorders: New insights into pathogenic mechanisms. *Nat Rev Genet* 2009;10(11):769–782. [PMID: 19823194] (Reviews genes that cause motor neuron disease.)

Miller RG, Mitchell JD, Lyon M, Moore DH. Riluzole for amyotrophic lateral sclerosis (ALS)/motor neuron disease (MND). *Cochrane Database Syst Rev* 2007(1):CD001447. [PMID: 17253460] (This meta-analysis of data reported in clinical trials of riluzole for ALS concludes that the drug extends survival by 2–3 months.)

Miller RG, et al. Practice parameter update: The care of the patient with amyotrophic lateral sclerosis: Drug, nutritional, and respiratory therapies (an evidence-based review). Report of the Quality Standards Subcommittee of the American Academy of Neurology. *Neurology* 2009;73(15):1218–1226. [PMID: 19822872] (Evidence-based review from the American Academy of Neurology that provides specific guidelines for the drug, nutritional, and respiratory therapies in ALS.)

Miller RG, et al. Practice parameter update: The care of the patient with amyotrophic lateral sclerosis: Multidisciplinary care, symptom management, and cognitive/behavioral impairment (an evidence-based review). Report of the Quality Standards Subcommittee of the American Academy of Neurology. *Neurology* 2009;73(15):1227–1233. [PMID: 19822873] (Evidence-based review from the American Academy of Neurology that provides specific guidelines regarding multidisciplinary care, symptom management, and neuropsychological impairments in ALS.)

Mitsumoto H, Rabkin JG. Palliative care for patients with amyotrophic lateral sclerosis: "Prepare for the worst and hope for the best." *JAMA* 2007;298(2):207–216. [PMID: 17622602] (An excellent overview highlighting the importance of palliative care.)

Traub R, Mitsumoto H, Rowland LP. Research advances in amyotrophic lateral sclerosis, 2009 to 2010. *Curr Neurol Neurosci Rep* 2011;11(1):67–77. [PMID: 21080240] (An excellent review of ALS literature published in 2009–2010.)

LOWER MOTOR NEURON DISORDERS

1. Spinal Muscular Atrophy

ESSENTIALS OF DIAGNOSIS

▶ Subacute weakness with variable age at onset

▶ LMN dysfunction—weakness, wasting and fasciculations, areflexia or hyporeflexia

▶ Absence of cognitive and sensory changes

▶ SMN gene mutation

▶ General Considerations

Spinal muscular atrophy (SMA) is a common autosomal-recessive motor neuron disease with an estimated incidence of 8 per 100,000 people. SMA has been subclassified according to severity. SMA I (Werdnig Hoffmann disease) begins within the first 6 months of life and is a frequent cause of floppy infant syndrome. Affected infants never sit independently and usually die before 2 years of age. In contrast, SMA II (intermediate or chronic infantile disease) starts between ages 6 and 18 months, and affected children develop the ability to sit unsupported. Survival is variable; most patients live into their twenties or thirties. In SMA III (Kugelberg-Welander or chronic juvenile disease), patients develop symptoms after age 18 months, usually manifesting as difficulty climbing stairs or impaired walking, and have normal life expectancies.

SMA is caused by *SMN1* mutations located at chromosome 5q11. The gene product, SMN, is required for the assembly of spliceosomal small nuclear ribonucleoproteins, which in turn are involved in messenger RNA processing.

▶ Clinical Findings

A. Symptoms and Signs

As in ALS, extraocular muscles are spared in SMA. Facial weakness is mild or absent, but tongue fasciculations are seen in nearly all patients. Postural tremor is common. Respiratory muscles are affected. Weakness of axial muscles can lead to scoliosis, which may further impair respiration. Pulmonary insufficiency and pneumonia are common complications.

B. Diagnostic Studies

Routine laboratory studies often reveal mildly elevated serum creatine kinase, typically one to two times the upper limit of normal. A serum creatine kinase level that is more than 10 times normal suggests myopathy. Electromyography reveals spontaneous activity (fibrillations and positive sharp waves). Fasciculations are more common in SMA II and III than in SMA I. Reduced recruitment and long-duration, high-amplitude motor unit action potentials are prominent. The diagnosis is definitively confirmed by the identification of *SMN1* gene mutation.

▶ Treatment

Treatment of SMA is limited to symptomatic management. Therapies for restrictive lung disease, gastrointestinal dysmotility (dysphagia and constipation), and skeletal deformities caused by muscle weakness are important interventions that can prolong life expectancy and improve quality of life.

Iannaccone ST. Modern management of spinal muscular atrophy. *J Child Neurol* 2007;22(8):974–978. [PMID: 17761652] (A review focusing on recent advances in the pathogenesis and treatment of SMA.)

2. Monomelic Amyotrophic Lateral Sclerosis

ESSENTIALS OF DIAGNOSIS

▶ Subacute weakness, typically in young men

▶ Weakness, wasting, and fasciculations in one limb (usually an arm)

▶ Absence of sensory involvement

▶ Normal tendon reflexes

Monomelic ALS (also called *Hirayama disease, monomelic atrophy*, or *benign focal atrophy*) is a focal motor neuron disease that causes the weakness of one arm, although there are a few cases of single leg involvement. The disease affects men more often than women (5:1 ratio), with onset typically in the late teens or twenties. Weakness progresses slowly over 1–3 years before stabilizing. Sensory examination is usually normal, but mild sensory abnormalities may be present in the dorsum of the hand. Tendon reflexes are typically normal, and UMN signs are absent. Ischemia of the anterior horn has been postulated to cause the disorder.

Nerve conduction studies and electromyography reveal normal sensory nerve functions, but neurogenic changes consistent with LMN disease are observed in the affected limb and, to a lesser extent, in the unaffected limbs. MRI of the spine or CT-myelogram may reveal spinal cord atrophy in the lower cervical or upper thoracic cord. No specific treatment has proven to be effective for the disorder.

3. Kennedy Disease

ESSENTIALS OF DIAGNOSIS

▶ Subacute weakness in men

▶ Onset in the third through fifth decades

▶ LMN dysfunction in limb and facial muscles

▶ Facial fasciculation, particularly prominent in the chin

▶ Gynecomastia and impotence

▶ Nerve conduction studies and electromyographic studies showing neurogenic changes, including sensory nerve abnormalities

▶ Elevated serum creatine kinase

▶ Genetic testing showing abnormal expansions of a CAG trinucleotide repeat in the androgen receptor gene confirms the diagnosis

Kennedy disease (X-linked spinobulbar atrophy) is an X-linked recessive disease that usually presents as progressive weakness in men in their twenties to forties. Limb muscle weakness is more prominent proximally than distally. Bulbar muscles are affected. Facial, tongue, and mastication muscles are often weak; dysarthria and dysphagia are late manifestations. Fasciculations around the mouth and particularly in the chin are prominent. Gynecomastia and impotence are caused by androgen receptor defects.

Nerve conduction studies reveal absent or low-amplitude sensory nerve action potentials, and electromyography shows neurogenic abnormalities. Although Kennedy disease is primarily a motor neuron disorder, serum creatine kinase is usually elevated to 900–8000 U/L. The disease is caused by expansions of a CAG trinucleotide repeat in the androgen receptor gene; therefore, the diagnosis can be confirmed by genetic testing. Treatment is limited to supportive therapy.

Finsterer J. Perspectives of Kennedy's disease. *J Neurol Sci* 2010;298:1–10. [PID: 20846673] (A comprehensive review of this X-linked spinobulbar atrophy.)

UPPER MOTOR NEURON DISORDERS

1. Hereditary Spastic Paraparesis

ESSENTIALS OF DIAGNOSIS

▶ Slowly progressive gait disturbance (spastic paraparesis)

▶ Autosomal-dominant, autosomal-recessive, or X-linked recessive inheritance

Hereditary spastic paraparesis (HSP) is a genetically heterogeneous syndrome manifesting as insidiously progressive gait disturbance. HSP has been classified into 44 genetically distinct forms, including autosomal-dominant, autosomal-recessive, and X-linked recessive types (see Table 20–2). Age at onset is variable. *Uncomplicated* or *pure HSP* refers to spastic leg weakness with hyperreflexia and Babinski signs, and, in some patients, urinary urgency, frequency, or hesitancy as well as mild loss of vibratory sensation in the feet. Rectal and sexual dysfunction is rarely associated with uncomplicated HSP. *Complicated HSP* describes conditions in which spastic paraparesis is accompanied by such neurologic abnormalities as optic atrophy, retinopathy, seizures, mental retardation, dementia, extrapyramidal abnormalities, and peripheral neuropathy.

Routine laboratory studies are usually normal in patients with HSP. MRI scans of the brain are usually unremarkable. MRI of the thoracic or lumbar spinal cord may reveal atrophy. Somatosensory evoked potentials sometimes show delayed conductions with stimulation of the legs. Magnetostimulation of the corticospinal tract typically demonstrates reduced conduction velocities and amplitude of evoked potentials in the legs.

Although genetic testing for HSP is available commercially, causative genes have been identified in less than half of the genetic subtypes.

Treatment for HSP is symptomatic. Antispasticity medications include oral or intrathecal baclofen, and oral tizanidine hydrochloride. Oxybutynin, 5 mg two to three times a day, or extended-release oxybutynin, 5–30 mg once a day, can reduce urinary urgency. Physical therapy can reduce deconditioning.

Salinas S, Proukakis C, Crosby A, Warner TT. Hereditary spastic paraplegia: Clinical features and pathogenetic mechanisms. *Lancet Neurol* 2008;7(12):1127–1138. [PMID: 19007737] (An overview of this increasingly complex subject.)

2. Primary Lateral Sclerosis

ESSENTIALS OF DIAGNOSIS

► Slowly progressive spastic quadriparesis
► Onset after age 40
► Absence of LMN signs and cognitive or sensory manifestations
► Absence of positive family history

Primary lateral sclerosis (PLS), a diagnosis of exclusion, is a pure UMN disorder. ALS beginning with UMN manifestations would be indistinguishable from early PLS. Although some clinicians think that PLS is a variant of ALS, patients with PLS sometimes have bladder symptoms, which are atypical for ALS. In addition, electromyographic findings are usually abnormal in ALS (even in the absence of LMN signs) but are normal in PLS. Multiple sclerosis presenting with spastic paraparesis may resemble PLS, but the distinction should be evident based on brain lesions on MRI, oligoclonal bands in CSF, and abnormal evoked potentials. Although HSP can be distinguished by the presence of affected relatives, isolated patients with autosomal-recessive or X-linked recessive disease may be difficult to distinguish from patients with PLS.

Gordon PH, et al. The natural history of primary lateral sclerosis. *Neurology* 2006;66(5):647–653. [PMID: 16534101] (This paper highlights the difficulty in distinguishing PLS from ALS during the first 4 years after symptom onset.)

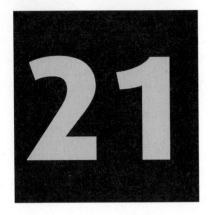

Autonomic Disorders

21

Louis H. Weimer, MD

▼ DYSAUTONOMIA

▶ General Considerations

Impairment throughout the nervous system by diverse processes—mass lesions, infections, strokes, multiple sclerosis plaques, seizures, and degenerative conditions—can produce autonomic symptoms. A much smaller number of disorders specifically targets autonomic structures, resulting in disordered autonomic control (dysautonomia).

The opposing sympathetic "fight-or-flight" and parasympathetic "rest-and-digest" systems comprise the autonomic nervous system. In most organs, dual control maintains unconscious, normal function. The systems are highly complex, however, with components in the cerebral cortex, limbic system, brainstem, spinal cord, autonomic ganglia, peripheral nerves, and specialized special sense and effector end organs. Sympathetic centers are located in the thoracic spinal cord and parasympathetic centers in the brainstem and the sacral spinal cord. The enteric nervous system of the gastrointestinal (GI) tract is considered by many to be an additional autonomous nervous system "mind of the gut." Acetylcholine and norepinephrine are only two of a multitude of neurotransmitters that play important roles in autonomic control. Serotonin, for example, is a major enteric motor neuron neurotransmitter.

▶ Clinical Findings

A. Symptoms and Signs

Many autonomic symptoms (Table 21–1) are nonspecific, and the diagnosis of dysautonomia can be missed when symptoms are atypical or each symptom is considered in isolation. For example, orthostatic hypotension—a significant decrease in blood pressure (BP) upon standing—can cause isolated postural pure vertigo, occipital headache, neck and shoulder "coat-hanger pattern" neck ache, cognitive changes, and fatigue in the absence of light-headedness. Inquiring about exacerbating conditions or medications can

help distinguish orthostatic hypotension from other paroxysmal processes. Exacerbating conditions include:

1. Warm environment, hot bath, and fever
2. Large meals (carbohydrate load)
3. Valsalva maneuver
4. Volume depletion
5. Rapid postural change
6. Alcohol

Orthostatic hypotension is also aggravated in the post-exercise period, in the early morning, and after rising from prolonged bed rest.

Among the many medications that may exacerbate orthostatic hypotension are the following:

1. Tricyclic antidepressants, atropine, propantheline, bethanechol
2. β-Adrenergic blockers (eg, propranolol and others)
3. α_1-Adrenergic antagonists (eg, phentolamine, phenoxybenzamine, guanabenz)
4. Agents with α_2-adrenergic activity (eg, clonidine, prazosin, methyldopa, terazosin, doxazosin)
5. Ganglionic blockers (eg, guanethidine, hexamethonium, mecamylamine)
6. Antihypertensive agents (eg, calcium channel blockers, hydralazine, diuretics, angiotensin-converting enzyme inhibitors)
7. Erectile dysfunction agents (alprostadil, sildenafil, tadalafil, vardenafil)
8. Other agents, including antipsychotics (neuroleptics and newer atypical agents), antiparkinsonian agents, disopyramide, nitrates, antihistamines, narcotics, and pyridostigmine, prostatic hypertrophy agents (finasteride, dutasteride, tamsulosin)

Table 21–1. Common Symptoms of Dysautonomia

	Autonomic Symptoms
Secretomotor	Dry eyes and mouth (sicca syndrome), requiring frequent sips of water
Visual	Blurred vision, sensitivity to light or glare, poor night vision
Upper GI	Postprandial bloating, fullness, nausea, dizziness, sweating, orthostatic hypotension
Lower GI	Constipation, nocturnal or intermittent diarrhea, incontinence or urgency
Genitourinary	Urinary retention, difficulty with initiation, frequency, incomplete emptying, incontinence
Sexual	Erectile failure, ejaculatory dysfunction, retrograde ejaculation into bladder, dyspareunia, decreased vaginal lubrication
Sudomotor	Reduced or loss of sweating ability (distally in polyneuropathies); excessive, paroxysmal, or inappropriate sweating (eg, gustatory); mixed pattern of loss and excessive areas of sweating; heat intolerance; loss of fingertip wrinkling in water and goose bumps
Vasomotor	Distal color changes, change in skin appearance, persistently cold extremities, Raynaud phenomenon, loss of skin wrinkling in water, heat intolerance
Orthostatic	Dizziness or light-headedness, weakness, fatigue, cognitive changes or confusion, slurred speech, visual disturbance, vertigo, neck or shoulder discomfort, anxiety, palpitations, pallor, nausea, syncope
Other	Unexplained syncope

GI = gastrointestinal.

Table 21–2. Examination Findings in Dysautonomia

	Clinical Findings
Eyes	Dry, red eyes; ptosis; pupillary dysfunction Adie pupil—dilated, slow light response Horner syndrome—miosis, ptosis, ipsilateral anhidrosis
Mucosa	Dry eyes, mouth Schirmer test—decreased tear production
Skin	Dry, scaly, pale skin; dry socks; areas of excessive sweating
Vasomotor	Mottled extremities, flushing color change, Raynaud phenomenon, excessively warm or cold skin
Cardiovascular	Orthostatic hypotension, orthostatic tachycardia (heart rate increment ≥ 30 beats/min or absolute value ≥ 120 beats/min)
Other	Disordered temperature regulation

Signs of autonomic dysfunction depend on lesion location. Some readily identifiable signs are listed in Table 21–2. Orthostatic hypotension is a sign of advanced autonomic failure. BP determinations should be obtained after the patient has been supine for at least 15 minutes. Initially, BP and heart rate are recorded while the patient is supine. The patient then stands without delay, while keeping the BP cuff at heart level (arm raised). An active exercise reflex is induced that acutely lowers BP. Normally, BP returns to baseline levels within 45–120 seconds; a longer delay is sometimes seen in patients with BP control disorders. Consensus criteria identify a drop of 20 mm Hg in systolic pressure and 10 mm Hg in diastolic pressure as significant, but most treatment centers require at least a 30-mm Hg systolic drop for diagnosis of orthostatic hypotension. A false-positive diagnosis can be made if BP is rechecked too early. Note should also be made of induced symptoms.

Orthostatic hypotension is a clinical sign and not a disease. Many elderly patients have measurable but asymptomatic BP declines that require no treatment other than instruction about exacerbating conditions. Coincident neurologic signs should be identified, including sensory peripheral neuropathy, parkinsonism, dementia, and cerebellar signs.

B. Autonomic Function Testing

1. General considerations—Unlike other anatomic systems, such as sensory and motor, most autonomic system functions cannot be assessed directly, but responses of complex reflexes can be measured after controlled perturbations. Numerous techniques are described, but only a few are considered suitable for routine clinical application (Table 21–3). Tests of cardiovagal heart rate variability (parasympathetic), adrenergic vasoconstriction (sympathetic), and sudomotor (sympathetic cholinergic, sweating) function are the most commonly performed. Devices that noninvasively record beat-to-beat BP without the need for invasive lines are common. Some measures can be performed with limited equipment, but formal evaluation of autonomic function in a dedicated laboratory is sometimes desirable (Table 21–4). Plasma catecholamine levels are sometimes useful, but are generally less sensitive than other measures discussed and rarely provide a specific diagnosis.

2. Indications for laboratory evaluation—Formal autonomic testing is especially valuable when suspicious symptoms are present but overt clinical signs (eg, orthostatic hypotension) are lacking. Common indications for laboratory testing are listed in Table 21–4.

3. Patient preparation—Many endogenous and environmental factors can confound autonomic testing. Patients should be normovolemic, comfortable, and free of anxiety,

Table 21–3. Commonly Performed Tests of Autonomic Function

Autonomic Function	Diagnostic Test
Cardiovagal heart rate variability	Heart rate (HR) response to deep breathing HR response to Valsalva (Valsalva ratio) HR response to standing (30:15 ratio)
Adrenergic vasoconstriction	Blood pressure (BP) Valsalva maneuver response (beat-to-beat waveform) BP response to standing or passive tilt
Sudomotor function	Quantitative sudomotor axon reflex test (QSART, QSweat) Thermoregulatory sweat testing Silastic skin imprinting Sympathetic skin response
Other	Supine and upright catecholamine levels Urodynamic studies Gastric and intestinal motility studies, manometry Schirmer test of tear production

and should have recuperated from any acute illness or prolonged bedrest. Compressive garments, if normally worn, are removed. Caffeine, nicotine, vigorous exercise, and alcohol should be avoided on the day of testing. Medications that affect sympathetic or parasympathetic activity or raise or lower BP should be discontinued, ideally 24–48 hours prior to testing, unless deemed medically unsafe by the referring physician.

Weimer LH. Autonomic testing: Clinical applications and common techniques. *Neurologist* 2010;16(4):215–222. [PMID: 20592565] (Review of testing aims and specific clinical measures.)

Table 21–4. Indications for Formal Autonomic Testing

Evaluation of questionable symptoms of dysautonomia
Confirmation of generalized autonomic failure:
• Autonomic neuropathy
• Multiple system atrophy
• Other degenerative causes of autonomic failure
Grading of disease severity
Confirmation that a process is limited to one system
Characterization of orthostatic intolerance syndrome
Assessment of treatment effectiveness
Assessment of disease progression
Confirmation of small-fiber neuropathy

▼ TREATMENT OF ORTHOSTATIC HYPOTENSION

Numerous pharmacologic and nonpharmacologic measures are used in the treatment of orthostatic hypotension. The primary goal is to prevent syncope and minimize symptoms, not to eliminate hypotension completely. In patients with mild hypotension, adequate precautions and avoidance of the numerous precipitating factors (see earlier discussion) may be adequate. However, symptoms of hypoperfusion other than imminent syncope should be targets of treatment. These include postural neck and shoulder fatigue, often termed "coat-hanger pattern headache" from local muscle ischemia; occipital headache; vertigo; and cognitive slowing.

▶ Nonpharmacologic Measures

Helpful initial measures include raising the head of the bed 4–6 in with blocks to nocturnally stimulate baroreceptors and decrease diuresis. Patients should be instructed to utilize postures such as leg crossing, squatting, and stooping, unless precluded by other neurologic impairment; avoid prolonged motionless standing; and arise from a prone or supine position in stages. Isotonic exercise and avoidance of straining, coughing, and isometric exercise may be beneficial. Compressive garments are less effective than generally assumed and should include abdominal compression for meaningful effect, often making them too cumbersome to expect compliance. Abdominal binders may be helpful. Small meals that are low in carbohydrates are beneficial in patients with postprandial hypotension. An increase in salt and fluid intake may be adequate to reduce mild symptomatic orthostatic hypotension, and both sodium chloride tablets and water supplements have been independently shown to be beneficial. Reconsideration of prescribed BP-lowering agents is prudent. However, excessive supine hypertension is also a concern.

▶ Pharmacotherapy

A. First-Line Agents

If nonpharmacologic interventions are insufficient, first-line medications include fludrocortisone, starting at 0.05–0.1 mg/day, the α-adrenergic agonist midodrine, or both. The dose of midodrine, the only medication currently approved by the Food and Drug Administration for treatment of orthostatic hypotension, is 2.5–10 mg three times a day, but not after 5 PM. Scalp piloerection and itching are common physiologic and not allergic responses.

Anemia exacerbates orthostatic hypotension, and correcting iron deficiency or boosting hematocrit with erythropoietin is beneficial in some patients. Oral or nasal vasopressin analogs may also be beneficial, especially at night. Supine hypertension is frequent and of controversial risk, but, when severe, may require small doses of a short-acting antihypertensive agent.

B. Second-Line Agents

Second-line agents are sometimes effective when earlier agents have failed; these include pyridostigmine and octreotide. Other possibly effective agents include serotonin reuptake inhibitors, the β-blockers pindolol and xamoterol, clonidine, yohimbine, and the norepinephrine precursor, L-threo-3,4-dihydroxyphenylserine (L-DOPS).

Freeman R. Treatment of orthostatic hypotension. *Semin Neurol* 2003;23:435–442. [PMID: 15088264] (Authoritative general overview of treatment of orthostatic hypotension.)

Shannon JR, et al. Water drinking as a treatment for orthostatic syndromes. *Am J Med* 2002;112:355–360. [PMID: 11904109] (Study demonstrating benefit of simply increasing water intake in patients with orthostatic hypotension.)

Vagaonescu TD, et al. Hypertensive cardiovascular damage in patients with primary autonomic failure. *Lancet* 2000;355:725–726. [PMID: 10703810] (Increased prevalence of left ventricular hypertrophy in patients with autonomic failure compared with controls suggests that cardiac injury occurs, likely from nocturnal hypertension.)

DISORDERS ASSOCIATED WITH AUTONOMIC FAILURE

NEURODEGENERATIVE DISORDERS & PARKINSONIAN SYNDROMES

ESSENTIALS OF DIAGNOSIS

▶ Parkinsonism and autonomic failure are features of several disorders

▶ Severe autonomic failure, stridor, sleep apnea, dystonia, and poor L-dopa response are characteristic of multiple system atrophy

▶ Autonomic failure sometimes occurs in Parkinson disease

▶ Severe autonomic failure in isolation occurs in pure autonomic failure

▶ General Considerations

Clinically important autonomic failure is an apparent and potentially disabling finding in several neurodegenerative disorders, especially multiple system atrophy, Parkinson disease with autonomic failure, diffuse Lewy body dementia, and pure autonomic failure. Many other common and uncommon disorders have lesser degrees of autonomic failure, notably typical Parkinson disease. Most disorders in this group begin after age 50 and are insidious in onset and progression. For more detailed discussion of these disorders, refer to Chapter 15.

▶ Clinical Findings

A. Symptoms and Signs

1. Multiple system atrophy—Shy-Drager syndrome, a progressive disorder that causes prominent autonomic failure, is one form of a larger group of disorders, termed *multiple system atrophy*, that share pathologic and clinical features, notably autonomic failure, parkinsonism, and cerebellar dysfunction. Other characteristic features include respiratory stridor, sleep apnea, dystonia, and incontinence. Autonomic dysfunction is often the presenting feature, and virtually all patients with multiple system atrophy develop signs of dysautonomia during the course of the disease, including severe postural hypotension, impotence, bladder and bowel dysfunction, and reduced or paradoxical sweating.

2. Idiopathic Parkinson disease—Patients with idiopathic Parkinson disease often have symptoms of autonomic dysfunction, most commonly constipation. Symptomatic orthostatic hypotension is uncommon, but a subset of patients have severe autonomic failure and are separately designated as having *Parkinson disease with autonomic failure*.

3. Pure autonomic failure—A separate disorder, pure autonomic failure (PAF), is also known as *Bradbury-Eggleston syndrome* and *idiopathic orthostatic hypotension*. In patients with this form of dysautonomia, other neurologic abnormalities are absent. Although many autonomic symptoms are present, orthostatic hypotension is the most disabling, often producing recurrent syncope. In patients with severe PAF, sitting or a large meal may be sufficient to provoke hypotensive symptoms. Lewy bodies, a pathologic hallmark of Parkinson disease, are present in autonomic ganglia and in areas within the central nervous system. The relationship between Parkinson disease and PAF is unclear. *Diffuse Lewy body disease* with dementia may also produce autonomic failure of varying severity.

B. Diagnostic Studies

Several tests are employed to differentiate these overlapping disorders, but neuropathologic evaluation is the only definitive method. Autonomic testing, positron emission tomography (PET) or magnetic resonance imaging (MRI) scan patterns, L-dopa response, and sleep studies may aid the clinical diagnosis. Plasma catecholamine levels are low in both multiple system atrophy and PAF.

▶ Differential Diagnosis

Diffuse Lewy body dementia can also produce parkinsonism, autonomic dysfunction, and prominent hallucinations. Creutzfeldt-Jakob disease may cause autonomic failure, but the course is rapidly progressive. Autonomic peripheral neuropathy must also be considered.

▶ Treatment & Prognosis

Treatment of these disorders is detailed in Chapter 15. As noted, prognosis varies among these disorders. Multiple system atrophy is a relentlessly progressive disease that results in death, usually within several years. In contrast, PAF is a slowly progressive disorder with a longer life expectancy. The prognosis is likely worse for patients who have Parkinson disease with autonomic failure compared to typical patients with Parkinson disease.

Kaufmann H, Biaggioni I. Autonomic failure in neurodegenerative disorders. *Semin Neurol* 2003;23:351–363. [PMID: 15088256] (Thorough but straightforward overview of present clinical, pathologic, and experimental knowledge.)

ACUTE & SUBACUTE AUTONOMIC NEUROPATHIES

1. Guillain-Barré Syndrome

ESSENTIALS OF DIAGNOSIS

- ▶ Abnormal cardiac rhythms raise suspicion of autonomic involvement
- ▶ Autonomic failure increases mortality and correlates with outcome
- ▶ Resting tachycardia is a common early indicator of dysautonomia; close monitoring is essential in suspicious cases

▶ General Considerations

Guillain-Barré syndrome commonly affects autonomic peripheral pathways and is an important cause of cardiovascular disturbances, tachyarrhythmias, bradyarrhythmias, and sudden death. Autonomic involvement has been reported in up to two thirds of patients, and fatal cardiovascular complications now rival respiratory complications and thromboembolism as important causes of mortality. A detailed discussion of this disorder is presented in Chapter 19.

▶ Clinical Findings

Dysfunction can manifest as autonomic failure or overactivity, and it correlates with weakness severity, elevated catecholamines, and respiratory failure. Bursts of paroxysmal sweating, episodic hypertensive episodes, and a characteristic resting tachycardia are caused by autonomic overactivity or loss of normal suppression. Tachyarrhythmias are common and demand close monitoring; numerous subtypes are described. Care must be taken to exclude treatable causes of dysrhythmia such as hypoxia, electrolyte disturbance, sepsis, and cardiac ischemia. Bradycardia or even frank asystole is

less frequent but can sometimes be triggered by tracheal suctioning and Valsalva-like maneuvers. Rarely, temporary cardiac pacing is necessary. Large swings in BP are not uncommon, and rarely there is progression to frank cardiovascular collapse. Medication effects are often magnified because of denervation and supersensitive receptor activity. Consequently, conventional doses of vasoactive medications can produce unusually large and potentially dangerous responses. Urinary retention, pupil dysfunction, GI dysmotility, and ileus are underappreciated.

Baseline electrocardiographic recording is essential, and some clinicians recommend cardiac telemetry and initial sequential supine and upright BP measures for all patients with Guillain-Barré syndrome. If potential complications are detected, transfer to an intensive care unit for continual heart rate and BP monitoring is indicated. Unfortunately, it is difficult to predict in advance which patients should be intensively monitored. Abnormalities on formal autonomic testing slowly improve over time, paralleling motor recovery.

▶ Treatment & Prognosis

Short-acting medications given in small doses are preferred in weak, ventilated patients. Medications reported to cause significant hypotension in patients with Guillain-Barré syndrome include phentolamine, nitroglycerin, hexamethonium, edrophonium, morphine, and furosemide. Excessive hypertension has been associated with phenylephrine, ephedrine, dopamine, and isoprenaline. Complications appear to diminish as overall improvement occurs. Monitoring BP when upright, maintaining blood volume, watching for arrhythmias during procedures, and avoiding unnecessary vasoactive drugs are prudent measures. Aspects of treatment are discussed in more detail in Chapter 19.

The link between mortality and autonomic neuropathy in patients with Guillain-Barré syndrome demands close observation. Small-fiber sensory and autonomic nerve abnormalities correlate with overall prognosis and outcome.

Burns TM, et al. Adynamic ileus in severe Guillain-Barré syndrome. *Muscle Nerve* 2001;24:963–965. [PMID: 11410925] (Description of one of several autonomic complications that is less rare than is generally thought.)

Pan CL, et al. Cutaneous innervation in Guillain-Barré syndrome: Pathology and clinical correlations. *Brain* 2003;126:386–397. [PMID: 12538405] (Series documenting high frequency of small-fiber sensory and autonomic involvement by skin biopsy and autonomic function testing and correlation with outcome and disease severity.)

2. Acute Autonomic Neuropathy (Acute Pandysautonomia)

▶ General Considerations

Acute or subacute autonomic neuropathy (acute pandysautonomia) primarily but not exclusively affects peripheral autonomic fibers. The disorder is analogous to Guillain-Barré syndrome, but distinct. Diagnosis is frequently delayed due to lack of recognition, which reduces the potential for timely, beneficial treatment.

Pathogenesis

The disorder is presumed to be immune mediated. A large minority (41%) of patients has antibodies to ganglionic acetylcholine receptor (AChR) α_3 subunits, which are distinct from neuromuscular junction AChR subunits (α_1). There is strong clinical and experimental evidence that the ganglionic acetylcholine receptor antibodies are pathogenic in patients with positive antibody titers.

Clinical Findings

A. Symptoms and Signs

Roughly half of cases are preceded by a viral prodrome, including herpes simplex, mononucleosis, rubella, and nondescript febrile illnesses. The neuropathy is monophasic, with acute or subacute onset and progression over several weeks. Patients typically develop generalized autonomic failure, including orthostatic hypotension, anhidrosis, Adie pupils, dry eyes and mouth, urinary retention, and GI dysfunction. Acute signs such as ileus may develop into lesser degrees of dysmotility, including bloating, early satiety, nausea, vomiting, and alternating diarrhea and constipation. Predominantly adrenergic and cholinergic variants are sometimes seen, but pandysautonomia is most common. The restricted cholinergic form (acute cholinergic neuropathy) is characterized by dry eyes and mouth, ileus and other GI dysmotility, bladder dysfunction, hypohidrosis (sweating loss), unreactive pupils, fixed heart rate, and sexual dysfunction, but not orthostatic hypotension or syncope.

B. Diagnostic Studies

Abnormalities on formal autonomic testing are prominent. The lack of orthostatic hypotension in patients with the cholinergic form of the disorder makes laboratory testing especially valuable in establishing the diagnosis. Nerve conduction studies typically show normal findings or minor sensory abnormalities. Ganglionic acetylcholine receptor antibody testing is commercially available.

Differential Diagnosis

A paraneoplastic form, which develops over a similar time course, is indistinguishable on clinical or laboratory grounds prior to tumor discovery. True Guillain-Barré syndrome is distinguished by weakness and areflexia; elevated cerebrospinal fluid protein is seen in both disorders. An attenuated form of this disorder may underlie some cases of orthostatic intolerance, discussed later. Botulism (cholinergic), diphtheria, and acute intermittent porphyria are other diagnostic considerations.

Treatment

Supportive care and symptomatic treatment of the involved systems is a primary aim, especially reducing the degree of symptomatic orthostatic hypotension and managing GI dysmotility. Some patients require temporary intravenous or gastric or jejunal tube feedings. Because of the probable immune mechanisms, steroids, plasmapheresis, and intravenous immunoglobulin have all been used, with anecdotal reports of benefit.

Prognosis

Recovery generally occurs but is often slow and incomplete, with less motor and sensory improvement than in patients with Guillain-Barré syndrome. Acute treatment may improve outcome, but no controlled studies are available. One third of patients make a good functional recovery; one third have a partial recovery with persistent symptoms, including orthostatic hypotension; and the remainder of patients do not improve. GI dysfunction and orthostatic hypotension are usually the most debilitating manifestations.

Freeman R. Autonomic peripheral neuropathy. *Lancet* 2005; 365(9466):1259–1270. [PMID: 15811460] (Excellent review of diagnosis, pathogenesis, and management of autonomic neuropathy.)

Sakakibara R, et al. Micturition disturbance in acute idiopathic autonomic neuropathy. *J Neurol Neurosurg Psychiatry* 2004;75:287–291. [PMID: 14742606] (Description of aspects of urinary function and clinical features.)

3. Paraneoplastic Syndromes

ESSENTIALS OF DIAGNOSIS

▶ Subacute onset of dysautonomia should prompt a search for an occult neoplasm; small cell lung cancer is the most common association

▶ Some syndromes are clinically indistinguishable from idiopathic forms

▶ Intestinal pseudo-obstruction can mimic an acute abdomen

General Considerations

A paraneoplastic syndrome can be the first manifestation of an underlying tumor (see Chapter 13). Several paraneoplastic syndromes have prominent autonomic involvement.

Clinical Syndromes

A. Lambert-Eaton Myasthenic Syndrome

Lambert-Eaton myasthenic syndrome is an acquired disorder of presynaptic neuromuscular junction transmission.

Roughly half of affected patients have an associated neoplasm, about 80% of which are small cell lung cancer. In addition to proximal weakness and reduced or absent deep tendon reflexes, 80% of patients have dysautonomia. Cholinergic-mediated complaints are most common, including, in order of frequency, dry mouth, impotence, constipation, blurred vision, altered sweating, and orthostatic hypotension. In roughly 20% of patients, autonomic symptoms are severe. Laboratory evidence of dysautonomia is seen on autonomic testing. For more detailed discussion of this syndrome, see Chapter 22.

B. Subacute Sensory Neuronopathy

Symptoms in subacute sensory neuronopathy are usually subacute in onset, but some patients have abrupt onset. The disorder is most common in patients with small cell lung cancer, and antineuronal nuclear antibodies (ANNA-1, anti-Hu) are often present. Patients have dysesthesias, lancinating pains, and numbness; in addition, paraneoplastic autonomic neuropathy is present in roughly 30% of antibody-positive patients. Other symptoms include postural hypotension, GI dysmotility (pseudo-obstruction), impotence, pupil dysfunction, urinary retention, and dry mouth.

C. Paraneoplastic Autonomic Neuropathy

Subacute autonomic neuropathy can occur in patients with small cell lung cancer or other tumors, with or without somatic neuropathy and with several antibodies other than ANNA-1, including AChR antibodies, discussed earlier. Formal autonomic testing reveals abnormal findings in involved systems. Improvement in autonomic function sometimes follows treatment for the underlying cancer.

D. Enteric Neuronopathy

Enteric neuronopathy causes intestinal pseudo-obstruction and marked derangement of function on gastric and intestinal motility studies. Neurons of the enteric nervous system are the presumed target of immunologic attack. GI symptoms usually precede the tumor discovery, on average by 9 months, but can also follow the cancer. Symptoms include abrupt onset of progressive constipation, crampy abdominal pain, and vomiting, which can be severe enough to mimic an acute bowel obstruction. Physiologic studies demonstrate delayed gastric emptying and GI dysmotility and hypomotility. Symptoms and signs of more widespread autonomic involvement are often present and are similar but less severe than those in other paraneoplastic autonomic neuropathies. The associated malignancy is most often small cell lung cancer; some patients have ANNA-1 antibodies. GI dysfunction is often refractory to pharmacologic manipulation or surgical intervention. Symptoms occasionally remit spontaneously or after chemotherapy or radiation treatments.

Camdessanche JP, et al. Paraneoplastic peripheral neuropathy associated with anti-Hu antibodies. A clinical and electrophysiological study of 20 patients. *Brain* 2002;125:166–175. [PMID: 11834602] (Large series including autonomic neuropathy screening.)

De Giorgio R, et al. Inflammatory neuropathies of the enteric nervous system. *Gastroenterology* 2004;126(7):1872–1883. [PMID: 15188182] (Excellent review of and most recent discussion of current concepts, diagnostic considerations, and treatment.)

CHRONIC AUTONOMIC NEUROPATHIES

Most of the more than 200 known causes of peripheral neuropathy have some degree of autonomic involvement, but the dysfunction is usually limited to distal sweating and vasomotor control. A few causes can lead to severe or targeted autonomic dysfunction.

1. Diabetic Autonomic Neuropathy

 ESSENTIALS OF DIAGNOSIS

▶ Can affect virtually all organ systems
▶ Somatic and autonomic peripheral neuropathy may occur without other end-organ damage
▶ Orthostatic hypotension is a late, severe finding

▶ General Considerations

Diabetic autonomic neuropathy (DAN) is a common and dangerous complication of diabetes mellitus types 1 and 2 that greatly affects quality of life and life expectancy of patients with the disease. Clinical symptoms generally develop many years after onset of diabetes; however, subclinical DAN may be evident within 1–2 years of disease onset, even in the absence of other diabetic complications or overt sensorimotor peripheral neuropathy.

▶ Clinical Findings
A. Symptoms and Signs

Clinical manifestations are heterogeneous and diverse; few organ systems are spared. Because, in part, of the long length and vulnerability of the vagus nerve, cardiovascular autonomic neuropathy is a common form of DAN, contributing to orthostatic hypotension, exercise intolerance, cardiovascular lability, asymptomatic cardiac ischemia, and reduced survival. Symptoms, however, are not generally noted until impairment is sufficiently severe to cause orthostatic hypotension or frank syncope. A characteristic resting tachycardia is a frequent finding.

GI symptoms in diabetic patients are frequently caused by autonomic neuropathy. Dysphagia for solid food, gastric acid blunting, and impaired gastric emptying (gastroparesis) may result from dysfunction of the vagus nerve or intrinsic enteric neurons. Common complaints include early satiety, loss of appetite, nausea and vomiting, bloating, and epigastric discomfort. If severe, gastroparesis may lead to recurrent bouts of vomiting of undigested food and creation of bezoars. Milder forms may delay the anticipated postprandial glucose surge and lead to unexpected treatment-induced hypoglycemia, giving the appearance of erratic diabetes control. Episodic diarrhea, especially prominent at night, also occurs, but constipation is much more common. Fecal incontinence can occur.

Large meals, especially those high in carbohydrate load, cause a postprandial drop in BP (postprandial hypotension) that may be symptomatic and may be mistaken for hypoglycemia. Erectile dysfunction, common in individuals with diabetes, is often the initial autonomic complication. Bladder dysfunction is seen in up to half of diabetic patients. Impaired bladder sensation is usually the earliest symptom and leads to increased bladder size and a reduced urge to micturate. Later, efferent parasympathetic disease leads to hesitancy, weak stream, and incomplete bladder emptying. Eventually incontinence may ensue.

Sudomotor (sweating) dysfunction occurs early but is usually asymptomatic until marked. Impaired microvascular skin blood flow is similarly disordered, resulting in dry, cold, shiny, hairless distal skin areas that often have reduced pain and temperature sensation. When loss of sudomotor function is severe, less-affected areas attempt to compensate, resulting in areas of hyperhidrosis or perceived excessive sweating. Loss of sudomotor function may also result in insufficient body cooling and heat intolerance. Inappropriate gustatory cranial sweating is sometimes seen.

B. Diagnostic Studies and Special Tests

An autonomic testing battery can identify and grade the severity of DAN. Organ-specific tests include studies of GI motility and gastric emptying time, urodynamic studies, and impotency evaluations.

▶ Differential Diagnosis

Although DAN is the most common cause of chronic autonomic neuropathy, other entities should be considered, including amyloid, idiopathic, immune-mediated, and hereditary neuropathies; Addison disease; pheochromocytoma; and collagen vascular diseases.

▶ Treatment & Prognosis

Tight glycemic control, the only effective preventive treatment, may slow nerve damage. No other preventive treatment has shown benefit.

DAN negatively affects prognosis and survival in patients with diabetes. A controlled study found an 8-year mortality rate of 23% in diabetic patients with measurable cardiovascular autonomic neuropathy and no other initial complications.

Vinik AI, et al. Diabetic autonomic neuropathy. *Diabetes Care* 2003;26:1553–2579. [PMID: 12716821] (Comprehensive review of clinical features and pathologic mechanisms.)

2. Other Chronic Autonomic Neuropathies

A. Amyloidosis-Related Neuropathy

Amyloidosis, both hereditary and acquired, frequently causes significant autonomic neuropathy, with symptoms and findings similar to those seen in DAN, but often more severe. A painful distal sensory neuropathy is often coincident, and carpal tunnel syndrome commonly results from amyloid deposition. The diagnostic workup includes a careful family history and search for amyloid deposits. Fat pad and rectal biopsy are less invasive and more productive procedures than muscle or nerve biopsy. Genetic testing is available for many of the hereditary forms of amyloidosis. Multiple myeloma or monoclonal gammopathy is frequently present in patients with acquired forms of the disease.

Chemotherapy in combination with bone marrow or autologous stem cell transplantation is a promising and accepted treatment in patients with acquired forms of the disease. Reports show a beneficial effect on autonomic function and sensorimotor neuropathy, and halting of disease progression by orthotopic liver transplantation.

B. Toxic and Medication-Induced Neuropathies

Among the medications that affect autonomic function are the chemotherapeutic agents cisplatin, vincristine, paclitaxel, and docetaxel; and the antiarrhythmic agent amiodarone. Chronic ethanol exposure can also cause autonomic neuropathy. Arsenic, organic mercury, thallium, Vacor, acrylamide, podophyllotoxin, and hexacarbon toxicity are less commonly encountered causes.

C. Infection-Related Neuropathies

HIV infection can cause symptomatic autonomic neuropathy. Chagas disease causes a predominantly cholinergic neuropathy, with prominent esophageal dysmotility. Leprosy is a common cause of peripheral and autonomic neuropathy in endemic areas. Both syphilis and Lyme disease can affect autonomic systems and peripheral and cranial nerves. The Argyll-Robertson pupil, a miotic pupil that accommodates but fails to react to light, is seen not only in patients with neurosyphilis, but also in those with diabetes, sarcoidosis, and multiple sclerosis.

D. Immune-Mediated Neuropathies

Many immune-mediated neuropathies begin subacutely and were discussed earlier. Some develop more chronically and may respond to plasmapheresis. Autonomic neuropathy is seen in association with a variety of collagen vascular disorders, most notably Sjögren syndrome, but also systemic lupus erythematosus, mixed connective tissue disease, rheumatoid arthritis, and inflammatory bowel disease.

E. Hereditary Autonomic Neuropathies

In addition to hereditary amyloidosis, a number of inherited conditions can affect autonomic nerves. Most impair sensory nerves as well. Hereditary sensory and autonomic neuropathies (HSANs) are genetically separable from the hereditary motor-sensory neuropathies (HMSNs; eg, Charcot-Marie-Tooth disease). Most HSANs have childhood or infantile onset and known gene defects. Riley-Day syndrome (familial dysautonomia) is one notable form (HSAN3) that produces marked autonomic dysfunction (see Chapter 19). Porphyria and Fabry disease (α-galactosidase A deficiency) also may compromise autonomic nerves. Dopamine β-hydroxylase deficiency causes severe orthostatic hypotension and nearly undetectable norepinephrine levels.

3. Small-Fiber Neuropathy

The most common cause of predominant or isolated disease of small-diameter sensory and autonomic nerves, termed small-fiber neuropathy, is diabetes mellitus. Many cases of small-fiber neuropathy remain idiopathic, however, despite a thorough neuropathy workup (see Chapter 19). As in diabetes, patients have distal pain, paresthesias, and autonomic signs. In some cases isolated glucose intolerance is present, but not overt diabetes.

Klein CM, et al. The spectrum of autoimmune autonomic neuropathies. *Ann Neurol* 2003;53:752–758. [PMID: 12783421] (Clinical features and associated antibodies in 18 patients with autonomic neuropathy and AChR antibodies, showing correlation of antibody titers with disease severity.)

Low PA, et al. Autonomic dysfunction in peripheral nerve disease. *Muscle Nerve* 2003;27:646–661. [PMID: 12766975] (Detailed overview of clinical features, diagnosis, and treatment of acute and chronic autonomic neuropathies.)

Sandroni P, et al. Idiopathic autonomic neuropathy: Comparison of cases seropositive and seronegative for ganglionic acetylcholine receptor antibody. *Arch Neurol* 2004;61:44–48. [PMID: 14732619] (Comparison of clinical features of AChR antibodies, finding more prominent cholinergic signs in antibody-positive patients.)

Shimojima Y, et al. Ten-year follow-up of peripheral nerve function in patients with familial amyloid polyneuropathy after liver transplantation. *J Neurol* 2008;255(8):1220–1225. [PMID: 18484233] (Report of halting disease progression after 10 years.)

Toth C, Zochodne DW. Other autonomic neuropathies. *Semin Neurol* 2003;23:373–380. [PMID: 15088258] (Review of autonomic neuropathies other than DAN.)

Vernino S, et al. Autoantibodies to ganglionic acetylcholine receptors in autoimmune autonomic neuropathies. *N Engl J Med* 2000;343:847–855. [PMID: 10995864] (Primary report of AChR antibodies and autonomic neuropathy.)

ORTHOSTATIC INTOLERANCE & POSTURAL ORTHOSTATIC TACHYCARDIA SYNDROME

ESSENTIALS OF DIAGNOSIS

▶ Posturally triggered symptoms

▶ Postural tachycardia without identifiable cause

▶ Frequently, subacute onset

▶ Must be differentiated from chronic fatigue and panic disorder

▶ General Considerations

Any disorder that leads to a posturally related drop in BP (orthostatic hypotension) can be considered a form of orthostatic intolerance (OI), but today the latter term implies a separate, distinct group of disorders in which orthostatic symptoms occur without a concomitant drop in systemic BP. Postural orthostatic tachycardia syndrome (POTS) is synonymous with this entity. Orthostatic intolerance/POTS is the most common reason for referral to many treatment centers specializing in autonomic dysfunction.

▶ Pathogenesis

Underlying mechanisms are heterogeneous and include excessive venous pooling, autonomic neuropathy, idiopathic hypovolemia, α-adrenergic receptor supersensitivity, and primary central nervous system dysregulation. A defect in a norepinephrine transporter gene has been found in a clinically indistinguishable familial form.

▶ Clinical Findings

A. Symptoms and Signs

Symptoms are postural in nature and not continual or situational. Orthostatic tachycardia is a hallmark of OI but is also seen in secondary causes of orthostatic symptoms, which must be excluded before a primary diagnosis of OI can be made. The degree of tachycardia is defined as a heart-rate increment of 30 beats/min or greater on tilt or standing, or an absolute value of 120 beats/min or greater and development of orthostatic complaints within 5 minutes, despite a preserved systemic BP. In addition to symptoms of sympathetic activation, patients also often have light-headedness, fatigue, feeling of weakness, cognitive blunting, visual blurring, palpitations, anxiety, or pallor. Acute exacerbations usually respond better to volume expansion than to β-blockade or anxiety medications. Some patients have subacute onset, in many cases associated with a preceding viral illness. Antibodies to AChR, discussed earlier, are found in 10% of patients, consistent in some with a *forme fruste* of acute autonomic neuropathy; many patients have distal loss of vasomotor control, trophic skin changes, and posturally triggered bluish distal leg swelling. Symptoms may be cyclic or catamenial and are five times more frequent in women than in men. Neurocardiogenic syncope is also common.

B. Diagnostic Studies

Autonomic testing and tilt table studies are helpful in documenting the orthostatic tachycardia and characterizing the nature of the underlying mechanism. Catecholamine levels may show an excessive increase on upright tilting.

▶ Differential Diagnosis

Patients are often dismissed as having either chronic fatigue syndrome or panic disorder. Mitral valve prolapse is detectable in many patients with OI. Low-grade Chiari malformations were popularized in the press as a cause of OI, but the association is not yet established. Detection of reflex syncope by tilt table testing may lead to a diagnosis of benign syncope, while overlooking the primary underlying process.

▶ Treatment & Prognosis

Treatment is similar to that of orthostatic hypotension, discussed earlier, but with some distinct differences. Patients experiencing an acute episode may benefit from a fluid bolus. β-Blockers offer a tempting and sometimes beneficial approach to blunt the tachycardia but often make symptoms worse if the tachycardia is compensatory. Attempts to raise BP are often helpful (see Treatment of Orthostatic Hypotension, earlier). Despite being designated as a "benign" condition, OI causes severely disabling symptoms in many patients.

Shannon JR, et al. Orthostatic intolerance and tachycardia associated with norepinephrine-transporter deficiency. *N Engl J Med* 2000;342:541–549. [PMID: 10684912] (Discovery of genetic basis of clinically indistinguishable OI in a set of twins. The defect has not been found in sporadic cases.)

Weimer LH, Williams O. Syncope and orthostatic intolerance. *Med Clin North Am* 2003;87:835–865. [PMID: 12834151] (General review of syncope, orthostatic hypotension, and OI from a neurologic perspective.)

SUDOMOTOR (SWEATING) DISORDERS

▶ General Considerations

Eccrine sweat glands prevent overheating, and disorders that lead to excessive or inadequate function are termed, respectively, *hyperhidrosis* and *hypohidrosis*. Combinations of loss of function in some areas and compensatory heightened function in preserved areas are seen in many disorders that cause autonomic failure. Some disorders cause isolated sudomotor dysfunction.

▶ Clinical Findings

Essential hyperhidrosis is a relatively common and often familial disorder characterized by isolated, inappropriate sweating. Profuse sweating in minimally hot surroundings or anxiety-producing situations can occur in the palms, soles, and axillae, or more diffusely. Although not medically dangerous unless dehydration or electrolyte loss ensues, the condition can be socially debilitating. No specific laboratory test or marker aids diagnosis, and other autonomic functions are normal.

Hypohidrosis and anhidrosis occur with both autonomic peripheral neuropathy and central nervous system disorders. Isolated idiopathic anhidrosis can be seen without other autonomic dysfunction; Ross syndrome is characterized by presence of an Adie tonic pupil and areflexia. Many dermatologic conditions affect sweat gland function. Rare congenital states in which sweat glands are absent lead to life-threatening overheating (anhidrotic ectodermal dysplasia).

▶ Differential Diagnosis

Hyperhidrosis also occurs in pheochromocytoma, thyrotoxicosis, pituitary and hypothalamic dysfunction, anxiety disorders, menopause, carcinoid syndrome, and drug withdrawal. Medications that can enhance sweating include serotonin reuptake inhibitors, opioids, calcium channel blockers, and acyclovir. Anticholinergic drugs, including tricyclic antidepressants, oxybutynin, and phenothiazines, reduce sweating but generally do so asymptomatically and not to a degree that would aid in treatment of hyperhidrosis. Autonomic testing can document the lack of involvement of other autonomic functions. Asymmetric sweating suggests a focal structural lesion.

▶ Treatment

Hypohidrosis rarely requires treatment other than avoidance of overheating. Hyperhidrosis is much more bothersome and is difficult to treat. Extrastrength topical antiperspirants, such as 6–25% aluminum chloride hexahydrate (Drysol), are the first-line therapy in patients with axillary sweating; however, the skin on the palms and soles is often too thick to benefit from this treatment. Tap water iontophoresis is a noninvasive and safe means to blunt sweating, but effects are temporary and frequent home treatments are necessary. Anxiolytic medications are occasionally helpful. Intradermal botulinum toxin is a minimally invasive way to temporarily disable sweat glands in focal hyperhidrosis; hand and foot weakness is a potential complication. In refractory cases, endoscopic sympathectomy has been widely used and has a good safety profile. Heightened cranial sweating is a complication but is usually less objectionable than in the presurgical state.

Cheshire WP, Freeman R. Disorders of sweating. *Semin Neurol* 2003;23:399–406. [PMID: 15088261] (Overview of causes and treatment of hypohidrosis and hyperhidrosis.)

AUTONOMIC SYMPTOMS IN SPINAL CORD INJURY

Spinal cord injury at the midthoracic level (T6) often produces autonomic dysreflexia. Signals proximal to the lesion, including vagal nerve function, are intact; circuits below the injury are removed from normal inhibitory control. Consequently, despite a lack of voluntary control of bladder, bowel, and sexual function, excessive bursts of undesirable reflex function can be triggered by innocuous stimulation of various organs or by certain medications. Marked decreases in heart rate, spikes in BP, sweating, flushing, piloerection (goose bumps), and headaches are triggered. Marked orthostatic hypotension, which can be symptomatic even with sitting, is frequent in patients with spinal cord injury, and the severity of symptoms is exacerbated by a prolonged bedridden state. Detailed discussion of spinal cord injury and spinal disorders is presented in Chapters 14 and 15.

Myasthenia Gravis & Other Disorders of the Neuromuscular Junction

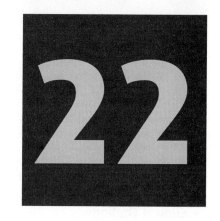

Shanna Kathlyn Patterson, MD, Petra Kaufmann, MD, MSc,
& Marisa Schiller Sosinsky, MD

NEUROMUSCULAR TRANSMISSION

The neuromuscular junction is the synaptic connection formed between a motor neuron axon and the muscle fiber it innervates. The transmitter used at the neuromuscular junction, acetylcholine, is stored in the presynaptic motor nerve terminals. The postsynaptic muscle membrane has many folds in which receptors for acetylcholine are located. When a motor nerve action potential reaches the presynaptic nerve terminal, there is a resultant increase in calcium conductance through voltage-gated calcium channels. This increase in intracellular calcium leads to the fusion of acetylcholine-filled presynaptic vesicles with the plasma membrane of the motor nerve terminal. Acetylcholine is subsequently released into the synaptic cleft by exocytosis.

The acetylcholine diffuses across the synapse and binds to the acetylcholine receptors on the postsynaptic muscle membrane. The binding of acetylcholine to these receptors facilitates increased conduction of sodium and potassium. This leads to transient depolarization of the postjunctional muscle membrane known as an *end-plate potential*. This depolarization allows for the generation and propagation of action potentials in the postsynaptic muscle cell. These processes initiate a chain of events in the muscle cell that culminates in muscle contraction. Disorders of the neuromuscular junction result from a disruption of this series of events.

MYASTHENIA GRAVIS (AUTOIMMUNE MYASTHENIA)

ESSENTIALS OF DIAGNOSIS

- ▶ Fluctuating, fatigable weakness of commonly used muscles
- ▶ Often involves ocular, bulbar, and respiratory muscles
- ▶ Can be associated with thymoma or thymic hyperplasia
- ▶ Presence of circulating antibodies to the acetylcholine receptor (most patients)

▶ General Considerations

Myasthenia gravis (MG), the most common of the neuromuscular junction disorders, is an acquired, predominantly antibody-mediated autoimmune disease. In this disorder, antibodies are targeted against the nicotinic acetylcholine receptor (AChR) at the neuromuscular junction, resulting in an overall reduction in the number of AChRs and damage to the postsynaptic membrane.

The prevalence of autoimmune MG is estimated at 1 case in 10,000–20,000 people. Women are affected more often in the second and third decades of life, and men more often in the fifth and sixth decades. Associated autoimmune diseases are present in approximately 5% of patients, and comorbid thyroid disease occurs in more than 10%.

▶ Pathogenesis

In generalized MG, AChR antibodies are detected in up to 90% of patients, whereas in purely ocular MG, only about 50% of patients are antibody positive. Three subtypes of AChR antibodies have been identified: binding, blocking, and modulating. All of these lead to ACh receptor loss on the postsynaptic membrane via accelerated receptor degradation or receptor blockade. ACh receptor modulation is caused by antibodies that cross-link AChRs and facilitate endocytosis, resulting in receptor loss on the postsynaptic membrane. In addition, complement-mediated damage to the postsynaptic membrane results in fewer membrane folds and widened synaptic clefts.

Antibodies to epitopes other than the AChR have been identified in patients with MG. These include antibodies to another postsynaptic neuromuscular junction protein, muscle-specific kinase (MuSK), found in about 40% of MG patients who do not have AChR antibodies. MuSK antibodies have been shown to disrupt neuromuscular junction function by adversely affecting the maintenance of AChR clustering at the muscle endplate, thus leading to reduced numbers of functional AChRs. In patients who have neither AChR nor

MuSK antibodies, so-called seronegative MG, antibodies to striated muscle proteins, such as titin and the ryanodine receptor, are sometimes detected. It is unclear how these other antibodies lead to clinical disease.

The antibody production is a T-cell–mediated process thought to be associated with thymic dysfunction. Thymic lymphofollicular hyperplasia occurs in 70% of MG patients. Thymoma, an epithelial tumor of the thymus, occurs in 10% of patients with MG. Of the previously mentioned muscle autoantibodies, thymoma is associated with antibodies against the AChR, titin, and the ryanodine receptor. In this subpopulation the disease can be thought of as a paraneoplastic disorder (see Chapter 13).

▶ **Clinical Findings**

A. Symptoms and Signs

MG is clinically characterized by fluctuating, fatigable weakness of commonly used muscles. Hallmark features include ptosis, diplopia, dysarthria, dysphagia, and respiratory and limb muscle weakness. About half of patients present with ocular findings. The ocular muscle weakness is usually bilateral and asymmetric and results in diplopia, ptosis, or both. Notably, the pupil is spared. Eventually, almost all patients with MG develop ocular symptoms, and in some the disease is limited to the extraocular muscles.

Within the first year of disease onset, up to 75% of patients develop generalized symptoms. Bulbar symptoms are common and include dysarthria, dysphagia, facial weakness, and weakness of mastication. Because of palatal weakness, patients often have nasal speech and can regurgitate liquids through the nose. Bulbar manifestations are often the most disabling symptoms. Limb and trunk weakness is common in a proximal greater than distal distribution. Frequently, the arms are more affected than the legs. The quadriceps, triceps, and neck extensor muscles appear to be preferentially involved. A hallmark of myasthenic weakness is its fluctuating and fatigable nature. It may increase throughout the day, worsen with sustained activity, and improve with rest.

The most serious of the symptoms is respiratory compromise caused by weakness of diaphragmatic and intercostal muscles. These respiratory symptoms, in conjunction with severe bulbar symptoms, can culminate in so-called *myasthenic crisis*, defined as respiratory failure requiring mechanical ventilation. This complication occurs in about 15–20% of patients with MG and may be precipitated by infection or aspiration.

In roughly one third of pregnant women MG is exacerbated by the pregnancy, with the greatest risk during the first trimester. In some patients, symptoms and signs improve during the second and third trimesters coincident with the relative immunosuppression that occurs during this phase of pregnancy. A high risk then returns during the postpartum period.

In addition to the effects on the mother, infants and children of mothers with myasthenia can develop transient or, rarely, permanent weakness. Approximately one third of infants of mothers with autoimmune MG have transitory *neonatal myasthenia*, with weakness appearing within the first 4 days of life and usually lasting for approximately 3 weeks. Infants with *neonatal myasthenia* often are poor feeders and have a weak cry. Weakness is the result of placental transfer of maternal antibodies to the fetal blood circulation, yet there is no clear association between neonatal weakness and maternal clinical status or antibody levels. In contrast to neonatal myasthenia, which is transient, permanent deficits can occur in a rare condition, known as *fetal AChR inactivation syndrome*. It has been proposed that this syndrome—characterized by facial weakness, high-arched palate, soft palate and pharyngeal weakness, conductive hearing loss, and cryptorchidism—is caused by elevated maternal antibodies against the fetal AChR subunit. These antibodies result in inactivation of the fetal AChR subunit during a critical period of muscle development. Serum testing for these antibodies is not widely available, and is currently only conducted in a specialized research laboratory setting.

B. Diagnostic Studies

1. Tensilon (edrophonium) test—This test evaluates the response to a short-acting cholinesterase inhibitor. The examiner must identify a clinical feature (most often ptosis) to observe. One milligram of edrophonium is given intravenously as a test dose. If no adverse effects are noted, a 3-mg dose is given. A clinical response should be seen within 30–60 seconds. If no response is seen, an additional 3 mg of edrophonium can be given and the patient examined again. If there is still no improvement, a final 3-mg dose can be given, for a total of 10 mg. If there is no clinical improvement after 2 minutes, the test is negative. Studies suggest a sensitivity of 70–95% for this test. Specificity is not as high; positive tests have been reported in a variety of conditions, including Lambert-Eaton myasthenic syndrome, botulism, snake envenomation, motor neuron disease, and multiple sclerosis.

Serious muscarinic cholinergic side effects can occur with the test, including increased oropharyngeal secretions and respiratory decompensation as well as bradycardia or asystole. Cardiac monitoring should be performed, and atropine should be available readily during the test.

When significant ptosis is present, myasthenic weakness can sometimes be evaluated by placing an ice pack over the closed ptotic eyelid for 2 minutes. The test is considered supportive of myasthenic weakness if the ptosis visibly improves. Cold temperature is thought to decrease cholinesterase activity and promote the efficiency of acetylcholine at eliciting depolarizations at the end plate. Similarly, one can evaluate for improved ptosis after 30 minutes of sleep.

2. Laboratory studies—Serologic testing should be performed in several steps. The first screening antibody should be the AChR-binding antibody, because it is the most sensitive. If it is negative, then an AChR-modulating antibody test increases the diagnostic yield. Testing for AChR-blocking antibodies does not increase sensitivity.

In patients who are seronegative for these antibodies, antibodies against MuSK may be present. Patients with thymoma may have antibodies to the muscle proteins ryanodine and titin. Of note, the absolute titers of these antibodies do not correlate well with disease course or severity.

3. Electrodiagnostic studies—Routine nerve conduction studies and electromyography usually do not identify dysfunction of the neuromuscular junction. Slow repetitive nerve stimulation is the most commonly used test to evaluate for MG. In this test, a nerve is stimulated 6–10 times at a rate of 2 or 3 Hz, and the compound muscle action potential (CMAP) is measured over the corresponding muscle. In normal individuals, no change occurs in the CMAP over time (see Chapter 2 for example). In patients with MG, however, there is a decrease of more than 10% in CMAP with the first four to five stimuli. Immediately following 10 seconds of maximal voluntary exercise, the decrement typically repairs toward normal. This is followed by postexercise exhaustion, with progressively greater decrement when stimulating at 1-minute intervals after maximal voluntary exercise (see Chapter 2). Low-frequency repetitive stimulation has low sensitivity; only 75% of patients with generalized MG and even fewer with only ocular or distal limb weakness have a positive test. In addition, repetitive nerve stimulation is not entirely specific for MG and can be positive in Lambert-Eaton myasthenic syndrome, and to a lesser degree in myositis or lower motor neuron disease. Abnormalities noted on repetitive nerve stimulation do not correlate well with the severity of weakness.

Single-fiber electromyography has a sensitivity of approximately 95% in MG. This test measures the variability in synaptic transmission time, otherwise known as "jitter," between two fibers innervated by the same axon. In MG, there is an increased variability of latencies among muscle fibers in a single motor unit. In addition, muscle fiber potential may be blocked if transmission at its neuromuscular junction fails completely. As with slow repetitive nerve stimulation, abnormalities seen on single-fiber electromyography are not specific to MG.

4. Imaging and other studies—Because of the association between MG and thymoma, all patients should be screened for this tumor using either a computed tomographic or magnetic resonance imaging scan of the chest. In addition, patients should be screened for common comorbid diseases such as thyroid disease or autoimmune diseases (eg, systemic lupus erythematosus, rheumatoid arthritis).

▶ Differential Diagnosis

For generalized MG, the differential diagnosis includes Lambert-Eaton myasthenic syndrome, botulism, and myopathy. For ocular myasthenia, alternative diagnoses include progressive external ophthalmoplegia, thyroid disease, and oculopharyngeal muscular dystrophy. Motor neuron disease, brainstem stroke, diphtheria, and botulism must be considered in patients with bulbar predominant myasthenia gravis.

▶ Treatment

A. Symptomatic Treatment

The mainstays of symptomatic treatment are the cholinesterase inhibitors, which increase the concentration of acetylcholine at the AChR (Table 22–1). Acetylcholinesterase inhibitors are most effective early in the disease when there are still adequate numbers of receptors present. In patients with mild disease, these agents may be used alone without immunosuppressive therapy. As the disease progresses,

Table 22–1. Cholinesterase Inhibitors Used in the Symptomatic Treatment of Myasthenia Gravis

Drug	Dosage	Adverse Effects
Pyridostigmine bromide	Up to 600 mg/day PO, with intervals and doses adjusted for symptoms (eg, 60–120 mg PO every 4-6 h)	**Common**—abdominal cramps, diarrhea, GI hypermotility, nausea, vomiting, diaphoresis, fasciculations, muscle cramps, increased bronchial secretions, increased salivation, miosis **Serious**—bradycardia, cholinergic crisis
Ambenonium[a]	5-25 mg PO 3-4 times a day, to maximum of 200 mg/day	**Common**—epigastric distress, general malaise with anxiety and vertigo, miosis, blurred vision, muscle fasciculations, cramps, sialorrhea, bronchorrhea, excessive lacrimal secretions, sweating, urinary urgency
Neostigmine[a]	Up to 150 mg/day PO, with intervals and doses adjusted for symptoms	**Common**—diaphoresis, diarrhea, flatulence, GI hypermotility, nausea, vomiting, increased salivation, muscle twitching **Serious**—anaphylaxis, bronchospasm, respiratory arrest, respiratory depression, cardiac arrhythmias, seizures

GI = gastrointestinal; PO = by mouth (orally).
[a]Ambenonium and neostigmine are used less commonly than pyridostigmine.

increasing doses may be required to achieve the same therapeutic effect. Pyridostigmine is usually given at least three to four times daily, but dose intervals need to be adjusted according to symptoms. A long-acting formulation is available and may be useful with overnight symptom control.

The main side effects of the cholinesterase inhibitors are related to excess levels of acetylcholine at nicotinic and muscarinic synapses. Muscarinic side effects include diarrhea, cramping, and excessive secretions that can worsen respiratory compromise. Nicotinic side effects include muscle fasciculations and increased blockade of neuromuscular transmission, which can lead to cholinergic crisis.

B. Immunosuppressive Treatment

1. Thymectomy—For patients with a neoplastic thymoma, surgical removal of the tumor is necessary to prevent tumor spread. For patients without thymoma, thymectomy increases the likelihood of remission. Data on the efficacy of thymectomy are confounded by factors such as variable surgical technique and lack of controlled trials. In most experienced centers, however, perioperative morbidity and mortality are very low and are outweighed by the chances for improvement in most cases. There is controversy about predictors of outcome, but thymus pathology, age, or disease severity does not reliably predict remission. Unless there are contraindications, thymectomy should be considered for patients of any age with MG. The procedure appears to be most effective when performed during the first 2 years of disease. Medical treatment of MG prior to surgery decreases the perioperative morbidity. Preoperative intravenous immunoglobulin (IVIG) or plasmapheresis is often used to stabilize patients with generalized MG.

There is debate about the best surgical procedure, and protocols have included extensive trans-sternal and transcervical approaches, as well as, more recently, endoscopic techniques and combination approaches. It has been suggested that more extensive resection of thymus tissue leads to higher remission rates, but this will remain a point of controversy until conclusive comparisons are available.

2. Medical therapy—For most patients, treatment includes inducing remission with the use of an immunosuppressant. Once remission is achieved, the immunosuppressant can be gradually tapered, but most patients need to continue at least a small dose of medication.

A. CORTICOSTEROIDS—These agents are the first-line immunosuppressive therapy for MG. Many patients have transient worsening of symptoms within the first 2 weeks of initiating such treatment. Corticosteroid therapy may therefore have to be initiated following stabilization with a course of plasmapheresis or intravenous immunoglobulin. Patients should be closely monitored when corticosteroid therapy is initiated, and hospitalization may be warranted.

Corticosteroids induce remission in up to 50% of patients, and up to 80% of all patients benefit from the therapy. Most patients improve within the first few weeks of treatment. Once remission is obtained, the corticosteroids are slowly tapered to the lowest dose possible that does not result in a flare-up of disease.

Complications of corticosteroids include impaired glucose tolerance, hypertension, cataracts, gastrointestinal ulcers, myopathy, avascular necrosis of the hip, osteoporosis, infection, and psychosis. Some of the risks can be reduced by implementation of a low-sodium, low-sugar diet, along with calcium supplementation and exercise. Fasting blood glucose should be checked periodically. Annual ophthalmological evaluations should be arranged to screen for glaucoma or cataracts. The osteoporosis risk can be reduced by prophylactic treatment (eg, alendronate sodium, 5 mg/day orally).

B. NONSTEROIDAL IMMUNOSUPPRESSION—Because of side effects from corticosteroids, clinicians often use so-called *steroid-sparing medications*, such as azathioprine (Table 22–2). At least 50% of patients appear to benefit from this medication. Most studies describe its use in conjunction with corticosteroids, not as monotherapy. Side effects are generally mild but can include bone marrow and hepatic toxicity; for this reason, blood counts and liver function need to be monitored. Azathioprine acts much more slowly than corticosteroids. Improvement may begin only after several months of treatment, and maximal improvement may require 1–2 years. Up to 20% of patients develop an idiosyncratic reaction to azathioprine during the first weeks of treatment, consisting of fever, chills, rash, and gastrointestinal symptoms. In these intolerant patients, azathioprine must be discontinued immediately.

Mycophenolate mofetil has been suggested as an adjunctive or corticosteroid-sparing therapy and perhaps as monotherapy. Side effects include gastrointestinal symptoms, hypertension, and peripheral edema. Patients should be advised to avoid ultraviolet-light exposure while taking this medication. The medication can also cause bone marrow suppression, and monitoring of blood counts is therefore indicated. The concurrent use of azathioprine and mycophenolate mofetil is not recommended. Preliminary studies had suggested benefit after 1–2 months, with a peak effect around 6 months. However, in controlled trials there was no benefit of mycophenolate mofetil over placebo. The use of mycophenolate mofetil for myasthenia gravis has therefore declined. Cyclosporine is used for patients with severe MG who cannot be managed with less toxic forms of therapy. Major side effects include renal toxicity and hypertension. Cyclophosphamide is an alkylating agent that has been used in patients with refractory disease. Side effects include severe bone marrow suppression, bladder toxicity, and risk of neoplasm. Treatment with cyclosporine or cyclophosphamide should be managed by a physician who is familiar with their adverse effects and monitoring requirements.

For all of these corticosteroid-sparing immunosuppressive drugs, there may be an increased long-term risk of lymphoma or other malignancies.

Table 22–2. Immunosuppressants Used in the Treatment of Myasthenia Gravis

Drug[a]	Dosage	Monitoring	Adverse Effects
Azathioprine	Increase gradually up to 2–3 mg/kg/day PO	Monitor CBC and liver function weekly during first month, twice monthly during second and third months, then monthly	**Common**—GI hypersensitivity, nausea, vomiting **Serious**—cancer (rare), hepatotoxicity, infection, leukopenia, thrombocytopenia, megaloblastic anemia, pancreatitis
Mycophenolate mofetil	1–1.5 g PO twice daily	Monitor CBC weekly during first month, twice monthly during second and third months, then monthly	**Common**—constipation, diarrhea, nausea, vomiting, headache **Serious**—confusion, tremor, GI bleeding, hypertension, peripheral edema, infection, sepsis, cancer (rare), myelosuppression
Cyclosporine	2.5 mg/kg/day PO divided twice daily; after 4 wk, dose may be increased by 0.5 mg/kg/day at 2-wk intervals, to maximum of 4 mg/kg/day	Monitor blood pressure, CBC, uric acid, potassium, lipids, magnesium, serum creatinine, and BUN every 2 wk during initial 3 mo of therapy and then monthly if patient is stable	**Common**—headache, hirsutism, nausea, diarrhea, tremor, gum hyperplasia **Serious**—anaphylaxis, seizure, hepatotoxicity, hyperkalemia (rare), hypomagnesemia, hypertension (frequent), infection, nephrotoxicity (frequent), hemolytic uremic syndrome (rare), paresthesia (rare), lymphoproliferative disorder (rare)

BUN = blood urea nitrogen; CBC = complete blood count; GI = gastrointestinal; PO = by mouth (orally).
[a]Not labeled by the Food and Drug Administration for use in myasthenia gravis.

c. Short-term treatments—Plasmapheresis and IVIG each induce rapid clinical improvement but have only short-term effects (Table 22–3). Both are often employed in the special situation of myasthenic crisis. In addition, either treatment can be used to stabilize patients prior to thymectomy or to treat exacerbations that occur during infection, surgery, or the tapering of a corticosteroid regimen.

Plasmapheresis usually produces clinical improvement within the first week, and benefits usually last for 1–2 months. Complications are uncommon but include hypotension, bradycardia, electrolyte imbalance, and infection.

IVIG has similar efficacy to plasmapheresis. Side effects include malaise, hypersensitivity, aseptic meningitis, and, rarely, renal insufficiency, stroke, and myocardial infarction.

Table 22–3. Short-Term Immunosuppressive Treatments for Myasthenia Gravis

Treatment	Regimen	Adverse Effects
Intravenous immunoglobulin (IVIG)[a]	2 g/kg per course divided over 5 daily treatments Consider premedication with diphenhydramine HCl (50 mg PO once) and acetaminophen (650 mg PO once), 30 min prior to IVIG treatment	**Common**—malaise, headache, chills, flushing, fever, tightness of the chest, nausea **Serious**—anaphylaxis; rash; thrombotic events, including stroke and myocardial infarction (risk lower with slow infusion: concentration < 5% and infusion rates < 0.5 mL/kg/h); renal dysfunction (higher risk with sucrose-containing products); hemolytic anemia; neutropenia; aseptic meningitis; transmission of infection (rare)
Plasmapheresis	Common regimen is 5 exchanges using an alternate-day schedule	**Common**—dizziness, nausea, vomiting, headache, citrate-induced hypocalcemia **Serious**—hemorrhage secondary to systemic anticoagulants; cardiovascular events due to fluid shifting; risk of transmitting infection when using replacement fluids containing plasma; allergic reactions leading to anaphylaxis; activation of coagulation, complement, and fibrinolytic cascades, or aggregation of platelets leading to intravascular coagulation, or both; problems with vascular access, including infection and sepsis

GI = gastrointestinal; HCl = hydrochloride; PO = by mouth (orally).
[a]Not labeled by the Food and Drug Administration for use in myasthenia gravis.

In addition, patients with immunoglobulin A deficiency can develop anaphylaxis. In most patients, however, IVIG is well tolerated.

There has been debate as to whether plasma exchange or IVIG is the preferred short-term immunotherapy for myasthenia gravis. In practice, the choice of therapy for acute disease is often dependent on feasibility and on resources available in a given situation.

C. Treatment of Myasthenic Crisis

Myasthenic crisis is defined as an exacerbation of weakness that leads to respiratory failure requiring mechanical ventilation. For patients with myasthenic exacerbation involving respiratory and bulbar symptoms, hospitalization should be considered to closely monitor clinical status and pulmonary function. Once a patient is intubated, anticholinesterase medications should be discontinued because they can promote excessive secretions. Corticosteroids can actually prolong the duration of a crisis by exacerbating weakness or predisposing to infection. The mainstay of therapy for myasthenic crisis is therefore short-term immunotherapy, either plasmapheresis or IVIG.

D. Drugs That May Worsen Symptoms of Myasthenia Gravis

Several classes of drugs are associated with clinical worsening of existing MG, and a smaller group of drugs actually causes MG in occasional patients.

D-Penicillamine, interferon alpha, and bone marrow transplantation have all been implicated in causing MG. The mechanism is unclear, but there is evidence of an autoimmune basis for both penicillamine and interferon alpha. In most cases, the symptoms resolve with discontinuation of the medication.

Many other drugs are associated with myasthenic worsening (Table 22–4). Because any drug can potentially worsen symptoms, patients with MG should be warned about possible exacerbation with the use of prescription and over-the-counter medications.

▶ Prognosis

Eighty percent of patients with more focal disease eventually develop generalized MG. Progression to maximum severity typically occurs within the first 2 years of onset. Spontaneous, long-lasting remissions are uncommon, but have been reported in 10–20% of patients. For patients with disease limited to the ocular muscles, cholinesterase inhibitors, low-dose corticosteroids, or nonmedicinal therapy (eg, eyelid crutches) may be sufficient to control symptoms.

Most patients with generalized MG enjoy a normal and productive life when adequately treated. However, quality of life may be compromised as a result of both the limited efficacy and the side effects of available drugs. Patients with an underlying thymoma often have a more aggressive disease course.

Ciafaloni E, Massey JM. Myasthenia gravis and pregnancy. *Neurol Clin* 2004;22:771–782. [PMID 15474766]

Ciafaloni E, Nikhar NK, Massey JM, Sanders DB. Retrospective analysis of the use of cyclosporine in myasthenia gravis. *Neurology* 2000;55:448–450. [PMID 10932288] (An analysis of patients who took cyclosporine for an average of 3.5 years; clinical improvement was seen in 96%, with a median time to the best clinical response of 7 months, and corticosteroids were discontinued or decreased in 95% of patients taking them.)

Cole RN, Reddel SW, Gervasio OL, Phillips WD. Anti-MuSK patient antibodies disrupt the mouse neuromuscular junction. *Ann Neurol* 2008;57:782–789. [PMID 18384168] (Experimental design exploring the pathophysiologic mechanism of anti-MuSK antibodies in MG.)

De Baets M, Stassen MH. The role of antibodies in myasthenia gravis. *J Neurol Sci* 2002;202:5–11. [PMID 12220686] (Reviews the different types of autoantibodies present in patients with MG.)

Djelmis J, Sostarko M, Mayer D, Ivanisevic M. Myasthenia gravis in pregnancy: Report on 69 cases. *Eur J Obstet Gynecol Reprod Biol* 2002;104:21–25. [PMID 12128277] (This review of 69 pregnancies among 65 women with MG, in which 15% of patients showed worsening of disease in pregnancy and a further 16% in the puerperium, emphasizes that MG patients can have normal pregnancy and delivery, but the course is unpredictable.)

Drachman DB, Adams RN, Josifek LF, Self SG. Functional activities of autoantibodies to acetylcholine receptors and the clinical severity of myasthenia gravis. *N Engl J Med* 1982;207:769–775. [PMID 7110241] (A study measuring the ability of serum immunoglobulin from 49 myasthenia gravis patients to induce accelerated degeneration or blockade of the binding sites of acetylcholine receptors. This study also correlated the rate of receptor degradation with patients' clinical status.)

Evoli A, et al. Thymoma in patients with MG: Characteristics and long-term outcome. *Neurology* 2002;59:1844–1850. [PMID 12503581] (A retrospective study of 207 myasthenic patients who were operated on for thymoma, with at least 1-year follow-up from surgery; MG-associated thymoma was invasive in the majority of patients, MG was generally severe, and most patients remained dependent on immunosuppressive therapy.)

Table 22–4. Medications That Can Exacerbate Myasthenia Gravis

Antibiotics (many), most notably the aminoglycosides
β-Blockers
Calcium channel blockers
Chloroquine
D-Penicillamine
Iodinated contrast
Lithium
Nondepolarizing and depolarizing neuromuscular-blocking agents
Phenothiazines
Procainamide
Quinidine
Quinine

Gilchrist JM, Sachs GM. Electrodiagnostic studies in the management and prognosis of neuromuscular disorders. *Muscle Nerve* 2004;29:165–190. [PMID 14755481] (Reviews electrophysiologic techniques for the prognosis and management of disorders of neuromuscular transmission.)

Grob D, Brunner N, Namba T, Pagala M. Lifetime course of myasthenia gravis. *Muscle Nerve* 2008;37:141–149. [PMID 18059039] (A review of 1976 patients with myasthenia gravis between 1940 and 2000, describing the clinical course and the influence of age, gender, thymectomy, thymomectomy, and serum antibodies to the acetylcholine receptor.)

Gronseth GS, Barohn RJ. Practice parameter: Thymectomy for autoimmune myasthenia gravis (an evidence-based review): Report of the Quality Standards Subcommittee of the American Academy of Neurology. *Neurology* 2000;55:7–15. [PMID 10891896] (An evidence-based review of thymectomy for autoimmune MG.)

Kirmani JF, Yahia AM, Qureshi AI. Myasthenic crisis. *Curr Treat Options Neurol* 2004;26:3–15. [PMID: 14664765] (Reviews myasthenic crisis, a life-threatening complication that occurs in approximately 15–20% of patients with MG.)

Marx A, Muller-Hermelink HK, Strobel P. The role of thymomas in the development of myasthenia gravis. *Ann N Y Acad Sci* 2003;998:223–236. [PMID 14592880] (Reviews thymic pathology, which occurs in 80–90% of patients with MG.)

Meriggioli MN, et al. Mycophenolate mofetil for myasthenia gravis: An analysis of efficacy, safety, and tolerability. *Neurology* 2003;61:1438–1440. [PMID 14638974] (In this study of 85 patients taking mycophenolate mofetil, improvement was seen in 73% of subjects; side effects were observed in 27% but were sufficient to require discontinuation of the drug in only 6%.)

Oskoui M, et al. Fetal acetylcholine receptor inactivation syndrome and maternal myasthenia gravis. *Neurology* 2008;71: 2010–2012. [PMID: 19064884] (A case report of three brothers with permanent weakness and other deficits following in utero exposure to high levels of maternal antibodies against the fetal AChR subunit.)

Palace J, Vincent A, Beeson D. Myasthenia gravis: Diagnostic and management dilemmas. *Curr Opin Neurol* 2001;14:583–589. [PMID 11562569] (Reviews diagnostic tests that may help to confirm MG in patients without AChR antibodies and management dilemmas.)

Pascuzzi RM. Pearls and pitfalls in the diagnosis and management of neuromuscular junction disorders. *Semin Neurol* 2001;21:425–440. [PMID 11774058] (Clinical features and treatment issues in MG and other disorders of neuromuscular transmission.)

Pascuzzi RM. The edrophonium test. *Semin Neurol* 2003;23:83–88. [PMID 12870109] (Sensitivity and specificity of the test with respect to the diagnosis of MG.)

Richman DP, Agius MA. Treatment of autoimmune myasthenia gravis. *Neurology* 2003;61:1652–1661. [PMID 14694025]

Sanders DB, et al. An international, phase III, randomized trial of mycophenolate mofetil in myasthenia gravis. *Neurology* 2008; 71:400–406. [PMID 18434638] (A prospective, double-blind, placebo-controlled, phase III trial assessing the efficacy, safety, and tolerability of mycophenolate mofetil as treatment in patients with myasthenia gravis. Treatment with the medication was not superior to placebo in maintaining myasthenia control over a 36-week period.)

Sanders DB, et al. A trial of mycophenolate mofetil with prednisone as initial immunotherapy in myasthenia gravis. *Neurology* 2008;71:394–399. [PMID 18434639] (A randomized, double-blind trial comparing the treatment of myasthenia gravis with mycophenolate mofetil plus 20 mg prednisone, versus 20 mg prednisone alone. No benefit was demonstrated of the combination therapy over prednisone alone at the end of 12 weeks. The negative result of this study may be related to a greater than predicted benefit of the prednisone dose used, short study duration, or the absence of any benefit of mycophenolate mofetil in this population of myasthenia gravis patients.)

Sanders DB, El-Salem K, Massey JM, McConville J, Vincent A. Clinical aspects of MuSK antibody positive seronegative MG. *Neurology* 2003;60:1978–1980. [PMID 12821744] (Clinical characteristics of 12 patients with serum antibodies to muscle-specific receptor tyrosine kinase; all were women, with symptom onset between ages 21 and 59 years. Seven had prominent neck, shoulder, or respiratory muscle weakness and little or delayed ocular muscle involvement. The response to cholinesterase inhibitors was variable, and electromyographic findings suggested myopathy in several. None improved after thymectomy. All patients improved after plasma exchange, and most had a good response to selected immunotherapy.)

Vincent A, et al. Antibodies in myasthenia gravis and related disorders. *Ann N Y Acad Sci* 2003;998:324–335. [PMID 14592891]

Vincent A, McConville J, Faruggia ME, Newsom-Davis J. Seronegative myasthenia gravis. *Semin Neurol* 2004;24:125–133. [PMID 15229799]

CONGENITAL MYASTHENIA SYNDROMES

There are multiple congenital myasthenic syndromes, which are the result of genetic defects in presynaptic, synaptic, and postsynaptic proteins. Symptoms are present at birth or appear in early childhood. Weakness typically affects cranial muscles, and there is often an associated high-arched palate. Similarly affected relatives can often be identified. Cholinesterase inhibitors are helpful in the treatment of some of these syndromes only.

Engel AG, Ohno K, Since SM. Congenital myasthenic syndromes: Progress over the past decade. *Muscle Nerve* 2003;27:4–25. [PMID 12508290]

LAMBERT-EATON MYASTHENIC SYNDROME

ESSENTIALS OF DIAGNOSIS

▶ Weakness of proximal limb muscles, which may improve with exercise
▶ Autonomic dysfunction (may be severe)
▶ Strong association with small cell lung cancer

▶ General Considerations

Lambert-Eaton myasthenic syndrome (LEMS) is an autoimmune or paraneoplastic disease caused by a presynaptic abnormality of acetylcholine release. It is characterized by chronic fluctuating weakness of the proximal limb muscles, especially the legs. Approximately 60% of patients with LEMS have an associated small cell carcinoma of the lung or, less often, another type of malignancy. The diagnosis of LEMS often precedes clinical detection of the malignancy. In those who do not have an underlying malignancy, a concurrent autoimmune disease is common. The onset of the disease is often midlife or later, but it has also been reported in childhood. Younger patients are more likely to have underlying autoimmune disease as opposed to malignancy.

LEMS is caused by antibodies directed at P/Q-type voltage-gated calcium channels (VGCCs) and reduced neurotransmitter release at the neuromuscular junction and autonomic nerve terminals. LEMS in association with neoplasm is discussed further in Chapter 13.

▶ Clinical Findings

A. Symptoms and Signs

The onset of symptoms is usually insidious. Generalized fatigable weakness is the major symptom. Patients often complain of myalgia, muscle tenderness, and stiffness. There may be improvement in strength with exercise. Oculobulbar and respiratory symptoms are much less common than with MG, but patients with LEMS can present with respiratory compromise. Unlike patients with MG, those with LEMS may complain of a metallic taste, and often have autonomic dysfunction causing dry mouth, orthostasis, constipation, and impotence. On examination, the elicited weakness is often mild compared with the patient's complaints. Deep tendon reflexes are often hypoactive or absent but may be potentiated by brief contraction. Pupils may be dilated and weakly responsive to light secondary to autonomic dysfunction.

B. Laboratory and Electrodiagnostic Findings

Antibodies against P/Q-type VGCCs can be detected in over 90% of patients with LEMS. In addition, antibodies to N-type VGCCs can be found in up to 50% of patients; this percentage is higher in malignancy-associated LEMS.

Organ-specific autoantibodies (to thyroid, gastric parietal cells, or skeletal muscle) and non–organ-specific autoantibodies (antinuclear, antimitochondrial) are also found in patients with LEMS.

Electrodiagnostic studies help confirm the diagnosis and monitor disease progression. The compound muscle action potential (CMAP) is low in most muscles tested, and CMAP amplitude at rest is the best marker of disease severity. As in MG, most patients have a decrementing response to slow rates of repetitive stimulation. Following exercise or repetitive stimulation at 20–50 Hz, there is usually a marked facilitation, with doubling of the CMAP amplitude (see Figure 2–5). Of note, electrodiagnostic study findings in LEMS differ markedly from MG, and are useful in distinguishing these neuromuscular junction disorders.

Conventional needle electromyography demonstrates unstable motor unit action potentials that change configuration from impulse to impulse due to blocking of individual muscle fibers. When many muscle fibers are blocked, the motor units can be small, polyphasic, and of short duration. As with MG, increased jitter and impulse blocking are seen on single-fiber electromyography.

▶ Differential Diagnosis

The main alternative diagnosis to consider is MG. LEMS can often be distinguished from MG by its mild oculobulbar symptoms and often prominent autonomic symptoms and signs. In addition, electrodiagnostic abnormalities are often more prominent in LEMS than in MG despite the often more severe weakness in MG. LEMS is often misdiagnosed as a myopathy because of the predominantly proximal weakness.

▶ Treatment

The first step in management should be an evaluation for malignancy, especially in older patients or those with a history of smoking. If LEMS is associated with a malignancy, symptoms often improve dramatically with tumor removal.

If no malignancy is found at initial presentation, patients should undergo regular surveillance, because the presentation of LEMS can predate the detection of neoplasm by years. For those with no underlying neoplasm, or insufficient symptom control with tumor removal, pharmacotherapy is employed.

3,4-Diaminopyridine (3,4-DAP) improves muscle strength and autonomic symptoms in approximately 80% of patients with LEMS. By blocking voltage-gated potassium channels, the drug prolongs action potentials at motor nerve terminals. Perioral paresthesias are the most common side effect, but seizures can occur at high doses. 3,4-DAP is not approved by the Food and Drug Administration (FDA) in the United States but can be obtained for compassionate use.

Guanidine hydrochloride inhibits mitochondrial calcium uptake, facilitating the release of acetylcholine at the motor nerve terminal. Guanidine effectively increases strength in patients with LEMS, but its use is limited by side effects that include bone marrow suppression.

Unlike MG, LEMS is not very responsive to anticholinesterase drugs, which, however, do potentiate the effects of 3,4-DAP and guanidine, allowing the use of lower doses.

If the preceding symptomatic therapy is insufficient, immunosuppressive therapy can be attempted, but it is less effective in LEMS than in MG. If weakness is severe, plasmapheresis or high-dose IVIG often provides rapid, although usually transitory, improvement.

▶ Prognosis

Prognosis in patients with underlying malignancy is determined by the prognosis of that malignancy. Because LEMS is less responsive to immunosuppressive therapy than MG, most patients with LEMS have residual weakness even with optimal immunosuppression.

Sanders DB. Lambert-Eaton myasthenic syndrome: Diagnosis and treatment. *Ann N Y Acad Sci* 2003;998:500–508. [PMID 14592920] (A comprehensive review of pathophysiology, clinical features, and treatment.)

Sanders DB, Massey JM, Sanders LL, Edwards LJ. A randomized trial of 3,4-diaminopyridine in Lambert-Eaton myasthenic syndrome. *Neurology* 2000;54:603–607. [PMID 10680790] (Report of a study showing that 3,4-DAP is an effective and safe treatment for LEMS.)

Tim RW, Massey JM, Sanders DB. Lambert-Eaton myasthenic syndrome: Electrodiagnostic findings and response to treatment. *Neurology* 2000;54:2176–2178. [PMID 10851390] (In this study of 73 patients [31 with lung cancer, 29 with small cell], treatment with 3,4-DAP produced moderate to marked self-reported functional improvement in 79% of the 53 treated patients.)

BOTULISM

ESSENTIALS OF DIAGNOSIS

- ▶ History of ingestion of home-canned foods or honey (in infants)
- ▶ Rapid onset of ocular symptoms (diplopia, ptosis, blurry vision) and bulbar symptoms (dysarthria and dysphagia)
- ▶ "Descending" pattern of weakness from oculobulbar to limb involvement
- ▶ Dilated pupils

▶ General Considerations

Botulism is caused by ingesting the neurotoxin of the bacterium *Clostridium botulinum,* an obligate anaerobic, robust, spore-forming bacillus commonly found in soil. After absorption into the bloodstream, botulinum toxin binds irreversibly to the presynaptic nerve endings of the peripheral nervous system and cranial nerves. Once internalized, the toxin inhibits the release of acetylcholine through the cleavage of polypeptides essential for the docking of synaptic vesicles to the presynaptic membrane of the nerve terminal.

Food-borne botulism is caused by the ingestion of preformed toxin. The most frequent source is home-canned or home-processed low-acid foods. In the infant form of botulism, *C botulinum* spores enter and colonize the immature gastrointestinal tract and produce toxin. This is most often associated with the ingestion of honey. In wound botulism, the toxin is produced from *C botulinum* infection of a wound. Recently a number of cases of wound botulism in

intravenous drug users have been traced to contaminated drugs, suggesting a particular risk of botulism in this demographic. Inadvertent botulism has also been reported in patients treated with intramuscular injections of botulinum toxin.

▶ Clinical Findings

A. Symptoms and Signs

The initial symptoms of food-borne botulism (but not the wound-acquired form) may be gastrointestinal—nausea, vomiting, and diarrhea—and generally appear within 2–36 hours of ingestion. Constipation is more common once neurologic symptoms are present. The earliest neurologic symptoms are oculobulbar and include dry mouth, blurred vision, diplopia, dysarthria, dysphagia, and dysphonia. In contrast to most cases of Guillain-Barré syndrome, botulism is characterized by a descending paralysis. Weakness begins in the cranial nerves, followed by the upper extremities, respiratory muscles, and finally lower extremities. The weakness progresses from proximal to distal muscles. Respiratory weakness can be severe and require prolonged intubation. Botulism also affects autonomic synaptic transmission, resulting in constipation, postural hypotension, and urinary retention. On examination, pupils are unreactive and tendon reflexes are absent.

Most infantile cases occur before the age of 6 months, and the first signs may be constipation, weak cry, and poor feeding. Weakness then progresses over days, causing poor suck and head control, hypotonia, and deceased movement. Autonomic signs and symptoms include hypotension, tachycardia, and dry mouth.

The symptoms of wound botulism are similar to those of food-borne botulism except that gastrointestinal manifestations are usually absent, the incubation period is longer, and symptoms are gradual in onset.

B. Laboratory and Electrodiagnostic Findings

Both blood and stool can be sent for detection of the botulinum toxin. *C botulinum* itself can be detected in stool. If possible, a food sample should also be sent for identification of the toxin.

Electrodiagnostic studies can support the diagnosis of botulism and help rule out other possible diagnoses such as Guillain-Barré syndrome. The most consistent finding is a small CMAP in response to a supramaximal stimulus. As with LEMS, repetitive stimulation testing may show a decrement of the CMAP to low rates of stimulation and postexercise facilitation of the CMAP amplitude.

▶ Differential Diagnosis

Botulism must be distinguished from MG, LEMS, Guillain-Barré syndrome (particularly the Miller Fisher variant), tick paralysis, diphtheritic neuropathy, and intoxication (including paralytic shellfish poisoning and organophosphates).

▶ Treatment

The major treatment is intensive supportive care. Patients should be closely monitored for respiratory decompensation. If the ingestion is recent, removal of unabsorbed gut toxin can be considered. The Centers for Disease Control and Prevention can provide a trivalent botulinum antitoxin, which, however, must be given early while toxin is still in the blood. The antitoxin can decrease the severity of disease and overall mortality, but side effects include anaphylaxis. Human botulism immune globulin is an FDA-approved treatment of infant botulism, which was shown in a randomized clinical trial to reduce length of hospital stay in treated infants. This intravenous treatment neutralizes all circulating botulinum toxin and remains present in neutralizing amounts for several months.

▶ Prognosis

Although significantly reduced, mortality from botulism remains high at 5–10%. Type A toxin is associated with a more severe course and higher mortality than other toxins. Clinical recovery is often prolonged over months, because it requires the formation of new presynaptic end plates and neuromuscular junctions. Recovery of autonomic function may take longer than recovery of muscle strength. For those who survive, the recovery is generally complete.

Cherington M. Botulism: Update and review. *Semin Neurol* 2004;24:155–163. [PMID 15257512] (Review of botulism as both an old and an emerging disease; five clinical forms of botulism—food borne, wound, infant, hidden, and inadvertent—as well as the actions of botulinum toxins, electrodiagnostic methods, treatments, and possible future directions are discussed.)

Domingo RM, Haller JS, Gruenthal M. Infant botulism: Two recent cases and literature review. *J Child Neurol* 2008;23:1336–1346. [PMID 18984848] (This paper begins by providing a description of two cases of infant botulism in upstate New York, followed by a review of literature on infant botulism in the United States, including pathophysiology, clinical features, epidemiology, and treatment.)

Schroeter M, Alpers K, Van Treeck U, Frank C, Rosenkoetter N, Schaumann R. Outbreak of wound botulism in injecting drug users. *Epidemiol Infect* 2009;137:1602–1608. [PMID 19351433] (A description of 16 cases of wound botulism reported in North Rhine-Westphalia, Germany, between October and December of 2005. All patients were using intravenous drugs, and investigations indicated that contaminated drugs were the most probable source of infection.)

TICK PARALYSIS

Tick paralysis is a rare disease that usually affects children, with a higher prevalence among young girls, although older men exposed to ticks may also be affected. This disease has been associated with 43 different tick species globally. Most reported cases have been from Australia and North America, in particular the Rocky Mountain states, the Pacific Northwest, and the Southeast. In Australia the *Ixodes* species dominates, especially *I holocyclus* and *I cornuatus*. In North America members of the *Dermacentor* species, *D andersoni* and *D variabilis*, are most commonly involved.

Often a prodrome of gait instability is followed by ascending paralysis and hyporeflexia or areflexia. Bulbar structures are eventually affected, leading to dysphagia, dysarthria, facial paralysis, and ocular weakness. If the tick is not removed, fatal respiratory failure can develop. The engorged tick attached to the patient produces a neurotoxin that acts on the neuromuscular junction. Removal of the tick is usually followed by rapid improvement. This disease is most often confused with Guillain-Barré syndrome.

Felz MW, Smith CD, Swift TR. A six-year-old girl with tick paralysis. *N Engl J Med* 2000;342:90–94. [PMID 10631277]

Greenstein P. Tick paralysis. *Med Clin North Am* 2002;86:441–446. [PMID 11982312]

Vedanarayanan V, Sorey WH, Subramony SH. Tick paralysis. *Semin Neurol* 2004;24:181–184. [PMID 15257515] (Reviews the pathophysiology, clinical presentation, electrophysiology, and treatment of tick paralysis.)

Diseases of Muscle

23

Olajide Williams, MD

MYOPATHY

ESSENTIALS OF DIAGNOSIS

► Weakness greater proximally than distally (myopathic distribution)
► Normal sensation
► Normal sphincter function
► Relative preservation of deep tendon reflexes
► Muscle biopsy often definitive
► Genetic testing can confirm diagnosis of hereditary disorders caused by specific mutations

► General Considerations

Disorders in which there is a primary structural or functional impairment of muscle (myopathy) can result from a variety of inherited and acquired disorders (Table 23–1); however, patterns of weakness remain similar despite the broad spectrum of etiologies. These patterns, the age of onset (including motor milestones), and the evolution of muscle weakness assist in narrowing down the differential diagnosis of muscle disorders. In general, proximal greater than distal muscle weakness leads to difficulty arising from a chair or commode, climbing stairs, reaching up for objects, or combing one's hair. Specific patterns of proximal weakness may be seen in certain disorders discussed later in this chapter, and facial, extraocular, bulbar, cardiac, and respiratory muscles may sometimes be involved. Detailed family history, broad systemic review, and careful drug history are mandatory. Understanding of this complex group of diseases has been greatly enhanced by significant advances in molecular genetics and immunology.

► Clinical Findings

A. Symptoms and Signs

Muscle weakness and fatigability are the most frequent symptoms, and although fatigability is a common complaint in those with muscle diseases, excessive fatigability out of proportion to the degree of weakness should raise suspicion of a neuromuscular junction disorder. Muscle pain, stiffness, spasms, or cramps may occur with varying severity, depending on the nature of injury. Patients should be asked about the color of their urine, which, when dark red, suggests myoglobinuria. Double vision, difficulty swallowing, and shortness of breath may be present. Distribution of weakness may vary among diseases, with some muscles affected more than others. Typical patterns are outlined in Table 23–2.

Muscle tone is usually reduced and in infants may result in a "floppy infant." In exceptional cases such as those characterized by continuous overactivity of motor units, or dystrophies with early onset of contractures, muscle stiffness is seen. Myotonia is present in specific muscular dystrophies and ion channel disorders (channelopathies). Muscle atrophy is common, but in certain disorders there is pseudohypertrophy (especially of the calf muscles) from connective tissue and fat replacement. In severely weak muscles, tendon reflexes may be diminished or absent. Muscle tenderness may be prominent or absent. Systemic signs and symptoms of endocrine disorders such as thyroid disease may be evident, and a skin rash may offer diagnostic clues. In some congenital myopathies, dysmorphic features and skeletal abnormalities are present.

B. Laboratory Findings

Routine and advanced tests used in the evaluation of patients with suspected myositis are detailed in Table 23–3. Muscle enzymes such as creatine kinase (CK) may be markedly elevated, mildly elevated, or normal. CK is released from the sarcoplasmic reticulum into the serum after muscle injury. When the serum myoglobin level exceeds its renal threshold,

Table 23–1. Classification of Myopathies

Hereditary
Congenital myopathies
Muscular dystrophies
Myotonias and channelopathies
Primary metabolic myopathies
Mitochondrial myopathies

Acquired
Inflammatory myopathies
Drug-induced and toxic myopathies
Secondary metabolic myopathies
Endocrine myopathies
Infectious myopathies

the result is myoglobinuria, producing dark urine and a positive Hematest in the absence of red cells. Thyroid function tests should be performed; myositis-specific autoantibodies such as the anti–Jo-1 antibody may be found in inflammatory myopathies.

Elevated alanine aminotransferase, aspartate aminotransferase, and lactate dehydrogenase levels may occur in patients

Table 23–2. Patterns of Muscle Weakness in Myopathies

Pattern	Associated Myopathy
Neck extensor weakness (dropped head)	Polymyositis, inclusion body myositis (IBM), mitochondrial myopathies, nemaline-rod myopathy, metabolic myopathies, certain muscular dystrophies
Early involvement of respiratory muscles	Acid maltase deficiency, severe polymyositis
Predominant weakness of ocular and pharyngeal musculature	Oculopharyngeal dystrophy, mitochondrial myopathy
Limb-girdle weakness	Most common presentation of myopathies and nonspecific—includes inflammatory, drug-induced or toxic, and hereditary forms
Predominant distal weakness	IBM, myotonic dystrophy, Miyoshi and Nonaka distal myopathies
Distal forearm and proximal leg weakness	IBM
Bifacial, shoulder-girdle, and proximal arm weakness	Fascioscapulohumeral dystrophy
Shoulder-girdle and distal leg weakness	Scapuloperoneal form of fascioscapulohumeral dystrophy
Generalized weakness	Periodic paralysis, and end stage of most myopathies

Table 23–3. Laboratory and Diagnostic Studies Used in Evaluation of Myopathy

Routine Tests	Advanced Tests[a]
Creatine kinase level	HIV screening
Urinalysis and urine myoglobin	Angiotensin-converting enzyme level
Liver function tests	Arterial blood gas measurement
Thyroid function tests	Arterial lactate level
Routine chemistry panel (including calcium, phosphorus, magnesium)	Myositis-specific antibody testing
	Chest radiography
Erythrocyte sedimentation rate	Pulmonary function tests
Electrocardiography	Transthoracic echocardiography
Electromyography	Holter monitoring
	Genetic testing
	Muscle biopsy
	Muscle imaging techniques

[a]Depends on clinical profile.

with muscle diseases; a normal γ-glutamyl transpeptidase in this situation makes liver pathology an unlikely culprit. Serum creatinine and electrolytes should be measured, because chronic renal failure and hypokalemia are associated with muscle weakness. Parathyroid hormone levels should be obtained in patients with hypercalcemia. Erythrocyte sedimentation rate is useful when an overlap syndrome is suspected, or in the diagnosis of polymyalgia rheumatica. Elevated serum angiotensin-converting enzyme levels suggest sarcoidosis, and testing for HIV may be warranted.

Arterial blood gas measurement may reveal high carbon dioxide levels in patients with shortness of breath caused by respiratory muscle involvement, and pulmonary function tests may support this finding. Elevated arterial lactate levels can occur in mitochondrial disorders. Molecular genetic testing for specific mutations may be clinically indicated. In patients with myopathies that involve cardiac muscle, electrocardiography, echocardiography, and Holter monitoring should be performed when clinically indicated.

C. Imaging Studies

For routine purposes imaging studies are rarely indicated. In specific situations (eg, muscle infarction), or to help localize the optimal biopsy site, imaging techniques may be useful. Radionuclide scanning using technetium-labeled phosphates, indium-labeled antibodies, and gallium 67 citrate may assess the extent and severity of muscle involvement in inflammatory myopathies and may assist in biopsy site determination. Ultrasound is rapid and may assist in optimizing the biopsy site, especially in younger children. Magnetic resonance imaging (MRI) is useful in evaluating myopathies that cause muscle edema and can be used to assess the response to therapy in inflammatory myopathies.

D. Special Tests

Electromyography (EMG) and nerve conduction studies (NCSs) may confirm the presence of a muscle disorder and exclude defects in neuromuscular transmission, neuropathy, or anterior horn cell disease. For the evaluation of myopathy, quantitative EMG should be performed. Classic EMG findings include short-duration, small-amplitude motor unit potentials with early recruitment (so-called myopathic features). Spontaneous activity (positive sharp waves, fibrillations) may be present in varying amounts, depending on the etiology.

Muscle biopsy is limited by sampling error but remains the gold standard for establishing the diagnosis of a muscle disease (Figure 23–1). A muscle that is not too severely affected by the disease process is usually selected. Open biopsy is generally performed, but needle biopsy is occasionally preferred in children. The biopsy may include fascia or skin in specific cases. Biopsy of muscles sampled by needle EMG should be delayed by at least 1 month.

▶ Treatment

Treatment of muscle disorders usually involves a multidisciplinary team approach that includes neurologists, physiatrists, cardiologists, pulmonologists, geneticists, rheumatologists, and orthopedists. Pharmacotherapy is disease specific; refer to the discussion of individual disorders that follows.

▼ ACQUIRED MYOPATHIES

INFLAMMATORY MYOPATHIES

The incidence of these disorders is approximately 1 in 100,000 people. Inflammatory infiltrates are typically found at muscle biopsy. Inflammatory myopathies can be idiopathic,

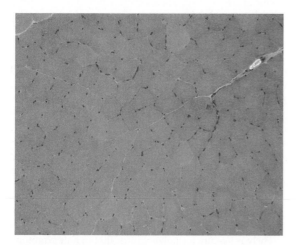

▲ Figure 23–1. Hematoxylin and eosin (H&E) stain of a biopsy specimen showing normal muscle fibers. (Used with permission from Arthur Hayes, MD, Columbia University.)

although evidence of a systemic connective tissue disorder is often found. They may also be associated with malignancy. Dermatomyositis affects both children and adults and females more than males. Polymyositis, on the other hand, is rare in childhood. Inclusion body myositis (IBM) usually presents after age 50 and affects men much more often than women and whites slightly more often than blacks. Different pathogenic mechanisms underlie these disorders: dermatomyositis results from a humoral process directed against intramuscular vasculature with complement-mediated tissue destruction. In polymyositis, no evidence of microangiopathy and muscle ischemia is seen, and T cells mediate an antigen-directed cytotoxicity. Myositis-specific antibodies are found in the serum of a few patients with polymyositis and dermatomyositis, but not IBM, and their presence effectively rules out the latter disorder.

1. Polymyositis

ESSENTIALS OF DIAGNOSIS

- ▶ Onset after age 30
- ▶ Myopathic distribution of weakness
- ▶ Prominent muscle pain and tenderness (one third of patients)
- ▶ Spontaneous activity on needle EMG
- ▶ Markedly elevated serum CK level
- ▶ Muscle biopsy evidence of endomysial infiltration of muscle by inflammatory cells provides definitive diagnosis

▶ General Considerations

Polymyositis may occur alone but is frequently associated with systemic autoimmune diseases (eg, primary biliary sclerosis, Crohn disease, celiac disease, Behçet disease, graft-versus-host disease, vasculitis, sarcoidosis, Hashimoto thyroiditis, psoriasis, and myasthenia gravis). It may be the first clinical sign of HIV infection. Other infectious causes, myotoxic drugs and toxins, endocrinopathies, and biochemical or hereditary muscle diseases need to be excluded. T cells are thought to govern the series of inflammatory events in polymyositis, unlike B cells, which are implicated in dermatomyositis.

▶ Clinical Findings

A. Symptoms and Signs

In polymyositis, a progressive limb-girdle pattern of symmetric weakness develops usually over weeks to months (rarely days). In some cases, weakness is preceded by an upper respiratory infection. Additional symptoms and signs occur when polymyositis is associated with systemic autoimmune diseases.

Shortness of breath may be the consequence of cardiac or pulmonary muscle involvement or interstitial lung disease (10% of patients). Patients with the antisynthetase syndrome, which is associated with antibodies to aminoacyl-tRNA synthetases (the most common of which is the myositis-specific antibody, anti-Jo-1 antibody), a group of intracytoplasmic enzymes that play a key role in protein synthesis, present with fevers, interstitial lung disease, Raynaud phenomenon, mechanic hand (hyperkeratosis and cracking of the skin over the palms and fingers), arthralgias, and pulmonary involvement; this syndrome may not be recognized initially as a manifestation of polymyositis or dermatomyositis. Cardiac involvement occurs in up to 40% of patients with polymyositis, causing conduction defects, tachyarrhythmias, dilated cardiomyopathy, congestive heart failure, and myocarditis. Dysphagia is a result of weakness of the oropharynx and distal esophagus. Facial muscle involvement is not rare. Palpation of involved muscles may reveal tenderness, especially early on in the disease. Myalgia may be a prominent symptom, although it is important to note that myalgia without weakness is not myositis. Weight loss, fatigue, and generalized malaise are common. The skin must be carefully examined for the presence of a rash, which may suggest dermatomyositis.

B. Laboratory Findings

The serum CK level may be normal even in patients with active disease, but is usually 50 times greater than the upper limit of normal. Levels of other muscle enzymes (eg, aldolase, aminotransferases, and lactate dehydrogenase) may also be elevated. When the CK level is high, it may be used to assess disease activity and response to treatment. Among the subset of patients with interstitial lung disease, half may have anti-Jo-1 antibodies. The presence of antinuclear antibodies (positive ANA titers in the blood) suggests associated systemic autoimmune disease.

C. Special Tests

A myopathic EMG with profuse spontaneous activity is usually seen. Nerve conduction studies show normal sensory nerve action potentials and low-amplitude motor responses when recording from weak muscles.

Echocardiography and radionucleotide scintigraphy may reveal wall motion abnormalities and a reduced ejection fraction. Patients with interstitial lung disease may have diffuse reticulonodular infiltrates or a "ground-glass" pattern on chest radiography.

Muscle biopsy is definitive and shows endomysial inflammatory infiltrates (Figure 23–2), necrosis of muscle fibers, and scattered atrophy and regeneration of muscle fibers.

▶ Treatment

Prednisone given initially in high doses intravenously, or orally depending on clinical severity, is the first-line treatment for

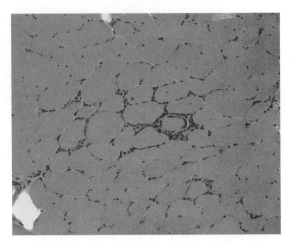

▲ **Figure 23–2.** H&E stain of a biopsy specimen from a patient with polymyositis, showing inflammatory infiltration in endomysial connective tissue around muscle fibers. (Used with permission from Arthur Hayes, MD, Columbia University.)

polymyositis. A maintenance dose of 1 mg/kg/day (not to exceed 100 mg/day) should be administered for at least 3 months. If a good response is seen (ie, objective increase in muscle strength, with or without declining CK levels), the dose should be tapered slowly and maintained at the lowest possible effective dose. If the clinical response is poor, the patient may be switched to azathioprine, 2–3 mg/kg/day divided two or three times a day, beginning with an initial dose of 50 mg/day and slowly titrating upward. Alternately, methotrexate can be given at a dose of 0.5–0.8 mg/kg/week intramuscularly or 15–25 mg/week orally. Mycophenolate mofetil, 1 g twice a day orally, can also be used. These agents may also be substituted for corticosteroids when steroid resistance is present or side effects preclude their continued use. Anti–Jo-1 antibody testing is advised in patients prior to methotrexate treatment, because this agent can cause pulmonary fibrosis. High-dose intravenous gamma globulin, 2 g/kg, may also be used in pulses. It is often preferred in immunodeficient patients or those in whom immunosuppression and corticosteroids are contraindicated. Cyclophosphamide, 1–2 mg/kg/day orally, is used in refractory cases. The results of plasma exchange have been disappointing. The duration of therapy for polymyositis with the above drugs is indefinite (usually 1–2 years), and stopping too soon frequently causes relapses. The possibility of a corticosteroid myopathy (discussed later) should always be kept in mind. Patients should also receive rehabilitation therapy to maximize their functional ability. Severe disease often requires multidisciplinary care.

There is no cure for polymyositis, although its symptoms can often be effectively treated with the above regimens. Clinical course may be one of remissions and relapses, but some patients may not respond adequately to treatment and develop significant disability. Rarely, in those with severe weakness, respiratory failure occurs from respiratory muscle involvement, and severe malnutrition follows involvement of swallowing muscles.

2. Dermatomyositis

ESSENTIALS OF DIAGNOSIS

▶ Onset in childhood or adulthood

▶ Myopathic distribution of weakness

▶ Characteristic skin lesions

▶ Prominent muscle pain and tenderness (one third of patients)

▶ Spontaneous activity on needle EMG

▶ Markedly elevated serum CK level

▶ Muscle biopsy evidence of perivascular and perimysial inflammatory infiltrates with perifascicular atrophy provides definitive diagnosis

▶ General Considerations

Dermatomyositis usually occurs alone but may be associated with systemic sclerosis, mixed connective tissue diseases (overlap syndrome), and malignancies (breast, lung, ovarian, gastric, Hodgkin lymphoma, colon) as a paraneoplastic manifestation. The increased incidence of malignancies occurs in the adult form of the disease. Fasciitis and skin changes similar to dermatomyositis can occur in eosinophilia-myalgia syndrome (a systemic syndrome characterized by high eosinophil white blood cell count and debilitating muscle pain that also affects the skin, fascia, peripheral nerves, blood vessels, heart, and lung) and in the syndrome of calciphylaxis seen in patients with end-stage renal disease, which can clinically mimic this disorder (see later discussion of chronic renal failure–related myopathies).

B cells are thought to govern the series of inflammatory events in dermatomyositis, unlike T cells, which are implicated in polymyositis.

▶ Clinical Findings

A. Symptoms and Signs

In general, the clinical manifestations of dermatomyositis are the same as those of polymyositis with the exception of the following characteristic skin lesions:

1. Heliotrope rash with eyelid edema and a facial rash

2. Gottron sign (erythema of knuckles accompanied by a raised violaceous scaly eruption)

3. Erythematous rash over the knees, elbows, malleoli, at the base of the neck and upper chest ("V" sign), or over upper back and shoulders (shawl sign) that worsens with sun exposure

4. Dilated capillary loops at the base of the fingernails

Mechanic-like hands are present in the antisynthetase syndrome (described under polymyositis), which can occur in dermatomyositis. In children, subcutaneous calcifications may extrude through the skin, causing ulceration and infection. Flexion contractures often occur in children with dermatomyositis, causing them to walk on their toes.

B. Laboratory Findings

Laboratory testing is the same as for polymyositis, and EMG findings are identical in the two disorders. Antibodies directed against the Mi-2 antigen are present almost exclusively in patients with dermatomyositis (although in only 15% of patients). Patients with this antibody usually have a "V" sign or "shawl" sign skin rash and are highly steroid sensitive. Muscle biopsy is definitive and shows perivascular or interfascicular inflammatory infiltrates, or both, with perifascicular atrophy (Figure 23–3). Deposition of C5b-9 complement membrane attack complex on small blood vessels precedes the appearance of inflammatory cells and structural changes in the muscles of patients with dermatomyositis.

▶ Treatment

Treatment and prognosis are generally similar to those of polymyositis, discussed earlier, although treatment with rituximab (2 infusions of 1 g each given 2 weeks apart), a chimeric

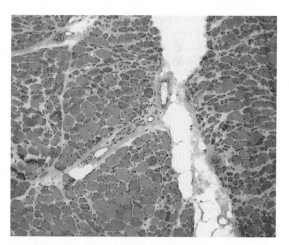

▲ **Figure 23–3.** H&E stain of a biopsy specimen from a patient with dermatomyositis, showing perivascular inflammatory infiltrates and perifascicular atrophy of myofibers; muscle fibers at the periphery of the muscle fascicles are smaller, whereas fibers located deeper are normal in size. (Used with permission from Arthur Hayes, MD, Columbia University.)

human/murine monoclonal antibody against CD-20 surface antigen expressed on B cells, has shown encouraging results in uncontrolled studies of dermatomyositis. However, the major differences in treatments when compared to polymyositis are related to skin involvement, which may require topical corticosteroids and practical steps such as high-protection sunscreen and protective clothing. In patients with cardiac or pulmonary involvement—markers of more severe disease—resistance to treatment and worse outcomes may occur.

3. Inclusion Body Myositis

ESSENTIALS OF DIAGNOSIS

▶ Onset usually after age 50

▶ Myopathic distribution of weakness

▶ Distal weakness (finger flexors and foot dorsiflexors) in approximately half of patients

▶ Weakness may be asymmetric with selective involvement (quadriceps, iliopsoas, triceps, biceps)

▶ Spontaneous activity on needle EMG

▶ Moderately elevated serum CK level

▶ General Considerations

IBM should be suspected in older patients with suspected polymyositis that is refractory to treatment, especially those with asymmetric or distal weakness. This disease may resemble amyotrophic lateral sclerosis, and 15% of cases are associated with systemic autoimmune disease. Some HIV-infected patients develop myopathy that clinically and histologically resembles IBM. A rare familial form exists that may be accompanied by leukoencephalopathy.

▶ Clinical Findings

A. Symptoms and Signs

The pattern and evolution of weakness help distinguish this disorder from polymyositis. IBM has an insidious, slowly progressive course that develops after age 50 and may lead to a delay in diagnosis by up to 6 years from onset. Characteristic patterns include:

1. Early distal weakness (wrist and finger flexors, foot dorsiflexors)

2. Early quadriceps weakness with early loss of patellar reflexes

3. Asymmetric weakness

Extraocular muscles are usually spared, but mild facial weakness and significant dysphagia can occur. Peripheral neuropathy is present in up to 30% of patients. Signs of systemic autoimmune disease occur in up to 15% of patients.

B. Laboratory Findings

Laboratory studies reveal normal or moderately elevated CK levels (up to 10 times the upper limit of normal). Serum autoantibodies are usually absent unless there is an associated autoimmune disease. Increased frequency of monoclonal gammopathy has been reported. EMG and nerve conduction studies may reveal mild axonal polyneuropathy and neurogenic-appearing motor units superimposed on predominantly "myopathic" features with abnormal spontaneous activity. Muscle biopsy shows variable endomysial inflammation, necrosis, neurogenic-appearing fiber atrophy, eosinophilic inclusions, and muscle fibers with one or more rimmed vacuoles (Figure 23–4A). These inclusion bodies contain β-amyloid, which can be revealed with Congo red staining under polarized light (Figure 23–4B). This finding has led to speculation that IBM is a degenerative disorder of muscle rather than an autoimmune inflammatory myopathy.

▶ Treatment

There is no cure for IBM and its course is often one of slow linear progression. Remissions are not typically seen and most patients accrue disability over time that can lead to severe functional impairment. Consistent with the notion that IBM may be a degenerative disorder rather than an autoimmune disease, response to corticosteroids and immunosuppressive therapy is generally poor despite anecdotal reports of partial response to these agents. Monthly infusions of high-dose intravenous immunoglobulin (2 g/kg) may be mildly effective by preventing disease progression or inducing mild improvement. Rehabilitation therapy helps to maximize functional status and prevent contractures.

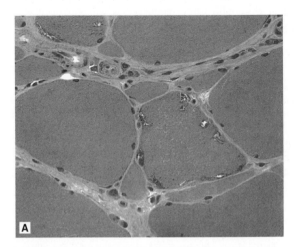

▲ **Figure 23–4A.** H&E stain of a biopsy specimen from a patient with inclusion body myositis, showing eosinophilic inclusions and muscle fibers containing rimmed vacuoles. (Used with permission from Arthur Hayes, MD, Columbia University.)

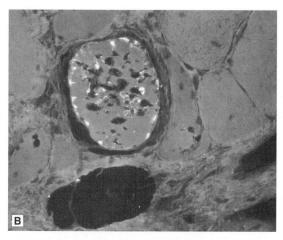

▲ Figure 23–4B. Inclusion body myositis. Vacuolated muscle fibers containing β-amyloid deposits revealed by Congo red staining under polarized light. (Used with permission from Arthur Hayes, MD, Columbia University.)

4. Sarcoid Myopathy

ESSENTIALS OF DIAGNOSIS

▶ Slowly progressive, symmetric proximal muscle weakness

▶ Often painless

▶ Muscle biopsy evidence of numerous noncaseating granulomas

▶ Often, pulmonary and extrapulmonary manifestations

Muscular involvement in sarcoidosis is usually asymptomatic, but progressive proximal weakness can occur. Weakness is usually insidious and symmetric but may be acute, subacute, focal, or multifocal, including involvement of bulbar and respiratory muscles. Symptoms may suggest dermatomyositis or IBM. Muscles may be atrophic, pseudohypertrophic, nodular, or tender to palpation. Pulmonary and other, extrapulmonary, manifestations are usually present, but isolated sarcoid myopathy can occur, and muscular signs and symptoms may be the presenting feature of sarcoidosis. Serum CK level may be normal or elevated.

Laboratory and radiographic evidence of systemic sarcoidosis usually accompanies the myopathy. Gallium 67 scintigraphy is useful for detecting inflammatory muscular involvement. EMG and nerve conduction studies can be normal or display myopathic features, with or without abnormal spontaneous activity. Superimposed sarcoid peripheral neuropathy may be present. Muscle biopsy typically reveals infiltration of inflammatory cells associated with noncaseating granulomas and segmental fiber necrosis. Most patients improve with corticosteroid therapy.

Amato AA, Griggs RC. Treatment of idiopathic inflammatory myopathies. *Curr Opin Neurol* 2003;16:569–575.[PMID: 14501840] (Reviews the results of therapeutic trials in inflammatory myopathies and offers an approach to treating patients with these disorders.)

Berger C, Sommer C, Meinck HM. Isolated sarcoid myopathy. *Muscle Nerve* 2002;26:553–556. [PMID: 12362424]

Bronner IM, et al. Polymyositis: An ongoing discussion about a disease entity. *Arch Neurol* 2004;61:132–135. [PMID: 14732633]

Chung L, Genovese MC, Fiorentino DF. A pilot trial of rituximab in the treatment of patients with dermatomyositis. *Arch Dermatol* 2007;143(6):763–767. [PMID: 17576943]

Dalakas MC. Therapeutic approaches in patients with inflammatory myopathies. *Semin Neurol* 2003;23:199–206. [PMID: 12894385] (Reviews treatment options that are currently available as well as new agents on the therapeutic horizon.)

Fathi M, et al. Interstitial lung disease, a common manifestation of newly diagnosed polymyositis and dermatomyositis. *Ann Rheum Dis* 2004;63:297–301. [PMID: 14962966]

Imbert-Masseau A, Hamidou M, Agard C, Grolleau JY, Chérin P. Antisynthetase syndrome. *Joint Bone Spine* 2003;70(3):161–168. [PMID: 12814758]

Laconis D. The utility of muscle biopsy. *Curr Neurol Neurosci Rep* 2004;4:81–86. [PMID: 14683634]

Mastaglia F, Garlepp M, Phillips B, Zilko P. Inflammatory myopathies: Clinical, diagnostic and therapeutic aspects. *Muscle Nerve* 2003;27:407–425. [PMID: 12661042] (An excellent clinical overview of dermatomyositis, polymyositis, and IBM.)

Tournadre A, Dubost JJ, Soubrier M. Treatment of inflammatory muscle disease in adults. *Joint Bone Spine* 2010;77(5):390–394. [PMID: 20627789]

Walter MC, et al. High-dose immunoglobulin therapy in sporadic inclusion body myositis: A double-blind, placebo-controlled study. *Neurology* 2000;247:22–28. [PMID: 10701893.]

INFECTIOUS MYOPATHIES

1. HIV-Associated Myopathy

ESSENTIALS OF DIAGNOSIS

▶ Progressive proximal muscle weakness

▶ Myalgias (usually present)

▶ Degree of immunosuppression does not correlate with development of muscle disease

▶ Ragged-red fibers on muscle biopsy suggest mitochondrial myopathy due to nucleoside reverse transcriptase inhibitors

▶ Concomitant HIV peripheral neuropathy (present in some patients)

General Considerations

Myopathies associated with HIV are uncommon. The degree of immunosuppression has not been shown to influence the development of muscle disease. These myopathies include mitochondrial myopathies related to antiretroviral therapy (nucleoside reverse transcriptase inhibitors, especially zidovudine [AZT]), polymyositis, IBM, microvasculitis, secondary infections causing myositis (pyomyositis, fungal myositis), rhabdomyolysis, and HIV-wasting syndrome. Human T-lymphotropic virus type 1 (HTLV-1)–related myositis can also occur with or without leukemia or myelopathy. Nemaline rods have also been found in muscle fibers of HIV-infected patients with myopathy.

Clinical Findings

A. Symptoms and Signs

Regardless of etiology, patients often present with progressive proximal muscle weakness and myalgias. Subacute or chronic evolution of muscle weakness can occur, depending on the severity and nature of the underlying cause. There are no clinical features that help distinguish between the different etiologies, and in some patients multiple etiologies are present at the same time. Peripheral neuropathy or myelopathy, or both, may also be present, masking or confounding myopathic signs. In patients with myositis caused by secondary bacterial or fungal infection, fever is present; if left untreated, these patients become septic. HIV-wasting syndrome is characterized by severe involuntary weight loss and generalized muscle atrophy, but mild proximal weakness and myalgia can also occur.

B. Laboratory and Diagnostic Findings

Laboratory and diagnostic studies help to distinguish the different myopathies encountered in HIV-positive patients (Table 23–4).

Treatment

Discontinuation of zidovudine should be done only if an alternate cause for the myopathy cannot be determined. Switching from zidovudine to dideoxyinosine (ddI) or dideoxycytidine (ddC) may be tried, but these agents are also associated with mitochondrial toxicity. Withdrawal of zidovudine does not always result in improvement, suggesting that HIV itself may be playing a more significant etiologic role. A trial of intravenous immunoglobulin may be beneficial if abundant spontaneous activity suggestive of an inflammatory myopathy is found during needle EMG of a patient with suspected zidovudine-related myopathy. For patients with HIV-associated myositis, antiretroviral therapy may be beneficial. In these patients, treatment with intravenous immunoglobulin may be effective and potentially safer than corticosteroids, with less risk of further immunosuppression. Pyomyositis should be treated with appropriate antibiotics and drainage when necessary. Anabolic steroids such as stanozolol and oxandrolone may reduce weight loss in patients with HIV-wasting syndrome, but do not appear to improve muscle strength.

Verma S, Misca E, Estanislao L, Simpson D. Neuromuscular complications in HIV. *Curr Neurol Neurosci Rep* 2004;4:62–67. [PMID: 14683631] (Reviews clinical manifestations, pathogenesis, diagnosis, and management of the neuromuscular complications of HIV, including myopathy.)

2. Other Viral Causes of Myositis

ESSENTIALS OF DIAGNOSIS

► Febrile illness
► Myalgias
► Muscle weakness
► Markedly elevated serum CK level

In addition to triggering polymyositis, viruses can cause acute and subacute inflammatory myopathies. HTLV-1 can cause a more chronic myopathy that resembles polymyositis

Table 23–4. HIV-Associated Myopathies: Laboratory and Diagnostic Findings

	Zidovudine-Related Myopathy	HIV-Related Inflammatory Myopathy	HIV-Wasting Syndrome
Serum CK level	Normal or mildly elevated (< 5-10 times upper limit of normal)	Moderately or markedly elevated (> 5-10 times upper limit of normal)	Normal
Serum lactate level	Often elevated	Often normal	Normal
EMG findings	Usually normal	Usually abnormal (spontaneous activity and myopathic motor units)	Normal
Muscle biopsy findings	Ragged-red fibers	Inflammation and necrosis	Atrophy of type 2 muscle fibers

CK = creatine kinase; EMG = electromyography; HIV = human immunodeficiency virus.

with or without myelopathy or polyneuropathy. Influenza and coxsackie viruses are the most common culprits. Respiratory syncytial virus and herpes simplex viruses have also been implicated. Clinical presentation is characterized by a febrile illness, myalgias, and weakness. Fever is usually absent in HTLV-1–associated polymyositis. The serum CK level is often markedly elevated, and myoglobinuria and renal failure can occur. Cardiopulmonary involvement is not uncommon, especially in adults, who generally have a less favorable prognosis than children. Prednisone, 60 mg/day, may benefit some patients with HTLV-1–associated polymyositis.

3. Bacterial Myositis

ESSENTIALS OF DIAGNOSIS

► Febrile illness
► Myalgias
► Focal or severe muscle weakness
► Elevated serum CK level

Risk factors for pyomyositis (muscle abscess) include HIV, diabetes mellitus, intravenous drug abuse, skin infections, malignancy, rheumatologic conditions, and muscle trauma. *Staphylococcus aureus* is the most commonly implicated organism, especially in patients living in tropical climates where incidence rates of pyomyositis are higher. Infections with streptococci, *Escherichia coli*, *Yersinia*, mycobacteria, *Mycoplasma*, and *Legionella* have also been reported. Non–HIV-infected patients may be more likely to have a gram-negative infection.

Bacterial myositis does not usually develop in the absence of primary infection at another site. Systemic signs of infection are often present, and patients may become septic if not treated early. Involved muscles are often hot, painful, and tender, and weakness may be focal or severe. The serum CK level is often elevated, and most patients have neutrophilic leukocytosis and an elevated erythrocyte sedimentation rate. However, leukocytosis and bacteremia tend to occur less frequently in those with HIV infection and pyomyositis.

Pyogenic abscesses can be localized by ultrasound, computed tomography, or MRI, for needle aspiration and diagnosis. Appropriate treatment with intravenous antibiotics is usually sufficient early in the course of the disease, but for more severe infections, drainage of the abscesses is required.

Crum NF. Bacterial pyomyositis in the United States. *Am J Med* 2004;117:420–428. [PMID: 15380499]

4. Parasitic Myositis

ESSENTIALS OF DIAGNOSIS

► Fever
► Myalgias
► Proximal muscle weakness
► Elevated serum CK level
► Often, prominent eosinophilia

Trichinosis, cysticercosis, and toxoplasmosis can cause inflammatory myopathy, and the incidence of these infections has increased in the era of AIDS. Myalgias, rather than frank weakness, are the most prominent symptoms, except in severe cases. Table 23–5 summarizes the clinical findings and treatment of these parasitic myopathies. For further discussion on AIDS-related toxoplasmosis, see Chapter 28).

Bale Jr JF. Cysticercosis. *Curr Treat Options Neurol* 2000;2:355–360. [PMID: 11096760]

DRUG-INDUCED OR TOXIC MYOPATHIES

Drugs can cause myopathy through a variety of mechanisms, as outlined in Table 23–6 and commonly used myotoxic drugs are listed in Table 23–7. The discussion that follows describes two of the more common drug-induced myopathies, as well as myopathies provoked by heavy alcohol consumption and critical illness.

CORTICOSTEROID MYOPATHY

ESSENTIALS OF DIAGNOSIS

► Slowly progressive proximal weakness (most common)
► Rapidly progressive weakness in some patients (rare)
► Follows long-term treatment with corticosteroid doses, eg, prednisone greater than 30 mg/day
► Cushingoid appearance
► Serum CK level usually normal
► Normal findings on EMG, or myopathic features without spontaneous activity
► Muscle biopsy evidence of type 2b fiber atrophy

Table 23–5. Parasitic Myopathies: Clinical Findings and Treatment

	Trichinosis	Cysticercosis	Toxoplasmosis
Clinical findings	Similar to polymyositis, although myalgias are more common than frank weakness Eye and respiratory muscle involvement can occur	Usually asymptomatic Myalgia may be present, although frank weakness is rare Extraocular muscles can be affected Muscle enlargement and nodularity may be present	Similar to polymyositis, although myalgias are more common than frank weakness, and rarely resembles dermatomyositis
Laboratory and imaging findings	Elevated serum CK level Eosinophilia	Usually normal serum CK level Eosinophilia Plain radiographs may show calcified cysts	Elevated serum CK level Markedly increased antitoxoplasmic antibodies (IgG, IgM)
EMG findings	Similar to polymyositis	Usually normal	Similar to polymyositis
Muscle biopsy findings	Definitive	Definitive but usually not necessary	Definitive
Treatment	Albendazole, 400 mg 3 times a day for 2 wk, treats larva and adult worm Prednisone, 1–1.5 mg/kg/day, ameliorates muscle weakness	Treatment is usually not required Albendazole, 15 mg/kg/day, has been used for symptomatic cases; however, this is controversial and potentially hazardous because of its propensity to aggravate symptoms Prednisone, 1–1.5 mg/kg/day, may attenuate acute inflammatory response	Pyrimethamine, 200 mg initial dose, followed by 50–100 mg/day, and sulfadiazine, 4–6 g/day, with folinic acid, 10–50 mg/day Plasmapheresis has been used successfully

CK = creatine kinase; EMG = electromyography; IgG = immunoglobulin G; IgM = immunoglobulin M.

▶ General Considerations

Corticosteroids are the most commonly implicated toxic causes of myopathy. Myotoxicity is linked mainly to fluorinated corticosteroids such as dexamethasone, betamethasone, and triamcinolone. High-dose inhaled fluticasone has caused myopathy in children. Rarely, chronic corticosteroid use may cause mitochondrial dysfunction and motor neuron involvement.

Table 23–6. Mechanisms of Drug-Induced Myopathy

Drug(s)	Mechanism
Cholesterol-lowering agents	Necrosis
Corticosteroids	Fiber atrophy
Diuretics	Metabolic disturbances (eg, hypokalemia)
D-penicillamine, l-tryptophan	Inflammation
Emetine, amiodarone, colchicine, and chloroquine	Vacuolar changes
Vaccine adjuvants containing aluminum hydroxide	Macrophagic myofasciitis
Valproic acid	Carnitine deficiency
Zidovudine	Mitochondrial dysfunction

▶ Clinical Findings

Two forms of corticosteroid myopathy have been clinically defined. The first, which is most often encountered, is a chronic, slowly progressive myopathy characterized by mild to moderate proximal muscle weakness, a cushingoid appearance, and chronic corticosteroid intake, usually at prednisone doses greater than 30 mg/day. In these patients, the serum CK level may be normal. EMG findings are normal or show myopathic features without spontaneous activity, distinguishing this disorder from polymyositis.

The second form of corticosteroid myopathy usually occurs in critically ill patients in intensive care units where other myotoxic agents, especially neuromuscular blocking drugs, are often used concomitantly, and patients are septic with multiorgan failure. Acute proximal and distal muscle weakness occurs, and facial and cardiopulmonary muscles are often affected. Extraocular muscles are usually spared. The serum CK level is commonly elevated, and EMG findings are often myopathic, with abnormal spontaneous activity, although in critically ill patients coexisting polyneuropathy may be seen (see section on myopathy in critical illness). Muscle biopsy specimens show atrophy of type 2b fibers.

Treatment

In patients with the chronic form, slow withdrawal of corticosteroids or reduction in dosage is recommended, in conjunction with rehabilitation therapy. Exercise may attenuate corticosteroid-induced muscle atrophy; however, this prescription should be individualized based on the patient's medical status and muscle function. In patients with the acute form, other myotoxic agents are eliminated, corticosteroids are rapidly tapered, and supportive care is provided. The use of nonfluorinated corticosteroids may reduce the risk of myopathy.

CHOLESTEROL-LOWERING AGENT MYOPATHY

ESSENTIALS OF DIAGNOSIS

- ▶ Exposure to cholesterol-lowering agents
- ▶ Myalgias
- ▶ Proximal muscle weakness

General Considerations

Every cholesterol-lowering agent, including statins, niacin, clofibrate, and gemfibrozil, has myotoxic effects. Cholesterol-lowering-agent myopathy (CLAM) occurs in 0.5% of patients when a single agent is used and in up to 5% with combination use. Statins (HMG CoA reductase inhibitors) are the most effective and most prescribed agents for lowering low-density lipoprotein cholesterol. They are generally well tolerated but produce a variety of muscle-related complaints, the most serious of which is myositis with rhabdomyolysis. The overall reported incidence of fatal rhabdomyolysis is 0.15 deaths per 1 million prescriptions, but available literature is confusing because of lack of clear definitions. To clarify this, the American Heart Association clinical advisory on the use and safety of statins defined four syndromes:

1. Statin myopathy—any muscle complaints related to these drugs
2. Myalgia—muscle pain without CK elevation
3. Myositis—muscle symptoms with CK elevations
4. Rhabdomyolysis—markedly elevated CK levels, usually greater than 10 times the upper limit of normal, with an elevated creatinine level consistent with pigment-induced nephropathy

How statins cause myopathy is unclear. Myotoxicity and rhabdomyolysis usually occur following at least 1 week of statin use, although rhabdomyolysis has occurred following a single dose of simvastatin.

Clinical Findings

Acute or insidious onset of myalgias occurs alone or in combination with proximal muscle weakness and myoglobulinuria, and symptoms may mimic polymyositis. The risk of myopathy is increased in patients with impaired hepatic and renal function, hypothyroidism, diabetes mellitus, and the concomitant use of myotoxic agents, such as fibric acid derivatives (gemfibrozil), niacin, cyclosporine, azole antifungals, macrolide antibiotics, zidovudine, nefazodone, verapamil, diltiazem, amiodarone, and excessive daily consumption of grapefruit juice (Table 23–7).

Muscle complaints may occur without CK elevation, and patients with CK elevations may not be symptomatic. Indeed, asymptomatic elevations of CK occur in 1% of patients taking statins. EMG may show abnormal spontaneous activity, including myotonic-like discharges, and myopathic features. Muscle biopsy findings in CLAM are generally nonspecific and include atrophy, inflammatory infiltrates, and necrosis. The presence of inflammatory infiltrates may represent an unmasking of polymyositis, and should prompt a search for underlying autoimmunity.

Treatment

The American Heart Association offers guidelines for managing muscle-related complaints in patients receiving statins (Table 23–8). In addition, coenzyme Q10 and vitamin D have been used in the treatment and prevention of statin myopathy, although limited studies supporting their efficacy exist.

Table 23–7. Commonly Used Myotoxic Agents

Drug	Type of Myopathy
Amiodarone	Painful vacuolar myopathy
Chloroquine	Painless vacuolar myopathy ± cardiac involvement
Colchicine	Painful vacuolar myopathy
Cyclosporine	Painful mitochondrial myopathy
D-penicillamine	Inflammatory myopathy (1%), usually affecting neuromuscular junction
Emetine (in ipecac)	Painful vacuolar myopathy
Imatinib	Inflammatory myopathy[a]
Interferon alpha	Inflammatory myopathy
Vaccines containing aluminum adjuvants	Macrophagic myofasciitis (with macrophage intracytoplasmic inclusions containing aluminum)
Valproic acid	Carnitine-related myopathy with mitochondrial changes
Vitamin E excess	Painful myopathy with muscle necrosis
Zidovudine	Mitochondrial myopathy

[a]A single case report.

Table 23–8. American Heart Association Expert Consensus Guidelines for the Management of Statin-Related Muscle Complaints

- No clinical or epidemiologic evidence permits differentiation among statins as to their myotoxicity potential.
- There is no absolute contraindication to combining a statin with an agent known to increase myopathy if benefits are likely to outweigh risks.
- If rhabdomyolysis occurs, discontinue agent. (Reports of successfully restarting at lower dose or switching to a different statin exist, but strong consideration should be given to switching agents.)
- Routine serum CK measurements in asymptomatic patients before and during treatment are not required, although some experts recommend obtaining a baseline measurement.
- There is no need to stop treatment if asymptomatic elevated serum CK is detected incidentally unless CK level exceeds 10 times upper limit of normal value. Some experts recommend monitoring if CK is incidentally detected to be greater than 5 times upper limit of normal value. Evaluate thyroid function in these patients.
- Consider discontinuation of statins before events that may exacerbate muscle injury (eg, surgical procedures or vigorous physical exertion, such as marathon running).
- Presence of tolerable myalgias without elevated CK level does not necessitate discontinuation.
- If myalgias are intolerable, discontinue agent. It may be possible to switch statins once patient becomes asymptomatic.
- Patients with severe myopathy having inflammatory features on biopsy and who fail to improve after discontinuation of the agent may improve with corticosteroid therapy.

CK = creatine kinase. (Data from Pasternak RC, Smith SC Jr, Bairey-Merz CN et al. ACC/AHA/NHLBI Clinical Advisory on the Use and Safety of Statins. Stroke. 2002;33(9):2337–41.)

Bannwarth B. Drug-induced myopathies. *Expert Opin Drug Saf* 2002;1:65–70. [PMID: 12904161] (A well-organized review of drug-induced myopathies with clinical and histopathologic emphasis.)

Gherardi RK, et al. Macrophagic myofasciitis lesions assess long-term persistence of vaccine-derived aluminium hydroxide in muscle. *Brain* 2001;124:1821–1831. [PMID: 11522584]

Harper CR, Jacobson TA. Evidence-based management of statin myopathy. *Curr Atheroscler Rep* 2010;12(5):322–330. [PMID: 20628837]

Jamil S, Iqbal P. Rhabdomyolysis induced by a single dose of a statin. *Heart* 2004;90:e3. [PMID: 14676266]

Lee P, Greenfield JR, Campbell LV. Vitamin D insufficiency—A novel mechanism of statin-induced myalgia? *Clin Endocrinol (Oxf)* 2009;71(1):154–155. [PMID: 19178510]

Mas E, Mori TA. Coenzyme Q(10) and statin myalgia: What is the evidence? *Curr Atheroscler Rep* 2010;12(6):407–413. [PMID: 20725809]

Mitsui T, et al. Chronic corticosteroid administration causes mitochondrial dysfunction in skeletal muscle. *J Neurol* 2002;249:1004–1009. [PMID: 12195445]

Mitsui T, et al. Motor neuron involvement in a patient with long-term corticosteroid administration. *Intern Med* 2003;42:862–866. [PMID: 14518677]

Rosenson RS. Current overview of statin-induced myopathy. *Am J Med* 2004;116:408–416. [PMID: 15006590] (Discusses myotoxic effects of statins and drug-drug interactions, and offers suggestions on statin selection for individual patients.)

Swert L, Wouters C, Zegher F. Myopathy in children receiving high-dose inhaled fluticasone. *N Engl J Med* 2004;350:1157–1159. [PMID: 15014196]

Thompson P, Clarkson P, Karas R. Statin-associated myopathy. *JAMA* 2003;289:1681–1690. [PMID: 12672737] (A comprehensive clinical review of statin-related muscle complaints with clear clinical guidelines.)

ALCOHOLIC MYOPATHY

 ESSENTIALS OF DIAGNOSIS

- ► Heavy alcohol consumption
- ► Acute or chronic muscle weakness

▶ General Considerations

Alcohol is associated with both an acute and a chronic myopathy (see Chapter 33). The acute form may be severe, with rhabdomyolysis and myoglobinuria. The chronic form may cause slowly progressive weakness or may be asymptomatic with an elevated CK level. Multiorgan damage, peripheral neuropathy, and malnutrition are frequent and may act synergistically with alcohol in causing muscle damage.

▶ Clinical Findings

Acute alcoholic myopathy is characterized by rapid (hours to days) onset of symptoms after a recent increase in alcohol consumption or binge drinking episode. Proximal weakness and pain usually predominate, but regional or focal involvement can occur. Serum CK level is elevated in most patients and in severe cases may lead to rhabdomyolysis. Hypophosphatemia and hypokalemia, frequently found in alcoholic patients, can also precipitate rhabdomyolysis and must be excluded. Motor hyperactivity during alcohol withdrawal can also cause a rise in serum CK level. EMG typically shows abnormal spontaneous activity with myopathic features. Muscle biopsy shows muscle necrosis with regenerating fibers.

Chronic alcoholic myopathy occurring in patients with chronic heavy alcohol consumption causes insidious, painless, proximal weakness, and, over time, atrophy. Myoglobinuria is typically absent, and serum CK level may be normal or mildly elevated. EMG and nerve conduction studies may reveal both myopathic and neuropathic changes. Muscle biopsy shows atrophy of type 2 muscle fibers without necrosis.

▶ Treatment

With abstinence from alcohol, weakness usually improves.

MYOPATHY IN CRITICAL ILLNESS

ESSENTIALS OF DIAGNOSIS

▶ Sepsis or multiorgan failure

▶ Exposure to corticosteroids or nondepolarizing neuromuscular blocking agents (common)

▶ Generalized muscle weakness

Muscle weakness in critically ill patients can be caused by a variety of insults that affect peripheral nerves, neuromuscular junctions, or muscles, alone or in combination. In the intensive care unit, three main types of myopathy, which often occur in combination, have been identified: critical illness myopathy, myopathy with selective loss of myosin filaments, and acute necrotizing myopathy.

Patients usually have sepsis and multiorgan failure and have often been exposed to corticosteroids or nondepolarizing neuromuscular blocking agents. Clinically, patients may present with difficultly being weaned off the ventilator, and they usually have profound muscle weakness. Sensory loss may reflect concurrent polyneuropathy, but most critically ill patients are not able to cooperate with a sensory examination.

Serum CK level is often normal. Routine EMG may not distinguish between neuropathy and myopathy because of insufficient motor units; special techniques such as direct muscle stimulation may be more discriminatory. Muscle biopsy may show preferential loss of myosin thick filaments.

Specific treatment is not available. Sepsis and multiorgan failure should be treated aggressively, and myotoxic agents, especially corticosteroids and neuromuscular blocking agents, should be avoided.

Trojaborg W, Weimer L, Hays A. Electrophysiologic studies in critical illness associated weakness: Myopathy or neuropathy—A reappraisal. *Clin Neurophysiol* 2001;112: 1586–1593. [PMID: 11514240]

SECONDARY METABOLIC & ENDOCRINE MYOPATHIES

ESSENTIALS OF DIAGNOSIS

▶ Systemic manifestations of specific metabolic or endocrine abnormalities

▶ Proximal muscle weakness

▶ Restoration of muscle strength with correction of metabolic or endocrine abnormality

HYPOKALEMIC MYOPATHY

Low serum potassium levels occur in various medical conditions and as a side effect of numerous medications, especially diuretics. Muscular symptoms are the most common manifestation of hypokalemia, and include weakness and myalgia. When serum potassium levels fall below 3.0 mEq/L, significant proximal weakness may be seen. If the potassium level falls further, below 2.5–2.0 mEq/L, structural muscle damage and rhabdomyolysis may occur. Cranial musculature is spared. Serum hyperosmolality in this setting predisposes to rhabdomyolysis. Electrocardiographic abnormalities include flattening and inversion of T waves, appearance of U waves, and ST segment depression. Muscle biopsy reveals vacuoles in muscle fibers. Potassium replacement is preventive and curative provided that irreversible renal failure has not occurred. For a discussion of hypokalemic periodic paralysis, see section on Channelopathies.

HYPOPHOSPHATEMIC MYOPATHY

Hypophosphatemia is often overlooked as a cause of muscle weakness. Low serum phosphate levels can occur in a variety of medical and iatrogenic settings (eg, diabetic ketoacidosis, alcoholism, intravenous hyperalimentation, use of phosphate-binding antacids). When severe and sustained (< 0.4 mM/L), hypophosphatemia can cause severe myopathy and rhabdomyolysis. Phosphorous replacement is preventive and curative provided that irreversible renal failure has not occurred.

CHRONIC RENAL FAILURE–RELATED MYOPATHIES

Uremic myopathy is much less common than uremic neuropathy. Its pathogenesis is unclear and may be related to secondary hyperparathyroidism or osteodystrophy. Hypophosphatemia can contribute to the myopathy, especially in patients who are being treated with aluminum hydroxide gel.

Calciphylaxis or calcific uremic arteriolopathy is a complication of chronic renal failure, characterized by medial calcification of small- to medium-sized arteries associated with ischemic necrosis of the skin and other organs. Predisposing conditions within the uremic milieu include elevated calcium and parathyroid hormone, and hyperphosphatemia with resultant increases in the calcium × phosphate product. Ischemic myopathy has been reported in this syndrome, which may mimic dermatomyositis. The prognosis for patients with this syndrome is poor; early aggressive lowering of calcium and phosphate levels, and parathyroidectomy may improve the outcome.

DIABETIC MUSCLE INFARCTION

This is a rare disorder characterized by ischemic infarction of the thigh (65% of patients) or calf muscle in patients with long-standing poorly controlled diabetes, and evidence of other end-organ damage. Acute or subacute focal pain and swelling are the presenting features, and recurrent infarction in the same or a contralateral muscle can occur. Serum CK level is sometimes elevated. MRI shows increased T2-weighted signal and edema in affected muscles. Muscle biopsy shows fiber necrosis and endomysial inflammation. Treatment consists of analgesics and immobilization of the involved limb.

Grigoriadis E, Fam AG, Starok M, Ang LC. Skeletal muscle infarction in diabetes mellitus. *J Rheumatol* 2000;27:1063–1068. [PMID: 10782838]

HYPOTHYROID MYOPATHY

▶ Clinical Findings

A. Symptoms and Signs

In addition to nonspecific constitutional symptoms, including hair loss, thick skin, and mental slowing (which may progress to myxedema coma), muscle weakness and cramping are often present in hypothyroidism. Prolonged or delayed relaxation of deep tendon reflexes is a characteristic finding, and myotonoid features (myotonia is a symptom manifested by the slow relaxation of a group of muscles following contraction; see Chapter 2) are seen in one quarter of patients. Proximal weakness develops insidiously and may be associated with pain and tenderness. An unusual finding is the presence of muscular enlargement or pseudohypertrophy, which can be seen in children (Debré-Sémélaigne syndrome, or "infant Hercules") and adults (Hoffman syndrome).

B. Laboratory Findings

Thyroid hormone levels are low. Serum CK level is often markedly elevated (10-fold to 100-fold), which may lead to an erroneous diagnosis of polymyositis.

C. Special Tests

EMG may show myopathic features with or without abnormal spontaneous activity. Muscle biopsy findings may be normal or show nonspecific fiber atrophy.

▶ Treatment

Patients generally respond well to thyroid hormone replacement.

HYPERTHYROID MYOPATHY

▶ General Considerations

There are many causes of the hyperthyroid state, including excessive exogenous thyroid hormone replacement, toxic goiter, and Graves disease. Most patients report weakness when asked, although this is not usually the presenting complaint. Graves ophthalmopathy is a progressive disorder of the extraocular muscles (thyroid ophthalmopathy), characterized by lid lag, lid retraction, proptosis, and ophthalmoplegia. It is important also to recognize distinguishing features of myasthenia gravis, which has an increased association with hyperthyroidism, because treatment of hyperthyroidism with β-blockers can dangerously worsen myasthenic weakness. Rarely, thyrotoxic periodic paralysis occurs (especially in Asians), presenting clinically in an identical manner to familial periodic paralysis (discussed later).

▶ Clinical Findings

A. Symptoms and Signs

Patients usually present insidiously with proximal weakness, prominent atrophy, and, often, hyperactive deep tendon reflexes. Occasionally, the presence of fasciculations suggests amyotrophic lateral sclerosis. Scapular winging and bulbar and ocular muscle weakness are sometimes present. Weakness may be painless, although occasional patients have myalgias.

B. Laboratory Findings

Excessive thyroid hormone levels are seen, and serum CK levels are usually normal.

C. Special Tests

EMG may reveal myopathic features with abnormal spontaneous activity, including fasciculations. Muscle biopsy findings are usually normal or show nonspecific fiber atrophy.

▶ Treatment

Achieving the euthyroid state usually leads to improvement of the myopathy. Patients with severe ophthalmopathy may require corticosteroids or surgical decompression.

HYPERPARATHYROID MYOPATHY

Myopathy related to parathyroid dysfunction is poorly understood, although phosphate depletion, calcium excess, and abnormal metabolism of vitamin D likely play a role.

▶ Clinical Findings

A. Symptoms and Signs

Patients may have proximal muscle weakness, atrophy, hyperactive deep tendon reflexes, and fasciculations, and in severe cases, this combination may resemble amyotrophic lateral sclerosis. Muscle cramps are occasionally present, and respiratory failure, presumably due to severe hypercalcemia, has been reported.

B. Laboratory Findings

Hypercalcemia and hypophosphatemia are usually present and may worsen clinical weakness. Parathyroid hormone levels are often very high. Serum CK levels are often normal.

C. Special Tests

EMG may show myopathic features without abnormal spontaneous activity. In some cases, peripheral neuropathy is superimposed. Muscle biopsy findings are usually normal or show nonspecific fiber atrophy.

▶ Treatment

In primary hyperparathyroidism, surgical removal of the oversecreting gland or adenoma often restores muscle strength. In secondary hyperparathyroidism resulting from chronic renal disease, treatment is more difficult, although administration of vitamin D and reduction in phosphorous intake may be beneficial.

VITAMIN D–RELATED MYOPATHY

A severe myopathy associated with vitamin D deficiency has been described. Symptoms include progressive proximal muscle weakness often associated with musculoskeletal pain involving the back, hips, or lower limbs and metabolic and radiographic findings consistent with osteomalacia. Low levels of 25-hydroxyvitamin D in the blood are seen, and oral treatment with vitamin D supplements may restore muscle strength in patients within 6 months.

Al-Said YA, et al. Severe proximal myopathy with remarkable recovery after vitamin D treatment. *Can J Neurol Sci* 2009;36(3):336–339. [PMID: 19534335]

CUSHING DISEASE

Cushing disease results from overproduction of adrenocorticotrophin, typically from a pituitary microadenoma. Cushing syndrome is characterized by truncal obesity, acne, hirsutism, hypertension, and impaired glucose tolerance; it is most commonly iatrogenic, resulting from therapeutic doses of synthetic glucocorticoids as well as Cushing disease. Myopathy in Cushing disease is identical to that seen in chronic corticosteroid myopathy (discussed earlier). Removal of the oversecreting gland often restores muscle strength.

Horak HA, Pourmand R. Endocrine myopathies. *Neurol Clin* 2000;18:203–213. [PMID: 10658176]

▼ PRIMARY METABOLIC MYOPATHIES

ESSENTIALS OF DIAGNOSIS

▶ Exercise intolerance
▶ Muscle weakness
▶ Muscle fatigability
▶ Myalgias and muscle cramps
▶ Myoglobinuria

Primary metabolic myopathies are rare conditions caused by a biochemical defect of skeletal muscle energy systems. The biochemical defect may involve carbohydrate metabolism (glycogen storage), lipid metabolism, mitochondria, or the purine nucleotide cycle. These conditions are featured in Table 23–9.

Most metabolic myopathies become symptomatic during activities that require increased muscle energy consumption such as exercise (exercise intolerance). Chief symptoms include muscle weakness or fatigability, myalgias, cramps, and myoglobinuria. Table 23–9 contrasts clinical features, diagnostic findings, and treatment of the most important of these disorders.

▶ Special Tests

The forearm ischemic exercise test (FIET) is useful for screening glycogen storage disorders such as myophosphorylase deficiency as well as myoadenylate deaminase deficiency. Prior to the test, baseline venous lactate and ammonia levels should be obtained. To perform the test, a blood pressure cuff is placed over the patient's upper arm and inflated to a pressure roughly 20 mm Hg greater than the systolic pressure that renders the forearm ischemic. The patient then immediately begins repetitive, rapid grip exercises (eg, squeezing a ball or hand ergometer) for as long as possible. The test is aborted if the patient develops a cramp or contracture during cuff inflation or exercise. When the patient fatigues, the cuff is released and blood is drawn at 1, 3, 5, 10, and 15 minutes postexercise for evaluation of elevated lactate and ammonia levels. The test should be performed with caution, however, because of the risk of compartment syndrome with ulnar nerve damage or severe rhabdomyolysis that may lead to renal failure.

Pourmand R. Metabolic myopathies: A diagnostic evaluation. *Neurol Clin* 2000;18:1–13. [PMID: 10658166] (Discusses the initial approach to the patient suspected of having a metabolic myopathy.)

▼ MITOCHONDRIAL MYOPATHIES

Defects in the mitochondrial respiratory chain (see Chapter 24), particularly complex IV deficiency and coenzyme Q10 deficiency, may impair energy production and

Table 23-9. Primary Metabolic Myopathies: Clinical Findings and Treatment

	Acid Maltase Deficiency	Myophosphorylase Deficiency	Phosphofructokinase Deficiency	CPT Deficiency	MAD Deficiency
Inheritance	Autosomal recessive	Autosomal recessive	Autosomal recessive	Autosomal recessive	Autosomal recessive
Clinical findings	Infantile form (Pompe disease)—generalized weakness and hypotonia, liver dysfunction, early death from cardiorespiratory failure Childhood form—delayed milestones, progressive proximal weakness, respiratory involvement, occasional cardiac involvement Adult form—respiratory involvement may be earliest manifestation; progressive proximal weakness; can mimic polymyositis	Exercise intolerance (shortly after exercise), with cramps, muscle stiffness, fatigability Muscle weakness in 30% of cases late in disease	Exercise intolerance (shortly after exercise), with cramps, muscle stiffness, fatigability Normal muscle strength Signs of anemia	Exercise intolerance (after prolonged sustained exercise or fasting), with cramps, muscle fatigability, and stiffness Normal muscle strength between attacks	Exertional myalgias and muscle fatigability, but syndrome is usually mild. An association with gout has been reported
Laboratory findings	Elevated serum CK level Reduced acid maltase levels in lymphocytes and urine	Elevated serum CK level Reduced or absent myophosphorylase activity in muscle Myoglobinuria	Elevated serum CK level Hemolytic anemia, with high bilirubin and reticulocytosis Myoglobinuria	Serum CK level usually normal but may be increased Occasionally, reduced CPT levels in liver and leukocytes Occasional myoglobinuria	Variable serum CK level Occasional myoglobinuria Occasionally, elevated serum uric acid levels
FIET results	Normal increase in lactate level	No increase in lactate level	No increase in lactate level	Normal increase in lactate level	Reduced ammonia rise with normal lactate rise
EMG findings	Myopathic features, often with abundant myotonic discharges and spontaneous activity that is most profuse in paraspinal musculature	Myopathic features ± abnormal spontaneous activity, electrically silent muscle cramps, significant decrement with repetitive nerve stimulation	Myopathic features ± abnormal spontaneous activity, electrically silent muscle cramps, significant decrement with repetitive nerve stimulation	Normal	Normal
Muscle biopsy findings	Vacuoles containing glycogen in muscle fibers Reduced acid maltase levels in muscle	PAS + subsarcolemmal vacuoles in muscle fibers Absent phosphorylase activity in muscle	PAS + subsarcolemmal vacuoles in muscle fibers Absent PFK in muscle	Normal except for reduced CPT activity in muscle	Absent MAD activity in muscle
Treatment	None	None	None	No specific treatment; patients should avoid prolonged fasting and prolonged exercise without carbohydrate loading	None

CK = creatine kinase; CPT = carnitine palmityltransferase; EMG = Electromyography; FIET = forearm ischemic exercise test; MAD = myoadenylate deaminase; PAS = periodic acid-Schiff stain; PFK = phosphofructokinase.

almost invariably involve skeletal muscle, causing exercise intolerance, cramps, and recurrent myoglobinuria, similar to the primary metabolic myopathies. In patients with coenzyme Q10 deficiency, complete recovery may occur with oral coenzyme Q10 supplementation at a dose of 150 mg/day.

MYOGLOBINURIA

ESSENTIALS OF DIAGNOSIS

► Muscle weakness

► Myalgia

► Elevated CK level

► Myoglobinuria (brownish to dark-red urine that tests positive for heme despite the absence of red blood cells)

The term *myoglobinuria* is often used interchangeably with rhabdomyolysis. It is caused by injury to skeletal muscle from a variety of insults (Table 23–10), leading to the release of potentially toxic substances, most notably myoglobin and CK, into the circulation.

Patients with myoglobinuria typically present with weakness, myalgias, and edema involving affected muscles. Urine is characteristically brownish to dark red and tests positive for heme by the dipstick test despite the absence of red blood cells on microscopic examination. The serum CK level is often greater than 50,000 IU/L. Acute myoglobinuric renal failure and life-threatening electrolyte disturbances are the most dreaded complications. In severe cases, treatment may require peritoneal dialysis or hemodialysis; patients with milder disease can be treated with aggressive hydration, alkalinization of urine with sodium bicarbonate, and correction of electrolyte disturbances. The underlying disorder should be specifically treated.

Allison RC, Bedsole DL. The other medical causes of rhabdomyolysis. *Am J Med Sci* 2003;326:79–88. [PMID: 12920439]

CHANNELOPATHIES

ESSENTIALS OF DIAGNOSIS

► Inherited disorder

► Weakness (episodic), myotonia, or both

► Precipitating factors are usually identifiable

Channelopathies are rare diseases caused by functional disturbances of ion channel proteins as a result of specific

Table 23–10. Causes of Myoglobinuria

Hereditary
Primary metabolic myopathies
Familial malignant hyperthermia (an inherited disease caused by rapid rise in body temperature and severe muscle contraction when affected individuals receive general anesthesia)
Dystrophinopathies

Acquired
Strenuous or unaccustomed physical exertion
Agitated delirium, restraints
Hyperthermia (including heat stroke and neuroleptic malignant syndrome; see Chapter 15)
Trauma (crush injuries, burns)
Prolonged tonic-clonic seizures
Severe hypokalemia, hypophosphatemia
Diabetic ketoacidosis, hyperosmolar nonketotic states
Infectious myositis
Polymyositis, dermatomyositis
Muscle infarction
Toxins (alcohol, cocaine, heroin, phencyclidine, amphetamine/methamphetamine)
Drugs (statins, succinylcholine)

mutations. These disorders include the familial periodic paralyses and disorders with myotonia. They should be considered in patients with attacks of episodic weakness.

These diseases tend to spare respiratory muscles and are rarely life threatening. Table 23–11 summarizes clinical features and treatment of these disorders.

Special Tests for Periodic Paralysis

In all forms of periodic paralysis, muscle biopsy may show vacuoles within muscle fibers during severe attacks. EMG findings may be normal between attacks or reveal myopathic features with or without myotonia in patients with periodic paralysis who develop fixed weakness. During attacks, EMG is abnormal. Specialized EMG protocols using controlled limb temperatures (cooling) and repetitive stimulation may also be useful in the interattack diagnostic evaluation of periodic paralysis.

Lehmann-Horn F, Jurkat-Rott K, Rudel R. Periodic paralysis: Understanding channelopathies. *Curr Neurol Neurosci Rep* 2002;2:61–69. [PMID: 11898585]

CONGENITAL MYOPATHIES

Congenital myopathies are primary muscle disorders caused by mutations of contractile and structural proteins that lead to structural abnormalities of muscle fibers and the

Table 23–11. Channelopathies: Clinical Findings and Treatment

	Hypokalemic Periodic Paralysis	Hyperkalemic Periodic Paralysis	Paramyotonia Congenita	Myotonia Congenita (Thomsen)	Generalized Myotonia (Becker)	Malignant Hyperthermia
Inheritance	Autosomal dominant	Autosomal dominant	Autosomal dominant	Autosomal dominant	Autosomal recessive	Autosomal dominant
Ion channel defect	Type 1 = calcium channel Type 2 = sodium channel	Sodium channel	Sodium channel	Chloride channel	Chloride channel	Calcium channel
Onset	Puberty to third decade	First decade	First decade	Childhood	Childhood	All ages
Clinical findings						
• Episodic attacks of weakness (presence, typical duration, severity)	Present; >2 h; often severe	Present; <2 h; seldom severe	May be present; >2 h; seldom severe	Absent	Absent	Absent
• Serum CK level during attack	Normal or mildly elevated	Elevated	Elevated	Usually normal	Mildly elevated	Markedly elevated
• Myotonia	Confined to eyelids	May be present	Present	Prominent	Prominent	Absent
• Muscle hypertrophy	Absent	Rarely present	Present	Present	Present	Absent
• Precipitating factors	Carbohydrate load, postexercise period, pregnancy, emotional stress, cold	Postexercise period, fasting, pregnancy, emotional stress, cold	During exercise, cold, pregnancy, emotional stress	"Warming up effect,"[a] postexercise period, emotional stress, pregnancy, anesthetics	"Warming up effect,"[a] postexercise period, emotional stress, pregnancy, anesthetics	Anesthetics, (increased prevalence in dystrophinopathies and central core myopathy)
Treatment	Potassium chloride, 0.25 mEq/kg PO (may repeat every 30 min until weakness subsides) Avoid IV potassium because of risk of uncontrollable hyperkalemia	Ingestion of glucose-rich carbohydrates Inhalation of a β-adrenergic agent (albuterol) Thiazide diuretic (eg, hydrochlorothiazide, 25 mg) may also abort an attack.	Glucose for severe cases Mexiletine for myotonia; begin 150 mg PO 2 times a day, to maximum of 1200 mg/day.	Mexiletine for myotonia; begin 150 mg PO 2 times a day, to maximum of 1200 mg/day. Phenytoin, 300 mg/day or quinine sulfate, 200–300 mg/day, is also useful.	Same as for myotonia congenita	Dantrolene Discontinuation of anesthesia Correction of acid-base disturbances Management of myoglobinuric renal failure
Prophylaxis	Acetazolamide; titrate up to 250 mg 3 times a day Dichlorphenamide, 25 mg 3 times a day Avoidance of precipitants	Acetazolamide; titrate up to 250 mg 3 times a day Avoidance of precipitants	Avoidance of precipitants	Avoidance of precipitants	Avoidance of precipitants	Avoidance of precipitants

CK = creatine kinase; PO = orally (by mouth); IV = intravenous.
[a] "Warming up effect" refers to myotonia that is worse on initiation of exercise, although ameliorated by the increasing vigor of movements.

accumulation of abnormal protein within them. These conditions can be distinguished from muscular dystrophies, which are caused by defects of the muscle membrane. Congenital myopathies usually manifest in infancy with delayed milestones or occur in the neonatal period (floppy infant syndrome) or, less commonly, in adulthood. They are usually familial, but sporadic cases do occur. Weakness may progress slowly or not at all. Cardiac involvement is present in some cases. Patients with central core myopathy, even in the absence of clinical weakness, are at risk for malignant hyperthermia during general anesthesia.

Table 23–12 summarizes clinical features and treatment of these disorders.

▼ MUSCULAR DYSTROPHIES

Muscular dystrophies are hereditary diseases that cause static or slowly progressive muscle weakness and characteristic histologic abnormalities, including extensive fibrosis, degeneration and regeneration of muscle, and proliferation of fatty and connective tissue. Weakness may be evident at birth or have a late adult onset.

Table 23–12. Congenital Myopathies: Clinical Findings and Treatment

	Central Core Myopathy	Nemaline Myopathy	Myotubular (Centronuclear) Myopathy
Inheritance	Autosomal dominant, with variable penetrance	Autosomal dominant, autosomal recessive, and sporadic	Three forms: • Neonatal X-linked recessive (most severe) • Late infantile–early childhood autosomal recessive • Late childhood–adult autosomal dominant
Clinical findings	Proximal weakness, hypotonia, absent reflexes, delayed milestones Up to one third of individuals with central cores have a normal examination Clubfeet, scoliosis, hip dislocation, and contractures of the fingers may be present Muscle cramps may occur after exercise	Six clinical forms, with ages of onset ranging from infancy to adulthood, and variable features—hypotonia, dysmorphism, skeletal abnormalities, including congenital dislocation of hip, cardiomyopathy, ophthalmoplegia, rigid spine, and dropped head sign	X-linked recessive neonatal form—severe hypotonia, weakness, poor suck and swallow, prominent respiratory failure; symptoms often present at birth Late infantile–early childhood form—mild to severely progressive course, with hypotonia, muscle weakness, delayed motor milestones, and skeletal abnormalities (long thin face, high-arched palate, scoliosis, club feet) Late childhood–adult form—mild limb-girdle weakness
Laboratory findings	Normal or slightly elevated serum CK level	Normal serum CK level Elevated ESR in adult form	Normal serum CK level
EMG findings	Normal or myopathic features	Myopathic features; as disease progresses, neurogenic features may be seen	Myopathic potentials, with abnormal spontaneous activity that may include bizarre high-frequency potentials and myotonia
Muscle biopsy findings	Well-circumscribed circular regions in center of most type 1 fibers	Modified trichrome stain shows dark-red-staining material in type 1 fibers that looks like short rods on longitudinal sections	Small myofibers with central nuclei resembling fetal myotubes
Treatment	Symptomatic; includes PT Avoid general anesthetic agents, especially halothane and succinylcholine Encourage patients to wear an identifying bracelet or necklace that indicates predisposition to malignant hyperthermia	Symptomatic; includes PT Orthopedic surgery to correct disabling deformities Susceptibility to malignant hyperthermia has been reported	Symptomatic; may include respiratory support and gastric feeding in addition to PT Orthopedic surgery may be required

CK = creatine kinase; EMG = Electromyography; ESR = erythrocyte sedimentation rate; PT = physical therapy.

CONGENITAL MUSCULAR DYSTROPHIES

ESSENTIALS OF DIAGNOSIS

► Weakness at birth

► Hypotonia

► Muscle biopsy evidence of changes consistent with muscular dystrophy

▶ General Considerations

Congenital muscular dystrophies can be separated into two groups: those associated with mental retardation and those associated with normal mental development. MRI is important for delineating the extent of central nervous system involvement and brain development. Table 23–13 contrasts the clinical features of these disorders. There is no specific treatment for the congenital muscular dystrophies, and management focuses on supportive care and rehabilitation therapy.

DUCHENNE MUSCULAR DYSTROPHY

ESSENTIALS OF DIAGNOSIS

► Typically affects males

► Positive family history (X-linked recessive inheritance)

► Onset before 5 years of age, with delayed motor milestones

► Proximal muscle weakness, positive Gowers sign, and calf muscle pseudohypertrophy (common)

► Elevated CK level (10-fold increase)

► Severely reduced or absent dystrophin in muscle biopsy or genetic testing provides definitive diagnosis

▶ General Considerations

Duchenne muscular dystrophy is the most common and severe form of childhood muscular dystrophy, with an incidence of 1 in 3500 male births. Most cases are X-linked recessive, although 30% involve spontaneous new mutations.

▶ Clinical Findings

A. Symptoms and Signs

No obvious abnormalities are seen at birth; however, delayed motor milestones may be apparent after the first year of life. Weakness progresses, causing children to fall frequently, and calves become enlarged (pseudohypertrophy). Contraction of Achilles tendons forces children to walk on their toes or on the balls of their feet. At this stage, patients employ Gowers maneuver to stand up from the floor: they rise from the floor by climbing up the thighs with their hands. Lordosis and severe scoliosis are common. Between the ages of 7 and 12 years, most patients lose their ability to walk and become wheelchair dependent. Mental retardation occurs in 10% of patients. Acute gastric dilation causing intestinal pseudo-obstruction may be present. Fatty infiltration of the heart and respiratory infections often lead to death, which typically occurs by the end of the second decade. Life-threatening vulnerability to malignant hyperthermia from anesthesia (halothane, succinylcholine) exists. Up to 8% of female carriers manifest mild proximal muscle weakness.

B. Laboratory and Diagnostic Findings

Most patients have abnormalities on electrocardiography. Striking elevation of CK level (> 50–100 times normal) is often seen in the first 3 years and may decline, although typically not below 10 times the upper limit of normal. EMG shows myopathic features, and muscle biopsy shows dystrophic changes. Diagnosis is confirmed by demonstrating severely reduced or absent dystrophin in a muscle biopsy specimen or a mutation in the dystrophin gene.

▶ Treatment

Prednisone, 0.75 mg/kg/day, can produce a significant increase in muscle strength and prolong ambulation up to 3 years. If side effects require it, a decrease in dosage as low as 0.3 mg/kg/day may still provide significant benefit. Deflazacort, 0.9 mg/kg/day, a new corticosteroid with potentially fewer side effects, may be preferred in countries in which it is available (currently this drug is not available in the United States). Physical therapy, bracing, orthoses, and orthopedic surgery are often required.

BECKER MUSCULAR DYSTROPHY

ESSENTIALS OF DIAGNOSIS

► Typically affects males

► Positive family history (X-linked recessive)

► Onset after 12 years of age

► Proximal muscle weakness and calf muscle pseudo-hypertrophy (common)

► Elevated CK level (at least fivefold)

► Muscle biopsy evidence of decreased or structurally abnormal dystrophin or genetic testing provides definitive diagnosis

Table 23-13. Congenital Muscular Dystrophies: Clinical and Laboratory Findings

	Disorders With Normal Mental Development		
	Merosin (Laminin-2)–Deficient CMD	Fukutin-Related Proteinopathy	Ullrich CMD
Inheritance	Autosomal recessive	Autosomal recessive	Autosomal recessive
Clinical findings	Variable severity. Onset at birth. Hypotonia, contractures, and respiratory and feeding difficulties	Similar to merosin-deficient CMD	Generalized muscle weakness, distal joint hyperextensibility, proximal contractures, kyphoscoliosis
CNS involvement	Abnormal white matter signal on MRI. Occipital pachygyria or agyria (5%)	Occasional structural abnormalities with cerebellar cysts	None
Laboratory findings	Serum CK level may be elevated. Almost-complete laminin-2 deficiency on IH/WB	Serum CK level may be elevated. α-Dystroglycan with diminished molecular weight on WB and secondary reductions in laminin-2 on IH/WB	Serum CK level may be elevated. Deficient collagen VI on IH

	Disorders With Abnormal Brain Development and Mental Retardation		
	Fukuyama CMD	Muscle-Eye-Brain Disease	Walker-Warburg Syndrome
Inheritance	Autosomal recessive (Japanese)	Autosomal recessive	Autosomal recessive
Clinical findings	Onset at birth. Hypotonia, poor swallowing, profound delay in motor development that precludes independent walking, seizures, severe mental retardation. Death by age 10 y	Similar to Fukuyama CMD, with additional ocular abnormalities (eg, retinal hypoplasia, ocular atrophy)	Severe weakness, ocular and CNS involvement. Lethal prenatally or within first years of life
CNS involvement	Lissencephaly, pachygyria, cerebellar hypoplasia	Similar to Fukuyama CMD, with additional eye malformations	Similar to Fukuyama CMD, with additional eye malformations, hydrocephalus, encephalocele, fusion of hemispheres, and absence of corpus callosum
Laboratory findings	Similar to Fukutin-related proteinopathy	Similar to Fukutin-related proteinopathy	Similar to Fukutin-related proteinopathy

CK = creatine kinase; CMD = congenital muscular dystrophy; CNS = central nervous system; IH = immunohistochemistry; MRI = magnetic resonance imaging; WB = Western blot. Adapted from Kirschner J, Bonnemann CG. The congenital and limb-girdle muscular dystrophies. *Arch Neurol* 2004;61:189–199.

This disorder is a milder allelic form of dystrophinopathy, with decreased or altered dystrophin rather than absence. Onset is usually after 12 years of age, and delayed onset after the fourth decade is occasionally seen. Limb-girdle weakness is typical, and cardiac involvement may occur. Mental retardation is rare. Life expectancy is reduced; however, most patients survive into the fourth or fifth decade. The clinical approach is similar to that in Duchenne muscular dystrophy.

MYOTONIC DYSTROPHY

ESSENTIALS OF DIAGNOSIS

▶ Variable onset from infancy to adult life

▶ Positive family history (autosomal-dominant inheritance)

▶ Weakness of facial, bulbar, and distal greater than proximal muscles

▶ Clinical myotonia (myotonia of grip or percussion myotonia)

▶ EMG evidence of myotonia

▶ Associated systemic problems (diabetes mellitus, cardiac arrhythmias, cataracts, frontal baldness, testicular atrophy)

▶ Genetic testing provides definitive diagnosis

▶ General Considerations

Myotonic dystrophy is the most prevalent form of muscular dystrophy in adults. It is a trinucleotide expansion disorder. Both myotonic dystrophy type 1 (DM1) and myotonic dystrophy type 2 (DM2) are transmitted by an autosomal-dominant inheritance. *DMPK* (dystrophia-myotonica protein kinase) gene on chromosome 19 is the gene affected in DM1, and *ZnFP9* (zinc finger protein 9) gene on chromosome 3 is the gene affected in DM2.

Trinucleotide repeats are found throughout the human genome and are normally stable through generations of the same pedigree. The number of repeats varies among healthy individuals, and their function is largely unknown. When expansion occurs, the DNA fragment becomes unstable, and above a critical threshold these expansions can be associated with disease.

A direct correlation exists between the number of trinucleotide repeats and the age of onset and severity of disease. This phenomenon is seen with succeeding generations, who experience this disease earlier and more severely due to the tendency for the expansion to grow during meiosis

(anticipation). Mothers with more than 100 repeats are at greater risk of having a child with the severe infantile form than are mothers with a smaller expansion. Because a marked increase in the trinucleotide repeat region seems to occur during maternal transmission, the mother is the parent affected in cases of congenital myotonic dystrophy (weakness present at birth).

▶ Clinical Findings

A. Symptoms and Signs

Onset of disease may occur in any decade, including the neonatal period. Slowly progressive weakness of facial and sternocleidomastoid muscles occurs in association with frontal balding, ptosis, and temporalis wasting that produces a hatchet-faced appearance. Bulbar and neck muscle weakness is often present. Unlike most myopathies, this disease tends to affect distal muscles more severely than proximal muscles, and patients typically develop hand weakness and foot drops. Myotonia is a characteristic finding and can be elicited by percussion of the thenar muscles or tongue; a sustained involuntary contraction is seen. Most patients have cardiac involvement (heart block and cardiomyopathy), raising the risk of sudden death. Diaphragmatic and intercostal muscle weakness, insulin resistance, hypogonadism, and cataracts also occur, and hypersomnia is common. Nausea, vomiting, and early satiety may be a result of slow gastric emptying.

B. Laboratory and Diagnostic Findings

The serum CK level may be normal or mildly elevated (threefold). Up to 90% of patients have electrocardiographic abnormalities. EMG shows myotonic discharges and myopathic features. Serum glucose may be elevated, and slit-lamp examinations may be required to detect cataracts. DNA analysis (including prenatal) provides definitive diagnosis. Genetic counseling is important.

▶ Treatment

No specific treatment is available other than for the management of complicating systemic disease. Orthotic devices are helpful as are drugs to suppress myotonia, such as phenytoin, 300 mg/day. Phenytoin is preferred to quinine and procainamide in the treatment of myotonic dystrophy because it has fewer adverse effects on cardiac conduction. Careful follow-up of patients with cardiac conduction abnormalities is warranted, and pacemaker insertion may eventually become necessary. Patients with myotonic dystrophy are at risk for developing malignant hyperthermia during anesthesia.

FASCIOSCAPULOHUMERAL DYSTROPHY

ESSENTIALS OF DIAGNOSIS

- ▶ Positive family history (autosomal-dominant inheritance); occasional sporadic cases
- ▶ Onset of disease in facial or shoulder-girdle muscles, with weakness and wasting
- ▶ Variable involvement of humeral, hip-girdle, and distal leg muscles
- ▶ Usually asymmetric at onset
- ▶ Muscle biopsy evidence of nonspecific muscular dystrophy
- ▶ Genetic testing provides definitive diagnosis

▶ General Considerations

Fascioscapulohumeral dystrophy (FSHD) is an autosomal-dominant disorder, although sporadic cases occur. It has an estimated prevalence of 1 in 20,000 people. FSHD is usually slowly progressive and can be extremely variable in its severity and age of onset (infancy to middle age). Extramuscular manifestations occur with variable frequency and include mental impairment, hearing loss, retinal vasculopathy, and cardiac involvement. About 85–95% of patients with clinically defined FSHD have a demonstrable 4q35 deletion, but the gene or genes that are affected in FSHD are still unknown.

▶ Clinical Findings

A. Symptoms and Signs

Onset usually occurs in childhood or adolescence but can be delayed until the fifth decade. Weakness preferentially affects the facial and shoulder-girdle muscles. Patients are typically unable to whistle, smile, or fully close their eyes, and some are said to sleep with their eyes open. Extraocular muscles are typically spared. Scapular winging is common and becomes more evident when the patient attempts to elevate the arms laterally. Pelvic-girdle weakness is present in approximately 20% of patients; however, the anterior compartment (anterior tibialis and peroneus muscles) is more often affected (scapuloperoneal variety). Respiratory insufficiency is rare, and most patients have a normal life expectancy.

B. Laboratory and Diagnostic Findings

The serum CK level may be normal or mildly elevated, and EMG shows myopathic features. Muscle biopsy evidence is nonspecific, with myopathic changes and variable inflammation. Genetic testing to confirm the diagnosis is available.

▶ Treatment

Treatment is symptomatic, consisting of orthotic devices, braces, walking aids that may include a wheelchair, and physical therapy. Scapular fixation surgery may be beneficial.

Moxely RT, et al. Practice parameter: Corticosteroid treatment of Duchenne dystrophy. *Neurology* 2005;64:13–20. [PMID: 15642897] (Practice parameter on corticosteroid treatment of Duchenne dystrophy by the American Academy of Neurology and Child Neurology Society.)

Mummery CJ, Copeland SA, Rose MR. Scapular fixation in muscular dystrophy. *Cochrane Database Syst Rev* 2003;3:CD003278. [PMID: 12917959]

LIMB-GIRDLE MUSCULAR DYSTROPHY

ESSENTIALS OF DIAGNOSIS

- ▶ Positive family history (autosomal-dominant or autosomal-recessive inheritance)
- ▶ Onset of weakness and wasting in pelvic or shoulder-girdle muscles
- ▶ Elevated serum CK level in recessive cases
- ▶ Muscle biopsy evidence of lack of staining for the particular proteins (sarcoglycans, calpain, dysferlin, or caveolin)
- ▶ Genetic testing, when available, provides definitive diagnosis

▶ General Considerations

The term *limb-girdle muscular dystrophy* is reserved for noncongenital muscular dystrophies not due to dystrophin deficiency with progressive proximal weakness. Autosomal-dominant (LGMD-1) and autosomal-recessive (LGMD-2) forms exist, and increasing numbers of distinct forms continue to be described. These disorders are caused by different protein deficiencies, such as the sarcogylcans (dystrophin-associated proteins), calpain, dysferlin, and caveolin.

▶ Clinical Findings

A. Symptoms and Signs

Onset may occur in early childhood or adulthood. Progression and distribution of weakness is equally variable among patients and genetic subtypes. Slowly progressive pelvic and shoulder-girdle weakness is often seen, and cardiomyopathy can occur. Calf pseudohypertrophy is a frequent but not invariable finding, and early contractures may be seen in some autosomal-dominant forms. Considerable clinical overlap with the dystrophinopathies may occur.

B. Laboratory and Diagnostic Findings

The serum CK level is often elevated, especially in dysferlinopathies (LGMD-2B), in which it tends to be very high. Muscle biopsy with special staining for sarcoglycan, calpain, dysferlin, and caveolin may help distinguish these disorders. Mutation analysis is not commercially available for most of these disorders, and the correlation between clinical phenotype and the gene mutations is not robust.

▶ **Treatment**

Treatment of these disorders is symptomatic.

Kirschner J, Bonnemann CG. The congenital and limb-girdle muscular dystrophies. *Arch Neurol* 2004;61:189–199. [PMID: 14967765] (A detailed review of limb-girdle and congenital dystrophies, with emphasis on the molecular genetics and clinical phenotypes.)

EMERY-DREIFUSS MUSCULAR DYSTROPHY

ESSENTIALS OF DIAGNOSIS

▶ Positive family history (X-linked recessive inheritance)

▶ Prominent early contractures

▶ Weakness and atrophy of humeral and peroneal muscles

▶ Cardiac conduction defects and cardiomyopathy

▶ Genetic testing provides definitive diagnosis

Emery-Dreifuss muscular dystrophy is an X-linked recessive disease that typically presents in early childhood and adolescence. The classic triad of symptoms consists of prominent early contractures (elbows, fingers, knees, ankles, and spine), weakness and atrophy of humeral and peroneal muscles, and

cardiac conduction defects that can lead to syncope or sudden death. The serum CK level may be elevated, and muscle biopsy specimens show nonspecific dystrophic changes. DNA or gene product (emerin) analysis is needed for precise diagnosis. Cardiac surveillance and timely pacemaker insertion is an essential part of disease management. Treatment is otherwise symptomatic.

OCULOPHARYNGEAL MUSCULAR DYSTROPHY

ESSENTIALS OF DIAGNOSIS

▶ Positive family history (autosomal-dominant inheritance)

▶ Late onset (fourth to sixth decade)

▶ Ptosis

▶ Dysphagia

▶ Ophthalmoplegia and mild proximal weakness, later in the disease course

▶ Genetic testing provides definitive diagnosis

Oculopharyngeal muscular dystrophy is an autosomal-dominant disorder with onset in the fourth to sixth decade. It is caused by GCG repeat expansions in exon 1 of the poly(A) binding protein 2 gene (*PABP2*).

Clinical features include ptosis, dysphagia, and mild proximal limb weakness. Extraocular muscle weakness is variable, and this disorder must be distinguished from myasthenia gravis and other disorders with progressive external ophthalmoplegia. The serum CK level may be normal or mildly elevated, and EMG may reveal myopathic features. Muscle biopsy findings typically show rimmed vacuoles and tubular filaments within nuclei. Treatment is symptomatic, requiring special glasses or surgical correction for ptosis, and when severe, cricopharyngeal myotomy for dysphagia.

Fan X, Rouleau GA. Progress in understanding the pathogenesis of oculopharyngeal muscular dystrophy. *Can J Neurol Sci* 2003;30:8–14. [PMID: 12619777]

Mitochondrial Diseases

24

Michio Hirano, MD

▶ General Considerations

Mitochondria are essential cellular organelles that convert metabolites of carbohydrates, lipids, and proteins into a usable form of energy—adenosine triphosphate (ATP). By convention, the term *mitochondrial diseases* refers to disorders caused by defects in the respiratory chain, the terminal mitochondrial pathway responsible for generating ATP; oxidative phosphorylation; or both.

In mammals, respiratory chain enzymes are unique because they are the products of two genomes—nuclear DNA (nDNA) and mitochondrial DNA (mtDNA). The dual genetic origin of the respiratory chain contributes to the clinical heterogeneity of mitochondrial diseases. Because of their phenotypic diversity and complex multisystemic presentations, mitochondrial diseases can be difficult to diagnose. Most often, mitochondrial diseases affect brain and skeletal muscle and are therefore called *mitochondrial encephalomyopathies* (Table 24–1). Central nervous system manifestations of mitochondrial diseases include dementia, strokes at a young age, seizures, myoclonus, migraine-like headaches, optic neuropathy, and hearing loss. Myopathic involvement often presents as ptosis and progressive ophthalmoparesis, oropharyngeal weakness, and limb myopathy. Endocrinopathies and cardiopathies are common in mitochondrial diseases. Gastrointestinal, hematologic, renal, and psychiatric manifestations are also observed.

A. Biochemical Functions of Mitochondria

Mitochondria perform multiple biochemical functions, including breakdown of fatty acids through β-oxidation and catabolism of pyruvate derived from glycogen via the Krebs or citric acid cycle (Figure 24–1). These two metabolic pathways liberate electrons that are transported through four respiratory chain enzymes (complexes I–IV) embedded within the inner membrane of mitochondria. The transport of electrons through these enzyme complexes generates, across the inner membrane, a proton gradient that drives the synthesis of ATP at complex V (oxidation-phosphorylation).

B. Genetics of Mitochondrial Disorders

According to the endosymbiont hypothesis, mitochondria evolved from protobacteria that carried not only the capacity to generate ATP by oxidative phosphorylation, but also genetic material that has evolved into mtDNA. MtDNA is a small (16,569 base-pair) circular molecule that contains only 37 genes (encoding 13 polypeptides, 22 transfer RNAs [tRNAs], and 2 ribosomal RNAs [rRNAs]). All of the mtDNA-encoded genes as well as an even larger number of nDNA genes are required to maintain normal respiratory chain function; therefore, mutations in either genome can cause mitochondrial diseases.

MtDNA does not conform to the same rules of inheritance that govern nDNA. An important principle of mtDNA genetics is **heteroplasmy**. Each mitochondrion contains 2–10 copies of mtDNA, and in turn each cell contains multiple mitochondria; therefore, there are numerous copies of mtDNA in each cell. Alterations of mtDNA may be present in some of the mtDNA molecules (heteroplasmy) or in all of the molecules (homoplasmy). As a consequence of heteroplasmy, the proportion of a deleterious mtDNA mutation can vary widely. An individual who harbors a large proportion of mutant mtDNA will be more severely afflicted by the mitochondrial dysfunction than a person with a low percentage of the same mutation;

Table 24–1. Typical Features of Mitochondrial Diseases

Central Nervous System	**Cardiac**
Migraine headaches	Hypertrophic cardiomyopathy
Sensorineural hearing loss	Cardiac conduction block
Seizures	**Gastrointestinal**
Cognitive dysfunction	Dysphagia
Ataxia	Gastroparesis
Myoclonus	Intestinal pseudo-obstruction
Extrapyramidal signs	Hepatopathy
Ophthalmologic (optic atrophy, pigmentary retinopathy)	**Endocrine**
Neuromuscular	Diabetes mellitus
Progressive external	Growth hormone deficiency
ophthalmoplegia (PEO)	Hypothyroidism
Ptosis	Hypoparathyroidism
Exercise intolerance	**Renal**
Peripheral neuropathy	Tubular acidosis
Psychiatric	Steroid-resistant nephrotic syndrome
Affective disorders	
Schizophrenia-like symptoms	

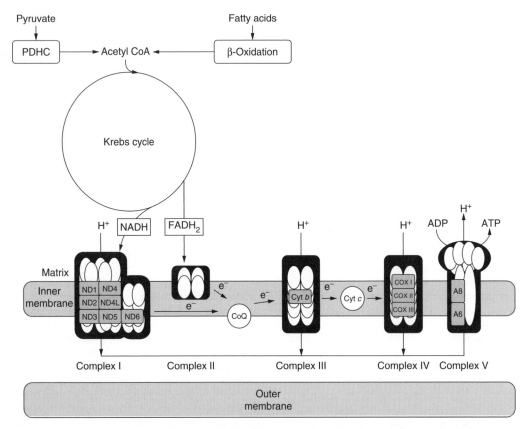

▲ **Figure 24–1.** Schematic representation of mitochondrial metabolism. Respiratory chain components or complexes encoded by nuclear DNA are white ovals; subunits encoded by mitochondrial DNA are gray rectangles. ADP = adenosine diphosphate; ATP = adenosine triphosphate; CoA = coenzyme A; CoQ = coenzyme Q; Cyt b and c = cytochrome b and c; FADH$_2$ = flavin adenine dinucleotide (reduced form); NADH = nicotinamide adenine dinucleotide (reduced form); PDHC = pyruvate dehydrogenase complex; I, II, III, IV, V = respiratory chain enzyme complexes.

therefore, there is a spectrum of clinical severity among patients with a given mitochondrial mutation.

A second factor that can influence the expression of mtDNA defects in a person is the **tissue distribution** of that mutation. The best example of tissue distribution variation is large-scale mtDNA deletions. Infants with a high proportion of deleted mtDNA in blood can develop Pearson syndrome of sideroblastic anemia, often accompanied by exocrine pancreatic dysfunction. Presumably, these infants have a high proportion of deleted mtDNA in bone marrow stem cells. Some children survive the anemia with blood transfusions and subsequently recover because the stem cells with a high proportion of deleted mtDNA are under a negative selection bias. Later in life, however, those children may develop Kearns-Sayre syndrome (KSS), a multisystem mitochondrial disorder, characterized by ophthalmoplegia, pigmentary retinopathy, and cardiac conduction block. Thus, variable tissue distribution broadens the clinical spectrum of pathogenic mtDNA mutations.

The third factor that determines clinical manifestations of mtDNA mutation is tissue **threshold effect**. Cells with high metabolic activities are severely and adversely affected by mtDNA mutations; therefore, these disorders tend to affect disproportionately brain and muscle.

A fourth unusual characteristic of mtDNA is **maternal inheritance**. During the formation of the zygote, the mtDNA is derived exclusively from the oocyte. Thus, mtDNA is transmitted vertically in a nonmendelian fashion from the mother to both male and female progeny. This inheritance pattern is important to recognize in determining whether a family is likely to harbor mtDNA mutations. A caveat to this principle is the fact that maternal relatives who have a lower percentage of the mtDNA mutation may have fewer symptoms (oligosymptomatic) than the proband, or they may even be asymptomatic.

DiMauro S, Schon EA. Mitochondrial disorders in the nervous system. *Annu Rev Neurosci* 2008;31:91–123. [PMID: 18333761] (An excellent overview of mitochondrial diseases.)

▶ Epidemiology

Epidemiologic evidence suggests that the mitochondrial diseases caused by mtDNA mutations are not rare and that the prevalence of mitochondrial diseases caused by nDNA mutations is probably higher than that of mtDNA defects. In fact, in western Sweden, based on a combination of biochemical, histologic, and genetic criteria, the prevalence of mitochondrial diseases in preschool children was estimated at 1 case in 11,000. A similar prevalence, 1 in 10,800, of symptomatic adults with mtDNA mutations has been observed in adults in the northeast of England.

Schaefer AM, et al. Prevalence of mitochondrial DNA disease in adults. *Ann Neurol* 2008;63(1):35–39. [PMID: 17886296] (Nicely reviews current knowledge regarding the epidemiology of mitochondrial diseases in adults.)

▼ MITOCHONDRIAL DNA MUTATIONS

To date, more than 200 distinct point mutations and hundreds of deletions of mtDNA have been identified. Because of this diversity of mtDNA mutations, as well as heteroplasmy and tissue distribution, the associated clinical phenotypes are heterogeneous. Nevertheless, specific clinically recognizable syndromes occur frequently.

KEARNS-SAYRE SYNDROME & CHRONIC PROGRESSIVE EXTERNAL OPHTHALMOPLEGIA

ESSENTIALS OF DIAGNOSIS

Kearns-Sayre Syndrome (KSS)
- ▶ Ophthalmoparesis and ptosis
- ▶ Pigmentary retinopathy
- ▶ Onset before age 20, plus at least one of the following—cardiac conduction block, ataxia, increased CSF protein
- ▶ Muscle biopsy demonstrating ragged-red fibers, identification of a single deletion of mtDNA, or both

Chronic Progressive External Ophthalmoplegia (CPEO)
- ▶ Ophthalmoparesis and ptosis
- ▶ Variable involvement of facial, oropharyngeal, and limb muscles
- ▶ Muscle biopsy demonstrating ragged-red fibers, identification of a single deletion of mtDNA, or both

▶ General Considerations

Ptosis and ophthalmoparesis are the central features of CPEO and KSS, a more severe multisystemic disorder. The incidences of these conditions are unknown; however, hundreds of cases have been reported.

▶ Clinical Findings

CPEO is a pure myopathy characterized by weakness of extraocular muscle manifesting as ptosis and ophthalmoparesis. Other muscles may be affected, causing weakness of the face, oropharynx, and limbs. In contrast, KSS is a multisystem disorder with juvenile or young-adult onset that produces extraocular muscle weakness, pigmentary degeneration of the retina, and variable combinations of cardiac conduction block, elevated CSF protein concentration (> 100 mg/dL), and cerebellar ataxia. Patients with KSS are often short and thin and may have diabetes mellitus, hypoparathyroidism, cardiomyopathy, and renal disease. Typically, the disorder is sporadic and is caused by a single large-scale deletion of mtDNA. The mtDNA mutation is rarely detectable in blood; muscle biopsy is therefore necessary to screen for ragged-red fibers and to identify the molecular defect.

Differential Diagnosis

KSS and CPEO must be differentiated from other disorders that cause ophthalmoparesis, such as myasthenia gravis, oculopharyngeal myopathy, myotonic dystrophy, and other mitochondrial myopathies with progressive external ophthalmoplegia (PEO), including autosomal-dominant or autosomal-recessive variants (see later discussion).

Treatment

Management of these disorders is symptomatic. Cardiac conduction block is present in most patients with KSS, and progression to a complete heart block can cause death; therefore, placement of a cardiac pacemaker can be lifesaving. Surgical correction of ptosis can be functionally and cosmetically beneficial. Prism eyeglasses can alleviate diplopia. Coenzyme Q_{10}, 50–200 mg three times a day, and L-carnitine, 300–1000 mg three times a day, have been used to improve mitochondrial function. Antioxidants, including vitamins A, C, and E; β-carotene; and α-lipoic acid have been used without clear objective benefits. Patients often take B-complex vitamins, as they are cofactors for several mitochondrial enzymes. Because deficiency of cerebral folate has been observed in KSS, folinic acid has been administered and ataxia improved in at least one patient.

Prognosis

The prognosis for patients with KSS or CPEO is difficult to determine because of the variable tissue distribution of deleted mtDNA in both disorders. Severe central nervous system involvement can cause debilitating ataxia, mental impairment, and spasticity. Retinal pigmentary degeneration causes loss of vision, particularly loss of night (dim light) vision. Dysphagia due to pharyngeal and upper esophageal pathology is a common complication.

MELAS SYNDROME

ESSENTIALS OF DIAGNOSIS

▶ Stroke-like episodes typically before age 40
▶ Encephalopathy manifesting as dementia, seizures, or both
▶ Mitochondrial dysfunction evident as lactic acidosis, ragged-red fibers in muscle, or both
▶ Identification of a pathogenic mtDNA mutation

General Considerations

MELAS (mitochondrial encephalomyopathy, lactic acidosis, and stroke-like episodes) syndrome is a maternally inherited disorder that is clinically defined by the following features:
(1) stroke-like episodes occurring at a young age (typically before age 40); (2) encephalopathy manifesting as seizures, dementia, or both; and (3) mitochondrial dysfunction as evidenced by lactic acidosis, ragged-red fibers, or both. The incidence of MELAS syndrome is uncertain; the prevalence of the most common MELAS mtDNA mutation ranges from 1.4–236 per 100,000 people.

Pathogenesis

The mtDNA m.3243A>G mutation in the $tRNA^{Leu(UUR)}$ gene has been identified in about 80% of patients with MELAS syndrome. At least 29 additional mtDNA point mutations have been identified as causes of MELAS. Most of the MELAS-associated mtDNA mutations are in tRNA genes and therefore impair mitochondrial protein synthesis. The cause of the stroke-like episodes is unknown. Small arterioles and capillaries in the brains of patients with MELAS have an overabundance of mitochondria, which may impair blood flow, autoregulation, or both. Alternatively, the stroke-like episodes may be due to metabolic disarray in neurons.

Clinical Findings

In addition to the previously listed findings, which distinguish MELAS syndrome, at least two of the following clinical features should be present: normal early development, recurrent headaches, or recurrent vomiting. Other commonly encountered manifestations include myopathic weakness, exercise intolerance, myoclonus, ataxia, short stature, and hearing loss. It is uncommon for more than one family member to have the full MELAS syndrome; in most pedigrees, maternal relatives of a MELAS patient are oligosymptomatic or asymptomatic.

Although in patients with MELAS syndrome the stroke-like episodes can be clinically indistinguishable from ischemic strokes, magnetic resonance imaging of the brain in these patients typically shows cortical lesions that do not conform to territories supplied by a large vessel. The presence of lactic acidosis and muscle biopsy showing ragged-red fibers provides evidence of mitochondrial dysfunction. Usually, the diagnosis can be confirmed by identification of a pathogenic mtDNA mutation in blood.

Differential Diagnosis

When a patient with MELAS presents with an acute stroke-like episode, the differential diagnosis includes other causes of stroke in a young person: heart disease, carotid or vertebral artery disorders, sickle cell anemia, vasculopathies, lipoprotein disorders, cancer, venous thrombosis, moyamoya disease, complicated migraine, and homocystinuria. Because there is often an antecedent history of migraine headache and of headache with the acute stroke, patients with mitochondrial myopathy, encephalopathy, lactic acidosis, and stroke-like episodes might be diagnosed as having migraine with prolonged aura, basilar migraine, or hemiplegic migraine.

Treatment

No treatment for the genetic defect is available. Anecdotal reports suggest that corticosteroids may be beneficial in treating acute strokes in patients with MELAS syndrome. Seizures respond to conventional anticonvulsant therapy; most clinicians avoid valproic acid because this drug may cause carnitine deficiency. Aggressive treatment of epilepsy in MELAS syndrome is recommended, because the acute metabolic stress of seizures may cause neuronal injury. Hearing loss caused by isolated cochlear dysfunction has been successfully treated with cochlear implantation. Nutritional supplements similar to those used in KSS and CPEO are often taken by patients with MELAS syndrome. Open-label pilot studies suggest that L-arginine may reduce the severity of acute strokes and recurrence of strokes in MELAS.

MERRF SYNDROME

ESSENTIALS OF DIAGNOSIS

▶ Myoclonus
▶ Epilepsy
▶ Ataxia
▶ Muscle biopsy demonstrating ragged-red fibers or identification of a pathogenic mtDNA mutation

General Considerations

MERRF (myoclonus with epilepsy and ragged-red fibers) syndrome is maternally inherited. The incidence is unknown; however, the prevalence of the most common MERRF mutation is probably less than 1 case in 100,000 people.

Clinical Findings

The disease is defined by myoclonus, seizures, ataxia, and the presence of ragged-red fibers on muscle biopsy. Other common clinical manifestations are hearing loss, dementia, peripheral neuropathy, short stature, exercise intolerance, lipomas, and lactic acidosis.

Although most patients with MERRF syndrome have a history of affected maternally related family members, not all may have the full syndrome. The diagnosis is typically confirmed by identifying a pathogenic mtDNA mutation in a blood sample. An A-to-G mutation at nucleotide 8344 (m.8344A>G) of the mtDNA $tRNA^{Lys}$ gene has been found in about 80% of MERRF patients tested. Other mtDNA mutations have been identified.

Differential Diagnosis

The differential diagnosis of syndromes characterized by myoclonus, epilepsy, and ataxia includes Unverricht-Lundborg disease, Lafora body disease, neuronal ceroid lipofuscinosis, and sialidosis.

Treatment

The seizures of MERRF can be treated with conventional anticonvulsant therapy. No controlled studies have compared the efficacy of different antiepilepsy regimens. Patients usually take nutritional supplements, as previously described for KSS and CPEO.

NARP SYNDROME & MATERNALLY INHERITED LEIGH SYNDROME

ESSENTIALS OF DIAGNOSIS

Neuropathy, Ataxia, and Retinitis Pigmentosa (NARP) Syndrome
▶ Peripheral neuropathy
▶ Ataxia
▶ Retinitis pigmentosa
▶ Identification of a pathogenic mtDNA mutation
Maternally Inherited Leigh Syndrome (MILS)
▶ Maternal inheritance
▶ Subacute encephalopathy affecting deep gray matter structures
▶ Evidence of mitochondrial dysfunction (defect of respiratory chain activity and mtDNA mutation)

Clinical Findings

Patients with NARP syndrome have peripheral neuropathy that usually affects sensory more than motor nerves. In contrast to MELAS and MERRF syndromes, which result from mtDNA point mutations in tRNA genes and are therefore disorders of mitochondrial protein synthesis, NARP results from mtDNA point mutations in a polypeptide coding gene, subunit 6 of complex V (*ATPase 6*). Most patients with these syndromes harbor either an m.8993T>G or m.8993T>C mutation in the *ATPase 6* gene. In NARP patients, the heteroplasmic level is 70–90%, whereas individuals with the more severe MILS phenotype have greater than 90% mutation, demonstrating a clear relationship between mutation load and clinical phenotype. Curiously, in NARP patients, skeletal muscle biopsies do not show ragged-red fibers, which are typically seen in MELAS and MERRF.

Infants or young children with very high proportions of the NARP *ATPase 6* mutations (eg, > 90%) will develop MILS, a devastating encephalomyopathy characterized by psychomotor regression, seizures, lactic acidosis, and subacute necrotizing lesions in the basal ganglia and other midline gray matter structures in the brain and brainstem. Magnetic resonance imaging of the brain reveals characteristic symmetric lesions of the periaqueductal region of the midbrain and pons and in the medulla adjacent to the fourth ventricle. Other parts of the central nervous system and peripheral nerves may also be affected. The lesions are a combination of cell necrosis, demyelination, and vascular proliferation.

The incidences of NARP and MILS are unknown. The prevalence of these mtDNA mutations appears to be less than 1 case in 100,000 adults.

Differential Diagnosis

The differential diagnosis of NARP includes Refsum disease, abetalipoproteinemia, and other mitochondrial diseases. MILS resulting from an *ATPase 6* mutation must be distinguished from other forms of Leigh syndrome (see later discussion).

Treatment & Prognosis

Treatment of these syndromes is limited to symptomatic therapy and nutritional supplements. Similar to other diseases caused by mtDNA mutations, the prognosis in NARP and MILS depends on the level of heteroplasmy; hence, patients with MILS have a worse outcome than those with NARP.

LEBER HEREDITARY OPTIC NEUROPATHY

ESSENTIALS OF DIAGNOSIS

► Subacute painless optic neuropathy
► Maternal inheritance
► Peripapillary telangiectasias and cardiac preexcitation (frequently present)
► Identification of a pathogenic mtDNA mutation in most patients

General Considerations

Leber hereditary optic neuropathy (LHON) is another maternally inherited disorder that curiously affects men (60–90%) more than women. Penetrance rates of the LHON mutations are uncertain; however, some reports estimate that symptoms appear in 20–83% of men and 4–32% of women at risk.

Three point mutations of mtDNA, all in genes encoding subunits of complex I, cause approximately 90% of LHON cases. The most common LHON mutation is an A-to-G transition at nucleotide 11778 (A11778G) in the gene encoding subunit 4 of complex I (NADH dehydrogenase 4; *ND4*). The other two mutations are G3460A in *ND1* and T14484C. In most LHON patients, the mtDNA mutations are homoplasmic.

In the northeast of England, the minimum point prevalence of vision loss resulting from LHON was estimated to be 3.2 per 100,000 adults, whereas the point prevalence of the

three most frequent LHON mutations was 11.8 per 100,000 adults. Thus, LHON may be the most common genetic mitochondrial disease.

Clinical Findings

LHON usually presents as subacute to acute loss of central or cecocentral vision as a result of a painless optic neuropathy in one eye followed by loss of vision in the other eye weeks or months later. The age at onset is typically 18–35 years. The presence of tortuous blood vessels adjacent to the optic nerve (peripapillary telangiectasias) can be a clue to the diagnosis. Wolff-Parkinson-White cardiac preexcitation is often observed in LHON patients. Skeletal muscle is not affected clinically and, accordingly, ragged-red fibers are not observed.

Differential Diagnosis

LHON must be distinguished from other forms of bilateral optic neuropathy, including demyelinating disease, toxic-nutritional optic neuropathy, autosomal-dominant or autosomal-recessive optic neuropathy, glaucoma, ischemic optic neuropathy, and compressive lesions.

Treatment & Prognosis

No treatment is of proven value. Antioxidants and other nutritional supplements are frequently used. Unaffected carriers of LHON mutation are generally counseled to avoid tobacco and alcohol use.

Vision loss in LHON may be severe and generally remains stable. In a minority of patients, there is later improvement, which is usually mild. The probability of improvement varies with the particular LHON mutation.

SPORADIC EXERCISE INTOLERANCE

ESSENTIALS OF DIAGNOSIS

► Exercise intolerance with normal cardiac and pulmonary functions
► Recurrent myoglobinuria or weakness
► Absence of family history
► Mitochondrial dysfunction evident as ragged-red fibers, lactic acidosis, respiratory chain enzyme defect, or mtDNA mutation

An expanding group of mtDNA mutations in protein-coding genes is associated with pure skeletal myopathies that present with exercise intolerance and, in some cases, weakness, myoglobinuria, or both. The mtDNA mutations are isolated to skeletal muscle and are not present in matrilineal relatives of patients, indicating an origin in somatic tissues, probably early in embryogenesis. The incidence of sporadic exercise intolerance due to mtDNA mutation is unknown but is probably very low.

MtDNA mutations in polypeptide-coding genes, particularly cytochrome *b*, have been identified in skeletal muscle of patients with exercise intolerance. Patients with exercise intolerance due to mtDNA mutation may develop fixed muscle weakness or, rarely, manifestations in other tissues, depending on the distribution of the genetic defect.

Diagnostic considerations include other metabolic myopathies, hypothyroidism, muscular dystrophies, inflammatory myopathies, chronic fatigue syndrome, fibromyalgia, and depression.

As with other mitochondrial diseases, treatment is limited to symptomatic therapies (eg, avoiding strenuous exercise that may provoke myoglobinuria) and nutritional supplements.

Carelli V, et al. Retinal ganglion cell neurodegeneration in mitochondrial inherited disorders. *Biochim Biophys Acta* 2009; 1787(5):518–528. [PMID: 19268652] (A comprehensive review of mitochondrial optic neuropathies, including LHON.)

Hirano M. Kearns-Sayre syndrome. In: Gilman S, ed. Medlink. Available at: http://www.medlink.com. Accessed November 30, 2010.

Hirano M. MELAS. In: Gilman S, ed. Medlink. Available at: http://www.medlink.com. Accessed November 30, 2010.

Hirano M. Myoclonus epilepsy ragged-red fibers. In: Gilman S, ed. Medlink. Available at: http://www.medlink.com. Accessed November 30, 2010.

NUCLEAR DNA MUTATIONS

The vast majority of the proteins in mitochondria are encoded in nDNA; therefore, it is not surprising that nDNA mutations cause many mitochondrial diseases. As a general rule, symptoms begin in infancy or childhood (Table 24–2). The most common clinical presentation is Leigh syndrome. Clinical manifestations may be tissue specific or generalized. Diagnosis depends on the clinical findings plus biochemical and DNA analyses.

Mutations encoding structural subunits of complexes I–V have been identified in a small number of patients, mainly those with Leigh syndrome (see Table 24–2). Autosomal-recessive Leigh syndrome or other encephalomyopathies are also associated with deficiency of complex I–V due to defects in genes encoding assembly factors for these enzymes.

A growing number of autosomal diseases, defects of intergenomic communication, have been associated with mtDNA depletion and multiple deletions. Autosomal-dominant or autosomal-recessive PEO with multiple mtDNA deletions is characterized by ptosis and progressive ophthalmoplegia, beginning in early adulthood, and are most commonly due to mutations in the *POLG* gene encoding mtDNA polymerase gamma. *POLG* mutations also cause other clinical phenotypes, including sensory ataxic neuropathy dysarthria neuropathy ophthalmoplegia

(SANDO), autosomal-recessive ataxia, and the severe infantile-onset hepatocerebral disorder called Alpers syndrome, which is associated with the depletion of mtDNA. In addition to hepatocerebral diseases, mtDNA depletion syndrome may present as a pure myopathy or spinal muscular-atrophy–like disorder. Mitochondrial neurogastrointestinal encephalomyopathy (MNGIE) is an autosomal-recessive disorder manifesting as ptosis, PEO, severe gastrointestinal dysmotility, cachexia, peripheral neuropathy, and leukoencephalopathy; it is associated with depletion, multiple deletions, and point mutations of mtDNA. MNGIE is caused by mutations in the gene encoding thymidine phosphorylase, a cytosolic enzyme that contributes to the regulation of nucleotide pools in the mitochondria. Deficiency of coenzyme Q_{10} (CoQ_{10}) has been associated with infantile-onset multisystemic diseases (mainly encephalopathy and kidney disease), cerebellar ataxias, and encephalomyopathies. Primary CoQ_{10} deficiencies are due to mutation in nuclear DNA genes required for CoQ_{10} biosynthesis, while secondary forms are due to mutations in other genes. Both primary and secondary CoQ_{10} deficiencies are important to recognize, because the disorders often improve with CoQ_{10} supplementation.

Quinzii CM, Hirano M. Coenzyme Q and mitochondrial disease. *Dev Disabil Res Rev* 2010;16(2):183–188. [PMID: 20818733] (A review of primary and secondary CoQ_{10} deficiencies.)

Saneto RP, Naviaux RK. Polymerase gamma disease through the ages. *Dev Disabil Res Rev* 2010;16(2):163–174. [PMID: 20818731] (A review of the spectrum of diseases associated with *POLG* mutations, which are the most frequent autosomal causes of mitochondrial disorders.)

Zeviani M, Lamperti C, DiMauro. Disorders of nuclear-mitochondrial intergenomic signaling. In: Gilman S, ed. Medlink. Available at: http://www.medlink.com. Accessed November 30, 2010. (A summary of the autosomal disorders with pathogenic instability of mtDNA.)

OTHER MITOCHONDRIAL DISORDERS

NUCLEOSIDE REVERSE-TRANSCRIPTASE INHIBITOR–INDUCED MYOPATHY

A rare iatrogenic form of mtDNA depletion has been observed in patients with HIV. These patients developed myopathy with ragged-red fibers while receiving zidovudine (AZT), a nucleoside reverse-transcriptase inhibitor that inhibits polymerase gamma. The manifestations resolve after discontinuation of the drug.

Koczor CA, Lewis W. Nucleoside reverse transcriptase inhibitor toxicity and mitochondrial DNA. *Expert Opin Drug Metab Toxicol* 2010;6:1493–1504. [PMID: 20929279] (A review of the mitochondrial toxicity of nucleoside reverse transcriptase inhibitors.)

Table 24-2. Clinical Syndromes Associated With Nuclear DNA Mutations

Syndrome	Clinical Findings
Leigh syndrome	Onset typically in infancy or childhood, but can occur in adulthood
• Infantile onset	Typically occurs before age 6 mo in a previously normal infant Developmental arrest or regression, hypotonia, feeding difficulty, respiratory abnormalities, vision loss, oculomotor palsies, and nystagmus MRI scan of brain shows symmetric lesions of basal ganglia and midline brainstem
• Childhood onset	Similar to infantile-onset patients, but PEO, dystonia, or ataxia may be prominent
Fatal infantile myopathy with COX deficiency	Diffuse weakness, hypotonia, and respiratory insufficiency due to myopathy Sometimes, renal tubular acidosis (de Toni-Debré-Fanconi syndrome)
Reversible infantile myopathy with COX deficiency	Diffuse weakness, hypotonia, and respiratory insufficiency due to myopathy Spontaneous improvement by age 2–3 y
Autosomal-dominant progressive external ophthalmoplegia (adPEO)	Ptosis and PEO generally beginning in young adulthood Ragged-red and COX-deficient fibers in skeletal muscle Multiple Δ-mtDNA Proximal limb weakness, respiratory insufficiency, depression, peripheral neuropathy, sensorineural hearing loss, cataracts, and endocrinopathies
Mitochondrial neurogastrointestinal encephalomyopathy (MNGIE)	Ptosis and PEO Gastrointestinal dysmotility Demyelinating peripheral neuropathy Cachexia Leukoencephalopathy on MRI scan
Autosomal-recessive cardiomyopathy ophthalmoplegia (ARCO)	Ptosis and PEO Proximal muscle weakness Hypertrophic cardiomyopathy
Infantile mtDNA depletion syndrome	
• Myopathic form	Feeding difficulty, failure to thrive, hypotonia, weakness, and occasionally PEO Elevated serum creatine kinase level (2–30 times upper limit of normal) Myopathy with COX-deficient fibers and sometimes ragged-red fibers
• Hepatopathy	Liver failure manifesting as persistent vomiting, failure to thrive, hypotonia, and hypoglycemia
• Alpers syndrome	Normal early development followed by rapid episodic psychomotor regression, intractable seizures, and liver disease
• Navaho neurohepatopathy (NHH)	Four of the following 6 criteria or 3 plus a positive family history of NHH: • Sensory neuropathy • Motor neuropathy • Corneal anesthesia, ulcers, or scars • Liver disease • Documented metabolic or immunologic derangement • Central nervous system demyelination

COX = cytochrome *c* oxidase; MRI = magnetic resonance imaging; PEO = progressive external ophthalmoplegia.

AMINOGLYCOSIDE-INDUCED DEAFNESS

An example of an interaction between genetic and environmental factors, aminoglycoside-induced deafness usually occurs in patients harboring an m.1555A>G mtDNA mutation in the *12S* rRNA gene. These patients develop sensorineural hearing loss when exposed to aminoglycoside antibiotics. However, the mutation can also cause nonsyndromic deafness without aminoglycoside therapy. Conversely, aminoglycosides can cause deafness without the m.1555A>G mtDNA mutation.

Fischel-Ghodsian N. Mitochondrial deafness. *Ear Hear* 2003;24: 303–313. [PMID: 12923421] (A summary of hearing loss in mitochondrial diseases.)

Neurologic Intensive Care

Santiago Ortega-Gutierrez, MD, & Alan Z. Segal, MD

25

INCREASED INTRACRANIAL PRESSURE

ESSENTIALS OF DIAGNOSIS

▶ Headache, nausea, and vomiting, with progression to obtundation and coma with or without localizing signs

▶ Brain imaging showing a space-occupying lesion, edema, blood, or hydrocephalus

▶ General Considerations

Increased intracranial pressure (ICP) is a pathologic state common to a variety of serious neurologic illnesses, all of which are characterized by the addition of volume to the intracranial vault. According to the Monro Kellie doctrine, the intracranial contents include brain, blood, and cerebrospinal fluid (CSF), all of which are relatively incompressible. Expansion of any one of these compartments must take place at the expense of the others and therefore will produce an increase in ICP. The normal ICP range oscillates between 5 and 20 cm H_2O or 3–15 mm Hg. Because elevations beyond these levels can rapidly lead to brain injury and death, rapid acute identification and treatment of the primary cause of elevated ICP is paramount.

▶ Clinical Findings

The most appropriate way to diagnose increased ICP is to measure it directly. A depressed level of consciousness in all its stages and reflex hypertension are probably the most consistent clinical signs. In principle they both reflect the effects of globally reduced cerebral blood flow. Marked hypertension with bradycardia and irregular respiration is characteristic of the *Kocher-Cushing reflex* due to a rapid rise in ICP in the posterior fossa and impending cerebral herniation. However,

in clinical practice, hypertension is most commonly associated with initial tachycardia before the bradycardic effect.

Headache, nausea, projectile vomiting, fourth and sixth cranial nerve palsies, and pupillary dilatation are also frequent signs seen in patients with increased ICP. Nevertheless, they do not correlate well with the severity of the disease. Although papilledema is a specific indicator of intracranial hypertension, it is present only in a minority of patients.

Localized mass lesions or diffuse increase in ICP can cause coma due to herniation of brain structures beyond the confines of the supratentorial-infratentorial compartments. Supratentorial lesions are associated with uncal and central herniation depending on the location of the lesion. Infratentorial structural lesions may also cause herniation, either transtentorially upward, producing midbrain compression, or downward through the foramen magnum with distortion of the medulla by the cerebellar tonsils. These syndromes must be recognized and rapidly managed medically and surgically as appropriate (Table 25–1).

Imaging guidance (midline shift, effaced basal cisterns, loss of gray white matter differentiation, and hydrocephalus) may also assist in the identification of patients with a suspected increase in ICP, but significant ICP elevations may occur without these findings. Computed tomography (CT) of head is the initial preferred test, followed by MRI or vascular imaging depending on the clinical suspicion and patient stability (Figure 25–1).

Increases in ICP may result from an increase in brain volume due to edema, a focal space-occupying cerebral or extracerebral mass, increases in venous pressure transmitted from the thorax, or an increase in CSF volume caused by obstruction (Table 25–2). In addition to the mechanical compression and distortion of brain tissue, ICP elevations cause global hypoxic-ischemic injury as a result of critical reduction in cerebral perfusion pressure (CPP) and cerebral blood flow (CBF).

The gold standard for **invasive** ICP monitoring remains the ventricular catheter with external pressure transducer, known as a *ventriculostomy* or an external ventricular drain

Table 25–1. Herniation Syndrome

Type	Lesion	Injured Structure	Clinical Presentation
Uncal	Hemispheric or lateral middle fossa mass	Ipsilateral CN III compression and cerebral peduncle	**Initially:** ipsilateral pupil dilated with preserved or sluggish reaction to light **Advanced stage:** complete internal and external ophthalmoplegia, hemiparesis (50% ipsilateral and 50% contralateral)
Central	Supratentorial diffuse brain edema, hemorrhage, or midline brain tumors	Initial obstructive hydrocephalus and displacement of thalamus and hypothalamus	**Initially:** decreased consciousness, small reactive pupils, normal eye movements **Advanced stage:** unreactive mid-position pupils, ophthalmoplegia, flexor ("decorticate") posturing
Midbrain compression	Advanced stage of uncal, central, or upward infratentorial herniation	Midbrain and upper pons	Extensor ("decerebrate") posturing, midposition pupils, sometimes irregular and loss of pupillary, oculocephalic, and oculovestibular reflexes
Foramen magnum herniation	Infratentorial lesions or end-stage transtentorial herniation	Medulla-lower pons and cerebellar tonsils.	Absent brainstem reflexes; flaccid paralysis; respirations ataxic, irregular, and slow and subsequently ceasing
Subfalcine herniation	Frontal or temporal lesions	Bilateral pericallosal and callosomarginal arteries	**Initially:** asymptomatic or increased tone in the lower extremities **Advanced stage:** leg weakness and abulia

CN = cranial nerve.

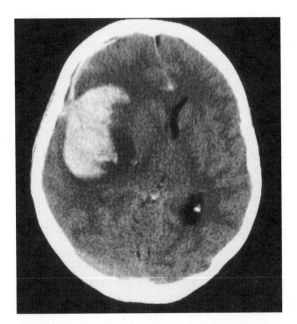

▲ **Figure 25–1.** CT of the head showing large acute intracranial hemorrhage causing significant midline shift and subfalcine and uncal herniation.

(EVD). It is primarily used in situations in which therapeutic CSF drainage is desirable in addition to global ICP monitoring. The main complications of an EVD are hemorrhage and infection, which become increasingly likely after day 5. CSF cultures may be routinely obtained from an EVD as a means of monitoring for intercurrent infection.

When no CSF diversion is desired or there is suspicion of compartmental ICP increase, a *parenchymal fiberoptic monitor* is generally used. It carries a very low risk for infection (<1%), but its accuracy decreases over time, and no recalibration can be done after insertion. Other types of ICP monitors include *epidural transducers* and *subarachnoid bolts.* Although each is associated with a low infection risk, they are less accurate, and many neurologic intensive care units have abandoned their use (Figure 25–2).

Currently, there is no **noninvasive** method that can provide accurate, continuous, online measurement of ICP. Transcranial Doppler (TCD) ultrasonography can indirectly reflect elevated ICP by altering vascular resistance in a characteristic pattern. The pulsatility index is equal to the difference between systolic and diastolic flow velocities divided by the mean flow velocity. When resistance to flow increases, as occurs in elevated ICP, the pulsatility index increases as well.

Multimodal assessment of cerebral physiology can include the combination of TCD ultrasonography, neuroimaging, ICP, cerebral perfusion and CBF monitoring, brain tissue oxygen tension probes, brain microdialysis, evoked potentials, and continuous electroencephalography.

Table 25–2. Causes of Increased Intracranial Pressure

Mechanism	Disease or Injury
Brain swelling	Head injury, anoxia, hepatic failure, hypertensive encephalopathy, Reye syndrome
Cerebral mass lesions	Neoplasms (gliomas, metastases), cerebral infarction, intracerebral hemorrhage, abscess (bacterial or other)
Extracerebral mass lesions	Meningeal neoplasms, subdural or epidural hematoma
Elevated venous pressure	Congestive heart failure, superior mediastinal obstruction, cerebral or jugular venous thrombosis
Obstruction to flow of cerebrospinal fluid	Communicating or noncommunicating hydrocephalus

▶ Treatment

The proper management of all critically brain-injured patients begins with general care management designed to optimize oxygenation and CBF and to minimize factors that can aggravate neuronal injury or trigger ICP elevations (Table 25–3).

A. General ICP Management

1. Patient positioning—Head position should be maintained at 20–30 degrees of elevation to maximize venous return. The head must be in the neutral position, unconstrained by tape and bandages, as head turning and neck constriction may impair jugular venous drainage and raise ICP.

2. Initial fluid management—The optimal goal of fluid management in patients with elevated ICP is to achieve a state of initial euvolemia. When serum osmolality is decreased, water will move into brain cells and worsen cerebral edema. Therefore, free water or hypotonic fluids should not be administered to these patients.

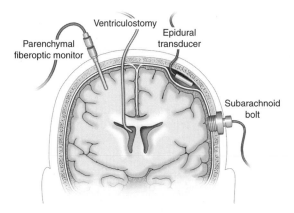

Ventriculostomy
Epidural transducer
Parenchymal fiberoptic monitor
Subarachnoid bolt

▲ **Figure 25–2.** Types of invasive intracranial pressure monitors.

3. Hyperventilation and optimization of mechanical ventilation—Hyperventilation can rapidly reduce ICP and is useful in the acute setting for patients with signs of brain herniation. Because hyperventilation causes generalized vasoconstriction, it reduces CBF and therefore ICP. Although the time and duration of hyperventilation that can be used safely and effectively is uncertain, most experts recommend hyperventilation to a PCO_2 of approximately 30–35 mm Hg for no longer than 30 minutes.

4. Treatment of fever or induction of hypothermia—Treatment of fever is paramount in any brain injury and is particularly important in the setting of increased ICP. Acetaminophen and cooling blankets are initial options, but more aggressive hypothermia can be achieved with specialized central intravenous lines or surface cooling devices.

5. Blood pressure control—Management of blood pressure in the setting of increased ICP must focus on maintenance of CPP. Although there is variability in the ischemic threshold among patients, CPP must be kept higher than 60 mm Hg to deliver optimal brain tissue oxygenation. At its upper limit, CPP should usually be kept under 110–120 mm Hg to avoid further increasing ICP by creating a state of hyperperfusion. Labetalol and nicardipine are favored in these patients for their short half-life and lack of ICP side effects.

6. Corticosteroids—These agents have a limited role in the treatment of elevated ICP. They reduce vasogenic edema related to neoplasm or infection, but they are not beneficial against cytotoxic edema produced by ischemic stroke, intracerebral hemorrhage, or head trauma.

B. Pharmacotherapy and Surgical Management

1. Ventriculostomy—Drainage of CSF with an external ventricular catheter allows reduction in ventricular size in the setting of hydrocephalus but also may be employed in the absence of ventricular enlargement in a noncompliant brain in patients suffering from high-grade subarachnoid hemorrhage, space-occupying lesion with mass effect, severe intraventricular hemorrhage, or traumatic brain injury.

Table 25–3. ICP Management Protocol

ICP > 20 mm Hg for > 10 minutes (EVD is open and draining, patient is not coughing or getting suctioned).
Step 1: Surgical Decompression
• Decompressive craniectomy/craniotomy is the most effective way of reducing intracranial hypertension. If surgery is not an option, proceed to the following medical steps.
Step 2: Sedation With Short-Acting Agents
(Patients should be on mechanical ventilation.) The very first step in medically addressing an ICP crisis is sedation.
If hemodynamically stable (no hypotension)
IV propofol: repeat 20 mg IV every 20 s up to 1–2 mg/kg for initial bolus; maintenance 0.3–3 mg/kg/h.
OR
If hemodynamically unstable (hypotensive, poor cardiac output, intravascular volume depletion)
IV midazolam: load 0.01–0.05 mg/kg over 2 min, maintenance 0.02–0.2 mg/kg/min
AND
Consider adding an analgesic agent:
IV fentanyl: IV bolus 25–100 µg followed by maintenance 1–3 µg/kg/h
Step 3: Hyperventilation and Order Osmotic Agents
• **Hyperventilation** with a $Paco_2$ goal 30–35 mm Hg during the acute phase.
• **Mannitol:** 1–1.5 g/kg IV bag infused over 30 min, every 6 h as needed. Osm < 360, Osm gap < 10.
• **Hypertonic saline:** 30 mL of 23.4% IV push over 5 min, every 4–6 h as needed. Serum sodium < 160.
Step 4: Barbiturate Coma
Pentobarbital: load 10 mg/kg IV infusion over 1 h, maintenance 1–3 mg/kg/h, target 1–2 bursts per 10 s suppression on continuous EEG. As alternative give 50-mg boluses every 5–10 min until ICP is controlled.
Step 5: Therapeutic Hypothermia
Target temperature = 32–34°C using either surface cooling or endovascular cooling device.
• Shivering needs to be aggressively treated for three reasons:
• Shivering prevents the core body temperature from falling and leads to prolonged time to achieve the target temperature.
• Shivering can increase the ICP and further worsen the intracranial hypertension.
• Shivering can increase the brain metabolism and increase the risk of developing brain hypoxia and cellular metabolic distress.
• Anti-shivering methods:
• Skin counter-warming: warm, forced air blankets and mattress
• IV magnesium (IV bolus 60–80 mg/kg then maintenance 2 g/h) may reduce the shivering threshold but is not effective as a single agent
• Buspirone 20–30 mg via NGT after crushing TID
• IV dexmedetomidine 0.4–1.5 µg/kg/h
• IV meperidine 0.4 mg/kg IV every 4–6 h
• IV propofol 50–100 mg rapid IV push, maintenance 0.3–3 mg/kg/h
• IV clonidine 1–3 µg/kg prn

EVD = external ventricular device; EEG = electroencephalogram; ICP = intracranial pressure; NGT = nasogastric tube; Osm = osmolality.

2. Surgical decompression—Surgical decompression of an intracranial space-occupying lesion can have immediate impact on ICP elevations refractory to medical therapies, often with durable effects.

3. Sedation—Sedation improves ICP by reducing the cerebral metabolic rate (CMR) and CBF, decreasing agitation, and minimizing cough and Valsalva responses. In some settings, it should be considered as a first step of ICP management once the patient is intubated.

Propofol is an intravenous sedative with rapid onset and offset, making it excellent for short-term use. It decreases CMR, CBF, and, consequently, ICP. It also possesses antiepileptic and free radical scavenging properties. Because of its short half-life, propofol allows frequent opportunities to waken patients and assess their neurologic status. Propofol may cause hypotension and myocardial dysfunction, and with prolonged use it can cause hepatic dysfunction, metabolic acidosis, or an excess of fat calories resulting from its lipid base: *propofol infusion syndrome*. With prolonged use, its rapid offset is lost.

Other options for sedation and analgesia include benzodiazepines such as lorazepam or midazolam and opioids such as morphine or fentanyl. Their effect on CBF and CMR is modest, and so they are usually considered adjunctive medications for acute ICP crises.

4. Hyperosmolar therapy—This medication works by the basic principle that fluid will move through a semipermeable membrane (eg, blood–brain barrier) from an area of low osmolarity to an area of high osmolarity. Therefore, an increase in plasma osmolarity decreases brain parenchymal fluid volume.

5. Barbiturate coma—Barbiturates are usually reserved for refractory ICP cases not responding to the above therapies. For ICP management, they primarily decrease CMR, leading to a decrease in CBF, CBV, and thus ICP. Although any barbiturate can be given, *pentobarbital* is the most commonly used, administered initially as 50-mg boluses every 10 minutes until ICP is controlled or 5–10 mg/kg bolus followed by continuous infusion titrated by burst suppression on electroencephalogram. Barbiturates are associated with high morbidity and mortality due to hypotension and cardiodepression (usually requiring vasopressor and inotropic support), metabolic acidosis, ileus, and liver failure.

Kincaid MS, Lam AM. Monitoring and managing intracranial pressure. *Crit Care Neurol Contin* 2006;12:93–108.

Wartenberg KE, Schmidt JM, Mayer SA. Multimodality monitoring in neurocritical care. *Crit Care Clin* 2007;23:507–538. [PMID: 17900483]

Wolfe T, Torbey M. Management of intracranial pressure. *Curr Neurol Neurosci Rep* 2009;9:477–485. [PMID: 19818235]

HYPOXIC-ISCHEMIC ENCEPHALOPATHY AFTER CARDIAC ARREST

ESSENTIALS OF DIAGNOSIS

▶ Caused by decreased cerebral blood flow or oxygenation

▶ Mild deprivation produces an amnestic syndrome

▶ Severe deprivation produces stupor, coma, and myoclonic jerks

▶ General Considerations

Cardiovascular disease is the leading cause of mortality and morbidity in the United States, causing more than one third of all deaths. The majority of these deaths follow sudden cardiac arrest outside of the health care setting. The advent of basic and advanced cardiac life support training has allowed more patients to survive initial resuscitation and to be admitted to intensive care units. Despite the modest success of the initial resuscitation, the functional outcome of survivors remains poor as a result of hypoxic-ischemic encephalopathy. Despite multiple large randomized studies using various neuroprotective strategies, only hypothermia shows a clear outcome benefit among cardiac arrest survivors.

▶ Clinical Findings

A. Symptoms and Signs

Consciousness is lost within seconds of cessation of cerebral blood flow, and most patients are initially comatose after resuscitation from cardiac arrest. The most severely affected patients remain comatose, progress to a minimally conscious or vegetative state, or become brain dead. The longer the duration of coma, the less likely that the patient will awaken and more likely that there will be severe neurologic deficits.

Patients who sustain brief anoxic damage may manifest only transient confusion and amnesia, whereas more severely affected individuals may have a permanent global amnestic syndrome. If hypotension is the main abnormality, patients may show areas of border-zone cerebral infarction, which may produce cortical blindness or bilateral arm weakness with sparing of the hands, or quadriparesis, sparing the face and feet (known as the "man in the barrel" syndrome). Paraplegia may follow infarction of the spinal cord in the thoracic border-zone region.

Myoclonus (asynchronous jerking of one or more limbs) is frequently observed after anoxia.

A subset of patients may become alert only to show relapse, with delayed postanoxic encephalopathy. This phenomenon is seen most often in cases of carbon monoxide poisoning. The basal ganglia may be severely affected, and such patients may show apathy, confusion, abnormal movements disorders such as chorea, and dysarthria.

ICP is not generally elevated after cardiac arrest, but, when it occurs, it is associated with widespread cerebral edema and portends a poor prognosis, including brain herniation.

B. Diagnostic Studies

Three markers during the acute phase of cardiac arrest have shown to have prognostic value. Elevated serum levels of neuron-specific enolase and S-100 are correlated with poor prognosis. Elevated levels of creatine kinase BB in the CSF 48–72 hours after cardiac arrest also predict poor outcome.

Computed tomography (CT) scanning is usually normal within the first 24 hours of anoxic injury. After 24–48 hours of severe anoxia, a loss of distinction between gray matter and white matter at the level of cortex and basal ganglia reflects cytotoxic edema.

Magnetic resonance imaging (MRI) with diffusion-weighted imaging (DWI) demonstrates hyperintensity of the cortical ribbon consistent with acute laminar necrosis. Border-zone infarction, occurring in the setting of a primarily hypotensive rather than a hypoxic event, may also be demonstrated on CT or MRI.

Electroencephalogram (EEG) patterns including periodic phenomena, burst suppression, electrocerebral silence, and so-called *alpha coma* carry a nearly uniformly poor prognosis. EEG is essential in seizure detection, which occurs in up to 40% of patients. It should be considered in patients with unexplained coma, with or without convulsive activity, after cardiac arrest.

Somatosensory-evoked potentials (SSEPs) also have prognostic value after cardiac arrest. Absent short-latency SSEP bilaterally carries a sensitivity of 42% and a positive predictive value of 100% in identifying patients who will never awaken.

Treatment

After return of spontaneous circulation, induction of *mild hypothermia* as early as possible improves functional outcome after cardiac arrest. Cooling to 32–34°C (89.6–93.2°F) should be achieved within the first 4–6 hours and should be maintained for a period of 12–24 hours. Initially, ice packs are placed in the axillae and around the torso and limbs, and cooling blankets are applied both under and over the patient. In the intensive care unit, both endovascular and commercial surface cooling devices are applied. Continuous temperature monitoring and feedback enable precise temperature control. Sedation and the use of shivering protocols, requiring paralysis with a neuromuscular blockade (eg, vecuronium) when severe, are important. Shivering increases systemic metabolic demand and hypercapnia, worsens postischemic metabolic failure, and negates the benefits of hypothermia. Hypothermia is maintained for approximately 24 hours, and rewarming is accomplished slowly and passively to avoid rebound ICP response and potassium disarrangements that could trigger fatal arrhythmias.

Myoclonus can be treated with benzodiazepines or valproic acid, and seizure activity should be managed according to standard epilepsy protocols.

Prognosis

Patients who are arousable or fully alert within 12 hours of cardiac arrest generally have a favorable prognosis. Conversely, at 12–24 hours postarrest, coma with absent brainstem reflexes (corneal and pupillary light reflexes and eye movement responses) is uniformly associated with a vegetative or fatal outcome. Patients with a favorable prognosis have motor responses of withdrawal or better on day 1, along with eye opening to noise or spontaneously. At day 3, spontaneous eye movements should be normal, and by day 7, the patient should be able to obey commands (Figure 25–3).

Clinicians should be careful when interpreting early findings on physical examination to ensure that no confounding, potentially reversible factors (eg, seizures) exist. Also, with hypothermia, the neurologic examination loses its prognostic value because most of these patients are receiving sedatives, paralytics, or neurodepressants. Finally, as noted, diagnostic tools possess a very high positive predictive value but very low sensitivity.

Bernard SA, et al. Treatment of comatose survivors of out-of-hospital cardiac arrest with induced hypothermia. *N Engl J Med* 2002;346:557–563. [PMID: 11856794]

Hirsch K, et al. Management of brain injury after cardiac arrest. *Continuum Lifelong Learning Neurol* 2009;15:100–120.

Kandiah P, Ortega-Gutierrez S, Torbey MT. Biomarkers and neuroimaging of brain injury after cardiac arrest. *Semin Neurol* 2006;26:413–421. [PMID: 16969742]

Tirschwell D. Coma in the intensive care unit: Predicting awakening following cardiac and respiratory arrest. *Continuum Lifelong Learning Neurol* 2006;12:46–69.

NEUROMUSCULAR WEAKNESS IN CRITICAL ILLNESS

ESSENTIALS OF DIAGNOSIS

▶ Critically ill patient with diffuse muscle weakness and diminished or absent deep tendon reflexes, sometimes with signs of impending respiratory failure

▶ Often occurs with use of neuromuscular junction-blocking agents or corticosteroids, or both

▶ Elevated cerebrospinal fluid protein suggests possible Guillain-Barré syndrome

General Considerations

A variety of neurologic disorders cause acute generalized weakness that requires critical care. Serious dysfunction of the neuromuscular system may lead to hypoventilation and hypercapnia, with respiratory failure requiring mechanical ventilation.

Clinical Findings

The pattern of weakness may be helpful in localizing the underlying disorder. *Guillain-Barré syndrome (GBS),* an acute monophasic immune-mediated symmetrically progressive polyneuropathy often provoked by a preceding infection, usually presents as an ascending paralysis starting in the lower extremities (see Chapter 19). Approximately one third of patients with GBS admitted to the ICU require mechanical ventilation, and 10–20% develop severe dysautonomia requiring close hemodynamic monitoring. Patients with *critical illness polyneuropathy* (CIP) and *acute necrotizing myopathy* also develop generalized weakness and absent or diminished deep tendon reflexes. Proximal musculature may be more adversely affected, but distal weakness is common. Sensation may be impaired but is often difficult to assess in critically ill patients. Cranial nerves are not typically affected except for bilateral facial weakness, which may be difficult to recognize in a ventilated patient. *Myasthenic crisis* is usually triggered by acute illness or new medication (see Chapter 22).

It is crucial to recognize signs of respiratory weakness and the need for intubation and mechanical ventilation before an

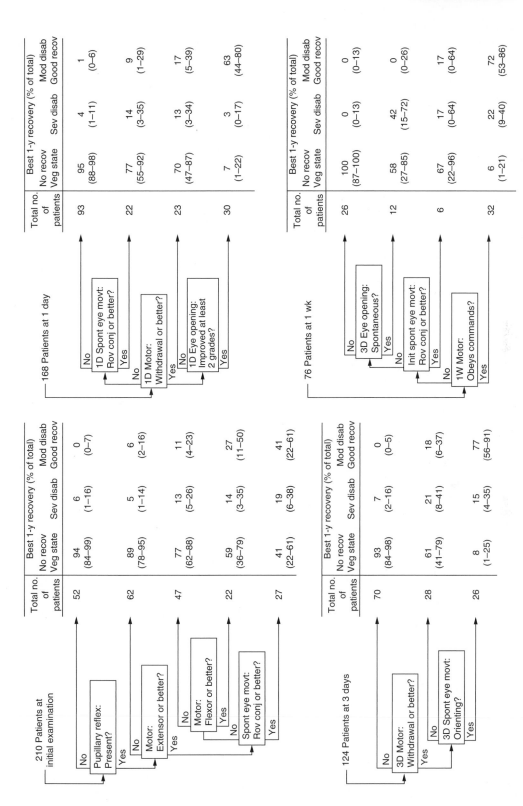

▲ **Figure 25-3.** Guidelines for prognosis in patients with hypoxic-ischemic coma after cardiopulmonary arrest. 1D = one-day; 3D = three-day; 1W Motor = 1-week motor; Init Spont Eye Movt = initial spontaneous eye movement; Mod Disab Good Recov = moderate disability with good recovery; No Recov Veg State = no recovery/vegetative state; Rov Conj = roving conjugate; Sev Disab = severe disability; Spont Eye Movt = spontaneous eye movement. (Adapted with permission from Levy DE, et al. Predicting outcome from hypoxic-ischemic coma. *JAMA* 1985;253:1420.)

acute decompensation. Delayed intubation contributes to the development of aspiration pneumonia (Table 25–4).

Differential Diagnosis & Laboratory Testing

Diagnostic considerations in diffusely weak critically ill patients include GBS, CIP, and acute quadriplegic myopathy (AQM). Patients who have been exposed to neuromuscular junction-blocking agents are at risk for prolonged effects of these agents. Paralytics (most commonly, but not uniformly,

vecuronium) have also been implicated as a specific cause of AQM associated with degeneration of thick (myosin) filaments. Corticosteroids may add a component of steroid myopathy and can compound the effects of paralytics in causing AQM. Interestingly, even without exogenous corticosteroids, it has been suggested that critically ill patients may release endogenous glucocorticoids, which may put them at risk for AQM.

Electromyography shows signs of denervation and abnormal compound muscle action potentials. Nerve conduction studies may confirm axonal neuropathy but are often unreliable in this setting. Serum creatine kinase levels are normal in patients with CIP or steroid myopathy and are typically but not invariably elevated in AQM. Definitive diagnosis of these syndromes is made by nerve and muscle biopsy. Because light microscopy of muscle may show similar findings of muscle breakdown in both CIP and AQM, electron microscopy may be needed to specifically diagnose myosin fiber loss.

In GBS, lumbar puncture can identify an elevated CSF protein concentration. It is important to diagnose GBS, because it requires treatment with intravenous immunoglobulin or plasmapheresis.

Table 25–4. Signs of Impending Neuromuscular Respiratory Failure

Sign	Red Flag Sign
Clinical	
Progressive quadriparesis	Quadriplegia, inability to lift head off bed
Bulbar involvement	Dysphagia, weak voice, bifacial weakness
Weak cough	Trouble expelling secretions, "wet" voice
Respiratory complaint	
Dyspnea	Complaints of respiratory fatigue
Tachypnea	Inability to speak in full sentences or count to 20
Orthopnea	Nocturnal desaturations, prefers to sit up
Accessory muscle use	Use of neck and abdominal muscles
Abdominal paradox	Inward motion of abdomen with inspiration
Signs of distress	
Tachycardia	Restlessness
Diaphoresis	Staccato speech
Monitoring	
Vital capacity testing (bedside)	Vital capacity < 15-20 mL/kg, falling, drop by 30%
Arterial oxygen saturation	Desaturation (late sign)
Arterial blood gas: PaCO2	Hypercapnia = hypoventilation (late sign)
Chest radiographs	Atelectasis, pneumonia

Treatment & Prognosis

The suggestion that patients with CIP might benefit from intravenous immunoglobulin treatment has never been substantiated. Both CIP and AQM eventually resolve spontaneously, but there may be prolonged periods of paralysis (up to 6 months or more). Because management consists of physical therapy for both syndromes, muscle biopsy is reserved for specific settings. As a preventative strategy, paralytic agents should be used judiciously and sparingly, particularly in combination with high-dose corticosteroids.

Dhar R. Neuromuscular respiratory failure. *Continuum Lifelong Learning Neurol* 2009;15:40–67.

Sander HW, Golden M, Danon MJ. Quadriplegic areflexic ICU illness: Selective thick filament loss and normal nerve histology. *Muscle Nerve* 2002;26:499–505. [PMID: 12362415]

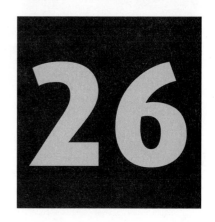

Bacterial, Fungal, & Parasitic Infections of the Nervous System

Barbara S. Koppel, MD, & Todd Hayano, MS

Infection can affect the function of the nervous system by damaging the brain or its lining (meningoencephalitis, abscess, subdural empyema), spinal cord (myelitis, cord compression), lumbosacral plexus, muscles, and nerves. At least 1% of hospital admissions relate to infection of the central nervous system (CNS), primarily bacterial meningitis.

▼ BACTERIAL INFECTIONS

BACTERIAL MENINGITIS

ESSENTIALS OF DIAGNOSIS

▶ Acute onset of headache, stiff neck, confusion, lethargy or coma, and fever

▶ Petechial rash implicates meningococcal cause

▶ Most likely organism depends on patient's age, immune status including vaccination history, and special risk factors of exposure, surgeries, drug use

▶ Cerebrospinal fluid (CSF) analysis: high opening pressure, decreased glucose (normal 0.6 CSF/serum), more than 10 white blood cells (WBCs)/µL (predominantly polymorphonuclear neutrophils) and increased protein

▶ Encapsulated organisms visualized by Gram stain

▶ General Considerations

Bacterial meningitis in adults has an incidence rate of 4–6 cases per 100,000 in the United States and can be much higher in developing countries. It is associated with morbidity in up to 30%, the most serious being cerebral edema with depression of consciousness, stroke, septic shock, and cognitive impairment in up to 25% of survivors; mortality rates up to 20% have been reported. Time to begin treatment is of the

essence; when antibiotics are initiated after 6 hours (generally due to delay caused by obtaining imaging before performing lumbar puncture), prognosis is much worse. Therefore, emergency management of meningitis now includes the initiation of corticosteroids before antibiotics and allowing empiric antibiotics to be given even before obtaining cerebrospinal fluid for culture if there will be any delay (after obtaining blood cultures). As valuable as the lumbar puncture is to definitely prove bacterial meningitis and to isolate and culture the causative organism, clinical clues can be substituted and the causative organism can be predicted based on the patient's age, history of vaccination against common agents (eg, *Haemophilus influenzae*, *Streptococcus pneumoniae*, or *Neisseria meningitidis*), immune state (alcoholic, postsplenectomy, steroid dependent), and other special risk factors, including epidemic exposure and recent dental or surgical procedure. Common organisms and their treatment are reviewed in Tables 26–1 and 26–2.

▶ Pathogenesis

Most bacteria enter CSF as a result of colonization of the nasopharynx with hematogenous spread to the choroid plexus (site of CSF production) or capillaries to enter the parenchyma, subarachnoid spaces, and then reproduce, releasing proinflammatory cytokines in the meninges. These cytokines, such as tumor necrosis factor and interleukin-1, break down the blood–brain barrier, leading to edema and cell death. The capsule helps evade complement-mediated efforts to kill and phagocytose the bacteria, and vesicles released by the outer membrane of bacteria divert the immune response. Occlusion of the arachnoid granulations in sinuses contributes to more cerebral edema. Special entry mechanisms include thrombosed veins in the presence of extracranial infection such as otitis or mastoiditis, which allow retrograde transmission of infection. After head trauma or nasal, sinus, or cranial surgery, violation of the dura allows a passageway for bacterial entry, with those colonizing the skin or sinuses responsible for meningitis. Similarly, injection

Table 26–1. Antibiotic Treatment of Bacterial Meningitis

Causative Organism	Drug (2-wk course)	Dosage[a]	
		Children	Adults
Neisseria meningitides (gram-negative pairs)	Penicillin G	50,000 U/kg q 4 h Neonates: 0.15-0.2 mU/kg/d (q 8-12 h)	24 million units q day (q 4-6 h)
	or Ampicillin	75 mg/kg q 6 h, Neonates: 50 mg/kg q 8 h	3 g q 4 h
	Ceftriaxone (PCN resistant)	40-75 mg/kg q 12 h	2 g q 12 h
	or Cefotaxime or ceftizoxime	50-75 mg/kg q 6 h Neonates: 50-75 q 12 h	2-3 g q 6 h
• Chemoprophylaxis of close contacts of patient[b]	Rifampin (oral)	5-10 mg/kg q 12 h for 2 days	600 mg q 12 h for 2 days
	or Ciprofloxacin (oral)	Not approved	500 mg for 1 dose
Streptococcus pneumoniae (gram-positive pairs)			
• Penicillin sensitive	Penicillin G	50,000 U/kg q 4 h	4 million units q 4 h
	or Ceftriaxone	40-75 mg/kg q 12 h	2 g q 12 h
• Highly penicillin resistant	Vancomycin	15 mg/kg q 6 h or IT 10 mg/day	1-3 g q 6-12 h or 20 mg/day IT
	plus 3rd-generation cephalosporin	As for ceftriaxone	As for ceftriaxone
	or Meropenem	—	1-2 g q 8 h
Haemophilus influenzae type B (gram-negative cocci)	Ampicillin	200-300 mg/kg q 4 h	12 g q 4 h
	or Ceftriaxone	40-50 mg/kg q 12 h	2 g q 12 h
	or Cefotaxime	200 mg/kg q 4-6 h	12 g q 4 h
Listeria monocytogenes[c] (gram-positive rods)	Ampicillin *plus*	75 mg/kg q 6 h	2-3 g q 4 h
	Ceftriaxone *or*	50-75 mg/kg q 12 h	2 g q 12 h
	Gentamicin	—	8mg/kg day (renal adjusted)
	Trimethoprim-sulfamethoxazole	10 mg/kg q 12 h	20 mg/kg q 6 h
Staphylococcus aureus (gram-positive cocci)	Oxacillin *or*	35-50 mg/kg q 4 h	1-3 g q 4 h
	Nafcillin	35-50 mg/kg q 4 h	2-3 g q 4 h
Staphylococcal epidermidis	Vancomycin[c]	15 mg/kg q 6 h IVT or 0.5 mg/kg/day IT	1-3 g q q 8-12 h IVT or 20 mg/day IT
• Methicillin-resistant *S aureus* (MRSA)	Linezolid *or*	7.5 mg/kg q 8 h IVT	600-1200 mg q 12 h
	Quinupristin-dalfopristin	2 mg/day IT	—
Pseudomonas aeruginosa (gram-negative rods)	Ceftazidime	45-50 mg/kg q 8 h	2 g q 8 h
Other gram-negative bacilli[d]	Ceftriaxone *or*	50-50 mg/kg q 12 h	2 g q 12 h
	Cefotaxime *or*	50 mg/kg q 6-8 h	2 g q 6 h
	Meropenem	50 mg/kg q 8 h	1 g q 8 h
Group B *Streptococcus* (gram-positive ovoid or cocci)	Ampicillin *or* Penicillin G *or*	50 mg/kg q 4 h	2-3 g q 4 h
	Vancomycin (monitor levels)	15 mg/kg q 6 h	1 g q 12 h
Unknown pathogens	Vancomycin	15 mg/kg q 6 h Neonates: 20-30 mg/kg/d	15-20 mg/kg q 8 h
	plus Ceftazidime	45-50 mg/kg q 8 h	2 g q 8 h

IT = intrathecal; IVT = intraventricular; q = every.

[a]All therapy is intravenous unless indicated.

[b]Pregnant contacts of patients with *N meningitides* should receive azithromycin, 500 mg orally, or ceftriaxone, 250 mg intramuscularly (one time only).

[c]Duration of therapy for *L monocytogenes* is 3 weeks, and for staphylococcal infection, with vancomycin, is 1 week or 5 days after becoming afebrile.

[d]Includes *Enterobacteria, Klebsiella, Acinetobacter.*

Table 26–2. Empiric Antibiotic Treatment of Age-Associated Pathogens

Age of Patient	Causative Organism	Antibiotic	Alternative
Neonate	Group B *Streptococcus, Listeria, Escherichia coli*	Ampicillin plus 3rd-generation cephalosporin	Chloramphenicol plus gentamicin
3 mo–18 y	*Neisseria meningitides, Streptococcus pneumoniae, Haemophilus influenzae*	3rd-generation cephalosporin; vancomycin if resistant	Meropenem
18–50 y	*S pneumoniae, N meningitides, H influenzae*	3rd-generation cephalosporin	Meropenem
> 50 y	*S pneumoniae,* gram-negative bacilli, *Listeria monocytogenes*	Ampicillin plus 3rd-generation cephalosporin, plus gentamicin	Ampicillin plus fluoroquinolone

of epidural corticosteroids or anesthesia, spinal cord or deep brain stimulators, and lumbar or ventricular drains will cause meningitis with organisms that colonize the skin. Foreign bodies such as cochlear implants, Ommaya reservoirs, or ventriculoperitoneal shunts can become infected after even transient bacteremia.

Although meningitis refers only to inflammation of the lining of the brain, its devastating effects are the result of inflammation within the brain and secondary effects of edema, thrombosed veins, and blockage of CSF resorption. Hydrocephalous can be the result, or increased intracranial pressure and herniation. Stroke may be the consequence of large vessel arteritis as they cross through the exudate at the base of the brain. Abscess formation is another serious sequela of meningitis.

▶ Prevention

Vaccination programs against common pathogens such as *H influenzae* and *N meningitidis* were expanded to infants in 1990, and in 2000, *S pneumoniae* was added, although fewer than half of adults over 65 have received it. Despite efforts to prolong a vaccine's efficacy by covalent binding to a protein carrier, effectiveness usually wanes after 1 year, especially in infants, requiring adherence to a schedule of vaccination throughout childhood. This effort led to a significant decline in the incidence of meningitis (both unexplained and due to the above organisms) in the United States and all areas with good rates of vaccination. Median age of infection increased from 15 months to 25 years with more patients over age 60. In addition, all patients undergoing splenectomy should have vaccination against pneumococcus.

Using double gloves during neurosurgery and changing gloves before handling a ventricular catheter have reduced nosocomial infection, as has limiting manipulation of CSF and surgical wound drains, and time of drain to under 5 days. Topical antibiotics may lower craniotomy and dural implant chronic infection.

Other prevention efforts include screening and treatment of group B *Streptococcus*–infected women prepartum to avoid neonatal meningitis. Use of maintenance antibiotics in

immunocompromised patients lowers fungal and parasitic meningitis, and efforts to eliminate food contamination have lowered the incidence of neonatal meningitis due to *Listeria*.

Prophylactic antibiotics before dental work or other surgical procedures are no longer recommended for mitral valve prolapse unless the patient has had bacterial endocarditis in the past.

▶ Clinical Findings

A. Symptoms and Signs

Classic symptoms include headache, fever (in 80–95%), stiff neck to flexion but not lateral rotation, and altered mentation; two of these four are present in almost all patients, while the classic triad of fever, altered mental status, and nuchal rigidity is only found in about 45% of patients. Symptoms develop acutely in hours to days in bacterial meningitis, allowing differentiation from more subacute or chronic causes such as tuberculous or fungal meningitis. Cognitive dysfunction may progress from confusion and irritability with difficulty concentrating, to stupor or coma. Babies with meningitis generally do not have neck stiffness, but will have fever (although they can be hypothermic), inconsolable crying, irritability, poor feeding, and bulging fontanelles, and can develop lethargy or coma. Nuchal rigidity is only 30% sensitive. Kernig sign (ie, pain or resistance when the examiner attempts to extend the patient's knee while the hip is flexed) and Brudzinski sign (ie, hip flexion when the examiner bends the patient's neck forward) are attempts to guard from pain induced by stretching of inflamed meninges and as such will disappear in comatose patients who no longer respond to pain.

Signs of increased intracranial pressure include depressed consciousness, nausea, vomiting, and papilledema on fundoscopic examination. Infants will have bulging fontanelles acutely, and babies with hydrocephalous will have increased head circumference. Focal signs occur as a consequence of cerebral infarct or transtentorial herniation. Fluctuating signs may occur with unwitnessed seizures followed by postictal ("Todd") paresis. When deterioration of consciousness and seizures accompanies signs of stroke that do not fit an arterial territory, supperative venous thrombophlebitis may be responsible. Rarely, focal signs precede meningitic symptoms, for example, an abscess that ruptures into the ventricular or subarachnoid space.

Cranial nerve palsies are the result of inflammation affecting nerves as they traverse the meninges; abducens palsy can additionally occur as a result of increased intracranial pressure. Third nerve palsy, with pupillary or extraocular muscle dysfunction (in either order), may indicate transtentorial herniation. The eighth nerve is the most commonly affected cranial nerve.

Focal or generalized seizures result from the diffuse microvascular effects of meningeal inflammation, from coexisting abscess or subdural empyema, or more rarely from toxins released systemically by some organisms, such as *Shigella*.

Acute meningitis progresses over hours or days. Symptoms may persist for at least 4 weeks, even with appropriate treatment. Cognitive impairment, including slowness of performance of usual activities, is present in 25% of survivors.

Meningococcal meningitis is accompanied by a petechial rash on the trunk, legs, and mucous membranes.

Risk factors for meningitis include recent neurosurgery or procedures with potential to penetrate the dura or to induce bacteremia (dental cleaning, injection drug use), age, presence of HIV, and geographic location in areas with low vaccination rates or failure to receive pneumococcal vaccination. Neonatal meningitis is now more often caused by *Escherichia coli* than group B *Streptococcus*.

B. Laboratory Findings

Confirmation of meningitis depends on analysis of the CSF, which usually appears cloudy or turbulent in bacterial meningitis. If it is impossible to obtain spinal fluid from the lumbar interspaces because of local infection, uncorrectable coagulopathy, failed attempts under fluoroscopy, or fear of herniation due to expanding masses (especially in the posterior fossa), other useful means of confirming bacterial meningitis include raised levels of inflammatory markers such as procalcitonin (> 2 ng/mL) and C-reactive protein (> 40 mg/L), erythrocyte sedimentation rate, and discovering the pathogenic organism by blood cultures or culturing of suspected originating sites (lungs, sinuses, nasopharynx). Of note, in one survey of 301 patients, a mass lesion that would make lumbar puncture dangerous was found in up to 5% of patients and was predicted by focal signs, depressed sensorium, papilledema, and recent seizure activity.

Opening pressure is elevated (> 180 mm H_2O in adults, 110 mm in infants, and 150 mm in children) with very high levels (> 400 mm) in up to 40%, especially those with decreased alertness. Pleocytosis of 100–10,000 WBCs/μL is present, usually 80–95% neutrophilic, although lymphocytes or monocytes may predominate. Absence of pleocytosis is associated with poor outcome, and is seen in 5–10% of patients. Rupture of a brain abscess causes extreme pleocytosis. Protein concentration is elevated (> 50 mg/dL) and is greater than 200 mg/dL in 50% of patients. CSF glucose that is less than 30% of simultaneously obtained serum glucose is present in 70% of cases, although the normal ratio is 0.6.

Culture is very important, especially with the emergence of resistant strains of common organisms. Using expectations based on circumstances, the Gram stain result will dictate initial treatment. Gram stain is positive in 70–85% of patients, especially those with *S pneumoniae*, *N meningitides*, and gram-negative bacilli. The first collected tube is likely to be contaminated and should not be used for culture. Prior use of antibiotics lowers the likelihood of positive cultures, but bacterial antigen panels for pathogens such as *N meningitides*, *S pneumoniae*, *E coli*, *H influenzae*, and group B streptococci have a sensitivity of 10–50%. Polymerase chain reaction analysis is becoming more widely available for bacteria determination. Culture of blood, sputum, or fluid from nasopharynx and wounds can provide diagnostic help.

C. Imaging Studies

Contrast-enhanced computed tomography (CT) and magnetic resonance imaging (MRI) show meningeal enhancement (Figure 26–1), occasional sulcal effacement (beginning with the sylvian fissures) due to cerebral edema, and any parameningeal infection such as subdural empyema or mastoiditis. Imaging also has a role in diagnosing late complications of

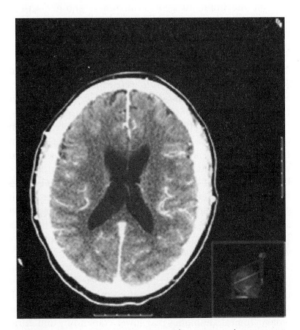

▲ **Figure 26–1.** Meningitis. CT with contrast demonstrating leptomeningeal enhancement and moderate hydrocephalus in a patient with meningitis due to *Strep viridans*. (Used with permission from Maria Chiechi, MD.)

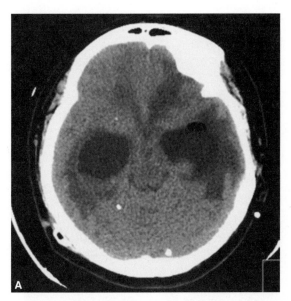
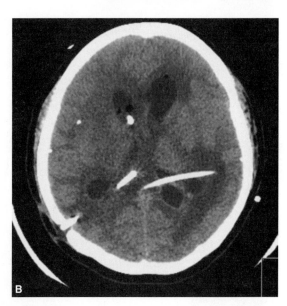

▲ **Figure 26–2.** Ventriculitis. **(A)** Axial CT showing hydrocephalous with air and **(B)** multiple shunts in ventricles, and calcified cysticerci. Hydrocephalous was a consequence of blockage by intraventricular cysticercosis and fatal ventriculitis developed eventually. (Used with permission from Maria Chiechi, MD.)

meningitis, such as hydrocephalus (Figure 26–2), ventriculitis (Figure 26–2) or ependymitis, abscess (Figure 26–3), stroke, and subdural empyema (Figure 26–4). In cases of recurrent meningitis, thin cuts through the base of the skull may reveal a basilar skull fracture, sinus compromise, or other potential breach of the dura. Subdural effusions that resolve spontaneously are common in *H influenzae* meningitis.

▶ Differential Diagnosis

Meningitis is broadly classified into aseptic and septic forms, based on the absence or presence of bacteria. Bacterial infection is acute, whereas fungal and tuberculous meningitis can be subacute or insidious. The latter are more likely to have lymphocytic predominance in CSF, with CSF glucose level closer to normal. Viral meningitis shares symptoms of headache, fever, stiff neck, and photophobia, which tend to be milder than those of bacterial meningitis, but with clear consciousness and absence of seizures and focal deficits. (For further discussion of viral meningitis, see Chapter 27.) Conversely, viral encephalitis (herpes simplex, West Nile, or other) may present with fever, seizures, and altered mental status, similar to bacterial meningitis. Other organisms that can produce nonbacterial meningitis include spirochetes, parasites, rickettsiae, and mycoplasma.

Chemical meningitis can complicate the introduction of any foreign fluid (or blood) into the subarachnoid space, including povidone-iodine used to clean the skin prior to lumbar puncture, intrathecal chemotherapeutic drugs, and contrast dye for myelography. Sarcoidosis, lymphoma, carcinoma, collagen vascular disease, and other autoimmune disorders also

can provoke meningitis. Meningitis secondary to medications such as nonsteroidal anti-inflammatory or anticonvulsant agents is milder. Rarely, glucose-transport deficiency causes hypoglycorrhachia in neonates, but without pleocytosis.

Abrupt onset of headache and nuchal rigidity is suggestive of subarachnoid hemorrhage.

▶ Complications

Mortality is 21% for patients infected with *S pneumoniae*, 3% for *N meningitides* (especially in those with the Waterhouse-Friderichsen reaction of thrombocytopenia, disseminated intravascular coagulation, and shock), 15% for *Listeria monocytogenes*, 7% for group B *Streptococcus*, and 6% for *H influenzae*.

Morbidity, including permanent neurologic deficit, is found in 14% of children, especially those from underdeveloped areas who recover from meningitis. Use of dexamethasone has lowerd the incidence of sensorineural hearing loss, which still affects 10–20% of survivors (5% have total deafness). Incidence is highest in cases of pneumococcal meningitis (especially those who had very high intracranial pressure). Blindness, static encephalopathy, or focal deficits are present in 5%. Fifty percent of neonates surviving group B streptococcal meningitis have permanent sequelae. Although 31% of patients with bacterial meningitis have seizures during the acute phase, only the 5% who have permanent neurologic deficits develop epilepsy. *S pneumoniae* infection in adults has a higher complication rate than other organisms. Blindness from prolonged papilledema can occur in patients with prolonged intracranial pressure elevation.

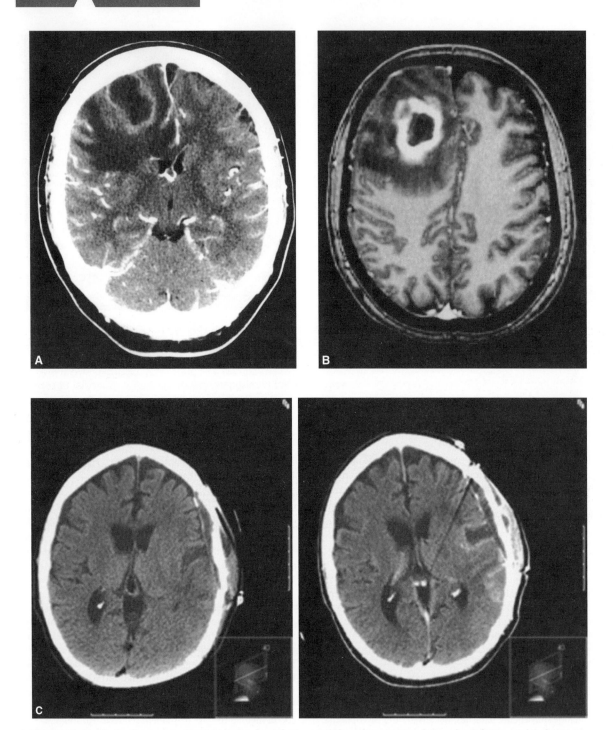

▲ **Figure 26–3.** Brain abscess. Contrast-enhanced axial CT scan **(A)** and contrast-enhanced axial T1-weighted MRI scan **(B)** show a ring-enhancing mass in the right frontal lobe with surrounding vasogenic edema in the same patient. **(C)** CT without and with contrast 1 month postoperative for brain abscess, showing enhancing extra-axial collection below craniotomy defect and left parietal parenchymal enhancement consistent with ongoing inflammation or cerebritis. (Used with permission from Maria Chiechi, MD.)

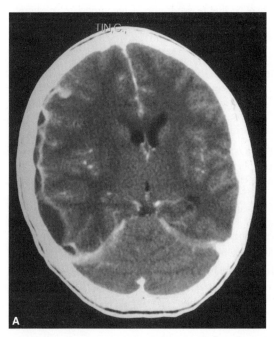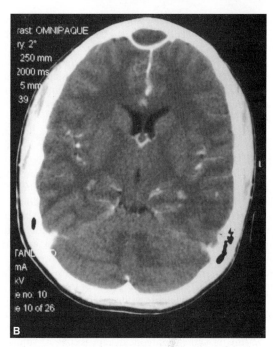

▲ **Figure 26–4.** Subdural empyema and cranial epidural abscess. **(A)** Contrast-enhanced axial CT scan shows a low-density subdural collection over the convexity of the right cerebral hemisphere. **(B)** Contrast-enhanced axial CT scan shows a low-density frontal midline epidural collection. (Used with permission from John Loh, MD.)

Stroke occurs in up to 20% of patients with pneumococcal meningitis, which is attributed to inflammatory reactions in large vessels passing through the sticky exudate at the base of the brain. Recently, a delayed syndrome of stroke, with thrombosis of deep vessels, has been described and may be due to hypercoagulopathy exacerbated by corticosteroids.

Septic shock and disseminated intravascular coagulopathy contribute to the mortality of meningitis. Hyperglycemia is present in up to one quarter of patients with meningitis and may be a nonspecific response to central blood-glucose regulation or reflect the higher incidence of meningitis in diabetic patients, who have a predilection for pneumococcal meningitis.

Rarely, subdural empyema, epidural abscess, and parenchymal brain abscess evolve, even in patients treated with antibiotics. Hydrocephalous can be the consequence of obstructed reabsorption of CSF in the arachnoid villi, especially when there is very high protein or much inflammation in the CSF.

▶ Treatment

A. Antibiotic Therapy

Treatment must be urgently initiated, although pretreatment with 10 mg dexamethasone (followed by 10 mg every 6 hours for 4 days) should be given one half hour before antibiotics, if possible. It should not be initiated after the first 2 days of therapy, as it will impede antibiotic entry. The empiric antibiotic choice depends on whether the organism is community or hospital acquired, and on local sensitivity patterns (see Tables 26–1 and 26–2). A third- or fourth-generation cephalosporin such as cefotaxime or ceftriaxone, plus ampicillin is indicated for infants and elderly patients, and vancomycin for patients whose meningitis may have spread from the skin or scalp.

Extremely ill-appearing patients should receive antiviral coverage for herpes encephalitis in addition to antibacterial therapy when the diagnosis of bacterial meningitis is in doubt. Until another organism is identified (including by Gram stain) or tuberculosis cultures are negative, which takes 4 weeks, antitubercular therapy is also prudent in patients at high risk such as those with AIDS or other immunosuppressed states. To ensure adequate treatment of *Listeria* meningitis in very ill patients, gentamicin should be given with ampicillin.

The treatment of choice for the most common adult cause of meningitis, *S pneumoniae*, is penicillin, with increasing doses in patients with more resistant strains, which are present in up to 34% of pathogens in the United States. For the most resistant strains, meropenem, with a third- or fourth-generation cephalosporin, plus vancomycin or a fluoroquinolone can be substituted. Penicillin resistance can cross over to cephalosporins (14% of *S pneumoniae* are resistant to ceftriaxone) and carbapenems; thus, timely sensitivity reporting is necessary for all bacterial cultures, with some strains tolerant of vancomycin also. The ratio of an antibiotic's minimal inhibitory concentration (MIC) to CSF concentration is an important variable if the organism is sensitive to that antibiotic.

Duration of treatment varies with the pathogen, from 5–7 days for *N meningitidis*, 10–14 days for *S pneumoniae*, and 3–4 weeks for *L monocytogenes*.

Rifampin is used in meningococcal infection to eliminate nasopharyngeal carrier status or reduce the risk of meningitis in close contacts of the patient. Patients with meningococcal meningitis are the only ones requiring respiratory isolation for 24 hours.

Drugs such as ertapenem, gemifloxacin or moxifloxacin, and daptomycin (an oxazolidinone) also show promise for treating meningitis.

The breakdown of the blood–brain barrier in the presence of inflamed meninges aids antibiotic penetration into CSF, although there is theoretical concern that the addition of corticosteroids may prematurely restore the barrier. Although failure to enter the CNS is considered especially problematic in the case of vancomycin, this was not proven by measurement of lower CSF:serum levels in one study. However, some guidelines recommend higher doses of vancomycin and other antibiotics toward the end of the course of treatment.

Repeat lumbar puncture at the end of therapy is no longer standard practice, although in patients with pneumococcal meningitis a repeat spinal tap after 48 hours is indicated to be sure the chosen antibiotic therapy is correct. Although protein elevation, hypoglycorrachia, and pleocytosis may remain abnormal at 48 hours, the culture should become negative if successful choice of antibiotic was initiated.

B. Management of Complications

1. Corticosteroid therapy—Studies in both children and adults demonstrate the efficacy of glucocorticosteroids for reducing mortality (from 34–14% in pneumococcal meningitis) and morbidity (from 25–15%) including deafness, stroke, and other sequelae of meningitis. Beneficial effects are limited to organisms with a polysaccharide capsule (gram positive), especially *S pneumoniae*. A standard regimen of dexamethasone (in adults, 10 mg every 6 hours for 4 days; in children, 0.15 mg/kg every 6 hours for 4 days) should be started a half hour before the first dose of antibiotics (if the patient is stable) to help prevent the inflammatory response as bacteria die. Complications of corticosteroid use include progression of undiagnosed tuberculous infection. For unclear reasons, outcomes are also worse in HIV-infected patients who receive corticosteroid therapy. Monitoring for hyperglycemia is prudent.

2. Transtentorial herniation—Although an infrequent complication, transtentorial herniation can be fatal. It is managed in the standard manner with hyperventilation, mannitol, and drainage of CSF from intraventricular catheters. Fluid management can be difficult; the clinician must balance the need for adequate blood pressure with that of avoiding increased intracranial pressure. Transcranial Doppler ultrasound can identify decreased cerebral perfusion.

3. Metabolic derangement—Hyponatremia is more common than hypernatremia (20% as opposed to 7% of cases) and may be due to syndrome of inappropriate antidiuretic hormone (SIADH), cerebral salt wasting, or fluid mismanagement. Fluid restriction is detrimental, so in correcting sodium levels it is more important to support the patient's volume.

4. Septic shock—This development requires especially careful management, using traditional plasma expanders, catecholamines such as dobutamine, and sulfonylurea, which acts as a vasopressin K_{ATP} channel inhibitor of vascular smooth muscle. Acidosis must be corrected to avoid hyperpnea.

5. Coma/seizures—Coma can result from nonconvulsive status epilepticus, the identification and treatment of which requires electroencephalography. Although seizures occur in up to 31% of all infections and increase mortality (OR 17.6), remote seizures after meningitis only occur in about 7% of children. Prophylactic anticonvulsants are not indicated when monitoring (close clinical observation or electrophysiologic) is available.

6. Suppurative thrombophlebitis—This complication can be treated with anticoagulation, especially if the sagittal sinus is thrombosed or there are no other drainage channels, unless there is significant hemorrhage.

▶ Prognosis

Prognosis is excellent with early diagnosis and treatment of bacterial meningitis (ie, antibiotics and corticosteroids started < 4 hours after presentation to hospital). Approximately 15% of survivors of nonmeningococcal meningitis have sequelae. Neurologic deficits are seldom seen in meningococcal meningitis survivors, but mortality, which is 3% overall, is very high in patients with the Waterhouse-Friderichsen reaction of thrombocytopenia, disseminated intravascular coagulation, and shock.

Assiri AM, et al. Corticosteroid administration and outcome of adolescents and adults with acute bacterial meningitis: A meta-analysis. *Mayo Clin Proc* 2009;84(5):403–409. [PMID: 19411436] (Describes rationale, risks, and outcome of supplementing antibacterial treatment with corticosteroids in 1261 patients from four trials published between 1999 and 2007.)

Hall-Baker PA, et al. Summary of notifiable diseases—United States, 2007. *MMWR Morb Mortal Wkly Rep* 2009;56(53):1–94. [PMID: 18354374] (Provides trends and most recent numbers of cases of reportable types of meningitis.)

Miranda J, Tunkel AR. Strategies and new developments in the management of bacterial meningitis. *Infect Dis Clin* 2009;23(4): 925–943. [PMID: 19909891] (A practical list of current and potential antibiotics and adjunctive therapies for meningitis.)

Roos KL. Pearls: Infectious diseases. *Semin Neurol* 2010;30:71–73. [PMID: 20127585] (Brief bullet points of clinical manifestations of meningitis and CSF findings.)

Safdieh JE, et al. Bacterial and fungal meningitis in patients with cancer. *Neurology* 2008;70(12):943–937. [PMID: 18347316] (Seventy-nine positive CSF cultures were found in 77 cancer patients, 78% having had prior neurosurgical procedures. Classic meningeal symptoms were lacking and CSF showed less inflammation.)

Schut ES, et al. Delayed cerebral thrombosis after initial good recovery from pneumococcal meningitis. *Neurology* 2009;73:1988–1995. [PMID: 19890068] (Stroke in deep penetrating vessels occurred more than a week after recovery from pneumococcal meningitis in six patients, without inflammatory reactions seen in the two patients studied on autopsy. Possible causes were corticosteroid-induced hypercoagulable state or incomplete vasculitis.)

Schut ES, et al. Hyperglycemia in bacterial meningitis: A prospective cohort study. *BMC Infect Dis* 2009;9:57–64. [PMID: 19426501] (Review of 696 episodes of meningitis stratified by blood glucose level with discussion of etiologies and implications for prognosis.)

Tan LKK, Carlone GM, Borrow R. Current contents: Advances in the development of vaccines against *Neisseria meningitides*. *N Engl J Med* 2010;362:1511–1520 [PMID: 20410516] (Review of history and recent development, physiology, and efficacy of vaccination programs against this organism.)

Thigpen MC, Whitney CG, Messonnier NE et al. Bacterial meningitis in the United States,1998–2007. *N Engl J Med* 2011;364:1511–1520 [PMID: 21612470] (Surveillance of eight regions of the United States detected 3188 patients with bacterial meningitis during the period, representing a 31 percent decline over the study period, especially amongst children. Median age advanced over the years from 30.3 to 41.9 towards the end. Mortality rate was unchanged (14.8%), higher with advancing age)

van de Beek D, de Gans J, Tunkel AR, Wijdicks EFM. Community-acquired bacterial meningitis in adults. *N Engl J Med* 2006;354:44–53. [PMID: 20071704] (Evidence- based review of optimal approach to diagnosis, and antibiotic and ancillary treatment of bacterial meningitis.)

van de Beek D, Drake JM, Tunkel AR. Nosocomial bacterial meningitis. *N Engl J Med* 2010;362:146–154. [PMID: 19943708] (Very practical review of causes [neurosurgical, trauma, procedures] of meningitis and how to prevent and treat.)

van de Beek D, et al. Adjunctive dexamethasone in bacterial meningitis: A meta-analysis of individual patient data. *Lancet Neurol* 2010;9(3):254–263. [PMID: 20138011] (Meta-analysis of five trials [2029 patients] showing that adding dexamethasone to the antibiotic treatment of bacterial meningitis failed to show reduction in death, severe neurologic sequelae, or severe deafness, but there was mild reduction in hearing loss compared to placebo [24% compared to 29%]).

BACTERIAL BRAIN ABSCESS

ESSENTIALS OF DIAGNOSIS

► Acts as an expanding mass, producing headache, lethargy, and signs of elevated intracranial pressure

► Few systemic signs—fever, increased erythrocyte sedimentation rate (ESR), neutrophilic reaction rare

► Seizures (common)

► Arises from contiguous spread from nearby infection, such as mastoiditis, penetrating head trauma, open skull fracture, intracranial foreign body; or hematogenous spread from infection elsewhere in body

▶ General Considerations

Parenchymal brain infection arises from hematogenous spread of infected material, especially from the mouth after dental work, which often results in multiple abscesses. Especially at risk are patients with congenital heart disease or valve infection. Abscess can also be the result of contiguous spread following meningitis or infection in nearby structures such as the nasopharynx and sinuses (frontal lobe), or middle ear and mastoid (temporal lobe or cerebellum), and it can follow penetrating head trauma, open skull fracture, or intracranial placement of a foreign body (ventricular drain, shunt, intracranial pressure monitor).

▶ Pathogenesis

Abscesses begin with local cerebritis, causing necrosis and surrounding edema. Fibroblasts form a thick capsule outside the abscess. Other than seizures, which are a common presenting problem, symptoms arise gradually from pressure on nearby structures or, rarely, suddenly from arteritis or stroke.

▶ Prevention

Elimination of infection outside the CNS before it can spread to the brain is the ideal form of prevention. Extra caution during neurosurgical procedures, such as changing sterile gloves before placement of and immediate removal of drains or intraventricular catheters, at the first sign of bacteremia may prevent the spread of infection from skin or blood to brain. Vaccination against common pathogens, such as *S pneumoniae* in patients undergoing splenectomy or cochlear implant placement or suffering from sickle cell disease, *H influenzae* in babies and children, and *N meningitidis* in young adults, is very effective. However, infection remains possible with an organism of differing serotype than those in the vaccine, so it is not a guarantee of permanent protection.

▶ Clinical Findings

A. Symptoms and Signs

The manifestations of an abscess reflect its location(s). Cortical signs evolve slowly over days to weeks and include personality change, aphasia, hemiparesis, hemisensory loss, and visual field defects. Infratentorial signs include ataxia, nystagmus, cranial nerve dysfunction, nausea, and vomiting. More diffuse signs, sometimes evolving over weeks, include headache in about 75% of patients, fever in more than 50%, and deterioration of mental status in 50%. Obtundation or coma may be due to increased intracranial pressure, often caused by obstructive hydrocephalus or rarely after rupture of an abscess into the ventricles causes meningitis. Papilledema is often present. Seizures, even status epilepticus, are common. Hypothalamic dysfunction may lead to diabetes insipidus, or temperature dysregulation. Hyponatremia from syndrome of inappropriate antidiuretic hormone sometimes occurs. Neonates develop fontanelle distention or increased head circumference.

Clues to the originating source of infection can be obtained by examination of the skin, ears, teeth, and heart. Risk factors include congenital heart disease, diabetes, alcohol abuse, recent tattoos, immunosuppression, and poor dentition.

B. Laboratory Findings

Systemic abnormalities are unusual, although some elevation of ESR and mild leukocytosis are present in half of patients. Blood cultures can reveal the organism, especially in patients with endocarditis. Attempts should be made to discover the organism from culture of peripheral infected sites, such as decubitus ulcers. CSF changes are nonspecific, rarely yielding the organism in a brain abscess, and because lumbar puncture can risk herniation, it should be avoided. Open biopsy can usually be safely performed if the abscess is located near the brain surface. When the abscess is deep, needle aspiration under stereotactic guidance may be necessary. Because many cultures are sterile, polymerase chain reaction (PCR) with DNA sequencing may prove useful in establishing the presence of an organism, but cannot guide the antibiotic choice. Instead, each hospital's unique biograms with recent sensitivity results for common pathogens may help once PCR establishes which organism to treat.

In abscesses causing tolerable symptoms (ie, not in danger of herniation), empiric antibiotics, using imaging to measure capsule thickness and overall size, can be safely administered, with adjustments made for the effect of corticosteroid therapy on capsule size and surrounding edema. Periodic reexamination for treatment failure is mandatory.

B. Imaging Studies

CT scan reveals poorly defined low-density lesions that do not initially enhance (see Figure 26–3A). MRI is the most sensitive test for abscess (see Figure 26–3B). Typical findings include hypointense areas of necrosis (abscess) surrounded by hyperintense signal (edema) on T2-weighted or fluid-attenuated inversion recovery (FLAIR) images. On diffusion-weighted imaging (DWI), abscess is hyperintense, with reduced apparent diffusion coefficient (ADC) compared to lesions that are not pus containing (eg, cystic tumor). Contrast enhancement with gadolinium outlines the capsule, but must be avoided in renal failure in order to prevent nephrogenic systemic fibrosis. Venous compromise can be seen with magnetic resonance venography. In abscess, unlike tumor or multiple sclerosis, the thinnest section of the capsule tends to be on the side away from the ventricle, and the inner rim of the capsule is smooth, as opposed to irregular. After about 2 weeks an enhancing rim forms, representing the beginning of capsule formation (see Figure 26–3C). Imaging may also show complications such as infarction.

▶ Differential Diagnosis

The main differential diagnosis of this "space-occupying lesion" is neoplasm, either primary or metastatic. Nonbacterial abscess (eg, fungal, parasitic such as toxoplasmosis) occurs, especially in diabetic or immunocompromised hosts. Other considerations include subacute stroke, radiation necrosis, resolving hematoma, herpes encephalitis, and acute disseminated encephalomyelitis.

▶ Complications

Death occurs in 10–15% of adults and 25% of children, even in the antibiotic era. Transtentorial or central herniation is a complication of temporal lobe or large frontal abscess, and cerebellar abscess can lead to brainstem herniation. Hydrocephalus occurs if the abscess occludes the fourth ventricle. Meningitis or ventriculitis follows abscess eruption into the CSF.

Relapse occurs in 5–10% of patients after completed courses of appropriate antibiotics.

Epilepsy may be a permanent consequence of infection, occurring in 3% of newly diagnosed epilepsies in Rochester, Minnesota, and 5.2% in Ecuador.

▶ Treatment

A. Medical Therapy

Once the pathogenic organism has been established or suspected based on individual patient risk factors such as recent surgery, presence of diabetes, or injection drug use, the choice of antibiotic treatment is the same as for organisms mentioned in the discussion of bacterial meningitis (Table 26–3). However, intravenous antibiotic therapy must be continued for 4–6 weeks or longer, as determined by a decrease in the size of the abscess, seen on imaging. Carbapenems, fluoroquinolones, and aztreonam all have good penetration into the CNS, but dose adjustment for weight and renal function is necessary to avoid CNS toxicity such as seizures or tremor. Aminoglycoside delivery into an abscess or the ventricular system by Ommaya reservoir is sometimes attempted. Tuberculous abscess requires treatment with four drugs: pyrazinamide, ethambutol, isoniazid, and rifabutin. Corticosteroids may slow antibiotic delivery and capsule formation; their use should be limited to short periods when reduction in edema or elevated intracranial pressure is mandatory.

B. Surgical Therapy

Neurosurgical intervention takes two forms: biopsy and abscess removal. Needle biopsy, or aspiration if in a late stage of cerebritis, helps determine the causative organism and correct antibiotic treatment, and once a capsule has formed may help antibiotic penetration into it. Judgment is required to see if biopsy or resection is safe, and in cases where the abscess is located deep in the brain, stereotactic guidance is always

Table 26–3. Antibiotic Treatment of Brain Abscess

Infection Source	Causative Organism	Antibiotic
Ear, mastoid, sinus	Streptococcal species, *Pseudomonas*, anaerobes, Enterobacteriaceae	Metronidazole, 7.5 mg IV q 6 h *plus* Cefepime, 2 g IV q 6 h *or* Meropenem, 2 g IV q 8 h
Lung	*S pneumoniae*	Same as above
Teeth, mouth	Anaerobic streptococci, *Eikenella*, *Prevotella*, and *Actinomyces*	Metronidazole, 7.5 mg/kg IV q 12 h *plus* Penicillin G, 4 million units IV q 4 h *or* ceftizoxime, 3 g IV q 6 h
Postoperative infection, decubiti, furuncles	*Staphylococcus aureus* or *S epidermidis* Methicillin-resistant *S aureus* (MRSA)	Cefepime, 2 g IV q 8 h *or* Nafcillin or oxacillin, 2 g IV q 4 h Linezolid, 600 mg IV q 12 h

IV = intravenously; q = every.

recommended. Removal of the abscess is required in only a limited number of cases: loculated abscesses, those enlarging on appropriate antibiotic therapy, or those causing herniation. Although abscesses at risk of rupturing into the ventricle because they are separated only by ependyma theoretically should be removed, their deep location makes surgery technically difficult; therefore, small periventricular abscesses can usually be treated with antibiotics alone. At times, temporary external drainage is useful, although the thickness of the necrotic tissue does not lend itself to easy flow. Adjunctive surgery for otitis, mastoiditis, sinusitis, or chronic CSF leak is often required, especially when the abscess or meningitis recurs. If an abscess is located in a place that obstructs ventricular flow, such as near the fourth ventricle, hydrocephalus may require temporary drainage or permanent shunting.

 Prognosis

Prognosis is generally good, with 10% mortality in developed countries. Survivors have up to a 25% incidence of focal deficits and a highly variable rate of epilepsy. In children, especially those with cyanotic congenital heart disease, there is a 15% incidence of static encephalopathy. Prognosis is worse in patients older than 60 years and in those with multiple lesions, ruptured abscess, or decreased state of consciousness on presentation.

Chandra PS, et al. Surgery for medically intractable epilepsy due to post-infectious etiologies. *Epilepsia* 2010;51:1097–1100. [PMID: 20345935] (Brain abscess is one of several postinfectious causes of epilepsy that responds to resection of gliosis in 28 patients operated on over 2 years.)

Goodkin HP, Harper MB, Pomeroy SL. Intracerebral abscess in children: Historical trends at Children's Hospital Boston. *Pediatrics* 2004;113:1765–1770. [PMID: 15173504] (Review of intracerebral abscess in 54 children between 1981 and 2000, emphasizing predisposing factors, bacterial causes, and outcomes.)

Shachor-Meyouhas Y, et al. Brain abscess in children—Epidemiology, predisposing factors and management in the modern medicine era. *Acta Paediatr* 2010;99:1163–1167. [PMID: 20222876] (Review of recent developments in childhood brain abscess.)

Singh G, Prabhakar S. The association between central nervous system (CNS) infections and epilepsy: Epidemiological approaches and microbiological and epileptological perspectives. *Epilepsia* 2008;49(Suppl 6):2–7. [PMID: 18754954] (A summary of the relationship between symptomatic epilepsy and infection, including malaria, meningitis, parastic infection, and viral causes.)

Ziai WC, Lewin III JJ. Update in the diagnosis and management of central nervous system infections. *Neurol Clin* 2008;26: 427–468. [PMID: 18514821] (Broad review of all infections with detailed recommendations of diagnosis and management.)

SUBDURAL EMPYEMA

ESSENTIALS OF DIAGNOSIS

- ▶ Rapid and unilateral spread of pus over the brain surface
- ▶ crosses boundaries between fossae
- ▶ Headache, localized tenderness, fever, focal seizures, progressive cortical signs; if untreated, coma, herniation
- ▶ Arises from nearby sinus infection or after thrombosis of venous sinus, penetrating trauma, skull fracture

General Considerations

Subdural empyema, an infected collection situated beneath the skull and dura, is a rare complication of frontal or ethmoid sinusitis, meningitis, and osteomyelitis that can be life-threatening. It can also follow venous sinus thrombosis, skull fracture, penetrating trauma, or craniotomy. Prompt recognition and treatment of sinusitis and CSF leak can prevent infection in the subdural space.

▶ Clinical Findings

A. Symptoms and Signs

Initial extracranial infection (eg, otitis media, sinusitis) is followed in days to weeks by increased localized pain or headache, recurrent fever, and the development of cortical signs, especially seizures. Seizures are usually partial with some secondary generalization. Depressed sensorium occurs eventually, along with hemiparesis and cranial nerve deficits, including papilledema. Development of stroke or brain abscess occurs if the problem is unrecognized for prolonged periods.

B. Laboratory Findings

Lumbar puncture, although not recommended owing to the risk of herniation and insufficient yield, reveals increased protein concentration, mild lymphocytic pleocytosis, and normal glucose level, but rarely grows any organisms on culture. Direct smear and culture results obtained surgically may reveal organisms.

C. Imaging Studies

CT should be performed with contrast, which reveals enhancement of the margins of the low-density collection overlying (and molding) the cortex (see Figure 26–4A). MRI shows a collection, hyperintense on T1-weighted and isointense to CSF on T2-weighted images, lying outside the brain. In contrast to epidural abscess, subdural infection can spread across fossae boundaries.

▶ Differential Diagnosis

Subdural hematoma, meningioma, granuloma (eg, sarcoidosis), and mycobacterial infection make up the differential diagnosis.

▶ Complications

Herniation and death are rare, except in patients in whom the condition goes unrecognized. Chronic epilepsy is also rare.

▶ Treatment & Prognosis

Surgical drainage is always indicated, rarely by trephination (burr hole), as craniotomy is required to dislodge organized fibrous and granulation tissue. Debridement of the initial source (eg, mastoid, sinus) is also recommended to prevent recurrence. Antibiotics are chosen based on culture results and continued for 4–6 weeks, depending on clinical and radiographic response. With early intervention complete recovery is the norm.

Foerster BR, et al. Intracranial infections: Clinical and imaging characteristics. *Acta Radiol* 2007;48(8):875–893. [PMID: 17924219] (Anatomic predilection and characteristic imaging findings for several types of infection are reviewed. Magnetic resonance spectroscopy and diffusion features are given, including high signal in subdural and low or isointense signal in epidural on apparent diffusion coefficient map.)

Mat Nayan SA, et al. Two surgical methods used in 90 patients with intracranial subdural empyema. *J Clin Neurosci* 2009;16(12):1567–1571. [PMID: 19793660] (Open drainage had better outcome than burr hole and drainage; both required 6 weeks of antibiotics).

Tsou T-P, et al. Microbiology and epidemiology of brain abscess and subdural empyema in a medical center: A 10-year experience. *J Microbiol Immunol Infect* 2009;42:405–412. [PMID: 20182670] (Subdural empyema incidence did not change from 1998–2007 in a Taiwan hospital, and 4 of 10 were the consequence of bacterial meningitis, with variable infective agents.)

Wanna GB, et al. Contemporary management of intracranial complications of otitis media. *Otol Neurotol* 2010;31(1):111–117. [PMID: 19887978] (Surgical and medical approach to infection spreading from the ear and mastoid.)

EPIDURAL ABSCESS

1. Cranial Epidural Abscess

ESSENTIALS OF DIAGNOSIS

- ▶ Developes continuously to post-operative infection or osteomyelitis secondary to chronic sinus or middle ear infection
- ▶ Location outside the arachnoid and dura, extent bounded by fossae
- ▶ Gradenigo syndrome (ipsilateral cranial nerve V, VI palsies) occurs when petrous bone is involved
- ▶ Less cortical symptomatology (seizure, focal deficit) than subdural empyema or brain abscess

▶ Pathogenesis

Many epidural abscesses are due to multiple organisms, most commonly streptococci, followed by staphylococci and anaerobes, although nosocomial infections are often caused by *Pseudomonas* or other gram-negative bacteria.

▶ Clinical Findings

A. Symptoms and Signs

Cranial epidural abscess resembles subdural empyema, except that symptoms develop more insidiously and herniation is less likely. Involvement of the base of the skull produces specific syndromes, which are summarized in Table 26–4.

Table 26–4. Syndromes Associated With Skull Base Infection

Syndrome	Cranial Nerves Affected	Clinical Findings	Site of Lesion	Source of Infection
Foix-Jefferson	III, IV, V-1, V-2, V-3(?), VI	Eye pain, ophthalmoparesis, hemifacial numbness, exophthalmos	Cavernous sinus	Ethmoid or sphenoid sinusitis, mucormycosis
Cavernous sinus/ Supraorbital syndrome	III, IV, V-1, VI	Same, except numbness limited to V-I (forehead)	Cavernous sinus, lateral wall	Same as above
Gradenigo	V, VI	Diplopia, (horizontal) facial neuralgia	Petrous bone, tip	Otitis, mastoiditis
No eponym	VII, VIII	Facial weakness, ear pain, deafness	Petrous bone	Otitis media
Vernet	IX-XI	Dysphagia, pharyngeal numbness, hoarseness, trapezius weakness, temporal lobe seizures	Base of skull, jugular foramen	Otitis externa, mastoiditis
Villaret	IX-XII	Same as for Vernet syndrome, plus tongue weakness, sympathetic ptosis, miosis, enophthalmos	Base of skull, retroparotid space	Retropharyngeal abscess or retroparotid lymphadenitis

B. Imaging Studies

CT or MRI scan shows a lens-shaped hypodense area with irregular enhancement at the rim, respecting divisions of anterior, middle and posterior cranial fossa. Bony infection can be seen nearby (see Figure 26–4B).

▶ Treatment

Surgery (trephination, less often craniotomy) is necessary to obtain material for culture and to relieve pressure. Antibiotic therapy, broad spectrum until culture results are obtained, is outlined in Table 26–5.

2. Spinal Epidural Abscess

ESSENTIALS OF DIAGNOSIS

▶ Arises as contiguous spread from disk infection, vertebral body osteomyelitis, infected deep decubiti, surgery, trauma, or injection of epidural anesthesia or corticosteroids; or hematogenous spread during sepsis

▶ Chronic or acute onset of symptoms

▶ Weakness and sensory loss below the level of the lesion (spinal cord compression)

▶ Paraplegia and pain/temperature loss below the level of the lesion, with preserved proprioception (anterior spinal artery infarction)

▶ General Considerations

Infection of the spine is a rare cause of neck and back pain that accounts for about 3 per 10,000 hospital admissions.

Diskitis has an incidence of 0.1–2 cases per 100,000 per year. It may lead to cord compression. Although the extensive involvement of subdural space over many vertebral levels implies that this infection is actually an empyema, it is most commonly called an abscess.

▶ Pathogenesis

Posterior abscesses are in the vertical sleeve between the dura and the vertebral column, allowing extension over several levels, with bacteria arriving from hematogenous spread, nearby structures that are infected (eg, psoas muscle abscess), or after iatrogenic disruption of the dura. However up to 40% of cases have no identifiable source. There is a predisposition for abscess to develop at sites of prior trauma or surgery, related to devascularization of the area. Anterior epidural abscesses arise from disk or vertebral body infection, and rarely can complicate bacterial meningitis. Epidural abscess formation can result from invasive procedures such as spine surgery, including placement of pumps for baclofen or morphine infusion, epidural anesthesia to support childbirth or pelvic surgery, vertebroplasty or facet joint injection, or even lumbar puncture. Although pain is usually present for days to weeks, an acute evolution of neurologic deficit (ie, occurring over hours) is often the result of spinal cord infarction and is therefore irreversible. Infarction can be caused by thrombophlebitis or profound cord compression. The more common chronic evolution is associated with the deposition of granulation tissue and pus, and is usually reversible if surgically decompressed. Bone destruction leading to kyphosis (gibbus formation) can also contribute to cord stretching and dysfunction.

Populations at increased risk of this infection are diabetics; alcoholics; injection drug users; those with end-stage renal or hepatic disease, or with chronic urinary tract infections; smokers; and the immunosuppressed.

Table 26–5. Antibiotic Treatment of Parameningeal Infection[a]

Infection Source	Causative Organism	Antibiotic	
		First Choice	Alternative
Ear, mastoid	Anaerobes,[b] Pseudomonas aeruainosa, Proteus mirabilis, Staphylococcus aureus	Penicillin G, 2–4 million units IV q 4–6 h plus Fluoroquinolone[c] plus Metronidazole, 15 mg/kg IV q 12 h, or, if allergic to penicillin, chloramphenicol, 500 mg IV q 6 h	Cefepime, 2 g IV q 12 h or Ceftizoxime, 3 g IV q 8 h or Meropenem, 2 g IV q 8 h
Paranasal and ethmoid sinuses	Peptostreptococcus species, Streptococcus viridans, Streptococcus anainosus, Haemophilus influenzae	Penicillin G, 2–4 million units IV q 4–6 h plus Metronidazole, 15 mg/kg IV q 12 h	Ceftriaxone, 2 g IV q 12 h plus Metronidazole, 15 mg/kg IV q 12 h
Teeth, mouth	Bacteroides species, Prevotella species, Gemella haemolysans	Ceftizoxime, 3 g IV q 6 h	Ceftriaxone, 2 g IV q 12 h plus Metronidazole, 15 mg/kg IV q 12 h
Postoperative or trauma	S aureus S epidermidis, Enterobacteriaceae, MRSA	Vancomycin, 1 g IV q 12 h plus 3rd- or 4th-generation cephalosporin	Linezolid, 600 mg IV q 12 h
Elsewhere in body	Variable bacteria	Use culture, sensitivity results from source	Follow culture, sensitivity

IV = intravenously; MRSA = methicillin-resistant S aureus; q = every.
[a]Includes subdural empyema, cranial or spinal epidural abscess, and suppurative thrombophlebitis.
[b]Anaerobes, such as Bacillus fragilis, Fusobacterium species, Veillonella, Actinomyces, Propionibacterium acnes, and Eubacterium, are rarely cultured and often polymicrobial.
[c]Fluoroquinolones include ciprofloxacin, 400 mg IV q 12 h; moxifloxacin, 400 mg/day IV; levofloxacin, 500 mg/day IV; and gatifloxacin, 400 mg/day IV.

Staphylococcal infection, spread from the skin in more than 50% of cases, is responsible for most cases, but more chronic abscess can be caused by tuberculous infection. Fungal infections (especially Aspergillus) are also encountered. Less commonly encountered bacteria include Pneumococcus; gram-negative organisms such as E coli, Brucella, Pseudomonas, and Salmonella; and anaerobes such as Fusobacterium, Actinomyces, Proteus, and Nocardia species. Predilection for location in the thoracic spine relates to the wide epidural space found in this region and to retrograde transmission of infection from the pelvis through the valveless venous (Batson) plexus and, in the case of Aspergillus, to direct spread from adjacent pulmonary or mediastinal infection.

▶ Clinical Findings

A. Symptoms and Signs

Only a minority of patients have all three of the classic triad of pain, fever, and neurologic deficit; of these pain is the most common symptom, present in about 75% of patients, and is at the site of disk or vertebral bone involvement. Fever

is present in half and neurologic deficit in one third, usually following several days of pain. Lesions of the thoracic spine cause paraparesis and sensory loss below the lesion, or rarely dermatomal pain and numbness due to root compression. Within the spinal canal, dorsal locations were more associated with paraplegia or quadriplegia than ventral in one series of 104 patients. If the abscess is cervical, arm pain or weakness is a rare complication. Bladder symptoms include frequency, urgency, and incontinence of small amounts, but not a constant dribbling. Constipation is common. If the abscess is lumbar, with conus medullaris or cauda equina involvement, urinary signs include overflow incontinence and absent pelvic sensation. Sexual dysfunction occurs with a lesion at any level. Symptoms are reviewed in Table 26–6.

B. Laboratory Findings

Elevated WBC count, ESR, and C-reactive protein level are common. Skin testing with purified protein derivative (PPD) is usually positive in cases of mycobacterial infection. CSF shows increased protein concentration and white cell count, with normal glucose level. During lumbar puncture it

Table 26–6. Clinical Findings in Spinal Epidural Abscess

| Characteristic | Cervical | Location | | |
		Thoracic	Lumbar	Sacral
Pain[a]	Arms	Bandlike chest	Groin, legs	Leg, pelvis
Numbness	Radicular (pin), sensory level	Sensory level, dermatomal (rare)	Sensory level, dermatomal	Legs, vagina, penis
Weakness	Below neck, arm, and hand	Legs	Legs	Feet
Bladder signs	UMN	UMN	LMN	LMN
Reflexes[b]	↓ in arms, ↑ in legs	↑ in legs	↓ in legs	↓ in ankles

↓ = decreased; ↑ = increased; LMN = lower motor neuron; UMN = upper motor neuron.
[a]Pain is accompanied by tenderness in corresponding spine region.
[b]Babinski sign is present in all but lumbosacral abscesses.

is essential to avoid introducing material from an epidural abscess into the subarachnoid space. CT-guided biopsy of the abscess can provide tissue to culture to determine the organism.

C. Imaging Studies

Bacterial epidural abscess usually involves at least two adjacent vertebrae, with destruction of the disk (Figure 26–5) and occasional vertebral osteomyelitis; conversely, malignancy rarely crosses to adjacent vertebrae in this way. MRI with contrast is 90% sensitive and specific, and shows decreased signal in the intervertebral disk space with loss of end plates adjacent to the infected disk and enhancement in the subarachnoid space over one or more levels. Adjacent bone may show low signal areas, end plate and cortical destruction on T1-weighted images, and high signal in the disk or vertebral body on T2-weighted images. Bone marrow edema and soft tissue extension are detected by fat suppression techniques. Where MRI is not available, CT with delayed imaging after intravenous contrast shows similar findings. CT plus intrathecal administration of metrizamide has replaced traditional pantopaque myelography, as there is no need for C1–C2 puncture to show the upper limit of an abscess, but it is still invasive. Bone destruction is better visualized on CT than MRI; when advanced it can be seen on plain radiographs as well. Nuclear imaging shows increased uptake in vertebral osteomyelitis, but this is indistinguishable from tumor. Gallium scan can reveal a paraspinal source of infection.

▶ Differential Diagnosis

Metastatic tumor, epidermal lipomatosis, and osteoporotic compression fracture comprise the main differential diagnosis of spinal epidural abscess. They can be distinguished from abscess, which usually is accompanied by fever and leukocytosis, in addition to signs of cord compression. Herniation of a disk usually causes radicular pain, but if cord compression

occurs its onset is more rapid than that of abscess. Rarely, parasitic infection with *Schistosoma* or *Echinococcus* can mimic a bacterial abscess. Viral and bacterial intramedullary infection must also be considered.

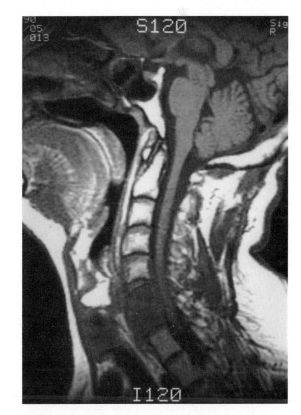

▲ **Figure 26–5.** C6–C7 spondylodiskitis. Sagittal T1-weighted image shows low T1-signal infiltration of the C6–C7 disk space and adjacent vertebral bodies associated with a moderately large ventral epidural mass deforming the spinal cord. (Used with permission from John Loh, MD.)

Complications

Reversibility of paralysis and other deficits correlates with the length of time they took to develop. In patients whose deficits progress over the course of hours, paraplegia is usually permanent because of spinal cord infarction. Death is rare, although paraplegia shortens mortality overall.

Prevention

Improved surgical techniques such as using double gloves and changing them before placing epidural catheters can lower the incidence of postoperative infection.

Treatment

Discovering the organism from blood culture or using CT-guided aspiration to obtain tissue to culture prior to decompressive surgery facilitates the choice of appropriate antibiotic. In patients who have pus apparent on imaging, drainage plus antibiotics is usually sufficient. Decompression is required in patients whose neurologic examination is deteriorating and in patients with chronic infection that is not responding to antibiotics. Postoperative (nosocomial) infection should be assumed to be methicillin-resistant and may require intraventricular vancomycin, 20 mg/day for adults and 10 mg/day for children.

Darouiche RO. Spinal epidural abscess. *N Engl J Med* 2006; 355(19):2012–2020. [PMID: 17093252] (An article in the Current Concepts series that reviews diagnosis and treatment schema, with excellent graphic explanations.)

Karikari IO, et al. Management of a spontaneous spinal epidural abscess: A single-center 10-year experience. *Neurosurgery* 2009; 65(5):919–924. [PMID: 19834405] (One hundred four patients treated over 10 years are reviewed, conservative management being used in 61%, but early surgery, including CT-guided aspiration, is recommended due to better outcome.)

Okada Y, et al. Clinical and radiological outcome of surgery for pyogenic and tuberculous spondylitis: Comparisons of surgical techniques and disease types. *J Neurosurg Spine* 2009;11(5):620–627. [PMID: 19929368] (In 52 patients, the half with pyogenic spondylitis did better than those with tuberculous infection, whose time to recovery was much longer and who had more residual neurologic deficits. The patients who underwent anterior decompression and fusion did better than those treated by posterior approach. Those who had instrumentation placed instead of bone autograph had less residual kyphosis.)

O'Toole JE, Eicholz KM, Fessler RG. Surgical site infection rates after minimally invasive spinal surgery. *J Neurosurg Spine* 2009;11(4):471–476. [PMID: 19929344] (Review of large surgical databases found three postoperative surgical site infections in 1338 procedures, for a rate of 0.1% for decompressions and 0.74% for fusion/fixation, which is much better than the incidence when an open rather than tubular retractor system is used.)

Sendi P, et al. Spinal epidural abscess in clinical practice. *QJM* 2008;101(1):1–12. [PMID: 17982180] (Comprehensive review of the subject.)

INTRACRANIAL SUPPURATIVE THROMBOPHLEBITIS

ESSENTIALS OF DIAGNOSIS

▶ May occur as a complication of facial cellulitis, otitis, sinusitis, or meningitis in children

▶ Life-threatening complication: increased intracranial pressure secondary to venous sinus occlusion (rare)

Pathogenesis

The deep and superficial veins and dural venous sinuses are susceptible to infection because of the lack of valves, which allows blood flow in both directions. Thus, cavernous sinus phlebitis can cause orbital infection, ethmoid sinusitis can cause cranial infarcts, and mastoiditis or otitis can cause transverse sinus infarction. Contiguous infection can lead to reactive (sterile) venulitis as well.

Clinical Findings

A. Symptoms and Signs

Focal findings, including partial seizures, reflect the location of the vein or sinus involved, eg, cavernous sinus thrombosis causes third, fourth, and sixth cranial nerve palsies, with absence of sensation in the first division of the trigeminal nerve (and orbital displacement), (see Table 26–4), frontal cortical vein thrombosis causes hemiparesis, or aphasia. Elevated intracranial pressure, obtundation, visual blurring, and sixth nerve paresis can occur in extensive venous or sagittal sinus thrombosis due to lack of venous drainage. Headache and stuttering stroke-like progression of focal deficits are also seen. Pharyngeal or tonsillar infection in young adults can cause jugular vein phlebitis.

B. Imaging Studies

Venous infarcts can be inferred from loss of sulci near the appropriate sinus, occasionally accompanied by petechial hemorrhage. If a large sinus is involved, more extensive edema is seen. CT with contrast can show filling voids in the sinuses or dural enhancement. MRI is a more sensitive method for visualizing ischemic changes than CT, which often shows only the secondary hemorrhage. Magnetic resonance venography (MRV) is especially useful. Thrombus is initially isointense on T1-weighted MR and becomes hyperintense to brain over days. DWI is hyperintesne due to the increased water content in the necrotic tissue. When MRV is unavailable, catheter cerebral angiography is required to make the diagnosis.

Differential Diagnosis

In the cavernous sinus, vascular abnormalities such as fistula, tumor, sarcoidosis, Tolosa-Hunt inflammatory syndrome,

Herpes zoster ophthalmicus, and diabetic cranial nerve infarct can present similarly to infection. In the neck, dissection of arteries may resemble thrombophlebitis. Trauma due to catheters may also resemble thrombophlebitis.

Complications

Stroke, hemorrhage, herniation, and seizures are the most common complications. Long-standing papilledema can lead to optic atrophy and decreased vision. Cavernous sinus thrombosis even in the antibiotic era has a mortality rate of 20–30%, with blindness or cranial nerve palsies remaining in up to 75% of survivors.

Treatment

Prolonged antibiotic therapy directed at the organism present at the originating site of infection is given for up to 8 weeks (see Tables 26–1, 26–3, and 26–5). Anticoagulation is dangerous because of the risk of hemorrhage in the infected area, but may be necessary in cases without adequate collateral channels such as sagittal sinus thrombosis. Increased intracranial pressure should be treated with elevation of the head, mannitol infusion (1 g/kg), and hyperventilation if necessary; corticosteroids are unlikely to be helpful. Ventriculoperitoneal shunt is occasionally required if hydrocephalus develops after thrombosis of the superior sagittal sinus. As in noninfectious venous thrombosis, long-term anticoagulation is used, but has not been tested in controlled trials. No evidence of increased risk of hematoma formation has been associated with anticoagulation.

Ito E, et al. Cavernous sinus thrombophlebitis caused by *Porphyromonas gingivalis* with abscess formation extending to the orbital cavity. *Neurol Med Chir (Tokyo)* 2009;49(8): 370–373. [PMID: 19707005] (Case report with excellent imaging and description of cavernous sinus abnormalities, including pathophysiology of thrombosis.)

MALIGNANT OTITIS EXTERNA

General Considerations

Adults with diabetes or immunosuppression are at highest risk for this infection, which spreads from the external auditory canal to the temporal bone, temporomandibular joint, or mastoid, and from there into the petrous bone.

Clinical Findings

A. Symptoms and Signs

Severe ear pain followed by symptoms of compression of the facial nerve occurs first in 30% of patients. Occasionally the fifth and sixth nerves are involved at the apex. Other foraminal involvement will affect cranial nerves passing through, such as the glossopharyngeal, vagal, and spinal accessory

nerves with involvement of the jugular foramen and the hypoglossal nerve in the hypoglossal canal.

Pathogenesis

Chronic ear infection (4–6 weeks) spreads from the external ear canal to involve the bone. The most common cause is *Pseudomonas aeruginosa*.

Diagnosis

CT shows bony destruction, and often pus drains from the ear canal, which should be cultured even if local antibiotic therapy has been ongoing.

Treatment and Prognosis

Surgical debridement is necessary, even when culturing pus draining from the ear allows selection of appropriate antibiotics. At least 2–3 weeks of parenteral antibiotic followed by prolonged oral antibiotics are necessary. Prognosis is guarded, with residual cranial nerve deficits being common.

Chen CN, et al. Outcomes of malignant external otitis: Survival vs mortality. *Acta Otolaryngol* 2009;22:1–6. [PMID: 19466617] (Twenty-six diabetic patients with mean age of 63 collected from 1993–2005 are described, of whom 11 had cranial nerve dysfunction [38% facial nerve]. Three patients developed intracranial involvement. Most cases were caused by *Pseudomonas*, followed by *Klebsiella* and fungi).

CHRONIC & RECURRENT MENINGITIS

ESSENTIALS OF DIAGNOSIS

► Chronic meningitis—symptoms that last more than 4 weeks

► Recurrent meningitis—acute symptoms that return more than twice, with periods of complete recovery in between

► Both aseptic and septic causes

General Considerations

Ten percent of all cases of meningitis are chronic; even fewer are recurrent. Chronic meningitis shares all the symptoms of acute meningitis, but to a lesser degree, and may fluctuate or improve spontaneously. In severely immunosuppressed patients who cannot mount a strong inflammatory response, chronic meningitis may result from virulent bacterial organisms that are usually associated with acute meningitis. Persistent or recurrent headache following meningitis does not always have an infectious origin, and may even be a "low-pressure" headache brought on by repeated lumbar punctures creating a CSF leak.

▶ Pathogenesis

Chronic meningitis often results from ongoing infection (Table 26–7), especially in patients with skull fracture or prior neurosurgery; chemical causes such as epidermoid cyst rupture or instillation of chemotherapy; malignancies; autoimmune disease; or bacterial infection of lower virulence (Table 26–8). Recurrent bacterial meningitis is associated with defects in the protective barriers to the meninges, including congential cranial or spinal sinus tracts, basilar skull fracture, or following CNS surgery.

▶ Prevention

Control of systemic illness such as lupus erythematosus with immunosuppressive treatment lowers the incidence of chronic autoimmune meningitis (discussed later). Radiation and chemotherapy can prevent carcinomatous causes of meningitis. Vaccination with bacille Calmette-Guérin (BCG) may reduce the incidence of tuberculous meningitis, and pneumococcal vaccine limits recurrent infection in at-risk patients. Avoidance of repeat exposure to medications known to induce aseptic meningitis, especially nonsteroidal anti-inflammatory agents that may be used without prescription, limits drug-induced meningitis in sensitive patients.

▶ Clinical Findings

A. Symptoms and Signs

Meningeal signs, fever, encephalopathy, and rarely focal signs are present to varying degrees in patients with chronic or recurrent meningitis. Slow, spontaneous resolution may occur. In recurrent meningitis, examination for dermal sinus tracts or a history of basilar skull fracture can reveal the source of infection.

Table 26–7. Infectious Causes of Chronic Meningitis

Cause	CSF		Special Considerations/Laboratory Studies/Treatment[a]
	Cells	Glucose	
Bacterial			
Actinomyces	Neu	Low	Atypical—fungal-like; gram positive; penicillin
Brucella suis, melitensis, abortus	Lym	Low	Contracted from contact with swine, sheep, goats, and cattle; doxycycline plus gentamicin (TMP-SMX < 8 y)
Nocardia	Neu	Low	Atypical—fungal; abscess; acid-fast; TMP-SMX, imipenem
Fungal			
Cryptococcus	Lym	Low	Serum and CSF Ag and Ab, India ink stain
Coccidioides	Lym	Low-normal	Geographic distribution: southwest US/Mexico
Histoplasmosis	Mono	Normal-slightly low	Ab in CSF/CF or RIA Geographic distribution near river valleys
Mycobacterial			
Mycobacterium tuberculosis	Neu (early), Lym	Low	+PPD, PCR, acid-fast stain, > 25 mL for culture
Mycobacterium avium intracellulare	Lym	Low	Blood and CSF culture
Rickettsial			
Rickettsia	Lym	Low	Relapsing; serum Ab; doxycycline
Treponemal			Stage of infection affects CSF; atraumatic lumbar puncture required
Treponema pallidum (syphilitic)	Lym	Low	+ VDRL or RPR, oligoclonal bands; penicillin
Borrelia burgdorferi	Lym	Low	Anti-B burgdorferi Ab in CSF > serum; ELISA; ceftriaxone
Leptospira	Lym, Neu	Low	Serum agglutination, culture, enzyme immunoassay, ELISA
Viral			
HIV	Lym	Normal	Oligoclonal bands and elevated IgG index
Cytomegalovirus	Lym, Neu	Low	Serum and CSF Ab, PCR, culture
Herpes simplex 1 or 2	Lym or endothelial	Normal to Low	(Mollaret meningitis) PCR
Enteroviruses	Lym	Low	Exposure, children > adults
Epstein-Barr	Lym	Normal	Seroconversion
Lymphocytic choriomeningitis	Lym	Normal to Low	Seroconversion, thrombocytopenia
West Nile	Neu	Normal to Low	With polio-like syndrome

Ab = antibody; Ag = antigen; CSF = cerebrospinal fluid; CF = complement fixation; ELISA = enzyme-linked immunosorbent assay; Eos = eosinophil; Lym = lymphocyte; Neu = neutrophil; PCR = polymerase chain reaction; PPD = purified protein derivative; RIA = radioimmunoassay; RPR = rapid plasma reagin; VDRL = Venereal Disease Research Laboratory; + = positive.
[a]See also Table 26–1.

Table 26–8. Noninfectious Causes of "Aseptic" Meningitis (Lymphocytic Pleocytosis)

Cause	CSF Cells	CSF Glucose	Special Considerations/Laboratory Studies/Treatment
Inflammatory			
Sarcoidosis	Lym	Low	ACE levels, uveitis, diabetes insipidus; radiographic imaging-enhancing lesions
Behçet syndrome	Lym, Neu	Normal	Mucous membrane lesions, sometimes uveitis, arthritis; IgG
Systemic lupus erythematosus, Sjögren syndrome	Lym, Neu	Normal	+ANA, +dsDNA, antiSMAb
Postvaccine or post-*Mycoplasma* response	Lym	Normal	History; cold agglutinins
Vogt-Koyanagi-Harada syndrome	Lym	Normal	Uveitis
Wegener granulomatosis	Lym (mild)	Normal	Sinus involvement, +cANCA in serum CSF protein elevated, IgG present
Malignancy			
Non-CNS tumors (carcinomatosis)	Lym, Neu	Low	Cytology, look for primary neoplasm, enhanced MRI
Lymphomatosis	Lym	Low	Cytology, immunomarkers in CSF
Gliomatosis (primary or CNS tumor)	Lym	Low	Meningeal biopsy
Chemical			
Subarachnoid hemorrhage	Neu, Lym	Low	Hydrocephalus can occur 1 wk after event
Cyst rupture	Lym, Eos	Low	Reaction to keratin; craniopharyngioma; epidermoid
Lead or arsenic poisoning	Lym	Normal	Encephalopathy, ↑ intracranial pressure; ↑ protein
Intrathecal injection of dye, medication, or cleansing agent	Lym, Eos	Low or normal	History of procedure; distinguish from nosocomial meningitis
Medication related			
Antibiotics, NSAIDs, antiepileptic drugs	Lym, Eos, Neu	Normal	Rechallenge to prove cause
Intravenous immunoglobulin	Lym, Neu	Normal	History
Serum sickness	Neu, Lym	Normal	Circulating immune complexes
Unknown			
Hypertrophic pachymeningitis	Lym or normal	Normal	Dural biopsy diagnostic, corticosteroid treatment
Benign lymphocytic meningitis	Lym	Low or normal	Possible herpes virus

ACE = angiotensin-converting enzyme; ANA = antinuclear antibody; cANCA = cytoplasmic antineutrophil cytoplasmic antibody; CNS = central nervous system; CSF = cerebrospinal fluid; dsDNA = double-stranded DNA; Eos = eosinophil; IgG = immunoglobulin G; Lym = lymphocyte; cANCA = circulating anti-neutrophil cytoplasmic antibody, MRI = magnetic resonance imaging; Neu = neutrophil; NSAIDs = nonsteroidal anti-inflammatory drugs; SMAb = smooth muscle antibody; + = positive; ↑ = increased. Normal CSF:Serum glucose ratio = 0.6.

B. Laboratory Findings

Investigation into the patient's immune status, using anergy panels or measurement of complement level and T4 (helper) cell count, uncovers increased susceptibility to recurrent infection. CSF analysis can show low or normal glucose level, mild to moderate pleocytosis, and elevated protein concentration (extremely so in tuberculous or malignancy-related meningitis). CSF characteristics of some causes of chronic meningitis and ancillary test results are listed in Tables 26–7 and 26–8.

C. Imaging Studies

CT or MRI scans of the brain with contrast may reveal a parameningeal source of infection, sarcoidosis or other granulomata, and tumor such as craniopharyngioma or epidermoid cyst (which can cause recurrent chemical meningitis by releasing cyst contents). Intrathecal isotope or dye injection with collection of drained liquid on pledgets in the nose or ears can establish the presence of a CSF leak, but not identify the path taken, which requires imaging through the suspected area using fine cuts.

▶ Differential Diagnosis

Infectious causes of chronic or recurrent meningitis include less virulent or partially treated bacterial, viral, fungal, and protozoan infections. Mycobacterial infection causes a subacute meningitis. Mollaret meningitis, a unique recurrent, benign, aseptic meningitis with epithelial and lymphocytic cells in the CSF, is attributed to Herpes simplex type 2. Recurrent meningitis also arises from untreated parameningeal infection, violation of the blood–brain barrier, or fistula to the skin. Recurrent headache may be postural after lumbar puncture. These and other causes are listed in Tables 26–7 and 26–8.

Treatment

Infectious causes are treated with appropriate antibiotics, as outlined in earlier discussions (see Tables 26–1, 26–2, 26–5, and 26–7; fungal infections are treated as outlined in Table 26–9, later). Once appropriate treatment for infection is under way or a noninfectious cause has been discovered, corticosteroids can sometimes provide symptomatic relief.

Abu Khattab M, et al. Herpes simplex virus type 2 (Mollaret's) meningitis: A case report. *Int J Infect Dis* 2009;13(6):e476–e479. [PMID: 19329344] (Description of pathophysiology of this type of recurrent meningitis.)

Neufeld MY, Treves TA, Chistik V, Korczyn AD. Postmeningitis headache. *Headache* 1999;39:132–134. [PMID: 15613206] (Almost half of 70 patients with persistent headache following treated bacterial or aseptic meningitis developed recurrent headaches, some of which were migrainous in nature.)

TUBERCULOSIS & OTHER GRANULOMATOUS INFECTIONS

CNS TUBERCULOSIS

The incidence of CNS and systemic tuberculosis is falling: The US Centers for Disease Control and Prevention (CDC) in 2009 reported 11,540 cases, but worldwide the infection rate is much higher. The causative organism, *Mycobacterium tuberculosis*, is described as "acid fast" because the lipid content of the cell wall acquires stain that is not then dissolvable by alcohol; it is red on Ziehl-Nielsen stain, leading to the nickname "red snapper." Three forms of tuberculous infection of the CNS are discussed here: tuberculous meningitis, tuberculoma or tuberculous abscess, and Pott disease, vertebral bone infection with potential for spinal cord compression.

1. Tuberculous Meningitis

ESSENTIALS OF DIAGNOSIS

► Intracranial involvement with (in decreasing frequency) meningitis, vasculopathy, hydrocephalus, and mass lesion (tuberculoma or abscess)

► Spinal cord involvement from adjacent vertebral body infection (Pott disease), arachnoiditis, intramedullary tuberculoma, and chronic meningitis

► Morbidity and mortality as high as 30% due to delayed recognition and treatment

► Fewer than 50% of patients have positive skin test (PPD, Mantoux) results

General Considerations

Tuberculous meningitis arises from hematogenous spread of infection to the brain parenchyma, forming small tuberculomas that rupture into the subarachnoid space or ventricle, in the initial weeks following airborne mycobacterial acquisition. Less often there is spread from nearby otitis or skull infection. In other patients, instead of a subacute pattern of meningitis, after many years of asymptomatic infection, a ruptured tuberculoma may cause fulminant meningitis. Stroke may result from arteritis in the large vessels passing through the infected adhesive material at the base of the brain. If meningeal fibrosis occludes the arachnoid villi, communicating hydrocephalous slowly develops, or if subependymal fibrosis interferes with CSF flow through the ventricles, acute hydrocephalous may result.

Prevention

Vaccination with bacille Calmette-Guérin (BCG) offers incomplete protection from CNS infection (52–84%), but is recommended in areas of high prevalence.

Clinical Findings

A. Symptoms and Signs

Systemic symptoms—headache, anorexia, low-grade fever, and overall "poor health"—can be present for many weeks before meningeal signs such as neck stiffness develop. Cranial nerve involvement, especially of the sixth nerve, is present at the time of diagnosis in one third of patients. Gradual cognitive impairment may progress to coma. Seizures are more common in children. Hyponatremia, found in about half of meningitis patients, may contribute to obtundation and seizures. Increased intracranial pressure in adults leads to nausea and vomiting in about 25–43% of patients (more often in children), with papilledema in 10–15%. Infants have bulging fontanelles. Focal signs are usually attributable to stroke. A family history of tuberculosis, usually pulmonary but occasionally in the skin, lymph nodes, or elsewhere, is found in 25% of children with tuberculous meningitis or tuberculoma. Without treatment, the average duration of meningitis symptoms to death is approximately 3 weeks, although some cases are more fulminant.

B. Laboratory Findings

CSF analysis shows WBC counts ranging from 50–1000 cells/µL, with a mean of 235 cells/µL. Lymphocytes predominate, although neutrophils are seen early in the disease course in many patients. Elderly and immunocompromised patients have fewer WBCs in the CSF, which may even be acellular. Glucose level is usually less than half of the serum level, or 30 mg/dL, but may be normal, and protein concentration is elevated, often greater than 150 mg/dL. Elevated lactate levels correlate adversely with prognosis. Adenosine deaminase levels, although elevated, are not specific for tuberculosis.

Results of CSF smear are positive in fewer than 25% of patients. Culture, which requires at least 2 weeks, is positive only half of the time, even with use of large volumes of CSF, multiple lumbar punctures, and special media. Eight weeks of no growth are required to confirm a negative culture. Therefore, nucleic acid amplification (polymerase chain reaction) tests such as AMPLICOR or Gen-Probe MTD, which have a sensitivity of 90% and specificity of 80%, should be performed on all patients suspected of harboring mycobacterial infection. However, culture remains the only definite way of monitoring antibiotic sensitivity. Multidrug-resistant isolates are present in 5–9% of isolates in two series, with risk factors of HIV infection, history of previous treatment for tuberculosis, and being homeless or from endemic areas of infection. The Beijing genotype strain is hypervirulent and usually multidrug resistant, but "superresistant" has not been separately reported in recent series of CNS infection.

C. Imaging Studies

CT and MRI scans show hydrocephalus in 80% of children and up to 23% of adults. Basal meningeal enhancement is present (Figure 26–6), and thick "en plaque" meninges are

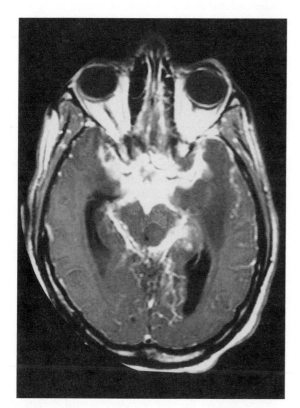

▲ **Figure 26–6.** Tuberculous meningitis. Contrast-enhanced axial T1-weighted MRI scan shows marked enhancement of the basal cisterns and mild obstructive hydrocephalus. (Used with permission from John Loh, MD.)

sometimes seen even without contrast administration in the basal cisterns. Scan findings are normal in up to 30% of patients with meningitis. Chest radiograph demonstrates the existence of tuberculous infection by apical scarring, hilar lymphadenopathy, infiltrates, or miliary tuberculosis in 40–50% of patients.

▶ Complications

Morbidity rates are 25–50% in children and higher than 10% in adults. Sequelae include seizures, developmental delay, stroke (25–40%), and hydrocephalus (50% of adults; 85% of children). Syndrome of inappropriate antidiuretic hormone (SIADH) and hyponatremia increase the risk of seizure and brain edema. Syringomyelia occasionally develops many years after tuberculous meningitis, probably as a result of spinal cord vasculitis. Fatality rates of 2–20% are cited, even in countries with access to diagnostic facilities and chemotherapeutic drugs, including directly observed therapy. Patients who are older than 60 years and those who are immunodeficient are at increased risk. Optic atrophy can complicate TB infection or its treatment. Complications of antibiotic therapy include isoniazid-induced neuropathy, ethambutol-induced optic neuritis or other visual dysfunction, streptomycin-induced ototoxicity and vestibular toxicity, and cycloserine-induced seizures. Thirty percent of severely immunosuppressed patients can develop immune reconstitution inflammatory syndrome, which is treated with corticosteroids. To prevent this complication, the treatment of HIV infection with antiviral therapy may be postponed until the tuberculous infection is controlled, usually in several weeks.

▶ Treatment

In the United States, the CDC currently recommends a three-drug regimen of oral antibiotics, including daily isoniazid, 10–20 mg/kg (generally 300 mg in adults); rifampin, 10–20 mg/kg (600 mg); and pyrazinamide, 15–30 mg/kg (maximum, 2 g/day). British guidelines add ethambutol, 15–25 mg/kg/day, for at least 2 months, followed by isoniazid and rifampin for 4 more months. The World Health Organization (WHO) recommends the same regimen, plus streptomycin, 20–40 mg/kg/day (maximum, 1 g/day) for 4 weeks, then 7 months of therapy with isoniazid or rifampin. In immunosuppressed patients, or those with multidrug-resistant organisms, streptomycin 15 mg/kg IM daily, para-aminosalicyclic acid, ethionamide, cycloserine, capreomycin, kanamycin, amikacin, or clofazimine can be added, and continued for at least 6–9 months. Such prolonged courses of therapy are required because of poor penetration into the CNS and the fact that ethambutol and streptomycin are bacteriostatic, not bactericidal. Isoniazid must be given with pyridoxine (vitamin B_6) 50 mg daily to prevent peripheral nerve damage.

Dexamethasone, 0.5–1.5 mg/kg/day, has been effective in reducing mortality in adults and children, although the reduction in morbidity has been variable. The drug is initially administered intravenously, followed by orally, with taper to complete the course after 8 weeks. Efficacy is related to reduction in cytokines and inflammatory response to infection.

Be NA, et al. Pathogenesis of central nervous system tuberculosis. *Curr Mol Med* 2009;9(2):94–99. [PMID: 19275620] (Review of tuberculous infection, including molecular aspects of the organism that affect invasion of the central nervous system and virulence.)

Caws M, et al. Beijing genotype of *Mycobacterium tuberculosis* is significantly associated with human immunodeficiency virus infection and multidrug resistance in cases of tuberculous meningitis. *J Clin Microbiol* 2006;44(11):3934–3939. [PMID: 16971650] (Analysis of 222 CSF isolates from Vietnamese patients with tuberculous meningitis demonstrated resistance to two medications [INH, rifampin] in 31% of HIV-positive and 19.5% HIV-negative patients, and to three medications [INH, rifampin and streptomycin] in 11.5% positive and 3.4% negative, and to four drugs [as above plus ethambutol] in 3.8%.)

Centers for Disease Control and Prevention: Decrease in reported tuberculosis cases—United States, 2009. *MMWR Morbid Mortal Weekly Rep* 2010;59(10):289–294 [PMID: 20300055] (Unexplained decrease of 11.4% in rate of tuberculosis infection from 2008–2009, with foreign-born cases remaining 11 times higher than US-born patients.)

Thwaites GE, et al. Dexamethasone for the treatment of tuberculous meningitis in adolescents and adults. *N Engl J Med* 2004;351:1741–1751. [PMID: 15496623] (A placebo-controlled study of 545 patients demonstrated a reduction of 0.69 relative risk of death, but no decrease in disability. This is probably because complications due to stroke were not prevented, even as complications of communicating hydrocephalus were relieved.)

Thwaites G, et al; British Infection Society. British Infection Society guidelines for the diagnosis and treatment of tuberculosis of the central nervous system in adults and children. *J Infect* 2009;59(3):167–187. [PMID: 19643501] (Summary of antimycobacterial treatment of meningitis, tuberculoma, and spinal infection using four antimicrobial agents for 2 months, then two for 10 more months, and simultaneously using corticosteroids in all cases. HIV should be tested for and treated.)

2. Tuberculoma & Tuberculous Abscess

ESSENTIALS OF DIAGNOSIS

► Seizures, progressive focal symptoms and signs, or cognitive dysfunction

▶ General Considerations

The term *tuberculoma* describes a tumor-like mass that evolves from intraparenchymal deposits of mycobacteria. These lesions, which can become calcified, comprise the most common focal intracranial mass seen in patients in developing countries. Tuberculous abscess occurs when the center of a tuberculoma becomes necrotic and cystic. These abscesses are often larger than tuberculomas and multiloculated.

▶ Clinical Findings

A. Symptoms and Signs

Patients with tuberculomas present with seizures and focal signs or, in cases of multiple lesions, increased intracranial pressure and diffuse cognitive dysfunction. Multiple lesions are often present, ranging in size from 1 mm to 5 cm. Abscesses tend to enlarge more rapidly than tuberculomas. Evidence of prior pulmonary involvement can often be seen on chest radiographs, even in patients without a known history of prior tuberculosis.

B. Laboratory Findings

CSF analysis shows normal or slightly elevated protein concentration if the mass is near the meninges. If the mass ruptures into the ventricles, a marked pleocytosis and protein elevation will be present. Stereotactic biopsy or surgical removal may show acid-fast bacilli. PCR using DNA amplification technique is more sensitive.

C. Imaging Studies

Tuberculomas can occur anywhere in the brain. Solitary lesions are present in 31% of patients, and calcified lesions in 10%, with enhancement patterns ranging from ring to diffuse enhancement (Figure 26–7). MRI shows a hypointense core and hyperintense rim on T2-weighted or FLAIR images, and hypointense or isointense (to brain) lesion on T1-weighted images (Figure 26–8), which correlates with necrosis and increased cellularity. Before the lesion becomes encapsulated, hypodensity with no enhancement is seen. Hydrocephalus is present in 37% of patients. Abscesses cause a greater mass effect and surrounding edema, and are hypodense on CT and hyperintense on T2-weighted MRI scans.

▶ Differential Diagnosis

Neoplasm, brain abscess, and other CNS infections (especially cysticercal) make up the differential diagnosis of tuberculoma. Unless surgery is required, tuberculomas can be differentiated from cysticercosis by monitoring the therapeutic response to antituberculous therapy.

▶ Treatment & Prognosis

Treatment includes the same antimycobacterial drugs and doses described for tuberculous meningitis earlier; however, more prolonged courses, determined by radiographic response, are required. In one series, 18% of patients

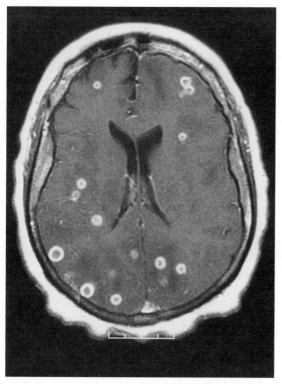

▲ **Figure 26–7.** Tuberculous granulomata. Contrast-enhanced axial T1-weighted MRI scan shows multiple, small parenchymal ring-enhancing lesions. (Used with permission from John Loh, MD.)

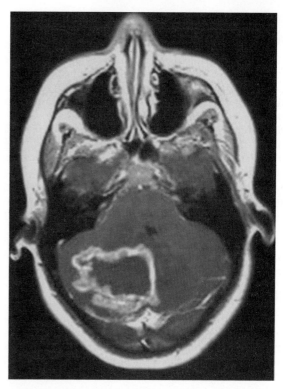

▲ **Figure 26–8.** Tuberculoma. Axial T1-weighted MRI scan shows a large, thick-walled, ring-enhancing mass in the cerebellum. (Used with permission from John Loh, MD.)

responded in 9 months, and some resolution was seen in 71% of patients in 18 months. If no response is seen after 8 weeks, antimicrobial agents should be changed. Large lesions (> 4 cm in diameter) have a worse response to medication and may require surgery. Permanent ventriculoperitoneal shunting may also be needed for persistent hydrocephalus. When lesions are small or treated early, prognosis for complete recovery is good.

Garg RK, et al. Neurological complications of miliary tuberculosis. *Clin Neurol Neurosurg* 2010;112(3):188–192. [PMID: 20031301] (Twenty-seven of 60 miliary tuberculosis patients had tuberculomas, representing half of those with tuberculous meningitis.)

Wasay M, et al. Prognostic indicators in patients with intracranial tuberculoma: A review of 102 cases. *J Pak Med Assoc* 2004;54(7):401. [PMID: 15134209] (Half of this series had meningitis; 25% had evidence of tuberculosis on chest x-ray; 66% had multiple lesions, mean 4.5 per patient; and 37% had hydrocephalus. Patients with coma and miliary tuberculosis on presentation were more likely to have poor recovery.)

3. Spinal Tuberculosis (Pott Disease)

 ESSENTIALS OF DIAGNOSIS

▶ Slow-growing granulomatous infection arising from vertebral body infection (most often thoracolumbar) that invades the epidural space

▶ Distinguished from vertebral metastatic cancer by involvement of adjacent vertebral bodies, with collapse and kyphosis

▶ Occasional calcification of paraspinal granulomata

▶ General Considerations

Pott disease, also referred to as spinal tuberculosis, is a slow-growing granulomatous infection that arises in a vertebral body, which subsequently invades the epidural space. The most common site of infection is the thoracolumbar spine.

▶ Clinical Findings

A. Symptoms and Signs

Patients have back pain, fever, and generalized malaise that progresses over weeks to months, with eventual neurologic deficit appropriate for the level involved. Thoracic lesions cause paraparesis with hyperreflexia in the legs, sensory loss below the lesion, bilateral Babinski signs, and urinary symptoms of urgency and frequency. Lumbar lesions affect roots of the cauda equina, with urinary symptoms of overflow incontinence and leg pain, sensory loss, or weakness in radicular distributions. Complete, irreversible paraplegia with spared posterior column function results from infarction in the territory of the anterior spinal artery. Compression of dorsal roots at any level of infection produces radiating pain and numbness in a dermatomal pattern. Gibbus formation due to thoracic vertebral body infection and collapse leads to severe kyphosis with spinal instability that can also compress the cord.

B. Laboratory Findings

CSF analysis shows elevated protein concentration and the presence of lymphocytes with variable degrees of hypoglycorrhachia. Biopsy material contains granulomatous debris and organisms that can be seen on acid-fast (Ziehl-Nielsen) stain.

C. Imaging Studies

MRI shows hypointense areas in vertebral bodies on T1-weighted images, hyperintense images in disk spaces on T2-weighted images, and enhancement of infected bone, along with a mass extending over several segments, producing cord deviation. CT findings are similar, with striking bony end plate destruction (which is absent in neoplasm). The disk between adjacent infected vertebral bodies is destroyed by bacterial infection, but can be spared by tuberculous infection. Tuberculous infection generally involves adjacent vertebral bodies, unlike neoplasm. Tuberculous psoas abscesses are more likely than bacterial infection to calcify.

▶ Differential Diagnosis

Metastatic tumor and bacterial and parasitic spinal cord infection must be considered in the differential diagnosis of Pott disease.

▶ Treatment

The treatment of choice is antituberculous therapy specific to culture and sensitivity results, using the same medications outlined for tuberculous meningitis. Corticosteroids are beneficial. If stabilization is required, surgery with installation of Harrington rods or pedicle screws can be performed. Debridement is occasionally required, even in patients with a stable spine. Hyperbaric oxygen therapy along with antibiotics may offer faster resolution but has not been well studied.

Jain AK, et al. Kyphosis in spinal tuberculosis—Prevention and correction. *Indian J Orthop* 2010;44(2):127–136. [PMID: 20418999] (Thoracic vertebral involvement is most likely to cause kyphosis, although it can follow reversal of lordosis in cervical and lumbar locations. Complications include pain, reduced respiratory vital capacity, and paraplegia. Correction involves removal of the vertebral body and fusion from both front and back, using instruments [pedicle screws and rods] or bone graft.)

LEPROSY *(MYCOBACTERIUM LEPRAE)*

Leprosy is discussed in Chapter 19.

▼ INFECTIOUS TOXINS

In situations where CNS symptoms occur without active infection invading tissue, toxins secreted remotely by bacteria may be responsible. Examples include shiga toxin causing thrombocytopenic purpura with coma and fluctuating focal neurologic signs, hemolytic uremia syndrome following *E coli* infection, paralysis from diphtheria (discussed in Chapter 19), and paralysis caused by *Clostridium botulinium* (discussed in Chapter 22).

TETANUS

ESSENTIALS OF DIAGNOSIS

- ▶ Localized or generalized muscle stiffness
- ▶ Superimposed paroxysmal tonic spasms (tetanospasms)
- ▶ Autonomic instability
- ▶ Normal mental status

▶ General Considerations

Tetanus is caused by a neurotoxin produced at the site of injury by *Clostridium tetani*, an anaerobic, gram-positive bacillus. Spores of *C tetani* are present in soil worldwide. Portals of entry resulting in human disease include traumatic and surgical wounds, injection sites (especially among parenteral drug abusers), skin ulcers, burns, and infected umbilical cords. Tissue necrosis and suppuration allow the bacteria to germinate and produce the toxin (tetanospasmin), which is taken up by peripheral nerve terminals and ascends intra-axonally to the spinal cord or brainstem. Tetanospasmin blocks inhibitory interneurons, resulting in excessive discharge of motor neurons and, in severe cases, autonomic dysfunction. In the United States, 50–70 cases of tetanus are reported yearly, most from acute or chronic wounds. In developing countries lacking adequate vaccination programs, 1 million cases of neonatal tetanus occur annually as a result of nonsterile birthing technique.

Prevention

Acute immunization of infants and children with DPT (diphtheria and tetanus toxoids and pertussis adsorbed) is recommended at 2, 4, 6, and 15 months, and 4–6 years, with booster immunization every 10 years thereafter. Passive immunization with human tetanus immune globulin (HTIG) is recommended for tetanus-prone wounds (eg, wounds contaminated by dirt, feces, or saliva; puncture or missile wounds; avulsions; burns) in patients with uncertain immunization history.

Clinical Findings

A. Symptoms and Signs

The usual incubation period from injury to first symptoms is 7–21 days. Trismus ("lockjaw") and stiffness of the neck and paraspinal muscles are prominent early symptoms, spreading as the disease progresses to the limbs. Stiffness of facial muscles produces *risus sardonicus*, and paraspinal rigidity can produce opisthotonus. Superimposed paroxysmal painful tonic spasms (tetanospasms) occur spontaneously or are triggered by tactile stimuli or sound. Pharyngeal muscle spasm causes dysphagia, and laryngeal and respiratory muscle spasms cause asphyxia. Autonomic dysfunction can cause fever, blood pressure swings, severe diaphoresis, and cardiac arrhythmia even when body spasms are controlled. Most patients remain mentally clear. Partially immunized subjects can develop localized tetanus confined to the injured limb or to cephalic muscles after a head injury or otitis.

B. Laboratory Findings

CSF analysis shows normal findings. There are no specific laboratory tests to confirm the diagnosis, which is based on the characteristic signs. A wound may not be apparent, and even when it is present, *C tetani* may not be identified.

Differential Diagnosis

Diagnostic considerations include neuroleptic-induced dystonia, meningitis, dental abscess, status epilepticus, subarachnoid hemorrhage, hypocalcemic tetany, ethanol, sedative or opiate withdrawal, strychnine poisoning, black widow spider bite, stiff-person syndrome, and rabies.

Treatment

Patients should be treated in an intensive care unit. The wound is debrided after administration of HTIG (human tetanus immune globulin, 3000–6000 units) into one limb and tetanus toxoid into another. (Tetanus toxoid is required

because infection with *C tetani* does not confer its own immunity.) Because penicillin use can exacerbate spasms as it antagonizes the inhibitory neurotransmitter γ-aminobutyric acid, metronidazole, 2 g/day for 7–10 days, is the antimicrobial of choice. Patients with tetanospasms require ventilatory support and, because endotracheal intubation provokes spasms, tracheostomy is usually indicated. Benzodiazepines, often titrated to very high doses, are given to control spasms and provide sedation, but neuromuscular blockade (eg, vecuronium, 6–8 mg/h) may be necessary in patients with severe spasms. Infusion of magnesium sulfate may be useful as well. In patients with autonomic instability, labetalol, 0.25–1.0 mg/min, can be given for hypertension, and verapamil is used for tachycardia. Pressors may be necessary for hypotension, and bradycardia may require a pacemaker.

Prognosis

The disease may progress for 2 weeks even after administration of antitoxin, and severe tetanus may require several weeks more for recovery. Mortality is up to 25% even in modern intensive care units. Complications include bone fractures, dehydration, pneumonia, and pulmonary emboli.

Saltoglu N, et al. Prognostic factors affecting deaths from adult tetanus. *Clin Microbiol Infect* 2004;10:229–233. [PMID: 15008944] (Fifty-three cases from a hospital in Adana, Turkey, demonstrated a high mortality rate, 52.8%, that related to the length of the incubation period, higher in those with generalized tetanus, fever, tachycardia, and postoperative tetanus, and was not lowered by tetanus antiserum or human immunoglobulin, but was worse in those who did not receive vaccination.)

Thwaites CL, et al. Magnesium sulphate for treatment of severe tetanus: A randomised controlled trial. *Lancet* 2006;368(9545):1398–1399. [PMID: 17055945] (Use of one week of intravenous magnesium did not lower the need for mechanical ventilation but did reduce requirements for midazolam or pipecuronium to control muscle spasms in 97 of 256 treated Vietnamese patients.)

FUNGAL INFECTIONS

ESSENTIALS OF DIAGNOSIS

► Fungal meningitis—onset is more insidious and symptoms are less pronounced than septic meningitis

► CSF analysis showing elevated opening pressure, 20–1000 WBCs (predominantly lymphocytes or monocytes), mild or markedly depressed glucose, and elevated protein

► Immunosuppression is a major predisposing condition

General Considerations

Fungal infections are an infrequent cause of CNS infection in the United States, but may produce severe cases of meningitis, as well as necrotic abscesses. *Cryptococcus neoformans* is the most common pathogen, followed by *Candida*, *Coccidioides immitis*, and *Histoplasma*.

A history of possible geographic or occupational exposure aids in diagnosis of these infections. For example, *Cryptococcus* infection is caused by exposure to pigeon feces. Infection caused by *Coccidioides* occurs in residents of or travelers to the southwestern United States, Mexico, and Central America. *Histoplasma* infection may occur after exposure to contaminated soil in the Ohio, Mississippi, or other river valleys and in the Caribbean and Latin America. *Aspergillus* infection occurs in the spine by direct spread from pulmonary infection and can cause hemorrhagic abscess in the brain. Other rarely reported fungal infections are caused by *Pseudoallescheria boydii*; *Paracoccidioides brasiliensis*; *Phaeohyphomycosis* (or black yeasts), such as *Cladophialophora bantiana*; *Exophiala dermatitidis*, *Ramichloridium mackenziei*, and *Cladosporium*.

Most cases of cryptococcal meningitis represent reemergence of existing infection in immunosuppressed patients, especially those with AIDS, when CD4 cell counts fall below 200 cells/μL. Other causes of immunosuppression, such as use of antirejection drugs in organ transplant recipients, chemotherapy-induced neutropenia, diabetes mellitus, malignancy, alcoholism, corticosteroid use, pregnancy, or prematurity, all predispose to recrudescence of latent infection. Coccidioidal chronic meningitis, in contrast, usually appears as a new primary infection.

Pathogenesis

Fungi are ubiquitous, existing in the form of mold (tubular with branching or single hyphae) and yeast (thick walled, one cell). Spores are inhaled or invade through the skin, mucous membranes, sinuses, or wounds. Immunocompetent hosts can suffer chronic meningitis from *Coccidioides*, but most fungal infections occur in T-cell immunodeficient hosts. Other at-risk patients include those exposed to large amounts of bat or bird guano (*Cryptococcus*), heroin users, patients requiring chronic antibiotics or very young patients (*Candida*), uncontrolled diabetics or those with IV drug use or burns (*Mucor*), and those exposed to dirt containing *Aspergillus* or *Coccidioides*.

Clinical Findings

A. Symptoms and Signs

Headache, which may become severe, develops over weeks or months. Meningeal signs, fever, and altered mental state are usually less frequent and less pronounced in fungal than in bacterial or tuberculous meningitis, although encephalopathy is found in nearly half of patients. Coma implies severe intracranial hypertension, hydrocephalus, or hyponatremia due to inappropriate antidiuretic hormone (ADH) secretion. Papilledema, diplopia, and focal findings are seen in 10% of patients. Seizures and stroke are occasional complications. Fever is usually low grade.

Candida, *Aspergillus*, and rarely *Blastomycosis* infections tend to invade the brain more often than they cause meningitis, where they cause microabscesses.

Mucormycosis, resulting from infection with Zygomycetes fungus (eg, *Rhizopus*, *Rhizomucor*, or *Absidia*) is often seen in neutropenic or diabetic patients with hyperglycemic ketoacidosis or in normal hosts who have smoked contaminated marijuana. This fungal infection causes orbital cellulitis and nasal destruction, followed by cavernous sinus thrombosis and frontal abscess that is highly necrotic.

Aspergillus can produce sudden focal symptoms as a result of hemorrhage into a mass. Lung infection can invade adjacent vertebrae to cause cord compression.

Coccidioidal meningitis is difficult to treat and has significant morbidity (hydrocephalus, vasculitis, abscess, or infarct) and mortality.

B. Laboratory Findings

Diagnosis is made by CSF examination, which shows moderately low glucose and high protein content, and more than 20 WBCs/μL, mostly lymphocytes. Coccidioidomycosis may produce eosinophils or neutrophils in CSF. Neutrophilic predominance can also be found in histoplasmosis, blastomycosis, and infections caused by *Candida*, *Aspergillus*, Zygomycetes, or *P boydii*. Special stains may reveal the organism; for example, India ink shows encapsulated, round, budding cells in cryptococcal infection.

Some organisms can be reliably detected using antigen tests: *C neoformans* with latex agglutination, *Histoplasma* with radioimmunoassay or enzyme immunoassay, and *Blastomyces* using enzyme immunoassay. Most fungal antibodies are detectable in CSF by complement fixation as well as radioimmunoassay. CSF titers that rise or fall can be used to follow disease progression or response to therapy. Serum titers greater than 1:16 imply active infection. Cross-reaction of antibodies may be misleading. Antibodies against *Coccidioides* are more likely to be present in serum than in CSF.

Large volumes (> 15 mL) of CSF aid in culture, but prolonged growth and repeated lumbar punctures may still be required. Brain or meningeal biopsy is occasionally necessary.

All patients with fungal meningitis should receive HIV testing and, if negative, also be evaluated for malignancy.

C. Imaging Studies

Imaging can show hydrocephalus, caused by ependymitis or blockage of subarachnoid space. Meningeal enhancement is almost always present, especially in the basilar meninges (Figure 26–9). Small areas of cryptococcoma can be present adjacent to ventricles and subsequently disappear with medical treatment. MRI with contrast can reveal candidal

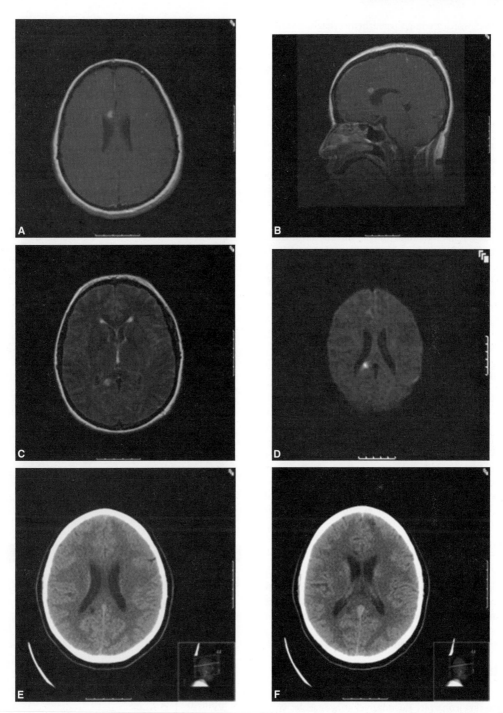

▲ **Figure 26–9.** Cryptococcal meningitis and cryptococcoma. **(A)** Contrast-enhanced T1-weighted MRI shows mild meningeal enhancement, with toruloma near frontal horn of right lateral ventricle. **(B)** Sagittal T1-weighted image shows focus of abnormal enhancement in anterior body of corpous callosum. **(C)** Axial FLAIR MRI shows focus of increased signal in right splenium of corpus callosum. **(D)** Diffusion-weighted image of same lesion. **(E)** CT scan without and **(F)** with contrast, 2 months later, shows nonenhancing CSF density focus in right splenium near lateral ventricle representing healed cryptococcoma. (Used with permission from Maria Chiechi, MD.)

microabscesses, which are ring shaped, hemorrhagic, and usually multiple and widespread in the brain. Less common are infarcts due to vasculitis. Hemorrhage is a common finding in patients with *Aspergillus* infection. Necrosis with infarction is seen in those with *Zygomycetes* infection. *Blastomyces* infection causes epidural abscess as well as intracranial abscess.

D. Special Tests

In immunocompetent patients, skin anergy panels may reveal prior exposure to fungi, especially *Coccidioides* and *Candida*. Chest radiographs can document another site of infection, which may warrant bronchial lavage or sputum collection.

▶ Differential Diagnosis

Other disorders that resemble fungal meningitis include chronic meningitis with less virulent organisms such as *Brucella* or *Francisella tularensis*, and meningitis that is usually acute but is indolent in the immunocompromised patient. Carcinomatous, autoimmune, chemical, and medication-induced meningitis, as well as sarcoidosis, Behçet syndrome, and Vogt-Koyanagi-Harada disease are other considerations. A "fungoma" in patients with aspergillosis or *Mucor* infection can resemble a neoplasm or bacterial abscess.

▶ Complications

Complications include cranial nerve palsies, arteritis with infarct or vasculitis, hydrocephalus, intracranial infection, syndrome of inappropriate antidiuretic hormone, seizures, and dementia. Neurologic complications occur in up to 40% of patients with cryptococcal meningitis and 50–75% of patients with coccidioidal or histoplasmal meningitis. Only 25% of aspergillomas and Zygomycetes abscesses can be cured, even with surgery. Mortality is very high in fungal meningitis without effective treatment, especially in immunocompromised patients who cannot reverse their state.

▶ Prevention

Prevention is not vaccine-based. Instead, prevention involves educating high-risk people to avoid potentially infected sites such as archeologic digs, construction sites where spores become airborne from disrupted soil, bird cages or air-conditioning units where pigeon feces accumulate, caves containing bat feces, and certain river valleys.

▶ Treatment

Antifungal agents fall into five classes: polyene, (amphotericin); azoles (ketoconazole, fluconazole, itraconazole, voriconazole, posaconazole, and experimental ravuconazole); pyrimidine analog (flucytosine); echinocandins (caspofungin, micarfungin, and the investigational anidulafungin); and allylamin (terbinafine). Most work by disrupting aspects of the fungal cell membrane or wall formation; 5-flucytosine (5-FC) interferes with pyrimidine metabolism in the nucleus.

Nocardia, which has features of both fungus and bacteria in its structure, is treated with antibiotics such as trimethoprim-sulfamethoxazole or imipenem and amikacin. In immunosuppressed patients, after initial treatment of any fungal infection, maintenance with fluconazole, 200 mg/day orally, is continued until the CD4+ lymphocyte count recovers to 100 cells/µL or higher. Treatment of *Candida* often requires the removal of infected catheters or drains.

Standard treatment regimens are outlined in Table 26–9.

Supportive management includes control of elevated intracranial pressure by repeated lumbar puncture or ventricular drain. Although it acts as a potential locus of future infection, in some cases of hydrocephalus, conversion to a permanent shunt is necessary.

Bariola JR, et al. Blastomycosis of the central nervous system: A multicenter review of diagnosis and treatment in the modern era. *Clin Infect Dis* 2010;50(6):797–804. [PMID: 20166817] (Eighteen percent mortality is found in 22 cases collected over 18 years; treatment consisted of amphotericin followed by chronic azole use.)

Blair JE. Coccidioidal meningitis: Update on epidemiology, clinical features, diagnosis, and management. *Curr Infect Dis Rep* 2009;11(4):289–295. [PMID: 19545498] (Review of significant CNS sequalae of this infection, including hydrocephalus, vasculitis, infarct and brain abscess, and problems with triazole antifungal treatment.)

Denning DW, Hope WW. Therapy for fungal infections. *Trends Microbiol* 2010;18(5):195–204. [PMID: 20207544] (Guidelines for management of fungal infection, including that of CNS.)

Drake KW, Adam RD. Coccidioidal meningitis and brain abscesses: Analysis of 71 cases at a referral center. *Neurology* 2009;73(21):1780–1786. [PMID: 19933980] (Epidemiology and antibody testing of serum and CSF in 71 patients with meningitis seen in Tucson, Arizona.)

Redmond A, Dancer C, Woods ML. Fungal infections of the central nervous system: A review of fungal pathogens and treatments. *Neurol India* 2007;55(3):251–259. [PMID: 17921654] (Reviews epidemiology, immunology, and treatment of fungal infections.)

▼ SPIROCHETAL INFECTIONS

SYPHILIS

ESSENTIALS OF DIAGNOSIS

- ▶ Optic, vestibulocochlear, and facial nerve involvement (common)
- ▶ Chronic meningitis any time after the first year of infection
- ▶ CSF analysis showing 100–1000 lymphocytes/µL, increased protein, oligoclonal bands, and positive serologic tests
- ▶ Late neurologic presentations—Argyll-Robertson pupils, dementia, tabes dorsalis, and stroke

Table 26–9. Treatment of Fungal Infection

Causative Organism	Antifungal Drug[a]
Aspergillus sp	Itraconazole, 200 mg/day/IV or 200 mg po (suspension or tablet) *or* Voriconazole, 4 mg/kg IV bid × 7 days then 200 mg PO q 12 h × 12 wk *or* Caspofungin, 70 mg day 1 then 50 mg/day × 10
Candida	Amphotericin B, 1 mg/kg/day IV, plus 5-FC, 1 mg/kg PO q 6 h *or* Voriconazole, 4 mg/kg[b] IV q 12 h, or 200 mg PO q 12 h for 8 wk Caspofungin, 60 mg/day[b] IV for 8 wk
Cryptococcus	Amphotericin B,[c] 1 mg/kg/day IV, plus 5-FC, 1 mg/kg PO q 6 h Same for 2 wk, then fluconazole,[d] 400 mg/day for 10 wk
Coccidioides	Same as for *Cryptococcus* for prolonged course. Intrathecal amphotericin may be required Fluconazole, 6 mg/kg/day PO in children, 400–600 mg/day PO in adults *or* Itraconazole, 200 mg PO with meals *or* Ketoconazole, 800–1200 mg/day
Histoplasma	Amphotericin B, 0.6 mg/kg/day, followed by ketoconazole, 200 mg, or itraconazole, 200 mg/day in immunosuppressed patients

5-FC = 5-flucytosine; IV = intravenously; PO = orally (by mouth); q = every.
[a]Therapeutic course is 4–6 weeks unless otherwise indicated. Treatment is continued if cerebrospinal fluid (CSF) is not sterile or serum latex agglutination for organism is not near zero.
[b]Loading dose is 1.5 times daily dose given first day. 5-FC cannot be given alone, due to resistance and bone marrow toxicity.
[c]Amphotericin is available in lipid formulation, 5 mg/kg/day IV for 6 weeks, then 3 times a week for 4 weeks. Intrathecal delivery is by Ommaya reservoir or barbotage (mixing drug with CSF and reinstilling).
[d]Fluconazole has many drug interactions.

▶ General Considerations

Syphilis, an infectious disease caused by the spirochete *Treponema pallidum*, can infect almost any body organ or tissue. Symptoms of both primary and secondary syphilis (disseminated rash) can resolve in the absence of antibiotic treatment, leading to potential development of neurosyphilis in about 25% of infected patients.

T pallidum is most often transmitted during sexual contact. In 2007, 11,466 primary and secondary, and a total of 40,920 all stages of syphilis cases were reported in the United States, representing a decline since the AIDS-related peak in the 1990s. Placental transmission from mother to fetus after the 10th week of pregnancy results in congenital syphilis. This condition, which is avoidable by screening pregnant women, occurs in about 500 infants annually in the United States.

▶ Pathogenesis

The corkscrew-shaped spirochete arrives in the CNS through the meninges. Well-known syndromes reflect involvement of the frontal lobes (general paresis and dementia), upper brainstem (Argyll-Robertson pupils), or spinal cord (tabes dorsalis). Although atrophy and tract degeneration are evident, the exact pathophysiologic mechanism of these slowly evolving conditions is unclear, as there is little inflammatory response. Rarely, an inflammatory mass or gumma develops after many years, with symptoms, including seizures, corresponding to the location.

▶ Clinical Findings

A. Symptoms and Signs

Various neurologic manifestations are associated with the stage of infection. Primary syphilis occurs within 21 days of exposure and is manifested by a painless genital ulcer (chancre), which heals spontaneously in 3–6 weeks. During this stage, asymptomatic CNS seeding occurs in up to 25% of patients. The CNS may be involved at any subsequent stage of syphilis. Syphilitic meningitis occurs any time after healing of the chancre, usually 4–10 weeks later. During this stage (secondary syphilis), a highly variable, potentially infectious rash that tends to involve the palms and soles accompanies meningeal signs such as photophobia and headache. Five percent of patients develop symptoms of cranial nerve dysfunction, especially of vestibular or auditory nerves. Uveitis and stroke also occur; any young person with stroke lacking prominent vascular risk factors should be screened for syphilis. The disease then becomes latent for many years, but CSF analysis reveals ongoing infection. Eventually, symptoms of tertiary syphilis emerge; several of these merit discussion here.

1. Meningovascular lues—Stroke in the setting of chronic meningitis occurs from 3–50 years after infection in 10% of patients (earlier in patients with AIDS). Focal symptoms progress over days, often after several weeks of headache or personality change. Angiography is consistent with vasculitis involving large and small vessels.

2. Tabes dorsalis—Demyelination of the posterior columns of the spinal cord causes lightning-like back and leg pain, jabbing pains in the spine, gastric crisis, and Lhérmitte sign (a feeling of electricity going down the back upon flexion of the neck). In addition, impotence, urinary or fecal incontinence, and constipation occur. Position and vibratory sense are absent in the feet or legs (and less often, pin sensation is impaired), and tendon reflexes are absent in the legs. Sensory loss leads to joint destruction of the knees or ankles (Charcot joints). Sensory ataxia causes Romberg sign (unsteadiness with eye closure) and foot-slapping gait. The bladder is atonic. Tabes dorsalis occurs in up to 10% of patients with untreated syphilis.

3. General paresis (dementia paralytica)—Symptoms of general paresis develop at least 10 years after infection in about 5% of patients with neurosyphilis. Chronic meningoencephalitis causes psychosis, dementia with poor judgment, "manic" behavior, and late generalized paralysis. Despite its inclusion in the list of treatable dementias, symptoms respond to antibiotics only if treated before atrophy and neuronal destruction have occurred.

4. Gumma—Focal signs such as seizures or frontal dysfunction result from this granulomatous lesion, which formerly developed in 15% of patients 1–46 years after infection but now is exceedingly rare. All recent reports involve HIV-infected patients.

5. Other signs and symptoms—Hydrocephalus, either communicating or obstructive, may result from occlusion of CSF pathways after meningitis or obstruction due to granular ependymitis of the fourth ventricle. Congenital syphilis causes bone pain, keratitis, and eighth nerve dysfunction (vertigo, which may be induced by noise, as well as deafness). Visual loss due to uveitis or optic atrophy occurs. Argyll-Robertson pupils that react to accommodation but not to light may be present even without visual disturbance.

B. Laboratory Findings

Diagnosis of syphilis relies on serologic study, which is summarized in Table 26–10.

1. Serologic tests—Screening tests include VDRL (Venereal Disease Research Laboratory) and RPR (rapid plasma reagin), which use a lipoidal antigen response that can be very sensitive but not completely specific, with cross-reaction known to occur with cardiolipin antibodies and mycobacterial antibodies in up to 2% of cases. False-negative results are rare, except in very high titers producing a "prozone reaction" that requires dilution before processing. Fluorescent treponemal assay (FTA), *T pallidum* hemagglutination assay (TPHA), and enzyme-linked immunosorbent assay (ELISA) antibody tests are more specific than VDRL or RPR tests and are confirmatory. Titers are not useful for following disease progression or response to treatment. VDRL and RPR titers decrease as

Table 26–10. Serologic and CSF Studies in Syphilis

Type of Syphilis	Nonspecific Nontreponemal (Reagenic) Tests[a]	Specific Treponemal (Fluorescent Antibody) Tests[b]	Other Tests
Primary	> 1:4	Positive	—
Secondary	> 1:4	Positive	—
Treated or late	Negative after 1 y[c]	Stays positive for life (specific, not sensitive, cannot use to follow patient response to therapy)	—
Neurosyphilis	Useful in CSF (positive result rules in, specific but less sensitive)	Too sensitive to be useful in CSF (but negative result rules out neurosyphilis)	Oligoclonal bands, monocytes, polymerase chain reaction

CSF = cerebrospinal fluid.
[a]VDRL, rapid plasma reagin (RPR), and immunoglobulin G (IgG) tests.
[b]Fluorescent treponemal antibody, absorbed (TA-Abs); *Treponema pallidum* hemagglutination assay (TPHA); microhemagglutination–*T pallidum* (MHA-TP).
[c]Persistent positive VDRL implies reinfection, false-positive result, or treatment failure. One quarter of untreated patients become negative. Screen with reagenic tests (VDRL, RPR, IgG) and confirm with specific treponemal tests (FTA-Abs, TPHA, MHA-TP). Use change in titer or RPR or VDRL to follow response to therapy. Fourfold change in titer is meaningful.

infection advances over years, leading to false-negative results in older patients. Similarly, serology is unreliable in immuno-suppressed HIV-positive patients; in these patients, a lumbar puncture must be performed.

2. Microscopic examination—The spirochete is too small to be seen with light microscopy and is also rarely seen with darkfield analysis.

3. Spinal fluid analysis—In routine primary and second-ary syphilis, CSF analysis is not recommended (CDC guide-lines). If neurologic or ophthalmic signs are present, or there is any evidence of tertiary syphilis (aortitis, gumma, etc.), CSF analysis is indicated. If serum titers fail to decrease sig-nificantly (ie, twofold) 8 weeks after completion of treat-ment, or the patient is coinfected with HIV, CSF analysis is required. Lymphocytic or monocytic pleocytosis can persist throughout the course of syphilis infection, with several hundred cells present in the secondary, meningeal stage. Glucose level is usually normal or mildly decreased, CSF protein concentration may be elevated as high as 100 mg/dL, and oligoclonal bands are often present. Patients with AIDS who are treated for neurosyphilis should undergo a repeat lumbar puncture at 6 months to identify those not respond-ing to standard courses of antibiotics. Lymphocytes can be present in chronic HIV infection at any stage.

VDRL of CSF is 100% specific, assuming the lumbar puncture is atraumatic (ie, < 15 red blood cells/μL), but only 50% sensitive; CSF FTA is 30% specific but almost 100% sensitive, which is too high to allow it to be a screening test for neurosyphilis. In addition, fluorescent treponemal antibody absorption (FTA-ABS) testing of CSF is not yet standardized and cannot be quantified, other than to express the brilliance of the fluorescence from 1–4+. Microhemagglutination tests (MHA-TP) can be checked for titers. This leads to the general interpretation that a *positive* CSF VDRL means the patient *does* have neurosyphilis, but a *negative* CSF VDRL *does not rule it out*, whereas a *negative* CSF FTA *does rule out* neuro-syphilis, but a *positive* CSF FTA *does not make that diagnosis*. Because the FTA will remain positive throughout the patient's life, even after treatment, it should not be used to follow a patient's response to treatment.

C. Imaging Studies

Meningeal inflammation on enhanced CT or MRI scan is suspicious for meningovascular lues. MRI visualization of a gumma has been reported rarely. Magnetic resonance angiog-raphy or routine angiography can demonstrate vascular occlusion.

▶ Treatment

Table 26–11 outlines treatment for various types of syphilis. Treatment of primary, secondary, and early latent (< 1 year) syphilis consists of one intramuscular injection of benzathine penicillin, 2.4 million units, or 2 weeks of oral doxycycline, 100 mg twice a day, in patients who are allergic to penicillin.

Currently under investigation, azithromycin, 500 mg/day for 3 days, may prove useful in treatment of primary or second-ary syphilis. Success (eradication of the infection and pre-vention of progression to tertiary syphilis) is determined by twofold lowering or disappearance of serum titers when tested 3 months after completion of therapy determines success.

Patients with late latent syphilis (> 1 year), syphilis of unknown duration, and tertiary syphilis require the same dose of penicillin, repeated each week for 3 weeks, or oral doxycycline, 100 mg twice a day for 28 days. Neurosyphilis (or ocular or auditory involvement) requires intravenous treatment with penicillin G, 3–4 million units every 4 hours for 2 weeks, to achieve treponemicidal levels in the CNS. In patients who are unable or unwilling to receive intravenous therapy, oral probenecid, 500 mg four times a day, can aug-ment CNS levels of procaine penicillin, 2.4 million units daily given intramuscularly for 2 weeks, but the failure rate is higher. Intravenous ceftriaxone, 1 g/day for 2 weeks, has a 20% failure rate. In penicillin-allergic patients, desensitiza-tion is recommended rather than substitution, as only peni-cillin is reliably treponemicidal. A 1-month course of oral doxycycline, 100 mg twice a day, or minocycline, 100 mg twice a day, can be substituted if necessary. Antimicrobial success is assumed if there is a fourfold drop in serum titer, although HIV-positive patients should have a repeat lumbar puncture after 6 months to ensure successful treatment. Some experts recommend following a course of intravenous therapy with three weekly penicillin intramuscular injec-tions, similar to initial treatment.

Symptoms of general paresis and tabes almost never respond to antibiotic treatment and require symptomatic treatment such as antipsychotics or behavioral therapy.

▶ Prognosis

The prognosis is excellent for patients with syphilitic menin-gitis and in all stages prior to end-organ involvement. Some complications, such as stroke or deafness, are irreversible, even with treatment.

Halperin JJ. A tale of two spirochetes: Lyme disease and syph-ilis. *Neurol Clin* 2010;28(1):277–291. [PMID: 2019932386] (Comparative summary of syphilis and Lyme disease with description of clinical signs, laboratory testing, and treatment.)

Timmermans M, Carr J. Neurosyphilis in the modern era. *J Neurol Neurosurg Psychiatry* 2004;75:1727–1730. [PMID: 15548491] (Over a 10-year period, 161 patients with neurosyphilis were diagnosed by positive FTA-ABS in CSF; 82 patients had demen-tia or delirium, 24 had stroke, 15 had tabes dorsalis, and 14 had seizures. CSF VDRL result was positive in 73%.)

Workowski KA, Berman SM. Centers for Disease Control and Prevention sexually transmitted diseases treatment guidelines. *Clin Infect Dis* 2007;44(Suppl 3):S73–S76. [PMID: 17342670] (Diagnosis, including when to do lumbar puncture, and treat-ment recommendations from the CDC.)

Table 26–11. Syphilis and Neurosyphilis: Clinical Findings and Treatment

Type of Syphilis	Symptoms and Signs	Imaging Features	Treatment	Response
Primary	Painless chancre	—	Bnz PenG 2.4 million units IM for 1 dose, or doxycycline, 100 mg PO q 12 h for 14 days	—
Secondary				
Asymptomatic	None	—	—	—
Syphilitic meningitis	Headache, stroke, CN II and VIII palsy, stiff neck, uveitis, diffuse rash	Meningeal enhancement	PenG 3–4 million units IV q 4 h for 10 days, or ceftriaxone, 1 g/day IM for 14 days, or Pro PenG 2.4 million U/day IM for 14 days with probenecid, 500 mg PO 4 times a day	Curative or minimal deficit
Early latent (< 1 y)	Positive serum VDRL	Normal	Bnz PenG 2.4 million units IM for 1 dose	Curative
Late latent (> 1 y)	Persistent positive VDRL	Normal	Bnz PenG 2.4 million units IM q wk for 3 doses	Curative
Tertiary				
Meningovascular meningitis	↑ ICP, headache, CN VII and VIII palsy	Meningeal enhancement	PenG[a] 3–4 million units IV q 4 h for 14 days, or ceftriaxone, 1 g/day IV for 14 days	Reversible
Cerebrovascular	Acute focal signs, often MCA territory	Infarct ± enhancement	Same as for meningovascular meningitis	Reversible
Gumma	Slowly progressive focal signs; ± ↑ ICP	Mass lesion	Same as for meningovascular meningitis	Stabilized
Spinal myelitis (acute)	Myelopathy, sensory level, paraesthesias	MRI shows spinal cord enhancement	Same as for meningovascular meningitis; some authorities recommend continuing for 21 days	Stabilized or improved
Tabes dorsalis (chronic)	Electric pain, ataxia, Argyll-Robertson pupils, areflexia, poor proprioception, Charcot joints, optic atrophy	Atrophy in spinal cord	Same as for meningovascular meningitis. Additional symptomatic therapy with gabapentin, amitriptyline, baclofen	Poor
General paresis (dementia paralytica)	Dementia, mania, seizures, personality change	Meningoencephalitis	Same as for spinal meningitis; symptomatic antipsychotics as needed	Poor
Optic atrophy	Pale disks, poor vision	Optic atrophy	No treatment	Poor
Congenital	Deafness, dementia, deformed bones and teeth, tabes (rare)	Atrophy	PenG 50,000 U/kg IV q 8–12 h for 10 days	Reversible (with early diagnosis)

Bnz PenG = benzathine penicillin G; CN = cranial nerve; ↑ ICP = intracranial pressure; IM = intramuscular; IV = intravenous; MCA = middle cerebral artery; MRI = magnetic resonance imaging; N/A = not applicable; PenG = penicillin G; PO = orally (per os); Pro PenG = procaine penicillin G; VDRL = Venereal Disease Research Laboratory; ±, may or may not be present; q = every.
[a]All penicillin-allergic tertiary cases and pregnant women should undergo desensitization. HIV-infected patients may require a longer course of treatment.

NONSEXUALLY TRANSMITTED TREPONEMATOSES

Other spirochetal infections, such as yaws (*Treponema pertenue*) and pinta (*Treponema carateum*), only rarely affect the nervous system, although myalgias and headache may be prominent features late in the disease course.

LEPTOSPIROSIS

Leptospirosis is an acute and often severe infection that affects the liver and other organs, and is caused by the spirochete *Leptospira interrogans*, which affects rats, dogs, cattle, and swine, among other animals. Humans may contract the infection by consuming food contaminated by urine of a reservoir animal, or from infected soil or water.

Symptoms of leptospirosis vary from those of aseptic meningitis, with conjunctivitis, chills, fever, headache, and meningismus, to septicemia with liver and cardiac failure. All symptoms start 1–2 weeks after exposure and may recur after resolution. Analysis of CSF (initially acellular) eventually shows some monocytes and an elevated protein concentration, with seroconversion manifested as immune complexes and IgM antibody to *Leptospira* subtypes. Occasionally the organism can be grown in culture.

If recognized early, treatment consists of high doses of intravenous penicillin G or doxycycline, oral or intravenous, in doses similar to those used for treatment of syphilis. Most patients recover with no therapy. In older patients with liver disease, mortality can reach 50%.

LYME DISEASE (NEUROBORRELIOSIS)

ESSENTIALS OF DIAGNOSIS

▶ Erythema migrans, a target-shaped, expanding, red rash at site of the tick bite in first stage

▶ Early lymphocytic meningitis and facial nerve palsy

▶ Early involvement of heart, joints, and muscles

▶ Late-stage painful radiculitis, patchy polyneuropathy, encephalopathy

▶ General Considerations

Borrelia burgdorferi, the spirochete responsible for US cases of Lyme disease and European cases of tickborne meningoradiculitis (Bannwarth disease), was isolated from the adult *Ixodes* tick in 1983. Currently, approximately 27,000 cases are reported to the CDC each year, with most occurring in the spring and summer. *Borrelia* species are bacteria with corkscrew-like flagella that are used for host attachment and continuous feeding to survive. Virulence of the spirochete depends on the proteins making up the flagella, which dictate the degree of attachment to the host's surface. Many strains of *Borrelia* are found in different regions of the world, including *B garinii*, *B lone starii*, and *B miyamati*. Vectors of the *Ixodes* family, including *I scapularis* (formerly *dammini*), *pacificus*, *ricinus*, *persulcatus*, and *holocyclus*, and hosts, including deer, white-footed mice, cattle, lizards, dogs, birds, and other rodents, vary by location.

▶ Prevention

As the vaccine initially marketed is no longer available for humans, prevention requires simple measures to reduce exposure. These include landscaping or use of acaricides to treat grassy areas, avoiding areas of forest or vegetation that could hide the most common intermediate host, the white-footed deer mouse, as well as deer. When outside in endemic areas, insecticides and clothing such as long-sleeved shirts, socks, and long pants reduce the opportunity for a tick bite. Because the transmission rate is proportional to the time the tick is in place, with at least 24 hours considered necessary for transmission, daily checks for the presence of ticks and their gentle removal are recommended. (This probably explains the relatively low rate of infection in small children whose parents have the opportunity to discover ticks during daily baths.) A typical tiny *Ixodes* tick does not need to be analyzed, because absence of a spirochete may mean that it has already been injected into the patient. Chemoprophylaxis with one dose of doxycycline at the time of the tick bite may help prevent further infection.

▶ Clinical Findings

A. Symptoms and Signs

1. Early localized infection (stage 1)—The earliest symptom of infection is typically a red rash with white center (target shaped), at least 5 cms, which begins to expand at the site of prior tick attachment, after about a week. The rash is sometimes more homogeneous and may include a central intensification rather than clearing. This rash, termed *erythema migrans*, is not always visible to the patient, so careful examination of the belt line, back of the neck, and ankles is necessary. A flulike illness follows.

2. Early disseminated infection (stage 2)—Neurologic involvement results from hematogenous seeding of the CNS 2–4 weeks after inoculation. Infected individuals develop flulike illness causing headache, mild neck stiffness, myalgias, and prominent, persistent fatigue. Approximately 1 month later, patients may develop arthralgias (60% of which involve the knee), meningeal signs, carditis with conduction blocks, conjunctivitis, and cranial nerve palsies, especially of the facial nerve.

3. Late persistent infection (stage 3)—Late symptoms (occurring after 3 months) include radicular pain, which may respond to antibiotics; uveitis; encephalopathy; and, in treated adult patients, axonal neuropathy with mild patchy sensory loss, paresthesias, and variable weakness. Myelopathy and spinal cord compression are rare. The neuropathy does not respond to further courses of antibiotics, as it represents a toxic perineuronal immune reaction. Peripheral neuropathies resulting from neuroborreliosis are further detailed in Chapter 19.

In Europe, infection with *B garinii* or *B burgdorferi* can cause persistent leukoencephalitis with dementia, urinary incontinence, and spastic paraparesis.

The neuropsychiatric *post-Lyme syndrome* is unlikely to be due to ongoing infection, but the term has been used to describe persistent symptoms occurring in patients previously treated with standard courses of antibiotics (often repeatedly). These symptoms include difficulty concentrating, poor cognitive function, diffuse myalgias, and easy fatiguability. Such symptoms are much rarer than the public presumes. Instead, depression or chronic fatigue may account for most.

Other conditions anecdotally attributed to Lyme disease include cerebellitis, intracranial aneurysm, parkinsonism, benign intracranial hypertension (especially in children who have had a high CSF protein concentration), vasculitis-induced stroke, and acute hearing loss. Systemic disease appearing years later includes arthritis and acrodermatitis chronicum atrophicans.

B. Laboratory Findings

Laboratory abnormalities in Lyme disease, which consist of serologic responses in the blood or CSF, although usually appearing at 2 weeks, may take up to 3 months to develop. The spirochete is very difficult to culture, although it may sometimes be obtained from a punch biopsy of the rash.

Serologic tests should be ordered in at-risk patients (ie, those who have been outdoors in areas where Lyme disease is endemic, such as the northeastern, north-central, and mid-Atlantic regions of the United States). The disease is now widespread, however, with reports of cases in nearly every state and the District of Columbia. Serologic tests include enzyme-linked immunosorbent assay (ELISA), and immunofluorescence antibody (IFA). Specimens that test positive or equivocal by ELISA or IFA require Western immunoblot confirmation. Specific bands, at least two and up to eight, are present on IgM; the bands develop 2–4 weeks after onset of the erythematous rash, become strongest at 6–8 weeks, and gradually decline. IgG bands appear 6–8 weeks after the appearance of the rash, peak at 4–6 months, and may persist for the patient's life. A rapid test suitable for office use analyzes recombinant protein in an immunochromatographic format for the initial test, but confirmation with the more specific Western immunoblot is still required. A fourfold increase in titers confirms the presence of recent infection. False-positive responses reflect autoimmune collagen-vascular diseases, other infections, or prior Lyme infection. False-negative responses, which occur in up to 10% of confirmed cases, can be the result of appropriate early treatment that prevents antibodies from developing.

The antibody response to Lyme infection takes some time to develop, making CSF antibody unreliable for establishing diagnosis of cerebral infection. For this reason, a formula using ratios of CSF to serum, known as the anti-*Borrelia* antibody index, has been successfully substituted, as it rules out nonspecific causes of elevated antibody titers in CSF. It is calculated by taking the ratio of Lyme IgG in CSF/IgG in serum to total IgG in CSF/serum, with a positive result as greater than 2. Pleocytosis with monocytes and lymphocytes can last as long as meningeal reaction persists, sometimes for months, although CSF will be negative early and late in infection. Low CSF glucose level is unusual, but protein elevation, up to 300 mg%, is common. Free antibodies are present in CSF in only about half of cases, and immune complexes in a few additional cases. Polymerase chain reaction analysis of CSF is positive in 40–50% of patients with meningitis. Surrogate evidence of infection includes the presence of OspA antigen from the spirochete membrane, found in 25% of patients and the chemokine CXCL13, which is not specific to Lyme infection. False-positive antibody tests as a result of previous infection or traumatic lumbar puncture are avoided by using this antigen test. CSF may contain nonspecific inflammatory markers such as oligoclonal bands or specific intrathecally produced antibodies to *Borrelia*, as evidenced by titers that are higher in CSF than in serum.

C. Imaging Studies

In patients with cognitive dysfunction, single-photon emission computed tomography (SPECT) scans can show decreased frontal metabolism, and MRI can show white matter lesions reminiscent of multiple sclerosis.

D. Special Tests

In selected patients, ancillary tests for sequelae of Lyme disease include nerve conduction studies, which show decreased amplitude of evoked motor and sensory responses consistent with axonal neuropathy, or delayed F waves, consistent with proximal nerve or radicular dysfunction. Neuropsychological tests sometimes show slowed responses or memory loss.

▶ Differential Diagnosis

Other diseases of white matter, including multiple sclerosis, progressive multifocal leukoencephalopathy, and acute disseminated encephalomyelitis, are included in the differential diagnosis. Transverse myelitis following viral or mycoplasmal infection may reproduce spinal cord symptoms.

▶ Complications

Neurologic complications are more prominent in European cases and include chronic encephalopathy and myelopathy. Chronic radicular pain and neuropathy are rarely seen in Europe, but are often reported in the United States, as is cognitive and emotional dysfunction. Rarely, vasculitis causes permanent white matter pathology. "Post-Lyme encephalopathy" does not respond to long-term antibiotics and is not considered an infection.

▶ Treatment

Facial palsy in patients without meningeal signs or with negative findings on CSF analysis can be treated as early-stage Lyme disease, using 14–21 days of oral doxycycline, 100 mg twice a day, or amoxicillin, 500 mg three times a day. Patients with severe headache or radiculopathy with CSF abnormalities should receive treatment for neuroborreliosis, which requires antibiotic levels sufficient to provide sustained bactericidal activity in the CSF. This is achievable using intravenous ceftriaxone, 2 g once daily, or intravenous cefotaxime, 2 g every 8 hours, for at least 2 weeks. Parenteral penicillin G, 18–24 million U/day in divided doses, is also effective if given within the first 5 weeks of symptom onset. For patients who are allergic to penicillin or those without access to prolonged parenteral therapy, oral doxycycline, 100–200 mg twice daily for 10–28 days, or minocycline can be substituted, with appropriate warnings to avoid sun exposure. Doxycycline should not be given to pregnant women or children younger than 8 years because of its effects on teeth and bone. Children should receive 4 weeks of treatment with ceftriaxone, 75–100 mg/kg/day, or cefotaxime, 150 mg/kg/day, or penicillin G, 200,000–400,000 U/kg/day in six divided doses.

Clinical response to antibiotic therapy may take several weeks and may be incomplete. Headache can be treated with nonsteroidal anti-inflammatory medications; as prolonged antibiotic penetration of the CNS is required to eradicate the infection, corticosteroids should be avoided because of possible interference with the bactericidal activity of antibiotics. In chronically ill patients, corticosteroids can be used to control inflammation not only of joints but also of the CNS.

In patients with severe symptoms, including seizures and headache that do not respond to the previously mentioned antibiotics, there may be coinfection with other *Borrelia* strains such as *B miyamati*.

The existence of a chronic form of CNS Lyme infection is highly controversial, but a cult-like group of believers continues to endorse months or years of intravenous antibiotic therapy despite many studies that fail to establish a relationship of infection to nonspecific symptoms of pain, depression, fatigue, and poor cognitive function. Retreatment with antibiotics for patients with post-Lyme syndrome has been shown to reduce fatigue, but not to improve cognitive dysfunction or pain. Treatment should be directed at symptom relief, using antidepressants, and modafinil for fatigue, instead of antibiotics.

▶ Prognosis

With prompt antibiotic treatment, patients recover fully, especially from facial palsy. No immunologic protection is gained from infection; recurrent cases sometimes occur.

Bacon RM, Kugeler KJ, Mead PS; Centers for Disease Control and Prevention (CDC). Surveillance for Lyme disease—United States, 1992–2006. *MMWR Morb Mortal Wkly Rep* 2008;57(SS10):1–9. [PMID: 18830214] (There were 248,074 cases reported in these 15 years, most in summer months, with neurologic signs in 12%.)

Cerar D, et al. Subjective symptoms after treatment of early Lyme disease. *Am J Med* 2010;123(1):79–86. [PMID: 20102996] (In a prospective study of 230 treated European patients, the rate of development of late nonspecific symptoms such as pain did not differ between Lyme patients and controls.)

Halperin JJ. A tale of two spirochetes: Lyme disease and syphilis. *Neurol Clin* 2010;28(1):277–291. [PMID: 2019932386] (Description of acquisition and diagnosis of Lyme disease with pitfalls of laboratory testing and controversies of treatment, especially lack of evidence for late Lyme encephalopathy.)

Pachner AR, Steiner I. Lyme neuroborreliosis: Infection, immunity, and inflammation. *Lancet Neurol* 2007;6:544–552. [PMID: 17509489] (Clinical signs, laboratory diagnosis, and rational treatment are reviewed.)

Roos KL, Berger JR. Is the presence of antibodies in CSF sufficient to make a diagnosis of Lyme disease? *Neurology* 2007;69:949–950. [PMID: 17785661] (Editorial succinctly summarizing clinical and laboratory features of Lyme with emphasis on serologies and CSF antibody production's special contribution, and who should receive treatment.)

▼ RICKETTSIAL, PROTOZOAL, & HELMINTHIC INFECTIONS

RICKETTSIAL & OTHER ARTHROPOD-BORNE INFECTIONS

ESSENTIALS OF DIAGNOSIS

- ▶ Transmitted by ticks, or rarely mites, fleas, lice
- ▶ Flulike illness with fever, headache, and often rash
- ▶ Variable encephalopathic features

▶ General Considerations

Rickettsial diseases are known for the rash that precedes headache, fever, and other symptoms, but those that cause typhus tend to have encephalopathic features and a lower incidence of rash. Some recently identified diseases caused by organisms that are also considered members of the *Rickettsia* family are reviewed in Table 26–12. These diseases include monocytic or granulocytic ehrlichiosis, bacillary angiomatosis in immunosuppressed patients and cat-scratch disease in normal hosts, trench fever, Q fever, and scrub typhus. Ticks provide the vector for all but the *Bartonella*-related diseases, which are transmitted by fleas or lice, and scrub typhus, which is transmitted by mites.

Although not a member of the rickettsial group, the piroplasms *Babesia microti* and *Babesia divergens*, which cause babesiosis, are also transmitted by ticks and occur as copathogens in patients who have Lyme disease accompanied by anemia and thrombocytopenia. Tick paralysis, which is not caused by a microorganism, is discussed in Chapter 22.

▶ Epidemiology

Rocky Mountain spotted fever (RMSF), despite its name, is not limited to the Rocky Mountains and in fact is most prevalent in the mid-Atlantic and southeastern states. It also occurs in Alaska and Central America. Similar illnesses, caused by related organisms and presenting with fever, rash, and multiple organ failure, are found throughout the world. In some cases the rash consists of macules, petechiae, and purpura (eg, RMSF, typhus); in others it contains vesicles (rickettsial pox).

Human granulocytic and monocytic ehrlichiosis, tick-borne infections caused by *Ehrlichia chaffeensis* and *E phagocytophila*, respectively, can be acquired at the same time and from the same tick as borreliosis. They are endemic in the northeastern and midwestern United States, as well as Texas and California.

▶ Clinical Findings

A. Symptoms and Signs

1. Rocky mountain spotted fever—Clinical features of RMSF, including neurologic symptoms, reflect endothelial

Table 26–12. Arthropod-Borne Infections Causing Neurologic Symptoms

Disease	Causative Organism	Vector[a]	Intermediate Host(s)	Geographic Distribution	Neurologic Findings
Babesiosis	*Babesia microti* and *divergens*	*Ixodes scapularis* and *ricinus*	Cattle, rodent	Worldwide	Headache, depression, fatigue, DIC
Boutonneuse fever[b]	*Rickettsia conorii*	*Rhipicephalus sanguineus*	Rodent	Africa, Europe, Middle East, Asia	Headache
Bubonic plague	*Yersinia pestis*	*Pulex irritons*	Rat, cat, human	Worldwide	Rare meningitis
Cat-scratch disease, bacillary angiomatosis[d]	*Bartonella henselae*[c]	Cat flea	Cat	Worldwide	Fever, adenopathy, skin lesions
Ehrlichiosis (human monocytotropic)	*Ehrlichia chaffeensis*	*Amblylomma americanum, Dermacentor variabilis*	Rodent, deer	Southern United States	Headache, delirium, dementia; decreased sodium, platelets, and white cells; morulae in neutrophils
Ehrlichiosis (human granulo-cytotropic)	*Ehrlichia phagocyte-phila*	*I scapularis*	Mice, deer	Eastern and Northern United States, California	Plexopathy, demylinating polyneuropathy, rhabdomyolysis
Lyme disease	*Borrelia burgdorferi*	*I scapularis*	Deer, mice	Worldwide	Aseptic meningitis, cranial nerve palsy (facial), meningoencephalitis, radiculoneuritis, encephalopathy
Q fever	*Coxiella burnetii*[e]	Tick or direct animal contact	Cow, goat, sheep, cat, bird, python	Farm, leather, abattoir workers	Aseptic meningitis, encephalitis (< 1%), flulike illness, seizures, optic neuritis
Relapsing fever	*Borrelia species*	*Ornithodoros*	Bird, rodent	Worldwide; western United States	Headache, rare cranial nerve palsy
Rocky Mountain spotted fever	*Rickettsia rickettsii*	*Dermatocentor*	Dog, rodent, oppossum, rabbit	United States, South America	Headache, myalgia, seizure, insomnia, lethargy, delirium, coma
Trench fever	*Bartonella quintana*	*Pediculus humanus*	Vole	Europe, United States	Headache, back and eye pain
Tularemia	*Francisella tularensis*	*Dermacentor*[f]	Wild or domestic animals	Northern hemisphere	Headache, DIC, malaise
Typhus: Murine	*Rickettsia typhi*	*Xenopsilla cheopsis*	Rat	Southwestern United States, South America	Headache (mild)
Typhus: Scrub	*Orientia tstutsugamushi*	*Leptotromibidium* sp	Rat, mouse, shrew, vole	Asia, India, Australia	Headache, backache, conjunctivitis, meningitis, encephalitis

DIC = disseminated intravascular coagulation.
[a]All vectors are ticks except *X cheopis,* a flea; *P humanus,* a louse; and *L sanguineus* and *Leptotrombidium* species, which are mites.
[b]Synonyms for Boutonneuse reflect originating locale and include Mediterranean, Marseilles, African, Kenya, and India tick fever.
[c]*C burnetii* was formerly classified as *Rickesttsia burnetii.* There is no rash.
[d]Bacillary angiomatosis is found in immunodeficient hosts.
[e]*Bartonella* is a member of the rickettsiae family.
[f]Rabbit ticks include *D variabilis, D andersoni, A americanum; Ixodes* and *Haemaphysalis* species are involved with other animals, and other arthropods have been known to transmit.

damage, which causes hemorrhage, thrombosis, inflammation, and, in the CNS, breakdown of the blood–brain barrier. Antibody formation to endothelium and phospholipid membranes of red blood cells contributes further to vasculitis of the skin, heart, kidneys, and brain. Headache is a prominent finding, and fever is variably present with chills, muscle aches, prostration, and, in severe cases, altered mental status. Patients with milder disease complain of photophobia or insomnia and appear restless or confused. The rash, which is petechial or even purpuric, may be localized, present only near the bite, on the palms and soles, or diffuse. Symptoms begin up to 2 weeks after the bite and persist for 2–3 weeks. Mortality in untreated patients is 20%. Similar neurologic findings are present in the other spotted fevers, with the additional finding of a black scab formed at the site of the tick bite.

2. Typhus-like diseases—Patients with these diseases present with severe headache along with fever that can fluctuate, like that of malaria, but without rash. Symptoms recur, due to either reinfection or waning immunity. Scrub typhus, which is transmitted by chiggers that inject *Orientia tsutsugamushi*, can produce seizures. Focal findings resembling herpes encephalitis may complicate Q fever, which has a relapsing pattern and is caused by inhalation of *Rickettsia* rather than being transmitted by tick bite.

3. Ehrlichiosis—Infection produces symptoms of a flulike illness, prevalent during summer months. Encephalitis can be severe. It can complicate Lyme disease and be transmitted by the same tick bite.

4. Babesiosis—The piroplasm *Babesia bartonella* causes headache and seizures.

5. Cat-scratch disease—Infection with *Bartonella henselae* and, less often, with *Bartonella quintana* manifests as a papule at the site of a scratch from a kitten or cat, or a fleabite. This is followed by regional adenopathy 1–2 weeks later, and occasionally by conjunctivitis, fever, and malaise, and is usually self-limited over the next 2 months. Confusion, leading to coma, can emerge 1–6 weeks after the adenopathy. Seizures occur in 80% of patients; status epilepticus is especially common in children. Painless optic neuritis or retinitis causes loss of vision, especially for color. Focal findings of hemiparesis, unilateral tremor, ataxia, or chorea are sometimes present.

In immunosuppressed patients, including those with AIDS, bacillary angiomatosis can be caused by *B henselae*. At the site of bacterial entry, small-vessel proliferation produces a lesion reminiscent of Kaposi sarcoma. Other signs include personality change, dementia, and psychiatric symptoms.

B. Laboratory Findings

Laboratory confirmation can be made by staining a skin biopsy specimen obtained from the rash site or by detection of serum antibodies to *R rickettsii*, *Bartonella* sp, and other bacteria that are tick-borne. Polymerase chain reaction

amplification provides more timely diagnosis. CSF analysis shows normal glucose, elevated protein concentration, and a few WBCs, although in 20–30% of patients with *B henselae* infection, CSF analysis exhibits mononuclear pleocytosis. (Lumbar puncture should be avoided in patients in whom bleeding time is prolonged.)

C. Imaging Studies

Imaging can show infarcts, meningeal enhancement, or diffuse edema. In scrub typhus and typhus-like diseases caused by *B henselae*, the CT scan or angiogram is usually normal, suggesting that vasculitis without frank infarction is responsible for the symptoms.

D. Special Tests

The electroencephalogram shows slowing or periodic lateralizing epileptiform discharges.

▶ Treatment
A. General Approach

Treatment of all rickettsial infections consists of intravenous or oral doxycycline, 200 mg every 12 hours for 3 days, then 100 mg every 12 hours for 4 days, or a quinolone such as ciprofloxacin or ofloxacin, 400 mg every 12 hours intravenously or orally. Alternately, chloramphenicol, 12.5–20 mg/kg or 500 mg intravenously or orally every 6 hours for 7 days, can be administered in patients infected with organisms resistant to the drug or those unable to take doxycycline, such as pregnant women. Azithromycin has been effective in vitro; it should be started promptly and should be continued for either 7 days or until 2 days after fever resolves.

B. Specific Infections

Erlichiosis is treated with tetracycline, 25 mg/kg/day in four divided doses, or doxycycline, 100 mg twice a day in adults or 3 mg/kg every 12 hours in children over age 8 for 14 days. Treatment of cat-scratch disease consists of intravenous doxycycline, 200 mg every 12 hours for 3 days, then 100 mg every 12 hours for 4–8 weeks. Alternatives include administration of a quinolone such as ciprofloxacin (400 mg intravenously or 500 mg orally every 12 hours), gatifloxacin (400 mg intravenously or orally every 24 hours), levofloxacin (500 mg intravenously or orally every 24 hours), or moxifloxacin (400 mg intravenously or orally every 24 hours), or azithromycin (500 mg intravenously or 250 mg orally every 24 hours) for the same period. Chloramphenicol can be used in doses noted in the preceding paragraph.

Babesiosis is treated with 7 days of azithromycin, 500 mg on day 1 and then 250 mg daily, with atovaquone, 750 mg twice a day in adults, or clindamycin 20-40 mg/kg/day, plus quinine, 25 mg/kg/day, in children. Red blood cell exchange transfusion is used in patients with more than 5% parasitemia or life-threatening signs.

Bacillary angiomatosis, also caused by *B henselae* or *B quintana*, is treated with oral erythromycin, 500 mg every 6 hours, or oral doxycycline, 100 mg every 12 hours for 14 days.

Chapman A, et al; Centers for Disease Control and Prevention. Diagnosis and management of tickborne rickettsial diseases: Rocky Mountain spotted fever, ehrlichioses, and anaplasmosis—United States: A practical guide for physicians and other health care professionals. *MMWR Recomm Rep* 2006;55 (RR 4):1–27 [PMID: 16572105] (Comprehensive surveillance and review of the diagnosis and management of several rickettsial diseases, including photographs of the ticks that carry these diseases).

Dworkin MS, et al. Tick-borne relapsing fever. *Infect Dis Clin North Am* 2008;22(3):449–468. [PMID: 18755384] (Discusses rickettsial infections and its management.)

Hendershot EF, Sexton DJ. Scrub typhus and rickettsial diseases in international travelers: A review. *Curr Infect Dis Rep* 2009;11(1):66–72. [PMID: 19094827] (Clinical presentation of 16 rickettsial illnesses are described, and therapies. Absence of rash is not important in diagnosis.)

PROTOZOAL INFECTIONS

1. Amebic Infections

ESSENTIALS OF DIAGNOSIS

▶ Meningoencephalitis, mass lesions, or cysts in the brain and spinal cord

▶ Exposure in warm freshwater lakes or swimming pools

▶ Rapid symptom onset (3 days after exposure), usually fatal

▶ General Considerations

Pathogenic free-living amebas are ubiquitous and can cause three syndromes: meningoencephalitis, granulomatous encephalitis and other granulomatous lesions (especially of skin), and keratitis. Primary amebic meningoencephalitis in children and young adults is caused by the ameboflagellate *Naegleria fowleri*, and in immunocompromised patients, by *Balamuthia mandrillaris* (formerly called *Leptomyxid ameba*) or *Acanthamoeba* species. Granulomatous amebic encephalitis is caused by *Acanthamoeba*. Infection occurs worldwide.

N fowleri is a thermophilic organism that is found in warm or polluted waters, such as freshwater lakes, unchlorinated swimming pools, and rarely in soil or dust. Similarly, *Acanthamoeba* species live as trophozoites in fresh or brackish water, hot springs, poorly disinfected contact lens or medical solutions, and as cysts in soil. The reservoir of *B mandrillaris* is unknown.

▶ Clinical Findings

A. Symptoms and Signs

N fowleri enters the CNS through the cribiform plate producing a necrotizing meningitis that is usually fatal after incubation periods of 2–15 days. Fever, headache, lethargy, rhinitis, and pharyngitis are followed within 2 days by vomiting, disorientation, and nuchal rigidity; coma and death usually occur by the fifth or sixth day of illness. This syndrome is clinically indistinguishable from acute bacterial meningoencephalitis.

Acanthamoeba, such as *A castellanii* and *A culbertsoni*, and *B mandrillaris* cause slow (over months) granuloma production in the skin, nasal or ocular membranes, lungs, brain, and other organs after entering through the lungs, skin, or eyes. Encephalitis usually manifests as fluctuating cognitive dysfunction, along with meningeal and focal signs reflecting the area of cyst location. Strokes may occur due to endothelial disruption during prolonged meningitis.

B. Laboratory Findings

CSF and skin biopsy are helpful by ruling out infection due to bacteria and fungi even though the ameba itself rarely stains positively. CSF contains lymphocytes, erythrocytes, and eosinophils, which may be difficult to see in fresh samples. Refrigeration interferes with culture of ameba. Exact serotyping by monoclonal or polyclonal antibodies is available at the CDC, but patients usually die before antibodies are detectable. On surgical specimens, the ameboid trophozoites of *Naegleria* are distributed perivascularly with many nearby polymorphonuclear cells, whereas the cysts or trophozoite forms of *Acanthamoeba* and *B mandrillaris* are accompanied by mononuclear cells, hemorrhage, and vasculitis.

B. Imaging Studies

Nonspecific multiple, patchy enhancing lesions with minimal mass effect evolve to ring-enhancing lesions. There is decreased signal intensity on T1-weighted MRI scans and increased signal on T2-weighted images. Eventual calcification on CT may be seen in patients who survive 3 months.

▶ Treatment & Prognosis

Although there is no known effective treatment, several drugs have been tried with rare partial success using albendazole combined with other antibiotics. Surgery and corticosteroids are not helpful. Prognosis is dismal, with almost 100% fatality rates.

Khan NA. *Acanthamoeba* invasion of the central nervous system. *Int J Parasitol* 2007;37(2):131–138. [PMID: 17207487] (Brain entry through the olfactory nerve or bronchi, as well as skin, is facilitated by transporter mechanisms that affect the blood–brain barrier, and may be targets for therapy.)

Lackner P, et al. Acute granulomatous *Acanthamoeba* encephalitis in an immunocompetent patient. *Neurocrit Care* 2010;12(1):91–94. [PMID: 19847677] (A 17-year-old developed *A lenticulatus* meningoencephalitis after disruption of ethmoid sinuses and survived after treatment with many months of meropenem, linezolide, fluconazole, and moxifloxacin.)

Marano C, Freedman DO. Global health surveillance and travelers' health. *Curr Opin Infect Dis* 2009;22(5):423–429. [PMID: 19726984] (Use of GeoSentinel surveillance systems allows rapid information to be disseminated that is useful in assessing which illness may be affecting specific patients who have travelled outside of their home country, and offering advice for prevention and protection from these illnesses).

Singhal T, et al. Successful treatment of *Acanthamoeba* meningitis with combination oral antimicrobials. *Pediatr Infect Dis J* 2001;20:623–627. [PMID: 11419508] (Two of three children responded to trimethoprim-sulfamethoxazole, rifampin, and ketoconazole treatment of *Acanthamoeba*.)

2. Toxoplasmosis

In HIV-seropositive patients, opportunistic infection emerges as cell-mediated immunity wanes, and in those not receiving appropriate chemoprophylaxis, toxoplasmosis is the most common opportunistic infection encountered in the CNS. Avoidance of cat feces and proper cooking of meat can reduce the risk of infection in naive patients, but most cases of toxoplasmosis in HIV patients represent reactivation. Permanent sequelae are highly unusual, but herniation and death can occur in rapidly progressive cases. Chapter 28 discusses toxoplasmosis and other complications of HIV infection in detail.

3. Malaria

ESSENTIALS OF DIAGNOSIS

▶ Chills, fever, and diaphoresis lasting 4–6 hours, recurring every other or every third day
▶ Cerebral malaria—severe headache, confusion, seizures, high fever, coma, and death in up to 40% of patients

▶ General Considerations

Human malaria is caused by four species of the genus *Plasmodium*—*P vivax*, *P malariae*, *P ovale*, and *P falciparum*—but only the usually causes cerebral malaria. The disease has been entirely eradicated outside of tropical regions, but is still a major health problem in Africa, the Caribbean, Central and South America, the Middle East, India, Asia, and Oceania. *P falciparum* (the predominant species in Africa) causes diffuse encephalopathy with seizures or status epilepticus. In 2008, worldwide, malaria caused more than 300 million clinical episodes with almost 1 million deaths, 90% in African children or pregnant women. In 2008, in the

United States, 1298 cases of malaria were reported, 39% due to *P falciparum*, almost all in returning travelers or recent immigrants. In the 6 weeks following Haiti's earthquake in January 2010, 11 cases were reported.

▶ Pathogenesis

Malaria parasites are spread between humans by female *Anopheles* mosquitoes or, rarely, are acquired by blood transfusion or maternal transmission. The mosquito ingests blood containing the parasite in gametocyte form. The sporozoite that subsequently develops is inoculated into the next human when the mosquito feeds. The parasites multiply in the liver and then in red blood cells, where successive broods cause red cells to rupture, releasing daughter parasites. Severity of infection is judged by the percentage of red blood cells containing parasites; a rate of 5–10% is present in severe infection, and 20% usually is fatal.

Cerebral malaria is defined by the World Health Organization as follows: (1) demonstration of parasitemia with *P falciparum* (although *P vivax* and *P knowlesi* cases have been reported); (2) presence of coma; (3) exclusion of other causes of coma, including hypoglycemia; and (4) favorable response to antimalarial therapy. Most CNS damage is due to hypoxia as a result of sequestration of parasite-containing red blood cells, which adhere to the endothelium of brain capillaries and venules, where the red cells form rosettes, "ring" hemorrhages, and granulomatous nodules (Dürck granuloma). In addition, filling of venules by parasites causes diffuse cerebral edema, which may lead to herniation. Cytokine and chemokine release by immune reaction to infection, especially TNF-α, can also lead to direct toxicity to neurons and astrocytes. Eventual memory deficits and poor school performance may be a result of repeated hypoglycemia or hippocampal damage from seizures or coma.

▶ Prevention

Avoiding exposure to the carrier mosquito is the best preventive measure. This may be accomplished using insect-treated nets for sleeping, long-sleeved clothing, screens or air conditioning, and insecticide. Prophylactic use of antiprotozoal drugs does not provide complete protection (see later discussion). Vaccination is still in Phase 1 trials.

▶ Clinical Findings

A. Symptoms and Signs

Typical malaria infection causes sequential phases of shaking chills, fever of 41°C (105.8°F) or more, and marked diaphoresis over a 4- to 6-hour period. Secondary symptoms may include fatigue, headache, dizziness, nausea or diarrhea, myalgias, arthralgias, backache, and dry cough. Attacks resulting from *P vivax*, *P ovale*, or *P falciparum* follow a tertian pattern, recurring every other day, and those due to *P malariae* a quartan periodicity, recurring every third day.

Between attacks, the patient is generally well or feels tired. Splenomegaly and mild hepatomegaly appear after 4 days of continuous acute symptoms. The uncomplicated and untreated primary malaria attack usually lasts 2–4 weeks (*P malariae* attacks last about twice as long). Relapses may occur before infection terminates spontaneously.

Cerebral malaria presents with a rapid onset of unconsciousness and no localizing signs; seizures are especially frequent in children. It may also present as psychomotor agitation or acute psychotic behavior; patients become restless, confused, and disoriented, or develop violent behavior or hallucinatory delirium.

B. Laboratory Findings

Microscopic examination of thick and thin blood films, using Giemsa or Wright stains, confirms the diagnosis. Serologic tests are not used, as antibodies only become detectable 8–10 days after disease onset, and their presence cannot distinguish between current and past infection.

▶ Differential Diagnosis

Other causes of febrile illness include influenza, urinary tract infection, typhoid fever, infectious hepatitis, dengue, chikungunya, kala azar, amebic liver abscess, leptospirosis, and relapsing fever from rickettsial infection, the last sharing a recurring pattern of fever with malaria.

▶ Complications

Complications from severe *P falciparum* malaria other than cerebral malaria include disseminated intravascular coagulation, hemoglobinuria, renal failure due to acute tubular necrosis, electrolyte imbalance and hypoglycemia, metabolic acidosis, pulmonary edema, gram-negative sepsis, jaundice or liver failure, severe anemia, seizures, and shock. Hemolysis can follow quinine administration, causing "black water fever."

Mortality is high in cerebral malaria, even in treated patients (14–40%), but most survivors of coma do not suffer persistent sequalae. Weakness, deafness, epilepsy, and cortical blindness occur in 10% of survivors. More subtle complications of cognitive dysfunction and school failure are quite common.

▶ Treatment & Chemoprophylaxis

Travelers should be advised that prophylactic measures do not provide complete protection from malaria; attacks may start up to 8 weeks after stopping prophylaxis. Chemoprophylaxis generally consists of chloroquine, 500 mg (salt), in adults and 8 mg/kg syrup in children; mefloquine, 250 mg (salt), in adults and weight-based from one-quarter tablet to one tablet in children from 30–90 lb, given once a week; daily doxycycline, 100 mg, or the combination atovaquone, 250 mg, plus proguanil, 100 mg, in adults, and pediatric tablets, weight-based, in children, which have to be started before visiting the area and continued for several weeks after return, although the duration of the combination medication is shorter. Chemoprophylaxis is not used for residents of these areas, due to cost and side effects generated by prolonged use. In addition, protocols change based on the development of chloroquine resistance in geographic areas. It is recommended that the latest guidelines be used, which are available by calling the Malaria Hot Line (770) 488-7788 or (770) 488-7100 after hours, or by checking the CDC website: http://www.cdc.gov/malaria/diagnosis_treatment/treatment.htm.

Guidelines for treatment offered by the CDC, using only medications available in the United States are summarized in Table 26–13. Parasitologic confirmation is not required, although measuring the density of parasitemia, in addition to determining severity, provides evidence of treatment response when checked sequentially. Antimicrobial resistance is assumed if parasitemia is not reduced rapidly (clinical response takes 2–3 days). Patients suspected of *P falciparum* infection should be hospitalized in anticipation of the severe complications described above. Indications for parenteral treatment are (1) failure to ingest or retain drugs, (2) cerebral malaria, (3) multiple complications, and (4) peripheral parasitemia of 5% or higher. After completion of the treatment course, blood smears should be checked weekly for 4 weeks to ensure that there is no recrudescence of infection.

Supportive measures include rehydration with great caution, especially in the first 24 hours, because overhydration may cause noncardiogenic pulmonary edema. Seizures require medication initially, although prolonged use of antiepileptics is not required. Dialysis may be necessary for renal failure. The patient's temperature should be kept below 38.5°C (101.3°F) with acetaminophen. Patients with clinically significant disseminated intravascular coagulation should be treated with fresh whole blood, clotting factors, or platelets and avoidance of corticosteroids, aspirin, anti-inflammatory agents, dextran, norepinephrine, and heparin. Admission to an intensive care unit is mandated when complications of coma, anemia, renal failure, pulmonary edema, or disseminated intravascular coagulation are present.

Centers for Disease Control. Preventing Malaria in Travelers: A Guide for Travelers in Malaria-Risk Areas. Available at: http://wwwn.cdc.gov/travel/contentdiseases.aspx#malaria; or Malaria Hotline (770) 488–7788; or Parasitic Drug Help Line (877) 252–1200. (A brochure for members of the public that gives guidelines for prophylaxis and treatment, based on geographic location; additional information about malaria can also be obtained from the CDC website: http://www.cdc.gov/malaria/html.)

Crawley J, et al. Malaria in children. *Lancet* 2010;375(9724):1468–1481. [PMID: 20417858] (Reviews the overall approach to managing malaria, especially due to *P falciparum* and *P vivax*, including prevention and artemisin-based antibiotic use.)

Table 26–13. Treatment of Malaria

Type	Drug Regimen
Uncomplicated malaria	Chloroquine phosphate, PO, 1 g (600 mg base), followed by 500 mg (300 mg base) at 6, 24, and 48 h
Plasmodium vivax or *P ovale*	Same *plus* Primaquine phosphate, 52.6 mg (30 mg base) PO daily for 14 days; not used in G6PD-deficient patients
Chloroquine resistant	Quinine sulfate,[a] PO, 650 mg (500 mg base) q 8 h *plus* Doxycycline,[b] PO, 200 mg q 12 h for 3 days, then 100 mg q 12 h for 4 days (IM or SC if needed) Quinidine gluconate, 10 mg base/kg (15 mg salt) IV over 1–2 h, followed by 0.0125 mg base or 0.02 mg salt/kg/min for 24 h, or 1–1.5 mg/kg/h, unless prophylaxis given in previous 48 h
Parasitemia < 1%	Change to oral quinine sulfate, as above for chloroquine-resistant disease, for 3 days if African or South American or 7 days if Southeast Asian—acquired *plus* Doxycycline or tetracycline, 100 mg IV or PO q 12 h for 7 days

G6PD = glucose-6-phosphate dehydrogenase; IM = intramuscularly; IV = intravenously; PO = orally (by mouth); SC = subcutaneously.
[a]Quinine and chloroquine can be given SC or IM if needed. Ongoing monitoring for hypoglycemia, widened QRS complex, prolonged QT interval required.
[b]In pregnancy or childhood, clindamycin, 600 mg IV q 8 h or 300 mg PO q 12 h, substituted for doxycycline and tetracycline which harm teeth.

Kihara M, et al. Impaired everyday memory associated with encephalopathy of severe malaria: The role of seizures and hippocampal damage. *Malar J* 2009;8:273–281. [PMID: 19951424] (Neuropsychological testing in 152 children establishes cognitive deficits after cerebral malaria, and relation to seizures versus coma and hypoglycemia is discussed.)

Kilama W, Ntoumi F. Malaria: A research agenda for the eradication era. *Lancet* 2009;374(9700):1480–1482. [PMID: 19880004] (New developments in the management of malaria, including diagnostic techniques, medications, and prevention methodology.)

Mali S, et al. Malaria surveillance—United States, 2006. *MMWR Surveil Summ* 2009;58:SS02:1–16. [PMID: 18566568] (A listing of cases due to all forms of malaria reported in 2006 in the United States, with details for the deaths, laboratory testing, and treatment.)

4. Trypanosomiasis: African Variant (Sleeping Sickness)

 ESSENTIALS OF DIAGNOSIS

▶ Transmitted by tsetse fly bite in sub-Saharan Africa
▶ Insidious encephalopathy follows a lymphatic stage, leading to death in several years if untreated

▶ General Considerations

African trypanosomiasis is caused by the extracellular flagellated protozoa *Trypanosoma brucei gambiense* (in West and Central Africa) and *rhodesiense* (in East Africa); both are transmitted by bites of the tsetse fly, which inhabits shaded areas along rivers. Inflammation occurs at the site of inoculation on the host, forming a chancre. The trypanosomes enter the lymphatic system, and a hemolymphatic form of the disease persists for weeks to months, followed by meningoencephalitis with disrupted sleep cycles.

In Africa, approximately 100,000 people die of the disease each year. Americans returning from East African game parks are at risk, but on average only one case is reported each year in the United States.

▶ Pathogenesis

Demyelination and inflammatory changes are cytokine and prostaglandin mediated and most marked in white matter and periventricular areas. Hypothalamic damage is responsible for neuroendocrine abnormalities and diencephalic damage for sleep dysfunction.

▶ Clinical Findings

A. Symptoms and Signs

The Rhodesian form of trypanosomiasis is a more compressed version of the *T b gambiense* disease, with chancre (often not noticed in the Gambian form), followed 3–10 days later by the hemolymphatic stage, and a few weeks later by encephalitis. The Gambian form has an insidious hemolymphatic phase that lasts months and an encephalitic stage that can last years.

The hemolymphatic stage is characterized by episodes of high fever, severe headache, arthralgias, myalgias, rash, and malaise, recurring at about 2-week intervals corresponding to waves of parasitemia. Most patients develop large, painless lymphadenopathy. Myocardial involvement may lead to death before encephalitis in *T b rhodesiense* infection. The early signs of encephalitis are insomnia or disruption of the circadian pattern of sleep cycle, anorexia, personality change, apathy, and headache. Tremors and disturbances of speech, gait, and tendon reflexes develop, with eventual somnolence and coma. Patients become severely emaciated. Death often results from secondary infection.

B. Laboratory Findings

Nonspecific findings include anemia, increased erythrocyte sedimentation rate, thrombocytopenia, and increased serum globulin. Eosinophilia is not seen. Definitive diagnosis requires identification of motile organisms in wet films and Giemsa- or Wright-stained blood smears or wet films of aspirates of chancres, lymph nodes, bone marrow, or CSF. Cultures of CSF, blood, bone marrow, or tissue can be done in liquid culture medium or mouse inoculation. Serology is available for *T b gambiense* only and is not reliable. Serum proteomic testing is very sensitive and specific, and may replace PCR and antigen testing, which are not widely available.

CSF is clear, with elevated opening pressure, up to 2000 cells/mm³/μL, normal glucose level, and elevated protein concentration. To detect the organism, CSF should be examined within 20 minutes (to avoid parasitic lysis), but absence of visualization of trypanosomes does not exclude the diagnosis. A field-adapted agglutination test (sensitivity about 96%, specificity high) can detect circulating and CSF antigen to determine the IgM index, which is especially beneficial in late infection when parasitemia and systemic circulating antibodies become undetectable. Mott cells are large eosinophilic plasma cells seen rarely.

B. Imaging Studies

MRI scan of one patient showed initial basal ganglia, midbrain, internal capsule, and periventricular nonenhancing hyperintensities followed 1 year later by decreased signal in the same regions, with cerebral atrophy.

C. Special Tests

Electroencephalography shows excessive delta activity (slowing), and polysomnographic monitoring shows severe alterations of the sequence of sleep stages involving slow-wave sleep and paradoxical rapid-eye movement sleep with overall disruption of the circadian rhythm of sleep.

▶ Differential Diagnosis

Sleeping sickness, despite occurring in similar tropical climates, is readily differentiated from other protozoan infections such as malaria, but it may resemble the postencephalitic form of Parkinson disease or the rare prion disease responsible

for fatal familial insomnia (see Chapter 29). Paraneoplastic limbic encephalitis resulting from leukemia and lymphoma as well as arbovirus encephalitides should be considered, along with catatonic forms of psychosis.

▶ Prevention

Use of protective clothing and insect repellant in regions where tsetse flies live is recommended. Medications to protect against infection are not useful. Early detection of CNS involvement, using CSF analysis, can prevent severe damage. There is no vaccine planned as the organism mutates rapidly, although previous infection provides some immunity.

▶ Treatment

Detection of the organism is required before treatment because of the toxicity of all therapies used to treat this infection. Medication choice, reviewed in Table 26–14, varies with the stage of illness.

> Priotto G, et al. Nifurtimox-eflornithine combination therapy for second-stage African *Trypanosoma brucei gambiense* trypanosomiasis: A multicentre, randomized, phase III, non-inferiority trial. *Lancet* 2009;374(9683):56–64 [PMID: 19559476] (Latest WHO-recommended therapy combinations, with less toxicity and more efficacy than older medications.)

5. Trypanosomiasis: American Variant (Chagas Disease)

ESSENTIALS OF DIAGNOSIS

▶ Transmitted by the reduviid ("kissing," "assassin") bug, blood transfusion, or transplacentally

▶ Heart failure, dysphagia, constipation, and (rarely) meningoencephalitis

▶ Encephalitis, brain abscess common in AIDS patients

▶ General Considerations

American trypanosomiasis, also called *Chagas disease*, is caused by the flagellated protozoan, *Trypanosoma cruzi*, found primarily in Central and South America. It is transmitted by bites of infected reduviid bugs, through fecal contamination of mucous membranes or conjunctiva, by blood transfusion, or transplacentally. The parasite invades cells of myocardium, smooth muscle, and CNS, and, assuming the leishmanial form, provokes cellular destruction, inflammation, and fibrosis.

Worldwide, 16–25 million people are estimated to be infected, with 50,000 annual deaths, mainly among the rural poor. Chagas disease is the most important cause of heart

Table 26–14. Antimicrobial Treatment of Trypanosomal Infection

Disease/Stage	Drug Regimen
T b gambiense (West African Sleeping Sickness)	
Early stage (hemolymphatic)	Pentamidine, 4 mg/kg IM or IV daily × 10 days *or* Suramin,[a] test dose 100 mg IV, then 1 g IV on days 1, 3, 7, 14, and 21 *or* Eflornithine, 100 mg/kg IV q 6 h for 14 days, followed by 300 mg/kg/day PO for 3–4 wk
Late stage (CNS)	Eflornithine as above *or* Eflornithine 200 mg q 12 h IV × 7 days plus nifurtimox 5 mg/kg q 8 h × 10 days Melarsoprol,[a] 2.0–3.6 mg/kg IV on days 1, 2, 3, 10, 11, 12, plus 19–21 if high CSF WBC *or* 2.16 mg/kg daily for 12 days *plus* corticosteroids, any form *plus* Suramin 100–200 mg (test dose) IV, followed by 20 mg/kg q 5 days for 12 injections
T b rhodesiense	
East African Sleeping Sickness Early stage (hemolymphatic)	Suramin,[a] test dose 100 mg IV, then 1 g or 20 mg/kg on days 1, 3, 7, 14, and 21 *or* Pentamidine, 4 mg/kg IM q 24 h for 7–10 days *or* Eflornithine, 100 mg/kg IV q 6 h for 14 days, followed by 300 mg/kg/day for 3–4 wk
Late stage (CNS)	Melarsoprol,[a] 2–3.6 mg/kg IV q 24 h for 3 days; repeat in 1 wk and in 2 or 3 wk Give with prednisolone
Chagas disease	Nifurtimox • Adults: 2 mg/kg PO q 6 h for 3–4 mo • Children < 10 y: 4–5 mg/kg PO q 6 h for 4 mo Benznidazole, 3.5 mg/kg PO q 12 h for 2 mo (only available through the CDC in United States)

CNS = central nervous system; IM = intramuscularly; IV = intravenously; PO = orally (by mouth); q = every.
[a]Suramin, melarsoprol, and nifurtimox are only available from the Parasitic Disease Drug Service, Centers for Disease Control and Prevention, Atlanta, GA 30333; (404) 639-3670 or 639-2888. Alternatively, melarsoprol may be given according to a schedule of four daily injections, increasing from 1.2–3.6 mg/kg, repeated q 7 days. Toxicity (encephalopathy and neuropathy) is seen in 5–20% of patients; corticosteroids help alleviate.

disease in many South American countries; up to 70% of infected persons are asymptomatic.

▶ Clinical Findings

A. Symptoms and Signs

The parasite often produces an inflammatory reaction at its site of entry, either in the eye or in the skin, followed by fever, malaise, headache, hepatomegaly, mild splenomegaly, and generalized lymphadenopathy. Acute myocarditis develops in about 10% of patients. Meningoencephalitis, often fatal, is seen only in children usually under age 2.

The latent period (intermediate phase) may last for 10–30 years. The chronic phase usually manifests as cardiac disease, starting in the third or fourth decade and characterized by arrhythmias, including ventricular fibrillation, congestive heart failure, ventricular aneurysm, and systemic, pulmonary, or brain embolization originating from mural thrombi. Stroke has occurred in patients with normal hearts, suggesting CNS vasculitis. Destruction of the autonomic ganglia regulating esophageal and intestinal motility leads to constipation, obstipation, and megaesophagus. Neuronitis causes sensory loss in an axonal pattern. Dementia and encephalopathy may occur rarely, but neurologic findings in the chronic stage are usually found only in immunocompromised patients, especially those with advanced HIV infection. Diffuse meningoencephalitis, necrotizing encephalitis, and intracranial abscess have all been reported.

B. Laboratory Findings

Motile trypanosomes are detected in the blood in most patients with acute and congenital disease, and in 40% of those with chronic disease, amastigotes can be found in tissue aspirates or biopsies of skin lesions. Lumbar puncture is nonspecific but may reveal the parasite; intracranial biopsy may be required to confirm diagnosis. Histopathologic evaluation reveals areas of hemorrhagic necrotic encephalitis, with prominent obliterative angiitis, and amastigote forms of *T cruzi* can be seen within glial cells, macrophages, and endothelial cells on light and electron microscopy.

C. Imaging Studies

Cranial CT scan shows single or multiple contrast-enhancing lesions, surrounded by edema. The appearance is similar to toxoplasmosis or CNS lymphoma.

▶ Prevention

As in all tropical diseases, prevention involves vector control. In this case, no vaccination program exists yet (despite genome sequencing for *T cruzi* being accomplished).

▶ Treatment

Table 26–14 summarizes pharmacotherapy for Chagas disease. Treatment is often ineffective, and the available drugs, nifurtimox and benznidazole, are potentially toxic. In chronic disease, treatment may cause parasitemia to disappear but has no effect on cardiac function.

Side effects of nifurtimox include gastrointestinal complaints, weight loss, tremors, peripheral neuropathy, and, rarely, hallucinations, pulmonary infiltrates, and convulsions. Benznidazole (not available in the United States) has side effects of granulocytopenia, rash, and peripheral neuropathy. Supportive cardiac medications include amiodarone as an antiarrhythmic drug, cardiac pacemakers or defibrillators, and angiotensin-converting enzyme inhibitors (not digoxin) for congestive heart failure.

Córdova E, et al. Neurological manifestations of Chagas' disease. *Neurol Res* 2010;32(3):238–244. [PMID: 20406601] (A literature review of the subject demonstrates meningoencephalitis in patients under 2 and "neuritis" in older patients, with the highest mortality rates in immunosuppressed patients suffering recurrent disease.)

HELMINTHIC INFECTIONS

Eosinophilic meningitis, although representing only 2% of all cases of meningitis, is the most common presentation of helminthic infection, but mass lesions in the brain and spinal cord due to migrating worms are also found. The helminth family includes tapeworms (cestodes), such as *Taenia solium* and *Echinococcus granulosus*; flukes (trematodes), such as *Schistosoma* and *Paragonimus*; and roundworms (nematodes),

such as *Trichinella spiralis*, *Toxocara canis*, *Toxocara cati*, *Angiostrongylus cantonensis*, *Gnathostoma spinigerum*, and *Strongyloides stercoralis*.

These organisms variably cause muscle infection (*Trichinella*, *Toxocara*), meningitis (*Gnathostoma*, *Strongyloides*, *Angiostrongylus*), or the most serious complication, cystic masses in brain or spinal cord (*Cysticercus*, *Schistosoma*, *Echinococcus*). Risk factors for parasitic infections are close contact with domestic and farm animals, poor sanitation that allows water to be contaminated by human fecal waste, and swimming, which allows schistosomiasis to enter through the skin. Eosinophilia is present, and parasites are occasionally detectable in stool. Eosinophilic meningitis, with eosinophils accounting for more than 10% of CSF white count, is a feature of most helminthic infections. Noninfectious causes include clonal leukemia or drug- or device-induced reactions.

1. Cysticercosis

ESSENTIALS OF DIAGNOSIS

- ▶ Neurocysticercosis, caused by the larval form of pork tapeworm, *T solium*
- ▶ Common cause of epilepsy
- ▶ Small parenchymal, subarachnoid, or intraventricular cysts
- ▶ Meningitis caused by reaction to death of the parasite

▶ General Considerations

Neurocysticercosis is the most common CNS parasitic disease, with 50 million cases worldwide. Epilepsy in the developing world is often due to this infection. Travel and immigration from endemic areas such as Mexico and India have led to an increasing number of cases seen in the United States; 10% of seizures evaluated in a Los Angeles hospital emergency department were attributed to cysticercosis. In addition to epilepsy, neurocysticercosis causes hydrocephalus, basal meningitis, and lesions in the brain or spinal cord (< 5% all masses).

▶ Pathogenesis

Humans are the definitive host of this tapeworm, whose scolex attaches to the intestinal wall and sheds eggs, which can then be ingested by pigs via contaminated water or vegetables that have been fertilized by human fecal material ("night soil"). The pig is the intermediate host, and humans are accidental intermediate hosts who acquire the parasite in the larval stage by ingestion of undercooked pork containing it in the muscle. After attachment in the intestine, larvae migrate to the eye and brain among other organs. The racemose form of infection consists of grapelike clusters within the subarachnoid or ventricular space, causing obstruction of CSF. Transient neurologic symptoms, including headache, vertigo, and other brainstem signs, or sudden increase in intracranial pressure can occur when the live worm moves inside the ventricular system. Death of the parasite provokes an intense inflammatory reaction with meningitis. After death of the larvae, the granulomata calcify. Calcifications are usually small and asymptomatic (other than seizures) and can be solitary or multiple.

▶ Prevention

Interruption of the cestode life cycle by public health measures ensuring proper water sanitation has caused a decline in cases from developed areas. Cooks who may be infected must be treated and trained in hygiene procedures to avoid fecal contamination of food. Avoiding human waste use as fertilizer interrupts acquisition in those who don't eat pork.

▶ Clinical Findings

A. Symptoms and Signs

Calcified cysts are often asymptomatic or produce seizures, which are focal or generalized. As the larvae die, meningeal signs including headache, due to the meningeal reaction to cyst death, which can be intense but rarely lasts more than 2 weeks. Visual scotomata are present with retinal involvement. Increased intracranial pressure with headache, poor

upgaze, and obtundation can occur in obstructive hydrocephalus (20% of cases) when intraventricular or subarachnoid cysts block CSF circulation. Grapelike clusters of cysts sharing membranes (racemose form) are occasionally fatal. Mass effect of very large cysts produces focal dysfunction.

B. Laboratory Findings

ELISA serology and PCR are reliable tests, although not usually necessary, for diagnosis. During meningitis, CSF analysis shows eosinophils and monocytes, rarely more than 300 cells/mm^3, and normal glucose and protein concentration.

C. Imaging Studies

Cysts, some or all calcified, and containing a scolex, are seen on CT and MRI scans, especially with FLAIR sequences (Figure 26–10). They enhance during the period of dying. Diagnosis is based on this characteristic CT finding, combined with a history of traveling or living in an endemic area.

▶ Differential Diagnosis

Brain tumors, especially oligodendroglioma, tuberculoma, and other infection, comprise the differential diagnosis. Arachnoid cysts are not usually confused with cysticercosis, as they do not calcify.

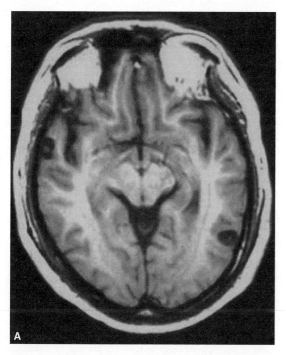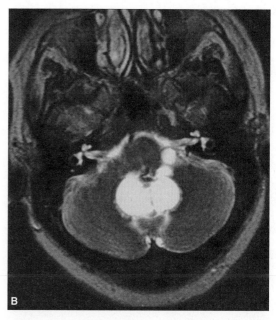

▲ **Figure 26–10.** Cysticercosis. **(A)** Axial T1-weighted MRI scan shows small cortical cysts, each containing a slightly hyperintense scolex. **(B)** Intraventricular cysticercosis, different patient. Axial T2-weighted MRI scan shows several high T2-signal cysts in the fourth ventricle, extending out the left lateral recess. (Used with permission from John Loh, MD.)

▶ Complications

Hydrocephalus (see Figure 26–2) and increased intracranial pressure have a 2-year mortality rate of 50%. Even after the death of all worms, epilepsy can persist, and can be treated surgically with hippocampal, not lesion, resection in younger patients. Stroke is a rare complication. Poor cognitive function and dementia can be demonstrated on neuropsychologic testing in many patients.

▶ Treatment

Cysticidal treatment remains controversial with some studies demonstrating decrease in seizures after treatment with corticosteroids alone and some with antiparasitic agents alone. Discovery of active infection during screening does not predict symptom development, and enhancement of a lesion implies it is already dying. (Calcified lesions represent dead cysts.) Anticonvulsants are recommended, at least during the first several months after symptomatic seizures and during periods of cysticidal therapy, which consists of albendazole, 15 mg/kg (400 mg) orally every 12 hours for 10 days, with corticosteroids added prophylactically to prevent seizures (reduced by 41% in one series) and minimize meningeal reactions. Controlled trials demonstrated better response to albendazole than praziquantel. The benefit of cysticidal therapy is questionable, as spontaneous resolution of cysts occurs in two thirds of patients. Conversely, all cysts are not eliminated by this therapy. When retinal lesions are present, no cysticidal therapy should be given, as resultant inflammation on death of the cysticercus can lead to scarring and blindness. Surgical decompression is required only in patients with giant, symptomatic, or intraventricular cysts. Ventriculoperitoneal shunts may be necessary.

Abba K, Ramaratnam S, Ranganathan LN. Anthelmintics for people with neurocysticercosis. *Cochrane Database Syst Rev* 2010;3:CD000215. [PMID: 20238309] (Confusing results of decreased seizure recurrence when albendazole is used to treat nonviable cysts, and no effect on seizure frequency but decrease in number of lesions with therapy of viable cysts. Addition of dexamethasone to anthelminthic did not affect frequency of headache during treatment in one trial.)

Ciampi de Andrade D, et al. Cognitive impairment and dementia in neurocysticercosis: A cross-sectional controlled study. *Neurology* 2010;74(16):1288–1295. [PMID: 20404310] (Forty patients with active neurocysticercosis were studied in a battery of cognitive tests. Dementia was present in 12.5%, unrelated to antiepileptic medication or seizure frequency. Impairment of verbal and nonverbal memory, fluency, construction, and executive function was widespread and unrelated to cyst location.)

DelBrutto OH, et al. Meta-analysis: Cysticidal drugs for neurocysticercosis: Albendazole and praziquantel. *Ann Intern Med* 2006;145(1):43–51. [PMID: 16818928] (Eleven randomized trials from 1979–2005; 464 patients with cystic and 478 with enhancing lesions were reviewed. Cysticidal therapy led to complete resolution in 44% of patients and seizure recurrence was lower (14% instead of 37%), including generalized seizure rate (67% reduced) with treatment.)

2. Schistosomiasis (Bilharziasis)

ESSENTIALS OF DIAGNOSIS

- ▶ Acquired by swimming or working in fresh water, such as rice fields
- ▶ Occurs mainly in sub-Saharan Africa, the Caribbean (except Puerto Rico), South America
- ▶ Seizures result from granuloma in the brain
- ▶ Myelopathy or radiculopathy result from spinal cord or cauda equina involvement
- ▶ Hepatic encephalopathy in patients with severe liver involvement

▶ General Considerations

Schistosomiasis is caused by the trematode *Schistosoma*, of which five major species affect humans: *S mansoni*, *S japonicum*, *S haematobium*, *S intercalatum*, and *S mekongi*. The life cycle of the parasite is complex; the intermediate hosts are small water-living organisms such as snails. The parasite enters humans through the skin or through consumption of raw snails, and eventually ova reach sites such as liver, brain, and spinal cord. *S japonicum* tends to localize in the cerebral hemispheres and *S mansoni* in the spinal cord. Prevalence rates in endemic areas, determined by testing stool samples, range from 25–100%, but most cases are asymptomatic. Worldwide, 200 million people have infection, most outside of the nervous system.

▶ Prevention

Public health measures to purify water supplies and improve sanitation decrease the incidence of schistosomiasis. Eliminating the intermediate host with molluscicides or lining irrigation pipes with concrete that the snails cannot cross is also effective.

▶ Clinical Findings

A. Symptoms and Signs

Skin itching and erythema may mark the infection site. Focal signs in the brain or spinal cord reflect the location of the granuloma, which is usually solitary. There is a predilection for the lumbar region of the spinal canal, where radicular signs of pain and numbness predominate, but abscess anywhere within the spinal cord can produce signs of weakness and loss of sensation below that level, with dysfunction of bladder and bowel. Increased intracranial pressure may occur if multiple or large lesions are present or obstruction of CSF circulation occurs. Fluctuating consciousness or depressed sensorium, tremor, and asterixis are signs of hepatic encephalopathy, which may follow liver infestation.

B. Laboratory Findings

Eosinophilia is not present in patients with chronic infection. Results of serologic testing may be negative, but antibodies to soluble egg antigen are detected in 56% of samples, and are 95% specific. In endemic areas, high background rates of infection make this unreliable. In the chronic state that produces neurologic symptoms, stool and urine samples rarely contain the parasite or eggs. Mild pleocytosis and protein elevation are found in CSF.

C. Imaging Studies

MRI is the best modality for identifying infection, especially of the spinal cord, although calcifications may be present on CT scan of the brain. Thickened nerve roots and heterogeneous enhancement can be seen on MRI T1 images of the spinal cord and cauda equina.

▶ Treatment

Praziquantel, 20 mg/kg orally every 12 hours for two doses, or oxamniquine, 50 mg/kg orally for one dose (South American studies), or 20 mg/kg daily for five doses (African studies) are all useful. Corticosteroids should accompany treatment and may need to be continued for several months.

3. Echinococcosis (Hydatid Cyst)

ESSENTIALS OF DIAGNOSIS

- ▶ Cysts may be present in the liver (65%), lungs (25%), bones, CNS (rare)
- ▶ Seizures, cranial nerve palsies, focal cerebral signs, and hydrocephalus

▶ General Considerations

The cestode *E granulosus* or, rarely, *E multilocularis* is found in dogs, foxes, sheep, cats, and other animals. Eliminating the parasite from dogs by frequent treatment (or separating dogs from cattle) eliminates the intermediate host. Avoiding ingestion of water or vegetables that may be contaminated with dog feces, and avoiding close contact with dogs whose tongues may carry eggs of *Echinococcus* help limit human exposure.

▶ Clinical Findings

Most cases are asymptomatic. If cysts are large enough, they will cause seizures or focal signs that reflect their location. Hydrocephalus occurs if intraventricular cysts reach sufficient size to block CSF flow. Symptoms generally arise within 8 months of infection.

ELISA and Western immunoblot tests are sensitive and specific. Eosinophilia in the blood relates to parasitic infection in general. CSF does not contain eosinophils.

MRI is better than CT for detecting lesions in brain and spinal cord. Cysts are more often unilocular than multilocular. They do not enhance and lack surrounding edema. Sometimes the protoscolice or "hydatid sand" may be visualized inside the wall. Liver involvement is detectable by ultrasound.

▶ Treatment

Treatment is generally surgery, with care not to spill the cyst contents at time of removal. Some surgeons instill a cysticidal agent such as ethanol or hypertonic saline before removing the cyst. After removal, albendazole, 400 mg orally every 12 hours, or oral mebendazole, 50 mg/kg/day, is given until radiographic studies confirm cure.

4. Gnathostomiasis

The nematode *G spinigerum* is responsible for eosinophilic meningitis, often with red blood cells found in CSF as well. Paraplegia is present in patients with myelitis, although painful radiculitis is more common. Rarely altered mental status, even coma, occurs in encephalitis. Symptoms can move from one cranial nerve or spinal root to another. The organism is occasionally seen in the eye. Treatment is surgical, followed by albendazole.

5. Lung Fluke Infection

Paragonimus westermani, a large trematode, is endemic in Africa, Central and South America, India, and the Far East. The fluke initially infects the lungs, causing an abnormal chest radiograph in 80% of patients. Cerebral symptoms may resemble embolic stroke, tumor, or chronic epilepsy. Treatment is surgical, followed by praziquantel, 25 mg/kg orally every 8 hours for 2 days, or bithionol, 50 mg/kg orally every 48 hours for 10 days.

6. Trichinella

ESSENTIALS OF DIAGNOSIS

- ▶ *T spiralis* causes a flulike syndrome (myalgias) as muscles are infected, with weakness only in extreme cases
- ▶ Most infections are acquired from pork; 15% are from wild animals, especially in Africa

▶ General Considerations

The larva of *T spiralis* is found in muscles of swine and infects humans via ingestion of infected, undercooked meat. The nematode matures 2 days after ingestion, mates in the intestine, and releases larvae that spread through the circulation, ending their journey in the most active muscles, such as those in limbs, diaphragm, lumbar spine, and jaw. Once in the muscle, the larva grows for 6 weeks and surrounds itself with a cyst, which calcifies in 6 months. Reinfection is possible despite antibody formation. Only 44 cases of trichinosis were reported annually in the 1980s in the United States, with autopsy inspections revealing a prevalence of 2% in 1970. Recent outbreaks reported are traced to wild animal consumption or pork acquired directly from unregulated farms instead of USDA-inspected slaughterhouses.

► Prevention

Inspection for trichinosis in slaughterhouses and elimination of raw meat from table scraps or garbage found in feed has virtually eliminated the problem in domestic cases; ingestion of bear, wild boar, and other game or uninspected fresh meat accounts for most cases now. Cooking meat to a temperature of 57°C (134.6°F) or freezing to −15°C (5°F) kills the parasite.

► Clinical Findings

A. Signs and Symptoms

Infected patients are usually asymptomatic; 10–100 parasites per gram of muscle are required to produce symptoms. Incubation usually lasts 10 days but varies from 1–43 days. Gastroenteritis occurs in 15% of patients and is followed by fever, chills, headache, swelling of the eyelids, conjunctival and subungual hemorrhage, myalgias, and myositis, with weakness in extreme cases. A heavy burden of infection can also cause rash and respiratory, cardiac, and meningeal symptoms. Death is extremely rare.

B. Laboratory Findings

All patients have eosinophilia (> 6%), with leukocytosis in the majority. Positive ELISA with elevated titers of IgG antibodies indicates recent infection; somewhat less sensitive results are obtained using indirect immunofluorescence. Muscle breakdown is measured by levels of creatine kinase or lactic dehydrogenase in serum. Biopsy is rarely required.

C. Imaging Studies

Muscle radiographs may show the presence of calcified cysts if obtained more than 6 months after ingestion of the organism.

► Differential Diagnosis

Muscle pain due to collagen-vascular diseases such as polymyositis have a much longer-time course. Influenza and other viral infections with prominent myalgias may imitate trichinosis.

► Treatment

Treatment is ineffective after the larvae arrive in muscle, but exposed people can be given mebendazole (200–400 mg three times a day for 3 days, then 400–500 mg three times a day for 10 days) or albendazole (400 mg twice a day for 8–14 days), with corticosteroids for symptom relief (required in cases of heart or brain infection).

7. Other Infections

Angiostrongyloides causes meningitis, radiculomyeloencephalitis with cranial nerve involvement, and hemorrhage. *Toxocara* infection can be acquired from cats or dogs, and also causes meningitis. *Baylisascaris* is carried by raccoons and also causes eosinophilic meningitis or lesions that cause edema or hydrocephalus.

Graeff-Teixeira C, daSilva ACA, Yoshimura K. Update on eosinophilic meningoencephalitis and its clinical relevance. *Clin Microbiol Rev* 2009;22(2):322–348. [PMID: 19366917] (An excellent, complete discussion of several parasites with pictures, life cycle, clinical and radiographic features, and treatment of several worms, including angiostrongyliasis, gnathostomiasis, toxocariasis, cysticercosis, schistosomiasis, baylisascariasis, and paragonimiasis among others.)

Viral Infections of the Nervous System

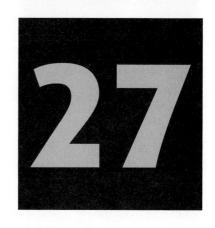

Jeffrey Sevigny, MD, Jennifer Frontera, MD,
& James M. Noble, MD, MS

ACUTE VIRAL ENCEPHALITIS

ESSENTIALS OF DIAGNOSIS

▶ Clinical triad of fever, headache, and altered mental status

▶ Cerebrospinal fluid (CSF) analysis showing mildly elevated opening pressure, lymphocytic pleocytosis, normal glucose, and mildly elevated protein

▶ CSF virus-specific polymerase chain reaction (PCR) and antibody (IgM and IgG) testing is useful for supporting diagnosis

▶ General Considerations

Viral encephalitis is an inflammation of the brain parenchyma caused by a viral vector. Direct infection of neurons accounts for the majority of cases. Viral encephalitis occurs in the context of active infection, whereas a postinfectious encephalitis may present with a similar clinical picture but as an autoimmune response to an antecedent non–central nervous system infection. It is estimated that several thousand cases of viral encephalitis occur annually in the United States, but good epidemiologic data are lacking. Well over 100 viruses can cause encephalitis. In the United States, herpes simplex virus type 1 (HSV-1), arthropod-borne viruses (arboviruses, especially West Nile virus), and enteroviruses are the most common causes among adults. Table 27–1 outlines the epidemiology and clinical features of selected viruses that cause encephalitis.

▶ Clinical Findings

A. Symptoms and Signs

Acute or subacute onset of fever, headache, and altered mental status are the cardinal features of acute viral encephalitis. The altered mental state may range from mild delirium to frank coma. Personality change, perceptional disturbance (illusions and hallucinations), and disorientation are common and can be the heralding symptoms. A myriad of other neurologic signs and symptoms, reflecting the area of brain affected, often accompanies the syndrome. Most commonly associated with encephalitis is evidence of meningeal inflammation (meningoencephalitis), which may manifest with Kernig or Brudzinski signs. Less common syndromes include rhombencephalitis (involvement of the brainstem) or encephalomyelitis (spinal cord involvement), which can be concomitantly involved in patients with encephalitis. Additional clinical features related to involved areas include aphasia, ataxia, hemiparesis, movement disorders, visual field defects, cranial nerve deficits, focal seizures (with or without secondary generalization), and pathologic reflexes.

General physical symptoms of upper respiratory tract infection (mumps, enterovirus) or gastrointestinal infection (enterovirus) and signs such as an exanthem (enterovirus, measles, rubella, herpesviruses), parotitis or orchitis (mumps or lymphocytic choriomeningitis), or the presence of mosquito (arboviruses), tick (Powassan, Colorado tick virus), or animal (rabies) bites can provide clues to the type of pathogen involved.

B. Laboratory Findings

CSF analysis shows pleocytosis ranging from 5–1000 cells/mm^3 in 95% of patients. During the first 48 hours of infection, the pleocytosis tends to be predominantly polymorphonuclear cells, changing to lymphocytes over several days. CSF glucose level may be normal or mildly decreased, the protein concentration moderately elevated (50–500 mg/dL), and opening pressure mildly high (20–30 cm H$_2$O). The immunoglobulin G (IgG) synthesis rate is typically elevated, indicating the intrathecal production of immunoglobulins, but is not specific to a cause. Xanthochromia and red blood cells are commonly seen with HSV-1 encephalitis. CSF obtained early in the infection or from immunocompromised patients may be relatively normal despite striking neurologic findings.

Table 27–1. Viral Encephalitis: Epidemiology of Selected Causes

Virus	Time of Year	Geographic Distribution	Frequency (US)	Clinical Findings
Herpesviruses				
HSV-1	Any	Worldwide	1000s/y; most common cause of sporadic encephalitis in United States	Predilection for orbitofrontal and temporal lobes Personality changes, cognitive impairment, focal neurologic deficits (aphasia, quadrantanopsia, hemiparesis), and seizures common Up to 30% mortality and high morbidity even among patients treated with acyclovir Cases of chronic and recurrent encephalitis reported
HSV-2	Any	Worldwide	Uncommon	Usual cause of encephalitis in neonates In adults, presentation is similar to HSV-1 but course is usually milder Meningitis, radiculitis, and myelitis are more likely complications in adults
CMV	Any	Worldwide	Rare	Acute or subacute onset Retinitis, polyradiculitis, myelitis, or multifocal neuropathy may accompany encephalitis Usually occurs in setting of systemic infection; therefore, serum PCR amplification for CMV DNA should be positive Immunocompromised are at risk (eg, AIDS; see Chapter 28)
EBV	Any	Worldwide	Rare	May be accompanied by optic neuritis, myelitis, polyradiculitis, or cerebellitis Cerebellitis and meningitis are more common complications
VZV	Any	Worldwide	Rare	Encephalitis, myelitis, or cerebellitis are rare Infarcts from small- or large-vessel CNS vasculitis are much more common, occurring during or within weeks of zoster rash Elderly or immunocompromised (eg, AIDS) are at risk
HHV-6	Any	Worldwide	Unknown	Course seems to simulate HSV-1 Most cases reported in transplant recipients receiving immunosuppressive therapy
Arthropod-Borne Viruses				
Eastern equine	Mosquito season	Atlantic and Gulf Coasts	0–15/y	Fulminant onset with predilection for basal ganglia and thalamus High morbidity, mortality, and risk of neurologic sequelae Children and elderly are at higher risk
Western equine	Mosquito season	Western US	0–40/y	Milder symptoms than with other arbovirus infections Low morbidity and mortality Children appear to be at highest risk
St Louis	Mosquito season	Entire US	2–250/y; occasional epidemic	Meningitis is more common in children; encephalitis in older adults Usually abrupt onset with spectrum of symptoms from mild to severe Tremor and myoclonus, reflecting predilection for basal ganglia involvement Myopathy is common
California serotypes (La Crosse)	Mosquito season	Eastern and central US	30–160/y	Meningitis is probably more common Symptoms and MRI findings may simulate HSV-1 Seizures are common Low mortality Children are at highest risk
West Nile encephalitis	Mosquito season	Entire but primarily western US	100–1000s/y (since 1999)	Neuromuscular weakness in 50% of meningoencephalitis patients (acute flaccid paralysis/poliomyelitis-like syndrome, Guillain-Barré-like syndrome, or generalized myeloradiculitis) Movement disorders can occur along with meningoencephalitis Also transmitted via tissue transplantation, blood transfusions, or in utero Extremes of age are at greatest risk

(Continued)

Table 27–1. Viral Encephalitis: Epidemiology of Selected Causes (*Continued*)

Powassan	May–December	Northeast US	<10/y	Tick-borne encephalitis transmitted via *Ixodes cookie* (woodchuck tick) Fulminant course that can simulate HSV-1 encephalitis High morbidity, mortality, and risk of neurologic sequelae
Colorado tick fever	Spring, fall	Rocky Mountains	<50/y	Caused by *Dermacentor andersoni* tick Meningitis is more common than encephalitis Typically a biphasic fever; constitutional signs and symptoms, leukopenia, and thrombocytopenia Erythrocytes may harbor persistent bacterial infection
Japanese encephalitis	Summer, fall	Most of Asia, parts of Russia	>10,000/y	Not endemic to United States but most common cause of encephalitis worldwide
Enteroviruses				
71 serotypes, including coxsackie-viruses, poliovirus, echoviruses	Fall, winter	Worldwide	100s/y (US)	Up to 10% of cases of encephalitis are attributable to enteroviruses Usually mild course, associated with other systemic features (eg, rash, pharyngitis, diarrhea), and low morbidity, mortality, and neurologic sequelae Poliomyelitis is very rare in United States; usually presents with asymmetric flaccid paralysis or bulbar signs Encephalitis, transverse myelitis, and cerebellitis are rare
Other Viral Causes				
Adenovirus	Winter, spring	Worldwide	Uncommon	Usually occurs in setting of severe respiratory disease Outbreaks reported among children Immunocompromised may be at higher risk
Mumps	Winter, spring	Worldwide	Rare	Encephalitis is mild Myelitis, optic neuritis, or peripheral neuritis may coexist Prodromal symptoms include respiratory symptoms, parotitis, orchitis, pancreatitis, thyroiditis
Measles	Winter, spring	Worldwide	Rare	Encephalitis is believed to result from immune response to infection rather than virus itself Prodromal symptoms include exanthem and other URI symptoms
Rubella	Winter, spring	Worldwide	Rare	Adults are at higher risk Prodromal symptoms including exanthema and other URI symptoms not always present
Rabies	Any	Worldwide	<5/y	Variable incubation period (1 wk–1 y) from exposure to encephalitis Phase 1—constitutional symptoms and paresthesias and fasciculations around inoculation site Phase 2—frank encephalitis with delirium, hallucinations, seizures, paresis, and autonomic dysfunction Phase 3—bulbar dysfunction Usually fatal once early symptoms develop Rarely, presentation simulates Guillain-Barré syndrome
Nipah	Any	Southeast Asia, Australia	Epidemics	Causes CNS and systemic endothelial infection, leading to vasculitis, thrombosis, and ischemia in addition to encephalitis Epidemics are centered around pig-farming villages

CMV = cytomegalovirus; CNS = central nervous system; EBV = Epstein-Barr virus; HHV = human herpesvirus; HSV = herpes simplex virus; MRI = magnetic resonance imaging; PCR = polymerase chain reaction; URI = upper respiratory infection; VZV = varicella-zoster virus.

Viruses associated with exceptional CSF abnormalities are profiled in Table 27–2.

Polymerase chain reaction (PCR) technology is now readily available for most encephalitis-causing viruses and can be used to support a clinical diagnosis during the acute phase of the illness. The sensitivity and specificity of PCR on CSF varies considerably for each virus. Furthermore, the utility of these tests is abrogated when CSF is obtained in the

Table 27–2. Variant Spinal Fluid Profiles in Viral Meningitis and Encephalitis

Viral Disease	Very Elevated Lymphocytosis	PMN Pleocytosis	Low Glucose	Elevated RBCs or Xanthochromia
Lymphocytic choriomeningitis			X	
Eastern equine encephalitis		X		
Echovirus 9 (enterovirus)		X		
Mumps	X		X	
HSV-1			X	X
Varicella-zoster			X	
Colorado tick fever				X
California serotypes encephalitis				X

HSV-1 = herpes simplex virus types 1; PMN = polymorphonuclear neutrophil; RBC = red blood cell.

subacute phase or after antiviral medications have been administered.

Virus-specific antibody (serology) testing of CSF and blood should be performed in all patients suspected of having a viral infection when PCR is not available, is of unproven diagnostic value, or is negative. An elevated virus-specific immunoglobulin M (IgM) antibody titer (1–3 weeks after symptoms onset), an elevated CSF-to-serum IgG titer ratio (4–8 weeks after symptoms onset), or a trebling of the acute-to-convalescent virus-specific IgG antibody titer enables a retrospective diagnosis of viral infection. Because abnormal blood serology signifies exposure to a virus whereas abnormal CSF serology implies CNS involvement, CSF serology is always preferable. Table 27–3 outlines useful laboratory tests for selected viruses.

Other blood tests may show nonspecific abnormalities, including leukocytosis and hyponatremia. CSF, throat, nasal, and rectal viral cultures have a low yield in isolating and identifying a viral isolate.

C. Diagnostic Studies

Magnetic resonance imaging (MRI) of the brain with gadolinium enhancement is the preferred imaging test for suspected encephalitis. Typical findings include increased signal on T2-weighted images in both gray and white matter. Infected areas and the meninges usually enhance with gadolinium. For most causes of encephalitis the findings do not suggest a specific viral etiology. However, abnormalities localized in the temporal and orbitofrontal areas strongly suggest HSV encephalitis. Hemorrhage in these areas may be demonstrated by gradient echo sequencing.

Electroencephalography may show various degrees of generalized slowing or other nonspecific abnormalities. In the case of HSV, however, focal electroencephalographic changes may be seen, such as periodic lateralizing epileptiform discharges (PLEDs), focal temporal lobe spikes, or slow waves.

Table 27–3. Laboratory Tests for Selected Viral Infections of the Nervous System

Virus	Laboratory Test
Adenovirus	Acute phase—IgM antibody titer; virus culture from pharynx, stool, or conjunctiva in proper clinical setting; or CSF PCR Chronic phase—trebling of acute to convalescent IgG antibody titer
Arboviruses California serotypes Eastern equine Powassan St Louis West Nile Western equine	Acute phase—PCR experimental but available for some viruses Subacute phase—IgM antibody titer Chronic phase—trebling of acute to convalescent IgG antibody titer or elevated CSF-to-serum IgG antibody ratio[a]
Colorado tick fever	Virus isolation from RBCs
Enteroviruses	Acute phase—CSF PCR detects most serotypes; CSF (and stool and throat) culture
Herpesviruses CMV EBV HSV-1 and HSV-2 VZV	Acute phase—CSF PCR Subacute phase—IgM antibody titer Chronic phase—trebling of acute to convalescent IgG antibody titer or elevated CSF-to-serum IgG antibody ratio
Lymphocytic Choriomeningitis Virus	Acute phase—IgM antibody titer or PCR

CMV = cytomegalovirus; CSF = cerebrospinal fluid; EBV = Epstein-Barr virus; HSV-1 and -2 = herpes simplex virus types 1 and 2; IgG = immunoglobulin G; IgM = immunoglobulin M; PCR = polymerase chain reaction; RBCs = red blood cells; VZV = varicella-zoster virus.
[a]There is significant assay cross-reactivity among the viruses.

Table 27–4. Differential Diagnosis of Viral Meningitis and Encephalitis

Bacterial	*Taenia solium* (cysticercosis)
Partially treated bacterial meningitis	*Plasmodium falciparum* (cerebral malaria)
Parameningeal bacterial infection	*Trichinella spiralis*
Leptospira species	**Drug Reaction**
Borrelia burgdorferi (Lyme disease)	NSAIDs
Mycobacterium tuberculosis	Antibiotics (trimethoprim-sulfamethoxazole,
Treponema pallidum (syphilis)	penicillin, isoniazid)
Mycoplasma pneumoniae	Ranitidine
Rickettsia species	Pyridium
Ehrlichia species	Anti-CD3 monoclonal antibody
Brucella species	Azathioprine
Chlamydia species	Intravenous immunoglobulin
Bartonella	**Autoimmune**
Legionella	Sarcoidosis
Whipple disease (*Tropheryma whippelii*)	Behçet syndrome
Listeria monocytogenes	Lupus erythematosus
Nocardia species	Vogt-Koyanagi-Harada syndrome
Actinomyces species	Acute disseminated encephalomyelitis
Fungal	β-Amyloid-related angiitis
Cryptococcus neoformans	**Carcinomatous**
Coccidioides immitis	Lymphoma
Histoplasma capsulatum	Leukemia
Mucormycosis	Metastasis
Candida species	Ruptured intracranial cystic tumors (dermoid,
Aspergillus species	epidermoid, craniopharyngioma)
Blastomyces dermatitidis	**Vascular**
Sporothrix schenckii	Cerebral vasculitis
Parasitic	Migrainous syndromes with pleocytosis
Angiostrongylus cantonensis	Dural venous sinus thrombosis
Toxoplasma gondii	

NSAIDs = nonsteroidal anti-inflammatory drugs.

Any unexplained case of presumed encephalitis warrants a brain biopsy. Brain biopsy of the affected area can help discriminate viral encephalitis from other causes of nonviral CNS pathology (eg, acute disseminated encephalomyelitis) and, with the appropriate stains, can positively identify the causative virus in most viral encephalitides. Table 27–4 lists nonviral causes of encephalitis that should be considered when formulating a differential diagnosis.

▶ Treatment

Acyclovir, 10 mg/kg intravenously every 8 hours, reduces morbidity and mortality associated with HSV encephalitis and therefore should be initiated as soon as the diagnosis of encephalitis is considered. Dosing should be adjusted for renal insufficiency. Acyclovir is also effective in patients with varicella-zoster virus vasculitis-encephalitis. Both ganciclovir, 5 mg/kg intravenously every 12 hours, and foscarnet, 90–120 mg/kg/day, have demonstrated efficacy in the treatment of cytomegalovirus infections of the central nervous system. Immunocompromised patients with HHV-6

encephalitis should be treated with ganciclovir or foscarnet. High-risk exposures to B virus (*Cercopithecine herpesvirus* 1 associated with macaque monkeys) should be treated with oral valacyclovir 1 g given 3 times daily. Suspected cases of rabies must be immediately treated with human rabies immune globulin and rabies vaccine, which appears to be 100% effective in preventing encephalitis if given before the onset of symptoms. Treatment of West Nile encephalitis remains supportive. Finally, arboviral and tick-transmitted infections are reportable to either local health officials or the Centers for Disease Control and Prevention.

▶ Prognosis

Symptoms of acute encephalitis usually last from a few days to weeks, but recovery can occur slowly over months, and long-term neurologic deficits can persist for years. Frequent sequelae include personality change, cognitive impairment including short-term memory loss and impaired concentration, headache, anxiety, irritability, tremor, dizziness, and fatigue. Focal neurologic injury sustained during encephalitis can later become a nidus for localization-related epilepsy. In HSV encephalitis, age younger than 30 years, short duration of symptoms (< 4 days), and good neurologic function (Glasgow coma scale score > 6) at the time of treatment are predictors of good outcome.

Berger JR, Houff SA. Neurological infections: The year of PML and influenza. *Lancet Neurol* 2010;9(1):14–17. [PMID: 20083028]

Cohen JI, et al. Recommendations for prevention of and therapy for exposure to B virus (*Cercopithecine herpesvirus* 1). *Clin Infect Dis* 2002;35(10):1191–1203. [PMID: 12410479]

Gilden DH, et al. Neurologic complications of the reactivation of varicella-zoster virus. *N Engl J Med* 2000;342:635–645. [PMID: 10699164]

Gyure KA. West Nile virus infections. *J Neuropathol Exp Neurol* 2009;68(10):1053–1060. [PMID: 19918117]

Granerod J, Crowcroft NS. The epidemiology of acute encephalitis. *Neuropsychol Rehabil* 2007;17(4–5):406–428. [PMID: 17676528]

Sejvar JJ, Uyeki TM. Neurologic complications of 2009 influenza A (H1N1). Heightened attention on an ongoing question. *Neurology* 2010;74:1020–1021. [PMID: 20200340]

Solomon T. Flavivirus encephalitis. *N Engl J Med* 2004;351:370–378. [PMID: 15269317]

Tunkel AR, et al. The management of encephalitis: Clinical practice guidelines by the Infectious Diseases Society of America. *Clin Infect Dis* 2008;47(3):303–327. [PMID: 18582201]

Tyler K. West Nile virus infection in the United States. *Arch Neurol* 2004;61:1190–1195. [PMID: 15313835]

Whitley RJ, Gnann JW. Viral encephalitis: Familiar infections and emerging pathogens. *Lancet* 2002;359(9305):507–513. [PMID: 11853816]

Web Site

http://www.cdc.gov/ncidod/dvbid/. (Centers for Disease Control and Prevention site on vector-borne diseases.)

VIRAL MENINGITIS

ESSENTIALS OF DIAGNOSIS

► Acute onset of fever, headache, and nuchal rigidity in the absence of focal neurologic deficit

► CSF analysis showing lymphocytic pleocytosis, normal glucose, and mildly elevated protein

► Self-limiting and without neurologic sequelae (most patients)

▶ General Considerations

Viral meningitis, which falls within the category of the more broadly termed *aseptic meningitides*, is caused by a systemic viral infection whose infectivity within the central nervous

Table 27–5. Viral Causes of Aseptic Meningitis

Common
Coxsackievirus B (enterovirus)
Echovirus (enterovirus)
HIV
HSV-2
West Nile (arbovirus)
Less Common
Coxsackievirus A (enterovirus)
La Crosse (California subgroup, arbovirus)
Lymphocytic choriomeningitis virus
Other enterovirus serotypes
St Louis virus (arbovirus)
Rare
Adenovirus
Eastern equine virus (arbovirus)
Mumps
Parvovirus B19
Western equine virus (arbovirus)
H1N1 influenza (swine flu; despite pandemic 2009-2010)

HIV = human immunodeficiency virus; HSV-2 = herpes simplex virus type 2.

system is restricted to the meninges, ependyma, and subarachnoid space. This disorder is common yet clearly underdiagnosed; more than 35,000 people are admitted to US hospitals annually with presumed diagnoses.

In adults, nonpolio enteroviruses (coxsackievirus and enteropathic human orphan virus [echovirus]), arthropod-borne viruses (especially West Nile since 1999), and herpes simplex virus type 2 (HSV-2) appear to cause most cases (Table 27–5). In many cases the viral agent is never isolated but instead presumed based on season of infection, exposures (eg, swimming pools; laboratory animals, rodents, and insects; sick contacts; travel), and the existence of concomitant systemic symptoms (eg, rash, parotitis, diarrhea, or pharyngitis). Nonviral causes of aseptic meningitis are listed in Table 27–5.

▶ Clinical Findings

A. Symptoms and Signs

Fever, headache, and nuchal rigidity are the cardinal symptoms. Common associated symptoms include general malaise, myalgia, nausea, vomiting, photophobia, diarrhea, and rash (Table 27–6). Deep tendon reflexes may be transiently increased; otherwise, the examination is notable for the absence of abnormal findings on the neurologic examination.

B. Laboratory Findings

CSF analysis is characterized by lymphocytic pleocytosis (10–1000 cells/mm³), mild elevation of protein concentration,

Table 27–6. Clinical Considerations for Selected Causes of Viral Meningitis

Virus	Season	Associated Symptoms	Miscellaneous
Adenovirus	Winter, spring	URT symptoms, pneumonitis, conjunctivitis, encephalitis	—
Enteroviruses			Most common cause of viral meningitis
Echovirus	Summer, fall	Maculopapular rash	
Coxsackievirus A	Summer, fall	Hand-foot-mouth disease, herpangina	
Coxsackievirus B	Summer, fall	Myocarditis, pericarditis, pleurodynia	
HIV	Year-round	Mononucleosis-like syndrome	HIV test indicated in any individual with viral meningitis and HIV risk factors
HSV-2	Year-round	Herpetic rash in genital area, sometimes accompanied by polyradiculitis	A common cause of recurrent viral meningitis in adults
Lymphocytic choriomeningitis virus	Any, particularly cooler months	Upper respiratory, parotitis, leukopenia	Associated with animal exposure (laboratory mice, hamsters)
Mumps	Spring	URI symptoms, parotitis, orchitis	Rare in United States

HIV = human immunodeficiency virus; HSV-2 = herpes simplex virus type 2; URI = upper respiratory infection.

and normal glucose level. In the hyperacute stage, polymorphonuclear granulocytosis may predominate.

Virus-specific PCR, antibody titers, and culture should be obtained, as discussed in the preceding section on viral encephalitis, to support the clinical diagnosis.

Other serum analysis is often not helpful during the acute infection. Saliva, throat washings, and stool can be examined for virus, although the diagnostic yield is low except for some enteroviruses.

Brain imaging (computed tomography [CT] and MRI) rarely reveals diagnostic clues, although leptomeningeal enhancement may be seen.

▶ **Treatment**

Viral meningitis is a self-limited disease that requires only supportive treatment with analgesics, antiemetics, and intravenous hydration. The exceptions are HIV and HSV-2, in which treatment (antiretroviral therapy and acyclovir, respectively) may be initiated, although probably without direct influence on the course of meningitis itself. Full recovery usually occurs within 1–2 weeks.

Khetsuriani N, et al. Viral meningitis–associated hospitalizations in the United States, 1988–1999. *Neuroepidemiology* 2003;22:345–352. [PMID: 14557685]

Romero JR, Newland JG. Viral meningitis and encephalitis: Traditional and emerging viral agents. *Semin Pediatr Infect Dis* 2003;14:72–82. [PMID: 12881794]

Rotbart HA. Viral meningitis. *Semin Neurol* 2000;20:277–292. [PMID: 11051293]

ACUTE VIRAL MYELITIS

 ESSENTIALS OF DIAGNOSIS

▶ Acute onset of weakness, sensory loss, and autonomic dysfunction (urinary retention) in the absence of other cortical findings

▶ CSF analysis showing mild to moderate lymphocytic pleocytosis, elevated protein, and normal or mildly decreased glucose

▶ **General Considerations**

Myelitis refers to an inflammation of the spinal cord. The pathogenesis of viral myelitis is similar to viral encephalitis, and most viruses that cause encephalitis also cause myelitis. Myelitis can concomitantly occur with radiculitis (termed myeloradiculitis) and rarely encephalitis (encephalomyeloradiculitis), or both (encephalomyeloradiculitis). As with encephalitis, the clinician must determine whether the myelitis is caused by a direct viral infection, an immune-mediated response to an antecedent viral infection (postinfection myelitis), a primary immune-mediated process (eg, multiple sclerosis or lupus), or some other process (Table 27–7). Good epidemiologic data on viral myelitis are lacking, in part because it is relatively uncommon and because the underlying cause of most cases is not often determined. Table 27–8 lists the most common viruses.

Table 27–7. Differential Diagnosis of Acute Myelopathy

Infectious
Bacterial—Lyme disease, *Listeria monocytogenes*, *Mycoplasma*, epidural abscess
Fungal—cryptococcal abscess
Parasitic—*Toxoplasma* abscess

Autoimmune
Multiple sclerosis and Devic disease
Systemic lupus erythematosus
Sjögren syndrome
Sarcoidosis
Postinfectious myelitis
Postvaccination response

Structural
Compression from spinal disease (degenerative, infectious, inflammatory), nucleus pulposus herniation, or osteophyte complex formation

Vascular
Spinal cord infarction (embolism, vascular malformation, vasculitis, fibrocartilaginous embolism)

Tumors
Primary spinal cord tumor
Metastatic spinal tumor

Other
Idiopathic
Contusion

Table 27–8. Viral Causes of Acute Myelitis

Herpesvirus
HSV-2
Varicella-zoster virus
HSV-1
Epstein-Barr virus
Cytomegalovirus
Human herpesvirus 6

Enterovirus
Poliovirus
Enterovirus 70
Echovirus
Coxsackievirus

Arbovirus
West Nile virus

Other
Mumps
HIV
Dengue

HSV-1 and -2 = herpes simplex virus types 1 and 2.

▶ Clinical Findings

A. Symptoms and Signs

Weakness, sensory loss below the level of the lesion, and autonomic dysfunction are the cardinal features of most causes of viral myelitis. The clinical syndrome depends on the extent and location of the cord lesion: any level of the cord can be affected; multiple contiguous (or even noncontiguous) levels can be involved; and the lesion(s) can be either partial or complete on the axial plane of the spinal cord. When the complete axial plane of the cord is involved (transverse myelitis), all sensory and motor modalities below the lesion are affected. When only a portion of the axial cord is involved (partial myelitis), a Brown-Séquard syndrome can result. In general, viruses are more likely to cause a complete (transverse) myelitis while other causes (eg, multiple sclerosis) tend to be incomplete (partial). In either case, nerve roots exiting from the area of the myelitis may also be involved, causing a radiculitis. In the acute phase, tone of the affected limbs is decreased and reflexes may be absent or diminished. A careful examination to pinprick can demarcate a sensory level, usually one to two levels below the actual cord lesion. Anal sphincter tone, cremaster reflex, anal wink, and bulbocavernosus response are lost or diminished. Urinary retention and bowel dysfunction are the rule, and autonomic instability is common. In the chronic phase, spasticity with pathologic reflexes in the affected limbs develops.

A distinctive syndrome of lower motor neuron weakness (poliomyelitis) occurs with poliovirus and has been reported with West Nile virus and enterovirus serotype 71. Paralytic poliomyelitis occurs within days of an acute viral syndrome that includes meningitis. The onset of weakness is acute and usually asymmetric, with legs being affected more commonly than the thoracic, abdominal, or bulbar muscles. The tone is diminished and the reflexes are lost in the affected area(s); bladder dysfunction is common during the acute phase; and sensory modalities are spared.

B. Diagnostic Studies

CSF analysis demonstrates mild to moderate lymphocytic pleocytosis (10–1000 cells/mm³), elevated protein concentration (100–500 mg/dL), and normal or mildly depressed glucose level. Markedly elevated protein level (> 500 mg/dL) suggests spinal block (Froin syndrome) from cord swelling. The IgG synthesis rate is typically elevated, indicating the intrathecal production of immunoglobulin, but is not specific to a cause. Virus-specific PCR and antibody titer should be performed. (Refer to the discussion of viral encephalitis, earlier.) An extensive workup should be undertaken to assess for other causes of myelitis (see Table 27–7).

MRI of the spine is mandatory. Affected areas typically appear swollen, enhance with gadolinium on T1-weighted images, and display high signal on T2-weighted images. The entire axial plane is usually affected, in contrast to nonviral causes of acute myelitis. It is uncommon for both brain and spinal cord to be involved in most viral infections, in contrast to postinfectious or autoimmune myelitis. Therefore, when the cause of myelitis is unknown, abnormal findings in the brain or optic nerves may help narrow the virus differential or suggest an alternative cause such as multiple sclerosis or acute disseminated encephalomyelitis.

▶ Treatment

Antiviral treatment needs to be tailored to the specific causative virus, when known. If Epstein-Barr virus, varicella-zoster virus, or HSV-1 or HSV-2 is suspected, acyclovir (10 mg/kg intravenously every 8 hours) should be administered. If cytomegalovirus is suspected, ganciclovir (5 mg/kg intravenously every 12 hours) or foscarnet (90–120 mg/kg/day), or both, should be administered. There is no evidence supporting the use of glucocorticoids for viral myelitis; however, their use is indicated when the pathogenesis is unknown and immune-mediated processes are considered in the differential. Spasticity that typically ensues in the chronic phase can be alleviated with baclofen, benzodiazepines, and tizanidine.

Anderson O. Myelitis. *Curr Opin Neurol* 2000:13;311–316. [PMID: 10871257]

John TJ. Spinal cord disease in West Nile virus infection. *N Engl J Med* 2003;348:564–566. [PMID: 12575663]

Majid A, et al. Epstein-Barr virus myeloradiculitis and encephalomyeloradiculitis. *Brain* 2002;125:159–565. [PMID: 11834601]

Transverse Myelitis Consortium Working Group. Proposed diagnostic criteria and nosology of acute transverse myelitis. *Neurology* 2002;59:499–505. [PMID: 12236201]

RADICULITIS & GANGLIONITIS

ESSENTIALS OF DIAGNOSIS

Herpes Zoster
▶ Sudden onset of pain followed by vesicular eruption in a dermatomal distribution
▶ Involvement of the ophthalmic division of the trigeminal nerve (zoster ophthalmicus) is an ophthalmologic emergency
▶ Postherpetic neuralgia—defined by pain persisting more than 30 days

▶ General Considerations

Radiculitis is an inflammation of the nerve root or proximal cranial nerve. When the ganglion is affected—for example, the geniculate ganglion of the facial nerve or a dorsal root ganglion—the more specific term *ganglionitis* may be used. Herpes zoster, or shingles, is by far the most common ganglionitis, with approximately 500,000 cases occurring annually in the United States alone. It is caused by the reactivation

of varicella-zoster virus within a dorsal root or cranial nerve ganglion, where the virus lies dormant after a primary exposure in childhood. An attenuation of virus-specific T-cell immunity—from advancing age, immunosuppressive therapy, or neoplastic diseases—and exposure to varicella-zoster virus before the age of 1 year places a person at risk for developing zoster. Zoster is uncommon among immunocompetent persons younger than 50 years of age. Radiculitis or ganglionitis from other infectious causes is uncommon but has been described with several other viruses, including HSV-2, Epstein-Barr virus, cytomegalovirus, and rarely West Nile virus. The focus of this section is on herpes zoster.

▶ Clinical Findings

A. Symptoms and Signs

Zoster is characterized by sudden onset of a sharp, burning, lancinating pain with a vesicular or bullous eruption that conforms to one or more dermatomes. Pain usually precedes the rash by 3–5 days. A thoracic dermatome is affected in over 50% of cases; trigeminal, usually the ophthalmic division (zoster ophthalmicus), cervical, lumbar, and sacral dermatomes each account for approximately 10% of cases; and rarely the facial nerve is involved (see later discussion). Multiple contiguous or noncontiguous dermatomes may be involved, especially among immunosuppressed patients. Sensory examination is notable for decreased sensation and allodynia (pain from a nonnoxious stimulus).

Three relatively uncommon variants of zoster have been recognized. One is zoster with concomitant limb or diaphragm weakness (zoster paresis), signifying involvement of the corresponding ventral root; a second is noneruptive zoster (zoster sine herpete); and a third is the Ramsay Hunt syndrome, which occurs when the geniculate ganglion of the facial nerve is affected and manifests with peripheral facial weakness, usually with an ipsilateral eruption involving the external ear, hard palate, or anterior tongue.

Other viral causes of radiculitis typically present with weakness (signifying ventral root involvement) that may be accompanied by sensory impairment, rash, or eruption. Lumbar and sacral roots are most commonly involved, and multiple contiguous or noncontiguous roots may be affected (polyradiculitis). Guillain-Barré syndrome can occur in some acute viral infections (and not necessarily in the postinfectious period), including HIV, West Nile virus, and rarely rabies.

B. Diagnostic Studies

In most patients, diagnosis of herpes zoster can be easily made on clinical grounds without further workup. MRI with gadolinium may show enhancement of the affected root. CSF analysis may show mild lymphocytic-predominant pleocytosis. Varicella-zoster DNA can be amplified in the CSF during the acute stage. Direct fluorescent antibody testing of the vesicular fluid to detect varicella-zoster virus antigen can confirm the diagnosis. Further workup for HIV or other causes of immunosuppression is warranted in patients with unexplained zoster who are younger than 50 years of age.

Nonzoster causes of radiculitis require a workup similar to that described for viral myelitis. Blood and CSF should be examined for virus-specific PCR and antibody, and MRI of the entire neuroaxis is usually warranted.

▶ **Treatment**

Pain relief with nonsteroidal anti-inflammatory drugs or narcotics is necessary in most cases. Antiviral therapy with acyclovir (800 mg orally five times daily), famciclovir (500 mg orally three times daily), or valacyclovir (1000 mg orally three time daily) for 7–10 days may help reduce pain, shorten the course, and prevent postherpetic neuralgia, particularly if given within 3 days of eruption onset. Concomitant treatment with prednisone (60 mg orally for 7 days followed by 14-day taper) may shorten the duration of symptoms but does not appear to reduce the risk of postherpetic neuralgia.

Zoster ophthalmicus is considered an ophthalmologic emergency. Antiviral treatment should be administered immediately, with consideration for intravenous acyclovir, 10 mg/kg every 8 hours. Some authors describe similar response rates to oral acyclovir, valacyclovir, and famciclovir. A slit-lamp examination should be performed (preferably by an ophthalmologist) to evaluate for potentially vision-threatening keratitis, episcleritis, and iritis.

Cytomegalovirus polyradiculitis, which should be suspected in any patient with AIDS, is a neurologic emergency and requires immediate treatment with ganciclovir, 5 mg/kg every 12 hours, or foscarnet, 90–120 mg/kg/day, or both. (See Chapter 28 for further discussion.)

▶ **Prognosis & Complications**

Pain that persists more than 30 days after the onset of the eruption is deemed *postherpetic neuralgia*. Age is an important risk factor, and roughly 40% of those older than 60 years will develop this condition. The pain can be unrelenting and disabling and is often resistant to any form of treatment. Lidocaine patches (5%) or capsaicin cream applied to the rash and a trial of carbamazepine, amitriptyline, phenytoin, gabapentin, prednisone, or opiates are usually the first line of treatment. In extreme cases, nerve block, radiofrequency ablation, deep brain or spinal cord stimulation, surgical excision, or administration of intrathecal corticosteroids should be considered.

Ischemic stroke, cranial neuropathy (especially of the oculomotor nerve), and retinal necrosis rarely occur during or shortly after an episode of acute zoster. The presumed mechanism in most cases is virus-induced vasculitis. Patients with HIV or AIDS appear to be at greatest risk. (See the discussion of varicella-zoster vasculitis in Chapter 28.)

Eberhardt O, et al. HSV-2 sacral radiculitis (Elsberg syndrome). *Neurology* 2004;63:758–759. [PMID: 15326269]

Gnann JW, Whitley RJ. Clinical practice. Herpes zoster. *N Engl J Med* 2002;347:340–346. [PMID: 12151472]

Majid A, et al. Epstein-Barr virus myeloradiculitis and encephalomyeloradiculitis. *Brain* 2002;125(pt 1):159–165. [PMID: 11834601]

Pavan-Langston D. Herpes zoster antivirals and pain management. *Ophthalmology* 2008;115(2 Suppl):S13–S20. [PMID: 18243927]

Sweeney CJ, Gilden DH. Ramsay Hunt syndrome. *J Neurol Neurosurg Psychiatry* 2001;71:149–154. [PMID: 11459884]

CHRONIC VIRAL INFECTIONS

1. Subacute Sclerosing Panencephalitis

 ESSENTIALS OF DIAGNOSIS

- ▶ Caused by a defective measles virus
- ▶ Symptoms manifest 6–10 years after primary infection
- ▶ Characterized by rapidly progressive cognitive decline, ataxia, and myoclonic jerks
- ▶ Measles IgG antibody in CSF confirms the diagnosis

This progressive encephalitis is caused by persistent central nervous system infection of a defective measles virus. It is an uncommon disease, with an estimated 4–11 cases per 100,000 measles infections, and is largely relegated to areas of low vaccination rates such as the Middle East where 360 cases of measles/100,000 persons occur before 1 year of age. On rare occasions, subacute sclerosing panencephalitis (SSPE) can occur in persons previously appropriately vaccinated in early childhood but with presumably incomplete host response to the vaccination. Most cases of SSPE occur in children, typically between age 8 and 11 years and at least 6 years after measles infection; some studies suggest the highest rates being among those with primary measles infection before 2 years of age. Evidence does not support measles vaccination as a cause of SSPE. Symptoms begin with a subacute onset of cognitive impairment and behavioral changes including psychosis. Myoclonic jerks and ataxia appear shortly thereafter, and mental status continues to deteriorate to frank dementia. A myriad of other neurologic signs and symptoms may also be present, including weakness, rigidity, spasticity, dystonia, autonomic instability, and pathologic reflexes. Chorioretinitis, papilledema, and optic atrophy may occur, and on rare occasions may be the presenting illness. In the late stage of the disease, the myoclonic jerks disappear and patients become bedbound in a state of spastic, akinetic mutism. An adult-onset form, mostly affecting men, has been identified, with mean age of onset of 20 years and a much longer latency period. This syndrome may first present with visual symptoms followed by the typical course outlined above.

CSF analysis may show mild pleocytosis and elevated protein concentration. Invariably, CSF IgG level and IgG synthesis rate are elevated and oligoclonal bands are present, all attributable to the intrathecal production of antimeasles antibody. A CSF measles IgG antibody titer greater than 1:4, a serum antibody titer greater than 1:256, or a CSF-to-serum titer ratio greater than 1:200 supports the diagnosis of SSPE. Measles RNA has been detected in the CSF by PCR techniques in several patients with SSPE.

The electroencephalogram profile evolves over the course of the disease. The early symptomatic and terminal phases are characterized by generalized slowing. The middle stage of the disease has a nearly pathognomonic profile of slow-wave complexes, which are periodic bursts (4–6 seconds) of high-voltage polyphasic delta waves that coincide with the myoclonic jerks.

MRI of the brain reveals increased signal, predominantly affecting the subcortical white matter, on T2-weighted images. The occipital-parietal area is usually affected early, but eventually the entire cerebrum is involved. Gray matter eventually becomes affected, while U fibers are generally spared.

Death ensues within 3 years of symptom onset in many patients; children and those adults with rapid clinical progression have the most rapidly declining courses. Late-stage patients may persist without change for years; there have been rare reports of spontaneous long-term remissions, now thought to comprise about 5% of all cases.

About one third of patients treated with combination weekly intrathecal α-interferon and daily oral isoprinosine respond with slower disease progression, disease stabilization, or, on rare occasions, modest clinical improvement. Thus it is suggested that all patients be treated with this combination therapy at least initially. However, no studies have shown mortality benefit. Myoclonic seizures can be controlled with sodium valproate. Spasticity can be alleviated with tizanidine, baclofen, or benzodiazepines.

Garg RK. Subacute sclerosing panencephalitis. *Postgrad Med J* 2002;78:63–70. [PMID: 11807185]

Gutierrez J, Issacson RS, Koppel BS. Subacute sclerosing panencephalitis: An update. *Dev Med Child Neurol* 2010;52(10):901–907. [PMID: 20561004]

2. Human T-Cell Lymphotrophic Virus–Associated Myelopathy

ESSENTIALS OF DIAGNOSIS

▶ Chronic and slowly progressive myelopathy
▶ Presence of human T-cell lymphotrophic virus (HTLV) IgG antibody in CSF confirms diagnosis

Formerly known as *tropical spastic paraparesis*, HTLV-associated myelopathy is a chronic progressive myelopathy that results from persistent infection of the central nervous system by HTLV type 1 (HTLV-1) or, rarely, type 2 (HTLV-2). HTLV-1 infection is endemic in scattered populations around the world, particularly in the Caribbean basin (West Indies, parts of Central and South America, and southeastern United States), Japan, West and Central Africa, and Brazil. Patients are also encountered in areas with high concentrations of immigrants with childhood exposure in these countries. The seroprevalence is as high as 30% in certain populations, but fortunately less than 5% will develop neurologic complications. A slowly progressive demyelinating myelopathy is the most common neurologic sequela, although meningitis and polymyositis have been described. Rapid decline superimposed on a prior typical slowly progressive course should raise suspicion of a secondary process; HTLV-associated leukemia can co-occur in these patients, and on rare occasions patients will present with neurologic complications. Women are affected more often than men; symptoms typically begin in the fourth decade. The virus is contracted through sexual contact, mother-to-child transmission (usually through breast-feeding), transfusion of blood products, or sharing of contaminated needles (parenteral drug users). The infection is lifelong once acquired.

Symptoms are insidious in onset and include lower back pain, leg weakness and stiffness resulting in gait impairment, and leg paresthesias. When specifically asked, most patients report changes in urinary habits and loss of libido or impotence. Arms are not usually involved until late in the course. Classic myelopathic signs are found on examination: spasticity; weakness; pathologic reflexes, including extensor plantar reflexes (Babinski sign); and spastic gait. Sensory impairment is relatively mild, and a distinct sensory level is uncommon. Less frequent findings include cerebellar ataxia, optic atrophy, tremor, cranial or peripheral neuropathy, meningitis, muscular atrophy, or polymyositis.

The diagnosis is made by the detection of CSF IgG antibody to HTLV-1 or HTLV-2 in the appropriate clinical setting. CSF analysis may show mild lymphocytic pleocytosis, elevated protein concentration, high IgG synthesis rate, and oligoclonal bands. MRI of the spine may be normal or show areas of spinal cord atrophy. Nonspecific white matter lesions may also be found in the brain. In the workup, other causes of chronic progressive spastic paresis, particularly HIV-associated myelopathy, should be considered.

There is no effective treatment for HTLV-associated myelopathy. Studies of corticosteroids and interferon therapies are limited to small or open-label trials, but overall do not suggest sustained benefit; antiretroviral medications including zidovudine and lamivudine have also not shown benefit. Treatment is largely supportive or symptom based. Spasticity can be alleviated with baclofen, benzodiazepines, and tizanidine, complemented by physical therapy. Modest improvement in gait and bladder function has been reported with the anabolic steroid danazol. Special attention needs to be paid to maintaining adequate bowel and bladder function. In most cases the disease is slowly progressive, and most patients are still able to ambulate up to 10 years after symptom onset.

Araújo A, Hall WW. Human T-lymphotropic virus type II and neurological disease. *Ann Neurol* 2004;56:10–19. [PMID: 15236397]

Araújo A, Lima MA, Silva MT. Human T-lymphotropic virus 1 neurologic disease. *Curr Treat Options Neurol* 2008;10(3): 193–200. [PMID: 18579023]

Gonçalves DU, et al. Epidemiology, treatment, and prevention of human T-cell leukemia virus type 1-associated diseases. *Clin Microbiol Rev* 2010;23(3):577–589. [PMID: 20610824]

3. Progressive Multifocal Leukoencephalopathy

This subacute demyelinating disease is caused by a cerebral infection by JC virus with specific pathology related to glial cell lysis. Although most US adults have been exposed to JC virus, the lifetime prevalence of progressive multifocal leuko-encephalopathy (PML) in the pre-HIV era was 4.4 per 100,000 persons, mostly in patients with an underlying disorder affecting cell-mediated immunity. Today most cases of PML occur in the setting of HIV and AIDS. PML has also been reported in patients who are immunosuppressed as a result of hematologic malignancies, idiopathic CD4 lymphocytopenia, and autoimmune disorders. Several medications have been associated with increased risk of PML including natalizumab for multiple sclerosis, with approximately 1.56 in 1000 developing PML after 24 infusions. Rituximab has also been associated with PML, but many of these patients receive treatment for lymphoproliferative disorders, making distinction of the disease and treatment as specific risk factors difficult. Chronic corticosteroid use has also been associated with PML.

Irrespective of the underlying immunologic disorder, PML presents with the subacute onset of cognitive and focal neurologic deficits. (For a full description of clinical and diagnostic features, see Chapter 28.) In many cases the disease progresses until death, usually within a matter of months. Despite anecdotal reports, cidofovir and cytarabine have not proven effective in controlled studies. Studies investigating mirtazapine and mefloquine as potential therapeutic agents are ongoing.

Durable remissions among HIV patients can occur, and this has become increasingly more common with widespread use of combined antiretroviral therapy in HIV. Current data suggest 50% survival at 1 year, with some cases reported up to 188 months; those with the longest survival had CD4 counts consistent with immune reconstitution.

Patients treated with natalizumab and suspected PML should have natalizumab discontinued immediately. Most surviving patients have been treated with either plasma exchange or immunoabsorption in the immediate period. Immune reconstitution inflammatory syndrome nearly always occurs thereafter, can be clinically indistinguishable from PML reactivation but with a greater degree of contrast enhancement on MRI, and may require repeated courses of intravenous corticosteroids. Treatment in this manner has been associated with a 71% survival rate.

Tan CS, Koralnik IJ. Progressive multifocal leukoencephalopathy and other disorders caused by JC virus: Clinical features and pathogenesis. *Lancet Neurol* 2010;9(4):425–437. [PMID: 20298966]

Clifford DB, DeLuca A, Simpson DM, Arendt G, Giovannoni G, Nath A. Natalizumab-associated progressive multifocal leuko-encephalopathy in patients with multiple sclerosis: Lessons from 28 cases. *Lancet Neurol* 2010;9(4):438–446. [PMID: 20298967]

HIV Neurology

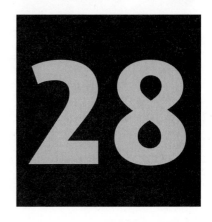

Ned Sacktor, MD, Jeffrey Rumbaugh, MD,
Jeffrey Sevigny, MD, & Lydia B. Estanislao, MD

HIV is a retrovirus belonging to the subfamily Lentivirus (slow virus), so-called because of the long latency period between primary infection and the CD4+ T-cell depletion that characterizes AIDS. During this latency period, the immune system becomes dysregulated and a chronic proinflammatory state develops, manifesting with hypergammaglobulinemia and an increased secretion of several cytokines. Many neurologic complications, particularly those occurring before the onset of AIDS, are attributable to immune-mediated processes. Without virologic control, eventually all components of the immune system (particularly the cellular response) become deficient, enabling opportunistic infections and malignancies to develop.

It is estimated that at least one third of those with HIV/AIDS are afflicted with an HIV-associated neurologic condition. The epidemiology of these complications has been dramatically altered since the widespread use of combination antiretroviral therapy (CART) in 1996 and the prudent use of other chemoprophylactic agents such as fluconazole and sulfamethoxazole-trimethoprim. In general, the incidence of neurologic complications has declined. But with improved survival, the prevalence of many appears to be rising. Consequently, neurologists are increasingly likely to see a patient with HIV/AIDS for a chronic HIV-associated illness or a non–HIV-related neurologic condition rather than for an acute, life-threatening HIV-related illness.

When approaching an HIV-infected patient, the neurologist must keep in mind the following principles: the entire neuroaxis, from brain to muscle, can be affected; the rule of parsimony is often violated, and more than one process may underlie the clinical picture; and the types of complications tend to be related to duration of HIV infection and degree of immunosuppression (Table 28–1). Early-stage (CD4+ > 500/µL) neurologic complications, such as those occurring during primary infection, usually result from HIV itself or as a consequence of an immune-mediated process; middle-stage (CD4+ 200–500/µL) complications tend to result from immune-mediated processes or medication toxicity; and

late-stage (CD4+ < 200/µL) complications tend to result from opportunistic infections, immune-mediated processes, or medication toxicity. Tantamount to developing a workable differential diagnosis is obtaining a thorough history, and some essential features are outlined in Table 28–2.

CENTRAL NERVOUS SYSTEM DISORDERS ASSOCIATED WITH HIV

CRYPTOCOCCAL MENINGITIS

ESSENTIALS OF DIAGNOSIS

- ▶ A late-stage complication of HIV infection
- ▶ Subacute onset of headache, general malaise, and fever followed by encephalopathy and cranial neuropathies from increased intracranial pressure
- ▶ Cryptococcal antigen and culture from cerebrospinal fluid (CSF) are diagnostic

▶ General Considerations

Cryptococcus is the most common cause of meningitis in HIV+ individuals. Cryptococcal meningitis is caused by the fungus *Cryptococcus neoformans*, an encapsulated yeast ubiquitously found in soil and avian droppings. After entering through the lungs, causing an asymptomatic pneumonia, *Cryptococcus* disseminates hematogenously. The central nervous system (CNS) is the most common secondary site of infection, and it is believed that most AIDS patients with cryptococcemia will develop meningitis if not treated. Once seeded into the CNS, slowly progressive meningitis ensues. It occurs as a late complication of HIV infection, typically in those with a CD4+ T-lymphocyte count of fewer than 100 cells/µL. Among HIV+ individuals not on antiretroviral

Table 28–1. Common Neurologic Complications of HIV Classified by the Stage in Which Each Occurs

Early Stage (CD4$^+$ > 500)
HIV meningitis (acute conversion syndrome)
Shingles (varicella-zoster)
Acute inflammatory demyelinating polyneuropathy (AIDP)
Middle Stage (CD4$^+$ 200–500)[a]
Distal sensory polyneuropathy (DSP)
HIV-associated dementia (HIVD)
HIV-associated neuromuscular weakness syndrome
Mononeuropathy multiplex
HIV-associated myopathy
Late Stage (CD4$^+$ < 200)
CNS toxoplasmosis
Cryptococcal meningitis
Primary CNS lymphoma (PCNSL)
Progressive multifocal leukoencephalopathy
HIV-associated myelopathy
Varicella-zoster vasculitis
CMV ventriculitis or polyradiculitis (CD4$^+$ < 100)

CMV = cytomegalovirus; CNS = central nervous system.
[a]Complications occurring in the middle stage can also occur in the late stage.

therapy, such as newly diagnosed cases in resource-limited countries, it is one of the most common CNS opportunistic infections developing in 5–13% of individuals with AIDS.

▶ Clinical Findings

A. Symptoms and Signs

Nonspecific headache and fever are the cardinal features of cryptococcal meningitis. Nausea, vomiting, phonophobia, and photophobia (migraine symptoms) are rare early in the infection. The clinical course is usually slow and insidious over several weeks, and when the early symptoms go unheeded, encephalopathy, diplopia, visual obscuration, nausea, and vomiting develop, usually signifying the presence of increased intracranial pressure. Seizures and, to a

Table 28–2. Essential Clinical Information When Forming an HIV-Related Differential Diagnosis

Duration of HIV infection
History of HIV-related illnesses
CD4$^+$ cell count (current and nadir)
HIV RNA level
Medication use and adherence
• Antiretroviral agents, current and past
• Chemoprophylactic agents (sulfamethoxazole-trimethoprim, fluconazole, acyclovir)
Serum *Toxoplasma* IgG antibody status
Serum syphilis serology

lesser extent, stroke are associated with cryptococcal meningitis. Early in the infection there is a paucity of neurologic signs. Typical signs and symptoms of meningitis may be lacking because the immunosuppressed patient fails to mount a vigorous inflammatory response to the organism. However, both the meninges and the brain can be infected, so focal neurological findings may occur. As the infection advances and intracranial pressure increases, encephalopathy, cranial neuropathies (especially sixth nerve palsy), and papilledema develop. Given the protean features of early infection, atypical headache or other signs or symptoms referable to the CNS warrant a workup for cryptococcal meningitis. Rarely, cryptococcal meningitis presents with a fulminant syndrome.

B. Laboratory and Imaging Studies

CSF analysis provides a definitive diagnosis in most cases. A positive CSF culture for *Cryptococcus* or the presence of cryptococcal antigen establishes the diagnosis of cryptococcal meningitis. India ink preparations may not be as specific or sensitive (< 50%), but can be rapidly performed while these other tests are pending. Routine CSF indices usually reveal nonspecific abnormalities, including mild to moderate lymphocytic pleocytosis, elevated protein concentration, and a normal to moderately low glucose level. **Caveat:** CSF indices can be normal, or show just a mild mononuclear pleocytosis or mild elevation in protein, particularly in those with advanced AIDS; markedly abnormal indices warrant a search for an alternative or concomitant diagnosis. The opening pressure is usually high (> 250 mm H_2O) and should be measured in all patients suspected of having cryptococcal meningitis to provide guidance during treatment.

Serum cryptococcal antigen and fungal cultures are sensitive tests for cryptococcemia. When a lumbar puncture is contraindicated or CSF indices are normal, including the rare false-negative CSF cryptococcal antigen or culture, a positive serum antigen or culture supports a presumed diagnosis of cryptococcal meningitis. However, although a negative serum antigen test makes the diagnosis of cryptococcal meningitis unlikely, it does not rule it out.

A focal neurologic finding or encephalopathy warrants an imaging study prior to lumbar puncture. Neither computed tomographic (CT) scan nor magnetic resonance imaging (MRI), however, provides sufficient evidence to make a diagnosis of cryptococcal meningitis. MRI may show enlarged Virchow-Robin spaces or enhancement of the meninges. At least one imaging test, preferably with contrast, is indicated to exclude a cryptococcoma or other concomitant CNS process.

▶ Treatment

For patients with acute infection, induction treatment with amphotericin B, 0.7–1.0 mg/kg/day, is given intravenously and flucytosine 25 mg/kg orally every 6 hours for 2 weeks or until the CSF is sterile, whichever occurs later, followed by fluconazole, 400 mg/day orally, to complete at least a 10-week course. After induction treatment is completed, fluconazole, 200 mg/day orally, is continued as consolidation treatment. When to discontinue fluconazole is debatable. Some clinicians continue it indefinitely, whereas others consider discontinuing it once the immune system has reconstituted to a CD4 cell count greater than 200 cells/mm^3.

Management of increased intracranial pressure is critical to decrease mortality. When intracranial pressure is elevated, (> 25 cm H$_2$O) frequent lumbar punctures are indicated as long as brain imaging does not raise concern for impending herniation. Ventricular or lumbar shunting should be used for patients with prolonged or malignant increased intracranial pressure, even if the CSF is not sterile. Glucocorticoids are not indicated for cryptococcal meningitis. Hydrocephalus can be a late manifestation of cryptococcal meningitis requiring permanent shunt placement.

▶ Prognosis

A depressed level of consciousness or an opening pressure greater than 250 mm H$_2$O predicts a worse prognosis. The serum cryptococcal antigen titer is not necessarily associated with disease activity and need not be followed, but the CSF cryptococcal antigen titer will usually decrease with successful treatment. Although technically a curable infection, *Cryptococcus* may sequester in the CNS, leading to a recurrence of meningitis.

Saag MS, et al. Practice guidelines for the management of cryptococcal disease. Infectious Diseases Society of America. *Clin Infect Dis* 2000;30:710–718. [PMID: 10770733] (A National Institute of Allergy and Infectious Diseases [NIAID] Mycoses Study Group review of available data and their recommendations on the treatment of cryptococcal disease.)

Sloan DJ, et al. Treatment of cryptococcal meningitis in resource-limited settings. *Curr Opin Infect Dis* 2009;22:455–463. [PMID: 19587589] (An excellent review of treatment options for cryptococcal disease in resource-limited settings, where cryptococcal meningitis is still a very common problem.)

TOXOPLASMOSIS OF THE CENTRAL NERVOUS SYSTEM

ESSENTIALS OF DIAGNOSIS

▶ A late-stage complication of HIV infection

▶ Focal neurologic deficits, subacute encephalopathy, and fever

▶ Multiple ring-enhancing lesions on MRI

▶ Presence of serum *Toxoplasma* IgG antibody

▶ Clinical and radiologic improvement with pyrimethamine and either sulfadiazine or clindamycin

▶ General Considerations

CNS toxoplasmosis is the most common cause of a focal brain mass in HIV patients. It is a late complication of HIV, usually occurring only after the CD4$^+$ T-lymphocyte count falls below 200 cells/µL. Most cases occur as a recrudescence of a latent infection of the small, intracellular protozoa *Toxoplasma gondii*, which is acquired through ingesting uncooked meat, contaminated water, or cat feces. *T gondii* is not a ubiquitous organism; therefore, the prevalence of CNS toxoplasmosis reflects regional prevalence and virulence of the organism as well as culinary habits, feline exposure, immune status, and genetic predisposition of the host. The incidence of CNS toxoplasmosis has significantly declined with the widespread use of combination antiretroviral therapy (CART) and use of sulfamethoxazole-trimethoprim for prophylaxis against *Pneumocystis carinii* pneumonia.

▶ Clinical Findings

A. Symptoms and Signs

Headache, fever, focal neurologic deficit(s), and altered mental status are the most common symptoms. Acute symptomatic seizures occur in 25% of patients. Rarely, toxoplasmosis presents with ocular pain and visual loss (toxoplasmic retinochoroiditis) or myelopathic signs (spinal cord toxoplasmosis). Unilateral chorea or ballism has been reported with toxoplasmic abscesses in the contralateral basal ganglia.

B. Laboratory and Imaging Studies

A presumed clinical diagnosis is made by combining historical information with results from serum tests and brain imaging. A serum IgG antibody titer indicates exposure to *T gondii*, thus raising the clinical probability of CNS toxoplasmosis. A negative titer does not rule out toxoplasmosis infection, as the antibody response may be attenuated in advanced AIDS or may not yet be mounted in newly acquired (primary) *Toxoplasma* infection. The absolute titer value is not helpful, nor is the presence of an IgM titer. A current CD4$^+$ T-lymphocyte count should be obtained; greater than 300 cells/µL should suggest alternative diagnoses.

Lumbar puncture is often contraindicated; moreover, CSF analyses seldom assist in the diagnosis of CNS toxoplasmosis. Mild to moderate pleocytosis, elevated protein concentration, and normal to low glucose level are the usual findings. A CSF *Toxoplasma* antibody titer is not helpful. CSF analysis for *Toxoplasma* DNA by polymerase chain reaction (PCR) lacks sensitivity but is helpful in confirming the diagnosis when positive.

MRI and CT brain scan typically show multiple ring-enhancing, space-occupying lesions with surrounding vasogenic edema. *Toxoplasma* has a predilection for the basal ganglia and the gray-white junction of the hemispheres. Being more sensitive, MRI is the preferred imaging test. Rarely, the lesion is solitary, suggesting primary CNS lymphoma (PCNSL), or is hemorrhagic. Magnetic resonance spectroscopy; thallium brain single-photon emission computed tomography (SPECT), which can show decreased uptake with a toxoplasmosis abscess; and positron emission tomography (PET), along with *Toxoplasma* serologies can aid in discriminating CNS toxoplasmosis from PCNSL (Table 28–3).

Treatment

In general, space-occupying brain lesions in a patient with AIDS are presumed to be toxoplasmosis. Induction treatment of pyrimethamine (200 mg oral load, then 50 mg [< 60 kg] or 75 mg [> 60 kg] orally per day), sulfadiazine (1000 mg [< 60 kg] or 1500 mg [> 60 kg] orally every 6 hours], and leucovorin (10–25 mg/day orally) should be started immediately. For patients with sulfa allergies, clindamycin (600 mg orally every 6 hours) or, as second-line therapy, azithromycin (900–1200 mg/day orally) or atovaquone (1.5 mg orally every 12 hours) can substitute for sulfadiazine. Glucocorticosteroids should be avoided unless clinically warranted for life-threatening vasogenic edema, because both PCNSL and symptoms from CNS toxoplasmosis respond to their use, leaving the actual diagnosis in doubt.

Clinical and radiographic improvement should be seen within 2 weeks. If so, and if glucocorticosteroids were not used, a presumptive diagnosis of CNS toxoplasmosis can be made. If improvement is not seen within 2 weeks, strong consideration should be given to a diagnosis of PCNSL. Acute therapy should continue for 6 weeks or until the lesions no longer enhance, whichever is later. Because of the high risk of recurrence, maintenance therapy of pyrimethamine (50 mg/day) and sulfadiazine (500–1000 mg orally four times a day) or clindamycin (800 mg three times

a day) should be continued until the immune system has sufficiently reconstituted to a CD4 cell count greater than 200 cells/mm^3. Thereafter, sulfamethoxazole-trimethoprim prophylaxis should be considered.

When both glucocorticoids and toxoplasmosis treatment are administered, the patient should be tapered off glucocorticoids as quickly as possible, a workup for PCNSL should be completed, and management should continue as for presumed toxoplasmosis. If patients do not respond to the therapeutic trial of antitoxoplasmosis therapy, a biopsy should be performed to evaluate for other causes of mass lesions (eg, tumor, bacterial abscess, tuberculoma, cryptococcoma).

Prognosis

In most patients, a complete recovery should be expected. CNS toxoplasmosis can recur, particularly in the severely immunosuppressed. Such patients usually require a biopsy for definitive diagnosis and resistance testing. Remote seizures are also a common complication.

Antinori A, et al. Prevalence, associated factors, and prognostic determinants of AIDS-related toxoplasmic encephalitis in the era of advanced highly active antiretroviral therapy. *Clin Infect Dis* 2004;39:1681–1691. [PMID: 15578371] (Reviews clinical characteristics of patients with CNS toxoplasmosis in the current era of HIV treatment.)

Dedicoat M, Livesley N. Management of toxoplasmic encephalitis in HIV-infected adults (with an emphasis on resource-poor settings). *Cochrane Database Syst Rev* 2006;3:CD005420. [PMID: 16856096] (A comprehensive review of management guidelines for toxoplasmosis infection.)

Table 28–3. Comparison of CNS Toxoplasmosis and Primary CNS Lymphoma

	Toxoplasmosis	PCNSL
Location	Basal ganglia Gray-white junction	Periventricular
Number of lesions	Multiple	Solitary > multiple
Enhancement pattern	Ring	Heterogeneous or homogeneous
Edema	Moderate to marked	Variable
T2-weighted image (lesion relative to white matter)	Hyperintense	Isointense to hypointense
Diffusion-weighted image	Usually hypointense	Often hyperintense (positive)
MR perfusion	Decreased	Increased
MR spectroscopy	Markedly elevated lactate	Markedly elevated choline
SPECT thallium (lesion relative to white matter)	"Cold"—no thallium uptake	"Hot"—increased thallium uptake
Other	*Toxoplasma* IgG antibody positive (90% of patients)	EBV DNA amplified by PCR in CSF (most patients)

CSF = cerebrospinal fluid; EBV = Epstein-Barr virus; MR = magnetic resonance; PCNSL = primary CNS lymphoma; PCR = polymerase chain reaction; SPECT = single-photon emission computed tomography.

PRIMARY CNS LYMPHOMA

ESSENTIALS OF DIAGNOSIS

▶ A late-stage complication of HIV infection
▶ Focal neurologic deficits and subacute encephalopathy
▶ Enhancing mass lesions on MRI
▶ Epstein-Barr virus DNA (amplified by PCR) in CSF

▶ General Considerations

Primary CNS lymphoma (PCNSL) is second to CNS toxoplasmosis as a cause of a brain mass lesion among patients with late-stage HIV. In most cases it is a high-grade, B-cell line non-Hodgkin lymphoma mediated by Epstein-Barr virus (EBV). It occurs among patients with advanced AIDS, in whom the typical CD4+ T-lymphocyte count is less than 50 cells/μL. Since the widespread use of CART, the frequency of PCNSL has declined, probably occurring in less than 5% of patients with AIDS.

▶ Clinical Findings

A. Symptoms and Signs

PCNSL classically presents with subacute focal neurologic deficits, encephalopathy, headaches, and seizures. Fever is uncommon, in contrast to CNS toxoplasmosis. The lymphoma is usually isolated to the CNS; therefore, systemic manifestations are not seen.

B. Laboratory and Imaging Studies

If not contraindicated, lumbar puncture should be performed. CSF typically reveals mild, lymphocytic-predominant pleocytosis, normal to mildly elevated protein concentration, and normal glucose level. The most useful test is PCR amplification for EBV; CSF that tests positive for EBV DNA in the presence of a mass lesion that has increased thallium uptake on brain SPECT (see Table 28–3) strongly suggests the diagnosis of PCNSL. However, a negative test does not exclude the diagnosis and a positive test does not exclude a comorbid process such as toxoplasmosis. If enough cells are present, cytology and molecular analyses may be helpful. Serum tests are not helpful in establishing a diagnosis of PCNSL, but tests such as *Toxoplasma* IgG, cultures, and markers for other malignancies may help with the differential.

CT or MRI scans typically show an isolated enhancing lesion or, less often, multiple enhancing lesions, commonly involving the frontal lobes and the periventricular region (see Table 28–3). PCNSL may cross the midline through the corpus callosum. Enhancement tends to be heterogeneous rather than the ringlike appearance seen with toxoplasmosis. Vasogenic edema is variably present. MRI is the preferred test. Signal intensity on T2-weighted images is variable, but

is often bright on diffusion-weighted images. Perfusion-weighted images show areas of increased regional blood volumes, in contrast to the low-volume areas seen with toxoplasmosis. Thallium SPECT imaging, which shows increased uptake with PCNSL, and magnetic resonance spectroscopy can be helpful in discriminating lymphoma from toxoplasmosis (see Table 28–3). None of these imaging results, however, is pathognomonic of PCNSL.

Biopsy provides a definitive diagnosis and should be considered in all suspected cases in which treatment with anti-*Toxoplasma* agents has not led to rapid radiographic or clinical improvement.

▶ Treatment

Cerebral edema from PCNSL can be treated with steroids. Ancillary treatment with fractionated whole brain radiation therapy or chemotherapeutic agents such as methotrexate can also be used, but these decisions need to be made on a case-by-case basis in collaboration with an oncologist (see Chapter 12). Virologic control of HIV is equally if not more important; therefore, CART should be initiated in naïve patients and changed in those on treatment but with a detectable plasma HIV RNA level.

▶ Prognosis

Chemotherapy and whole brain radiation therapy may prolong survival, but without virologic control of HIV, postdiagnosis survival remains on the order of months. If virologic control can be established with CART, survival can be longer. In fact, virologic control rather than use of methotrexate or whole brain radiation after diagnosis appears to offer the best prognosis.

Hochberg FH, et al. Primary CNS lymphoma. *Nat Clin Pract Neurol* 2007;3:24–35. [PMID: 17205072] (A comprehensive review of our current understanding of primary CNS lymphoma.)

Skiest DJ, Crosby C. Survival is prolonged by highly active antiretroviral therapy in AIDS patients with primary central nervous system lymphoma. *AIDS* 2003;17:1787–1793. [PMID: 12891064] (Illustrates the importance of virologic control and immune reconstitution on survival in HIV patients with PCNSL.)

PROGRESSIVE MULTIFOCAL LEUKOENCEPHALOPATHY

ESSENTIALS OF DIAGNOSIS

▶ A late-stage complication of HIV infection
▶ Subacute onset of focal neurologic deficits and dementia
▶ MRI of brain showing increased signal on T2-weighted images in white matter, including U fibers
▶ JC virus DNA (amplified by PCR) in CSF

General Considerations

Progressive multifocal leukoencephalopathy (PML) is a subacute demyelinating infectious disease affecting the CNS. The causative agent is the JC virus, a ubiquitous virus to which approximately 80% of adults in the United States have developed antibodies from a prior exposure. A reactivation of the virus, either within the CNS or at extraneural sites such as the kidneys or lymphoid tissue with subsequent spread to the CNS, in the setting of an immune-compromised state leads to a productive infection within oligodendrocytes, resulting in their apoptosis and subsequent demyelination.

PML is considered a late complication of HIV. Typically the CD4+ T-lymphocyte count is less than 100 cells/μL, although cases have been reported with counts well over 500 cells/μL. Less than 5% of those with AIDS develop PML, and this number is declining with improved antiretroviral treatment.

Clinical Findings

A. Symptoms and Signs

Patients with PML present with subacute, progressive focal neurologic deficits. Hemiparesis, language disturbance, cognitive impairment, headache, visual field cut, ataxia, and sensory loss are the most common initial symptoms. Multiple deficits are the norm as the disease progresses. Rarely is the spinal cord involved, and the peripheral nervous system, including the cranial nerves, is always spared.

B. Laboratory and Imaging Studies

PCR amplification for JC DNA in CSF has a sensitivity of 65–90% and a specificity of 90–100%. A negative PCR result does not exclude the diagnosis (false negative). Blood analysis—for JC DNA by PCR and JC virus antibody—is typically positive and not necessarily associated with the neurologic disease, although negative tests may argue against the diagnosis of PML. Other CSF indices are either normal or show mild, nonspecific derangements.

MRI of the brain is the preferred imaging test. Solitary or multifocal white matter abnormalities represented by high-intensity T2-weighted images and low-intensity T1-weighted images are seen. Diffusion-weighted images may show bright signal in the affected areas, suggesting a spurious diagnosis of stroke. As the disease progresses, affected areas tend to coalesce, and eventually U fibers are involved. Mass effect, enhancement, or gray matter involvement is rare, whereas focal atrophy and volume loss is common. CT scan of the brain reveals areas of white matter hypodensity and atrophy.

Although clinical history, JC virus DNA (amplified by PCR) in CSF, and characteristic MRI abnormalities support a probable diagnosis of PML, they are rarely present en totem. Furthermore, white matter abnormalities on MRI are common in patients with HIV. When in doubt, a brain biopsy is indicated, targeting an abnormal area on MRI, to provide definitive diagnosis.

Treatment

CART should be initiated to reconstitute the immune system. It is uncertain whether specific regimens are more efficacious. For those using virologically effective CART at presentation, few options exist, but consideration should be given to adding CNS-penetrant antiretroviral agents. Other agents have not had proven efficacy.

Prognosis

Use of CART has led to a significant improvement in survival and even reports of complete remission. Reversal of neurologic deficits is uncommon. Being CART naïve, absence of severe neurologic deficits, a CD4+ count greater than 100 cells/μL at presentation, and the presence of enhancement on neuroimaging suggest a better prognosis.

Berenguer J, et al. Clinical course and prognostic factors of progressive multifocal leukoencephalopathy in patients treated with highly active antiretroviral therapy. Clin Infect Dis 2003;36:1047–1052. [PMID: 12684918] (Findings for this study highlight the variable clinical course and risk factors for death.)

Cinque P, et al. Progressive multifocal leukoencephalopathy in HIV-1 infection. Lancet Infect Dis 2009;9:625–636. [PMID: 19778765] (This comprehensive review highlights the diagnosis, clinical course, and treatment options for PML.)

HIV-ASSOCIATED NEUROCOGNITIVE DISORDER (HAND)

 ESSENTIALS OF DIAGNOSIS

▸ A mid- to late-stage complication of HIV infection

▸ Subacute to chronic onset of cognitive impairment, motor slowing (psychomotor retardation), and behavioral changes without focal neurologic deficit

▸ MRI of brain showing increased signal in subcortical white matter on T2-weighted images and presence of central atrophy

General Considerations

Within weeks of primary viremia, HIV invades the CNS, primarily via monocytes trafficking from the periphery. Monocytes, macrophages, and microglia are the principal cell types capable of supporting productive CNS infection, although HIV also nonproductively infects astrocytes. HIV does not infect neurons. A chronic encephalitis ensues, characterized by the pathologic features of perivascular monocytic infiltrates, microglial nodules, multinucleated giant cells, white matter pallor, astrocytosis, and neuronal pruning and dropout. Frank dementia develops only after years of sustained immunosuppression, and therefore is considered a late sequela of HIV infection. Milder forms of neurocognitive impairment may occur even without significant immunosuppression. Most of the damage to the nervous system does not result directly from HIV itself, but from neurotoxic HIV proteins and from upregulated production of immune and inflammatory mediators from the cells capable of productive infection, creating a milieu toxic to neurons and their supporting cells.

The incidence of HIV dementia (HIVD) (previously known as AIDS dementia complex) has declined dramatically since 1996, when CART was introduced, reflecting improved immune status among those with HIV. However, among those with advanced HIV infection, including those with resistance and poor adherence to CART, the prevalence can be as high as 5–10%. Nevertheless, the prevalence of milder forms of cognitive impairment (HIV-associated asymptomatic neurocognitive impairment and mild neurocognitive disorder) may be as high as 35–40%. Older HIV+ individuals greater than age 50 years are twice as likely to develop HIVD than younger HIV+ individuals. HAND is still the most common form of dementia worldwide in people under the age of 40, striking people in their prime adult working years, and thus having a large socioeconomic impact.

▶ Clinical Findings

A. Symptoms and Signs

HIVD is characterized by the triad of cognitive impairment, motor impairment, and behavioral changes resulting in a decline in performance of activities of daily living. Psychomotor retardation best describes the syndrome. Early cognitive symptoms involve executive function and include difficulty concentrating, impaired information processing, and poor mental flexibility. Memory is relatively spared until the later stages of the dementia; impaired memory reflects problems with retrieval rather than encoding, in contrast to Alzheimer disease. Language and visual-spatial systems are relatively preserved. Bradykinesia is a common and early sign. On examination, saccadic eye movements and rapid alternating limb movements are slow, whereas tone (often with cog-wheeling) may be increased. Chorea, athetosis, and dystonia are rare. Focal weakness suggests an alternative or additional diagnosis. One should keep in mind that HIV myelopathy may accompany HIVD, in which case signs referable to the spinal cord would be present. Behavioral symptoms mimic those seen in depression: social withdrawal, apathy, irritability, and blunted affect.

B. Laboratory and Imaging Studies

HIVD is a clinical diagnosis. Ancillary testing can support the diagnosis and exclude others. CSF usually shows a mild pleocytosis, mildly elevated protein concentration, and normal glucose level—a profile often found in neurologically asymptomatic HIV patients. Several serum and CSF markers of immune activation and HIV RNA levels are associated with HIVD in antiretroviral naïve HIV+ individuals, but their role in making a diagnosis or even predicting further neurologic impairment in CART-experienced HIV+ individuals remains dubious. Other causes of dementia need to be excluded, and the standard workup should include tests outlined in Table 28–4. Neuropsychological testing can demonstrate a pattern of impairment typical of HIVD as opposed to other dementias and can help quantify the severity of the deficits.

MRI typically reveals subcortical white matter T2-weighted hyperintensities and central atrophy. There may be preferential atrophy in the basal ganglia, particularly within the caudate. CT scan of the head reveals patchy white matter lucencies and cortical atrophy, which are nonspecific. The primary role of MRI in the evaluation of an HIV+ individual is to exclude a CNS focal lesion such as a CNS opportunistic infection, malignancy, or stroke.

Table 28–4. Initial Diagnostic Workup for HIV Patients With Subacute or Chronic Cognitive Impairment

	Diagnostic Workup
Serum	Thyroid function tests Liver function tests and ammonia Cryptococcal antigen CMV DNA by PCR RPR/FTA-ABS Metabolic profile Toxicology Vitamin B_{12} level CD4+ T-lymphocyte count HIV RNA level
CSF	Cell count and differential Protein level Glucose level VDRL (consider FTA-ABS) Cryptococcal antigen EBV DNA by PCR CMV DNA by PCR VZV DNA by PCR HSV DNA by PCR JC virus DNA by PCR Bacterial, fungal, and acid-fast bacilli culture ±HIV RNA level
Urine	Toxicology
Imaging	MRI of brain with gadolinium enhancement

CMV = cytomegalovirus; CSF = cerebrospinal fluid; EBV = Epstein-Barr virus; FTA-ABS = fluorescent treponemal antibody, absorbed (test); HIV = human immunodeficiency virus; HSV = herpes simplex virus; MRI = magnetic resonance imaging; PCR = polymerase chain reaction; RPR = rapid plasma reagin; VDRL = Venereal Disease Research Laboratory (test for syphilis); VZV = varicella-zoster virus.

Treatment

Treatment is aimed at lowering HIV RNA in plasma and CSF to undetectable levels and reconstituting the immune system. For patients not receiving any antiretroviral treatment, CART should be started. For those on CART and with undetectable plasma HIV RNA level but detectable CSF levels, consideration should be given to using a regimen of antiretroviral agents capable of penetrating the blood–brain barrier ([CNS-penetrant] zidovudine, stavudine, emtricitabine, abacavir, efavirenz, nevirapine, delavirdine, indinavir, lopinavir, darunavir, fosamprenavir, maraviroc, vicriviroc, and raltegravir). The establishment of techniques to maintain medication adherence is critical for effective virological suppression and treatment of HAND. If an HIV+ individual starting initial CART regimen develops new cognitive symptoms despite virological suppression, a CNS immune reconstitution inflammatory syndrome (CNS-IRIS) should be considered, as rare cases of IRIS in association with new cognitive problems have been reported. Selective serotonin reuptake inhibitors should be considered for patients displaying depressive symptoms. Treatment targeting the immune and inflammatory products believed to be the direct cause of CNS damage has yet to be developed.

Prognosis

Several studies have shown durable clinical improvement for years subsequent to CART treatment, which is likely a reflection of virologic control of HIV and an improved immune system. In the absence of CART, the dementia progresses with death ensuing in the course of months.

McArthur JC, et al. Human immunodeficiency virus–associated dementia: An evolving disease. *J Neurovirol* 2003;9:205–221. [PMID: 12707851] (Reviews how the clinical course and epidemiology has changed since the introduction of CART).

Nath A, et al. Evolution of HIV dementia with HIV infection. *Int Rev Psychiatry* 2008;20:25–31. [PMID: 18240060] (Reviews the latest trends in the diagnosis and treatment of HAND.)

HIV-ASSOCIATED MYELOPATHY

ESSENTIALS OF DIAGNOSIS

► A late-stage complication of HIV infection
► Insidious onset of urinary and erectile dysfunction, spastic paraparesis, and gait ataxia

General Considerations

HIV-associated myelopathy, also called *vacuolar myelopathy*, is a late-stage HIV complication presenting when the CD4+ cell count is less than 200 cells/μL. Before the widespread use of CART, 10% of patients with AIDS developed this condition; now the condition is far less common. Clinically and histopathologically, HIV myelopathy resembles the myelopathy associated with vitamin B_{12} deficiency, and studies suggest that an abnormality in the vitamin B_{12}–dependent transmethylation pathway underlies its etiology.

Clinical Findings

A. Symptoms and Signs

HIV-associated myelopathy is a chronic disorder with an insidious, often asymmetric onset characterized by urinary and erectile dysfunction, spastic paraparesis, and gait ataxia from posterior column involvement. Mild fleeting paresthesias in the legs and feet may be present. Because the thoracic segments of the cord are affected first, arms are spared until late in the disease.

Examination reveals a spastic paraparesis and attenuated vibratory and proprioception sensation in the toes, reflecting posterior column dysfunction. Pain and temperature sensation are relatively preserved. Additional signs include exaggerated ankle and patellar stretch reflexes, extensor plantar responses, gait spasticity, and a Romberg sign. As the disease progresses, similar signs and symptoms involve the arms. When HIV-related peripheral neuropathy co-occurs, all sensory modalities may be impaired and reflexes and tone may be diminished or lost.

B. Laboratory and Imaging Studies

HIV-associated myelopathy is a clinical diagnosis based on the insidious course, signs and symptoms referable to the spinal cord (particularly posterior columns), and the exclusion of other causes of spinal cord disease (Table 28–5). Serum tests do not contribute to the diagnosis, although they can exclude other causes of myelopathy. CSF indices may show mild pleocytosis and elevation in protein concentration. MRI of the

Table 28–5. Differential Diagnosis of Nonacute Myelopathy

HIV-mediated
Human T-lymphotrophic virus, type 1 or 2
Varicella-zoster virus
Herpes simplex virus, type 1 or 2
Neurosyphilis
Spinal or epidural abscess (pyogenic, *Mycobacterium tuberculosis*, *Toxoplasma*)
Intramedullary or extramedullary tumor
Structural spine disease (eg, spinal stenosis, spondylosis, herniated nucleus pulposus, metastatic tumor)
Vitamin B_{12} deficiency
Autoimmune disorders (multiple sclerosis, systemic lupus erythematosus)
Vascular (infarction, arteriovenous malformation)

spine may show cord atrophy and increased T2-weighted signal in the posterior columns. Somatosensory-evoked potentials may be helpful in subtle cases, showing prolongation of the tibial central conduction time. Acute onset of symptoms, the presence of a sensory level, CSF pleocytosis greater than 30 cells/mL or protein concentration greater than 100 mg/dL, or back pain warrants search for an alternative diagnosis.

▶ Treatment

Symptomatic management is the mainstay of treatment (Table 28–6). Anecdotal reports suggest modest improvement after virologic control with CART. Vitamin B_{12}, methionine, glucocorticoids, and intravenous gamma globulins are ineffective in improving symptoms or delaying progression.

HIV MENINGITIS

ESSENTIALS OF DIAGNOSIS

▶ A common cause of aseptic meningitis among patients with HIV

▶ Usually occurs at time of seroconversion

▶ Self-limited illness

This self-limited, monophasic aseptic meningitis occurs during primary HIV dissemination as part of the acute conversion syndrome or less commonly after cessation of antiretroviral therapy (retroviral rebound syndrome). The frequency of HIV meningitis is unknown but is presumed to be a relatively common but often undiagnosed condition overshadowed or ascribed to the concomitant multitude of flulike symptoms associated with acute conversion syndrome. HIV is believed to directly cause the meningitis. Rarely,

Table 28–6. Symptomatic Management of HIV-Associated Myelopathy

Symptom	Treatment
Weakness and spasticity; gait or ambulation difficulty	Physical therapy (strengthening exercises, range-of-motion exercises, gait training, etc) Antispasticity agents: Baclofen, titrated to 20 mg 3 times daily *or* Tizanidine HCl, titrated to 8 mg 3 times daily, not to exceed 36 mg/day
Urinary dysfunction	Urinary frequency—oxybutynin, 5 mg 2-3 times daily Urinary incontinence—imipramine, 25-75 mg at bedtime
Erectile dysfunction	Sildenafil (after consultation with urologist, and if no contraindications for use)

encephalitis may accompany the meningitis. Associated cranial neuropathies may also rarely be seen.

CSF indices are consistent with aseptic meningitis with a lymphocytic pleocytosis of 20–300 cells. HIV DNA can be amplified in the CSF, although its presence does not exclude other coincident causes. MRI may show enhancement of the meninges. Serum HIV test will usually still be negative.

No specific treatment for the meningitis is recommended. When encephalitis is present, acyclovir (10 mg/kg intravenously three times a day) should be initiated until herpes simplex virus encephalitis has been excluded, and consideration for the immediate use of CNS-penetrant antiretroviral agents should be given.

Serrano P, et al. Bilateral Bell palsy and acute HIV type 1 infection: Report of 2 cases and review. *Clin Infect Dis* 2007;44:e57–e61. [PMID: 17304442] (This report demonstrates the rare association between HIV meningitis and cranial neuropathies.)

Tambussi G, et al. Neurological symptoms during primary human immunodeficiency virus (HIV) infection correlate with high levels of HIV RNA in cerebrospinal fluid. *Clin Infect Dis* 2000;30:962–965. [PMID: 10880317] (A small study reporting that neurologic manifestations of acute HIV infection are associated with elevated CSF but not plasma HIV RNA levels.)

VARICELLA-ZOSTER VASCULITIS

ESSENTIALS OF DIAGNOSIS

▶ Small-vessel vasculitis isolated to the CNS

▶ Fever, headache, encephalopathy, and focal neurologic deficits, usually within weeks of antecedent zoster rash

▶ CSF analysis showing varicella-zoster virus (VZV) DNA (amplified by PCR), IgM VZV antibody, or an elevated CSF-to-serum VZV IgG antibody titer confirms diagnosis

Although classic dermatomal zoster (shingles) is a common complication in both early and late HIV infection, the CNS is only rarely affected. A small-vessel vasculitis or myelitis (see later discussion) can develop, usually in the late stages of HIV infection and within weeks to months of an antecedent zoster rash. Symptoms of VZV vasculitis include fever, headache, encephalopathy, cranial neuropathies (especially oculomotor palsy), focal stroke-like neurologic deficits, and seizures. The symptoms may develop acutely, fluctuate, or slowly progress, creating a confusing clinical picture.

CSF generally shows mild to moderate lymphocytic or monocytic pleocytosis, elevated protein concentration, and normal to low glucose level. CSF should be analyzed for both VZV DNA (via PCR) and antibody (IgM and IgG). The presence of VZV DNA or IgM antibody in CSF or an elevated

CSF-to-serum IgG antibody ratio confirms the diagnosis. MRI typically shows multiple areas of hyperintensity on T2- and diffusion-weighted images, suggestive of acute or subacute infarcts. Some of these areas may become hemorrhagic. Transcranial Doppler and magnetic resonance angiography may show asymmetric increased flow velocities and focal stenoses, respectively, particularly in the distal arteries. A brain and meningeal biopsy or conventional angiogram should be considered in suspected cases with negative serologic and PCR tests.

Acyclovir (10 mg/kg intravenously three times a day) should be administered without delay in all patients with suspected VZV vasculitis for at least 14 days. Acyclovir resistance can develop; therefore, foscarnet (90 mg/kg every 12 hours) should be considered in patients with previous exposure to acyclovir. Optimization of CART should also be undertaken.

Amlie-Lefond C, Jubelt B. Neurologic manifestations of varicella zoster virus infections. *Curr Neurol Neurosci Rep* 2009;9:430–434. [PMID: 19818229] (A good, recent review.)

CYTOMEGALOVIRUS ENCEPHALITIS

ESSENTIALS OF DIAGNOSIS

▶ A late-stage complication of HIV infection

▶ Subacute, progressive cognitive, and behavioral changes

▶ Cytomegalovirus (CMV) polyradiculitis and other focal neurologic deficits

▶ CSF analysis showing mild to moderate pleocytosis, elevated protein, and normal to low glucose

▶ PCR amplification for CMV DNA is sensitive and specific for CNS disease

This is a devastating infection occurring in the very late stages of AIDS with CD4 counts less than 50 cells/mm^3, but is now rarely seen in HIV+ individuals on CART. Two forms of encephalitis have been described: a ventriculoencephalitis, more common among those with HIV, and a micronodular encephalitis.

Ventriculoencephalitis typically presents with subacute cognitive and behavioral changes that progress to death over the course of weeks. CMV polyradiculitis and other focal cortical, cerebellar, or brainstem findings often accompany the neurologic syndrome. Systemic manifestations, including retinitis, invariably complicate the clinical picture.

CSF indices are variably abnormal, depending on the extent of the infection. A typical profile shows mild to moderate monocytic pleocytosis, elevated protein concentration, and low glucose level. However, significant polymorphonuclear-predominant pleocytosis and hypoglycorrhachia are seen when polyradiculitis is present. CSF analysis for CMV DNA by PCR amplification is sensitive and specific. Plasma CMV by PCR amplification should be obtained to support the presence of a systemic infection. The classic MRI finding of ependymal and periventricular enhancement is seen in approximately two thirds of patients with the ventriculoencephalitic form.

A combination of ganciclovir (5 mg/kg intravenously every 12 hours) and foscarnet (90 mg/kg every 12 hours) for 3–6 weeks should be initiated in all suspected cases. Lifelong maintenance therapy with valganciclovir (900 mg/day orally) and foscarnet should then be provided. Consultation with infectious disease specialists is mandatory to optimize antiretroviral therapy and direct further workup, which must include an ophthalmologic examination to evaluate for CMV retinitis. Prognosis is poor in most cases.

Griffiths P. Cytomegalovirus infection of the central nervous system. *Herpes* 2004;11(Suppl 2):95A–104A. [PMID: 15319096] (A nice review of the clinical, epidemiologic, and pathologic features of CMV encephalitis.)

▼ PERIPHERAL NERVOUS SYSTEM COMPLICATIONS (TABLE 28–7)

CYTOMEGALOVIRUS POLYRADICULOPATHY

ESSENTIALS OF DIAGNOSIS

▶ A late-stage complication of HIV infection

▶ Acute to subacute onset of back pain, sensory loss, leg weakness, and bladder or bowel dysfunction

▶ CMV DNA (amplified by PCR) in CSF is diagnostic

▶ General Considerations

CMV is the most common infectious cause of polyradiculopathy among patients with AIDS, but since the widespread use of CART, cases are rare. It occurs almost exclusively as a late complication, typically when the CD4$^+$ cell count is less than 50 cells/μL. An increasingly more common cause of polyradiculopathy is structural spine or disk disease, although rarer causes include herpes viruses (VZV, EBV, and herpes simplex types 1 and 2), syphilis, and lymphoma.

▶ Clinical Findings

A. Symptoms and Signs

Acute to subacute onset of radicular back pain, paresthesias, urinary dysfunction, and leg weakness are the usual symptoms. Symptoms tend to be asymmetric at onset and rapidly spread to other lumbar and sacral roots. Lower motor neuron signs of flaccid paraparesis and areflexia as

Table 28–7. Peripheral Nervous System Complications of HIV Infection

Neuroaxis	Complication	Clinical Findings	Diagnostic Studies	Treatment
Nerve root	CMV polyradiculopathy	Acute onset of lower extremity flaccid weakness, paresthesias ("saddle"), bowel and bladder dysfunction, and areflexia	CSF—polymorphonuclear pleocytosis and positive CMV PCR EMG/NCV—polyradiculopathy	Anti-CMV therapy for CMV polyradiculopathy; appropriate treatment for other causes
	Herpes zoster (VZV)[a]	Abrupt onset of pain conforming to 1 or more dermatomes followed by associated rash	Direct fluorescent antibody test on vesicular fluid to detect VZV antigen	Anti-VZV therapy
Nerve	Distal symmetric polyneuropathy	Subacute to insidious onset of painful paresthesias in a stocking and, in later stages, glove distribution; depressed distal reflexes	EMG/NCV—abnormal sensory nerve amplitudes, distal axonopathy	Analgesics (primary and adjuvant), neurotoxic drug withdrawal or dose reduction, virologic control
	Mononeuropathy multiplex	Acute or subacute onset of foot or wrist drop, facial weakness, focal pain	EMG/NCV—multifocal axonal neuropathy	Immunomodulating therapy; consider anti-CMV therapy in late-onset mononeuropathy multiplex
	Acute inflammatory demyelinating polyneuropathy (AIDP)	Acute or subacute onset of weakness and paresthesias, usually affecting legs first; areflexia	CSF—lymphocytic pleocytosis (10–50 cells/μL), high protein EMG/NCV—demyelinating neuropathy	Immunomodulating therapy (IVIG, plasmapheresis); consider anti-CMV therapy in patients with AIDP and CD4+ < 200 cells/mL
Nerve and muscle	HIV-associated neuromuscular weakness	Subacute onset of general weakness and malaise (nausea, vomiting, fatigue)	Serum—hyperlactatemia and acidemia EMG/NCV—axonal > demyelinating neuropathy; myopathy Nerve or muscle biopsy—mitochondrial abnormalities or mitochondrial DNA depletion	Nucleoside antiretroviral withdrawal; supportive therapy
Muscle	HIV-associated myopathy	Acute or subacute onset of focal or diffuse weakness	Serum—elevated CK EMG—muscle irritability, abnormal spontaneous activity Muscle biopsy—myofiber atrophy with inflammatory infiltrates	Nucleoside antiretroviral withdrawal, immunomodulating therapy, antibiotics

CK = creatine kinase; CMV = cytomegalovirus; CSF = cerebrospinal fluid (analysis); EMG = electromyography; IVIG = intravenous immunoglobulin; NCV = nerve conduction velocity; PCR = polymerase chain reaction; VZV = varicella-zoster virus.
[a]Refer to Chapter 27 for additional discussion of herpes zoster.

well as loss of all sensory modalities (often in a peroneal "saddle" distribution) and bowel and bladder dysfunction are found on examination. Myelopathic features are present when there is secondary involvement of the spinal cord (myeloradiculopathy).

B. Laboratory and Imaging Studies

Marked CSF polymorphonuclear pleocytosis, hypoglycorrhachia, and moderately elevated protein concentration support the diagnosis. The presence of CMV DNA (amplified by PCR) in CSF confirms the diagnosis. This test has a sensitivity and specificity greater than 90%; therefore, a negative PCR test for CMV DNA in CSF or even plasma (CMV is a systemic illness) strongly argues against the diagnosis. Electromyography reveals reduced numbers of motor units and abnormal

spontaneous activity in weak muscles. Nerve conduction velocities are only mildly abnormal. Severe and widespread proximal axonal pathology in lumbar nerve root segments is seen. MRI with gadolinium of the lumbosacral spine may show enhancement of nerve roots, indicating an active inflammatory process but not a specific cause.

In patients in whom CMV has been excluded, a workup for other causes of acute polyradiculopathy should include appropriate tests for herpes simplex (types 1 and 2), EBV, VZV, lymphoma, syphilis, and structural spine disease.

▶ Treatment

Antiviral therapy with ganciclovir (5 mg/kg intravenously every 12 hours) or foscarnet (90 mg/kg every 12 hours) for 3–6 weeks should be initiated in all suspected cases of CMV polyradiculopathy followed by lifelong maintenance therapy with valganciclovir and foscarnet. Consultation with an infectious disease specialist is also indicated to address other therapies (eg, monotherapy versus dual anti-CMV therapy and use of CART), duration of treatment, and to assess for other systemic damage from CMV.

▶ Prognosis

Prompt diagnosis and treatment is essential to avoid irreversible nerve root necrosis and permanent disability. CMV polyradiculopathy carries a high morbidity even when promptly treated. Untreated CMV polyradiculopathy carries a high mortality.

DISTAL SYMMETRIC POLYNEUROPATHY

ESSENTIALS OF DIAGNOSIS

- ▶ Occurs as a complication in the middle and late stages of HIV infection
- ▶ Caused by both HIV-mediated inflammatory processes and nucleoside reverse transcriptase inhibitors (NRTIs)
- ▶ Acute to insidious onset of paresthesias (usually painful) in stocking distribution

▶ General Considerations

Peripheral neuropathy is the leading cause of neurologic morbidity in the HIV population, affecting over 30% of patients with AIDS. Distal symmetric polyneuropathy (DSP) is the most common type (see Chapter 19). It is caused either by HIV-mediated inflammatory pathways (eg, upregulation of cytokines or from viral proteins) or by antiretroviral toxicity. Among the currently approved antiretroviral agents, the dideoxynucleoside analogues didanosine (ddI), zalcitabine (ddC), and stavudine (d4T) cause most cases of DSP, probably by impairing mitochondrial function, resulting in markedly diminished use of these antiretroviral drugs. Clinical and laboratory studies do not enable the clinician to discriminate between the two causes; however, antiretroviral-related DSP tends to have an acute or a subacute onset in relationship to initiation or escalation and may develop at any stage of HIV infection. In contrast, HIV-mediated DSP tends to have a more insidious course and occurs mostly among those with a CD4+ count less than 200 cells/μL.

▶ Clinical Findings

A. Symptoms and Signs

Both HIV-mediated and antiretroviral-related DSP have indistinguishable clinical syndromes of symmetric painful (burning or cramping) paresthesias and decreased sensation to pinprick and temperature in the stocking and, in advanced stages, glove distribution. Joint position sense is usually preserved; allodynia and hyperalgesia may be present; and ankle reflexes are absent or depressed compared with knee reflexes. Weakness of intrinsic muscles of the feet may occur late in the course.

B. Laboratory and Diagnostic Studies

Laboratory investigations are usually unrevealing, but it is prudent to screen for other common causes of neuropathy such as vitamin B_{12} deficiency, hepatitis C, and diabetes mellitus. CSF analysis is usually not necessary, except in atypical presentations (see Chapter 19).

Nerve conduction studies may show reduced amplitudes, mildly prolonged F waves, and absent sural nerve responses—nonspecific signs of axonal neuropathy. Electromyography may show active or chronic denervation with reinnervation in distal muscles. Electrophysiologic studies are normal in up to 20% of patients meeting clinical criteria for DSP; furthermore, these studies cannot discriminate between HIV-mediated and antiretroviral-related DSP. Nerve biopsy is rarely necessary except in patients with atypical disease features, but skin biopsy to look at the small nerve fibers can confirm the diagnosis.

▶ Treatment

Control of pain is the primary treatment goal for most patients with DSP, and the World Health Organization guidelines for management of cancer pain may be adapted for this purpose. In addition to the use of mild analgesics, gabapentin (titrated to 300–1200 mg orally three times a day), pregabalin (titrated to 50–100 mg orally three times a day), lamotrigine (titrated to 200 mg orally twice a day), amitriptyline (25–150 mg/day orally), or duloxetine (20–60 mg/day orally) can provide modest relief. Lidocaine patches or gel, or topical capsaicin may also be effective.

HIV-mediated DSP usually improves with sustained virologic control. In patients with antiretroviral-related DSP, reduction or avoidance of nucleosides without sacrificing virologic control may be sufficient to alleviate symptoms. When alternative nontoxic antiretroviral agents cannot be used without jeopardizing HIV control, symptomatic analgesic treatment with non-narcotic agents (eg, tramadol) or narcotic agents while continuing the toxic antiretroviral may be appropriate.

Brew BJ. The peripheral nerve complications of human immunodeficiency virus (HIV) infection. *Muscle Nerve* 2003;28:542–552. [PMID: 14571455] (An outstanding review.)

Gonzalez-Duarte, et al. Diagnosis and management of HIV-associated neuropathy. *Neurol Clin* 2008;26:821–832. [PMID: 18657728] (A recent review of the epidemiology, pathogenesis, clinical features, diagnosis, and treatment of HIV-associated peripheral neuropathy.)

MONONEUROPATHY MULTIPLEX

ESSENTIALS OF DIAGNOSIS

▶ Syndrome of multiple neuropathies with corresponding motor and sensory deficits
▶ Occurs at any stage of HIV infection
▶ Cause is usually infectious or immune mediated

Mononeuropathy multiplex is a relatively rare form of neuropathy in HIV infection. It manifests as multiple motor and sensory deficits in an asymmetric distribution. Involvement of the common peroneal nerve (foot drop), lateral femoral cutaneous nerve (meralgia paresthetica), facial nerve (facial weakness), and phrenic nerve (diaphragmatic paralysis) has been reported. Mononeuropathy multiplex may occur in early HIV disease, in which case immune-mediated mechanisms are implicated, or late HIV disease, in which case infectious etiologies such as CMV likely play a role. Other reported causes or cofactors include hepatitis B and C, lymphomatous infiltration of nerves, cryoglobulinemia, and vasculitis (for additional discussion, see Chapter 19).

Investigations for hepatitis B and C, CMV, cryoglobulinemia, diabetes, and lymphoma should be considered, particularly in patients with atypical or late-stage AIDS. Electrophysiology studies can confirm the clinical diagnosis but do not provide an etiology. They typically show signs of axonal damage, including reduced compound muscle action potential and sensory nerve action potential amplitudes on nerve conduction and neurogenic denervation in the distribution of involved nerves, on electromyography. In patients with progressive or polyphasic symptoms, a nerve biopsy for definitive diagnosis should be undertaken to exclude vasculitis, CMV, or lymphoma.

Treatment is tailored to the underlying etiology when known. Corticosteroids, plasmapheresis, or intravenous immunoglobulins may be beneficial in patients with severe symptoms when the cause is not known or in cases of vasculitic mononeuropathy multiplex. In late-onset mononeuropathy multiplex occurring in advanced HIV infection, empiric therapy for CMV may be considered (refer to CMV polyradiculopathy, earlier).

ACUTE INFLAMMATORY DEMYELINATING POLYNEUROPATHY

ESSENTIALS OF DIAGNOSIS

▶ Usually occurs shortly after seroconversion (early stage complication)
▶ Rapidly progressive ascending weakness
▶ CSF analysis showing pleocytosis and elevated protein

An uncommon disorder, acute inflammatory demyelinating polyneuropathy (AIDP) is generally seen shortly after seroconversion when the CD4+ cell count is greater than 500 cells/μL. It presents with rapidly progressive ascending weakness, minor sensory symptoms, and generalized areflexia. The disorder is presumed to be immune mediated, although the offending antibody has not been identified.

CSF analysis shows mild to moderate CSF lymphocytic pleocytosis, in contrast to the acellular CSF found in HIV-seronegative individuals with AIDP. In fact, the presence of more than 5 lymphocytes/mm³ in CSF in the setting of ascending flaccid paralysis should raise suspicion of undiagnosed HIV infection. Protein concentration may be mild to moderately elevated, depending on the timing of the lumbar puncture, but glucose levels are normal.

Electrophysiology studies demonstrate decreased motor and sensory nerve conduction velocities, conduction block, prolonged distal latencies, reduced compound muscle action potential and sensory nerve action potential amplitudes, and reduced motor unit recruitment proportional to the degree of weakness.

Treatment for AIDP in HIV-seropositive patients is the same as for seronegatives. Hospitalization is necessary for close observation, as the need for ventilatory support can occur rapidly. Intravenous immunoglobulin (IVIG; 0.4 mg/kg/day for 5 days) or plasmapheresis should be initiated at onset. Some clinicians advocate performing plasmapheresis followed by IVIG. Empiric CMV treatment with ganciclovir (5 mg/kg intravenously every 12 hours) or foscarnet (90 mg/kg every 12 hours) is warranted in patients with a CD4+ cell count less than 200 cells/μL until CMV polyradiculopathy is excluded.

Brew BJ. The peripheral nerve complications of human immunodeficiency virus (HIV) infection. *Muscle Nerve* 2003;28:542–552. [PMID: 14571455] (An outstanding review.)

HIV-ASSOCIATED NEUROMUSCULAR WEAKNESS SYNDROME

ESSENTIALS OF DIAGNOSIS

▶ Rapid onset of ascending weakness simulating AIDP in the setting of nucleoside antiretroviral use
▶ Elevated serum lactate

This syndrome presents with rapidly progressive weakness resembling AIDP but in the setting of hyperlactatemia or lactic acidosis. Nucleoside antiretroviral use is associated with most cases, and mitochondrial toxicity likely underlies the pathophysiology.

The neuromuscular features include ascending weakness that develops over days to weeks. Sensory symptoms are variably present. In some cases, the rapid development of motor weakness may lead to respiratory failure and death. Associated systemic symptoms include nausea, vomiting, fatigue, weight loss, abdominal distention, hepatomegaly, and lipoatrophy.

Elevated plasma lactate levels and acidemia are present. CSF analysis is normal, but evaluation is necessary to exclude other potential causes of acute ascending weakness, including CMV polyradiculopathy and AIDP. Electrophysiology studies typically show signs of axonal neuropathy, but demyelinating neuropathy and evidence of myopathy may also be seen. Mitochondrial abnormalities may be noted in some muscle biopsies.

The current management includes supportive treatment in a monitored setting, medical management of lactic acidosis, and withdrawal of nucleoside antiretroviral agents. Prognosis for recovery is variable. Nucleoside rechallenge is contraindicated.

Simpson D, et al. HIV-associated neuromuscular weakness syndrome. *AIDS* 2004;18:1403–1412. [PMID: 15199316] (A multicenter study describing the clinical features of the syndrome.)

HIV-ASSOCIATED MYOPATHY

ESSENTIALS OF DIAGNOSIS

▶ An uncommon complication that can occur at any stage of HIV infection

▶ Usually produces either focal of diffuse weakness and myalgias

▶ Cause is usually infectious or immune mediated

▶ Serum creatine kinase is usually elevated

HIV-associated myopathy may occur at any stage of HIV infection and from a variety of causes, including zidovudine (AZT) therapy, inflammatory myopathy (polymyositis), vasculitis, and infection (*Staphylococcus aureus*, *Mycobacterium*, CMV, and *Toxoplasma*). The presentation varies with the underlying cause, but slowly progressive, diffuse proximal weakness characterizes most immune, toxic, or metabolic causes, whereas subacute, focal weakness characterizes most infectious causes. Myalgias are present in 25–50% of patients.

Neurologic examination reveals focal or symmetric weakness, usually affecting proximal muscles. Muscle stretch reflexes are normal, unless there is a coexisting myelopathy or neuropathy. Muscles may be tender or, in chronic cases, atrophic.

Serum creatine kinase levels are variably elevated. Electromyography is sensitive and specific in the diagnosis of myopathy, showing abnormal motor unit action potentials that appear short in amplitude and brief in duration, and abnormal recruitment characterized by an early and full interference pattern. MRI of affected areas may be helpful by showing an abscess or focal area of inflammation in cases in which an infectious process is suspected. In most cases a muscle biopsy is essential in the diagnosis.

Treatment is tailored to the underlying cause. Corticosteroids or IVIG may provide benefit in immune-mediated and inflammatory myopathy. AZT should be discontinued if an alternative cause cannot be determined. HIV-associated myopathy is further discussed in Chapter 23.

Authier FJ, et al. Skeletal muscle involvement in human immunodeficiency virus-infected patients in the era of highly active antiretroviral therapy. *Muscle Nerve* 2005;32:247–260. [PMID: 15902690] (A comprehensive review of the types of muscle involvement in HIV infection.)

Verma S, Micsa E, Estanislao L, Simpson D. Neuromuscular complications in HIV. *Curr Neurol Neurosci Rep* 2004;4:62–67. [PMID: 14683631] (A general review.)

Prion Diseases

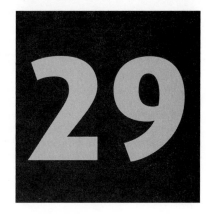

29

Lawrence S. Honig, MD, PhD

Prion diseases are a group of less common neurodegenerative disorders characterized by rapidly progressive dementia. Few other disorders resemble the clinical syndrome (Table 29–1). Prion diseases result from accumulation in the brain of an abnormal conformation of a cellular protein called prion protein (PrP). Prion diseases are unusual in that they may be sporadic, inherited, or transmissible (through infection by iatrogenic or oral intake exposures).

PrP is encoded by the prion gene (*PRNP*) on chromosome 20 and is a cell-surface glycoprotein of unclear function. It is expressed by a variety of cell types throughout the body. In the brain, normal cellular PrP (called PrP^c) is predominantly found in neurons and appears to play a role in synaptic function. In the disease state, PrP undergoes an abnormal post-translational change to produce a pathogenic conformation called either PrP^{sc} (scrapie inducing) or PrP^{res} (resistant to protease), which differs from PrP^c not in its amino acid sequence, but rather in its physical properties: the pathologic form includes a greater proportion of β-pleated sheet conformation, rendering the protein relatively insoluble and liable to the formation of protein deposits. What initiates a conformational shift from PrP^c to PrP^{res} is not understood; however, once present, PrP^{res} self-propagates by recruiting and converting the nonpathologic PrP^c to the PrP^{res} form. Recently, an additional molecular form of prion disease has been described in which there is an abnormal form of prion protein that is still partially sensitive to proteases.

Prion diseases occur in several clinically recognized human disorders, including Creutzfeldt-Jakob disease (CJD), variant Creutzfeldt-Jakob disease (vCJD), Gerstmann-Sträussler-Scheinker syndrome, fatal familial insomnia, and kuru. Prion diseases may have a sporadic, inherited, or transmissible pathogenesis.

CREUTZFELDT-JAKOB DISEASE

ESSENTIALS OF DIAGNOSIS

▶ Clinical triad of rapidly progressive dementia, myoclonus, and gait disorder—often accompanied by focal neurologic deficits

▶ CSF profile is acellular, but total protein, 14-3-3 protein, and tau may be elevated

▶ Magnetic resonance imaging (MRI) may show characteristic abnormalities on diffusion-weighted (DWI) and T2-weighted FLAIR images

▶ Brain biopsy provides definitive diagnosis

▶ General Considerations

The most common of the prion diseases, CJD can be subclassified as sporadic (sCJD), familial (fCJD), iatrogenic (iCJD), and variant (vCJD).

sCJD presumably results from post-translational structural protein changes, although spontaneous somatic *PRNP* gene mutation cannot be excluded. sCJD accounts for about 85% of all CJD cases and has an incidence of approximately 1–2 per 1 million people per year worldwide. Most patients who develop the disease are between the ages of 50 and 80 years. There are no clear modifiable or environmental risk factors, and there is no gender predilection. The only known genetic risk factor is homozygosity at codon 129 on the *PRNP* gene.

fCJD, a dominantly inherited condition resulting from one of about 20 recognized point mutations or insertions in the *PRNP* gene, represents approximately 10% of CJD cases.

Table 29–1. Differential Diagnoses of Rapidly Progressive Dementia With Abnormal Movements

Prion disease
Lewy body dementia
Voltage-gated potassium channel encephalitis
Other limbic encephalitides and paraneoplastic syndromes
Steroid-responsive encephalopathy (Hashimoto encephalopathy)
Herpes and other viral encephalitides (HIV, rabies, etc)
Toxic encephalopathies (eg, lithium intoxication)
Subacute sclerosing panencephalitis
Carcinomatous meningitis
Intravascular lymphomatosis

The phenotype of the disease is similar to sCJD, but onset is typically at an earlier age (eg, 30–50 years) and the disease course may be more protracted (eg, 1–10 years).

iCJD is a consequence of human-to-human transmission. Cases have been reported from a variety of transplants of nervous system–containing tissues, including corneal grafts, dura mater grafts, use of contaminated neurosurgical equipment, and human pituitary–derived growth hormone. There are no known cases of CJD transmission through transfusion of blood products, although such transmission has been found in four cases for variant CJD.

► Clinical Findings

A. Symptoms and Signs

Rapidly progressive dementia, focal neurologic deficits, and myoclonus are the classic clinical manifestations of sCJD. The earliest symptoms may be vague and constitutional (insomnia, anorexia, or fatigue) or psychiatric (depression, anxiety, emotional lability). Cognitive impairment (memory, concentration, aphasias, perceptual disorders), focal neurologic deficits (hemianopia, focal weakness, ataxia), and psychiatric abnormalities (hallucination and delusions) ensue shortly thereafter. Myoclonus, especially provoked by startle, is present in more than 80% of patients by the middle to late stages of the disease. The neurologic status deteriorates to akinetic mutism and then to death, typically within 1 year of clinical onset.

Other forms of CJD include Heidenhain variant in which initial symptoms are primarily visual-perceptual (visual hallucinations or illusions and cortical blindness) due to significant involvement of the occipital cortex. Some forms may present with prominent cerebellar involvement (Brownell-Oppenheimer variant), simulating Gerstmann-Sträussler-Scheinker syndrome, or with thalamic involvement (eg, sporadic fatal insomnia, which simulates fatal familial insomnia).

B. Diagnostic Studies

A probable diagnosis is based on clinical history and examination, and is supported by imaging and laboratory studies.

1. Cerebrospinal fluid (CSF) analysis—The CSF cell count and glucose level are typically normal, while the protein level may be mildly elevated. Elevations of CSF 14-3-3 protein and tau protein, neuronal proteins whose level in the CSF can increase following acute neuronal damage of various causes, may support the diagnosis of CJD if used in the proper clinical setting. Their presence does not exclude other diagnoses, and their absence does not exclude the diagnosis of CJD. Furthermore, these CSF tests are considerably less sensitive (50%) in more indolent cases of CJD, such as with vCJD or fCJD.

2. Electroencephalography—Findings are typically abnormal at some point in the course of disease. In sCJD, nonspecific background slowing is seen early in the disease; periodic, synchronous, biphasic or triphasic sharp wave complexes superimposed on a slow background rhythm are seen in the middle to late stages of the disease in up to 70% of patients, and a slow background rhythm is seen at the terminal stages. In the proper clinical setting the presence of periodic sharp wave complexes strongly supports the diagnosis of sCJD. Periodic sharp wave complexes are infrequently seen in iCJD and fCJD, and are not seen in vCJD.

3. Neuroimaging—MRI is the most sensitive noninvasive test to support the diagnosis of sCJD. Increased signal on diffusion-weighted imaging (DWI) sequences often occurs early in the disease. Signal abnormality may be particularly prominent in the cortical ribbon, caudate, and putamen. Increased signal on T2-weighted images, as seen on fluid-attenuated inversion recovery (FLAIR) sequences, may be found in the same brain regions, but appears to be a finding occurring later in disease course than DWI abnormalities.

4. Brain biopsy—Brain biopsy allows definitive diagnosis. Neuropathologic examination typically reveals spongiform change, which is a diffuse vacuolation of the neuropil, as well as prominent astrocytic gliosis and neuronal loss. Amyloid plaques consisting of prion protein are seen in rare cases. Biochemical tests on brain tissue are highly sensitive and specific for CJD and enable "typing" of the condition. The National Prion Disease Pathology Surveillance Center at Case Western Reserve University performs Western immunoblot analysis to detect the presence of abnormal PrP. Four different banding patterns, based on the glycosylation of the PrP, have been identified: types 1 and 2 are found with sCJD, type 3 is found with iCJD, and type 4 with vCJD (see below).

5. Genetic testing—DNA analysis can be performed on DNA from blood leukocytes or tissue to examine the *PRNP* gene for polymorphisms or mutations. For patients with a known family history of CJD, the presence of a known pathogenic mutation in the symptomatic patient is diagnostic.

VARIANT CREUTZFELDT-JAKOB DISEASE

This form of CJD was first recognized in 1996 in Great Britain when 10 cases of young-onset CJD with paresthesias and psychiatric symptoms were identified. A relationship of vCJD to

Table 29–2. Characteristics of Sporadic Versus New Variant Creutzfeldt-Jakob Disease

	sCJD	vCJD
Age at onset (median)	66 y; uncommon at age < 50 y	29 y; uncommon at age > 50 y
Duration of illness until death	~4 mo	~14 mo
Clinical symptoms	Dementia, early neurologic signs	Paresthesias, psychosis, late neurologic signs
Risk factor(s)	Homozygosity at codon 129	Methionine homozygosity at codon 129; exposure to BSE-tainted products (beef)
MRI findings	FLAIR sequences—high signal caudate and putamen DWI sequences—high signal caudate and putamen, or cortical ribbon, or both	FLAIR sequences—high signal posterior thalamus (pulvinar sign)
Elevated CSF 14-3-3 protein	~60–100% sensitivity	~50% sensitivity
EEG findings	Periodic sharp wave complexes	Nonspecific changes

BSE = bovine spongiform encephalopathy; CSF = cerebrospinal fluid; DWI = diffusion-weighted imaging; EEG = electroencephalographic; FLAIR = fluid-attenuated inversion recovery; MRI = magnetic resonance imaging; sCJD = sporadic Creutzfeldt-Jakob disease; vCJD = variant Creutzfeldt-Jakob disease.

an epidemic of bovine spongiform encephalopathy in cows was recognized, engendering much fear because it was the first set of cases in which a spongiform encephalopathy was transmitted from an animal species to humans. Over 200 cases worldwide have been reported, the great majority from the United Kingdom. Although bovine spongiform encephalopathy has been documented in a few cows in the United States that were imported from Canada, there have been no documented cases of vCJD originating from exposure to US bovine products.

▶ Clinical Findings

A. Symptoms and Signs

The syndrome is distinct from sCJD (Table 29–2). Affected individuals tend to be much younger (generally younger than age 40). Psychiatric symptoms (depression, anxiety, psychosis) are prominent early in the illness and are the presenting symptoms in 85% of patients. Painful paresthesias are common early in the disease, presumably resulting from thalamic involvement. Within months, more extensive neurologic findings may develop, including cognitive impairment, cerebellar ataxia, and abnormal movements (chorea, myoclonus, and dystonia). Both the neurologic and psychiatric symptoms progress relentlessly. They culminate in death on average 14 months after symptoms start, although some patients have had protracted clinical courses of years.

B. Diagnostic Studies

The CSF profile is usually normal except for elevated protein in some cases. CSF 14-3-3 protein is elevated in only 50% of patients. MRI is the most useful noninvasive test, showing increased signal on T2-weighted images in the posterior thalamus (pulvinar sign) in up to 90% of patients. Electroencephalography typically shows nonspecific abnormalities

such as background slowing. The periodic sharp wave complexes seen with sCJD are not present. Because the disease affects the lymphoreticular system, tonsil biopsy showing protease-resistant PrP may provide diagnostic information. A definitive diagnosis can be made by brain biopsy, with characteristic histopathologic change, and the presence of typical protease-resistant PrP protein on Western immunoblot analysis (type 4). Brain autopsy may show florid amyloid plaques in cerebral cortex and cerebellum, spongiform changes inclusive of the basal ganglia and thalamus, neuronal loss, and gliosis. No *PRNP* gene mutations have been identified in affected individuals, although all have been homozygous for methionine at codon 129.

GERSTMANN-STRÄUSSLER-SCHEINKER SYNDROME

ESSENTIALS OF DIAGNOSIS

▶ Most often familial (autosomal dominant)

▶ Ataxia and spasticity (prominent early features) and dementia (late in the disease)

▶ Normal CSF profile, lacking any clinically useful markers

▶ Neuropathology findings and DNA analysis provide definitive diagnosis

Gerstmann-Sträussler-Scheinker (GSS) syndrome is a prion disease characterized by ataxia and spasticity. Most cases are familial, inherited through an autosomal-dominant pattern and associated with mutations in codon 102, 105, 117, or 198 of the *PRNP* gene. GSS syndrome is rare, with an incidence of approximately 5 cases in 100 million people per year.

Individuals carrying a GSS mutation typically develop symptoms at age 40–70. There is heterogeneity of symptoms, depending on the mutation. In the most common form (codon 102 mutation), cerebellar ataxia and gait disturbance (ataxia, spasticity, rigidity) are the predominant symptoms. Dementia occurs late in the disease, and myoclonus is uncommon. In other forms, dementia (particularly with the codon 117 mutation), spasticity (codon 105 mutation), and parkinsonism (codons 117 and 198 mutations) are discriminating features. Typically, the illness progresses over 5–10 years, ending in death.

The diagnosis of GSS syndrome is based on family and clinical history. The CSF profile is usually unremarkable, and electroencephalography and MRI may show nonspecific abnormalities. Neuropathologic examination reveals findings similar to those of CJD, along with numerous amyloid plaques, particularly in the cerebellum. Neurofibrillary tangles are seen in some forms of the disease. Protease-resistant PrP can be demonstrated on Western immunoblot analysis. Definitive diagnosis is possible through DNA analysis for one of the *PRNP* gene mutations associated with the disease.

FATAL FAMILIAL INSOMNIA

ESSENTIALS OF DIAGNOSIS

▶ Most often familial (autosomal dominant)
▶ Prominent sleep disturbances and dysautonomia
▶ DNA genotype provides definitive diagnosis of inherited cases

Most cases of this very rare disease are familial (FFI), transmitted through an autosomal-dominant mutation occurring at PRNP codon 178 in the setting of methionine at codon 129. Some sporadic cases (now known as sFI) have also been reported. In both familial and sporadic forms, patients present between 40 and 60 years of age with progressive sleep disturbance and dysautonomia. Over the course of months, ataxia and dementia ensue. The sleep disturbance is characterized by a loss of the normal circadian sleep-activity pattern and manifests with insomnia, dreamlike confusional states during waking hours, and enacted dream states. Dysautonomia may be present with blood pressure and heart rate dysregulation, hyperhydrosis, hyperthermia, and excessive lacrimation.

The clinical and, in most cases, family history enables a probable diagnosis. CSF analysis is unremarkable, and abnormal levels of 14-3-3 protein are usually not detectable. Several endocrine disturbances have been reported. Electroencephalography shows abnormal sleep architecture, including a loss of the slow-wave and rapid-eye-movement phases of sleep as well as a total reduction in sleep time. The periodic sharp wave complexes seen in CJD are absent. MRI shows no distinctive abnormalities. A diagnosis may be missed on biopsy of cerebral cortex, because the pathology

seems to be relatively confined to the thalamus, particularly the anterior and dorsomedial nuclei. Affected tissue reveals protease-resistant PrP, neuronal loss, gliosis, and mild spongiform changes. Definitive diagnosis of FFI is possible through DNA sequencing of the *PRNP* gene.

KURU

Kuru was the first transmissible neurodegenerative disease to be identified in humans. Until 1968, this condition was endemic in New Guinea, transmitted from person to person during the preparation and consumption of human tissues of deceased individuals as part of ritual cannibalism. Following an incubation period of several years to several decades, symptoms progress in a somewhat predictable fashion over a span of 9–24 months, with early prominent ataxia and later dementia. Pathologic findings include spongiform changes, neuronal loss, astrogliosis, and protease-resistant PrP (especially in the cerebellum).

TREATMENT OF PRION DISEASES

Recent trials of quinacrine, a drug that in animal and in vitro studies prevents abnormal prion protein folding, have failed to show an effect on human disease. Because presently no effective treatment has been developed for any of the prion diseases, care is supportive, including hospice services. Death typically occurs within months to a few years from onset of symptoms. Prion diseases are reportable to the public health authorities. Autopsy is an important tool in the surveillance, study, and confirmation of cases. Genetic counseling is essential in patients whose disease has a suspected familial or genetic basis.

Du Plessis DG. Prion protein disease and neuropathology of prion disease. *Neuroimaging Clin N Am* 2008;18:163–182. [PMID 18319161]

Gambetti P, et al. A novel human disease with abnormal prion protein sensitive to proteases. *Ann Neurol* 2008;63:697–708. [PMID: 18571782]

Gambetti P, et al. Sporadic and familial CJD: Classification and characterisation. *Br Med Bull* 2003;66:213–239. [PMID: 14522861]

Heath CA, et al. Validation of diagnostic criteria for variant Creutzfeldt-Jakob disease. *Ann Neurol* 2010;67:761–770. [PMID: 20517937]

Johnson RT, Gibbs CJ Jr. Creutzfeldt-Jakob disease and related transmissible spongiform encephalopathies. *N Engl J Med* 1998;339:1994–2004. [PMID: 9869672]

Kovacs GG, Budka H. Molecular pathology of human prion disease. *Int J Mol Sci* 2009;10:976–999. [PMID: 19399233]

MacFarlane RG, et al. Neuroimaging findings in human prion disease. *J Neurol Neurosurg Psychiatry* 2007;78:665–670. [PMID: 17135459]

Van Everbroeck B, et al. Cerebrospinal fluid biomarkers in Creutzfeldt-Jakob disease. *Clin Neurol Neurosurg* 2005;107: 355–360. [PMID: 16023527]

Zerr I, et al. Updated clinical diagnostic criteria for sporadic Creutzfeldt-Jakob disease. *Brain* 2009;132:2659–2668. [PMID: 19773352]

Disorders of Cerebrospinal Fluid Dynamics

30

John C.M. Brust, MD

Increased intracranial pressure can be secondary to intracranial masses (eg, neoplasm, infection, hematoma, infarction), to generalized brain swelling (eg, anoxia/ischemia, Reye syndrome, hypertensive encephalopathy), or to increased venous pressure (eg, congestive heart failure, cerebral venous thrombosis). It can also be the result of impaired cerebrospinal fluid (CSF) circulation.

Disorders of CSF dynamics include obstructive hydrocephalus, normal pressure hydrocephalus, intracranial hypotension, and pseudotumor cerebri.

CSF pressure is normally 100–180 mm H_2O in adults and 30–60 mm H_2O in children. CSF volume ranges from 70–160 mL, and about 500 cc are formed each day; it thus turns over several times daily. It is principally made in the choroid plexus of the lateral, third, and fourth ventricles, and it exits the ventricles through the foramina of Magendie and Luschka, which connect the fourth ventricle with the subarachnoid space. CSF is principally absorbed through arachnoidal villi, which are invaginations of arachnoid membrane into the dural sinuses and veins of the cerebral convexities, the base of the brain, and the spinal nerve roots. When resorption cannot keep up with production, CSF pressure rises.

OBSTRUCTIVE HYDROCEPHALUS

ESSENTIALS OF DIAGNOSIS

▶ In infants: head enlargement, mental retardation, visual loss

▶ Acute in adults: headache, obtundation

▶ "Occult" in adults: unsteady or "magnetic" gait, altered mentation, urinary incontinence

▶ General Considerations

Obstructive, or tension, hydrocephalus is the result of obstruction of CSF flow either within the ventricles (including

the foramen of Monro connecting the third ventricle to the lateral ventricles and the midbrain aqueduct connecting the third ventricle to the fourth ventricle), at the foramina of Luschka and Magendie, or at the subarachnoid space at the base of the brain (the basal cisterns). (In the past a distinction was made between "communicating hydrocephalus," in which the ventricles remained in communication with subarachnoid space, and "noncommunicating hydrocephalus," in which they did not. This distinction is no longer considered meaningful, for in tension hydrocephalus obstruction is never total. Such an occurrence would be rapidly fatal.)

One or both foramina of Monro can be blocked by a third ventricular colloid cyst or other tumor. The aqueduct can be blocked by either congenital or acquired lesions, including mumps ependymitis, hemorrhage, or neoplasm. The foramina of Magendie and Luschka can be blocked by congenital failure of opening (Dandy-Walker syndrome), and the basal cisterns can be blocked by fibrosing posthemorrhagic or postinflammatory meningitis.

Controversial is whether tension hydrocephalus can result from obstruction of arachnoidal villi over the cerebral hemispheres. The weight of evidence is against such an occurrence. Radiographic enlargement of the subarachnoid spaces over and between the cerebral hemispheres is usually attributable to meningeal cysts or subdural hygromas.

In hydrocephalus secondary to nonprogressive disease, CSF absorption can equilibrate with CSF production; absorption increases because of increased CSF pressure, and production decreases because of compression of the choroid plexus. The result is a high-normal CSF pressure of 150–180 mm H_2O in the presence of continuing symptoms—so called "normal pressure hydrocephalus (NPH)."

▶ Clinical Findings

A. Symptoms and Signs

During the first few years of life, tension hydrocephalus causes head enlargement and, if untreated, mental retardation and visual loss. Hydrocephalus in the presence of closed cranial sutures does not enlarge the head, and the clinical picture depends on the degree of obstruction and the acuteness of the process.

With acute obstructive hydrocephalus (eg, following subarachnoid hemorrhage from a ruptured saccular aneurysm) headache and lethargy progress to coma. There may be papilledema, abducens palsy, hyperactive tendon reflexes, and signs of the causative lesion. Without treatment, brainstem reflexes are lost and death follows circulatory collapse.

Symptoms of "occult" obstructive hydrocephalus ("normal pressure hydrocephalus") develop more insidiously. There may be a history of subarachnoid hemorrhage, head trauma, or meningitis, but in many cases a cause, either present or remote, cannot be identified.

Occult hydrocephalus produces a triad of symptoms involving gait, mentation, and bladder function. In the great majority of patients gait disturbance appears first. There is impaired balance, and shuffling or "magnetic" gait can suggest parkinsonism but without tremor or bradykinesia. Backward falls are common, and eventually walking or even standing without assistance becomes impossible.

Mental symptoms rarely occur in the absence of gait disturbance, and unlike Alzheimer disease, which in its early stages tends to affect memory while preserving behavior and appearance, occult hydrocephalus produces mental symptoms suggestive of frontal lobe dysfunction: slow mental responses (abulia) and difficulty planning or sustaining activities. Urinary symptoms usually appear later in the course of illness, beginning with frequency and urgency and progressing to incontinence.

B. Laboratory Findings

Lumbar CSF pressure is usually normal or only mildly elevated, although monitoring of ventricular pressure sometimes reveals intermittent waves of higher pressure.

C. Imaging Studies

Computerized tomographic (CT) and magnetic resonance (MR) imaging in hydrocephalus, whether acute or occult, show ventricular enlargement disproportionate to sulcal widening. In elderly patients with concomitant diffuse brain atrophy (inappropriately sometimes called "hydrocephalus ex vacuo"), the findings on imaging can be ambiguous.

▶ Treatment & Prognosis

Treatment of acute hydrocephalus is by drainage of CSF through a ventricular catheter.

Treatment of occult hydrocephalus is with ventriculoatrial or ventriculoperitoneal shunting, but predicting which patients will have symptomatic improvement can be difficult. Favorable predictors are a history of subarachnoid hemorrhage or meningitis, ventricular enlargement without sulcal widening, CSF pressure above 155 mm H_2O, and improvement of gait following removal of 20–30 cc CSF by spinal tap.

Complications of shunting include postoperative subdural hematoma or hygroma, infection, shunt blockage within the ventricle, and overdrainage with orthostatic headache.

Bateman GA. The pathophysiology of idiopathic normal pressure hydrocephalus: Cerebral ischemia or altered venous hemodynamics? *Am J Neuroradiol* 2008;29(1):198–203. [PMID: 17925373] (Four decades after the first description of NPH, pathophysiologic mechanisms remain controversial.)

Eide PK, Sorteberg W. Diagnostic intracranial pressure monitoring and surgical management in idiopathic normal pressure hydrocephalus: A 6-year review of 214 patients. *Neurosurgery* 2010;66:80–91 [PMID: 20023540] (Increased intracranial pressure pulsatility predicts response to intraventricular shunting.)

INTRACRANIAL HYPOTENSION

ESSENTIALS OF DIAGNOSIS

► Orthostatic headache
► Low CSF pressure
► On MRI, dural gadolinium enhancement

▶ General Considerations

Lumbar puncture headache, caused by CSF leak at the needle site, occurs during standing, sometimes accompanied by stiff neck, nausea, and vomiting. It is promptly relieved by lying down. Repeat lumbar puncture sometimes shows mild pleocytosis, and MRI with gadolinium can show dural enhancement. The risk of lumbar puncture headache can be minimized by using a 22- or 24-gauge needle. The most effective treatment is a "blood patch"—injecting the patient's own blood into the spinal epidural space.

Spontaneous intracranial hypotension with similar symptoms can follow straining or trauma; in some cases no cause is apparent, but an arachnoidal tear is presumed. The great majority of tears, when identified, are at the level of the spine, especially thoracic.

▶ Clinical Findings
A. Symptoms and Signs

The most common symptom is headache in the upright position relieved by lying down. Headache can be steady or throbbing, and frontal, occipital, or diffuse. There may be nausea and vomiting. Cervical or interscapular pain can precede headache, and over weeks or months headache can become present during recumbency as well as standing.

Traction on intracranial structures can cause abducens paresis and visual blurring. Traction on nerve roots can cause radicular pain. Altered pressure within the inner ear can cause vertigo, tinnitus, or altered hearing.

B. Laboratory Findings

CSF pressure is low or even negative. CSF protein may be mildly elevated, and there may be lymphocytic pleocytosis or blood. CSF glucose is normal.

C. Imaging Studies

Normally a radioisotope such as indium-III, introduced intrathecally, is detected over the cerebral convexities within 24 hours. With CSF leaks, radioactivity is usually undetectable above the basal cisterns. There may be parathecal activity at the site of the leak.

Head MRI reveals diffuse dural enhancement with gadolinium, the result of compensatory increased intracranial blood volume. There may be reduction in size of the basal cisterns and subdural hygromas.

Myelography or CT/myelography may identify the site of the leak.

▶ Treatment

Sometimes the leak seals spontaneously during a few days of bed rest. Other times an extradural blood patch has a success rate of roughly 30% (much less than with post–lumbar puncture [LP] headache). For patients unresponsive to even multiple blood patches surgical repair is an option, but definitive localization of the leak can be difficult.

Mokri B. Low cerebrospinal fluid pressure syndromes. *Neurol Clin* 2004;22:55. [PMID: 15062528] (A comprehensive, practical review.)

PSEUDOTUMOR CEREBRI

 ESSENTIALS OF DIAGNOSIS

▶ Headache, diplopia, visual loss

▶ Elevated CSF pressure; normal CSF composition

▶ On imaging, no ventriculomegaly or mass

▶ General Considerations

Pseudotumor cerebri (PTC), a syndrome of increased intracranial pressure (ICP) without a space-occupying lesion, affects 0.9 per 100,000 people in the general population but 19 per 100,000 women 20–44 years of age who are 20% or more above ideal body weight. Women are nine times as often affected as men. The alternative term "benign intracranial hypertension" is a misnomer, for patients are at risk for permanent visual loss.

▶ Pathophysiology

A number of disorders are associated with PTC (Table 30–1). It is possible that their common pathophysiology is impaired

Table 30–1. Disorders Associated With Pseudotumor Cerebri

Idiopathic intracranial hypertension	**Increased CSF protein concentration**
	Guillain-Barré polyneuropathy
Drugs	Spinal oligodendroglioma
Vitamin A and isotretinoin	**Cerebral venous hypertension**
Tetracycline and related antibiotics	Venous sinus occlusion (hypercoagulable state, trauma, surgery, middle ear
Nitrofurantoin	infection)
Phenytoin	Arteriovenous malformation
Sulfonamides	Severe congestive heart failure
Quinolone antibiotics	Superior vena cava syndrome
Estrogen	**Hematologic**
Amiodarone	Iron deficiency anemia
Phenothiazines	Cryoglobulinemia
Cytarabine	Antiphospholipid antibody syndrome
Chlordecone	**Meningeal and infectious**
Cyclosporine	Chronic infectious and granulomatous meningitis (fungal, tuberculous,
Lithium carbonate	spirochetal, sarcoidosis)
Nalidixic acid	Carcinomatous and lymphomatous meningitis
Metabolic	Behçet disease
Corticosteroid therapy or withdrawal	Lyme disease
Cushing disease	HIV infection
Addison disease	Viral infections in children
Myxedema	**Other**
Hypoparathyroidism	Systemic lupus erythematosus
Menarche, pregnancy, oral contraceptives	Turner syndrome
Obesity and irregular menses	Sleep apnea
Polycystic ovary syndrome	

CSF resorption through the arachnoid villi into the venous sinuses. Such would be consistent with the normal ventricular size in PTC compared to the enlarged ventricles of obstructive hydrocephalus. In fact, venous sinus imaging in idiopathic PCT reveals a high incidence of transverse sinus stenosis.

Clinical Findings

A. Symptoms and Signs

Nearly all patients have headache, often daily and worse on awakening or with eye movement. Headaches may be throbbing with nausea and vomiting, and neck and back pain is sometimes present. Transient visual obscurations, unilateral or bilateral and lasting seconds, occur in 75% of patients. Pulsatile tinnitus and horizontal diplopia each occur in two thirds of patients. Constriction of the visual fields occurs early, and there can be rapid progression to blindness. Fifteen percent of patients reportedly have reduced visual acuity when first seen by a physician.

Papilledema (present in most but not all patients) is unilateral or bilateral. Goldman perimetry reveals enlargement of the physiologic blind spot and peripheral visual field constriction. Unilateral or bilateral lateral rectus palsy may be present. There are no symptoms or signs that cannot be attributed to increased intracranial pressure or papilledema.

B. Laboratory Findings

CSF pressure is 250 mm H_2O or greater. Values of 200–249 are equivocal except in children. CSF composition is normal.

C. Imaging Studies

CT or MRI shows normal-sized or small ventricles. The sella may be enlarged and filled with CSF ("empty sella syndrome"). No intracranial mass is evident. Magnetic resonance venography (MRV) may detect venous sinus stenosis and should be included in the workup of atypical patients with "idiopathic" PTC (men, children, nonobese women).

Differential Diagnosis

The principal diagnostic considerations are venous sinus obstruction, occult intracranial mass lesion, and chronic meningitis (including carcinomatous or lymphomatous). Choroid plexus papilloma can cause increased ICP when CSF production exceeds resorptive capacity.

Treatment & Prognosis

For obese patients treatment includes weight loss. Drugs that reduce CSF production include acetazolamide and

Table 30–2. Treatment of Pseudotumor Cerebri

Weight loss
Pharmacologic
Acetazolamide, 1–4 g/d in divided doses
Furosemide, 20–80 mg twice daily
Corticosteroids
Mannitol
Repeated LPs
Surgical
Optic nerve sheath decompression
Lumboperitoneal shunting
Venous sinus stenting

furosemide (Table 30–2). Most patients respond to these agents, but recurrence of symptoms is common when they are stopped. Corticosteroids can rapidly reduce ICP but are best reserved for emergency situations in which surgery is anticipated. The same applies to hypertonic mannitol. Lumbar puncture with CSF removal can similarly "buy time" when visual acuity is declining, but because of the rapid turnover of CSF, LP must be repeated frequently. CSF removal may be a necessary approach during the first half of pregnancy.

Surgical interventions to preserve vision include optic nerve sheath decompression and lumboperitoneal shunting. Each procedure reportedly produces visual improvement or stabilization in a majority of patients, but later deterioration requiring reintervention is common. In some centers venous sinus stenting is an option.

Arac A, et al. Efficacy of endovascular stenting in dural sinus stenosis for the treatment of idiopathic intracranial hypertension. *Neurosurg Focus* 2009;27(5):E14. [PMID: 19877792] (Reviewing 31 published cases, the authors conclude that a subgroup of patients with idiopathic intracranial hypertension have dural sinus stenosis and experience symptomatic resolution or improvement following endovascular stenting.)

Friedman DI. Pseudotumor cerebri. *Neurol Clin* 2004;22:99. [PMID: 15062530] (A review emphasizing diagnosis and treatment.)

Kesler A, et al. Idiopathic intracranial hypertension. Risk of recurrences. *Neurology* 2004;63:1737–1739. [PMID: 15534272] (Recurrences occurred in nearly 40% of patients with pseudotumor cerebri when acetazolamide was stopped.)

Randhawa S, Van Stavern GP. Idiopathic intracranial hypertension (pseudotumor cerebri). *Curr Opin Ophthalmol* 2008;19: 445–453. [PMID: 18854688] (An up-to-date review.)

Sleep Disorders

31

Anne Helena Remmes, MD

Sleep abnormalities occur in a large percentage of the population and typically are not addressed as part of a comprehensive medical evaluation. Sleepiness per se increases the risk of motor vehicle and workplace accidents, and decreases performance and quality of life. If not identified and treated appropriately, sleep disorders can result in, or exacerbate, medical and psychiatric disorders, including hypertension, coronary or cerebral vascular disease, obesity, and depression. Volitional sleep curtailment becomes a major problem as lives increase in complexity and the availability of late-night entertainment encourages late bedtimes. We sleep, on average, an hour less at night than we did 100 years ago, although our sleep need remains the same, around 8 hours a night.

Table 31–1 presents a markedly abbreviated list of the major sleep disorders.

SLEEP STAGES

Sleep consists of five discreet stages, each with unique properties. Most delta sleep occurs in the first third of the night; the second part of the night consists of alternating periods of rapid eye movement (REM) and stage 2 sleep.

Stage 1 consists of drowsiness or light sleep, with theta activity appearing in the electroencephalogram (EEG), and rolling eye movements. Stage 2 involves primarily theta activity. Stages 3 and 4 consist of slow wave or delta sleep, with high-amplitude, slow wave activity, and decreased arousability. REM (rapid eye movement) sleep is a stage of deep sleep, with EEG patterns that are similar to the waking EEG and periodic rapid eye movements.

SLEEP TESTING

Sleep patterns can be evaluated using a polysomnogram (PSG), the multiple sleep latency test (MSLT), sleep logs, or a combination of these methods. The PSG evaluates nocturnal sleep, including sleep architecture (progression of sleep from one stage to another through the night), oxygenation, airflow, and limb movements, and incorporates both EEG and

electrocardiogram (ECG) readings. The MSLT is administered the day after a nocturnal PSG. Four to five brief napping opportunities are conducted across the day to determine the extent of daytime sleepiness and to evaluate abnormalities of REM and other stages of sleep. Sleep logs provide a daily record of time in bed awake and asleep, and napping (volitional or "dozing").

Espana RA, Scammell TE. Sleep neurobiology for the clinician. *Sleep* 2004;27:811–820. [PMID: 15283019] (An overview of the principles of sleep mechanisms.)

Garbarino S, et al. The contributing role of sleepiness in highway accidents. *Sleep* 2001;24:203–206. [PMID: 11247057] (One of many articles on the dangers of sleepiness in our daily lives.)

INSOMNIA

ESSENTIALS OF DIAGNOSIS

▶ Difficulty falling or remaining asleep
▶ Daytime dysfunction as a result of poor-quality sleep

▶ General Considerations

Approximately 30% of the population of the United States has had transient insomnia, and 17% suffers from a chronic condition. **Primary insomnia** (idiopathic, psychophysiologic, or sleep state misperception syndrome) is an organic predisposition to fragile sleep, without a coexistent medical or psychiatric disorder. Idiopathic insomnia begins in childhood and persists through life with exacerbations and remissions; psychophysiologic insomnia typically is precipitated by a stressful life event or illness and persists thereafter. A patient with sleep state misperception syndrome is unable to accurately perceive sleep, in spite of normal sleep on a

Table 31–1. Abbreviated Classification of Major Sleep Disorders

Primary Insomnias
Idiopathic insomnia
Psychophysiologic insomnia
Sleep state misperception syndrome
Insomnias Secondary to Other Conditions
Medical or psychiatric disorders
Restless legs syndrome (RLS) or periodic limb movements of sleep (PLMS)
Use or withdrawal from illicit drugs, prescribed or over-the-counter medications, or alcohol
Obstructive sleep apnea/hypopnea syndrome (OSAHS)
Hypersomnias and Excessive Daytime Sleepiness
Insufficient sleep
OSAHS
Narcolepsy
Central nervous system hypersomnolence
Long sleep need
Circadian-mediated Dyssomnias
Jet lag
Shift work
Advanced sleep phase disorder
Delayed sleep phase disorder
Parasomnias
Rapid eye movement (REM) behavioral disorder
Sleepwalking
Sleep terrors

PSG. All patients with primary insomnia respond to the same treatment.

In contrast, **secondary insomnia** occurs in an individual as a consequence of significant ongoing psychic stress, a medical disorder, or another sleep disorder (eg, periodic limb movements of sleep, shift-work sleep disorder, jet lag, obstructive sleep apnea syndrome), or may coexist as a component of psychiatric disease. It can result from poor sleep hygiene or disruptive environmental conditions. Recreational drugs, medications (prescription and over the counter), alcohol, and caffeine may play a role. Untreated insomnia may result in serious social, occupational, and cognitive dysfunction, and is associated with increased risk for major depression.

▶ Clinical Findings
A. Symptoms and Signs

Insomnia is a self-reported condition. Primary insomnia can be differentiated from secondary insomnia by detailed questioning, including duration and pattern of the insomnia, current and prescribed medications, drug or alcohol use, medical and psychiatric disorders, and symptoms of other sleep disorders (snoring, leg irritability, or abnormal movements). A sleep log can identify dysfunctional sleep habits, such as napping or dozing during the day and variable bed/waking times.

Table 31–2. Behavioral Measures Used in the Treatment of Insomnia

Instruct patients to
• Regulate sleep period (uniform bedtime and rising time), 7 days a week.
• Disengage in a chair for 1 h before bed, reading something with good visual imagery that is neither boring nor too stimulating. During this time, there should be no phone calls, computer use, or interaction with others.
• Avoid clock-watching during the night.
• Get out of bed if not asleep in (estimated) 20–30 min.
• Seek exposure to sunlight within 2 h of waking in the morning.
• Avoid naps or dozing off during the day.

Patients with onset insomnia are unable to fall asleep at the beginning of the night. Those with maintenance insomnia have frequent or prolonged awakenings during the night or a complaint that sleep is superficial. In terminal insomnia, patients awaken an hour or two before the desired time (often a sign of depression).

B. Diagnostic Testing

Patients who do not respond to behavioral and appropriate pharmacologic treatment should have a PSG to rule out another primary sleep disorder and to document the severity of sleep disruption. Further appropriate testing may be necessary if the history and physical examination are suggestive of other medical or psychiatric disorders.

▶ Treatment

A combination of behavioral (Table 31–2), cognitive (muscle relaxation and guided visual imagery techniques), and pharmacologic (Table 31–3) treatment is likely to produce the best results. Although long-term pharmacologic treatment of insomnia is controversial, untreated insomnia can lead to a more severe and refractory condition than can chronic, appropriate use of hypnotic medication.

Léger D, et al. Medical and socio-professional impact of insomnia. *Sleep* 2002;25:625–629. [PMID: 12224841] (Outlines the consequences of sleepiness for society.)

Rosen R, Lewin D, Goldberg L, Woolfolk R. Psychophysiological insomnia: Combined effects of pharmacotherapy and relaxation-based treatments. *Sleep Med* 2000;1:279–288. [PMID: 11040460] (Medication alone is not the optimal treatment for insomnia; this article compares the effectiveness of various modes of treatment.)

Spiegel K, Tasali E, Penev P, VanCauter E. Sleep curtailment in healthy young men is associated with decreased leptin levels, elevated ghrelin levels and increased hunger and appetite. *Ann Intern Med* 2004;141:846–850. [PMID: 15583226] (Sleep intrinsically is necessary for health; this assessment of sleep curtailment and subsequent hunger improves understanding of the relationship between obesity and sleepiness.)

Table 31–3. Treatment of Insomnia

Class/Drug	Dose	Comments
Nonbenzodiazepines		
Zolpidem (Ambien)	5 mg, 10 mg	Elderly—5 mg is optimal dose Medication should be taken at bedtime to avoid sleepwalking or sleep-eating episodes
Zaleplon (Sonata)	5 mg, 10 mg	May be taken for nocturnal awakening, if 4 h of sleep period remain
Eszopiclone (Lunesta)	2 mg, 3 mg	Efficacy for onset as well as maintenance insomnia
Benzodiazepines		
Temazepam	7.5 mg, 15 mg, 30 mg, 60 mg	—
Clonazepam	0.25 mg, 0.5 mg, 1 mg	—
Tricyclic Antidepressants		
Sinequan	10 mg/mL	Used for sleep maintenance, not onset
Amitriptyline	10 mg, 20 mg	Administer 3-10 drops in water

NARCOLEPSY

ESSENTIALS OF DIAGNOSIS

► Daytime sleep attacks
► Abrupt episodes of weakness
► Paralysis on transitions to and from sleep
► Hallucinatory experiences

▶ General Considerations

Narcolepsy occurs in more than 200,000 Americans. The vast majority of cases are idiopathic, although there are reports of temporal association with hypothalamic-pituitary disorders (tumor, arteriovenous malformation, stroke). Symptoms may begin as early as 3 years of age, but more than 90% of patients develop the disorder in early adulthood. Symptoms persist throughout life and often are disabling. First-degree relatives have a 1–2% risk of developing narcolepsy.

▶ Pathogenesis

The cerebrospinal fluid of narcoleptics shows a low or absent level of hypocretin/orexin, a neuropeptide produced in cells of the hypothalamus that influences REM sleep.

▶ Clinical Findings

A. Symptoms and Signs

All the symptoms of the narcolepsy tetrad are a result of REM-associated phenomena appearing at inappropriate times. The primary symptom is abrupt, episodic, irresistible daytime sleep attacks with full wakefulness following the attacks. The attacks may occur in any situation, even during conversation, and last minutes or longer. "True" narcolepsy includes cataplexy, a sudden loss of muscle tone evoked by a sudden strong emotion (laughter, anger, startle). The cataplectic attack may be subtle (a loosening of the jaw, buckling of the knees, or a head bob), or there may be complete body collapse. Extraocular muscles are typically not involved. These episodes are brief and vary across the patient's life span, from several each day to 1–2 episodes in total.

Sleep paralysis at the onset or termination of sleep consists of a transient inability to move, speak, or open the eyes. Vivid, frightening hypnagogic (sleep onset) or hypnopompic (on awakening) hallucinatory experiences may occur in association with the sleep paralysis or alone. They are typically visual but may be auditory or tactile. These experiences may be reported as dreamlike, although the patient is aware of being awake. Narcoleptics report disturbed nocturnal sleep.

B. Diagnostic Testing

1. Blood tests—Genetic testing for HLA DR2/DQB1* 0602 may be useful in patients with symptoms suggestive of narcolepsy but not definitive. This HLA marker is found in 30% of patients without the disorder and may be absent in a narcoleptic patient without cataplexy.

2. Polysomnography and multiple sleep latency test—A full-night PSG rules out other causes of daytime sleepiness and documents a short onset to sleep and to the first REM period as well as fragmentation of sleep architecture. On MSLT, there is a short latency to sleep onset and to REM sleep in two or more naps. One week of sleep logs prior to the night of testing is useful, because severe sleep deprivation can produce confusing results.

Differential Diagnosis

Excessive daytime sleepiness is a nonspecific symptom of insufficient or poor-quality sleep. Sleep attacks, however, are unique in their abruptness, and the presence of cataplexy confirms the diagnosis of narcolepsy rather than another sleep disorder. Patients with severe sleep fragmentation for any reason (eg, sleep apnea, shift-work sleep disorder, jet lag) may have episodes of sleep paralysis on awakening and early-onset REM sleep on PSG, in addition to severe excessive daytime sleepiness. Clarification is made by careful history, PSG, and sleep logs.

Complications

Delay in diagnosis and treatment carries the risk of motor-vehicle accidents and self-injury from sleepiness and cataplexy. Narcolepsy can lead to poor school and work performance, reduced self-esteem, and reactive depression.

Treatment

A. Pharmacotherapy (Table 31–4)

With appropriate medication the response rate is excellent. Often a combination of a stimulant (eg, modafinil, which has a long onset and duration of action) with dextroamphetamine or methylphenidate (shorter onset and duration of action) provides optimal therapeutic response. Oxybutyrate taken at night is highly effective in patients with cataplexy and fragmented nocturnal sleep.

B. Behavioral Measures

Patients should be instructed to maintain regular sleep hours, take routine brief naps if required, and avoid frequent time-zone changes. Career counseling may be necessary to identify inappropriate job choices (shift work, transportation industry, extended periods of inactivity).

Ripley B, et al. CSF hypocretin/orexin levels in narcolepsy and other neurological conditions. *Neurology* 2001;57:2253–2258. [PMID: 11756606] (Hypocretin is essential to sleep-wake mechanisms; the authors relate hypocretin deficiencies to sleep and neurologic status.)

PARASOMNIAS

Several disorders occur during sleep that are not abnormalities of the primary sleep-wake mechanisms. They do not necessarily result in fragmented sleep or daytime sleepiness, but they have other undesirable consequences, such as the interjection of motor, verbal, or experiential phenomena into sleep. They are classified by the symptoms and the stage of sleep with which they are primarily associated.

1. REM Sleep Behavioral Disorder

ESSENTIALS OF DIAGNOSIS

- ▶ Violent jerking, thrashing, or shouting in sleep
- ▶ Accompanied by vivid dreams

REM sleep behavioral disorder (RBD) occurs in adults, predominantly men older than 50 years of age. Acute RBD episodes can be precipitated by stimulants, psychoactive medications, and alcohol withdrawal. Although 40–50% of cases are idiopathic and not associated with other pathology, there is an increased incidence of chronic RBD in patients with a variety of neurologic disorders, particularly Parkinson disease, progressive supranuclear palsy, multisystem atrophy, and narcolepsy.

RBD is characterized by loss of the atonia that normally accompanies REM sleep. The symptoms (body twitches, kicks, and vocalizations) occur during REM sleep, typically in the second half of the night. The patient appears to be enacting a combative dream and is at risk for serious injury to him- or herself or a bed partner. Due to the violent and potentially injurious nature of RBD, PSG testing with video to confirm the diagnosis is mandatory.

Violent behavior during sleep can accompany many disorders, and the differential diagnosis for RBD includes seizures, periodic limb movement disorder, sleep terrors, and obstructive sleep apnea syndrome.

Clonazepam, 0.5–2.0 mg at bedtime, is the most effective medication for this disorder, with excellent control in more than 85% of patients. The sleeping environment should be

Table 31–4. Treatment of Narcolepsy and Cataplexy

Symptom	Drug	Dose		
		AM	Noon	4 PM
Daytime sleepiness	Modafinil	100–200 mg	100–200 mg	—
	Methylphenidate	5–20 mg	5 mg	5 mg
	Dextroamphetamine	5–15 mg	5–15 mg	5 mg
Cataplexy or sleep paralysis	Oxybutyrate	9–15 g	—	—
	Protriptyline	15–40 mg	—	—

cleared of potentially dangerous objects should a breakthrough episode occur.

Matheson J, Saper C. REM sleep behavioral disorder, a dopaminergic deficiency disorder? *Neurology* 2003;61:1328–1329. [PMID: 14638948]

2. Sleepwalking

ESSENTIALS OF DIAGNOSIS

- ► Episodes of nocturnal walking and talking
- ► Occurs in the first third of the night
- ► Lack of recall of the event
- ► Absence of associated autonomic signs

► General Considerations

Sleepwalking occurs in the first third of the night, associated with non-REM sleep. It is characterized by lack of responsiveness to the environment.

Episodes are facilitated by events that increase slow wave sleep, such as jet lag, prior sleep deprivation, and fever, and are triggered by factors that fragment sleep (stress, pain, illness, obstructive sleep apnea syndrome, environmental stimuli). Occasional episodes are seen in 30–45% of healthy children. The peak age of occurrence is about 5 years, although the disorder may continue into puberty and, occasionally, adulthood. There is an increased familial association of sleepwalking with sleep terrors and deep sleepers. In children, sleepwalking is not associated with psychopathology. In adults it may coexist with psychiatric disorders.

► Clinical Findings

A. Symptoms and Signs

Characteristically, the patient sits up out of apparently deep sleep and appears awake but is unresponsive and may display automatic behaviors, such as pulling at night clothes or smoothing the hair. He or she may rise and ambulate in a calm, purposeful way, navigating obstructions and opening doors or windows. Although there is generally some clumsiness, complex tasks may be performed. There usually is no recall of the events or reports of associated dreaming. Events are generally brief (< 15 minutes) but may be prolonged and terminate spontaneously, typically with a return to either the patient's own or a parent's bed. Several events may occur per night.

B. Diagnostic Testing

Although no testing is necessary for infrequent prototypical events, unusual behaviors warrant a general PSG. The PSG documents an abrupt transition from deep sleep to a slow waking EEG pattern. The events observed and recorded in the laboratory may be incomplete because of the restrictions of the wires. There are no signs of autonomic arousal associated with these events.

► Differential Diagnosis

Sleepwalking events are stereotypic and not generally confused with other disorders, although seizure disorders (complex partial seizures or episodic nocturnal wanderings) may present with episodes of similar nocturnal activity. Seizures, however, can occur in any stage of sleep, and testing usually reveals epileptiform discharges associated with the events or during wakefulness.

► Complications

The potential for self-injury is of greatest concern. Patients may stumble and fall, risking head injuries; walk into traffic in the street; or open a window and step out, thinking it is a door. Attempts to intervene and awaken the patient during an event may lead to violent behavior, causing injury.

► Treatment

No attempt should be made to awaken the patient. Gentle redirection back to bed and protection from injury should allow the attack to terminate spontaneously. Parents should be assured that these events do not reflect psychiatric illness and that eventually they will be outgrown. Sufficient sleep with regular hours should be encouraged and the sleeping environment freed of potential dangers. Doors and windows should be locked or partially obstructed to deflect access. If the events are long or frequent, a low dose of short-acting benzodiazepine or tricyclic antidepressant at bedtime should be considered. Relaxation techniques may be useful.

3. Sleep Terrors (Night Terrors, Pavor Nocturnus)

ESSENTIALS OF DIAGNOSIS

- ► Abrupt arousal with a piercing scream
- ► Terrified behavior
- ► Lack of recall of the event
- ► Increased autonomic nervous system activity

► General Considerations

Sleep terrors are primarily a disorder of children, and in 90% of cases there is a family history of sleep terrors or somnambulism. The peak age of occurrence is 5–7 years, and it is rarely seen in adults. As with sleepwalkers, there is no associated psychopathology.

▶ Clinical Findings

A. Symptoms and Signs

A sleep terror is a terrifying experience for an uninitiated parent, although not for the child. The child suddenly sits up out of a deep sleep, appears to be awake, and emits a series of piercing screams. There are behavioral and physiologic signs of true terror, with increased cardiac and respiratory rates, sweating, and pupillary dilation. The episodes are brief (< 5 minutes), self-terminating, and the child has no recollection of the event on awakening, although there may be a vague frightening memory. Episodes may occur several times per night and may evolve into a sleepwalking episode. Like somnambulism, the events respond poorly to intervention, leading to increased terror and perhaps violent, injurious behavior.

B. Diagnostic Testing

Polysomnography is generally not necessary. The PSG findings will be similar to those of somnambulism, but with associated tachycardia, tachypnea, and decreased skin resistance (sweating) associated with the events.

▶ Differential Diagnosis

Dream anxiety attacks (nightmares) can be differentiated from sleep terrors by their usual appearance in the second half of the night when REM sleep occurs, by the patient's awareness of events as they occur, and by the recollection of a frightening dream on awakening. Nocturnal panic attacks typically are not associated with vocalizations, and the symptoms are present in the waking state.

▶ Treatment

The treatment of sleep terrors follows the same principles as that of sleepwalking. Parents should be educated as to the nature of the disorder and how to respond to the attacks. Low-dose tricyclic antidepressants at bedtime should be used when necessary.

4. Confusional Arousals (Nocturnal Sleep Drunkenness)

ESSENTIALS OF DIAGNOSIS

▶ Disorientation on awakening during the night
▶ Poor recall of events
▶ Slow reaction time

Confusional arousal is an elaboration of common "sleep inertia," which may be seen in anyone who is awakened from a deep sleep. It typically occurs in young children and gradually resolves over childhood. It may be seen occasionally in adults, particularly in deep sleepers or after insufficient sleep.

The child awakens confused, typically early in the night, vaguely aware of the surroundings, with no evident fright or attempt at ambulation. There may be some automatisms, such as inarticulate vocalizations or other inappropriate activity.

Compared with other arousal disorders, there is no appearance of fright, increased autonomic activity, or ambulation. Older adults with REM behavioral disorder may have some confusion associated with arousal, but this disorder occurs in the latter part of the night when REM sleep is more prominent and there is directed activity with vivid dream recall. Confusional arousals may occur in association with dementia, in substance abusers, in a variety of medical illnesses, and in the elderly.

Treatment is typically not necessary.

Mehlenbeck R, Spirito A, Owens J, Boergers J. The clinical presentation of partial arousal parasomnias. *Sleep Med* 2000;1:307–312. [PMID: 14638948] (Childhood arousal syndromes are fascinating, poorly understood phenomena; the clinical presentations in this article are apt.)

OBSTRUCTIVE SLEEP APNEA/HYPOPNEA SYNDROME

ESSENTIALS OF DIAGNOSIS

▶ Nocturnal snoring, gasping, or snorting
▶ Daytime sleepiness or poor concentration
▶ Constricted upper airway

▶ General Considerations

The spectrum of respiratory dysfunctional events during sleep includes snoring (vibration of the tissues of the upper airway), upper airway resistance syndrome (increased breathing effort without decrease in airflow or oxygenation), hypopnea (partial airway obstruction with decreased airflow and minimal oxyhemoglobin desaturation), and apnea (repetitive, periodic complete airway obstruction for more than 10 seconds, with decreased airflow and oxyhemoglobin desaturation and, when severe, cardiac acceleration or deceleration).

Each may cause a range of symptoms and result in significant sleep fragmentation and daytime sleepiness, even without oxyhemoglobin desaturation. Obstructive sleep apnea/hypopnea syndrome (OSAHS) is best known, but upper airway resistance syndrome and sleep-disruptive snoring are far more ubiquitous.

OSAHS is typically, but not uniformly, associated with snoring and increased respiratory effort. These respiratory events may occur hundreds of times a night, last 10–60 seconds or longer, and may result in oxygen desaturation and cardiac changes. OSAHS frequently occurs in obese patients, but it may occur in anyone, including children, with constriction of the upper airway for any reason (eg, congenital or juvenile rheumatoid arthritis–associated retrognathia, hypertrophic tonsils or nasal turbinates, hypothyroidism with macroglossia, upper airway myopathy, and acromegaly).

Patients with OSAHS have an increased risk of hypertension (40%), coronary artery disease, cardiac arrhythmia, stroke, and death from motor vehicle accidents due to daytime sleepiness. Young patients with simple snoring (without apnea) have an increased risk of early-onset hypertension.

▶ Clinical Findings

A. Symptoms and Signs

The nocturnal symptoms of OSAHS often are not perceived by the patient but are reported by a concerned or disturbed bed partner. There is observed snoring (which may be loud); arousals with snorting, coughing, or gasping; or episodes of arrested breathing, particularly when the patient is lying supine. The patient may be unaware of significant nocturnal symptoms but may report nocturia, esophageal reflux, restless sleep, or sweating.

The primary daytime symptoms of OSAHS, excessive daytime sleepiness, sleep "drunkenness" (extended grogginess after morning awakening), and cognitive impairment, are nonspecific symptoms related to poor-quality sleep. Patients may deny daytime sleepiness but on close probing may report an inability to remain awake when inactive, such as when watching television at night or when performing automatic tasks such as driving. There may be mood complaints (fatigue, depression, or irritability). About 50% of patients report dull, generalized morning headaches.

Obesity (basal metabolic index > 30 kg/m^2) is a primary indicator of apnea in men (apnea may exacerbate obesity). Neck circumference of more than 40 cm is highly correlated with apnea in both sexes.

In the upper airway examination, the clinician should look for

1. Nasal turbinate hypertrophy obstructing the nasal airway
2. Retrognathia and overbite
3. A high and narrow hard palate
4. Narrow maxilla
5. Macroglossia
6. Constricted retroglossal space
7. Erythematous, thick, or elongated soft palate and uvula
8. Tonsillar hypertrophy
9. Collapse of the lateral pharyngeal walls

B. Diagnostic Testing

Full-night polysomnography is indicated for any individual suspected of OSAHS. Anyone with unresponsive insomnia,

Table 31–5. Alternative Treatment Measures for Obstructive Sleep Apnea

Mandibular advancement with an appliance
Postural training with balls on back
Surgery; common procedures include
- Nasal turbinate decompression
- Decompression of soft palate and uvula (uvulopalatopharyngoplasty and laser-assisted uvulopalatoplasty)
- Decompression of base of tongue
- Tracheostomy or other more aggressive surgical techniques (in extreme cases)
- Atrial pacing (technique that has recently shown some promise)

chronic cluster headaches, or a refractory medical condition (eg, hyperthyroidism, hypertension, cardiac failure) should be considered for a PSG. Split-night studies (during which the first half of the night is used for diagnosis and the second half of the night for application and titration of continuous airway pressure) may be more convenient for the patient but may underestimate the apnea severity, compromising treatment, and such studies may miss other coexisting sleep disorders. Portable home-based studies are not recommended for the initial diagnosis.

▶ Treatment

The treatment of OSAHS depends on the severity of the disorder. The current gold standard for patients with moderate to severe apnea is continuous positive airway pressure. For patients with mild apnea, upper airway resistance syndrome, or sleep-disruptive snoring, the measures outlined in Table 31–5 are alternatives. Moderate apnea may respond to a combination of these measures, although follow-up studies are necessary to ensure control of the apnea.

In addition to directly addressing the apnea syndrome, an aggressive weight-loss program may be warranted in an overweight or obese patient. However, concurrent treatment of apnea is mandatory. Other treatment methods, such as nasal dilators, electrical stimulation of the upper airway, and various medications (stimulants, progestational agents, and serotonin agonists) have not proven effective.

Garrigue S, et al. Benefit of atrial pacing in sleep apnea syndrome. *N Engl J Med* 2002;346:404–411. [PMID: 11832528] (Although it has not become a "routine" practice, atrial pacing may be one hope of the future for apnea patients who are refractory to other treatment modalities.)

Lavie P, Hoffstein V. Sleep apnea syndrome: A possible contributing factor to resistant hypertension? *Sleep* 2001;24:721–725. [PMID: 11560187] (Sleep apnea sufferers are often unidentified and therefore unconcerned about the risk of the abnormal nocturnal respiratory events; the authors identify OSAS as a potential factor in the poor control of hypertension.)

PERIODIC LIMB MOVEMENTS OF SLEEP

ESSENTIALS OF DIAGNOSIS

► Brief jerks or flexor withdrawal of either leg

► Occurrence during stage 1 or 2 sleep

► Frequent co-occurrence with restless legs syndrome

► Nonrefreshing sleep or daytime cognitive dysfunction

Restless legs syndrome (RLS) is discussed in Chapter 15. Unlike RLS, periodic limb movements of sleep (PLMS) occurs during stage 1 or 2 sleep, sometimes causing arousal or fragmentation of sleep continuity, resulting in daytime sleepiness. Brief jerks or flexor withdrawals affect either leg, and may also involve the arms. Most patients with RLS have PLMS, but only a third with PLMS have RLS.

General polysomnographic findings include periodic limb movements during presleep wakefulness due to RLS, often prolonging sleep latency. Sleep is fragmented by periodic limb movements, with disruption of sleep architecture and brief arousals. The movement-associated arousals are typically evident as EEG changes but may be merely minor, brief changes in the cardiac rate.

Several conditions must be differentiated from PLMS. Nocturnal leg cramping is a common condition, involving acute, painful contraction of the large muscles of the calves. The cramps are not periodic, and they are of short duration. A sleep start (hypnic myoclonus) is a fairly prominent single body jerk that occurs at the transition between wake and sleep and is seen in normal individuals. During REM sleep there are brief, sharp twitches (fragmentary myoclonus) that are more prominent in the hands and repetitive but not rhythmic or periodic. Nocturnal seizures may manifest as minor focal twitches but may be associated with enuresis.

Treatment of PLMS is necessary when the movements interfere with sleep integrity or when coexisting RLS requires treatment. Various agents can relieve symptoms of both PLMS and RLS (Table 31–6). Dosing should occur at bedtime for PLMS and precede the expected appearance of symptoms for RLS (eg, prior to evening relaxation and at least 30 minutes before getting into bed at night). Patients should avoid stimulants (caffeine, drugs) and alcohol, exercise regularly but not excessively and not within 4 hours of bedtime, and maintain good sleep hygiene.

Comella C. Restless legs syndrome: Treatment with dopaminergic agents. *Neurology* 2002;58(Suppl 1):S87–S92. [PMID: 11909990] (Addresses the response of dopaminergic agents, which have become the first drug of choice in treating RLS and PLMS.)

Table 31–6. Treatment of Restless Legs Syndrome and Periodic Leg Movements of Sleep

Class/Drug	Dose (mg)
Dopamine Agonist	
Pramipexole	0.125–2
Ropinirole	0.25–4
Dopamine Precursor	
Levodopa/carbidopa	100/25 (regular or slow-release 200/500)
Antiepileptic Drug	
Gabapentin	100–800
Benzodiazepine	
Clonazepam	0.5–2.0
Temazepam	15–30
Opiate	
Morphine sulphate (extended release)	15–60
Oxycodone	10–40
Codeine	15–60

CIRCADIAN-MEDIATED DYSSOMNIAS

ESSENTIALS OF DIAGNOSIS

► Feeling "out of synch" with the environment

► Daytime sleepiness and cognitive dysfunction

► Mood problems (eg, irritability, depression)

Since we have been able to "light up" our lives 24 hours a day, circadian rhythm disorders have become an increasing problem. With an expanding global economy, commuting to another part of the world several times a month has become a commonplace work requirement. The result is excessive daytime sleepiness, nausea, a sense of confusion, and cognitive dysfunction. The major disorders that fall within the category of circadian-mediated dyssomnias are jet lag, shift-work sleep disorder, delayed sleep phase disorder, and advanced sleep phase disorder.

Jet lag occurs when a person travels across two or more time zones in a 24-hour period. This typically results in either inability to remain awake through the remainder of the day at one's final destination or an inability to fall asleep.

Shift-work sleep disorder can affect people who work regular evening or night shifts, or rotating shifts that require changing sleep times. For unknown reasons, this pattern is associated with increased risk of breast cancer.

Delayed sleep phase disorder describes the inability to fall asleep at "socially respectable" hours, the preferred sleep onset time being after midnight. Although this pattern is often normal sleep behavior in teenagers, it may persist into adulthood, resulting in chronic tardiness at school or work, or severe daytime sleepiness and cognitive problems due to insufficient sleep.

Advanced sleep phase disorder is seen in older adults, particularly after retirement or associated with medical illness. They grow sleepy and retire in the early evening and awaken in the early morning hours. The resulting social isolation can lead to depression.

▶ Treatment

Initial treatment measures include identifying the desired sleep hours and strictly regulating them, and providing exposure to light (eg, 10-lux light box or outside in daylight; inside in a bright atrium is not sufficient) at the beginning of the day or work shift, and exposure to late afternoon light for those with advanced sleep phase disorder. Some patients may require medication to facilitate sleep during the expected sleep phase and, if needed, to maintain wakefulness (modafinil) during the expected wake phase. Patients should be advised to wear dark glasses at appropriate times when out of synch with the ambient light-dark cycle.

Garbarino S, et al. Sleepiness and sleep disorders in shift workers: A study on a a group of Italian police officers. *Sleep* 2002;25:648–653. [PMID: 12224843]

Moore RY. A clock for the ages. *Science* 1999;284:2102–2103. [PMID: 10409066] (This article and the following provide a good introduction to the neurobiology of circadian rhythms.)

Turek F, Dugovic C, Zee P. Current understanding of the circadian clock and the clinical implications for neurological disorders. *Arch Neurol* 2001;58:1772–1778. [PMID: 11708983]

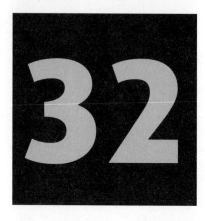

Systemic & Metabolic Disorders

Cheryl A. Jay, MD

NUTRITIONAL DEFICIENCIES

ESSENTIALS OF DIAGNOSIS

▶ Polyneuropathy (symmetric foot numbness, tingling, pain, with depressed or absent reflexes), occasionally with concomitant central nervous system (CNS) manifestations

▶ Associated with eating disorders, chronic gastrointestinal disease or surgery (including bariatric procedures), socioeconomic deprivation, alcoholism, and pregnancy

Several vitamin B deficiency states are associated with neurologic disease. Severe **vitamin B$_1$ (thiamine) deficiency** causes "wet" beriberi, with peripheral edema from cardiomyopathy, as well as peripheral neuropathy and Wernicke-Korsakoff syndrome. In the industrialized world, the neurologic manifestations are seen most often in the setting of alcoholism. They may also occur in cachexia as a result of advanced malignancies, HIV, or hyperemesis gravidarum, or when intravenous glucose, including parenteral nutrition, is administered to a malnourished patient, depleting available thiamine. Milder thiamine deficiency may cause peripheral neuropathy alone, known as "dry" beriberi. Serum thiamine levels do not accurately indicate thiamine status. Whole blood thiamine levels or erythrocyte transketolase activity is typically decreased, although thiamine supplementation (100 mg every 8–12 hours intravenously) can be administered empirically in most acute situations, followed by long-term oral maintenance (50–100 mg/day).

Vitamin B$_{12}$ (cyanocobalamin) deficiency causes neurologic disease, most commonly myeloneuropathy, and megaloblastic anemia as isolated syndromes or in combination. Dietary deficiency is relatively uncommon but can occur in strict vegans. More common causes include gastric disorders such as pernicious anemia, gastrectomy, bariatric surgery, atrophic gastritis, and achlorhydria; ileal disorders such as bacterial overgrowth, infestation with the fish tapeworm *Diphyllobothrium latum*, and surgery; and inflammatory bowel disease. Nitrous oxide inactivates cyanocobalamin, hence myeloneuropathy may complicate nitrous oxide abuse or, in patients with subclinical vitamin B$_{12}$ deficiency, therapeutic use. Vitamin B$_{12}$ deficiency is discussed further in Chapter 19.

Vitamin B$_6$ (pyridoxine) deficiency from severe malabsorption or as a consequence of therapy with isoniazid, cycloserine, hydralazine, or penicillamine can cause peripheral neuropathy. Daily pyridoxine therapy (25 mg/day orally) is standard in patients taking isoniazid. Excess pyridoxine intake can also cause sensory neuronopathy, which manifests clinically as sensory ataxia. **Niacin deficiency** (pellagra), rare in developed countries, causes dementia and neuropathy in association with dermatitis and diarrhea.

Neurologic disorders may complicate deficiencies of fat-soluble vitamins. **Vitamin A deficiency** causes night blindness and can lead to permanent blindness from corneal ulceration and scarring. Adults with **vitamin D deficiency** develop osteomalacia, with bone pain and proximal weakness. In addition to malabsorption, risk factors for vitamin D deficiency include decreased sun exposure (including institutionalization), many antiepileptic drugs, and obesity. **Vitamin E deficiency**, resulting from chronic fat malabsorption, abetalipoproteinemia, or as a familial disorder, causes neuropathy and cerebellar ataxia. **Vitamin K deficiency** does not have a recognized neurologic syndrome, although the resulting coagulopathy predisposes to subdural hematoma or intracerebral hemorrhage.

Copper deficiency, due to malabsorption or to excessive zinc consumption, can cause myeloneuropathy resembling that seen in cyanocobalamin deficiency. Muscle weakness and wasting develop in **protein-calorie malnutrition states** such as kwashiorkor, marasmus, and severe cachexia. Coexisting vitamin deficiencies (Table 32–1) likely contribute to neurologic impairment in this setting. Bariatric surgery for severe obesity may be complicated by neurologic disorders, including

Table 32–1. Vitamin Deficiencies: Neurologic and Systemic Features

Vitamin	Neurologic Features	Systemic Features
A (β-carotene)	Night blindness	Corneal ulceration
B₁ (thiamine)	Wernicke encephalopathy (classic triad of confusion, ataxia, and oculomotor abnormalities) Korsakoff amnestic syndrome Peripheral neuropathy	Congestive heart failure
B₃ (niacin, nicotinic acid)	Encephalopathy Polyneuropathy	Dermatitis Glossitis Diarrhea
B₆ (pyridoxine)	Peripheral neuropathy Seizures in neonates (and adults in setting of isoniazid overdose)	Seborrhea Glossitis Microcytic anemia
B₁₂ (cobalamin)	Myeloneuropathy (subacute combined degeneration) Cognitive impairment Optic neuropathy	Macrocytic anemia
D (calciferol)	Proximal muscle weakness	Bone pain
E (α-tocopherol)	Spinocerebellar syndromes Peripheral neuropathy	None

peripheral neuropathy. In many instances, this appears to be due to thiamine or cobalamin deficiency.

Kumar N. Neurologic presentations of nutritional deficiencies. *Neurol Clin* 2010;28:107 [PMID: 19932379] (Exhaustively referenced review, emphasizing these disorders in association with bariatric surgery, alcoholism, and in specific international settings.)

ELECTROLYTE DISORDERS

 ESSENTIALS OF DIAGNOSIS

▶ Metabolic encephalopathy (depressed or fluctuating level of consciousness with reactive pupils and no lateralizing signs), variably accompanied by neuromuscular disorders (cramps, weakness, fasciculations)

▶ Patients with chronic, mild electrolyte abnormalities may be asymptomatic; acute, severe disturbances are more likely to be accompanied by encephalopathy with or without neuromuscular signs

▶ Often reversible

1. Sodium Imbalances

Hypernatremia is most commonly caused by net water loss from impaired access to water, diarrhea, increased insensible losses, or less commonly diabetes insipidus, but may complicate

hypertonic saline therapy. Initial irritability and complaints of thirst give way to worsening metabolic encephalopathy progressing from mild drowsiness to coma as the sodium concentration continues to rise. Cellular water loss causes brain shrinkage, which can, in rare instances, tear bridging veins and cause parenchymal or subdural hemorrhage.

Hyponatremia is common, with a broad differential diagnosis organized by the patient's fluid status: hypovolemic (sodium loss from the kidney, gut, or excessive sweating), euvolemic (syndrome of inappropriate antidiuretic hormone secretion, hypocortisolism, hypothyroidism), or hypervolemic (fluid overload states such as heart failure, cirrhosis, or renal disease). The encephalopathy ranges from a mild confusional state sometimes accompanied by headache, vomiting, cramps, and fasciculations to coma and may be complicated further by seizures or cerebral edema. Hyponatremia should be considered in patients with altered mental status following surgery or after intense physical activity, such as long-distance running. The risk of permanent neurologic injury or death from hyponatremia is higher for women, especially before menopause.

Rapid correction or overcorrection of hyponatremia can cause central pontine myelinolysis, an osmotic demyelination syndrome. Typical clinical presentations include the locked-in state or coma with quadriparesis.

2. Potassium Imbalances

Renal insufficiency, hypocortisolism, or distribution of potassium to the extracellular space causes hyperkalemia. Muscle weakness is the predominant neurologic abnormality, and CNS manifestations are rare. The potentially fatal complication of hyperkalemia is malignant cardiac dysrhythmias. Renal loss from diuretics or mineralocorticoid excess, gastrointestinal loss from vomiting or diarrhea, inadequate intake or transcellular potassium shift into cells may lead to hypokalemia. Levels below 3 mEq/L cause muscle weakness and occasionally rhabdomyolysis. Severe hypokalemia with alkalosis can cause tetany. Cerebral symptoms are rare.

3. Calcium Imbalances

Calcium plays critical roles in neuronal and myocyte function, and thus central nervous system and neuromuscular dysfunction are prominent clinical features of calcium disorders. As with most electrolyte disorders, disturbances that evolve rapidly are more likely to be symptomatic than those that develop gradually.

Malignancy is a common cause of hypercalcemia and, conversely, hypercalcemia is a diagnostic consideration in an encephalopathic cancer patient. Outside the setting of known malignancy, primary hyperparathyroidism is an important diagnostic consideration, along with medications such as thiazide diuretics and vitamin D. Markedly elevated serum calcium causes lethargy and coma; in mild hypercalcemia, personality change or memory impairment can mimic psychiatric disease or dementia. Neuromuscular syndromes include cramps, proximal wasting, and weakness, with normal serum creatine kinase levels; electromyography and biopsy typically show myopathic features.

Hypocalcemia develops as a consequence of hypoparathyroid states (including thyroid or parathyroid surgery) severe renal failure, vitamin D deficiency, massive transfusion, or pancreatitis. Both cerebral and neuromuscular manifestations are characterized by irritability of neural tissues: seizures (including nonconvulsive status epilepticus), anxiety, agitated delirium, and tetany. Severe tetany causes tonic spasms involving the hand (carpopedal spasm), trunk (opisthotonus), or larynx (stridor). Computed tomographic (CT) scans of the brain in patients with long-standing hypoparathyroid states may show calcification in basal ganglia and less commonly in cerebellum, brainstem, and cortex. Occasional patients have chorea, rigidity, or other extrapyramidal dysfunction, but most are asymptomatic (and most basal ganglia calcification seen on CT scan of the brain is idiopathic, rather than indicative of hypoparathyroidism). Latent tetany may be induced by hyperventilation, ischemia (Trousseau sign), or tapping on the facial nerve (Chvostek sign). Calcium repletion reverses neurologic symptoms and signs.

4. Magnesium Imbalances

Hypermagnesemia is seen primarily in patients receiving intravenous magnesium sulfate treatment for pre-eclampsia or eclampsia, or in patients with renal failure who ingest excessive magnesium, in particular some antacids and laxatives. Whether severe hypermagnesemia impairs cerebral function remains a topic of debate, but neuromuscular function is clearly impaired. Depressed deep tendon reflexes may signal impending paralysis; lethargy may reflect hypoxemia and hypercarbia from severe muscle weakness rather than a primary effect on the brain.

Hypomagnesemia results from inadequate intake, impaired gastrointestinal absorption, or renal loss, as occurs with diuretics. Alcohol withdrawal is a common clinical setting for hypomagnesemia. Neurologic features resemble those of hypocalcemia: irritability, agitation, seizures, tremor, hyperreflexia, and latent or overt tetany. Hypomagnesemia decreases the activity, and possibly levels, of parathyroid hormone and should be considered in patients with symptomatic hypocalcemia who do not improve with calcium repletion.

5. Phosphorus Imbalances

Hyperphosphatemia is commonly caused by acute or chronic renal failure. Elevated phosphate does not directly lead to neurologic dysfunction, but can cause symptomatic hypocalcemia by binding calcium. Hypophosphatemia can occur as a consequence of malnutrition or increased renal losses. Weakness of cranial and limb muscles is a prominent symptom, particularly at serum levels below 1 mg/dL, and can manifest as respiratory failure or inability to wean from mechanical ventilation.

Castilla-Guerra L, et al. Electrolytes disturbances and seizures. *Epilepsia* 2006;47:1990. [PMID: 17201695] (Reviews disorders of sodium, calcium, and magnesium with an emphasis on seizures, but also consideration of other clinical features.)

Cooper MS, Gittoes NJL. Diagnosis and management of hypocalcaemia. *BMJ* 2008;336:1298. [PMID: 18535072] (Practical summary of the clinical aspects of hypocalcemia, in question and answer format.)

Lien Y-HH, Shapiro, JI. Hyponatremia: Clinical diagnosis and management. *Am J Med* 2007;120:653. [PMID: 17679119] (Covers the pathophysiology, differential diagnosis, and treatment of this common electrolyte disorder.)

Schaefer TJ, Wolford RW. Disorders of potassium. *Emerg Med Clin North Am* 2005;23:723. [PMID: 15982543] (Comprehensive, practical discussion of the differential diagnosis and management of hyper- and hypokalemia.)

Yee AH, Rabinstein AA. Neurologic presentations of acid-base imbalance, electrolyte abnormalities, and endocrine emergencies. *Neurol Clin* 2010;28:1. [PMID: 19932372] (Well-referenced survey of the neurologic manifestations of common metabolic disturbances and endocrinopathies.)

HYPERGLYCEMIA & HYPOGLYCEMIA

Diabetic ketoacidosis (DKA) and hyperosmolar hyperglycemic state (HHS) are acute metabolic complications of diabetes mellitus. Infection is a common precipitant. Hyperglycemia-induced osmotic diuresis causes severe volume depletion with deficits in sodium, potassium, phosphate, magnesium, and calcium. DKA classically occurs in type 1 diabetes mellitus and HHS in type 2 disease, although these associations are not invariate. DKA typically evolves over hours and HHS over days to weeks. Rapid, deep (Kussmaul) respirations are seen in DKA but not HHS. In both disorders, encephalopathy of varying degrees of severity is the predominant neurologic manifestation. Focal or generalized seizures and focal cerebral findings resembling stroke are more common in HHS than in DKA. A grave complication of insulin and fluid therapy is cerebral edema, although this appears to be less common with modern fluid and electrolyte management. A thorough search for infection (including of the CNS) should be conducted. Additionally, it should be recalled that stroke, seizure, head trauma, or other neurologic events may render patients unable to take prescribed hypoglycemic agents, thus causing hyperglycemia.

Mild hypoglycemia activates the autonomic nervous system, causing anxiety, dizziness, tremulousness, and sweating. If counter-regulatory mechanisms fail to raise glucose, inadequate brain glucose leads to neuroglycopenic manifestations of agitated delirium focal or generalized seizures, coma, and focal cerebral dysfunction such as hemiparesis. Risk factors include insulin therapy and prior hypoglycemic episodes. Neurologic symptoms and signs typically reverse quickly with prompt diagnosis and therapy, but prolonged hypoglycemia can lead to permanent brain dysfunction, ranging from hemiparesis to persistent vegetative state.

Guettier J-M, Gorden P. Hypoglycemia. *Endocrinol Metab Clin North Am* 2006;35:753. [PMID: 17127144] (Discusses risk factors, pathophysiology, etiologies outside the setting of diabetes, and treatment.)

Kitabchi AE, et al. Hyperglycemic crises in adult patients with diabetes. *Diabetes Care* 2009;32:1335. [PMID: 19564476] (Concise, clinically oriented review of DKA and HHS.)

HYPERTENSIVE ENCEPHALOPATHY & POSTERIOR REVERSIBLE ENCEPHALOPATHY SYNDROME

ESSENTIALS OF DIAGNOSIS

► Headache, altered mental status, visual dysfunction, seizures, papilledema, with severe hypertension (often with retinal hemorrhage, aortic dissection, myocardial ischemia, congestive heart failure, renal insufficiency)

► Also occurs with pre-eclampsia, after transplantation or chemotherapy, or accompanying autoimmune disorders, metabolic derangements, or some drugs

► Parieto-occipital white matter edema on magnetic resonance imaging (MRI) scan

End-organ damage involving the heart, kidney, or brain differentiates hypertensive urgencies from emergencies. Cerebral involvement typically evolves over hours with headache, visual dysfunction, altered mental status, seizures, and papilledema. Without treatment, there may be cerebral ischemia, hemorrhage, or both, with focal cerebral symptoms or signs. Other target organs may be simultaneously affected, but hypertensive encephalopathy can occur without associated extraneural end-organ involvement.

A similar syndrome of encephalopathy with prominent visual symptoms and signs and bilateral parieto-occipital edema on neuroimaging, particularly MRI, can complicate pre-eclampsia, a major global cause of maternal mortality. More recently, it has been described, sometimes without associated hypertension, after cancer chemotherapy or bone marrow, stem cell, or solid-organ transplantation; in autoimmune disorders such as systemic lupus erythematosus; with sepsis; and in association with thrombotic thrombocytopenic purpura, endocrinopathies, metabolic derangements, or medications. This clinicoradiologic picture of symptomatic vasogenic brain edema is referred to as posterior reversible encephalopathy syndrome (PRES).

► Clinical Findings

In 70–80% of patients, blood pressure is markedly elevated, and a typical clinical scenario is accelerated hypertension in a patient with essential hypertension. PRES may also complicate severe secondary hypertension from pheochromocytoma or drugs such as cocaine. Acute cerebral events such as head trauma, stroke, and CNS infection can also cause encephalopathy with elevated blood pressure. In some of these disorders, particularly ischemic stroke, aggressive antihypertensive therapy can worsen neurologic status.

Laboratory findings depend on the clinical context. In accelerated hypertension, studies may reveal acute renal failure, hematuria, or evidence of myocardial ischemia. PRES complicating pregnancy may be accompanied by proteinuria in pre-eclampsia, or there may be hemolysis, elevated liver enzymes, and low platelets (HELLP syndrome).

Neuroimaging is often obtained to identify ischemic or hemorrhagic stroke. MRI is superior to CT in demonstrating the bilateral hemispheric edema, most prominent in the parietal and occipital lobes (Figure 32–1) typical of PRES, although holohemispheric and cerebellar involvement may be seen. Depending on the parts of the brain involved, imaging findings may resemble arterial ischemia from bilateral posterior cerebral artery occlusion or venous ischemia from sinus thrombosis. The resulting visual symptoms often reverse with prompt antihypertensive therapy. Routine cerebrospinal fluid (CSF) studies are usually normal except for elevated pressure.

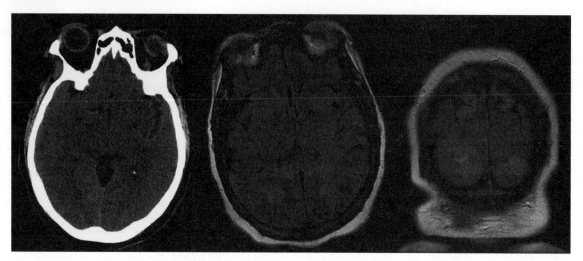

▲ **Figure 32–1.** CT and MRI in PRES. Noncontrast head CT (left) from a patient with severe hypertension and several hours of headache, visual impairment, and disorientation shows subtle swelling in both occipital lobes. Axial (center) and coronal (right) FLAIR MRI, performed several hours later, more clearly demonstrates the extent of edema.

▶ **Treatment**

First-line agents for PRES from acute hypertension (Table 32–2) are the β-blocker labetalol and calcium channel blocker nicardipine, given intravenously in a critical care setting with close hemodynamic monitoring. Sodium nitroprusside and nitroglycerin are not preferred agents to lower blood pressure in patients with PRES, due to concerns about adverse effects on cerebral blood flow. Angiotensin-converting enzyme inhibitors are contraindicated in pregnancy due to adverse effects on fetal kidneys. Seizures are managed in the usual manner, except in eclampsia, where intravenous magnesium has been shown to be superior to phenytoin. Encephalopathy may begin to reverse even before blood pressure returns to normal.

Neurologic deterioration, rather than the expected improvement, suggests that elevated blood pressure was secondary to a primary cerebral event or that PRES has progressed to cerebral ischemia or hemorrhage. Treated early, patients with PRES can recover fully.

Bartynski WS. Posterior reversible encephalopathy syndrome, part 1: Fundamental imaging and clinical features. *Am J Neuroradiol* 2008;29:1036. [PMID: 18356474] (Summarizes the clinical features, associated medical conditions, CT and MRI findings, and controversies regarding pathogenesis.)

Rhoney D, Peacock WF. Intravenous therapy for hypertensive emergencies, part 1. *Am J Health Syst Pharm* 2009;66:1343. [PMID: 19635770] (Reviews the clinical pharmacology of rapidly acting intravenous antihypertensive agents.)

Rhoney D, Peacock WF. Intravenous therapy for hypertensive emergencies, part 2. *Am J Health Syst Pharm* 2009;66:1448. [PMID: 19667001] (Discusses the use of specific intravenous antihypertensive agents by clinical setting, including stroke and pre-eclampsia.)

Servillo G, et al. Posterior reversible encephalopathy syndrome in intensive care medicine. *Intensive Care Med* 2007;33:230. [PMID: 17119920] (Reviews clinical and radiologic features, pathophysiology, and critical care management.)

Zeeman GG. Neurologic complications of pre-eclampsia. *Semin Perinatol* 2009;33:166. [PMID: 19464507] (Discusses the pathogenesis, clinical features, neuroimaging findings, and management of PRES in the context of pre-eclampsia.)

Table 32–2. Treatment of Hypertension in PRES

Drug	Dose	Cautions
Labetalol	Loading dose—20 mg IV over 2 min, 20–80 mg IV every 10 min Maintenance—2–3 mg/min IV	Asthma, bradycardia, heart block, severe congestive heart failure
Nicardipine	Initial rate—5 mg/h IV, increasing by 2.5 mg/h every 5 minutes to maximum of 15 mg/h	Aortic stenosis, cardiac conduction abnormalities, severe congestive heart failure

CARDIAC DISEASE

1. Cardiac Surgery

Heart surgery may be complicated by postoperative delirium, which has a broad differential diagnosis that includes metabolic disturbances, medication effects, stroke, and hypoxic-ischemic brain injury. Clinically evident ischemic stroke is more common than intracranial hemorrhage and complicates up to 5% of coronary bypass graft (CABG) procedures. Focal signs are usually evident in large-vessel infarctions. Multiple small-vessel infarctions, by contrast, may manifest as persistent unexplained encephalopathy, undiagnosed until neuroimaging, particularly MRI, is obtained. Hypotension or hypoxemia during or after surgery can cause hypoxic-ischemic encephalopathy of varying degrees. Even patients with completely uneventful intraoperative and postoperative courses sometimes complain of being "not quite right" months to years after surgery, with subtle but unequivocal abnormalities on neuropsychological testing. Microemboli to the brain may account for this phenomenon. Arterial filters to reduce embolization, higher intraoperative mean arterial pressure to avoid hypoperfusion, hypothermia for neuroprotection, and performing CABG procedures without cardiopulmonary bypass have been proposed to prevent cerebral complications, but are not in routine use.

In addition, patients undergoing sternotomy occasionally develop peripheral nerve injuries such as phrenic nerve damage with diaphragmatic paralysis, recurrent laryngeal nerve injury with hoarseness or poor cough, or brachial plexopathy with numbness, pain, and weakness in one or both hands. Saphenous vein harvest may result in injury to the saphenous nerve, with numbness and painful paresthesias in the medial lower leg and foot, without weakness.

2. Endocarditis

Neurologic complications develop in up to a third of patients with endocarditis and can be the presenting feature. Patients with focal cerebral dysfunction and known or suspected endocarditis require neuroimaging to distinguish among ischemic stroke, mycotic aneurysm rupture, or brain abscess. Patients who have subarachnoid or parenchymal hemorrhage identified by CT or CSF examination should undergo angiography to search for mycotic aneurysms. Many such aneurysms resolve with antibiotics alone, but surgical excision or endovascular procedures may be required. Cardioembolism in endocarditis may be clinically silent or manifest as transient ischemic attack or ischemic stroke. Antiplatelet or anticoagulant therapy is not routinely used, because of the risk of intracranial hemorrhage. Ischemic stroke in a patient with prosthetic valve endocarditis or requiring valve replacement for uncontrolled infection or other indication poses particular challenges in management. Intraoperative anticoagulation necessary for valve replacement increases the risk that a recent large-vessel infarction will undergo hemorrhagic transformation.

Brain abscess is more commonly multiple than single in patients with endocarditis and may manifest as headache, encephalopathy, or seizure, with or without focal cerebral dysfunction. Neurosurgical consultation should be obtained, although patients can often be managed medically.

An additional diagnostic consideration in patients with more diffuse impairment of brain function, headache, or both is bacterial meningitis from meningeal seeding. A patient with headache, normal mental status, and lymphocytic CSF pleocytosis without blood or xanthochromia may have aseptic meningitis from bacteremia or parameningeal infection. Patients with neck or back pain and radiculopathy or myelopathy may have spinal osteomyelitis, epidural abscess, or both, requiring emergent MRI of the spine and neurosurgical consultation.

3. Hypoxic-Ischemic Encephalopathy

Most individuals surviving cardiac arrest are comatose after resuscitation, and hospital discharge rates after cardiac arrest have remained low over the past several decades, despite advances in critical care. Brain injury is the leading cause of morbidity and mortality after cardiac arrest. Functionally significant degrees of recovery occur, but the most common outcome a year after arrest is the vegetative state or death.

This grim prognosis has triggered an extensive search for neuroprotective strategies. Controlled studies demonstrated improved outcome in comatose patients cooled within minutes to hours after ventricular fibrillation arrest to 32–34°C for 12–24 hours. Consequently, therapeutic hypothermia is now recommended after cardiac arrest, although the optimal method (surface or internal devices) for inducing and maintaining hypothermia, duration of cooling, and procedure for rewarming have yet to be determined.

Prognosis usually cannot be determined with confidence in the initial hours after cardiac arrest. Neurologic examination in the initial several days after cardiac arrest does predict outcome among patients who were not cooled. Absent pupillary and corneal reflexes and extensor posturing or no response to noxious stimuli at 72 hours postarrest portend a poor prognosis for significant neurologic recovery in adults who have not been treated with therapeutic hypothermia. Evidence that poor motor function at 3 days may be a less reliable prognostic marker in patients who have been cooled suggests that neurologic examination criteria should be used with caution in this setting. Hypotension, hypothermia, and sedative and neuromuscular blocking drugs are confounders when using the examination to determine prognosis.

Generalized tonic-clonic seizures or asynchronous multifocal myoclonus may develop after cardiac arrest and do not have prognostic value, but myoclonic status epilepticus is a poor prognostic sign.

Somatosensory-evoked potentials (SSEPs) are used in some centers to supplement the examination. Bilaterally absent N20 responses of median SSEPs predict poor outcome before therapeutic hypothermia, but it remains uncertain if this is the case in patients with hypoxic-ischemic encephalopathy who have been cooled.

Gottesmann RF, McKhann GM, Hogue CW. Neurologic complications of cardiac surgery. *Semin Neurol* 2008;28:703. [PMID: 19115176] (Organized by specific cardiac procedure and by type of neurologic injury, with an emphasis on cerebral disorders.)

Grocott HP, et al. "Other" neurologic complications after cardiac surgery. *Semin Cardiothorac Vasc Anesth* 2004;8:213. [PMID: 15375481] (Focuses on peripheral nerve injuries after cardiac surgery.)

Johnson MD, Johnson CD. Neurologic presentations of infective endocarditis. *Neurol Clin* 2010;28:311. [PMID: 19932388] (Covers the epidemiology, clinical syndromes, and common treatment dilemmas in patients with neurologic complications of endocarditis.)

Neumar RW, et al. Post-cardiac arrest syndrome: Epidemiology, pathophysiology, treatment, and prognostication. A consensus statement from the International Liaison Committee on Resuscitation (American Heart Association, Australian and New Zealand Council on Resuscitation, European Resuscitation Council, Heart and Stroke Foundation of Canada, InterAmerican Heart Foundation, Resuscitation Council of Asia, and the Resuscitation Council of Southern Africa); the American Heart Association Emergency Cardiovascular Care Committee; the Council on Cardiovascular Surgery and Anesthesia; the Council on Cardiopulmonary, Perioperative, and Critical Care; the Council on Clinical Cardiology; and the Stroke Council. *Circulation* 2008;118;2452. [PMID: 18948368] (Comprehensive review of postcardiac arrest care, including recommendation for hypothermia as standard treatment for patients with postarrest coma.)

Young GB. Neurologic prognosis after cardiac arrest. *N Engl J Med* 2009;361:605. [PMID: 19657124] (Discusses neurologic examination, electrodiagnostic studies, biochemical tests, and neuroimaging in postarrest coma, with an emphasis on the uncertainties in the setting of induced hypothermia.)

PULMONARY DISEASE

Neurologic symptoms in patients with acute or chronic respiratory failure are the result of hypoxia, hypercarbia, or both, even with adequate circulation. Severe hypoxia causes coma that may be accompanied by loss of pupillary, corneal, and other brainstem reflexes. With lesser degrees of hypoxia, wakefulness may be relatively preserved; patients may report lightheadedness or visual loss, or manifest impaired cognition. Recovery depends on the severity and duration of hypoxia. Hypercarbia in chronic respiratory failure can cause altered cognition and behavioral changes, sometimes associated with asterixis. Headache may be prominent, likely from cerebral vasodilation and occasionally associated with papilledema.

Symptoms of hyperventilation are those of hypocapnia and include dizziness, perioral and distal paresthesias, carpopedal spasm, and, occasionally, tetany.

Dreibelbis JE, Jozefowicz RF. Neurologic complications of respiratory disease. *Neurol Clin* 2010;28:37. [PMID: 19932374] (Concise review of clinical features and pathophysiology.)

LIVER DISEASE

ESSENTIALS OF DIAGNOSIS

▸ Altered mental status with or without asterixis, accompanying chronic liver failure with portal hypertension or acute hepatic failure

▸ Coexisting cerebral edema and increased intracranial pressure in patients with acute liver failure

▸ General Considerations

Hepatic encephalopathy can complicate chronic liver disease with cirrhosis as well as acute hepatic failure and is a worrisome prognostic sign in both situations. The diagnosis is perhaps less difficult in patients with portal hypertension who become confused or comatose after an obvious precipitant, such as hypokalemia, gastrointestinal hemorrhage, protein load, or sedative medications (including those used to manage ethanol withdrawal). Identifying early disease can be challenging. *Minimal, latent,* or *subclinical hepatic encephalopathy* is present in nearly 70% of cirrhotic patients, with adverse consequences for quality of life.

▸ Clinical Findings

The clinical picture is metabolic encephalopathy, with early inattention, confusion, and mood and personality changes. Subsequent disorientation, often with asterixis, progresses to impaired alertness and coma. Electroencephalography may show triphasic waves, but this abnormality, as well as asterixis, can accompany other metabolic encephalopathies.

▸ Differential Diagnosis

The differential diagnosis is broad and includes other metabolic derangements, medication effects, withdrawal states (including ethanol), CNS infection, and Wernicke-Korsakoff syndrome. Many patients with cirrhosis severe enough to cause hepatic encephalopathy also have coagulopathy from failure to synthesize coagulation factors, thrombocytopenia secondary to hypersplenism, or both. These increase the risk for subdural hematoma, even without a history of trauma.

▸ Treatment

Once other diagnostic possibilities have been excluded (with appropriate blood tests, CT scan of the brain, and lumbar puncture in selected patients), a precipitant for hepatic encephalopathy should be sought and managed as needed. Protein restriction and medications (Table 32–3) to facilitate the removal of ammoniagenic compounds from the gut are mainstays of therapy. Nonabsorbable disaccharides such as lactulose accomplish this by cathartic action and lowering colonic pH, which inhibits the growth of urease-producing

Table 32–3. Drug Treatment of Hepatic Encephalopathy in Chronic Liver Disease

Drug	Dose	Cautions
Lactulose	Start 30 mL PO (or NG) 2–4 times daily, titrated to several soft bowel movements per day	Caution in galactosemia or constipation Overdosage can cause severe diarrhea with subsequent electrolyte disturbances
Rifaximin	550 mg PO every 12 h	Consider *Clostridium difficile* if diarrhea develops on therapy

bacteria. Bacterial ammoniagenesis can also be decreased with antibiotics such as rifaximin or metronidazole, although peripheral neuropathy can complicate long-term therapy with the latter. Chronic neomycin therapy can be complicated by nephro- and ototoxicity.

Hepatic encephalopathy in patients with acute liver failure may be accompanied by cerebral edema and increased intracranial pressure. Intracranial pressure monitoring can guide hyperosmolar therapy, although controversy persists about the risks of invasive monitoring and the benefits of treatment to lower intracranial pressure.

Cash WJ, et al. Current concepts in the assessment and treatment of hepatic encephalopathy. *QJM* 2010;103:9. [PMID: 19903725] (Covers the pathophysiology and management of hepatic encephalopathy complicating cirrhosis.)

Wendon J, Lee W. Encephalopathy and cerebral edema in the setting of acute liver failure: Pathogenesis and management. *Neurocrit Care* 2008;9:97. [PMID: 18688582] (Concise discussion of putative pathophysiologic mechanisms and management options.)

RENOAL DISEASE

 ESSENTIALS OF DIAGNOSIS

▶ Metabolic encephalopathy in acute renal failure

▶ Dialysis dysequilibrium syndrome, dementia, and Wernicke encephalopathy as complications of dialysis

▶ Mononeuropathies as complications of arteriovenous shunt placement

▶ Distal symmetric polyneuropathy with or without restless legs syndrome in chronic renal failure

Acute complications of renal failure include encephalopathy syndromes associated with uremia and dialysis. Metabolic encephalopathy is the predominant neurologic feature of acute uremia, ranging from mildly impaired concentration and personality change to delirium and frank coma. Asterixis occurs, along with multifocal myoclonus or generalized seizures. The degree of azotemia does not always correlate with

the severity of cerebral dysfunction. Chronic renal insufficiency generally causes fewer symptoms than acute renal failure.

CT and CSF examination help exclude subdural hematoma or CNS infection, but otherwise reveal nonspecific findings such as cerebral atrophy or mildly elevated CSF protein. Electroencephalography shows low voltage and slowing, indicating generalized cerebral disturbance. Other causes of encephalopathy may coexist with renal failure. For example, cerebral aneurysms occur more often in patients with polycystic kidney disease, making subarachnoid hemorrhage an important diagnostic consideration when such patients develop altered mentation. Hypertension, diabetes mellitus, vasculitis, and other causes of end-stage renal disease may cause stroke or other acute cerebral disorders. Advanced renal failure increases the risk for CNS infections such as meningitis, particularly with *Listeria monocytogenes*.

Uremic encephalopathy is an indication for dialysis, but the procedure itself may produce neurologic complications. Dialysis disequilibrium syndrome results from rapid shifts in urea levels and cerebral edema, and manifests with headache, restlessness, and cramps, which can progress to frank delirium with myoclonus or seizures and increased intracranial pressure. It can complicate hemodialysis and peritoneal dialysis, and is less common with modern dialysis techniques. Other diagnostic considerations for altered mental status occurring during or after dialysis include electrolyte disturbances and Wernicke encephalopathy. Uremia-related platelet dysfunction and anticoagulants used during hemodialysis predispose patients to subdural hemorrhages, even without trauma.

Dialysis dementia was linked to aluminum exposure from oral aluminum hydroxide and dialysis solutions. The syndrome of dysarthria and dysphagia during and after dialysis, progressing to persistence of these symptoms with myoclonus, seizures, ataxia, and generalized cognitive impairment, has become rare with modifications in dialysate solutions and oral phosphate binders. Chronic kidney disease (CKD) is a risk factor for cognitive impairment, independent of other vascular risk factors, even in patients who do not require dialysis. Renal transplantation improves cognitive function.

Patients with restless legs syndrome (RLS) report creeping, crawling, and other uncomfortable sensations in the legs that improve with movement. Renal failure is a secondary

Table 32–4. Neurologic Complications of Renal Insufficiency

	Central Nervous System Features	Neuromuscular Features
Renal failure		
Acute	Encephalopathy Myoclonus, asterixis Seizures	Tetany (if associated hypocalcemia)
Chronic	Infection, especially *Listeria monocytogenes* meningitis Subdural hematoma Dementia Myoclonus, asterixis Restless legs syndrome	Neuropathy Myopathy
Dialysis	Dysequilibrium syndrome Dementia	Arteriovenous fistula—related mononeuropathies

cause of RLS, as are iron deficiency and peripheral neuropathy, which commonly accompany CKD.

Uremic polyneuropathy affects over half of dialysis patients. The clinical syndrome is distal symmetric polyneuropathy, similar to diabetic, alcoholic, or HIV neuropathies: gradual onset of numbness, pain, and paresthesias beginning in the feet, with absent or depressed ankle reflexes and sensory loss, especially vibration sense. Impotence, bladder and bowel dysfunction, orthostatic hypotension, and sudden cardiac death may signify dysautonomia, which occasionally occurs without associated distal symmetric polyneuropathy. Focal neuropathies complicating CKD include ischemic monomelic neuropathy after arteriovenous fistula placement and carpal tunnel syndrome. Other neuromuscular manifestations of CKD include uremic myopathy, which presents as proximal muscle wasting and weakness, particularly in the legs, with normal creatine kinase levels.

The neurologic complications of renal insufficiency are summarized in Table 32–4.

Brouns R, DeDeyn PP. Neurological complications in renal failure: A review. *Clin Neurol Neurosurg* 2004;107:1. [PMID: 15567546] (Extensively referenced, comprehensive review of central nervous system and neuromuscular disorders in renal failure.)

Krishnan AV, Kiernan MC. Neurologic complications of chronic kidney disease. *Nature Rev Neurol* 2009;5:542. [PMID: 19724248] (Surveys clinical features, pathophysiology, and management of common cerebral and neuromuscular complications of chronic kidney disease.)

PANCREATIC DISEASE

Patients with acute pancreatitis and a clinical picture of metabolic encephalopathy without other evident cause are said to have pancreatic encephalopathy. Hypocalcemia and hyperglycemia or hypoglycemia may accompany pancreatitis and should be considered in this setting. Alcohol withdrawal, liver disease, and Wernicke-Korsakoff syndrome are diagnostic possibilities among patients whose pancreatitis results from alcoholism. Blood–brain barrier disruption, increased cytokine production, cerebral microcirculatory disturbances, and hypoxemia have been postulated as possible pathogenetic mechanisms but remain unproven.

Zhang X-P, Tian H. Pathogenesis of pancreatic encephalopathy in severe acute pancreatitis. *Hepatobiliary Pancreat Dis Int* 2007;6:134. [PMID: 17374570] (Briefly summarizes clinical features, followed by a survey of hormonal, inflammatory, hemodynamic, and other putative mechanisms.)

ENDOCRINE DISORDERS

ESSENTIALS OF DIAGNOSIS

▶ Impaired cerebral or neuromuscular function (or both)

▶ Constitutional symptoms, disorders of other organ systems

▶ Global cognitive dysfunction, psychiatric syndromes, myopathic weakness, and polyneuropathy

1. Thyroid Disease

Hyperthyroidism can cause headache, mood disturbances, psychosis, cognitive impairment, tremor, or chorea, singly or in various combinations. Proximal muscle wasting and weakness are common, usually with normal creatine kinase, although rhabdomyolysis occasionally complicates thyroid storm (incompletely treated or undiagnosed hyperthyroidism combined with a trauma, infection, or other precipitant). Periodic paralysis sometimes develops, especially in Asian men. Symptomatic peripheral neuropathy may also occur. Patients whose hyperthyroidism is due to Graves disease may develop ophthalmopathy, with lid edema, proptosis, and ophthalmoparesis. Graves ophthalmopathy can be disfiguring and threaten vision because of corneal ulceration, increased intraocular pressure, or optic nerve compression. Neurologic manifestations of hyperthyroidism usually improve when patients become euthyroid with treatment. Graves ophthalmopathy is a notable exception and can occur even after proper therapy of the endocrinopathy, requiring additional treatment including steroids, orbital radiotherapy, or, occasionally, surgery.

Hypothyroidism causes encephalopathy, ranging in severity from mood disorders and cognitive slowing to myxedema coma, accompanied by hypothermia and hyponatremia. Myopathy is the most common neurologic manifestation. Patients report weakness, cramps, and myalgia. Examination shows proximal weakness, myoedema, and reflex abnormalities, specifically, delayed relaxation phase. Serum creatine kinase level may be elevated, even in asymptomatic patients. Hypothyroidism predisposes to carpal tunnel syndrome and other entrapment neuropathies, and can also cause polyneuropathy. Other neurologic syndromes include cerebellar ataxia, central and obstructive sleep apnea, and hearing loss. Neurologic improvement usually accompanies thyroid replacement, but recovery may be incomplete. Congenital hypothyroidism, or cretinism, with mental retardation, spasticity, and extrapyramidal dysfunction, results from maternal iodine deficiency, making it a common global cause of preventable brain disease.

In Hashimoto thyroiditis, transient hyperthyroidism is typically followed by hypothyroidism, as antithyroid antibodies result in immune-mediated damage to the gland. In addition to the neurologic manifestations of thyroid disease, Hashimoto thyroiditis is sometimes associated with myasthenia gravis, as is Graves disease, another autoimmune thyroid disorder. Hashimoto encephalopathy is a rare syndrome of diverse types of cerebral dysfunction, including behavioral abnormalities, strokelike syndromes, movement disorders, and seizures, associated with antithyroperoxidase or antithyroglobulin antibodies, and responding to corticosteroid therapy. Thyroid function tests may be normal or demonstrate hypo- or hyperthyroidism. CSF protein is often elevated, without pleocytosis, and there are no specific neuroimaging or neuropathologic findings. Whether the antithyroid antibodies are pathogenic or perhaps a marker of an autoimmune cerebral disorder is among many controversies surrounding Hashimoto encephalopathy.

The neurologic complications of thyroid disease and other endocrine disorders are summarized in Table 32–5.

2. Parathyroid Disease

Primary hyperparathyroidism, most commonly due to parathyroid adenoma, seldom progresses to the full triad of kidney stones, bone disease, and peptic ulcer ("stones, bones, and abdominal groans") because routine serum calcium determination allows earlier diagnosis. Cerebral and neuromuscular manifestations are those of hypercalcemia,

Table 32–5. Endocrine Disorders: Central Nervous System and Neuromuscular Features

Disorder	Central Nervous System Features	Neuromuscular Features
Hyperthyroidism	Anxiety, personality change, delirium, psychosis, coma Tremor, chorea	Proximal weakness (CK level is normal, except in thyroid storm) Periodic paralysis (Asian men are at particular risk) Ophthalmopathy, myasthenia gravis (Graves disease) Peripheral neuropathy
Hypothyroidism	Mental slowing, depression, psychosis, cognitive impairment Coma (in myxedema) Ataxia Central (and obstructive) sleep apnea	Proximal weakness (CK level is often elevated) Abnormal tendon reflexes (delayed relaxation phase) Predisposition to carpal tunnel syndrome and other entrapment neuropathies Myasthenia gravis (with Hashimoto thyroiditis) Peripheral neuropathy
Hyperparathyroidism	Impaired memory, mood disorders, delirium, psychosis Compressive myelopathy (brown tumor)	Proximal weakness (CK level is normal)
Hypoparathyroidism	Dementia, psychosis Seizures Chorea, tremor	Tetany
Hypercortisolism	Cognitive impairment, affective disorders Compressive myelopathy (epidural lipomatosis)	Proximal weakness (CK level is normal)
Adrenal insufficiency	Irritability, cognitive impairment	Proximal weakness (CK level is normal) Hyperkalemic periodic paralysis

discussed earlier, and often improve after parathyroidectomy. Although more commonly seen in secondary hyperparathyroidism from long-standing renal failure, brown tumors can also develop in primary hyperparathyroidism and cause compressive myelopathy, requiring emergent neurosurgical intervention.

Hypoparathyroidism may develop after thyroid or parathyroid surgery, causing hypocalcemia and hypophosphatemia. Neurologic manifestations are those of hypocalcemia, as previously discussed.

3. Adrenal Disease

Hypercortisolism, or Cushing syndrome, causes cognitive or affective disturbance, myopathy with normal creatine kinase, and, much less commonly, epidural lipomatosis with compressive radiculopathy or myelopathy. Adrenal insufficiency, or Addison syndrome, can also cause irritability and proximal weakness, as well as hyperkalemic periodic paralysis. Associated hyperkalemia, hyponatremia, hypoglycemia, or hypotension can provide an important clue to the underlying endocrine disorder.

Al-Khawaja D, Seex K, Eslick GD. Spinal epidural lipomatosis—A brief review. *J Clin Neurosci* 2008;15:1323. [PMID: 18954986] (Survey of reported cases, comparing the disorder in patients with associated endocrinopathy or corticosteroid therapy to those without evident cause.)

Alshekhlee A, Kaminski HJ, Ruff RL. Neuromuscular manifestations of endocrine disorders. *Neurol Clin* 2002;20:35. [PMID: 11754301] (Comprehensive review of the muscular complications of disorders of thyroid, parathyroid, adrenal, pituitary, and vitamin D metabolism.)

Anglin RE, Rosebush PI, Mazurek MF. The neuropsychiatric profile of Addison's disease: Revisiting a forgotten phenomenon. *J Neuropsychiatry Clin Neurosci* 2006;18:450. [PMID: 17135373] (Case report and discussion of associated changes in mental status.)

Fraser WD. Hyperparathyroidism. *Lancet* 2009;374:145. [PMID: 19595349] (Comprehensive review, highlighting the changing clinical presentations over time.)

Kaya RA, et al. Spinal cord compression caused by a brown tumor at the cervicothoracic junction. *Spine J* 2007;7:728. [PMID: 17998132] (Case report in a patient with renal failure with a concise summary of reported cases in primary and secondary hyperparathyroidism.)

Lovas K, Husebye ES. Addison's disease. *Lancet* 2005;365:2058. [PMID: 15950720] (Case presentation, discussion of clinical features, and historical review.)

Mistry N, Wass J, Turner MR. When to consider thyroid dysfunction in the neurology clinic. *Pract Neurol* 2009;9:145. [PMID: 19448057] (Clinically oriented discussion of central and neuromuscular disorders complicating thyroid disease, organized by neurologic syndrome.)

Newell-Price J, Bertagna X, Grossman AB, Nieman LK. Cushing's syndrome. *Lancet* 2006;367:1605. [PMID: 16698415] (Comprehensive review, from epidemiology and clinical manifestations to the challenges in diagnostic evaluation and management.)

Schiess N, Pardo CA. Hashimoto's encephalopathy. *Ann NY Acad Sci* 2008;1142:254. [PMID: 18990131] (Reviews the history, clinical features, and controversies surrounding the syndrome.)

Shoback D. Hypoparathyroidism. *N Engl J Med* 2008;359:391. [PMID: 18650515] (Case-driven review of the differential diagnosis and evaluation of the patient with hypocalcemia, including assessment of neuromuscular irritability.)

HEMATOLOGIC DISORDERS

ESSENTIALS OF DIAGNOSIS

▶ Ischemic (venous and arterial) and hemorrhagic stroke complicates many hematologic disorders

▶ Hyperviscosity syndrome (bleeding, visual dysfunction, focal cerebral disturbances) in hyperproteinemic states and myeloproliferative disorders

▶ Headache, fatigue, and syncope in anemia

▶ Increased risk for CNS infection, with subtle clinical features and unusual pathogens, in neutropenic states

1. Red Blood Cell Disorders

Patients with anemia from any cause experience headache and fatigue, but certain anemias are associated with additional neurologic features. Neurologic complications are common in sickle cell disease and include ischemic and hemorrhagic stroke, seizures, CNS infection, hearing loss, cognitive impairment, and, rarely, spinal cord infarction. Increased blood viscosity from sickled erythrocytes can occlude small or large vessels. Large-vessel stenosis from intimal fibrosis in sickle cell disease can lead to moyamoya disease, referring to the "puff of smoke" angiographic appearance from small-vessel collaterals. Exchange transfusions are effective secondary prophylaxis in patients with sickle cell disease who have had ischemic stroke and effective primary stroke prophylaxis when transcranial Doppler ultrasound identifies high velocities in major intracranial arteries. Subarachnoid and parenchymal hemorrhages also complicate sickle cell disease; in addition to moyamoya or hemorrhagic transformation of cerebral infarction, venous sinus thrombosis and ruptured aneurysm are diagnostic considerations. Patients with asplenia for any reason, including sickle cell disease, are at increased risk for infection with encapsulated organisms, including the meningeal pathogens *Streptococcus pneumoniae* and *Haemophilus influenzae*. Conductive and sensorineural hearing loss may occur from ear infection or ischemia. This and cerebral small-vessel disease likely contribute to learning disabilities.

Extramedullary hematopoiesis in thalassemia usually occurs in lymphoreticular tissues but can occasionally occur in the spinal epidural space, causing myelopathy or radiculopathy.

Treatment includes decompressive surgery, local radiation, corticosteroids, and transfusion in various combinations.

In polycythemia vera, ischemic and hemorrhagic strokes are feared complications. Cerebral ischemia, ascribed to increased blood viscosity, results from thrombosis in the veins and venous sinuses as well as cerebral arteries and arterioles. Veno-occlusive disease can be indolent with prominent headache prior to focal cerebral syndromes, followed later by venous ischemia, seizures, or hemorrhage. The triad of bleeding, visual symptoms, and focal cerebral signs suggests hyperviscosity syndrome, which can also occur in other myeloproliferative disorders such as essential thrombocytosis, and in hyperproteinemic states.

2. Thrombotic Microangiopathies

These disorders are characterized by thrombosis of small vessels within and outside the brain and include thrombotic thrombocytopenic purpura (TTP). The classic pentad consists of fever, renal insufficiency, thrombocytopenia, hemolytic anemia, and neurologic abnormalities, including headache, altered mentation, seizures, and various focal cerebral syndromes. The differential diagnosis includes disseminated intravascular coagulation, hemolytic-uremic syndrome, immune thrombocytopenic purpura, and heparin-induced thrombocytopenia. Plasmapheresis can be lifesaving in TTP.

3. White Blood Cell Disorders

Low white cell count or impaired function predisposes to infection, including the CNS. Granulocyte dysfunction, as occurs in cancer chemotherapy, increases vulnerability to bacterial infection. Impaired cell-mediated immunity complicating advanced HIV infection or chronic corticosteroid or cytotoxic therapy increases the risk for infection with unusual bacteria (including *Mycobacterium tuberculosis*), viruses, fungi, and protozoa. CNS infection causes significant morbidity and mortality in transplant recipients and other immunocompromised patients, who frequently present with subtle symptoms and signs. Early diagnosis depends on a high index of suspicion and low threshold for rapid, comprehensive evaluation with neuroimaging and CSF examination.

Acute leukemia is a common cause of hyperleukocytosis, or white blood cell count exceeding 100,000/mm³. Neurologic manifestations include headache, encephalopathy, ischemic or hemorrhagic stroke, or hyperviscosity syndrome. Other complications of leukemia include spinal, orbital, or dural mass lesions of myeloid leukemic blasts (chloromas) in acute myelogenous leukemia, leukemic infiltration of the leptomeninges, and chemotherapy-related CNS infections or neurotoxicity.

Monoclonal gammopathies complicating myeloma or Waldenström macroglobulinemia can cause peripheral neuropathy. Multiple myeloma involving the spine can cause radiculopathy, myelopathy, or both, requiring emergent intervention, including MRI, high-dose corticosteroids, radiotherapy, and neurosurgical consultation. Both of these hyperproteinemic states also cause hyperviscosity syndrome.

4. Coagulation Disorders

Genetic risk factors for venous thrombosis include deficiency of intrinsic anticoagulants, such as antithrombin 3 and proteins C and S, and procoagulant mutations in factor V Leiden or the G20210 prothrombin gene. Oral contraceptive medications are an important exogenous cause. Cerebral venous thrombosis presents as headache with encephalopathy, focal cerebral dysfunction, or seizure. Anticoagulation is usually necessary, despite the risk of hemorrhagic transformation in venous infarction. Arterial ischemic stroke in this setting suggests venous thromboembolism with patent foramen ovale or other right-to-left cardiac shunt (paradoxical embolism).

Coagulopathies may be inherited, such as hemophilia, or acquired (anticoagulation therapy, cirrhosis with synthetic failure) and predispose to hemorrhagic stroke, subdural hematoma, and cerebral and spinal epidural hematoma.

Adams BD, et al. Myeloproliferative disorders and the hyperviscosity syndrome. *Emerg Med Clin North Am* 2009;27:459. [PMID: 19646648] (Covers presenting features, evaluation, and acute management of symptomatic hyperviscosity due to hyperproteinemia, as well as myeloproliferative disorders.)

Austin S, Cohen H, Losseff N. Haematology and neurology. *J Neurol Neurosurg Psychiatry* 2007;78:334. [PMID: 17369588] (Update on blood disorders commonly seen in neurologic practice.)

Chamberlain MC. Leukemia and the nervous system. *Curr Onc Rep* 2005;7:66. [PMID: 15610689] (Covers the central and peripheral nervous system manifestations of the leukemias and their treatment.)

Kirkham FJ. Therapy insight: Stroke risk and its management in patients with sickle cell disease. *Nat Clin Pract Neurol* 2007;3:264. [PMID: 17479074] (Surveys the neurologic complications of sickle cell disease, with a detailed discussion of cerebrovascular disease and the role and limitations of transfusion for the primary and secondary prevention of ischemic stroke.)

Tsitsopoulos P, et al. Lumbar nerve root compression due to extramedullary hemopoiesis in a patient with thalassemia: Complete clinical regression with radiation therapy: Case report and review of the literature. *J Neurosurg Spine* 2007;6:156. [PMID: 17330584] (Describes a patient with radiculopathy managed successfully with radiation, followed by a review of reported cases involving the spine.)

BONE & JOINT DISORDERS

ESSENTIALS OF DIAGNOSIS

► Cranial neuropathy, myelopathy, radiculopathy, cauda equina syndrome, with head or spine pain
► Atlantoaxial instability is potentially life threatening

Paget disease of bone, a disorder of middle age and beyond, presents with bone pain and deformity or may be discovered on plain radiographs obtained for other reasons. Increased osteoclast activity causes disordered bone remodeling and structure. Neurologic complications include deafness or other cranial neuropathies from skull base disease, hydrocephalus from posterior fossa compression, and radiculopathy or myelopathy from spinal involvement. Serum alkaline phosphatase is usually elevated. Plain radiograph findings are often specific enough to establish the diagnosis, although biopsy may be necessary. Treatment consists of bisphosphonates or calcitonin; decompressive spine surgery may be necessary. Sarcomatous degeneration in pagetic bone is an ominous complication.

Fibrous dysplasia, a developmental disorder of bone, may involve one bone (monostotic) or several (polyostotic), including the skull and spine. Bone pain and pathologic fractures are common presentations. Patients, usually children and young adults, may present with a skull mass. Cranial nerve compression can cause visual impairment, hearing loss, or anosmia, and spinal disease causes scoliosis and occasionally cord compression. Plain films and CT may suggest the diagnosis, which can be established by biopsy. MRI should be obtained in patients with suspected cord compression. Treatment consists of bisphosphonates, mineral and vitamin D supplementation, and surgery.

Patients with **achondroplasia** may develop cervicomedullary compression due to bony abnormalities at the cranial–cervical junction. Clinical manifestations include posterior headache or neck pain, quadriparesis, bowel and bladder dysfunction, central and obstructive sleep apnea, and respiratory arrest. MRI (or CT) of the region can document the extent of compression in anticipation of decompressive surgery. Other neurologic complications include obstructive or communicating hydrocephalus, radiculopathy or neurogenic claudication from lumbar stenosis, and hearing loss from recurrent ear infections due to eustachian tube abnormalities. Neurologic complications may appear as early as infancy.

Ankylosing spondylitis, an inflammatory HLA B27–associated arthropathy primarily affecting spine and sacroiliac joints, typically becomes symptomatic in adolescents and young adults. In addition to spinal pain, microfractures, osteoporosis, and kyphosis, patients with ankylosing spondylitis are vulnerable to spinal fractures, even with minor trauma. Neurologic complications include atlantoaxial instability, myelopathy, and radiculopathy with or without associated fracture, and, in advanced disease, cauda equina syndrome. Characteristic plain radiographic features are usually sufficient to establish the diagnosis when combined with the history and examination. Medical management includes nonsteroidal anti-inflammatory drugs and bisphosphonates. Patients with root or cord symptoms or signs require spine MRI and surgery.

Atlantoaxial instability refers to excessive movement between C1 (atlas) and C2 (axis) due to ligamentous or bony abnormalities. Neck pain, quadriparesis, bowel and bladder dysfunction, limb weakness, and respiratory arrest may develop due to compression at the cervicomedullary junction. Among the many conditions associated with atlantoaxial instability are ankylosing spondylitis, rheumatoid arthritis (discussed later), trauma, and Down syndrome. Neurosurgical consultation should be obtained in patients with suspected or proven atlantoaxial instability.

Baujat G, et al. Achondroplasia. *Best Pract Res Clin Rheumatol* 2008;22:3. [PMID: 18328977] (Covers the genetics, pathophysiology, epidemiology, diagnosis, complications and management.)

Braun J, Sieper J. Ankylosing spondylitis. *Lancet* 2007;369:1379. [PMID: 17448825] (Comprehensive review, from epidemiology and pathogenesis to new therapeutic options.)

Collins MT. Spectrum and natural history of fibrous dysplasia of bone. *J Bone Miner Res* 2006;21(Suppl 2):P99. [PMID: 17229019] (Discusses clinical features, including compressive optic neuropathy and spinal involvement.)

Mundwiler ML, et al. Complications of the spine in ankylosing spondylitis with a focus on deformity correction. *Neurosurg Focus* 2008;24:E6. [PMID: 18290744] (Neurosurgical perspective on inflammatory and noninflammatory spine disease in ankylosing spondylitis.)

Ralston SH, Langston AL, Reid IR. Pathogenesis and management of Paget's disease of bone. *Lancet* 2008;372:155. [PMID: 18620951] (Comprehensive review of pathogenesis and clinical aspects of Paget disease.)

NEUROSARCOIDOSIS

ESSENTIALS OF DIAGNOSIS

▶ Any neurologic syndrome in a patient with an established diagnosis of sarcoidosis

▶ Cranial neuropathies, aseptic meningitis, CNS mass lesion, focal or diffuse neuropathies, or muscle disease of unclear cause in any patient

▶ Consider neurologic complications of immunosuppression and medications in patients being treated for established disease

▶ General Considerations

Sarcoidosis, an idiopathic multisystem granulomatous disorder, causes clinically evident neurologic disease in up to 10% of patients, although autopsy studies suggest that nervous system involvement is even more frequent. The literature includes reports of involvement across the entire neuroaxis: meningeal disease, cranial neuropathies, cerebral white matter lesions whose MRI appearance mimics multiple sclerosis or vasculitis, intra- or extra-axial granulomata affecting the brain or spinal cord, peripheral neuropathy, and myopathy. The diagnosis is particularly challenging when neurologic disease is the presenting feature.

Clinical Findings

Cranial neuropathies are the most common neurologic manifestation, with the facial nerve being most frequently affected, resembling Bell palsy. Eighth nerve involvement can threaten hearing. Dysfunction of the optic or third, fourth, or sixth cranial nerves may reflect meningeal disease or invasion or compression of nerves in the orbit by granuloma. Monophasic or recurrent aseptic meningitis or chronic meningitis, sometimes complicated by hydrocephalus, is associated with mononuclear pleocytosis, elevated protein concentration, and low or normal glucose level in CSF. Cerebral disease may involve the hypothalamus, with subsequent endocrinopathies, or present as an intracranial mass. Granulomata in or around the spinal cord cause myelopathy.

Sarcoidosis causes both mononeuropathy multiplex and distal symmetric polyneuropathy. Muscle involvement is more common pathologically than clinically, but occasionally causes proximal weakness.

The definitive diagnosis of sarcoidosis requires tissue diagnosis demonstrating noncaseating granuloma. In patients with known systemic disease, the diagnosis of neurosarcoidosis may be presumptive, based on compatible MRI and CSF findings. It is important to be vigilant for alternative diagnoses in patients who develop neurologic symptoms and signs while receiving chronic corticosteroid or other immunosuppressive therapy for systemic sarcoidosis, because of the increased risk for CNS infections. In patients without known sarcoidosis who develop an otherwise unexplained compatible neurologic syndrome, careful search for subtle systemic disease, especially in the lungs or skin, supplemented by gallium scanning and serum angiotensin-converting enzyme levels, may identify an extraneural site for tissue diagnosis.

Treatment

Neurosarcoidosis warrants therapy in most instances, although controlled data are lacking. Experience is greatest with corticosteroids, although cyclosporine, azathioprine, methotrexate, and other corticosteroid-sparing agents have been used with varying degrees of success. Drugs active against tumor necrosis factor-α, such as pentoxifylline, thalidomide, and infliximab, have been used with some success in sarcoidosis, systemic and neurologic, that has been refractory to corticosteroids and other agents. Hydrocephalus may require shunting. Seizures typically respond to antiepileptic drugs. Overall prognosis for patients with neurosarcoidosis is worse than for those with only systemic disease. Cranial neuropathies and aseptic meningitis have more favorable outcomes.

Joseph FG, Scolding NJ. Sarcoidosis of the nervous system. *Pract Neurol* 2007;7:234. [PMID: 17636138] (Reviews the protean clinical manifestations of neurosarcoid, with a helpful discussion of the common diagnostic and therapeutic dilemmas.)

Terushkin V, et al. Neurosarcoidosis: Presentations and management. *Neurologist* 2010;16:2. [PMID: 20065791] (Comprehensive review, including numerous brain and spine MRI scans demonstrating typical findings in neurosarcoidosis.)

VASCULITIS & CONNECTIVE TISSUE DISORDERS

ESSENTIALS OF DIAGNOSIS

- ► Encephalopathy, ischemic (arterial or venous) or hemorrhagic stroke, myelopathy, mononeuritis multiplex, or myopathy, associated with joint, skin, renal, or other extraneural disease
- ► Mild or asymptomatic distal symmetric polyneuropathy is commonly seen
- ► Consider neurologic complications of immunosuppression and organ failure in patients with long-standing vasculitis or connective tissue disorders

1. Vasculitis

Headache or visual symptoms beginning after age 50 should prompt consideration of **giant cell arteritis (GCA)**. Although less common than the related condition, polymyalgia rheumatica, GCA is the most common systemic vasculitis. Constitutional symptoms, including fever, are common. Granulomatous inflammation of carotid vessels, particularly external branches, causes many of the neurologic and ophthalmic symptoms, such as headache, visual loss, and jaw claudication. Examination may disclose tender, thickened temporal arteries. Visual loss is common, resulting from retinal or optic nerve ischemia, and visual loss in one eye presages the same in the fellow eye without treatment. Recognizing amaurosis fugax is critical, because fixed visual loss rarely improves in GCA. Less common manifestations include diplopia due to extraocular muscle ischemia, ischemic stroke from internal carotid or vertebral artery involvement, or peripheral nerve disorders. Anemia of chronic disease is common, and the erythrocyte sedimentation rate (ESR) exceeds 40–50 mm/h in over 80% of patients. C-reactive protein (CRP) may be elevated when ESR is normal. Temporal artery biopsy establishes the diagnosis, although skip lesions may cause false-negative results. Specimens of at least 20 mm in length are recommended and bilateral biopsies may be necessary, because long-term corticosteroid therapy is not without significant side effects.

Given the threat to vision, high-dose corticosteroids (prednisone 1 mg/kg/day or methylprednisolone 1000 mg/day intravenously) should be started immediately. Empiric therapy does not significantly decrease the yield of biopsies performed within a week of starting corticosteroid therapy. Systemic symptoms typically improve within days, with ESR normalizing within weeks. Ophthalmologic consultation is mandatory in patients with suspected GCA, for careful funduscopic examination and to obtain temporal artery biopsy. In most patients, corticosteroids can be gradually tapered over several years, guided by systemic symptoms, ESR, and CRP.

Another large-vessel vasculitis with a distinctly different demographic is **Takayasu arteritis**, which most commonly affects children and young adults but may begin as early as infancy or as late as age 50. Most patients are women, and most US cases occur in Asians. Another notable contrast to GCA is that Takayasu arteritis most commonly affects the aorta and its main branches. In addition to ischemia in the arms or legs or abdominal pain, half or more of patients experience dizziness, which may reflect subclavian steal, transient ischemic attack, or ischemic stroke. Renovascular hypertension predisposes to hemorrhagic stroke.

Kawasaki disease, a primarily medium-vessel vasculitis, most commonly affects infants and children. Fever and other systemic inflammatory signs such as conjunctivitis, rash, and lymphadenopathy are typically present. Coronary artery involvement may lead to myocardial ischemia; neurologic features include aseptic meningitis, facial weakness, seizures, and occasionally stroke.

Polyarteritis nodosa, a necrotizing arteritis of medium and small vessels, affects most organ systems and may be associated with hepatitis B or C infection. Renal and dermatologic involvement is a common systemic feature. Neuromuscular disorders (mononeuropathy multiplex, radiculopathy, plexopathy, or sensorimotor polyneuropathy) occur in over half of patients. Ischemic or hemorrhagic stroke occurs in about a quarter of patients.

Upper and lower respiratory tract granulomata, focal segmental glomerulonephritis, and necrotizing systemic vasculitis comprise the characteristic triad of **Wegener granulomatosis**, a small-vessel vasculitis. Cerebral syndromes include granulomatous invasion into the skull base, cranial neuropathies, ischemic or hemorrhagic stroke, and pachymeningitis. Peripheral nerve manifestations include distal symmetric polyneuropathy and mononeuritis multiplex. In the appropriate clinical context, antineutrophil cytoplasmic antibodies suggest the diagnosis, although biopsy may still be necessary.

Other systemic causes of vasculopathy include **infections** such as varicella-zoster virus and syphilis, cryoglobulinemia complicating hepatitis C infection, and **sympathomimetic drugs** such as cocaine, psychostimulants, and phenylpropanolamine.

Primary angiitis of the CNS, also called *granulomatous angiitis of the nervous system*, affects small- and medium-sized vessels of the brain and leptomeninges, without systemic involvement. Peak incidence occurs in the fourth through sixth decades; headache and encephalopathy are common presenting features. MRI, CSF, or angiography are often abnormal, but not in a specific manner. Brain and leptomeningeal biopsy is the gold standard test. Anecdotal evidence supports treatment with corticosteroids and other immunosuppressants.

2. Connective Tissue Disorders

The neurologic complications of **systemic lupus erythematosus** span the entire neuroaxis. Antiphospholipid or antineuronal antibodies, vasculitis, organ failure, and complications of therapy, including immunosuppression, cause neurologic disease. Pathogenesis remains obscure for some disorders. Chorea or transverse myelitis typically develops in early systemic lupus erythematosus, before the diagnosis is established. Acute cerebral syndromes, such as delirium, psychosis, and seizures, occur throughout the course, and may be associated in some instances with antibody-mediated neural injury, although complications of renal failure, immunosuppression, or other aspects of lupus and its treatment should be considered. Patients with arterial and venous stroke with serum antiphospholipid antibodies are at high risk for recurrence. Cranial neuropathies, polyneuropathy, and mononeuritis multiplex may develop. Proximal weakness may suggest an associated myositis, although corticosteroid and other medication-induced myopathies are additional considerations. High-dose corticosteroids are typically administered for acute encephalopathy. When there is evidence of vasculitis, cyclophosphamide may be appropriate. Aggressive anticoagulation, antiplatelet agents, or both, are indicated for patients with antiphospholipid antibody syndrome.

Neurologic complications of **rheumatoid arthritis** include neuromuscular disorders such as compression neuropathies, mononeuritis multiplex, and mild polyneuropathy and myopathy resulting from corticosteroids, immobility, or inflammatory myositis. A worrisome complication is spinal disease with atlantoaxial subluxation. Cervical pain may be the only early symptom, with myelopathy developing later, as a result of cord compression and ischemia. Upper cervical to occipital fusion may be necessary, although optimal timing of the procedure remains controversial, in part because coexisting osteoporosis and chronic immunosuppressant therapy make surgery difficult technically and impede wound healing.

In **Sjögren syndrome**, dry eyes and mouth result from immune-mediated injury to lacrimal and salivary glands. Neurologic syndromes may be the presenting feature and include cognitive and behavioral changes, demyelinating syndromes resembling multiple sclerosis, myelopathy, dorsal root ganglionopathy with sensory ataxia, and sensorimotor demyelinating neuropathy.

Chew SSL, Kerr NM, Danesh-Meyer HV. Giant cell arteritis. *J Clin Neurosci* 2009;16:1263. [PMID: 19586772] (Reviews the epidemiology, clinical features, and management of the most common systemic vasculitis.)

Cikes N. Central nervous system involvement in systemic connective tissue diseases. *Clin Neurol Neurosurg* 2006;108:311. [PMID: 16368184] (Covers neuromuscular, as well as central nervous system, complications of the major connective tissue disorders.)

Rossi CM, Di Comite G. The clinical spectrum of the neurological involvement in vasculitides. *J Neurol Sci* 2009;285:13. [PMID: 19497586] (Comprehensive review of nonsystemic and systemic vasculitides affecting the nervous system.)

DISORDERED TEMPERATURE REGULATION

 ESSENTIALS OF DIAGNOSIS

▶ Encephalopathy of varying degrees, including coma, at the extremes of core body temperature
▶ Risk factors include advanced age, disability, medications, endocrine disorders, infection, environmental exposure

1. Hyperthermia

In heat stress, discomfort and physiologic strain result from exposure to a hot environment, particularly with physical exertion. With continued heat exposure and volume depletion, heat stress gives way to heat exhaustion, with dizziness, presyncope or syncope, headache, weakness, and thirst. Heatstroke, defined as temperature higher than 40°C with cerebral dysfunction (agitation, delirium, seizures, coma), results from exposure to a hot environment (classic or nonexertional heatstroke) or strenuous physical activity (exertional heatstroke). Medication history is important in hyperthermic patients. Psychotropic agents and anticholinergic drugs are on the long list of medications that predispose patients to heatstroke. High fever following general anesthesia with inhalational anesthetics suggests malignant hyperthermia. Neuroleptic malignant syndrome or serotonin syndrome (covered later in this chapter) should be suspected in patients receiving dopamine-blocking antipsychotic or antiemetic agents, or serotonergic drugs.

Other features of hyperthermic states include hypotension, cardiac arrhythmias, rhabdomyolysis, kidney or liver failure, and disseminated intravascular coagulation. Ischemic or hemorrhagic stroke may thus contribute to cerebral dysfunction in hyperthermic patients.

▶ Treatment

Heatstroke is a medical emergency; removing the patient from the hot environment and rapidly lowering body temperature are critical. Evaporative cooling (tepid water applied to the skin and fans) or other external methods (cold water immersion or cooling blankets) usually suffice. Lowering skin temperature below 30°C may induce shivering and vasoconstriction, which slow further cooling. Occasional patients may require internal cooling interventions such as gastric or peritoneal lavage, enemas with iced fluids, or dialysis or cardiopulmonary bypass with cooling of fluids or blood. In addition to mechanical ventilation, fluid resuscitation, and blood pressure support, patients may require antiseizure medications and should be monitored for disseminated intravascular coagulation, renal and hepatic failure, and cerebral edema. Neurologic recovery during cooling is a favorable sign, but survivors may be left with persistent cerebral dysfunction.

2. Hypothermia

Brain death determination protocols include a minimal temperature criterion, because hypothermia can cause coma with loss of brainstem reflexes and isoelectric EEG, mimicking brain death. Shivering is prominent in mild hypothermia (32–35°C). In moderate hypothermia (28–32°C), altered mental status, dysarthria, and motor impairment are seen. Bradycardia, hypotension, and hypoventilation accompany deteriorating mental status in severe hypothermia (< 28°C). The clinical picture does not always correlate precisely with temperature, so measuring core temperature is important. Exposure to low temperature is the usual cause, but hypothermia may also develop in sepsis, severe hypothyroidism, and in Wernicke encephalopathy. Risk factors are similar to hyperthermia: advanced age, disability, environmental exposure, and medications. Laboratory studies may reveal electrolyte or acid-base disturbances, renal insufficiency, abnormal liver function tests, or coagulopathy. Cardiac arrhythmias and other electrocardiographic abnormalities should be anticipated.

▶ Treatment

External rewarming maneuvers may be passive (blankets) or active (heating blankets, warm water immersion); internal techniques include warm air, intravenous fluids, or body cavity lavage (gastric, bladder, colon, peritoneal, pleural). Intubation may be required for airway protection. Cardiopulmonary bypass may be necessary in severe hypothermia, particularly when complicated by cardiac dysrhythmias. Coexisting disorders such as drug intoxication or sepsis must also be managed. Patients being rewarmed should be watched closely for hypotension due to vasodilation and cardiac arrhythmias, which may be resistant to cardioversion and drugs. Age, etiology of hypothermia, and medical and neurologic comorbidities are important prognostic factors.

Aslam AF, et al. Hypothermia: Evaluation, electrocardiographic manifestations, and management. *Am J Med* 2006;119:297. [PMID: 16564768] (Covers clinical features, with a focus on cardiac manifestations and rewarming strategies.)

Sucholeiki R. Heatstroke. *Semin Neurol* 2005;25:307. [PMID: 16170743] (Reviews the spectrum of heat-related illnesses, with an emphasis on neurologic manifestations.)

MEDICATION-INDUCED NEUROLOGIC EFFECTS

ESSENTIALS OF DIAGNOSIS

▶ Cerebral symptoms (altered mental status, headache, aseptic meningitis, seizures, stroke, extrapyramidal syndromes, cerebellar disorders), visual or hearing loss, myelopathy, neuromuscular disorders

▶ Use of prescription or over-the-counter medications

▶ Onset shortly after starting a drug (or increasing the dose) or occasionally after long-term exposure

▶ Elderly patients are especially vulnerable

1. Altered Mental Status (Table 32-6)

Antidepressant, antipsychotic, sedative, anticonvulsant, and opioid medications exert their therapeutic benefits on the brain, so it is not surprising that cerebral side effects are common. Patients who are older, are taking multiple medications, or have preexisting brain disease are at increased risk. Clinical manifestations include cognitive impairment that can resemble dementia, affective symptoms, psychosis, or delirium. Coma may also develop, usually with preserved brainstem reflexes, although overdose with barbiturates or anticholinergic drugs can cause fixed and dilated pupils.

Patients with **neuroleptic malignant syndrome** develop fever, autonomic instability, delirium, and rigidity as a rare and potentially fatal complication of dopamine antagonists. Even more rarely, the syndrome can occur after stopping dopaminergic drugs used to manage Parkinson disease. Stopping the offending agent (or resuming dopaminergic drugs when their withdrawal causes neuroleptic malignant syndrome); avoiding other neuroleptics; aggressive supportive care, often in the intensive care unit; and monitoring and managing elevated serum creatine kinase are mainstays of treatment in all patients. The muscle relaxant

Table 32-6. Important Drug-Induced Causes of Altered Mental Status

	Clinical Features	Selected Drugs
Cognitive impairment	Memory impairment Slowed thinking	Antipsychotics, antidepressants Sedatives—benzodiazepines, barbiturates, others Opioids Anticonvulsants Anticholinergics β-Blockers
Affective disorders	Depression Euphoria	Sedatives, β-Blockers, interferons Corticosteroids, efavirenz, mefloquine, sympathomimetics
Psychosis	Delusions Hallucinations Preserved consciousness	Drugs of abuse—lysergic acid diethylamide, mescaline, phencyclidine, sympathomimetics Dopaminergics—levodopa, bromocriptine, pergolide, pramipexole, ropinirole, entacapone Others—corticosteroids, mefloquine, anticholinergics
Delirium	Disorientation Fluctuating alertness Inattention Agitation Paranoia	Antidepressants (including serotonin syndrome[a]), antipsychotics (including neuroleptic malignant syndrome[a]) Sedatives—benzodiazepines, barbiturates Anticonvulsants Anticholinergics Dopaminergics—amantadine, levodopa, bromocriptine, pergolide, pramipexole, ropinirole, entacapone Others—lithium, anticholinergics, mefloquine, nitrous oxide Withdrawal states—ethanol, sedatives
Coma	Unresponsiveness Symmetric, reactive pupils No lateralizing motor signs or reflex asymmetry	Antipsychotics, antidepressants, lithium Sedatives—benzodiazepines, barbiturates Opioids Anticonvulsants Drugs of abuse—ethanol, cocaine, amphetamines Others—acetaminophen, salicylates, antihistamines

[a]See text for further discussion.

dantrolene or dopamine agonist bromocriptine may be helpful in severely affected patients. (For additional discussion, see Chapter 15.)

Patients with the **serotonin syndrome** develop agitated delirium with fever, hemodynamic instability, and hyperkinetic movement disorders, particularly myoclonus, while taking one or more serotonergic drugs. In addition to selective serotonin reuptake inhibitor antidepressants, implicated drugs include meperidine, monoamine oxidase inhibitors, trazodone, and triptans. As with neuroleptic malignant syndrome, diagnosis depends on linking the clinical syndrome to a recent change in medication. There are no pathognomonic tests, although disseminated intravascular coagulation, rhabdomyolysis, and renal insufficiency may coexist. Differential diagnosis includes and is similar to neuroleptic malignant syndrome. Therapy consists of stopping the offending drugs and supportive care in a critical care setting.

2. Other Cerebral Syndromes (Table 32–7)

Phosphodiesterase 5 (PDE-5) inhibitors prescribed for erectile dysfunction, nitrates, dipyridamole, and proton pump inhibitors can cause headache, as can withdrawal from caffeine and overuse of acute headache agents. Pseudotumor cerebri, with headache and papilledema, complicates hypervitaminosis A and treatment with corticosteroids and some antibiotics. Various intrathecal, parenteral (immunoglobulin, muromonab), and oral agents (nonsteroidal anti-inflammatory drugs, some antibiotics) can cause drug-induced aseptic meningitis. When headache, fever, and neck stiffness are accompanied by lymphocytic CSF pleocytosis, viral meningitis is usually suspected. If offending medications are not recognized as the cause and thus continued, the illness persists, resembling chronic meningitis. In such instances the differential diagnosis includes

Table 32–7. Important Drug-Induced Cerebral Syndromes

	Clinical Features	Selected Drugs
Headache	Migraine or tension-type headache	Nitrates, proton pump inhibitors, dipyridamole, phosphodiesterase-5 inhibitors; withdrawal from caffeine; overuse of acute headache therapies (triptans, ergotamine derivatives, opioids, butalbital-containing combination analgesics)
	Pseudotumor cerebri	Oral contraceptives, corticosteroids, antibiotics (tetracycline, minocycline), vitamin A
Aseptic or chronic meningitis	Headache Meningismus Cerebrospinal fluid pleocytosis	Nonsteroidal anti-inflammatory drugs Antibiotics—trimethoprim-sulfamethoxazole, co-trimoxazole, ciprofloxacin, β-lactams Others—azathioprine, intravenous immunoglobulin, muromonab, carbamazepine, intrathecal medications, or contrast agents
Seizure	Single or multiple generalized seizures Status epilepticus	Antidepressants—bupropion; occurs with all classes Antipsychotics—clozapine; occurs with all classes Opioids—meperidine Local anesthetics Antibiotics—β-lactam antibiotics in renal failure Cancer chemotherapy Sympathomimetics—amphetamines, cocaine, phenylpropanolamine, pseudoephedrine Bronchodilators—aminophylline, theophylline Withdrawal states—ethanol, benzodiazepines, barbiturates
Stroke	Acute focal cerebral dysfunction, including coma	Oral contraceptives Sympathomimetics—amphetamines, cocaine, phenylpropanolamine, pseudoephedrine Serotonin agonists—triptans, ergotamine
Extrapyramidal syndromes	Akathisia Choreoathetosis Dystonia Tremor Myoclonus Parkinsonism Neuroleptic malignant syndrome[a] Serotonin syndrome[a]	Antipsychotics—typical and atypical Antidepressants—tricyclic antidepressants, selective serotonin reuptake inhibitors, trazodone Antiemetics—prochlorperazine, metoclopramide Sympathomimetics—amphetamines, cocaine, phenylpropanolamine, pseudoephedrine
Cerebellar dysfunction	Ataxia Nystagmus	Anticonvulsants—phenytoin, carbamazepine Sedatives—benzodiazepines, barbiturates Others—lithium, cyclosporine, cancer chemotherapy

[a]See text for further discussion.

tuberculous, fungal, and neoplastic meningitis, and autoimmune disorders. Occasional patients have polymorphonuclear or eosinophilic pleocytosis, suggesting bacterial or parasitic meningitis.

Antipsychotic and antidepressant agents lower seizure threshold. Most can still be prescribed safely in patients with epilepsy, although many clinicians avoid bupropion in patients who have had prior seizures. Penicillin is used to trigger seizures in animal models of epilepsy; β-lactam antibiotics occasionally cause seizures in humans, particularly at high doses with concomitant renal insufficiency. Abrupt discontinuation of chronic benzodiazepine or barbiturate therapy (or ethanol) can precipitate withdrawal seizures.

Oral contraceptive therapy increases the risk of ischemic stroke. Hemorrhagic and ischemic stroke can occur after the use of sympathomimetic agents, both legal (over-the-counter decongestants) and illicit (cocaine, methamphetamine). Extrapyramidal syndromes, such as hyperkinetic or akinetic movement disorders, complicate therapy with dopamine antagonist antipsychotics and antiemetics, and, less commonly, other psychotropic and illicit drugs. Cerebellar dysfunction, with nystagmus and ataxia, commonly occurs with anticonvulsant drugs, particularly phenytoin and carbamazepine, beginning in the upper levels of the therapeutic range.

3. Neuromuscular Syndromes (Table 32–8)

Polyneuropathy complicates therapy with many medications. Length-dependent sensory or sensorimotor neuropathies are the most common syndromes. Among antimicrobial drugs, isoniazid, metronidazole, dapsone, and the "d-drug" nucleoside antiretroviral agents zalcitabine (ddC), didanosine (ddI), and stavudine (d4T) cause neuropathy. The cancer chemotherapy agents vincristine, paclitaxel, and cisplatin also cause neuropathy. Symptoms may be more severe and rapidly progressive in patients with preexisting neuropathy resulting from diabetes, alcoholism, HIV infection, or other causes. The list of other drugs causing toxic neuropathy is long, and includes

amiodarone, phenytoin, colchicine, gold, disulfiram, and thalidomide. (For additional discussion of toxic neuropathies, see Chapter 19.)

Aminoglycosides are the classic drug class for which neuromuscular blockade is an unintended effect. Macrolide antibiotics have also been implicated, as have a variety of antiarrhythmic agents such as quinidine and phenytoin. They should be prescribed cautiously in patients with myasthenia gravis, and they occasionally unmask the illness in individuals not previously diagnosed.

Focal muscle injury may occur after intramuscular injection, and myopathy or frank rhabdomyolysis may complicate therapy with various drugs. Lipid-lowering drugs of all classes, but in particular statins, cause myopathy. Screening serum creatine kinase levels does not appear to be helpful, but a baseline measurement before starting therapy allows comparison if proximal muscle weakness or myoglobinuria develops. The nucleoside antiretroviral agent zidovudine can cause mitochondrial myopathy after long-term use (ie, more than 6 months). High-dose corticosteroids in critically ill patients can cause critical illness myopathy with quadriplegia often requiring prolonged mechanical ventilatory support. Chronic corticosteroid therapy can cause a milder myopathy, usually with normal creatine kinase level. Other agents that cause myopathy include acute or chronic ethanol ingestion, amiodarone, colchicine, ipecac, and penicillamine.

4. Other Neurologic Syndromes (Table 32–9)

Dysfunction of the retina or anterior (optic nerve) or posterior (occipital lobe) pathways causes visual impairment. Chloroquine causes retinopathy. Ethambutol, linezolid, and amiodarone cause optic neuropathy, and PDE-5 inhibitor use has been temporally related to the development of nonarteritic anterior ischemic optic neuropathy. Cyclosporine and tacrolimus have been linked to PRES. Tinnitus or vertigo in a patient taking nonsteroidal anti-inflammatory drugs (especially aspirin), aminoglycosides or other antibiotics,

Table 32–8. Selected Drug-Induced Neuromuscular Syndromes

	Clinical Features	Selected Drugs
Neuropathy	Numbness, weakness, pain—usually symmetric and distal Distal weakness Depressed or absent reflexes	Antibiotics—isoniazid, ethambutol, nitrofurantoin, metronidazole, dapsone Antiretrovirals—didanosine (ddI), zalcitabine (ddC), stavudine (d4T) Cancer chemotherapy—*Vinca* alkaloids, cisplatin, paclitaxel, docetaxel, suramin Others—amiodarone, ethanol, phenytoin, disulfiram, pyridoxine, colchicine, gold, thalidomide
Neuromuscular blockade	Generalized weakness Failure to wean from mechanical ventilation	Antibiotics—aminoglycosides, macrolides Cardiovascular agents—antiarrhythmics, β-blockers, calcium channel blockers Others—penicillamine, chloroquine, phenytoin, local anesthetics
Myopathy	Myalgia Proximal weakness Elevated creatine kinase Rhabdomyolysis	Cholesterol-lowering agents—statins, clofibrate, gemfibrozil, niacin Drugs of abuse—ethanol, cocaine, amphetamines, phencyclidine, heroin Others—amiodarone, zidovudine, ipecac, corticosteroids, penicillamine

Table 32–9. Other Selected Drug-Induced Neurologic Syndromes

	Clinical Features	Selected Drugs
Visual impairment	Retinopathy Optic neuropathy Cortical blindness	Chloroquine Ethambutol, linezolid, amiodarone, phosphodiesterase-5 inhibitors Cyclosporine, tacrolimus
Ototoxicity	Tinnitus Hearing loss Vertigo	Antibiotics—aminoglycosides, minocycline, erythromycin, metronidazole Chemotherapy—vincristine, cisplatin, bleomycin Others—loop diuretics, nonsteroidal anti-inflammatory drugs
Myelopathy	Spastic paraparesis or quadriparesis Sensory level Bowel, bladder, or sexual dysfunction	Intrathecal drugs—corticosteroids, baclofen, opioids, cancer chemotherapy, iodinated contrast agents Nitrous oxide Anticoagulants (epidural hematoma) Corticosteroids (vertebral compression or epidural lipoma)

loop diuretics, or cancer chemotherapy should prompt consideration of ototoxicity. Renal insufficiency increases the risk for vestibular and cochlear damage, which can be permanent if offending agents are not stopped quickly.

Spinal cord dysfunction occasionally complicates intrathecal administration of various medications. Compressive myelopathy can result from epidural hematoma in patients receiving anticoagulants or from epidural lipomatosis in the setting of chronic corticosteroid therapy.

Dalakas MC. Toxic and drug-induced myopathies. *J Neurol Neurosurg Psychiatry* 2009;80:832. [PMID: 19608783] (Practical review of clinical features and pathogenesis of myopathies caused by prescription and recreational drugs.)

Ferrari A. Headache: One of the most common and troublesome adverse reactions to drugs. *Curr Drug Saf* 2006;1:43. [PMID: 18690914] (Tabulates the frequency of headache associated with various drugs and drug classes.)

Haddad PM, Dursun SM. Neurological complications of psychiatric drugs: Clinical features and management. *Hum Psychopharmacol* 2008;23(Suppl 1):15. [PMID: 18098217] (Review emphasizing extrapyramidal symptoms, neuroleptic malignant syndrome, and serotonin syndrome.)

Hopkins S, Jolles S. Drug-induced aseptic meningitis. *Expert Opin Drug Saf* 2005;4:285. [PMID: 15794720] (Discusses implicated drugs and pathogenesis of this easily missed condition.)

Li J, Tripathi RC, Tripathi BJ. Drug-induced ocular disorders. *Drug Saf* 2008;31:127. [PMID: 18217789] (Reviews ophthalmologic side effects of medications, including retinopathy and optic neuropathy.)

Pratt RW, Weimer LH. Medication and toxin-induced peripheral neuropathy. *Semin Neurol* 2005;25:204. [PMID: 15937736] (Covers common drugs and toxins, organized by class, implicated as peripheral neurotoxins.)

Toledano R, Gil-Nagel A. Adverse effects of antiepileptic drugs. *Semin Neurol* 2008;28:317. [PMID: 18777478] (Readable review of acute, idiosyncratic, and long-term effects, as well as teratogenicity, carcinogenicity, and pharmocokinetic and pharmacodynamic interactions.)

Wills B, Erickson T. Drug- and toxin-associated seizures. *Med Clin North Am* 2005;89:1297. [PMID: 16227064] (Survey of pathogenetic mechanisms, implicated drugs, and management.)

BIOLOGIC NEUROTOXINS

1. Animal Neurotoxins (Table 32–10)

Snake venoms vary by species in targeting the neuromuscular junction, coagulation pathways, muscle, heart, and kidney. Sea snakes may leave no bite marks; venomous terrestrial snakebites often cause local pain and swelling. Hours after bites of sea and some terrestrial (elapid and a few viperid and crotalid species) snakes, paralysis develops, with respiratory failure and death. Systemic manifestations include coagulopathy, rhabdomyolysis, severe hypotension, acute renal failure, and secondary wound infections. Treatment consists of antivenom, wound care, and aggressive medical support, usually in an intensive care unit.

Spiders, scorpions, and ticks are among the insect envenomations with neurologic manifestations. *Latrodectus* species include the black widow spider, whose painful bite is followed by abdominal colic, diaphoresis, bradycardia, and muscle cramping. The local pain and swelling of a scorpion sting are followed by a cholinergic phase (colic, salivary, and bronchial hypersecretion, diaphoresis, bradycardia, and priapism), followed by an adrenergic state (hypertension, tachycardia, and agitation) and, occasionally, respiratory failure. Tick paralysis, a disorder of presynaptic neuromuscular blockade, causes ascending paralysis resembling Guillain-Barré syndrome, primarily in children. Careful removal of the tick, classically from the scalp where it may remain undetected for days or weeks, is usually followed by rapid clinical improvement when the disorder results from *Dermacentor* species endemic to North America. In general, antivenom use is more controversial, especially in adults, for many insect bites, compared with snakebites.

Table 32–10. Animal Neurotoxins

Syndrome	Neurologic Features	Comments
Snake bite (neurotoxic envenomation)[a]	Generalized weakness (with respiratory failure) Rhabdomyolysis	Terrestrial snakes: rattlesnakes, cobras, kraits, mambas, coral snakes Sea snakes
Scorpion sting[a]	Initial cholinergic phase: vomiting, diaphoresis, hypersalivation, bradycardia, shock, priapism Adrenergic phase: agitation, tachycardia, hypertension Generalized weakness (with respiratory failure)	
Black widow spider (*Latrodectus*) bite[a]	Similar to scorpion sting	
Tick paralysis	Ascending weakness (with respiratory failure)	Tick removal is curative
Algal Marine Toxins Ciguatera	Perioral paresthesias Reversed temperature sensation	Tropical regions Large predatory fish Sometimes fatal
Neurotoxic shellfish poisoning	Perioral paresthesias Reversed temperature sensation Gait disorder	Resembles ciguatera, but more transient New Zealand, Gulf of Mexico, Caribbean
Amnesic shellfish poisoning	Headache Short-term memory loss (may be permanent) Seizures, coma	Eastern North American, western United States Sometimes fatal
Paralytic shellfish poisoning	Perioral paresthesias Generalized weakness (with respiratory failure)	Northwestern and northeastern United States, North Sea, Japan, southern Chile Can be rapidly fatal
Other Marine Toxins Puffer fish poisoning	Perioral paresthesias Sense of doom Ascending paralysis (with respiratory failure)	Japan, China
Scombroid	Perioral paresthesias, pain Headache	Ingestion of spoiled fish

[a]Antivenom available.

Seafood consumption can cause poisoning with neurologic features from microbial toxins that accumulate up the food chain. Abdominal symptoms such as nausea, vomiting, cramps, and diarrhea are common, and are accompanied or followed by sensorimotor and other neurologic syndromes. **Ciguatera** fish poisoning is associated with the consumption of large predatory fish such as groupers and snappers from tropical regions, including Florida and Hawaii. Perioral paresthesias beginning within hours of ingestion are followed by limb dysesthesias with a characteristic temperature reversal in which cold stimuli are perceived as hot (and vice versa) and which may persist for days to weeks. A controlled study showed no benefit from mannitol. Treatment is otherwise supportive.

Neurotoxic shellfish poisoning is more transient than ciguatera. Brevetoxins produced by dinoflagellates off New Zealand and in the Gulf of Mexico and Caribbean open voltage-sensitive sodium channels. This shared mechanism of action with ciguatoxin parallels the similar but milder clinical syndrome, with paresthesias, diarrhea, and reversal of temperature sensation. **Paralytic shellfish poisoning** occurs after the consumption of mussels and other bivalves that have ingested dinoflagellates producing saxitoxin and related poisons. Symptoms begin within minutes to hours later and include numbness and weakness, progressing to generalized paralysis and death from respiratory arrest. A similar syndrome characterizes **puffer fish poisoning**. Bacteria in puffer fish skin and viscera produce tetrodotoxin. Despite preparation by chefs trained to remove these tissues carefully, deaths occur yearly in Japan, where the fish is a delicacy (fugu).

Amnesic shellfish poisoning occurs after the consumption of shellfish that have ingested *Pseudonitzchia* dinoflagellates that make domoic acid, an excitatory neurotoxin. Gastrointestinal symptoms are followed by dizziness, seizures, and short-term memory loss, which may be permanent. Included on the diagnosis of most seafood-poisoning syndromes is **scombroid** toxicity, in which improper handling of tuna, mackerel, mahi-mahi, and others leads to the production of histamine and related compounds by proliferating bacteria. The related histaminergic syndrome consists of flushing, perioral pain and tingling, gastrointestinal symptoms, headache, diaphoresis, hives, and conjunctival injection beginning within minutes to hours of exposure.

2. Botanical Neurotoxins

Plants are a rich source of pharmacologic agents, some of which target the nervous system; hence it is not surprising that ingestion of some botanicals, intentional or not, can have neurologic consequences. Tobacco, poison hemlock, and other plants contain nicotine, conine, and related alkaloids. Transcutaneous absorption among tobacco workers or accidental ingestion can cause symptoms and signs of muscarinic (miosis, lacrimation, salivation, bronchospasm, emesis, abdominal cramps, bradycardia, urination) or nicotinic (seizures, coma, weakness, fasciculations) overactivity (or both). *Datura stramonium* (jimson weed) causes central and peripheral anticholinergic symptoms. For further discussion, see Chapter 34.

Mycotoxins may be ingested accidentally by mushroom foragers or intentionally by individuals seeking their mind-altering properties. *Amanita phalloides* (death cap amanita) is a major cause of death by mushroom poisoning, resulting from liver failure with acute hepatic encephalopathy and increased intracranial pressure. *A muscaria* and *pantherina* (fly and panther amanita) contain glutamatergic isoxazoles that cause agitated delirium and ataxia. *Clitocybe* (funnel caps) and *Inocybe* species contain muscarine in sufficient quantities to cause an acute peripheral cholinergic syndrome of salivation, lacrimation, emesis, increased bronchial secretions, urination, and diarrhea with miosis and bronchospasm. *Gyromitra* species (false morels) cause self-limited gastrointestinal symptoms, occasionally followed by vertigo, delirium, and seizures. *Psilocybe*, *Panaeolus*, and *Conocybe* species (magic mushrooms) contain psilocybin and other hallucinogenic compounds. Ethanol intake within 72 hours of ingesting *Coprinus* species mushrooms (inky caps) leads to a disulfiram reaction, from acetaldehyde accumulation, of headache, paresthesias, flushing, nausea, and vomiting. More recently recognized mushroom toxidromes include rhabdomyolysis from *Tricholoma equestre* (yellow trich) and erythromelalgia (erythema and swelling in the distal extremities with severe burning pain) from *Clitocybe acromelalga* or *amoenolens* (poison dwarf bamboo mushrooms).

Diaz JH. Syndromic diagnosis and management of confirmed mushroom poisonings. *Crit Care Med* 2005;33:427. [PMID: 15699849] (Comprehensive, readable review of classic and newly recognized toxidromes following mushroom ingestion.)

Edlow JA, McGillicuddy DC. Tick paralysis. *Infect Dis Clin North Am* 2008;22:397. [PMID: 18755381] (Comprehensive review, including the history and a comparison of Australian and North American cases.)

Froberg B, Ibrahim D, Furbee RB. Plant poisoning. *Emerg Med Clin North Am* 2007;25:375. [PMID: 17482026] (Comprehensive review of botanical toxins, including images of source plants, mechanisms of toxicity, clinical manifestations, and management.)

Junghanss T, Bodio M. Medically important venomous animals: Biology, prevention, first aid, and clinical management. *Clin Infect Dis* 2006;43:1309. [PMID: 17051499] (Practical review of commonly encountered poisonous insects, snakes, fish, and coelenterates around the world.)

Sobel J, Painter J. Illnesses caused by marine toxins. *Clin Infect Dis* 2005;41:1290. [PMID: 16206104] (Concise discussion of seafood algal and bacterial toxins, as well as scombroid and puffer fish poisoning and emerging marine toxins.)

NEUROTOXICITY CAUSED BY HEAVY METALS & INDUSTRIAL COMPOUNDS

ESSENTIALS OF DIAGNOSIS

► Encephalopathy, extrapyramidal syndromes, peripheral neuropathy

► Dermatologic, hematologic, gastrointestinal disorders

► Associated with occupational or environmental (rare) exposure, substance abuse, attempted suicide or homicide

Heavy metals, organic chemicals, and other compounds can lead to acute and chronic syndromes involving the brain, neuromuscular system, or both. Cerebral manifestations include delirium, dementia, and other global encephalopathies as well as extrapyramidal syndromes. Neuromuscular disorders include peripheral neuropathies and, in the case of organophosphates, neuromuscular junction dysfunction.

1. Heavy Metals (Table 32–11)

Heavy metal intoxication should be considered in at-risk individuals, such as chemical industry workers, with encephalopathy, peripheral neuropathy, or both, particularly when associated with anorexia, anemia, gastrointestinal symptoms, and skin, nail, or gingival abnormalities. Exposure is commonly occupational or environmental, but heavy metal poisoning occasionally results from attempted homicide. Removing the patient from the source of exposure is critical and sometimes overlooked. Debate continues regarding the indications for and optimal use of chelating agents such as dimercaprol (British antilewisite), ethylenediaminetetraacetic acid, D-penicillamine, and succimer. Other individuals who may have been exposed should be screened.

Acute and subacute exposure to lead causes encephalopathy, particularly in children. In adults, motor neuropathy is the predominant neurologic syndrome. Elevated lead levels

Table 32–11. Heavy Metal Toxicity: Neurologic and Systemic Features

	Neurologic Features	Systemic Features
Lead	Encephalopathy (headache, seizures, cerebral edema, especially in children) Motor neuropathy, particularly in arms	Anemia (hypochromic, microcytic, with basophilic stippling) Constipation, cramps Gingival lead lines
Arsenic	Sensorimotor neuropathy (may resemble Guillain-Barré syndrome)	Gastroenteritis Dermatitis, Mees lines in nails Anemia (with basophilic stippling) Myoglobinuria, renal failure
Elemental mercury (acute)	Encephalopathy (psychosis, tremor)	Interstitial pneumonia, pulmonary edema Nausea, vomiting, abdominal pain Renal insufficiency
Elemental mercury (chronic)	Encephalopathy (behavioral changes, tremor) Sensorimotor neuropathy	Gastrointestinal symptoms Exfoliative dermatitis
Organic mercury (methylmercury)	Encephalopathy (dementia, psychosis, tremor, ataxia) with visual and hearing loss	Gastrointestinal symptoms
Thallium	Encephalopathy Sensorimotor neuropathy	Nausea, vomiting, diarrhea Alopecia Anemia Renal insufficiency Hepatitis
Manganese	Encephalopathy (psychosis, extrapyramidal syndrome)	

in blood and urine are typically accompanied by hypochromic, microcytic anemia.

Arsenic exposure causes encephalopathy, gastrointestinal symptoms, and sensorimotor neuropathy, which may evolve rapidly following acute exposure and mimic Guillain-Barré syndrome. With chronic exposure, neuropsychiatric abnormalities, skin changes, and painful neuropathy occur. Urine tests are more useful than blood levels because arsenic is cleared rapidly from the blood.

Acute elemental mercury exposure typically occurs by vapor inhalation; the resulting pulmonary, renal, and gastrointestinal dysfunction can cause metabolic encephalopathy. Chronic exposure, previously seen in felt hatmakers, causes behavioral changes ("mad as a hatter") and tremor. Inorganic mercury exposure appears also to be associated with development of sensorimotor polyneuropathy. Methylmercury, an organic mercury compound, readily crosses the blood–brain barrier, causing encephalopathy, visual and hearing impairment, ataxia, and tremor. Microbial methylation of mercury eventually leads to accumulation in large predatory fish. Dumping of industrial waste in Minamata Bay, Japan, caused numerous cases of methylmercury poisoning in adults and in children of exposed mothers.

Thallium intoxication causes toxic encephalopathy and small-fiber polyneuropathy that may be accompanied by dysautonomia. Alopecia, which develops as a late manifestation, can be a useful diagnostic clue. Manganese intoxication causes a toxic psychosis with residual dysarthria, tremor, and incoordination as well as an extrapyramidal syndrome of parkinsonism or dystonia.

2. Industrial Compounds

Hexacarbons, toluene, and other organic solvents enter the brain quickly, because of their high lipid solubility. Their volatility puts individuals working in poorly ventilated areas at particular risk; some agents are also used recreationally ("huffing"). Symptoms usually clear within hours to days once the patient is removed from the source of exposure. Chronic neuropsychiatric syndromes have been described in patients with long-term exposure, particularly to toluene. Peripheral neuropathy occurs as a complication of exposure to a few organic solvents, in particular, *n*-hexane, carbon disulfide, and methyl *n*-butyl ketone.

Organophosphates are cholinesterase inhibitors used in many pesticides. Ingestion, inhalation, or transcutaneous absorption leads to symptoms and signs referable to peripheral and central cholinergic overactivity. Muscarinic manifestations include increased bronchial secretions, sweating, bradycardia, abdominal cramps, and diarrhea. Activation of nicotinic synapses causes weakness and fasciculations. Cerebral effects include altered mentation and seizures. Airway management and ventilatory support are critical aspects of therapy, along with decontaminating the skin or gut, depending on the route of exposure. Muscarinic symptoms respond to atropine. Pralidoxime reactivates phosphorylated cholinesterases and treats nicotinic symptoms. Controversy continues regarding its benefits, but, if administered, it should be given after atropine. Neither drug reverses CNS symptoms.

Extraocular, bulbar, neck, limb, and respiratory weakness developing several days after organophosphate exposure may result from depolarizing neuromuscular blockade. Length-dependent sensorimotor neuropathy with prominent weakness developing weeks later, as acute autonomic and neuromuscular manifestations resolve, is known as organophosphate-induced delayed neurotoxicity. It occurs after exposure to some organophosphates, including triorthocresylphosphate, added during the Prohibition era to the patent medicine Jamaican ginger extract ("jake") to interfere with detection of its ethanol content. The persistent distal leg weakness was termed "jake leg."

Methanol or ethylene glycol ingestion causes encephalopathy with severe metabolic acidosis and can progress to multiorgan failure and death. Ingestion occurs accidentally, in attempted suicide, or in an effort to substitute for ethanol. Methanol is a component of windshield wiper fluid, canned heating products, and paint removers, and may contaminate moonshine liquor. Symptoms of methanol intoxication appear several hours, rather than immediately, after exposure because its metabolites, rather than the parent compound, are neurotoxic. Visual symptoms indicate toxicity of one such metabolite, formic acid. Encephalopathy, seizures, and coma may ensue, as well as delayed extrapyramidal syndromes. Ethylene glycol exposure frequently occurs by way of ingesting antifreeze, whose sweet taste and bright color make ethylene glycol poisoning a consideration in pediatric ingestions. Fomepizole competitively inhibits alcohol dehydrogenase, blocking the production of toxic metabolites, and is FDA approved for the treatment of poisoning with methanol or ethylene glycol.

Carbon monoxide binds tightly to heme, thus blocking the oxygen-carrying capability of hemoglobin. Exposure may be intentional or accidental, from automobile exhaust furnaces, ovens, or space heaters, and causes headache and dizziness when mild, and coma, seizures, and death when severe. Long-term complications include cognitive impairment, behavioral changes, and parkinsonism.

Cyanide intoxication manifests acutely as headache, agitation, seizures, and coma and is usually fatal. Parkinsonism and dystonia may develop as delayed syndromes among survivors.

Brent J. Fomepizole for ethylene glycol and methanol poisoning. *N Engl J Med* 2009;360:2216. [PMID: 19458366] (Case-based discussion, pathophysiology, evidence, and clinical use of the alcohol dehydrogenase inhibitor to manage these serious ingestions.)

Eicher T, Avery E. Toxic encephalopathies. *Neurol Clin* 2005;23:353. [PMID: 15757789] (Covers cerebral disorders resulting from heavy metals, solvents, pesticides, and biological neurotoxins.)

Ibrahim D, Froberg B, Wolf A. Heavy metal poisoning: Clinical presentations and pathophysiology. *Clin Lab Med* 2006;26:67. [PMID: 16567226] (Well-referenced and readable review, including illustrative cases and historical anecdotes.)

London Z, Albers JW. Toxic neuropathies associated with pharmaceutic and industrial agents. *Neurol Clin* 2007;25:257. [PMID: 17324727] (Survey of common toxic neuropathies, organized by clinical and electrodiagnostic syndrome.)

Alcoholism

John C.M. Brust, MD

ESSENTIALS OF DIAGNOSIS

▶ Psychic and physical dependence
▶ "Problem drinking"
▶ Intoxication and withdrawal
▶ Medical and neurological complications

▶ General Considerations

Definitions of alcoholism vary. At its broadest the term includes any kind of "problem drinking" (ie, applying not only to persons who are psychically or physically dependent on ethanol, but also to those who, even if abstinent most of the time, get into trouble when they drink). In addition to dependence per se, neurological problems associated with ethanol include intoxication, withdrawal, and an array of specific neurological disorders.

▶ Epidemiology

In the United States, 7% of all adults and 19% of adolescents are problem drinkers. Ethanol-related deaths exceed 100,000 each year, accounting for 5% of mortality in the United States.

▶ Pathogenesis

Ethanol affects many central nervous system (CNS) neurotransmitters, but its most important pharmacological action is to inhibit glutamatergic excitatory transmission and to facilitate GABAergic inhibitory transmission. These effects probably contribute to the clinical features of intoxication, withdrawal, and long-term toxicity.

ETHANOL INTOXICATION

ESSENTIALS OF DIAGNOSIS

▶ Disinhibition
▶ Stupor or coma
▶ Respiratory depression

▶ Epidemiology

Acute ethanol poisoning causes more than 1000 deaths per year in the United States. An additional 2500 deaths are attributable to ethanol taken with other drugs, usually sedatives.

▶ Clinical Findings

Ethanol is a CNS depressant, and early symptoms of intoxication often reflect cerebral disinhibition rather than stimulation. A number of factors influence the severity of intoxication, including the setting and the degree of a subject's tolerance, and the correlations of Table 33–1 are broad generalizations. A blood ethanol concentration (BEC) of 500 mg/dL would be fatal in 50% of individuals. Death comes from respiratory depression.

The term "pathologic intoxication" refers to sudden excitement with irrational or violent behavior, sometimes with delusions and hallucinations, after even small doses of ethanol. Episodes last minutes or hours, and upon awakening the subject is amnestic for what happened. The term "alcoholic blackout" refers to amnesia for periods of intoxication during which the subject appeared fully conscious.

▶ Differential Diagnosis

Stupor or coma in an alcoholic is too often dismissed as intoxication without consideration of potentially life-threatening

Table 33–1. Blood Ethanol Concentration and Symptoms

Blood Ethanol Concentration (mg/dL)	Symptoms
50–150	Euphoria or dysphoria; disinhibition; impaired concentration and judgment
150–250	Slurred speech, ataxic gait, diplopia, nausea, tachycardia, drowsiness, labile mood
300	Stupor alternating with combativeness, heavy breathing, vomiting
400	Coma
500	Respiratory depression, death

Table 33–2. Treatment of Ethanol Intoxication

For Hyperactive Patients
Isolation, calming environment
Avoidance of sedatives
Close observation
For Stuporous or Comatose Patients
If respiratory depression, artificial ventilation in an intensive care unit
If serum glucose level in doubt, IV 50% glucose
Thiamine, 100 mg, and multivitamins, IV or IM
Blood pressure monitoring; correction of hypovolemia or acid-base imbalance
Avoidance of stimulants
Avoidance of emetics or gastric lavage
Hemodialysis if patient is apneic, deeply comatose, or severely acidotic
Consideration of other causes of coma in an alcoholic

IM = intramuscularly; IV = intravenously.

alternatives. These include cerebral trauma, meningitis, hemorrhagic stroke, hypoglycemia, Wernicke encephalopathy, seizures, hepatic encephalopathy, and concomitant drug use.

▶ Treatment

Artificial ventilation is the mainstay of treatment for severe ethanol intoxication (Table 33–2). No pharmacological agent is available that accelerates ethanol metabolism; in a nonhabitual drinker a BEC of 400 mg/dL takes roughly 20 hours to return to zero. Hemodialysis or peritoneal dialysis can be considered for BECs greater than 500 mg/dL; for severe acidosis; for concomitant ingestion of methanol, ethylene glycol, or other dialyzable drugs; or for severely intoxicated children.

ETHANOL DEPENDENCE & WITHDRAWAL

ESSENTIALS OF DIAGNOSIS

- ▶ Tremor
- ▶ Seizure
- ▶ Hallucinosis
- ▶ Delirium tremens

▶ General Considerations

Hangover—headache, nausea, malaise, tremulousness, sweating—can occur in anybody after brief but excessive drinking. "Ethanol withdrawal" signifies physical dependence and is divided into early and late syndromes.

▶ Clinical Findings

Early withdrawal, occurring usually within a few days of the last drink, consists of tremor, hallucinations, and seizures, alone or in combination. Tremor, the most common withdrawal symptom, tends to appear in the morning after several days of heavy drinking and is promptly relieved by ethanol. With continued abstinence, tremor becomes more intense, accompanied by insomnia, agitation, sweating, nausea, tachypnea, and tachycardia. Mentation is usually intact, however. Tremulousness can persist for weeks or longer.

Alcoholic hallucinosis refers to illusions or hallucinations, usually visual but sometimes auditory or tactile. Formed images (insects, animals, people) are usually fragmentary, lasting seconds or minutes for several days. Delirium is not a feature, and insight varies. Infrequently, repeated bouts of hallucinosis evolve into a chronic state, with delusions resembling schizophrenia.

Ethanol can trigger seizures in any epileptic. The term *alcohol-related seizures* refers to seizures in which ethanol is presumed to be the sole cause. They typically occur during early withdrawal but sometimes are seen during active drinking or after days or even weeks of abstinence. Seizures are usually grand mal, occurring singly or in a brief cluster; status epilepticus is infrequent. Diagnosis requires a normal electroencephalogram (EEG) and computed tomography (CT) or magnetic resonance imaging (MRI).

In contrast to tremor, hallucinosis, and seizures, *delirium tremens* usually begins 48–72 hours after the last drink, often in patients who have been hospitalized for other reasons. The syndrome may follow early withdrawal symptoms or occur de novo. Tremor is accompanied by delirium (severe inattentiveness and usually agitation) and autonomic instability (fever, tachycardia, profuse sweating, and blood pressure swings). Hallucinations are inferred from the patient's behavior. Mortality is as high as 15%; death is usually due to other diseases such as pneumonia or sepsis but may be consequent to autonomic derangement.

▶ Differential Diagnosis

As with ethanol intoxication, other possible causes of altered mentation in an alcoholic must be kept in mind, especially cerebral trauma and meningitis.

▶ Treatment

Treatment of ethanol withdrawal includes prevention or reduction in early symptoms, prevention of *delirium tremens*, and management of *delirium tremens* after it occurs. Benzodiazepines, which have cross-tolerance with ethanol, are given orally for early symptoms with doses titrated to avoid both intoxication and tremor. After a few days, tapering of the dose can be attempted. Neuroleptics, which are not cross-tolerant with ethanol and which lower seizure threshold, are inappropriate even in patients with hallucinations. Seizures usually do not require therapy unless they recur or the causal role of ethanol is in doubt; in particular, phenytoin is of no value in preventing ethanol seizures. Status epilepticus, on the other hand, is treated conventionally. Long-term treatment of ethanol seizures is superfluous; abstainers do not need their medications, and drinkers do not take them. Epileptics whose seizures are triggered by ethanol do merit anticonvulsant therapy.

Once it appears, *delirium tremens* cannot be abruptly reversed by any agent. Parenteral benzodiazepine is given in titrated and sometimes extremely high doses to achieve calming. The disorder is a medical emergency best treated in an intensive care unit, with strict monitoring of vital signs and fluid and electrolyte balance (Table 33–3). Other ethanol-related disorders including hypoglycemia, pancreatitis, meningitis, and subdural hematoma can coexist with *delirium tremens*. Hepatic encephalopathy can be aggravated by sedative drugs, precipitating coma that outlasts pharmacotherapy.

WERNICKE-KORSAKOFF SYNDROME

ESSENTIALS OF DIAGNOSIS

- ▶ Wernicke syndrome: acute global confusional state, abnormal eye movements, ataxic gait
- ▶ Korsakoff syndrome: chronic amnestic disorder

▶ General Considerations

Wernicke and Korsakoff syndromes share the same pathology, namely, histologically distinctive lesions in the medial thalamus, hypothalamus, and periaqueductal gray matter of the midbrain. Clinically, however, they are distinct. Full-blown Wernicke syndrome is a triad of mental, eye movement, and gait abnormalities. Korsakoff syndrome is only a mental disorder, qualitatively different from Wernicke syndrome. Both are caused by thiamine deficiency.

Table 33–3. Treatment of Ethanol Withdrawal

Prevention or Reduction of Early Mild Symptoms
Chlordiazepoxide, 25–100 mg, or diazepam, 5–20 mg, PO every 8 h for first day, tapering over 3–6 days
Thiamine, 100 mg, and multivitamins
For More Severe Symptoms, Including Delirium Tremens
Diazepam, 10 mg IV, or lorazepam, 2 mg IV or IM, repeated every 5–15 min until calming and normalization of vital signs; maintenance doses every 1–4 h as needed
If refractory to benzodiazepines, phenobarbital, 260 mg IV, repeated in 30 min as needed
If refractory to phenobarbital, pentobarbital, 3–5 mg/kg IV, with endotracheal intubation and repeated doses to produce general anesthesia
Careful attention to fluid and electrolyte balance; several liters of saline per day, or even pressors, may be needed
Cooling blanket or alcohol sponges for high fever
Prevention or correction of hypoglycemia
Thiamine and multivitamins
Consideration of coexisting illness (eg, liver failure, pancreatitis, sepsis, meningitis, or subdural hematoma)

IM = intramuscularly; IV = intravenously; PO = orally (by mouth).
Reproduced with permission from Brust JCM. *Neurological Aspects of Substance Abuse,* 2nd ed. Butterworth-Heinemann; 2004, Elsevier.

▶ Clinical Features

In Wernicke syndrome a global confusional state evolves over days or weeks, with inattentiveness, indifference, decreased spontaneous speech, impaired memory, and lethargy, which, if untreated, can progress to coma. Importantly, autopsy studies reveal that the mental symptoms of Wernicke syndrome, including progression to coma, can occur in the absence of eye movement abnormalities or ataxia.

Abnormal eye movements include nystagmus, lateral rectus paresis, and horizontal gaze paresis, with later involvement of vertical eye movements progressing to complete ophthalmoplegia. Loss of pupillary reactivity is rare. Truncal ataxia may prevent standing or walking; dysarthria and limb ataxia are infrequent. Systemic signs of nutritional deficiency may be present, and autonomic signs, especially tachycardia and postural hypotension, are common. Fever usually indicates infection.

Korsakoff syndrome is a more purely amnestic disorder that most often emerges as the other mental symptoms of Wernicke syndrome respond to treatment. Amnesia is both anterograde and retrograde, with relative preservation of alertness, attentiveness, and behavior. Confabulation is neither invariable nor specific. Insight varies.

▶ Treatment & Prognosis

Untreated Wernicke syndrome is fatal. Treatment includes parenteral thiamine, 50–100 mg daily, plus multivitamins.

Autonomic instability calls for strict bed rest. Concomitant liver failure, infection, or withdrawal symptoms complicate management. Fluid and electrolyte abnormalities include possible hypomagnesemia. With replacement, ocular abnormalities usually improve within hours and resolve within a week, but there may be residual nystagmus. Gait ataxia may or may not improve, and residual Korsakoff amnesia is a common residual of the mental disorder.

OTHER NEUROLOGICAL COMPLICATIONS OF ALCOHOLISM

▶ Alcoholic Cerebellar Degeneration

Truncal ataxia in the absence of other features of Wernicke syndrome is common in alcoholics, and the disorder is less clearly the result of nutritional deficiency. Symptoms are of more gradual onset and less likely to respond to treatment. The responsible lesion consists of neuronal loss in the anterior cerebellar vermis. The role of direct ethanol toxicity in this disorder is uncertain.

▶ Alcoholic Polyneuropathy

Sensorimotor polyneuropathy is common in alcoholics. Distal limb paresthesias are usually the initial symptom, progressing to sensory loss and sometimes severe pain. Early signs are distal vibratory loss and absent ankle tendon reflexes. Weakness appears at any time and can be severe. Autonomic abnormalities, less common than with diabetic neuropathy, include urinary incontinence, hypotension, cardiac arrhythmia, and altered sweat patterns. Alcoholic polyneuropathy appears to be both nutritional and toxic in origin. Clinical and pathological studies suggest that pure thiamine deficiency neuropathy is motor dominant and acutely progressive, and primarily affects large-fiber axons, whereas pure alcoholic (toxic) neuropathy is sensory dominant and slowly progressive, and primarily affects small-fiber axons. Most patients have a combination of the two.

Alcoholic polyneuropathy stabilizes or improves with abstinence and nutritional supplements.

Alcoholics are prone to pressure palsies especially affecting the radial and peroneal nerves.

▶ Alcoholic Amblyopia

Demyelination of the optic nerves in alcoholics results in impaired vision that progresses over days or weeks, with bilateral central scotomas and temporal disc pallor. The disorder is mainly nutritional in origin, but ethanol toxicity, as well as compounds contained in tobacco smoke, could be contributory. Alcoholic amblyopia does not progress to total blindness, and improvement (often incomplete) follows abstinence and nutritional replacement.

▶ Pellagra

Inadequate nutrition in alcoholics includes vitamins in addition to thiamine, especially folate, deficiency of which causes macrocytic anemia, and nicotinic acid, deficiency of which causes pellagra, with dermatologic, gastrointestinal, and neurological symptoms. Altered mentation progresses over hours, days, or weeks to amnesia, psychosis, or delirium. Improvement follows treatment with nicotinic acid plus other vitamins.

▶ Alcoholic Liver Disease

Abnormal mental status in an alcoholic always raises the possibility of hepatic encephalopathy. Also encountered in patients with alcoholic cirrhosis is a syndrome of altered mentation, myoclonus, and myelopathy following portocaval shunting. Patients who have repeated bouts of hepatic coma sometimes develop acquired chronic hepatocerebral degeneration, a syndrome of dementia, ataxia, choreoathetosis, muscular rigidity, and asterixis.

▶ Hypoglycemia

Hypoglycemia in alcoholics is the result of starvation, lack of liver glycogen, and especially depletion of nicotinamide adenine dinucleotide (NAD) and impairment of gluconeogenesis. Coma or a seizure in an alcoholic should always raise the possibility of hypoglycemia and not be dismissed as intoxication or withdrawal.

▶ Alcoholic Ketoacidosis

Starvation, increased lipolysis, and impaired fatty acid oxidation during heavy drinking cause accumulation of lactic acid and β-hydroxybutyric acid. Symptoms include anorexia, vomiting, obtundation, and hyperventilation. Blood glucose may be low, normal, or moderately elevated. There is a large anion gap, but β-hydroxybutyrate is not detected by the nitroprusside test (Acetest). Treatment includes infusion of glucose (and thiamine), correction of dehydration or hypotension, correction of electrolyte imbalance, and, as needed, sodium bicarbonate.

▶ Infection

Alcoholics are immune suppressed, and infectious meningitis, including tuberculous, must be considered in the presence of seizures or altered mentation. Intoxication is a risk factor for human immunodeficiency virus infection.

▶ Trauma

Alcoholics are prone to trauma, and impaired blood clotting increases the likelihood of intracranial hematoma after head injury.

▶ Stroke

Numerous studies have identified a "J-shaped association" between ethanol consumption and the risk of ischemic stroke: compared to abstainers, low to moderate consumption reduces

Table 33–4. Clinical Features of Fetal Alcohol Syndrome

Features	Majority	Minority
Central nervous system	Mental retardation Microcephaly Hypotonia Poor coordination Hyperactivity	—
Growth and development	Impaired growth prenatally and postnatally for length and weight Diminished adipose tissue	—
Face Eyes	Short palpebral fissures	Ptosis Strabismus Epicanthal folds Myopia Microphthalmia Blepharophimosis Cataracts Retinal pigmentary abnormalities
Nose	Short, upturned Hypoplastic philtrum	—
Mouth	Thin vermilion lip borders Retrognathia in infancy Micrognathia or prognathia in adolescence	Prominent lateral palatine ridges Cleft lip or palate Small teeth with faulty enamel
Maxilla	Hypoplastic	—
Ears	—	Posteriorly rotated Poorly formed concha
Skeletal	—	Pectus excavatum or carinatum Syndactyly, clinodactyly, or camptodactyly Limited joint movements Nail hypoplasia Radioulnar synostosis Bifid xiphoid Scoliosis Klippel-Feil anomaly
Cardiac	—	Septal defects Great vessel abnormalities
Cutaneous	—	Abnormal palmar creases Hemangiomas Infantile hirsutism
Muscular	—	Diaphragmatic, inguinal, or umbilical hernias Diastasis recti
Urogenital	—	Labial hypoplasia Hypospadias Small rotated kidneys Hydronephrosis

Reproduced with permission from Brust JCM. *Neurological Aspects of Substance Abuse,* 2nd ed. Butterworth-Heinemann, 2004, Elsevier.

the risk and heavy consumption increases the risk. In the United States the relationship holds for men and women and for spirits, beer, and wine. Whether extra risk is temporally associated with binge drinking and whether special benefit is conferred by wine is less clear. Mechanisms for benefit and for risk are uncertain and probably multiple. Alcoholic cardiomyopathy predisposes to embolic stroke. Ethanol in any dose increases the risk for hemorrhagic stroke.

Myopathy

Ethanol causes myopathy with different degrees of severity. Some patients have elevated creatine kinase levels and electromyographic changes, with or without intermittent cramps or weakness. Some have progressive proximal weakness resembling polymyositis but improving with abstinence. Some have acute myoglobinuria with severe weakness, pain, swelling, and myoglobinuria. The cause is toxicity, not nutritional deficiency, and symptoms sometimes emerge during a binge. Alcoholic cardiomyopathy often coexists.

Marchiafava-Bignami Disease

The pathology of Marchiafava-Bignami disease—demyelination within the corpus callosum—is insufficient to explain the severity of symptoms, which include psychosis, aphasia, dementia, seizures, hemiparesis, and ataxia progressing to coma and death over a few months. Occurring almost exclusively in alcoholics, Marchiafava-Bignami disease is of unknown cause. MRI can detect the lesions, which sometimes spontaneously regress with clinical improvement.

Alcoholic Dementia

Both animal and human studies support the view that ethanol, by directly damaging neurons, can cause progressive mental decline in the absence of nutritional deficiency, brain trauma, or other indirect mechanisms. On the other hand, attempts to identify a safe dose threshold for alcoholic dementia found a "J-shaped association" similar to what is seen with ethanol and ischemic stroke: low to moderate ethanol consumption reduces the likelihood of dementia, both vascular and Alzheimer type. The mechanism for increased risk might be glutamatergic excitotoxicity. The mechanism of protection might be the antioxidant properties of congeners in alcoholic beverages and of ethanol itself.

Fetal Alcohol Syndrome

Delayed psychomotor development and congenital malformations are a consequence of ethanol ingestion during pregnancy. Fetal alcohol syndrome (FAS) consists of cerebral dysfunction, growth deficiency, and distinctive facial abnormalities; less often there are anomalies of the heart, skeleton, urogenital organs, skin, and muscles (Table 33–4). Mental retardation can be severe, and in some cases in utero exposure to ethanol causes mental deficiency and behavioral disturbance ("fetal alcohol effects"; FAE) in the absence of other features of FAS. The syndrome has been reproduced in animals, and a safe dose has not been identified. It is estimated that in the United States the combined incidence of FAS and FAE is nearly 1% of all live births. FAE may affect 1% of infants born to women who drink 1 oz of ethanol early in pregnancy. More than 30% of the children of heavy drinkers are affected by FAS, which is probably the leading teratogenic cause of mental retardation in the Western world.

TREATMENT OF CHRONIC ALCOHOLISM

The large number of approaches to treating alcoholism—psychotherapy, group psychotherapy, family or social network therapy, behavioral (aversion) therapy, pharmacotherapy, hospitalization, vocational rehabilitation, Alcoholics Anonymous—reflects their limited efficacy. The success rate of Alcoholics Anonymous is estimated to be 34%.

Only three drugs are FDA approved for the specific treatment of alcoholism. Disulfiram, by inhibiting aldehyde dehydrogenase, causes accumulation of acetaldehyde when ethanol is consumed, resulting in flushing, headache, nausea, vomiting, sweating, palpitations, hypotension, and weakness. Severe reactions last hours and can be fatal. In the United States nearly 200,000 patients are maintained on disulfiram, yet studies demonstrating long-term benefit are mostly flawed methodologically. Side effects of disulfiram unrelated to ethanol ingestion include altered mentation, seizures, ataxia, and peripheral neuropathy.

Following reports of efficacy in humans, the FDA approved the μ-opioid antagonist naltrexone for treating alcoholism. Treatment response is quite variable, and patients are more likely to reduce heavy drinking than to achieve full abstinence.

Available in Europe for over a decade, acamprosate was approved by the FDA for treating alcoholism in 2004. The drug blocks glutamate receptors, and in combination with psychosocial support it is effective in maintaining abstinence. Acamprosate and naltrexone can be taken together.

The use of sedative or tranquilizing drugs is controversial, as they carry the risk of dependency switching and of drug-ethanol interactions.

Abel EL. Fetal alcohol syndrome: Same old, same old. *Addiction* 2009;104:1274–1280. [PMID: 19624316] (A review of current thinking on the subject.)

Brust JCM. Ethanol and cognition: Indirect effects, neurotoxicity, and neuroprotection: A review. *Int J Environ Res Public Health* 2010;7:1540–1557. [PMID: 20617045] (Heavy alcohol consumption produces lasting cognitive impairment, whereas low to moderate consumption reduces the risk of dementia, including Alzheimer type. An up-to-date review.)

Collins MA, et al. Alcohol in moderation, cardioprotection, and neuroprotection: Epidemiological considerations and mechanistic studies. *Alcohol Clin Exp Res* 2009;33:206–219. [PMID: 19032583] (Reviews the evidence for the protective effects of mild to moderate alcohol consumption against coronary artery disease and ischemic stroke.)

Koike H, et al. Alcoholic neuropathy is clinicopathologically distinct from thiamine-deficiency neuropathy. *Ann Neurol* 2003;54:19. [PMID: 12838517] (A clinical, electrodiagnostic, and pathological study that demonstrates that ethanol toxicity and thiamine deficiency each cause a distinctive form of peripheral neuropathy.)

Kosten TR, O'Connor PG. Management of drug and alcohol withdrawal. *N Engl J Med* 2003;348:1786. [PMID: 12724485] (Comprehensive review of management options for ethanol, benzodiazepines, opiates, amphetamines, and cocaine.)

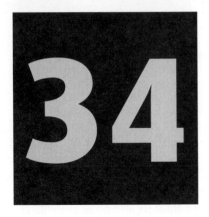

Drug Dependence

John C.M. Brust, MD

Drug dependence is of two types. Psychic dependence leads to craving and drug-seeking behavior. Physical dependence produces somatic withdrawal symptoms and signs. Psychic and physical dependence can coexist or occur alone. Addiction is psychic dependence.

Tolerance refers to the need for ever higher doses of a drug to achieve the desired effect. Sensitization ("reverse tolerance") refers to increased drug effects (including craving) with repeated administration.

Worldwide hundreds of different agents are used recreationally for their psychic properties. Broad categories of agents popular in North America and Europe are listed in Table 34–1. These agents differ in their addiction liability; in the symptoms and signs associated with intoxication, overdose, and withdrawal; and in the medical and neurological complications that sometimes follow their use.

DRUGS OF DEPENDENCE

▶ Opioids

Opioids include agonists, antagonists, and mixed agonist-antagonists (Table 34–2). At intended levels of intoxication, opioid agonists produce drowsy euphoria, miosis, analgesia, cough suppression, and often nausea, vomiting, pruritus, hypothermia, postural hypotension, constipation, and decreased libido. Parenteral or smoked heroin (the most widely abused opioid) produces a "rush"—a brief ecstatic feeling followed by euphoria and either relaxed "nodding" or garrulous hyperactivity.

Overdose causes the triad of coma, pinpoint pupils, and respiratory depression, and treatment consists of respiratory support and naloxone, 2 mg intravenously, repeated as needed up to 20 mg. If respiration is not depressed, smaller doses, 0.4–0.8 mg, are given to avoid the precipitation of withdrawal signs. Close observation is necessary, for naloxone is short acting.

Withdrawal from opioid agonists causes irritability, lacrimation, rhinorrhea, sweating, yawning, mydriasis, myalgia, muscle spasms, piloerection, nausea, vomiting, abdominal cramps, fever, hot flashes, tachycardia, hypertension, and orgasm. In adults, seizures and delirium are not features of opioid withdrawal, which is hardly ever life threatening. By contrast, seizures and myoclonus do occur with neonatal opioid withdrawal, which can be fatal if untreated. Treatment of opioid withdrawal is with titrated doses of methadone; for neonates paregoric is an alternative.

Effective therapy for opioid dependence consists of substitution with the long-acting opioid agonist methadone (a Schedule II drug, which can be administered to ambulatory patients only in federally approved methadone-maintenance treatment programs) or with the mixed agonist-antagonist buprenorphine (a Schedule III drug, which can be prescribed by appropriately registered private physicians).

▶ Psychostimulants

Psychostimulant drugs include amphetamine-like agents, cocaine, methylphenidate, and a number of compounds found in decongestants, diet pills, and "dietary supplements" (Table 34–3).

Intended effects include euphoria, increased motor activity, and increased endurance. Methylenedioxymethamphetamine (MDMA; "ecstasy") has properties that seem to bridge those of amphetamine and of hallucinogenic drugs such as mescaline. MDMA is a popular drug at "raves," in which frenetic dancing to loud music continues for hours at a time.

Table 34–1. Categories of Abused Drugs

Opioids
Psychostimulants
Hypnotics/sedatives
Marijuana
Hallucinogens
Inhalants
Phencyclidine
Anticholinergics
Tobacco

Cocaine is snorted intranasally, injected parenterally, or, as alkaloidal "crack," smoked. A smokable form of methamphetamine is called "ice." Parenteral or smoked cocaine or methamphetamine produces a rush clearly distinguishable from that of opioids. Repeated use leads to stereotypic activity progressing to bruxism or other dyskinesias and to paranoia

Table 34–2. Opioids Currently or Recently Available in the United States

Agonist
Powdered opium
Tincture of opium (laudanum)
Camphorated tincture of opium (paregoric)
Purified opium alkaloids (Pantopon)
Morphine (Morphine Sulfate Injection; MS Contin; Oramorph)
Heroin (legally available only for investigational use)
Methadone (Dolophine)
Fentanyl (Sublimaze; in Innovar; Duragesic Patch)
Sufentanil (Sufenta)
Alfentanil (Alfenta)
Oxymorphone (Numorphan)
Hydromorphone (Dilaudid)
Codeine
Dihydrocodeine (Synalgos)
Oxycodone (Oxy-Contin, and in mixtures, eg, Percodan, Percocet, Tylox)
Hydrocodone (in mixtures, eg, Hycodan, Lortab, Lorcet, Tussionex, Vicodin)
Levorphanol (Levo-Dromoran)
Meperidine (pethidine; Demerol, Pethadol)
Alphaprodine (Nisentil)
Propoxyphene (Darvon, and in Darvocet, Wygesic)
Diphenoxylate (in Lomotil)
Apomorphine

Antagonist
Naloxone (Narcan)
Naltrexone (Trexan)
Nalmefene (Revex)

Mixed Agonist-Antagonist
Pentazocine (Talwin, Talwin Nx, and in Talacen)
Butorphanol (Stadol)
Buprenorphine (Buprenex)
Nalbuphine (Nubain)

Table 34–3. Psychostimulants

Amphetamine (Benzedrine)
Dextroamphetamine (Dexedrine)
Amphetamine and dextroamphetamine (Biphetamine)
Methamphetamine (Methedrine; Desoxyn; Fetamin)
Methylenedioxymethamphetamine (MDMA; "Ecstasy")
Methylenedioxyethylamphetamine (MDEA)
Cocaine
Ephedrine
Pseudoephedrine
Methylphenidate (Ritalin)
Pemoline (Cylert)
Phenmetrazine (Preludin; Prelu-2)
Diethylpropion (Tenuate; Tepanil)
Benzphetamine (Didrex)
Fenfluramine (Pondimin) (withdrawn)
Dexfenfluramine (Redux) (withdrawn)
Phendimetrazine (Plegine; Bontril)
Phentermine (Ionamin; Wilpo; Adipex-P; Fastin)
Mazindol (Sanorex; Mazanor)
Phenylpropanolamine (Propadrine; Propagest; and in decongestants and diet pills) (withdrawn)
Propylhexedrine (Benzedrex nasal inhaler)
Naphazoline (Privine nasal solution; Naphcon ophthalmic solution)
Tetrahydrozoline (Tyzine nasal solution; Visine ophthalmic solution)
Oxymetazoline (Afrin nasal solution; OcuClear ophthalmic solution)
Xylometazoline (Otrivin nasal solution)
Phenoxazoline (nasal solutions)

progressing to hallucinatory psychosis. Overdose causes variable combinations of headache, chest pain, hypertension (sometimes severe), tachycardia, atrial or ventricular arrhythmia, fever, excitement, delirium, myoclonus, seizures, and myoglobinuria. Coma, shock, and death occur; malignant hyperthermia and disseminated intravascular coagulation are described. Treatment includes sedation, oxygen, bicarbonate, anticonvulsants, cooling, blood pressure lowering, cardiac monitoring, and respiratory and blood pressure support.

Psychostimulant withdrawal produces fatigue, hunger, and depression, but little in the way of objective signs. Suicidal ideation is the principal danger.

▶ Sedatives

Sedative drugs include barbiturates, benzodiazepines, and miscellaneous products (Table 34–4). Intended effects, overdose, and withdrawal resemble what is seen with ethanol. Respiratory depression is much milder with benzodiazepines than with barbiturates. Treatment of overdose is supportive. A specific benzodiazepine antagonist, flumazenil (Romazicon), has a brief duration of action and is therefore more useful in diagnosing overdose than in treating it. Withdrawal tremor and seizures can be prevented or treated with titrated doses of a barbiturate or a benzodiazepine. As with ethanol, delirium tremens is a medical emergency requiring intensive care.

Table 34–4. Sedatives/Hypnotics

Class	Drug
Barbiturates	
Long acting	Phenobarbital (Luminal, and in mixtures, eg, Bellergal, Donnatal, Gustase, Kinesed, Primatene, Quadrinal, Tedral)
	Mephobarbital (Mebaral)
	Barbital
	Primidone (Mysoline)
Intermediate acting	Amobarbital (Amytal, and in Tuinal)
	Aprobarbital (Alurate)
	Butabarbital (Butisol)
	Butalbital (only in mixtures, eg, Esgic, Fiorinal, Fioricet, Medigesic, Pacaps, Phrenilin, Repan, Sedapap, Tencet, Tencon)
Short acting	Hexobarbital
	Pentobarbital (Nembutal)
	Secobarbital (Seconal)
Ultra-short acting	Methohexital (Brevital)
	Thiamylal (Surital)
	Thiopental (Pentothal)
Benzodiazepines	
Promoted as tranquilizers	Alprazolam (Xanax)
	Chlorazepate (Tranxene)
	Chlordiazepoxide (Librium, others)
	Diazepam (Valium, others)
	Halazepam (Paxipam)
	Lorazepam (Ativan)
	Oxazepam (Serax, Zaxopam)
	Prazepam (Centrax)
Promoted as hypnotics	Estazolam (Prosom)
	Flurazepam (Dalmane)
	Quazepam (Doral)
	Temazepam (Restoril)
	Triazolam (Halcion)
Promoted as anticonvulsant	Clonazepam (Klonopin)
Promoted for anesthesia induction	Midazolam (Versed)
Nonbarbiturate, nonbenzodiazepine sedative-hypnotics	
	Buspirone (Buspar)
	Chloral hydrate (Noctec, others)
	Chlormezanone (Trancopal)
	Diphenhydramine (Benadryl, and in over-the-counter sleeping pills, eg, Miles Nervine, Nytol, Sleep-Eze, Sominex, Compoz)
	Ethchlorvynol (Placidyl)
	Ethinamate (Valmid, no longer produced in the US)
	Glutethimide (Doriden, after 1991 available only as generic)
	Hydroxyzine (Vistaril, Atarax, others)
	Meprobamate (Miltown, Equanil; in Equagesic with aspirin; in Deprol with benactyzine)
	Methaqualone (Quaalude, Sopar, no longer produced in the US)
	Methyprylon (Nodular, no longer produced in the US)
	Paraldehyde
	Triclofos (Triclos, no longer produced in the US)
	Zaleplon (Sonata)
	Zolpidem (Ambien, Stilnox, Niotal)

γ-Hydroxybutyric acid (GHB), normally present in the brain as a metabolite of the inhibitory neurotransmitter γ-aminobutyric acid (GABA), became a popular euphoriant during the 1990s both as a staple at rave parties and as a "date-rape" drug. GHB and two of its precursors, γ-butyrolactone and 1,4-butanediol, are sold under many different trade names.

Often taken with ethanol, they cause sedation and respiratory depression as well as agitation, hallucinations, and coma. Treatment is supportive. Dependence occurs, and withdrawal signs resemble those of ethanol and other sedatives.

▶ Marijuana

Marijuana consists of leaves and flowers of the hemp plant, *Cannabis sativa*, which contains numerous cannabinoid compounds, of which Δ-9-tetrahydrocannabinol (Δ-9-THC) is the principal psychoactive agent. Hashish, made from the plant resin, has particularly high concentrations of Δ-9-THC. Marijuana is pharmacologically active when eaten, but it is usually smoked. Intended effects include dreamy euphoria and jocularity; there may be disinhibition, depersonalization, subjective time-slowing, tachycardia, and postural hypotension. High doses cause auditory and visual hallucinations, confusion, and psychosis, but fatal overdose has not been documented. Withdrawal symptoms are mild, consisting of jitteriness and headache, but craving signifies psychic dependence.

▶ Hallucinogens

Hallucinogenic plants are used ritualistically and recreationally worldwide. In the United States, hallucinogenic agents include natural compounds from the peyote cactus and several mushroom species, as well as the synthetic drug lysergic acid diethylamide (LSD) (Table 34–5). Acute effects of these agents are perceptual (distortions or hallucinations, usually visual and elaborately formed), psychological (altered mood or depersonalization), and somatic (tremor, dizziness, and paresthesia). Paranoia or panic can follow use, and "flashbacks"—spontaneous recurrence of drug symptoms without taking the drug—can occur days to months after use. High doses of LSD cause hypertension, decreased alertness, seizures, and fatal accidents, but directly lethal overdose has not been documented. Treatment of overdose consists of a calm environment, reassurance, and, if necessary, a benzodiazepine. There are no withdrawal symptoms.

▶ Inhalants

Especially popular among children and adolescents, recreational inhalant use includes a wide array of products containing many different chemicals (Table 34–6). Desired effects resemble those of ethanol intoxication, but overdose can cause hallucinations and seizures as well as coma. Fatalities are attributed to cardiac arrhythmia, accidents, aspiration of vomitus, and suffocation during sniffing from plastic bags. Symptoms usually clear in a few hours; management includes respiratory and cardiac monitoring. Withdrawal produces little more than craving.

▶ Phencyclidine

Phencyclidine (PCP; "angel dust") is usually smoked. The related agents, ketamine and dextromethorphan, are also used recreationally. Symptoms of PCP intoxication are dose related (Table 34–7). Treatment of severe psychosis or delirium requires sedation with benzodiazepines and often restraints; calm reassurance is seldom effective. Antihypertensives, anticonvulsants, cooling, forced diuresis, and monitoring of cardiac, respiratory, and renal function may also be necessary. Neuroleptics, which can aggravate hypotension, seizures, and myoglobinuria, are best avoided. Psychic dependence occurs, but withdrawal signs (nervousness, tremor) are infrequent.

▶ Anticholinergics

Recreational use of anticholinergics includes ingestion of the plant *Datura stramonium* (popular among American adolescents) as well as the use of tricyclic antidepressant or antiparkinsonian drugs. Intoxication causes dry mouth, decreased sweating, tachycardia, fever, dilated unreactive pupils, and delirium with hallucinations, which can progress to myoclonus, seizures, coma, and death. Treatment includes physostigmine (0.5–3 mg, repeated as needed every 30 minutes to 2 hours), gastric lavage, cooling, bladder catheterization, and respiratory and cardiac monitoring. Anticonvulsants may be necessary. Neuroleptics, which have anticholinergic properties, are contraindicated. Withdrawal symptoms do not occur.

▶ Tobacco

The addictive chemical in tobacco is nicotine. Although signs of physical dependence are mild, craving can be intense.

Table 34–5. Hallucinogenic Compounds

Ergot-derived
D-Lysergic acid diethylamide (LSD)

Indolealkylamines
Psilocybin
Psilocin
N,N-dimethyltryptamine (DMT)
N,N-diethyltryptamine (DET)

Phenylalkylamines
Mescaline
2,4-Dimethoxy-4-methylamphetamine (DOM)
4-Bromo-2,5-dimethoxyamphetamine (DOB)
2,5-Dimethoxy-4-ethylamphetamine (DOET)
3-Methoxy-4,5-methylenedioxyamphetamine (MMDA)
3,4-Methylenedioxyamphetamine (MDA)

Table 34–6. Products Subject to Inhalant Abuse and Their Contents

Products	Contents
Aerosols (refrigerants, frying pan cleaners, antitussives, hair sprays, bronchodilators, shampoos, deodorants, antiseptics, pain killers)	Fluorinated hydrocarbons, propane, isobutane
Dry cleaning fluids, spot removers, furniture polish, degreasers	Chlorinated hydrocarbons, naphtha (gasoline hydrocarbons)
Glues, cements, rubber patching	Toluene, acetone, benzene, aliphatic acetates, *n*-hexane, cyclohexane, trichloroethylene, xylene, butyl alcohol, dichloroethylene, methylethylketone, methylethylisobutylketone, chloroform, ethanol, triorthocresyl phosphate
Lighter fluid	Aliphatic and aromatic hydrocarbons
Fire-extinguishing agents	Bromochlorodifluoromethane
Fingernail polish remover	Acetone, aliphatic acetates, benzene
Bottled fuel gas	Butane, propane
Typewriter correction fluid	Trichloroethane, trichloroethylene
Natural gas	Methane, ethane, propane, butane
Marker pens	Toluene, xylene
Mothballs	Naphthalene, paradichlorobenzene
Toilet deodorizers	Paradichlorobenzene
Paints, enamels, lacquers, lacquer and paint thinners	Toluene, methylene chloride, aliphatic acetates, benzene, ethanol
Petroleum (gasoline, naphtha gas, benzine)	Many aliphatic, aromatic, and other hydrocarbons (eg, olefins, naphthanes), including butane, hexane, pentane, benzene, toluene, and xylene; tetraethyl lead
Anesthetics (surgical supply, whipped cream dispensers)	Nitrous oxide, diethyl ether, halothane, chloroform, enflurane, isoflurane, trichloroethylene
"Room odorizers"	Amyl, butyl, and isobutyl nitrite

Reproduced with permission from Brust JCM. *Neurological Aspects of Substance Abuse,* 2nd ed. Butterworth-Heinemann, 2004, Elsevier.

A large majority of smokers would like to quit, and a large majority of them are unable to do so.

MEDICAL & NEUROLOGICAL COMPLICATIONS OF ABUSED SUBSTANCES

▶ Trauma

Trauma may accompany a drug's acute effects (eg, motor vehicle and other accidents in marijuana or inhalant users, violence in psychostimulant users, or self-mutilation in hallucinogen users). Sedatives are a major contributor to falls in the elderly. Trauma among users of illegal drugs, however, is more often the result of the illegal activities associated with their production and distribution.

▶ Infection

Parenteral drug users are subject to an array of local and systemic infections, including cellulitis, osteomyelitis, hepatitis, endocarditis, meningitis, brain abscess, tetanus, botulism, and malaria. Neurological complications are common. By 2008 in the United States, nonhomosexual drug abusers accounted for 26% of acquired immunodeficiency syndrome (AIDS), and male homosexual drug abusers accounted for another 6%. Parenteral drug abusers experience the same neurological complications of AIDS as do other groups. They are particularly susceptible to syphilis and tuberculosis (including drug-resistant forms).

Progressive myelopathy occurs in parenteral drug users infected with human T-lymphocytic virus infection, both HTLV-1 and HTLV-2.

▶ Seizures

Drug abusers may develop seizures indirectly (eg, as a result of CNS infection), as a manifestation of intoxication, or as an abstinence phenomenon. Sedatives, including benzodiazepines, cause withdrawal seizures. Other than in newborns, opioid withdrawal does not cause seizures. Opioids lower seizure threshold, but the appearance of seizures during

Table 34–7. Phencyclidine Poisoning: Approximate Order of Symptoms With Increasing Dose

Relaxation, euphoria
Anxiety, emotional lability, dysphoria, paranoia
Subjective time-slowing
Decreased sensory perception
Altered body image, sensory illusions
Amnesia
Agitation, bizarre or violent behavior
Analgesia
Synesthesias
Nystagmus
Miosis
Tachycardia, hypertension
Hyperpnea
Fever
Hypersalivation, sweating
Dysarthria, ataxia, vertigo
Psychosis (paranoid or catatonic)
Hallucinations
Dystonia, opisthotonus
Myoclonus
Rhabdomyolysis
Seizures
Stupor or coma with blank stare
Extensor posturing
Respiratory depression
Hypotension

Reproduced with permission from Brust JCM. *Neurological Aspects of Substance Abuse*, 2nd ed. Butterworth-Heinemann, 2004, Elsevier.

heroin overdose is so unusual as to warrant a search for another cause. Unlike other opioids, meperidine does cause seizures and myoclonus, a consequence of an active metabolite, normeperidine. Seizures are also common in parenteral users of pentazocine combined with the antihistamine tripelennamine ("Ts and blues").

Seizures in cocaine users can occur in the absence of other signs of toxicity. They are less frequent among users of amphetamine-like psychostimulants, including products containing phenylpropanolamine.

Stroke

Parenteral drug abusers are at risk for stroke related to systemic illness such as endocarditis, hepatitis, and AIDS. Heroin has also caused stroke in the absence of other apparent risk factors, perhaps through immunologic mechanisms. In some instances, ischemic stroke in opioid injectors has been the result of foreign material reaching the brain through acquired pulmonary arteriovenous shunts. Users of amphetamine-like psychostimulants are at risk for intracerebral hemorrhage following acute hypertension. They are also at risk for ischemic stroke secondary to immune-mediated vasculitis. More than

600 cases of cocaine-associated stroke have been reported, roughly half hemorrhagic and half ischemic. A principal cause of hemorrhagic stroke appears to be surges of high blood pressure; in many instances, underlying cerebral aneurysms or vascular malformations have been found at angiography. Most ischemic strokes are probably the result of direct vasoconstriction of cerebral vessels; cocaine has infrequently been associated with vasculitis. Intracerebral and subarachnoid hemorrhages have been described in MDMA users.

Because of their association with stroke, diet pills and decongestants containing phenylpropanolamine were banned by the US Food and Drug Administration. So were over-the-counter "food supplements" containing ephedra.

LSD and PCP are vasoconstrictive, and occlusive and hemorrhagic strokes have occurred in users.

Altered Mentation

Illicit drug users may develop lasting cognitive dysfunction secondary to head injury, infection (including AIDS), malnutrition, or concomitant ethanol abuse. Attributing cognitive or behavioral disturbance to the drugs themselves is more difficult, for baseline mental status is rarely known and many drug users have psychiatric comorbidity or are even self-medicating preexisting symptoms.

Opioids and hallucinogens probably do not directly cause permanent cognitive dysfunction; patients who have received methadone maintenance therapy for decades remain intellectually and behaviorally intact. On the other hand, magnetic resonance diffusion tensor imaging demonstrated decreased functional connectivity in limbic regions of subjects dependent on prescription opioids.

Although early reports of an "antimotivational syndrome" in marijuana users were probably exaggerated, heavy chronic marijuana use is associated with subtle cognitive impairment involving memory, executive function, and manual dexterity. Heavy marijuana use during adolescence appears to be an independent risk factor for schizophrenia.

Amphetamine, methamphetamine, and MDMA damage synaptic nerve endings, and chronic use probably causes lasting cognitive disturbance. Cocaine does not cause synaptic damage, but cognitive dysfunction is described, perhaps an indirect effect of widespread cerebral ischemia.

Cerebral white matter lesions and dementia are described in sniffers of products containing toluene.

Elderly smokers are at increased risk for cognitive decline and both vascular and Alzheimer dementia.

Fetal Effects

Determining the effects of illicit drugs on fetal development is confounded by concomitant exposure to ethanol or tobacco, malnutrition, lack of prenatal care, and inadequate home environment. Heroin (and other opioids, including methadone) causes a severe neonatal withdrawal syndrome, and some (but not all) investigators have found exposed infants to be small for gestational age, at risk for respiratory distress, and cognitively impaired later in life. In utero cocaine exposure causes diffuse or axial hypertonia during infancy, but signs usually clear by 24 months, and controlled studies have not identified later cognitive impairment. Whether exposure to other psychostimulants (including MDMA) is detrimental to later intellectual development is uncertain. Marijuana exposure is associated with decreased birthweight and length; late-appearing effects on executive function are subtle. Toluene and other inhalants are teratogenic.

▶ Miscellaneous Effects

A. Muscle, Nerve, and Spinal Cord

Rhabdomyolysis and renal failure have followed use of heroin, cocaine, other psychostimulants, and PCP. Peripheral neuropathy of Guillain-Barré type and brachial or lumbosacral plexopathy, probably immunologic in origin, have been described in heroin users. Severe sensorimotor polyneuropathy affects sniffers of products containing *n*-hexane. Myeloneuropathy indistinguishable from cobalamin deficiency occurs in nitrous oxide sniffers. An acute myelopathy, possibly vascular in origin, is described in heroin users.

B. Cerebrum

Severe irreversible parkinsonism occurred in Californians exposed to a meperidine analog contaminated with 1-methyl-4-phenyl-1,2,3,6-tetrahydropyridine (MPTP), a metabolite of which is toxic to neurons in the substantia nigra. Spongiform leukoencephalopathy causing dementia, quadriparesis, blindness, and often death is a consequence of "chasing the dragon"—inhaling the smoke of heroin heated on metal foil; the mechanism of toxicity is unclear.

C. Cerebellar

Ataxia and cerebellar white matter changes occur in toluene sniffers.

D. Hormonal

Marijuana inhibits luteinizing and follicle-stimulating hormones, causing reversible impotence and sterility in men and menstrual irregularity in women.

Anstey KJ, et al. Smoking as a risk factor for dementia and cognitive decline: A meta-analysis of prospective studies. *Am J Epidemiol* 2007;166:367–378. [PMID: 17573335] (A meta-analysis of 19 prospective studies concludes that elderly smokers are at increased risk for cognitive decline and dementia.)

Benowitz NL. Nicotine addiction. *N Engl J Med* 2010;362:2295–2303. [PMID: 20554984] (A review of the mechanisms underlying addiction to tobacco, with emphasis on genetics, vulnerability, and implications for treatment.)

Cami J, Farre M. Drug addiction. *N Engl J Med* 2003;349:975. [PMID: 12954747] (A review that emphasizes that addiction is a biological illness.)

De Win MML, et al. Sustained effects of ecstasy on the human brain: A prospective neuroimaging study in novel users. *Brain* 2008;131:2936–2945 [PMID: 18842607] (Novice users of methylenedioxymethamphetamine [MDMA; "ecstasy"] develop sustained cognitive impairment and abnormalities on neuroimaging.)

Le Bec PY, et al. Cannabis and psychosis: Search for a causal link through a critical and systematic review. *Encephale* 2009;35:377–385. [PMID: 19748375] (A meta-analysis of epidemiological studies providing evidence that marijuana use increases the risk for schizophrenia independently of several confounders.)

Upadhyay J, et al. Alterations in brain structure and functional connectivity in prescription opioid-dependent patients. *Brain* 2010;133:2098–2114. [PMID: 20558415] (This diffusion tensor imaging study showed reduced fractional anisotropy [FA] and functional connectivity in certain brain regions of subjects dependent on oxycodone, hydrocodone, or tramadol.)

Psychiatric Disorders

Eric R. Marcus, MD

The standard diagnostic manual in psychiatry is the American Psychiatric Association's *Diagnostic and Statistical Manual of Mental Disorders,* Fourth Edition (DSM-IV). This manual presents a categorical system with agreed-upon lists of symptoms. However, it is sometimes difficult for the clinician to identify the appropriate list when faced with a patient who has psychiatric symptoms. This chapter provides the information needed to organize a differential diagnosis for a patient with a neurologic disorder having psychiatric manifestations, which can then be elaborated and verified by consulting the DSM-IV.

▼ APPROACH TO THE PSYCHIATRIC PATIENT

The mental status examination can be performed by observing the patient's organization and expression of the information in his or her telling of the history. A major faculty to be observed is cognition, including logical thinking and memory.

Logical thinking includes especially the categorization, sequencing, and logical relationship of data, events, and ideas. The illness history should be told by the patient in a reasonably organized and understandably sequential form. Facts and feelings about facts should be relatively separate. The patient should be able to demonstrate the capacity for abstract thinking in his or her categorization of the facts of the narrative. The patient also should be able to flexibly move back and forth both sequentially and between the different levels of abstraction.

A cognitive function meriting special observation and perhaps specific examination is **reality testing**, which is absent in psychotic illnesses. Reality testing refers to the mind's ability to perform a comparison between sensory information and logical operations on the one hand versus emotional reactions on the other hand. The mind ought to have the ability to keep these two large categories of experience separate in conscious understanding and to base decisions about external reality on the sensory and the logical, even if that turns out to be wrong.

There are two modalities of experience in which psychosis commonly presents. The first is the modality of thinking. The second is the modality of sensory experience.

Loss of reality testing in the area of cognition is called a *delusion.* A psychotic idea is called a delusion. A delusion is an idea about which reality testing is lost. A *near-delusion* or *pseudodelusion* is an idea about which reality testing seems to be lost; however, upon subsequent questioning for an explanation, and with calming of emotionality, reality testing reappears. An overvalued idea is merely a favorite topic of great psychological meaning; reality testing is never in doubt.

The psychotic form of a sensory experience is called a *hallucination.* A hallucination is a real sensorial event in that the patient has a reality experience of sensation; there is no corresponding reality stimulus. If a voice is heard, the patient can describe it as being high or low, male or female, and single or multiple, as well as whether words were spoken, and if so what was said. Because there is no reality source for the sensory experience, the patient may have a delusional explanation for it. Reality testing is absent. The patient feels the voice has an origin in reality.

Hallucinosis occurs in patients who know they are hallucinating. There is a real sensorial event, without a reality stimulus, but reality testing is intact. Patients may say they are "crazy," because they are seeing things that are not there. By definition, they are not psychotic, but they do have a serious illness, usually a neurologic illness of the brain.

A *near-hallucination* or *pseudohallucination* is a sensory experience that upon questioning turns out not to be a real sensorial event in that the patient cannot describe the sensory qualities of the experience. Reality testing, which at first appeared absent, returns as questioning continues, particularly as the patient becomes calmer.

An *illusion* is merely a misperceived reality stimulus. There is a real sensorial event because there is a reality stimulus. Reality testing, although momentarily confused, returns immediately.

Observation of the patient's narrative can tell the clinician a great deal about **memory** function, as reflected in consistency of data information and its time sequencing.

Emotion is another major faculty observed and examined, including whether affect is modulated, controllable, and linked to cognition. When a devastating story of illness is told by the patient, an appropriate affect should be observable.

When one dominant affect influences all mental contents, it is called *mood*. Mood is observed both in its breadth and in its depth. As mood becomes more intense, its range of included topic areas broadens, and it is more deeply felt.

Attitude refers to a dominant emotional theme affecting interpersonal relationships. Attitude is observable in the narrative history as well as in the patient's developing relationship with the clinician.

Another category of mental faculty is **behavior**. The clinician observes whether or not impulse control of behavior is rigid or disinhibited. This affects the appropriateness of social interactions and, again, may be observable in language behavior and in social behavior with the clinician.

MAJOR PSYCHIATRIC ILLNESSES

The major psychotic illnesses, categorized as axis I disorders in the DSM-IV, include the organic brain syndromes, manic-depressive illness, and schizophrenia. Any of these illnesses may have psychotic or nonpsychotic forms.

Although all three categories have some organic basis, the term *organic brain syndrome* refers to illnesses that cause macrocellular damage to the brain, producing disorders such as dementia, delirium, and altered levels of consciousness. These are neurologic rather than psychiatric illnesses. Clinicians need to keep in mind, however, that psychiatric symptoms such as hallucinations, delusions, and mood changes may also be prominent features of neurologic disease. These neurologic disorders are specifically addressed in other chapters of this book. Memory dysfunction, especially recent memory, is the cardinal mental status feature of organic brain syndromes.

Suarez RE. *Quick Reference to the Diagnostic Criteria for the DSMIV-R*, 3rd ed. American Psychiatric Association; 2000. (A quick-look format for psychiatric diagnosis.)

MANIC-DEPRESSIVE ILLNESSES

ESSENTIALS OF DIAGNOSIS

▶ Cyclical alterations of mood (high, low, alternating, or mixed)

▶ Spectrum of illness ranging in severity from mild to severe

General Considerations

The manic-depressive illnesses comprise a group of disorders in which the patient is either depressed or manic, or both at the same time, or alternating. Any combination or sequence may be present. If the patient has both depression and mania, either at the same time or alternating, the patient is said to have a *bipolar disorder* or *bipolar form of manic-depressive illness.* Some of the different forms are listed as categories in the DSM-IV. The pathognomonic feature is that they are disorders of mood.

Epidemiology

Mood disorders are more common than any psychiatric illness except the organic brain syndromes. The general population is susceptible to an 8–25% or more incidence of major depression as a lifetime risk. Subpopulations of patients, such as those needing cardiac or gastroenterologic care, may have a prevalence of depression as high as 50%. The risk is higher in those with a genetic predisposition for mood disorders. Family histories of patients with a severe form of the illness usually show multiple affected relatives on both sides.

Increasing the risk in genetically predisposed individuals is any history of childhood abuse or abandonment. Emotional abuse, as in chronically critical and demeaning environments, either of childhood and/or adulthood, likewise increases risk. Major losses incurred at any age—of parents, spouse, loved ones, job, aspirations—all may precipitate a mood episode.

All age groups are vulnerable to the mood disorders, but groups undergoing rapid challenges of social growth and development, such as adolescents or the elderly, are the most vulnerable. Changes in the perception of one's body, in social status, and in locale (eg, going away to college or retiring) are major stresses to psychological adaptation. A major change that is perceived as good can be as stressful as one that is perceived as bad. Social change may be especially problematic when it is accompanied by physiologic change, as occurs during adolescence, postpartum, menopause, or old age. Crucial to the prognosis is the stability of the social environment, especially the positive and supportive emotional relationships in family, friendship circles, and employment.

Suicide is a risk in patients with mood disorders (both depression and mania). The highest rate of suicide occurs in depression, making this form of psychiatric illness particularly dangerous. In some forms of the illness, such as psychotic depression, the suicide rate in the untreated approaches 15%. Because treatment of psychotic depression differs from that of nonpsychotic depression, it is crucial for the clinician to identify this category of depression by probing for symptoms of impaired reality testing, as previously described.

1. Depression

ESSENTIALS OF DIAGNOSIS

▶ Persistent low mood affecting all, or almost all, mental contents and areas

▶ Retarded form—sadness, decreased pleasure, decreased appetite, decreased sleep, decreased sexual interest, slowing of thoughts, early morning awakening, and pessimism about the future

▶ Agitated form—anxiety, sadness, psychomotor agitation, difficulty concentrating, initial and middle insomnia

Depression occurs on a continuum from mild to intense, from acute to chronic, from one or two episodes to many episodes, and from complete recovery to no recovery. There is a particularly high incidence of depression in the medically ill, including the neurologically ill.

▶ Clinical Findings

The major mood manifestation of depression is sadness, although some patients present with anergy, even somnolence, and a poverty of thought rather than sad thoughts. In this form of depression, hopelessness, even if only about the patient's condition, is usually present. The sad hopelessness and despair may revolve around one central idea, which may or may not be of delusional proportions, but the mood usually affects all content areas of mentation in addition to the delusion. The patient has the same sad, despairing feelings about every topic (Table 35–1).

Two main categories of depression exist: an agitated form and a retarded form. In the agitated form, anxiety is high. A central depressive idea may predominate, and elaboration may be extensive. Sleep is highly disturbed, usually with initial insomnia, perhaps with frequent awakening, and

Table 35–1. DSM-IV Criteria for Major Depressive Episode

- Depressed mood most of the day, nearly every day
- Markedly diminished interest or pleasure
- Significant weight loss
- Insomnia or hypersomnia
- Psychomotor agitation or retardation
- Fatigue or loss of energy
- Feelings of worthlessness or inappropriate guilt
- Diminished ability to think or concentrate
- Recurrent thoughts of death or suicide

Reproduced with permission from American Psychiatric Association. *Diagnostic and Statistical Manual of Mental Disorders*, 4th ed, text revision, 2000.

classically with early morning awakening. When patients awaken, they are exhausted and anxious.

In the retarded form, patients seem slowed down, sometimes even drowsy or somnolent. Ideational content may be sparse and elaboration minimal. Sleep may be increased.

In both the retarded and the agitated forms, there is usually emotional display of sadness. Patients who have the agitated form are anxious and tearful, whereas those with the retarded form manifest sighing and glumness.

Chronic low-grade depressions seem mild by comparison with these more marked forms of depression but affect interpersonal relationships, work productivity, and enjoyment capacity over many years. They are thus debilitating illnesses. Patients with low-grade depression may respond to treatment, both medication and psychotherapy, sometimes rapidly and gratifyingly despite the chronicity of their disease.

Thinking may be affected, but when it is, the reason is the intrusion of mood-related content and, in severe forms, emotional organization that preempts logical organization of information. In organic mental syndromes, it may be difficult to follow what the patient says because of confusion about data. In mood disorders, it is usually easy to follow the patient because the data are obviously organized around the dominant mood. What the patient says makes sense, although the clinician may not believe that the facts of the narrative warrant the extreme emotional reaction.

Because depression is often felt in the body, patients may complain about an experience of a disordered bodily part or function (somatoform disorder) as the major manifestation of their illness. This experience manifests on a continuum ranging from hypochondriacal fears and worries to psychotic somatic delusion. The patient may then present to a general internist or neurologist rather than a psychiatrist. Many patients who commit suicide have seen their general internist in the preceding 3 months, making the diagnosis of depressive hypochondriasis and especially of somatic delusion a mandatory diagnostic capacity of all physicians.

Although the DSM-IV categorizes the somatoform disorders as a separate group of syndromes, in clinical practice, somatoform disorders are almost always a manifestation of depression.

▶ Treatment

The treatment of depression is most effective when a combination of medication and psychotherapy is prescribed (Table 35–2). Medications include the older but very effective tricyclic antidepressants, although these agents may have quinidine-like cardiac side effects. Among the newer antidepressants are selective serotonin reuptake inhibitors, which are somewhat more tolerable but may not be as efficacious for patients with the most severe forms of depression. Several newer and atypical antidepressants involve norepinephrine or dopamine pathways, or both. If the patient is highly agitated or anxious, a temporary comedication regimen can be used, consisting of antidepressants and minor tranquilizers.

Table 35–2. Pharmacotherapy of Mood Disorders

Drug Class	Generic Name	Trade Name	Acute Dose (per 24 h)	Maintenance Dose (per 24 h)	Side Effects
Tricyclic antidepressant	Nortriptyline	Pamelor	10–25 mg	75–150 mg	Anticholinergic effects—constipation, dry mouth, urinary hesitancy, orthostatic hypotension, increased intraocular pressure, tachyarrhythmia
	Imipramine	Tofranil	10–50 mg	100–300 mg	
	Desipramine	Norpramin	10–50 mg	100–200 mg	
	Amitriptyline	Elavil	10–50 mg	100–300 mg	
	Doxepin	Sinequan	25–50 mg	75–300 mg	
Selective serotonin reuptake inhibitor	Fluoxetine	Prozac	10–20 mg	10–60 mg	Nervousness, agitation, sedation, tremor, headache, decreased sexuality, nausea, headache, weight gain or loss
	Paroxetine	Paxil	20 mg	20–50 mg	
	Sertraline	Zoloft	50 mg	50–250 mg	
	Fluvoxamine	Luvox	50 mg	50–300 mg	
	Citalopram	Celexa	10 mg	10–60 mg	
	Escitalopram	Lexapro	10 mg	5–20 mg	
Atypical antidepressant	Venlafaxine	Effexor	25 mg, 3 times daily dosing	200–275 mg/day, divided dosing	Hypertension
	Bupropion	Wellbutrin	100 mg, once daily dosing	300 mg/day, divided dosing	Hypertensive seizures arrhythmias
Mood stabilizer	Lithium carbonate	Eskalith	—	300–1500 mg, divided dosing or at bedtime[a]	Tremor, nausea, diarrhea, dehydration, long-term renal and thyroid dysfunction[b]
	Sodium valproate	Depakote	—	Maximum 60 mg/kg/day in divided doses[a] or at bedtime	Weight gain, hair loss, tremor, hepatotoxicity, teratogenicity, pancreatitis[b]
	Carbamazepine	Tegretol	—	800–1200 mg/day in divided doses[a] or at bedtime	Bone marrow suppression, rash, dizziness, drowsiness, nausea, inappropriate secretion of antidiuretic hormone[b]
	Oxcarbazepine	Trileptal	—	150–600 mg, divided doses or at bedtime	

[a]Blood levels determine dose.
[b]Follow blood levels.

For patients with psychotic symptoms, concurrent treatment with an antipsychotic agent is mandatory. Electroconvulsive therapy is almost always quickly effective in delusional patients, and in those who are severely suicidal. This therapy is the preferred choice because of its rapid effect. Unilateral administration has greatly decreased side effects. Transmagnetic stimulation of the brain is a nonconvulsive method for the outpatient adjunctive treatment of depression. Outcome studies are mixed and varied.

Almost any form of psychotherapy is helpful as a cotreatment. Cognitive-behavioral therapy, which focuses on conscious negative thoughts; interpersonal therapy, which focuses on the strength and quality of social relationships; or psychodynamic therapy, which focuses on the emotional experience of illness and the preceding losses, may be equally effective. Different patients have different experiences of their illness, different morbidities of mental faculty function, and different capacities and tolerances for insight; therefore, psychotherapy needs to be tailored to the individual patient. Psychotherapy is especially indicated in patients who have a comorbid personality disorder.

Ebmeier KP, Donaghey C, Steele JD. Recent development and current controversies in depression. *Lancet* 2006;367:153–167. [PMID: 163413879] (A review of the spectrum of depression.)

2. Mania

 ESSENTIALS OF DIAGNOSIS

▶ Discrete episode of euphoric or irritable mood affecting all relationships and mental content

▶ Racing thoughts, inability to concentrate, initial and middle insomnia, early morning awakening

▶ Poor social judgment, grandiose ideas, excess spending or sexuality (or both)

Mania is a mood disorder in which patients are accelerated in their thinking, emotionality, and behavior. Mood is either euphoric or, less commonly, irritable or a combination of the two (Table 35–3). The illness varies from extreme and disorganizing to mild and focused, and from intermittent to chronic. Changes through the life course are usual although not necessarily the rule.

Clinical Findings

Severe mania involves acute agitation, disorganization, and psychotic hallucinations or delusions. It is a medical emergency, requiring hospitalization and rapid pharmacotherapy, because dangerous behavior and physical exhaustion can result in death. Patients in a severely manic state may neither drink, nor eat, nor sleep because their agitation is so great. Suicide is highly likely, particularly if patients are dysphoric and hallucinating. Moderately severe mania is the above symptoms without hallucinations or delusions.

Patients with mild chronic hypomania can look very productive on the surface but may be very dysfunctional when more thoughtful judgment is required. Mild chronic hypomania may wreak havoc on patients' close interpersonal relationships because the affect is unvarying, the mood may be irritable, focus is always on the patient, and the ability for differentiated concern and care of others may be superficial at best.

Treatment

Treatment of mania and hypomania consists of mood stabilizers, ranging from the classic agent, lithium, to many of the antiepileptic medications (see Table 35–2). In ambulatory patients, mood stabilizers are best administered initially at a low dose, which is increased slowly according to tolerance and effect. Side effects following small increases in dose often wear off, permitting the dose to be raised again. Mood stabilizers are first-line treatment for both manic and depressed bipolar patients.

Table 35–3. DSM-IV Diagnostic Criteria for Mania

A distinct period of abnormally and persistently elevated or irritable mood. During the period of mood disturbance the following symptoms appear:
- Inflated self-esteem or grandiosity
- Decreased need for sleep
- Increased rate and pressure of speech
- Flight of ideas, with subjective experience that thoughts are racing
- Distractibility
- Increased activity
- Excesses of behavior and lack of judgment in activities (ie, unrestrained buying sprees, sexual indiscretions, or risky business investments)

Reproduced with permission from American Psychiatric Association. *Diagnostic and Statistical Manual of Mental Disorders*, 4th ed, text revision, 2000.

One of the problems encountered by clinicians who prescribe medications to manic patients is that patients usually like the feeling of energy and power that comes with the illness, and they tend to minimize the problematic aspects of the illness because its first effects are on their social environment and only secondarily on themselves. Therefore, a supportive but confronting psychotherapy is required if the medication is to be accepted; that component is the job of the psychiatrist.

Psychotherapy is almost always required to help manic and hypomanic patients accept medication, repair social relationships, and stabilize self-esteem. Psychotherapies of many different types have in common the elements of support for self-esteem, confrontation of effects of behavior, and exploration of the grandiose euphoria and irritability. The goal is to make these usually pleasurable features of mania an unpleasant symptom by connecting the mood with behavior that results in consequences the patient does not like.

Swann AC, et al. Practical clues to early recognition of bipolar disorder: A primary care approach. *Prim Care Companion J Clin Psychiatry* 2005;7:15–21. [PMID: 15841189] (A review of the spectrum of depression.)

SCHIZOPHRENIA

 ESSENTIALS OF DIAGNOSIS

▶ Fragmentation of ideas and all products of concept formation and their expression

▶ Affects thinking, emotional experience, interpersonal relationships, and presentation of self in everyday life

▶ Behavior lacks logical, emotional, and interpersonal sense

▶ Fragmented hallucinations and delusions (common)

General Considerations

Similar to organic brain syndromes and manic-depressive illness, schizophrenia encompasses a group of related disorders. Unlike the organic brain syndromes, schizophrenic illnesses are probably microcellular rather than macrocellular brain diseases. Schizophrenic brain pathology may involve neurotransmitters, neuroreceptors, dendritic interconnections, cytoarchitectonics, or microcellular organs such as membranes or mitochondria. The exact physiology and etiology are unclear.

Schizophrenic illness carries a roughly 1% lifetime risk in all ethnic and socioeconomic groups studied. Adoption and twin studies show a strong genetic component, but as with other medical disorders such as hypertension, heritability is probably polygenetic rather than mendelian.

▶ Clinical Findings

Schizophrenia is a thinking disorder, the characteristic feature of which is fragmentation of mental function. The concept-organizing capacity of the brain and mind is impaired, and data cannot be assembled into coherent ideas. The illness affects all aspects of information processing. Cognition, emotional reactions, and behavior are fragmented; therefore, even the presentation of self in everyday life is fragmented and bizarre. The patient's narrative can be understood neither intellectually nor emotionally. Fragments of opposite ideas may appear contiguously and without explanation (Table 35–4).

Psychotic phenomena in schizophrenia are highly fragmented because of the thinking disorder. Hallucinations and delusions make no logical or emotional sense and show fragmentation of image, idea, sensory-emotional experience, and narrative explanation. The attempt by the patient's mind to represent this fragmentation graphically results in the bizarre, the horrific, and the cryptic.

In dealing with a schizophrenic patient, the examiner should be matter of fact, highly organized, specific, and patient.

The diagnosis is usually straightforward, and referral to a psychiatrist is mandatory because treatment of schizophrenia requires a comprehensive approach, and current pharmacotherapy is both complicated and rapidly changing.

Table 35–4. DSM-IV Criteria for Schizophrenia

- Disorganized thinking and speech, with fragmented logic, frequent derailment, or incoherence
- Auditory hallucinations that make little or no sense
- Grossly disorganized or catatonic behavior
- Fragmented delusions that are illogical
- Affect flattening, alogia, avolition

Reproduced with permission from American Psychiatric Association. *Diagnostic and Statistical Manual of Mental Disorders*, 4th ed, text revision, 2000.

▶ Treatment

The treatment of schizophrenia involves neuroleptic medications Table 35–5. Clozapine may be the most effective, but use is limited to psychiatrists because of the possibility of an agranulocytosis. Pharmacotherapy should be combined with an educational and organizing psychotherapy, a coordinated educational and organizing family therapy, and usually a day hospital, often after an initial acute hospitalization. The best care, therefore, is with a psychiatrist and perhaps even a specialist in schizophrenia.

▶ Prognosis

The course of untreated illness is said to be about one third with a single episode and no deterioration, one third with several episodes and little deterioration, and one third

Table 35–5. Pharmacotherapy of Schizophrenia

Drug Class	Generic Name	Trade Name	Acute Dose (per 24 h)[a]	Maintenance Dose (per 24 h)[a]	Side Effects
Phenothiazine	Chlorpromazine	Thorazine	25-100 mg PO	25-1000 mg PO	EPMD, hyperprolactinemia
	Perphenazine	Trilafon	2-4 mg PO	2-16 mg PO	EPMD
	Fluphenazine	Prolixin	2.5-10 mg PO; 5-10 mg IM	10-40 mg PO; 12.5-50 mg IM decanoate monthly	EPMD
	Mesoridazine	Serentil	50-100 mg PO	100-400 mg PO	—
	Trifluoperazine	Stelazine	1-5 mg PO	5-40 mg PO	EPMD
Butyrophenone	Haloperidol	Haldol	2-10 mg PO; 2-10 mg IM	1-20 mg PO; 50-100 mg IM decanoate monthly	EPMD
Thioxanthene	Thiothixene	Navane	2-5 mg PO	5-10 mg PO	EPMD
Atypical neuroleptic agent	Risperidone	Risperdal	1-4 mg PO	2-8 mg PO	Less EPMD; arrhythmias and diabetes type 2
	Olanzapine	Zyprexa	5-15 mg PO	5-20 mg PO	Less EPMD; arrhythmias and diabetes type 2
	Quetiapine	Seroquel	25 mg PO twice daily	50-600 mg PO daily	Less EPMD; arrhythmias and diabetes type 2

EPMD = extrapyramidal movement disorders; IM = intramuscularly; PO = orally (per os).
[a]Dose is per 24 hours unless otherwise specified.

with one or repeated episodes and severe deterioration. With active treatment about 80% of patients may achieve stability and some improvement.

ANXIETY DISORDERS

CHRONIC ANXIETY

ESSENTIALS OF DIAGNOSIS

- ▶ Chronic anxiety and worry that searches for mental content on which to focus
- ▶ Focus on physical complaints or on feared interpersonal disasters
- ▶ Minor annoyances experienced as major catastrophes
- ▶ Difficulty falling asleep

▶ General Considerations

Patients with anxiety disorders characteristically manifest an anxious affect and mild to moderately depressed mood. A feeling of peace or ease is missing, disorders of sleep are common, and personality adaptations may be exaggerated (Table 35–6).

The anxiety disorders are common disorders, the incidence and prevalence of which depends on diagnostic categories and severities. Because generalized anxiety disorders often show a mood component, usually depressive, and

---

Table 35–6. DSM-IV Criteria for Generalized Anxiety Disorder and Panic Attack

Generalized Anxiety Disorder
- Excessive anxiety and worry that is difficult to control
- Anxiety associated with restlessness, fatigue, irritability, or sleep disturbance

Panic Attack
A discreet period of intense fear or discomfort characterized by:
- Palpitations or accelerated heart rate
- Sweating
- Trembling or shaking
- Sensations of shortness of breath or choking
- Chest pain or discomfort
- Nausea or abdominal distress
- Feeling dizzy, unsteady, light-headed, or faint
- Derealization or depersonalization
- Fear of losing control or going crazy
- Fear of dying

Reproduced with permission from American Psychiatric Association. *Diagnostic and Statistical Manual of Mental Disorders*, 4th ed, text revision, 2000.

---

because family histories often reveal relatives who have mood disorders, the anxiety disorders, especially generalized anxiety disorder with or without panic disorder, may in large measure be a manifestation of mood disorders.

▶ Clinical Findings

The patient looks anxious and expresses anxious worries, usually with a depressive coloring. Psychomotor agitation may be present. Thinking and memory are intact. The patient may have somatic concerns about bodily damage, distortion, or illness.

▶ Treatment

The most effective treatment for patients with chronic anxiety disorders is pharmacotherapy consisting of antidepressants and mood stabilizers. Psychotherapy focusing on target areas of anxiety and background histories of feelings of safety and attachment is helpful.

PANIC ATTACKS

ESSENTIALS OF DIAGNOSIS

- ▶ Fear of imminent doom
- ▶ Physical symptoms of anxious distress

Panic attacks are the most acute form of anxiety. The feeling of anxiety is extreme, involving thoughts of death or disaster. Patients manifest a physiologic emergency reaction of rapid pulse, rapid breathing, air hunger, chest pain, trembling and sweating, and a feeling of depersonalization and derealization (see Table 35–6). Treatment consists of pharmacotherapy: either a selective serotonin reuptake inhibitor for prevention or a benzodiazepine (for acute treatment). Psychotherapy may be very helpful.

PERSONALITY DISORDERS

ESSENTIALS OF DIAGNOSIS

- ▶ Persistent attitude about self and others, varying in intensity, depending on the relationship to the other person but with unvarying content
- ▶ Spectrum of illness ranging from mild to so severe that it seems quasidelusional

▶ General Considerations

Patients with personality disorders have a psychological *attitude*, which is a preformed tendency to react with the

Table 35–7. Personality Disorders

Type	Description[a]
Paranoid	Lack of trust and suspiciousness
Narcissistic	Self-aggrandizement and denigration of others
Obsessive	Control of relationships with rigid categories of interaction and morality
Histrionic	Emotional lability and attention-getting displays
Infantile	Disorganizing emotionality and demandingness
Masochistic	Feelings of constant victimization

[a]Dominant attitude imposed on interpersonal relationships, including patient–physician encounter.

same emotional theme to all or most interpersonal situations. The same attitude appears over and over in the patient's experience of other people and events. Rigid, stereotyped reactions fail to adapt to subtleties and differences and changes in interpersonal and social situations (Table 35–7).

▶ Epidemiology

Because these disorders are exaggerations of normal personality, the categorization of them as pathologic according to severity is arbitrary and difficult to quantify. Epidemiology is, therefore, uncertain, especially as it involves less severely affected patients.

▶ Clinical Findings

A. Symptoms and Signs

Personality disorders are disturbances in stabilizing emotional reactions and adaptations that manifest especially in interpersonal relationships. In the personality disorders, social relationships are organized by an emotional theme or a limited array of related themes, expressed as attitudes about oneself in relationship to others. The imposition of the attitude on social reality varies from mild to severe. If severe, the theme affects all of the patient's interpersonal relationships, appears repeatedly in the narrative of his or her life history, and is observed in the physician–patient relationship.

Concurrent mood disorders may be present but hidden and should be diagnosed and treated aggressively. Personality disorders may interfere with the treatment of medical illness because the dominant theme influences the interactions with the clinician and the experience of treatment. Psychiatric consultation can be helpful in the acute management of personality reactions to medical treatment and in gaining the patient's cooperation.

B. Mental Status Examination

The basis of the mental status examination is the interpersonal interchange that is determined by the patient's emotional attitude. This attitude may range from patients who are mistrustful, to those who are constantly demanding and never satisfied, to those who are laudatory and praiseworthy even when things go wrong, to those who need to control every aspect of their treatment.

▶ Treatment

Because personality disorders are often destructive to intimate human relationships, as well as the physician–patient relationship, referral to a psychiatrist is advised. Pharmacotherapy may be most helpful if the patient has a comorbid mood or anxiety disorder, even if the mood disorder seems mild. For patients with major mood disorders, antidepressant or mood-stabilizing medication may be crucial. Intensity and rigidity are the hallmarks of patients with personality disorders and comorbid mood disorders.

Psychotherapy is integral to the effective treatment of personality disorders. Although both cognitive-behavioral and interpersonal therapists treat the acute forms of these disorders, usually only a psychodynamic approach effectively treats patients with chronic forms. Psychodynamic therapists and psychoanalysts are trained to use the physician–patient relationship for insight rather than to avoid or be overwhelmed by it.

Haas LG, et al. Management of the difficult patient. *Am Fam Physician* 2005;73:2063–2068. [PMID: 16342837] (Helpful tactics in managing difficult patients, often those with personality disorders.)

Neurologic Disorders of Childhood & Adolescence

Claudia A. Chiriboga, MD, MPH,
& Marc C. Patterson, MD, FRACP

It is sometimes said by adult practitioners that children are just small adults. Child neurologists recognize that adults are just large children, albeit with lesser potential. The knowledge of nervous system anatomy and physiology that is essential to accurate localization and diagnosis in adults must be complemented by a thorough understanding of the sequence and variability of normal development to attain the same goals in children. The challenge and promise of child neurology is that children have extraordinary potential for recovery and development in the face of insults that would devastate adults. They are subject to all of the groups of diseases that occur in adults, as well as many others that are unique to the developing brain. This chapter focuses on the essentials of the most prominent of these age-related encephalopathies.

▼ NEONATAL NEUROLOGIC DISORDERS

HYPOXIC-ISCHEMIC ENCEPHALOPATHY

ESSENTIALS OF DIAGNOSIS

▶ Acute brain damage resulting from a perinatal hypoxic-ischemic event

▶ Neurologic impairment ranging from jitteriness to deep coma

▶ General Considerations

Hypoxic-ischemic encephalopathy (HIE) can be the result of birth asphyxia or at-risk pregnancies, in which the fetus has prenatal problems that are independent of the delivery process. Suspicions of HIE may be based on fetal distress, low Apgar scores, and acidosis, but it is the clinical examination that is the most significant predictor of central nervous system (CNS) damage.

▶ Clinical Findings

A. Symptoms and Signs

Clinical manifestations of HIE differ between term and preterm infants. In term infants, three grades are identified: (1) *mild*, present in the first 24 hours and characterized by a hypervigilant jittery state; (2) *moderate*, characterized by lethargy or depressed sensorium and decreased spontaneous movements during the initial 24 hours (the infant is jittery when aroused); and (3) *severe*, characterized by obtundation or coma, seizures, hypotonia, absent reflexes, and depressed sucking and swallowing. The clinical expression of HIE is muted in preterm infants.

B. Laboratory Findings

Lactic acidemia (pH < 7.0) is usually seen at the time of birth. HIE is often associated with hypoxic damage to other systems (eg, renal shutdown or necrotizing enterocolitis).

C. Imaging Studies

Neuroimaging may show diffuse or focal ischemia (cortical or subcortical). Brief transient ischemia may result in infarction of the basal ganglia that clinically can result in the choreoathetoid form of cerebral palsy.

D. Special Tests

Electroencephalography is helpful in term infants in determining outcome: infants with normal electroencephalograms (EEGs) have a favorable prognosis; those with EEGs showing depressed background or burst-suppression patterns have an unfavorable one.

▶ Differential Diagnosis

The main differential diagnosis of HIE is neonatal sepsis, which should be suspected in all infants with presumptive HIE until proven otherwise. The placenta should be examined for signs of chorioamnionitis.

Complications

HIE increases the risk for intraventricular hemorrhage, syndrome of inappropriate antidiuretic hormone, and seizures.

Treatment

Supportive therapy includes fluid restriction (for syndrome of inappropriate antidiuretic hormone) and anticonvulsant medication. Phenobarbital (20-mg/kg loading dose) is still the first line of treatment for neonatal seizures. A second loading dose may be administered to a maximum of 40 mg/kg over 24 hours. Phenytoin (20-mg/kg loading dose) may be added if clinical seizures persist. The neuroprotective efficacy of cerebral hypothermia has been determined by several clinical trials that show reduced mortality and decrease in disability, but whether head or total body cooling is a superior method is not known.

Prognosis

Prognosis is favorable for infants with mild HIE, uncertain for those with moderate HIE, and generally poor in severe HIE. Moderate HIE may evolve in either direction within 48–72 hours; severe HIE often evolves into brain death.

Jacobs S, Hunt R, Tarnow-Mordi W, Inder T, Davis P. Cooling for newborns with hypoxic ischaemic encephalopathy. *Cochrane Database Syst Rev* 2007;17(4):CD003311. [PMID: 14583966] (Excellent systematic review of eight clinical trials showing the benefit of cooling in neonatal HIE.)

Scafidi J, Gallo V. New concepts in perinatal hypoxia ischemia encephalopathy. *Curr Neurol Neurosci Rep* 2008;8(2):130–138. [PMID: 18460281] (Update on mechanisms and neuroprotective strategies in HIE.)

INTRAVENTRICULAR HEMORRHAGE

ESSENTIALS OF DIAGNOSIS

▶ Germinal matrix hemorrhage of varying severity that can extend to ventricles or parenchyma

▶ Premature infants or asphyxiated term infants are at increased risk

General Considerations

The germinal matrix, thin vessels that surround the ventricles, matures during the last trimester of gestation. Spontaneous hemorrhage in the germinal matrix is common among premature infants and asphyxiated or cocaine-exposed infants. Intraventricular hemorrhage (IVH) is classified into four grades based on the distribution of hemorrhage observed on imaging studies: *grade 1*—germinal matrix hemorrhage only; *grade 2*—germinal matrix and intraventricular blood; *grade 3*—grade 2 plus hydrocephalus; and *grade 4*—parenchymal bleeding.

Clinical Findings

The disorder may be clinically silent or associated with seizures, hypotonia, and depressed mentation. Cerebrospinal fluid is hemorrhagic. Serial ultrasounds of the head, a bedside noninvasive imaging modality, readily identifies blood (echodensities) and ventricular size.

Differential Diagnosis

Sepsis, meningitis, encephalitis, and seizures may present with acute mental status changes.

Complications

About half of infants with grade 3 IVH present with progressive hydrocephalus; of those, about half (one fourth of total grade 3 infants) require surgical shunting.

Treatment

Progressive hydrocephalus that develops shortly after the onset of IVH is treated by removal of cerebrospinal fluid through repeated lumbar punctures or through an Ommaya-like reservoir. Such a device (eg, Leroy reservoir) may be placed if lumbar punctures are unsuccessful. Late progressive hydrocephalus (ie, hydrocephalus that develops 4–6 weeks after initial IVH) requires placement of a ventriculoperitoneal shunt when the infant is large enough (about 5 lb [2.3 kg]).

Prognosis

Infants with grade 1 or 2 IVH have a favorable prognosis; however, those with grade 3 or 4 have a high risk of neurodevelopmental sequelae.

Ballabh P. Intraventricular hemorrhage in premature infants: Mechanism of disease. *Pediatr Res* 2010;67(1):1–8. [PMID: 19816235] (An updated review of mechanism of IVH including novel imaging studies.)

Shooman D, Portess H, Sparrow O. A review of the current treatment methods for posthaemorrhagic hydrocephalus of infants. *Cerebrospinal Fluid Res* 2009;6:1. [PMID: 19183463] (An updated review on the treatment of hydrocephalus associated with IVH.)

PERIVENTRICULAR LEUKOENCEPHALOMALACIA

ESSENTIALS OF DIAGNOSIS

▶ Ischemia of the periventricular white matter region

▶ Premature infants are at increased risk

Premature infants are prone to developing ischemia in the periventricular white matter region (periventricular leuko-encephalomalacia [PVL]), site of deep arterial border zones, which is inhabited by preoligodendrocytes, immature cells that are inordinately sensitive to ischemic damage. Premature infants most at risk are those with significant lung disease and a pressure-passive vascular system. This type of vascular system has scant autoregulation so that changes in systemic blood pressure are transmitted in full to the brain (ie, the system is more prone to ischemia with low pressure [PVL] or bleeding with high pressure [IVH]).

Clinical manifestations in the newborn period are often absent. Later findings include cerebral palsy (spastic diparesis) and cognitive impairments.

Ultrasound of the head is helpful in identifying the lesions (echolucencies), which often coincide with IVH. Magnetic resonance imaging (MRI) of the brain obtained close to term is more sensitive in detecting PVL, manifested either as ventriculomegaly (from volume loss) or periventricular white matter signal changes.

The differential diagnosis is limited, especially in the setting of IVH and prematurity. Occasionally, congenital infections may be present with similar clinical and neuroimaging findings.

Treatment is palliative, and includes physical and occupational therapy. PVL is associated with spastic diparesis–type cerebral palsy and cognitive impairment. Because it is associated with cognitive impairment, ventriculomegaly carries a worse developmental prognosis.

Kinney HC. The near-term (late preterm) human brain and risk for periventricular leukomalacia: A review. *Semin Perinatol* 2006;30(2):81–88. [PMID: 16731282] (An updated review on PVL.)

NEONATAL STROKES

ESSENTIALS OF DIAGNOSIS

▶ May be clinically silent or present with focal seizures and scant weakness

▶ May be ischemic or hemorrhagic

Neonates are physiologically in a hypercoagulable state. Risk factors for newborn ischemic strokes include obstetric trauma, precipitous deliveries, HIE, placental infection and thrombi, cocaine exposure, factor V Leiden deficiency, and protein S, protein C, or antithrombin III deficiency. The middle cerebral artery is the most frequently affected vascular territory. Hemorrhagic strokes can result from obstetric trauma, coagulopathy, thrombocytopenia, and ruptured arteriovenous malformation. In over half of newborn strokes, no cause is identified.

Neonatal strokes may manifest as focal seizures but are often silent, because weakness in the newborn period may be subtle. Clinical manifestations often develop in infancy, with early handedness (before 1 year) and subsequent hemiparetic cerebral palsy. MRI is more sensitive than computed tomographic (CT) scan in detecting strokes.

Acutely, seizures are the main complication of neonatal strokes. Clinically significant increases in intracranial pressure rarely occur in newborns because of their open sutures and fontanel.

Procoagulant states usually require anticoagulation. Large hematomas only rarely require surgical evacuation. Strokes involving the middle cerebral artery are associated with varying degrees of hemiparesis, but language and cognition are spared.

Beslow LA, Jordan LC. Pediatric stroke: The importance of cerebral arteriopathy and vascular malformations. *Childs Nerv Syst* 2010;26(10):1263–1273. [PMID: 20625743] (Recent review of pediatric strokes with neuroimaging examples.)

Husson B, et al. Motor outcomes after neonatal arterial ischemic stroke related to early MRI data in a prospective study. *Pediatrics* 2010;126(4):912–918. [PMID: 20855393] (This study establishes the role of corticospinal involvement in predicting hemiparesis.)

Lynch JK. Epidemiology and classification of perinatal stroke. *Semin Fetal Neonatal Med* 2009;14(5):245–249. [PMID: 19664976]

▼ DEVELOPMENTAL DISORDERS

MENTAL RETARDATION

ESSENTIALS OF DIAGNOSIS

▶ General intellectual functioning below average (full-scale intelligence quotient [IQ] < 70)

▶ Impaired social, school, or work performance not better accounted for by other disability

▶ Onset before 18 years of age

▶ General Considerations

The prevalence of mental retardation varies from 1–10%, depending on the criteria used, efficiency of ascertainment, and population studied. Mental retardation is a significant public health problem, as well as a substantial burden for affected individuals and their families. It was formerly held that the likelihood of making a diagnosis in mental retardation was directly proportional to the severity of impairment. Advances in genetics have shown that many mild phenotypes can be assigned to specific mutations, and often, single genes can account for a variety of mental retardation phenotypes with variable systemic findings based on the precise location of the mutation in the DNA sequence.

Mental retardation is more common in boys than in girls, an imbalance accounted for by the frequency of X-linked mental retardation syndromes, of which more than 200 are recognized. The most frequent of these is the fragile X syndrome associated with triplet repeat expansion of the *FMR1* (familial mental retardation 1) gene.

▶ Pathogenesis

Mental retardation occurs when there is a widespread or diffuse malfunction of the cerebral cortex, rather than focal lesions. Most cases of mental retardation are likely to be chromosomal or genetic in origin. The best understood syndromes are associated with genes whose products are involved in key cellular and neuronal processes such as DNA transcription or protein glycosylation. Amplified expression of the response to teratogens may underlie the developmental anomalies of Down syndrome (trisomy 21). Acquired global insults, including HIE, meningoencephalitis, trauma (particularly nonaccidental), or poorly controlled seizures, can also cause mental retardation, usually in association with motor or sensory signs, or both.

▶ Clinical Findings

Patients show global impairment in cognitive function. Children who are severely retarded present with global developmental delay in infancy, but most children with mental retardation are not recognized until they begin school and are unable to keep up with their peers.

A. Symptoms and Signs

More severely affected children present with developmental delay, particularly language delay; those with milder impairment present with early school failure. Children often become frustrated by their inability to keep up with their peers and may develop behavioral disorders that distract the focus of caregivers from the primary problem.

B. Laboratory Findings

Standard laboratory tests are usually normal. It is particularly important to ensure that neonatal screening for phenylketonuria and hypothyroidism has been performed, and that there is no evidence of otherwise occult chronic disease or nutritional deficiency that can impair intellectual performance.

C. Imaging Studies

CT scans are usually normal in mildly affected individuals. MRI scans may show subtle developmental abnormalities, including dysgenesis of the corpus callosum in such children, and a variety of cortical malformations in more severe cases.

These range from lissencephaly and holoprosencephaly in the most profoundly affected children, to more subtle migrational defects. Children with secondary mental retardation show changes associated with the primary insult.

D. Special Tests

All children with suspected mental retardation must have formal tests of hearing and vision. If there is any suspicion of occult epilepsy, an EEG should be performed. Most authorities recommend high-resolution karyotyping and screening for fragile X syndrome (*FMR1* gene mutations). The extent to which metabolic and other genetic studies should be performed is controversial in the absence of definitive prospective studies.

Formal testing of intelligence using an age- and culturally appropriate instrument is essential for accurate diagnosis. It should be noted that standard developmental scales used in infants are heavily biased to motor function, and that developmental quotients do not correlate well with IQ.

▶ Differential Diagnosis

Mental retardation may be confused or coexist with visual and hearing impairment, pervasive developmental disorders, language-based developmental disorders, or a variety of inborn and acquired secondary causes, including inborn errors of metabolism, cerebral malformations, consequences of congenital infections, trauma, perinatal hypoxia, and ischemia.

▶ Complications

Individuals with unrecognized mental retardation are likely to be deprived of appropriate educational and psychosocial supports that allow them to realize their potential. The impaired communication skills typical of mental retardation may lead to common physical and psychiatric illnesses being overlooked until late in their course, with serious consequences. The possibility of treatable disorders, particularly depression, should always be considered in people with mental retardation whose function deteriorates without obvious explanation.

▶ Treatment

Early identification ensures that educational supports, either in specialized classrooms or in mainstream school settings with accommodations tailored to the individual student, can be instituted. Psychosocial support for the affected individual and the family is critical and should include long-term planning for the care of people with mental retardation beyond the capacity and life span of their parents.

▶ Prognosis

Most people with mental retardation are successfully integrated as productive members of society provided that appropriate support services are available. Life expectancy may be reduced as a consequence of underlying disorders or unrecognized illness.

Battaglia A, Carey JC. Diagnostic evaluation of developmental delay/mental retardation: An overview. *Am J Med Genet* 2003;117C:3–14. [PMID: 12561053] (Provides an overview of the workup of mental retardation.)

Kaufman L, Ayub M, Vincent JB. The genetic basis of non-syndromic intellectual disability: A review. *J Neurodev Disord* 2010;2(4):182–209. [PMID: 21124998] (An update on the genetics of mental retardation including autism.)

Xiang B, Li A, Valentin D, Nowak NJ, Zhao H, Li P. Analytical and clinical validity of whole-genome oligonucleotide array comparative genomic hybridization for pediatric patients with mental retardation and developmental delay. *Am J Med Genet A* 2008;146A(15):1942–1954. [PMID: 18627053] (Describes the utility [sensitivity and specificity] of comparative genomic hybridization in detecting etiologies of mental retardation and developmental delay.)

CEREBRAL PALSY

 ESSENTIALS OF DIAGNOSIS

▶ Nonprogressive disorder of perinatal onset
▶ Affects tone and posture
▶ May appear to worsen over time
▶ Identified before 2 years of age

▶ General Considerations

Cerebral palsy (CP) is a nonprogressive disorder of tone and posture that results from an acquired prenatal or postnatal (up to 30 days of life) insult that is not the result of an obvious congenital abnormality (eg, spina bifida). Numerous perinatal risk factors have been linked to CP, including prematurity, PVL, IVH, congenital infections such as TORCH (toxoplasmosis, other congenital infections [eg, syphilis], rubella, cytomegalovirus, and herpes simplex), trauma, neonatal infections or perinatal exposure to inflammatory cytokines, HIE, and stroke. Some authorities classify bilirubin encephalopathy (kernicterus) as a form of CP.

▶ Pathogenesis

The mechanisms implicated in the genesis of CP include ischemia, inflammation, and infection. HIE is a common identifiable cause of CP in term infants; however, in the vast majority of term infants with CP, no discernible obstetric cause is identified for the development of CP. High levels of cytokines in blood of term infants who develop quadriparetic spastic CP suggest that maternal inflammation (chorioamnionitis) plays a role in such cases.

▶ Clinical Findings

The neonatal examination is not predictive of CP; findings of CP become apparent during the first 2 years of life. CP can be classified based on type and distribution of tone abnormality (Table 36–1). Hypotonia often is the result of isolated hypoxic-ischemic damage to the basal ganglia, whereas diffuse insults that affect both cortical and subcortical structures result in hypertonia. Quadriparesis or tetraparesis denotes that both arms and legs are equally affected; diparesis denotes that legs are more affected than arms. Hemiparesis refers to unilateral weakness (see Table 36–1).

▶ Treatment

Management of children with CP requires a multidisciplinary approach. The treatment of spasticity should be individualized and can respond to physiotherapy, antispasmodic agents, botulinum toxin, bracing, orthopedic surgery, or neurosurgery (baclofen pump placement or dorsal rhizotomy).

▶ Prognosis

Spasticity often worsens over time, whereas hypotonia may improve with age. Some children outgrow CP; however, they remain at high risk of cognitive impairments and learning disability. CP is often associated with mental retardation, but

Table 36–1. Classification of Cerebral Palsy Based on Clinical Findings

Type of Cerebral Palsy	Clinical Manifestations
Hypotonic	
Quadriparesis or tetraparesis	Global decrease in muscle tone, axial and limbs; developmental delay, gross and fine motor
Diparesis or diplegia	Decreased muscle tone in legs, does not bear weight, gross motor delay
Hypotonia with choreoathetosis	Begins with isolated hypotonic cerebral palsy; choreoathetosis develops by age 2-3 y
Hypertonic or spastic	
Quadriparesis	Flexor posture of arms and legs, gross and fine motor delay, pseudobulbar palsy
Hemiparesis	Unilateral weakness and spasticity, hemiatrophy
Diparesis or diplegia	Spasticity of psoas, hamstring, and gastrocnemius; toe walking and scissoring; arms are less affected than legs
Dystonic	Facial rictus, simultaneous contraction of agonist and antagonist muscles, opisthotonus
Cerebellar ataxia	Unsteady wide-based gait, gross motor delay, coordination and balance problems (~3%)

severe motor deficits may be associated with normal intelligence. MRI is a useful tool to help establish an etiology and in assessing prognosis. Risk of developmental disability is greater in the presence of microcephaly.

Quality Standards Subcommittee of the American Academy of Neurology and the Practice Committee of the Child Neurology Society, et al. Practice parameter: Pharmacologic treatment of spasticity in children and adolescents with cerebral palsy (an evidence-based review): Report of the Quality Standards Subcommittee of the American Academy of Neurology and the Practice Committee of the Child Neurology Society. *Neurology* 2010;74(4):336–343. [PMID: 20101040] (Evidence-based medicine review of the treatment of spasticity.)

AUTISTIC DISORDER & PERVASIVE DEVELOPMENTAL DISORDER

ESSENTIALS OF DIAGNOSIS

▶ Impairments in each of the following domains, with onset before age 3 years:
- Social interaction (poor or absent eye contact; unusual postures, facial expressions, and peer relationships)
- Communication (delayed or absent spoken language, inability to converse or play normally)
- Restricted interests and repetitive behaviors (preoccupied with one or a few interests, inflexibility, stereotypies, and mannerisms)

▶ General Considerations

The term *pervasive developmental disorder* (PDD) is often used interchangeably with *autistic spectrum disorders* and describes individuals who show abnormal language development, impaired social interactions, restricted interests, and repetitive behaviors in the first few years of life. When the established criteria in all three domains (outlined in the preceding list) are satisfied, a diagnosis of autistic disorder can be made. If, however, the criteria are only partially satisfied, the diagnosis of "PDD, not otherwise specified" is used.

This group of disorders also includes Rett disorder, now known to be associated with mutations in the *MECP2* (methyl CpG–binding protein 2) gene; Asperger syndrome, diagnostic criteria of which match those for autistic disorder, except that language is preserved; and the rarely diagnosed entity of childhood disintegrative disorder. The latter diagnosis was first identified near the turn of the 20th century, and subsequent investigations have found that most children with this disorder have diagnosable progressive brain diseases. However, there are rare children with acquired deterioration of cognitive function of no extant cause in whom this diagnosis can be applied.

Recent studies suggest a marked increase in the prevalence of autistic disorders. The reason for this increase remains uncertain and controversial. More widespread education of physicians and other caregivers might have led to more frequent and appropriate application of the diagnostic criteria and more frequent recognition of the diagnosis. Some authors argue that environmental influences, including toxic exposures, have increased in recent years and may be etiologic culprits or cofactors in producing an increased number of children with these disorders. It seems likely that all of these factors play a part in specific individuals and populations.

▶ Pathogenesis

PDD is largely of genetic origin, probably polygenic in most cases, although associations exist with several monogenic disorders, most notably tuberous sclerosis complex. Recurrence rates in kindreds with an affected proband are high, and comorbid disorders are more common in first-degree relatives. As is the case in other age-related encephalopathies with multiple recognized etiologies (eg, infantile spasms), it seems likely that the PDD phenotype represents the final common pathway of response to a wide variety of developmental insults.

▶ Clinical Findings

A. Symptoms and Signs

Most children exhibit unusual social interactions and language delays, although a clear pattern of regression is observed in about one third of cases. Children may appear to learn new words while losing those previously used, the net result being a small, static vocabulary. Children typically treat others as objects rather than sentient beings and are intensely focused on a few limited interests. Sensitivity to environmental stimuli, particularly touch and texture, and inability to adapt to unfamiliar environments are typical. Some autistic individuals develop extraordinary skills in limited areas (autistic savants), such as calculation, memory, or artistic performance. Macrocephaly is common, and some authors have reported facial hypotonia as characteristic of PDD. The prevalence of epilepsy is increased in autistic spectrum disorders, and seizures should be managed appropriately.

B. Laboratory Findings

Inborn errors of metabolism and Duchenne muscular dystrophy can present with autistic features initially, leading some authors to advocate screening with creatine kinase and amino and organic acid panels. Many clinicians include karyotyping and screening for fragile X syndrome as part of the workup of PDD, although guidelines from professional organizations do not support such testing in the absence of specific clinical indications.

C. Imaging and Other Studies

Standard MRI scans are normal in most affected children, but volumetric studies show a variety of abnormalities, mainly in the cerebellum. The frequency of epilepsy and EEG abnormalities is increased in the autistic population.

D. Special Tests

Several instruments have been devised for the diagnosis of PDD, and many school districts require their use to confirm diagnoses before services are provided. The Autism Diagnostic Observational Scale (ADOS), widely regarded as the gold standard, mandates certified testers and requires several hours for administration, sometimes in more than one session. It is supplemented by the Autism Diagnostic Index, Revised (ADI-R), a checklist that is administered to parents and other caregivers.

▶ Differential Diagnosis

Mentally retarded individuals may have autistic features, and language-based developmental disorders and deafness should always be excluded. Virtually any static or slowly progressive encephalopathy of childhood can manifest autistic features. The most prominent of these are tuberous sclerosis complex and fragile X syndrome.

Diagnostic confusion can arise with the Landau-Kleffner syndrome of acquired verbal auditory agnosia, in which children with previously normal speech lose their expressive language and behave as if they are deaf. Such children may have unilateral or bilateral epileptiform discharges with or without overt seizures.

▶ Treatment

Various therapies have been advanced, including applied behavioral analysis and several other behavioral regimens. Risperidone, 2.5 mg/day for children 20–45 kg or 3.5 mg/day for those weighing more than 45 kg, is useful in symptomatic management of aberrant behaviors but does not appear to influence the developmental outcome.

The effective treatment of seizures or their spontaneous disappearance, particularly when the alternative diagnosis of Landau-Kleffner syndrome is entertained, may or may not be associated with improved language function. Several therapeutic approaches have been advocated, but no controlled studies are available to evaluate these claims. These approaches include antiepileptic drugs, corticosteroids, and, in extreme cases, aggressive management of isolated electrographic abnormalities (ie, those without clinical correlates) up to and including surgical procedures on the involved cortex.

▶ Prognosis

IQ is the best predictor of outcome; children whose IQ is lower than 50 fare significantly worse as adults than those with an IQ higher than 70. Nevertheless, most people with autism have significant impairments in communication and socialization that persist into adult life.

Johnson CP, Myers SM; American Academy of Pediatrics Council on Children With Disabilities. Identification and evaluation of children with autism spectrum disorders. *Pediatrics* 2007; 120(5):1183–1215. [PMID: 17967920] (A nice review of autistic spectrum disorders, including identifiable causes.)

LEARNING DISABILITIES

ESSENTIALS OF DIAGNOSIS

▶ Full-scale IQ in the normal range
▶ Significant impairment in one or more academic domains (reading, mathematics, written expression) as measured by standardized tests

▶ General Considerations

Children who are otherwise normal intellectually may perform poorly at school because of one or more specific learning disabilities. The most common of these is dyslexia, which occurs in as many as 20% of school-aged children. Successful management of these disorders is most likely when they are identified and treated early. The major risk is of school failure, with consequent limitation of progression to higher education and employment.

▶ Pathogenesis

The best understood learning disability is dyslexia, in which both anatomic abnormalities, and more recently functional aberrations, can be demonstrated by imaging studies. Functional MRI studies show decreased activation of the portion of the left occipitotemporal cortex involved with word form recognition and increased activation of the Broca region in dyslexic subjects compared with controls.

▶ Clinical Findings

Disproportionate difficulty with one or more academic skills (reading, spelling, writing, calculation) is evident despite clear efforts to learn. Children are typically frustrated by their difficulties and develop strategies to avoid the difficult tasks, occasionally manifesting school refusal or behavioral disorders.

Standard laboratory tests are normal, and standard MRI is usually normal. Volumetric MRI may show symmetry of planum temporale (normally asymmetric) in dyslexic children; functional MRI may show diminished activation of language areas. Criteria for a learning disability include specific defects (at least two standard deviations below the mean) in one or more academic domains on formal psychometric testing, with normal overall intelligence.

Differential Diagnosis

The differential diagnosis includes mental retardation, vision or hearing defects (unrecognized, often subtle), attention-deficit/hyperactivity disorder (ADHD), and progressive encephalopathies.

Treatment

Specific therapies directed at alternative approaches to learning are most effective if implemented early. For example, a phonics-based approach to learning with appropriate accommodations, including adequate time to complete assignments, can be successful in children with dyslexia.

Prognosis

Individuals with specific learning disabilities are capable of achieving academic and employment success when appropriate teaching techniques are used. Functional MRI has shown evidence of improved function that parallels clinical success. Some individuals achieve success despite lack of recognition of their disability, albeit at significant personal cost.

Demonet JF, Taylor MJ, Chaix Y. Developmental dyslexia. *Lancet* 2004;363:1451–1460. [PMID: 15121410] (Reviews recent advances in dyslexia from a European perspective.)

Shaywitz SE, Shaywitz BA. Paying attention to reading: The neurobiology of reading and dyslexia. *Dev Psychopathol* 2008; 20(4):1329–1349. [PMID: 18838044] (Overview from the US leaders in dyslexia research.)

ATTENTION-DEFICIT/HYPERACTIVITY DISORDER

ESSENTIALS OF DIAGNOSIS

- ► Onset before age 7 years
- ► Inattentiveness, hyperactivity, and impulsivity that interfere with learning or socialization, or both

General Considerations

ADHD is one of the most common behavioral disorders of childhood, affecting 3–10% of children of school age. The diagnosis is based on strict clinical criteria described in the *Diagnostic and Statistical Manual of Mental Disorders,* Fourth Edition (DSM-IV). Classification is based on salient behavioral features: hyperactive, impulsive, inattentive, or mixed. Boys are affected more often than girls. Most cases are idiopathic, familial, and associated with normal intelligence, but a minority of cases is associated with other brain disorders (eg, fragile X syndrome).

Pathogenesis

ADHD has been linked to perturbations in monoaminergic systems that serve frontostriatal systems involving arousal modulation and executive function (ie, dopamine [DA] and norepinephrine [NE]). Genetic influences on DA transporter and DA receptor (D_4) have been implicated in the pathogenesis of ADHD. Imaging studies show frontal lobe hypometabolism on functional MRI on tasks that tap executive function, as well as volumetric differences in prefrontal regions and striatum.

Clinical Findings

Impulsivity, hyperactivity, and inattention occur in varying combinations. Except where there is an underlying disorder, laboratory tests are normal.

Standardized behavioral questionnaires are helpful in confirming the diagnosis and gauging response to therapy. The Connors Behavioral Scale or Achenbach Child Behavioral Check List (CBCL) can be administered to parents, teachers, and other caregivers. Computer-based tests of continuous vigilance (eg, Test of Vigilance and Attention [TOVA]) are also useful in assessing response to treatment. Routine EEG is not warranted in children with attentional problems because seizures usually can be distinguished from ADHD on clinical grounds.

Differential Diagnosis

Absence seizures and complex partial seizures are rarely confused with ADHD. Bipolar disorder and generalized anxiety are the main disorders to consider. The rapid cycling observed in children with bipolar disorder, fidgetiness and inattention resulting from akathisia, and worry seen with anxiety are often confused with ADHD. Typically, children with these disorders do not respond or respond poorly to stimulant treatment. Obstructive sleep apnea has also been linked to classroom inattention.

Complications

Children with ADHD have higher rates of learning disabilities, especially children with the inattentive type. Comorbid disorders include bipolar disorder, oppositional defiant disorder, conduct disorder, and depression.

Treatment

Stimulants (either methylphenidate or amphetamines) are the first line of treatment. Table 36–2 outlines a treatment algorithm for ADHD. Numerous stimulant preparations are available that differ in their duration of action (Table 36–3). In 10–30% of children, stimulants may not be indicated, either because of lack of efficacy or side-effect profile. In such instances nonstimulant medications are advisable. Nonstimulant medications encompass the following categories: norepinephrine reuptake inhibitors (atomoxetine and

Table 36-2. Treatment Algorithm for Attention-Deficit/Hyperactivity Disorder

I. Try one stimulant at increasing doses over 4 wk; if no response switch to other stimulant (A, B; *or* B, A):
  A. Methylphenidate (short acting)
    Week 1: 5 mg 3 times daily (18 mg long acting)[a]
    Week 2: 10 mg 3 times daily
    Week 3: 15 mg 3 times daily
    Week 4: 20 mg 3 times daily (for children > 20 kg)
    or
  B. Amphetamine
    Week 1: 2.5 mg twice daily
    Week 2: 5 mg twice daily
    Week 3: 7.5 mg twice daily
    Week 4: 10 mg twice daily (for children > 20 kg)
II. If neither stimulant is effective, give
  A. Atomoxetine, 1–2 mg/kg/day once daily or divided twice daily; starting dose, 0.5 mg/kg/day
    or
  B. Bupropion, 3–5 mg/kg/day once daily or divided twice daily

[a]May use comparable dose of long-acting preparation.
Reproduced with permission from Pliszka SR, et al. A feasibility study of the children's medication algorithm project (CMAP) algorithm for the treatment of ADHD. *J Am Acad Child Adolesc Psychiatry* 2003;42:279–287.

bupropion); alpha agonists (clonidine, guanfacine); and tricyclic antidepressants. Nonstimulant medications are considered a second line of treatment. Only atomoxetine and guanfacine long-acting are FDA approved for ADHD. Because of liver toxicity, pemoline is no longer indicated for ADHD. Treatment is indicated if behavior or attentional difficulties are interfering with learning and affecting social interactions.

Prognosis

Hyperactivity and impulsivity improve with age; however, problems with attention, organization, and planning (eg, executive function) are usually lifelong disorders. Many adults require continuing pharmacotherapy.

Table 36-3. Available Stimulant Preparations Grouped by Duration of Action

Duration of Action	Methylphenidate	Amphetamine
Short	3–5 h, 3 times daily (Ritalin, Focalin)	4–6 h (Dexedrine, Dextrostat)
Intermediate	3–8 h, twice daily (Ritalin SR, Metadate ER, Methylin ER)	6–8 h (Adderall, Dexedrine spansule)
Long	8–12 h, once daily (Concerta, Ritalin LA, Metadate CD)	8–12 h (Adderall-XR)

Arnsten AF. The emerging neurobiology of attention deficit hyperactivity disorder: The key role of the prefrontal association cortex. *J Pediatr* 2009;154(5):I-S43. [PMID: 20596295] (An excellent update on the neurobiology of ADHD by an established expert in the field.)

Kelly AM, Margulies DS, Castellanos FX. Recent advances in structural and functional brain imaging studies of attention-deficit/hyperactivity disorder. *Curr Psychiatry Rep* 2007;9(5): 401–407. [PMID: 17915080] (Describes the structural and functional imaging findings linked to ADHD.)

GENETIC DISORDERS

The recent explosion of knowledge in human genetics has led to the identification of a rapidly growing number of genes involved in regulating the development of the nervous system, clarifying the basis of many previously poorly understood neurologic disorders in childhood. To date the dividends of this knowledge have been primarily diagnostic, but it is reasonable to anticipate that novel therapies will become available as disease mechanisms are elucidated. This section focuses on some of the more common neurogenetic disorders of children.

Gropman AL, Batshaw ML. Epigenetics, copy number variation, and other molecular mechanisms underlying neurodevelopmental disabilities: New insights and diagnostic approaches. *J Dev Behav Pediatr* 2010;31(7):582–591. [PMID: 20814257] (Describes role of epigenetic and genetic mechanisms in disorders associated with intellectual impairments that are amenable to diagnostic testing.)

Stankiewicz P. Beaudet AL. Use of array CGH in the evaluation of dysmorphology, malformations, developmental delay, and idiopathic mental retardation. *Curr Opin Genet & Dev* 2007; 17(3):182-92 [PMID: 17467974] (Describes the pros and cons of the utility of CGH in evaluating genetic diseases, specifically those with dysmorphic features and intellectual abnormalities.)

CHROMOSOMAL DISORDERS

 ESSENTIALS OF DIAGNOSIS

▶ Systemic disorders associated with net gain, loss, or disturbed structure of chromosomal material in all or only some tissues

▶ Dysmorphism (usually, but not invariably, present)

▶ Diagnosis requires chromosomal analysis by staining complemented by fluorescence in situ hybridization (FISH) or chromosomal microarray analysis (CMA) using microarray-based comparative genomic hybridization (CGH) of chromosomes in cultured cells (including lymphocytes, fibroblasts, and hair follicles) derived from one or more tissues

Chromosomal disorders disrupt the function of one or more genes, often leading to static encephalopathies of variable severity in combination with a variety of multisystem abnormalities.

1. Down Syndrome

One of the most frequent chromosomal disorders is Down syndrome. Most cases result from trisomy 21, the consequence of chromosomal nondisjunction during meiosis. A less frequent cause is translocation between chromosomes 14 and 21. It is critical to establish the diagnosis by chromosomal analysis of lymphocytes, because translocation-type Down syndrome can recur in future pregnancies if one of the parents is carrying a balanced translocation. Karyotyping of fibroblasts may be necessary to diagnose mosaic-type Down syndrome, whose manifestations are generally milder than the full-blown syndrome.

Findings include varying combinations of cardiac (endocardial cushion) defects, duodenal atresia, developmental delay and mental retardation, short stature, and characteristic dysmorphism, including brachycephaly, downslanting palpebral fissures, epicanthal folds, simian creases in the palms, and the presence of Brushfield spots on the iris in some children.

Complications of Down syndrome include cardiac failure, hypothyroidism, early-onset Alzheimer disease, and atlantoaxial subluxation. The last-mentioned complication puts these children at risk of cervical cord injury when participating in organized sports such as Special Olympics. Screening should include flexion and extension radiographs or MRI scans of the cervical spine.

Down syndrome also predisposes children to moyamoya disease. This proliferative arteriopathy causes acquired bilateral stenosis of the supraclinoid portions of the internal carotid arteries, leading to the development of fine collateral vessels in the basal ganglia that give the "puff of smoke" angiographic appearance for which the disorder is named. Children with moyamoya disease may experience ischemic or hemorrhagic strokes.

Life expectancy and quality of life in children with Down syndrome are directly related to intellectual function, complications, and access to medical care and support services. The proportion of people with Down syndrome surviving to later adulthood has continued to rise as care improves and individuals with less severe manifestations (including mosaicism) are accurately diagnosed. Essentially all individuals with Down syndrome who survive to the fifth decade or beyond develop Alzheimer disease.

2. Other Chromosomal Disorders

Other common chromosomal disorders are summarized in Table 36–4. New techniques, such as FISH studies for subtelomeric inversions and deletions, have allowed the recognition of subtle chromosomal abnormalities in as many as 5% of children with nonspecific mental retardation.

Table 36–4. Important Chromosomal Disorders

	Chromosomal Abnormality	Phenotype
Angelman syndrome	15q13 deletion (maternal allele), or uniparental disomy for paternal allele, or mutations in *UBE3A* gene	Microbrachycephaly, macrostomia, ataxia ("puppet movements"), mental retardation with severe language impairment; epilepsy
Fragile X syndrome	Excessive fragility of chromosomes cultured in folate-deficient medium; triplet repeat expansion in the *FMR1* gene	Mental retardation; tall stature; long face; large, soft ears; macro-orchidism after puberty; ataxia in older males
Klinefelter syndrome	47, XXY	Gynecomastia, hypogonadism, mental retardation
Prader-Willi syndrome	15q13 deletion (paternal allele), or uniparental disomy for maternal allele	Hypotonia, hernias, and failure to thrive in infancy; voracious appetite and obesity in childhood; mental retardation, hypogonadism, short stature
XYY syndrome	47,XYY	Tall stature, learning disabilities
Trisomy X	46,XXX	Varies from no phenotype to minor dysmorphism and tall stature with learning disabilities to mental retardation (rare)
Turner syndrome	45,X	Short stature, webbed neck, edema of hands and feet in neonates; mental retardation; full expression of X-linked recessive disorders (eg, Duchenne muscular dystrophy)
Williams syndrome	7q deletion (involves elastin gene)	Supravalvular aortic stenosis, neonatal hypercalcemia, elfin facies

Esbensen AJ. Health conditions associated with aging and end of life of adults with Down syndrome. *Int Rev Res Ment Retard* 2010; 39(C):107–126. [PMID: 21197120] (Non-neurological complications associated with aging patients with Down syndrome.)

Gardiner K, Herault Y, Lott IT, Antonarakis SE, Reeves RH, Dierssen M. Down syndrome: From understanding the neurobiology to therapy. *J Neurosci* 2010;30(45):14943–14945. [PMID: 21068296] (Interesting update on the topic.)

Menéndez M. Down syndrome, Alzheimer's disease and seizures. *Brain Dev* 2005;27(4):246–252. [PMID: 15862185] (Review of neurologic complications linked with Down syndrome as patients age.)

INBORN ERRORS OF METABOLISM

ESSENTIALS OF DIAGNOSIS

- ▶ Impaired homeostasis caused by absent or deficient gene product (classically an enzyme)
- ▶ Small-molecule disorders—manifest as neonatal encephalopathies or episodic functional decompensation precipitated by intercurrent infection or substrate loading
- ▶ Large-molecule disorders—cause slow neurodegeneration, with or without organomegaly, skeletal abnormalities (dysostosis multiplex), or dysmorphism
- ▶ Complex disorders—include features of both large- and small-molecule disorders
- ▶ Correct timing, handling, and analysis of samples is crucial for diagnosis; negative results of screening tests and absence of classic features do not rule out these disorders

▶ General Considerations

Inborn errors of metabolism (IEMs) are individually rare but collectively common. The incidence of lysosomal storage diseases (the classic large-molecule diseases) is about 1 in 8000 live births, and that of small-molecule diseases is about 16 in 100,000 births. Although only a few of these diseases have specific treatments, definitive diagnosis by biochemical or molecular methods is available for almost all, offering opportunities for prevention by genetic counseling or population screening. The latter approach has proven effective in dramatically reducing the burden of disorders such as phenylketonuria and Tay-Sachs disease. Table 36–5 offers a classification of IEMs, with examples.

Small-molecule diseases is the authors' term for disorders in which the substrates and products of the impaired metabolic pathways are amino or other organic acids or similar molecules involved in intermediary metabolism, energy generation, or neurotransmission. This family of IEMs contains the disorders amenable to specific therapy by dietary manipulation (eg, phenylalanine restriction in phenylketonuria) or cofactor therapy (eg, pyridoxine for pyridoxine dependency). The most severe phenotypes present as life-threatening emergencies in neonates. Milder forms present later in childhood or even adulthood with episodic decompensation precipitated by metabolic stressors such as the hypercatabolic state associated with febrile illness, or by a substrate load such as protein in a gastrointestinal hemorrhage.

Large-molecule diseases are those in which macromolecules (complex proteins, lipids, or carbohydrates) accumulate in cells and tissues, causing progressive neurodegeneration, with or without organomegaly, skeletal abnormalities (dysostosis multiplex), coarsening of facial features, and shortened life expectancy.

▶ Pathogenesis

IEMs classically result from deficiencies of enzyme function, through mutations affecting the enzyme itself, transport molecules, cofactors, or other facilitators of metabolic pathways. Substrate accumulates, either producing direct toxic effects or triggering a cascade of downstream effects, including activation of alternate pathways and impaired or aberrant intracellular and intercellular signaling. Product deficiency may in itself produce symptoms, as may substrate accumulation through loss of feedback inhibition. Variable expressivity of IEMs may reflect mutation-specific effects, the effects of modifier genes, or tissue heteroplasmy in disorders in which inheritance is mitochondrial.

▶ Clinical Findings

A. Symptoms and Signs

In patients with small-molecule diseases, intermittent coma, vomiting, seizures, or movement disorders can be provoked by substrate loads or intercurrent illness. Static encephalopathy also occurs, with mental retardation, behavioral disturbances, and physical signs (neurologic and systemic). Diagnostic clues may include characteristic odors (organic acidurias), rashes (biotinidase deficiency), abnormal hair (Menkes disease, urea cycle defects), neutropenia, and thrombocytopenia (organic acidurias). Large-molecule disorders cause progressive neurodegeneration with dementia and variable degrees of organomegaly, coarsening of facial features, and dysostosis multiplex.

B. Laboratory Findings

Findings are specific to the individual disorders; refer to Table 36–5.

C. Imaging Studies

CT and MRI scans are normal in many small-molecule diseases. Malformations are seen in some disorders (eg, agenesis of the corpus callosum in glycine encephalopathy, polymicrogyria in Zellweger syndrome). Diffuse white matter disease is found in IEMs that produce leukodystrophy (eg, X-linked adrenoleukodystrophy). Symmetric changes in the basal ganglia and brainstem are typical of disorders of energy generation (eg, Leigh disease).

Table 36–5. Inborn Errors of Metabolism

Major Division and Mechanism	Subgroup	Analytes	Examples
DNA Disorders			
DNA maintenance and transcription	Cell-cycle checkpoint regulation	Gene—*ATM*	Ataxia-telangiectasia
	Nucleotide excision repair	Genes—*XPA, XPD, CSA, CS*	Xeroderma pigmentosum, Cockayne syndrome
	Spliceosome function	Gene—*SMN*	Spinal muscular atrophy
Translation	Translation initiation	eIF2B	CACH
Small-Molecule Disorders			
Energy generation	OXPHOS defects	Lactate, pyruvate, carnitine	MELAS, MERRF, Kearns-Sayre syndrome
	Fatty-acid oxidation defects	Dicarboxylic acids, carnitine	MCAD
Intermediary metabolism	Urea cycle	Ammonia, orotic acid, citrulline, arginine	OTCD
	Amino acidopathies	Plasma and urine amino acids	Phenylketonuria
	Organic acidurias	Urine organic acids	Maple syrup urine disease
Neurotransmitter synthesis	Biogenic amine synthetic disorders	5-HIAA, serotonin	GTPCH
Large-Molecule Disorders			
Anabolism	Porphyrias	Porphyrins	Acute intermittent porphyria
	Sterol synthesis disorders	Cholesterol, 7-dehydrocholesterol	Smith-Lemli-Opitz syndrome, mevalonic aciduria
Catabolism			
Lysosomal storage diseases	Sphingolipidoses	Gangliosides, cerebrosides, lysosomal hydrolases	Tay-Sachs disease, Niemann-Pick disease
	Mucopolysaccharidoses	Glycosaminoglycans, lysosomal hydrolases	Hurler syndrome, Hunter syndrome
	Glycoproteinoses	Urine oligosaccharides, lysosomal hydrolases	Mannosidosis, fucosidosis, sialidosis
	Mucolipidoses	Glycosaminoglycans, urine oligosaccharides, serum and cellular lysosomal hydrolases	I-cell disease, pseudo-Hurler polydystrophy, mucolipidosis type 4
	NCLs	Urine dolichols, lysosomal hydrolases	NCL types 1–8
Peroxisomal biogenesis and protein importing	Peroxisomal disorders	Plasma very-long-chain fatty acids, plasma bile acids	Zellweger syndrome, X-linked adrenoleukodystrophy
Complex Diseases			
Cotranslational and post-translational glycosylation	Congenital disorders of glycosylation	Transferrin isoforms, coagulation factors, lysosomal enzymes, peptide hormones	CDG 1a (PMM deficiency)
Glycogen storage and mobilization	Glycogen storage diseases	Plasma glucose, uric acid, tissue glycogen	Acid maltase deficiency, McArdle disease, Tarui disease

CACH = childhood ataxia with central hypomyelination (vanishing white matter disease); CDG = congenital disorder of glycosylation; eIF2B = translation initiation factor 2B; GTPCH = GTP cyclohydrolase deficiency (dopa-responsive dystonia); 5-HIAA = 5-hydroxyindole acetic acid; MCAD = medium-chain acyl CoA dehydrogenase deficiency; MELAS = mitochondrial encephalomyelopathy with lactic acidosis and strokelike episodes; MERRF = mitochondrial encephalopathy with ragged-red fibers; NCLs = neuronal ceroid lipofuscinoses; OTCD = ornithine transcarbamylase deficiency; OXPHOS = oxidative phosphorylation; PMM = phosphomannomutase deficiency.

▶ Differential Diagnosis

IEMs can be confused (or coexist) with congenital malformations (peroxisomal disorders, disorders of O-linked glycosylation); infectious or immune-modulated disorders, including encephalitis; acute disseminated encephalomyelitis; multiple sclerosis; vasculitis; stroke (oxidative phosphorylation disorders, congenital disorders of glycosylation); nonaccidental trauma (glutaric aciduria type 1, Menkes disease); and neoplastic or paraneoplastic diseases.

▶ Complications

Many small-molecule and most large-molecule and complex diseases shorten life span and produce significant

Table 36–6. Treatment Options for Inborn Errors of Metabolism

Therapy	Example	Current Status
Substrate restriction	Phenylalanine-restricted diet in phenylketonuria	Standard of care; effective in maintaining normal function when closely followed
Substrate removal	Peritoneal dialysis for maple syrup urine disease	Effective short-term therapy
Substrate synthesis inhibition	Miglustat for lysosomal storage diseases (inhibits glucosylceramide synthase)	Approved therapy for selected patients with type 1 Gaucher disease; clinical trials in progress in Niemann-Pick diseases and type 3 Gaucher disease
Enzyme enhancement • Cofactor pharmacotherapy	Pyridoxine for pyridoxine-dependent seizures	Effective in controlling seizures; may not prevent developmental delays
• Chaperone therapy to enhance residual enzyme activity	Galactose infusions for cardiac variant of Fabry disease	Improves cardiac function; limited to patients with residual enzyme activity and suitable mutations
Enzyme replacement therapy	Imiglucerase infusions for type 1 Gaucher disease	Reverses systemic manifestations of disease; no effect on neurologic manifestations

neurologic and systemic disability specific to the disorder and mutation.

▶ Treatment

Dietary restriction, cofactor therapy, dialysis, and alternative energy sources are useful in the treatment of patients with small-molecule diseases. Enzyme replacement or enhancement therapy, stem cell transplantation, and experimental small-molecule therapies (substrate synthesis inhibition) are being employed for patients with large-molecule diseases. Examples are listed in Table 36–6.

▶ Prognosis

Normal life span and function are possible in patients with small-molecule diseases that are amenable to dietary or cofactor therapy when they are diagnosed and treated promptly; other small-molecule diseases produce varying degrees of disability and reduction of life span. Most large-molecule disorders are associated with progressive neurodegeneration and premature death.

Levy PA. Inborn errors of metabolism: Part 1: Overview. *Pediatr Rev* 2009;30(4):131–137. [PMID: 19339386] (Updated primer on the subject.)

Poll-The BT, Maillette de Buy Wenniger-Prick LJ, Barth PG, Duran M. The eye as a window to inborn errors of metabolism. *J Inherit Metab Dis* 2003;26:229–244. [PMID: 12889663] (A beautifully illustrated review of the ocular findings in IEMs.)

Shevell M. Metabolic evaluation in neurodevelopmental disabilities. *Ann Neurol* 2009;65(4):483–484. [PMID: 19399872] (Focuses on the association between inborn errors of metabolism, some of which have specific therapies, and neurodevelopmental disabilities.)

CONGENITAL BRAIN ANOMALIES

ESSENTIALS OF DIAGNOSIS

▶ Abnormalities of brain development that occur at different stages of embryogenesis

▶ Disorders arising from early stages of development are associated with more severe phenotypes (dysmorphic features and psychomotor retardation) and early death

These disorders are summarized in Table 36–7. In general, the earlier in gestation that the anomaly occurs, the more severe will be the clinical deficit. Etiology is mostly genetic or developmental in nature, but some congenital anomalies occur secondary to acquired disorders (infections, ischemia, exposure to drugs or radiation).

Affected children show developmental delay, mental retardation, and seizures. Seizures are especially common among children with any type of migrational disorder. Disorders of prosencephalic development are often associated with midline facial anomalies (nose and eyes).

MRI is the most sensitive imaging modality for identifying CNS malformations.

Barkovich AJ, Millen KJ, Dobyns WB. A developmental and genetic classification for midbrain-hindbrain malformations. *Brain* 2009;132:3199–3230. [PMID: 19933510] (Informative embryological review of brain development with illustrative examples and thoughtful classification.)

Table 36–7. Congenital Brain Anomalies

Type of Anomaly	Example	Clinical Findings/Associated Features
Neurulation Disorder of neural tube closure GA 7–28 d	Anencephaly	Complete failure of brain development and coverings Spinal cord and brainstem present Early demise
	Myeloschisis	Failure of closure of posterior neural tube; affects entire spine
	Encephalocele	Restricted failure of closure of anterior neuropore; brain protrudes through defect (70–80% are occipital)
	Spina bifida • Occulta (covered by skin) • Cystic (not covered by skin)	Restricted failure of closure of posterior neuropore T4–L2 lesion paraplegia with neurogenic bladder; S3–S5 lesions isolated neurogenic bladder Associated with Chiari II malformation
Prosencephalic Development Failure in development or cleavage of prosencephalon GA 5–7 wk	Aprosencephaly	Absent formation of telencephalon and diencephalon Rudimentary brainstem
	Holoprosencephaly	Failure of brain division into 2 hemispheres—alobar (complete), semilobar (posterior fusion) Fused thalami Associated with midline facial defects
Disorder of Proliferation Failure of neuronal proliferation GA 2–3 mo	Micrencephaly vera; radial microbrain	Small but well-formed brain due to fewer neurons Not due to destructive process Mental retardation, hyperactive behavior
Migrational Disorder Abnormal migration of neurons from ventricular zone GA 3–5 mo	Lissencephaly	Complete failure of migration Absent gyri (smooth brain) Type 1—spontaneous or linked with Miller-Dieker syndrome
	Schizencephaly	Type 2—seen with congenital muscular dystrophies Cleftlike defect lined with heterotopic cortex
	Double cortex	Half of neurons migrate to cortex, remaining neurons show a bandlike heterotopia (X linked)
	Focal dysplasia	Isolated area of migrational anomaly Frequent cause of seizures
	Neuronal heterotopias	Neurons localized in subependymal region, deep white matter (diffuse or nodular), and cortex Seen in metabolic and genetic disorders
GA 9–12 wk	Agenesis of corpus callosum	Complete or partial (posterior corpus callosum, only) Usually associated with other migrational anomalies and Chiari II malformation (see below)
Congenital Hydrocephalus		In utero or neonatal presentation Due to heterogeneous causes Genetic—X-linked aqueductal stenosis, Chiari or Dandy-Walker malformation Acquired (eg, TORCH infections) Mental retardation seen in two thirds of patients
Cerebellar Anomaly Hindbrain defect	Chiari I malformation	Herniation of cerebellar tonsils through foramen magnum Can lead to hydrocephalus, brainstem compression, and syringomyelia
	Chiari II malformation	Same as for Chiari I, plus beaking of tectum, medullary deformity Linked to spina bifida Symptomatic at birth or in early infancy
	Dandy-Walker syndrome	Cystic dilation of 4th ventricle Complete or partial agenesis of cerebellar vermis and hydrocephalus
	Joubert syndrome	Vermian hypoplasia, episodic hyperpnea, abnormal eye movements

GA = gestational age; TORCH = toxoplasmosis, other congenital infections (eg, syphilis), rubella, cytomegalovirus, and herpes simplex.

Table 36–8. Less Common Neurocutaneous Disorders

Disorder	Inheritance	Clinical Findings
Von Hippel-Lindau disease	Autosomal dominant, variable penetrance	Cerebellar and retinal hemangioblastomas; cystic lesions of kidneys, pancreas, and epididymis; renal cell carcinomas; pheochromocytomas (3–17%)
Hypomelanosis of Ito	Sporadic (often associated with chromosomal mosaicism)	Linear hypopigmentation in whorls, iris hypopigmentation, hemimegalencephaly, migrational disorders, seizures, mental retardation, dental anomalies
Sjögren-Larsson syndrome	Autosomal recessive	Ichthyosis, mental retardation, seizures, spasticity, juvenile macular dystrophy
Incontinentia pigmenti	X-linked dominant	Cerebral dysgenesis, microcephaly, seizures, mental retardation, macular dystrophy
Xeroderma pigmentosum	Autosomal recessive	Sun sensitivity, high risk of skin and eye neoplasms, hearing loss, neurodegeneration, mental retardation
Neurocutaneous melanosis	Spontaneous mutation	Giant hairy skin nevi, leptomeningeal melanosis with tendency to malignancy
Linear nevus sebaceus	Unknown	Yellow papules in linear patches, mental retardation, seizures

▼ NEUROCUTANEOUS DISORDERS

Among the most common neurocutaneous disorders are neurofibromatosis types 1 and 2, tuberous sclerosis complex, Sturge-Weber syndrome, and ataxia-telangiectasia, which are briefly discussed here. Other neurocutaneous disorders are summarized in Table 36–8.

NEUROFIBROMATOSIS TYPE 1

ESSENTIALS OF DIAGNOSIS

▶ Presence of six or more café au lait macules and Lisch nodules

▶ CNS tumors and neurofibromas (nodular and plexiform)

▶ Variable penetrance

▶ General Considerations

Neurofibromatosis type 1 (NF1) is characterized by skin and nervous system anomalies (central and peripheral). Diagnostic criteria are noted in Table 36–9. Lisch nodules (hamartomas of the iris) and axillary freckling are thought to be pathognomonic for NF1.

▶ Clinical Findings

CNS tumors include optic gliomas (usually bilateral), gliomas (especially of the thalamus and spinal cord), medulloblastomas, and hamartomas. Peripheral nerve tumors include schwannomas and neurofibromas. Neurofibromas can be nodular or plexiform. Dumbbell tumors of the nerve roots may compress the spinal cord. Scoliosis, common in neurofibromatosis, may be idiopathic or secondary to dural ectasias or spinal tumors (intramedullary or extramedullary).

Macrocephaly, learning impairments, and ADHD are common in children with NF1. Inheritance is autosomal dominant with a high rate of spontaneous mutations (over 50%).

MRI reveals hamartomas (observed as bright signal on T2-weighted or fluid-attenuated inversion recovery images) and brain or spinal cord tumors.

▶ Treatment

Plexiform neurofibromas may be highly deforming but do not require specific intervention unless they compress vital

Table 36–9. Diagnostic Criteria for Neurofibromatosis

Neurofibromatosis Type 1 (NF1)
Diagnosis requires 2 or more of the following:
• 6 or more café au lait macules (prepubertal children > 5 mm; postpubertal children > 15 mm)
• 2 or more neurofibromas or 1 plexiform neurofibroma
• Freckling in axillary region or groin
• 2 or more Lisch nodules (iris hamartomas)
• Distinctive bony lesion with sphenoid dysplasia or thinning long-bone cortex with or without pseudoarthrosis
• First-degree relative with NF1

Neurofibromatosis Type 2 (NF2)
Bilateral CN VIII nerve masses on neuroimaging
   or
First-degree relative with NF2 and either
Unilateral CN VIII nerve mass *or* 2 of the following:
• Neurofibroma
• Meningioma
• Glioma
• Schwannoma
• Juvenile posterior subcapsular lenticular opacity

Reproduced with permission from Mulvihill JJ, et al. NIH conference. Neurofibromatosis 1 (Recklinghausen disease) and neurofibromatosis 2 (bilateral acoustic neurofibromatosis). An update. *Ann Intern Med* 1990;113:39–52.

structures (eg, trachea) or undergo malignant transformation. Low-grade gliomas usually require no treatment and can be observed for progression. Depending on location and histopathology, other CNS tumors may require surgery, chemotherapy, irradiation, or a combination of these approaches.

 Prognosis

In children with NF1, CNS tumors behave less aggressively than comparable tumors in children without NF1.

Jett K, Friedman JM. Clinical and genetic aspects of neurofibromatosis 1. *Genet Med* 2010;12(1):1–11. [PMID: 20027112] (Updated review on the subject.)

NEUROFIBROMATOSIS TYPE 2

> ### ESSENTIALS OF DIAGNOSIS
>
> ▶ Bilateral acoustic neuromas
> ▶ Unilateral acoustic neuromas and an affected first-degree relative

Bilateral acoustic neuromas are the main diagnostic criteria for this neurocutaneous syndrome, but neurofibromas can affect other cranial nerves. Refer to Table 36–9 for diagnostic criteria for NF2.

Evans DG, et al. Management of the patient and family with neurofibromatosis 2: A consensus conference statement. *Br J Neurosurg* 2005;19:5–12. [PMID: 16147576] (Clearly described current management guidelines.)

Goutagny S, Kalamarides M. Meningiomas and neurofibromatosis. *J Neurooncol* 2010;99(3):341–347. [PMID: 20714782] (Reviews of NF2 clinical presentations.)

TUBEROUS SCLEROSIS COMPLEX

> ### ESSENTIALS OF DIAGNOSIS
>
> ▶ Cutaneous lesions (ash-leaf, adenoma sebaceum, and shagreen patch)
> ▶ Brain lesions (hamartomas, subependymal nodular heterotopias)
> ▶ Seizures and mental retardation of varying severity

 General Considerations

Tuberous sclerosis complex is a neurocutaneous disorder that affects the brain, skin, kidneys, and heart. Affected individuals may have normal intelligence or severe mental retardation. Seizures, the hallmark of the disorder, include infantile spasms; generalized tonic-clonic, tonic, partial, or myoclonic seizures; and drop attacks.

▶ **Clinical Findings**

Early-onset and severe or intractable seizures are associated with more severe mental retardation. Skin findings may be absent at birth but develop over time. The typical skin lesion is the ash-leaf lesion, a hypopigmented macule that may be difficult to see in fair-skinned children without a Wood lamp (ultraviolet light) examination. The shagreen patch is a leathery, brownish, elevated lesion usually located in the sacral region. Adenoma sebaceum, more accurately termed *angiofibromas*, are small cutaneous hamartomas located over the malar surface that become apparent by age 2–4 years. Subungual or periungual fibromas (Koenen tumors) are also found in children with tuberous sclerosis complex.

Eye findings include retinal hamartomas (phakomas) or mulberry lesions (retinal astrocytic hamartomas). Characteristic brain findings are hamartias or hamartomas and subependymal nodular heterotopias with secondary calcifications (so-called *candle wax drippings*). Hamartias are developmental malformations of glial-neuronal tissue that do not grow (eg, tubers), whereas hamartomas, composed of similar cells, undergo nonneoplastic growth. Tumors are seen in brain (subependymal giant cell astrocytoma), kidneys (renal cysts in children and angiomyolipoma in older patients), and heart (rhabdomyomas). Rapamycin has recently gained FDA approval for the treatment of unresectable subependymal giant cell astrocytoma. About half of cardiac rhabdomyomas are caused by tuberous sclerosis complex. Inheritance is autosomal dominant with variable penetrance; however, the disorder has a high rate of spontaneous mutations.

Orlova KA, Crino PB. The tuberous sclerosis complex. *Ann N Y Acad Sci* 2010;1184:87–105. [PMID: 20146692] (Comprehensive review describing phenotype and genotype issues.)

STURGE-WEBER SYNDROME

> ### ESSENTIALS OF DIAGNOSIS
>
> ▶ Port-wine nevus over trigeminal distribution
> ▶ Ipsilateral leptomeningeal angiomatosis
> ▶ Intractable seizures and mental retardation

 General Considerations

This disorder is characterized by a port-wine nevus over the trigeminal distribution, predominantly affecting the first division, ipsilateral leptomeningeal angiomatosis, contralateral hemiparesis; seizures, and mental retardation. Seizures are often partial but may be generalized or myoclonic. Congenital glaucoma (buphthalmos) is the rule when the nevus is located over the eye. Calcifications are seen usually in the parietal-occipital cortex by the end of the second decade (so-called *train-track sign*).

▶ Treatment

Patients with seizures that are refractory to anticonvulsant treatment may benefit from surgical removal of the affected lobe. The port-wine nevus may be treated with laser therapy. Treatment of glaucoma requires pharmacologic and often surgical intervention.

Puttgen KB, Lin DD. Neurocutaneous vascular syndromes. *Childs Nerv Syst* 2010;26(10):1407–1415. [PMID: 20582592] (Review of Sturge-Weber and PHACE syndromes.)

ATAXIA-TELANGIECTASIA

ESSENTIALS OF DIAGNOSIS

- ▶ Disorder of DNA repair
- ▶ Neurodegeneration (spinocerebellar and movement disorder)
- ▶ Sinopulmonary infections and lymphoproliferative neoplasms

▶ General Considerations

Ataxia-telangiectasia is discussed in detail in Chapter 16. The disorder is characterized by spinocerebellar degeneration (cerebellar ataxia, sensory neuropathy, and posterior column involvement) and chorea or dystonia. Children are prone to sinopulmonary infections, immune incompetence, and lymphoproliferative neoplasia. Oculomotor apraxia with head thrust is commonly observed. Oculocutaneous telangiectasia develops with the onset of ataxia at about 2–3 years of age. As the disease advances, MRI shows cerebellar atrophy.

α-Fetoprotein level is elevated after age 2 years in over 80% of affected individuals. Levels of immunoglobulins (IgA, IgE, IgG) are usually low. Inheritance is autosomal recessive. Ataxia-telangiectasia is caused by mutation of the *ATM* (ataxia telangiectasia mutation) gene, which results in spontaneous breakage of chromosomes.

▶ Treatment & Prognosis

Treatment is palliative and related primarily to the movement disorder. The disorder is associated with early mortality, due to either general decline in neurologic function or neoplasia.

Biton S, Barzilai A, Shiloh Y. The neurological phenotype of ataxia-telangiectasia: Solving a persistent puzzle. *DNA Repair (Amst)* 2008;7(7):1028–1038. [PMID: 18456574] (Good overview with an intriguing discussion of the neuropathology of ataxia-telangiectasia.)

INDEX

Note: Page numbers followed by "*f*" denote figures; those followed by "*t*" denote tables